Cancer Immunotherapy

Cancer Immunotherapy

Immune Suppression and Tumor Growth

Edited by

George C. Prendergast

The Lankenau Institute for Medical Research
Lankenau Cancer Center
Wynnewood, PA

Elizabeth M. Jaffee

The Sidney Kimmel Comprehensive
Cancer Center at Johns Hopkins Medical Institute
Bunting-Blaustein Cancer Research Building
Baltimore, MD

Amsterdam • Boston • Heidelberg • London • New York • Oxford
Paris • San Diego • San Francisco • Singapore • Sydney • Tokyo
Academic Press is an imprint of Elsevier

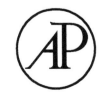

Academic Press is an imprint of Elsevier
525 B Street, Suite 1900, San Diego, CA 92101-4495, USA
32 Jamestown Road, London NW1 7BY, UK
225 Wyman Street, Waltham, MA 02451, USA

First edition 2007

British Library Cataloguing-in-Publication Data
A catalogue record for this book is available from the British Library

Library of Congress Cataloging-in-Publication Data
A catalog record for this book is available from the Library of Congress

ISBN: 978-0-12-394296-8

For information on all Academic Press publications
visit our website at elsevierdirect.com

Typeset by TNQ Books and Journals
www.tnq.co.in

Printed and bound in the United States of America
Transferred to Digital Printing, 2014

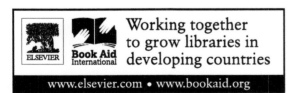

CONTENTS

CONTENTS

SECTION 2 • Principles of Cancer Immunobiology

SECTION 3 • Introduction to Cancer Therapeutics

SECTION 4 • Strategies of Passive and Active Immunotherapy

SECTION 5 • Improving Immunotherapeutic Responses

CONTENTS

x

SECTION 6 • Targeting Strategies to Defeat Immune Suppression

xiii

Paola Allavena
Humanitas Clinical and Research Center, Rozzano, Milan, Italy

Maria Libera Ascierto
Infectious Disease and Immunogenetics Section (IDIS), Department of Transfusion Medicine (DTM), FOCIS Center of Excellence, Clinical Center (CC) and Trans-National Institutes of Health (NIH) Center for Human Immunology (CHI), NIH, Bethesda, MD USA
Department of Internal Medicine (DiMI), University of Genoa, Genoa, Italy
Center of Excellence for Biomedical Research (CEBR), University of Genoa, Genoa, Italy

Davide Bedognetti
Infectious Disease and Immunogenetics Section (IDIS), Department of Transfusion Medicine (DTM), FOCIS Center of Excellence, Clinical Center (CC) and Trans-National Institutes of Health (NIH) Center for Human Immunology (CHI), NIH, Bethesda, MD USA
Department of Internal Medicine (DiMI), University of Genoa, Genoa, Italy

Daniel W. Beury
Dept. Biological Sciences, University of Maryland Baltimore County (UMBC), Baltimore, MD USA

Vincenzo Bronte
University Hospital and Department of Pathology, Immunology Section, Verona, Italy

Sjoerd H. van der Burg
Experimental Cancer Immunology and Therapy Group, Department of Clinical Oncology, Leiden University Medical Center, Leiden, The Netherlands

Zheng Cai
Department of Pathology and Lab Medicine, University of Pennsylvania Perelman School of Medicine, Philadelphia, PA USA

Margaret K. Callahan
Department of Medicine, Memorial Sloan-Kettering Cancer Center, New York, NY USA
Weill—Cornell Medical College, New York, NY USA

Bruce D. Car
Discovery Toxicology, Pharmaceutical Candidate Optimization, Bristol-Myers Squibb Co., Princeton, New Jersey USA

Gang Chen
Department of Oncology, Johns Hopkins University School of Medicine, The Sidney Kimmel Cancer Center at Johns Hopkins, Baltimore, MD USA

Mariacristina Chioda
Istituto Oncologico Veneto, Padova, Italy

Olesya Chornoguz
Dept. Biological Sciences, University of Maryland Baltimore County (UMBC), Baltimore, MD USA

Sandra Demaria
Department of Pathology, New York University School of Medicine, and NYU Langone Medical Center, New York, NY USA

Jiehui Deng
Department of Cancer Immunotherapeutics & Tumor Immunology, Beckman Research Institute and City of Hope Comprehensive Cancer Center, Duarte, CA USA

Julie Y. Djeu
H. Lee Moffitt Cancer Center, Tampa, FL USA

Sarah S. Donatelli
H. Lee Moffitt Cancer Center, Tampa, FL USA

Charles G. Drake
Department of Oncology, Johns Hopkins University, Baltimore, MD USA

Glenn Dranoff
Department of Medical Oncology and Cancer Vaccine Center, Dana-Farber Cancer Institute and Department of Medicine, Brigham and Women's Hospital and Harvard Medical School, Boston, MA USA

Nicholas M. Durham
Department of Oncology, Johns Hopkins University, Baltimore, MD USA

Laurence C. Eisenlohr
Department of Microbiology and Immunology, Kimmel Cancer Center, Thomas Jefferson University, Philadelphia, PA USA

Leisha A. Emens
Associate Professor of Oncology, Graduate Program in Pathobiology, Department of Oncology, Johns Hopkins University School of Medicine, The Sidney Kimmel Cancer Center at Johns Hopkins, Baltimore, MD USA

Benedetto Farsaci
Laboratory of Tumor Immunology and Biology, Center for Cancer Research, National Cancer Institute, National Institutes of Health, Bethesda, MD USA

Taylor Feehley
Committee on Immunology, Department of Pathology, The University of Chicago, Chicago, IL USA

Paola Filipazzi
Unit of Immunotherapy of Human Tumors, Fondazione IRCCS Istituto Nazionale dei Tumori, Milan, Italy

Maria Rosaria Galdiero
Humanitas Clinical and Research Center, Rozzano, Milan, Italy
Division of Allergy and Clinical Immunology, University of Naples, Naples, Italy

Gianfranco di Genova
Molecular Immunology Group, Cancer Sciences Unit, University of Southampton Faculty of Medicine, Southampton General Hospital, Southampton, United Kingdom

Paul B. Gilman
Lankenau Medical Center
Lankenau Institute for Medical Research, Wynnewood, PA USA

Mark I. Greene
Department of Pathology and Lab Medicine, University of Pennsylvania Perelman School of Medicine, Philadelphia, PA USA

John W. Greiner
Laboratory of Tumor Immunology and Biology, Center for Cancer Research, National Cancer Institute, National Institutes of Health, Bethesda, MD USA

James L. Gulley
Laboratory of Tumor Immunology and Biology, Center for Cancer Research, National Cancer Institute, National Institutes of Health, Bethesda, MD USA

Claire Hearnden
Adjuvant Research Group, School of Biochemistry and Immunology, Trinity Biomedical Sciences Institute, Trinity College Dublin, Dublin 2, Ireland

James W. Hodge
Laboratory of Tumor Immunology and Biology, Center for Cancer Research, National Cancer Institute, National Institutes of Health, Bethesda, MD USA

Veronica Huber
Unit of Immunotherapy of Human Tumors, Fondazione IRCCS Istituto Nazionale dei Tumori, Milan, Italy

Elizabeth M. Jaffee
The Dana and Albert "Cubby" Broccoli Professor of Oncology, Co-Director of the Gastrointestinal Cancers Program, Co-Director of the Skip Viragh Pancreatic Cancer Center, Associate Director for Translational Research, The Sidney Kimmel Cancer Center at Johns Hopkins, Baltimore, MD USA

Masahisa Jinushi
Research Center for Infection-Associated Cancer, Institute for Genetic Medicine, Hokkaido University, Sapporo, Japan

Richard Jove
Molecular Medicine, Beckman Research Institute and City of Hope Comprehensive Cancer Center, Duarte, CA USA

Michael H. Kershaw
Cancer Immunology Program, Peter MacCallum Cancer Centre, East Melbourne, Victoria, Australia
Sir Peter MacCallum Department of Oncology, University of Melbourne, Victoria, Australia

Robert Kiss
Laboratory of Toxicology, Faculty of Pharmacy, Université Libre de Bruxelles, Brussels, Belgium
R.K. and G.A.R. contributed equally to this chapter

Ilona Kryczek
Department of Surgery, University of Michigan School of Medicine, Ann Arbor, MI USA

Richard A. Lake
National Centre for Asbestos Related Diseases and Tumor Immunology Group, School of Medicine and Pharmacology, University of Western Australia, Sir Charles Gairdner Hospital, Nedlands, WA 6009, Australia

Bradley W. Lash
Lankenau Medical Center

Ed C. Lavelle
Adjuvant Research Group, School of Biochemistry and Immunology, Trinity Biomedical Sciences Institute, Trinity College Dublin, Dublin 2, Ireland

W. Joost Lesterhuis
National Centre for Asbestos Related Diseases and Tumor Immunology Group, School of Medicine and Pharmacology, University of Western Australia, Sir Charles Gairdner Hospital, Nedlands, WA 6009, Australia

Charles J. Link
NewLink Genetic Corporation, Ames, Iowa USA

Jing Liu
School of Life Sciences, University of Science and Technology of China, Hefei, Anhui China

Nancy Luckashenak
Department of Microbiology and Immunology, Kimmel Cancer Center, Thomas Jefferson University, Philadelphia, PA USA

Ravi A. Madan
Laboratory of Tumor Immunology and Biology, Center for Cancer Research, National Cancer Institute, National Institutes of Health, Bethesda, MD USA

Laura Mandik-Nayak
Lankenau Institute for Medical Research, Wynnewood, PA USA

Susanna Mandruzzato
Department of Surgery, Oncology and Gastroenterology, Oncology and Immunology Section, University of Padova, Italy

Alberto Mantovani
Humanitas Clinical and Research Center, Rozzano, Milan, Italy
Department of Biotechnology and Translational Medicine, University of Milan, Rozzano, Milan, Italy

Ilaria Marigo
Stem Cell Biology, Department of Medicine, Division of Experimental Medicine, Hammersmith Hospital, London, UK

Francesco M Marincola
Infectious Disease and Immunogenetics Section (IDIS), Department of Transfusion Medicine (DTM), FOCIS Center of Excellence, Clinical Center (CC) and Trans-National Institutes of Health (NIH) Center for Human Immunology (CHI), NIH, Bethesda, MD USA. Sidra Medical and Research Centre, Doha, Qatar

Veronique Mathieu
Laboratory of Toxicology, Faculty of Pharmacy, Université Libre de Bruxelles, Brussels, Belgium

Kenneth F. May, Jr.
Department of Medical Oncology and Cancer Vaccine Center, Dana-Farber Cancer Institute and Department of Medicine, Brigham and Women's Hospital and Harvard Medical School, Boston, MA USA

Andrew L. Mellor
Immunotherapy Center and Department of Medicine, Medical College of Georgia, Georgia Health Sciences University, Augusta, GA USA

Lauren M.F. Merlo
Lankenau Institute for Medical Research, Wynnewood, PA USA

Richard Metz
NewLink Genetics Corporation, Wynnewood, PA USA

Simone Mocellin
Department of Surgery, Oncology and Gastroenterology, Surgery Section, University of Padova, Italy

Richard A. Morgan
Surgery Branch, National Cancer Institute, National Institutes of Health, Bethesda, MD USA

Alexander J. Muller
Lankenau Institute for Medical Research, Wynnewood, PA USA

David H. Munn
Cancer Immunotherapy Program and Department of Pediatrics, Medical College of Georgia, Georgia Health Sciences University, Augusta, GA USA

Yasuhiro Nagai
Department of Pathology and Lab Medicine, University of Pennsylvania Perelman School of Medicine, Philadelphia, PA USA

Cathryn Nagler
Committee on Immunology, Department of Pathology, The University of Chicago, Chicago, IL USA

Amanda Norvell
Department of Biology, The College of New Jersey, Ewing NJ USA

Anna K. Nowak
National Centre for Asbestos Related Diseases and Tumor Immunology Group, School of Medicine and Pharmacology, University of Western Australia, Sir Charles Gairdner Hospital, Nedlands, WA 6009, Australia
Department of Medical Oncology, Sir Charles Gairdner Hospital Nedlands, WA, Australia

Takuya Ohtani
Department of Pathology and Lab Medicine, University of Pennsylvania Perelman School of Medicine, Philadelphia, PA USA

Suzanne Ostrand-Rosenberg
Dept. Biological Sciences, University of Maryland Baltimore County (UMBC), Baltimore, MD USA

Christian H Ottensmeier
Molecular Immunology Group, Cancer Sciences Unit, University of Southampton Faculty of Medicine, Southampton General Hospital, Southampton, United Kingdom

Claudia Palena
Laboratory of Tumor Immunology and Biology, Center for Cancer Research, National Cancer Institute, National Institutes of Health, Bethesda, MD USA

Katherine H. Parker
Dept. Biological Sciences, University of Maryland Baltimore County (UMBC), Baltimore, MD USA

Michael A. Postow
Department of Medicine, Memorial Sloan-Kettering Cancer Center, New York, NY USA
Weill–Cornell Medical College, New York, NY USA

George C. Prendergast
Lankenau Institute for Medical Research, Wynnewood, PA USA
Department of Pathology, Anatomy & Cell Biology
Kimmel Cancer Center, Jefferson Medical School, Thomas Jefferson University, Philadelphia, PA USA

Saul J. Priceman
Department of Cancer Immunotherapeutics & Tumor Immunology, Beckman Research Institute and City of Hope Comprehensive Cancer Center, Duarte, CA USA

Jenni Punt, VMD, PhD
Haverford College, Haverford, PA USA

Gabriel A. Rabinovich
Laboratorio de Inmunopatología, Instituto de Biología y Medicina Experimental (IBYME), Consejo Nacional de Investigaciones Científicas y Técnicas (CONICET), Buenos Aires, Argentina
Laboratorio de Glicómica Estructural y Funcional, IQUIBICEN-CONICET, Departamento de Química Biológica, Facultad de Ciencias Exactas y Naturales, Universidad de Buenos Aires, Ciudad de Buenos Aires, Argentina
R.K. and G.A.R. contributed equally to this chapter

W. Jay Ramsey
NewLink Genetic Corporation, Ames, Iowa USA

Licia Rivoltini
Unit of Immunotherapy of Human Tumors, Fondazione IRCCS Istituto Nazionale dei Tumori, Milan, Italy

Gabriela R. Rossi
NewLink Genetic Corporation, Ames, Iowa USA

Eva Sahakian
Department of Immunology and Malignant Hematology, H. Lee Moffitt Cancer Center & Research Institute, Tampa, FL USA

Arabinda Samanta
Department of Pathology and Lab Medicine, University of Pennsylvania Perelman School of Medicine, Philadelphia, PA USA

Marimo Sato-Matsushita
Infectious Disease and Immunogenetics Section (IDIS), Department of Transfusion Medicine (DTM), FOCIS Center of Excellence, Clinical Center (CC) and Trans-National Institutes of Health (NIH) Center for Human Immunology (CHI), NIH, Bethesda, MD USA
Institute of Medical Science, The University of Tokyo, Tokyo, Japan

Natalia Savelyeva
Molecular Immunology Group, Cancer Sciences Unit, University of Southampton Faculty of Medicine, Southampton General Hospital, Southampton, United Kingdom

Jeffrey Schlom
Laboratory of Tumor Immunology and Biology, Center for Cancer Research, National Cancer Institute, National Institutes of Health, Bethesda, MD USA

Antonio Sica
Humanitas Clinical and Research Center, Rozzano, Milan, Italy
DiSCAFF, University of Piemonte Orientale A. Avogadro, Novara, Italy

Pratima Sinha
Dept. Biological Sciences, University of Maryland Baltimore County (UMBC), Baltimore, MD USA

Courtney Smith
Lankenau Institute for Medical Research, Wynnewood, PA USA

Mark J. Smyth
Cancer Immunology Program, Peter MacCallum Cancer Centre, East Melbourne, Victoria, Australia
Sir Peter MacCallum Department of Oncology, University of Melbourne, Victoria, Australia

Eduardo M. Sotomayor
Department of Immunology and Malignant Hematology, H. Lee Moffitt Cancer Center & Research Institute, Tampa, FL USA

Freda K Stevenson
Molecular Immunology Group, Cancer Sciences Unit, University of Southampton Faculty of Medicine, Southampton General Hospital, Southampton, United Kingdom

Victoria Sundblad
Laboratorio de Inmunopatología, Instituto de Biología y Medicina Experimental (IBYME), Consejo Nacional de Investigaciones Científicas y Técnicas (CONICET), Buenos Aires, Argentina

Michele W.L. Teng
Cancer Immunology Program, Peter MacCallum Cancer Centre, East Melbourne, Victoria, Australia
Sir Peter MacCallum Department of Oncology, University of Melbourne, Victoria, Australia

Kwong-Yok Tsang
Laboratory of Tumor Immunology and Biology, Center for Cancer Research, National Cancer Institute, National Institutes of Health, Bethesda, MD USA

Hiromichi Tsuchiya
Department of Pathology and Lab Medicine, University of Pennsylvania Perelman School of Medicine, Philadelphia, PA USA

Nicholas N. Vahanian
NewLink Genetic Corporation, Ames, Iowa USA

Alejandro Villagra
Department of Immunology and Malignant Hematology, H. Lee Moffitt Cancer
Center & Research Institute, Tampa, FL USA

Ena Wang
Infectious Disease and Immunogenetics Section (IDIS), Department of Transfusion
Medicine (DTM), FOCIS Center of Excellence, Clinical Center (CC) and Trans-National
Institutes of Health (NIH) Center for Human Immunology (CHI), NIH, Bethesda, MD USA

Lin Wang
Central Laboratory, Union Hospital, Tongji Medical College, Huazhong University of Science
and Technology, Wuhan, China

Shuang Wei
Department of Surgery, University of Michigan School of Medicine, Ann Arbor, MI USA

Marij J.P. Welters
Experimental Cancer Immunology and Therapy Group, Department of Clinical Oncology,
Leiden University Medical Center, Leiden, The Netherlands

Richard A. Westhouse
Discovery Toxicology, Pharmaceutical Candidate Optimization, Bristol-Myers Squibb Co.,
Princeton, New Jersey USA

Karrune Woan
Department of Immunology and Malignant Hematology, H. Lee Moffitt Cancer
Center & Research Institute, Tampa, FL USA

Jedd D. Wolchok
Department of Medicine, Memorial Sloan-Kettering Cancer Center, New York, NY USA
Weill–Cornell Medical College, New York, NY USA
Ludwig Center for Cancer Immunotherapy, Immunology Program, New York, NY USA
The Ludwig Institute for Cancer Research, New York Branch, New York, NY USA

Hua Yu
Department of Cancer Immunotherapeutics & Tumor Immunology, Beckman Research
Institute and City of Hope Comprehensive Cancer Center, Duarte, CA USA

Hongtao Zhang
Department of Pathology and Lab Medicine, University of Pennsylvania Perelman School
of Medicine, Philadelphia, PA USA

Ende Zhao
Department of Surgery, University of Michigan School of Medicine, Ann Arbor, MI USA
Central Laboratory, Union Hospital, Tongji Medical College, Huazhong University of Science
and Technology, Wuhan, China

Zhiqiang Zhu
Department of Pathology and Lab Medicine, University of Pennsylvania Perelman School
of Medicine, Philadelphia, PA USA

Weiping Zou
Department of Surgery, University of Michigan School of Medicine, Ann Arbor, MI USA
Graduate Program in Immunology and Cancer Biology, University of Michigan School of
Medicine, Ann Arbor, MI USA
University of Michigan Comprehensive Cancer Center, University of Michigan School of
Medicine, Ann Arbor, MI USA

CHAPTER 1

Introduction

George C. Prendergast[1,2,3], **Elizabeth M. Jaffee**[4]
[1]Lankenau Institute for Medical Research, Wynnewood, PA USA
[2]Department of Pathology, Anatomy & Cell Biology
[3]Kimmel Cancer Center, Jefferson Medical School, Thomas Jefferson University, Philadelphia, PA USA
[4]The Sidney Kimmel Comprehensive Cancer Center at Johns Hopkins, Department of Oncology, The Johns Hopkins University, Baltimore, MD USA

I. SUMMARY

Immunological thought is exerting a growing effect in cancer research, correcting a divorce that occurred in the mainstream of the field decades ago as cancer genetics began to emerge as a dominant movement. During the past decade, a new general consensus has emerged among all cancer researchers that inflammation and immune escape play crucial causal roles in the development and progression of malignancy. This consensus is now driving a new synthesis of thought with great implications for cancer treatments of the future. In this book, we introduce new concepts and practices that will dramatically affect oncology by adding new immune modalities to present standards of care in surgery, radiotherapy and chemotherapy. We aim in particular to cross-fertilize ideas in the new area of immunochemotherapy, which strives to develop new combinations of immunological and pharmacological agents as cancer therapeutics. Specifically, our goals are to (1) highlight novel principles of immune suppression in cancer, which represent the major salient breakthroughs in the field of cancer immunology in the last decade, and to (2) discuss the latest thinking in how immunotherapeutic and chemotherapeutic agents might be combined, not only to defeat mechanisms of tumoral immune suppression but also to reprogram the inflammatory microenvironment of tumor cells to enhance the long-term outcomes of clinical intervention. Many immune-based therapies have focused on activating the immune system. However, it is now clear that these therapies are often thwarted by the ability of cancers to erect barricades that evade or suppress the immune system. Mechanistic insights into these barricades have enormous medical implications, not only to treat cancer but also many chronic infectious and age-associated diseases where relieving pathogenic immune tolerance is a key challenge. In this book, contributors with a wide diversity of perspectives and experience provide an introductory overview to the immune system; how tumors evolve to evade the immune system; the nature of various approaches used presently to treat cancer in the oncology clinic; and how these approaches might be enhanced by inhibiting important mechanisms of tumoral immune tolerance and suppression. The overarching aim of this treatise is to provide a conceptual foundation to create a more effective all-out attack on cancer. In this chapter, we offer a historical perspective on the development of immunological thought in cancer, a discussion of some of the fundamental challenges to be faced, and an overview of the chapters which frame and address these challenges.

Cancer Immunotherapy. http://dx.doi.org/10.1016/B978-0-12-394296-8.00001-4

1

II. HISTORICAL BACKGROUND

"I can't understand why people are frightened of new ideas. I'm frightened of the old ones."

— John Cage (1912–1992)

Starting about 1980, research investigations in cancer genetics and cell biology began to assume the prominence in cancer research that they now hold today. Hatched initially from studies of animal tumor viruses, the field of cancer genetics has contributed significantly to our understanding of the biologic pathways involved in tumor initiation and progression, and has identified specific targets for therapeutic intervention. With the discovery of cellular onco-genes, the once radical idea that cancer was a disease of normal cellular genes gone wrong not only came to be established as the dominant idea in the field but also to strongly influence how to develop new drugs to treat cancer, with the goal of attacking the products of those genes. At the same time, these developments outpaced other concepts of cancer as a systemic disease involving perturbations in the immune system. Now, after decades of mutual skepti-cism, a historically important consensus among cancer researchers is emerging about the causality of chronic inflammation and altered immunity in driving malignant development and progression. Ironically, this synthesis is having the effect of making the "new" genetic ideas of the past two decades about cancer seem somewhat dated: in particular, it is becoming apparent that the tumor cell-centric focus championed by cancer genetics is unlikely to give a full understanding of clinical disease, without knowing about the systemic and localized tissue conditions that surround and control the growth and activity of the tumor cell. Perhaps contributing to some consternation about the conceptual weight of the "new" ideas, few of the molecular therapeutics developed from them have had much major clinical impact (the Bcr-Abl kinase inhibitor Gleevec® still perhaps the most notable success among present molecular cancer therapeutics).

Among the earliest pathohistological descriptions of cancer, Virchow in the 1800s first noted the surfeit of inflammatory cells in many tumors. From this root, tumor immunologists have for many years struggled to fully understand the precise relationships between inflammation, immunity, and cancer, and to develop principles that can robustly impact the diagnosis, prognosis, and treatment of cancer. With the emergence of cancer genetics and tumor cell-centric concepts of disease as major conceptual drivers in the late 20th century, roles identified for tumor stromal cells and immunity in cancer became marginalized or simply ignored by many investigators. Indeed, old skepticisms about whether immunity was important or not in cancer have persisted until quite recently, as can be illustrated by the omissions of immune escape and inflammation as critical traits of cancer in influential reviews as recently as the turn of the new century [1]. However, since 2000 perspectives in the field have once again undergone a radical shift, with many cancer researchers now focusing intensely on how tumorigenesis and tumor dormancy versus progression are shaped by the stromal microen-vironment, inflammation, and alterations in the immune system. Indeed, a recent update to the prominent review cited above recognized the conceptual movement in this rapidly moving area of the field, including inflammation and immune escape as critical traits of cancer [2].

The restoration of immunological thought in the mainstream of cancer research is proceeding rapidly, creating a historically important synthesis that is seeding radically new approaches of immunochemotherapy and radioimmunotherapy [3]. Over the past 25 years, as a result of historical and scientific divisions, there have been limited communication, understanding, and collaboration between tumor immunologists, molecular geneticists, and cell biologists working in the field. On one hand, this situation has been exaggerated by what now seems like an overly narrow focus of geneticists and cell biologists on tumor cell-centric concepts of cancer, which continues to persist to some degree. On the other hand, immunologists have struggled to establish a clear understanding of how inflammation and immune cells can contribute to promoting or controlling cancer. Biases rooted to some extent in old controversies that have been transmitted to younger scientists entering each field have further limited communication and interaction between the two camps. Happily, in recent years many of these old issues have been put to rest, by experiments in modern transgenic animal model systems and by carefully controlled clinical observations, such that the key pathophysiological foundations of inflammation and immune dysfunction in cancer are now firmly established [4]. Contributing to the new perspective, there is a wider appreciation of both the critical role of the tumor microenvironment in malignant development and the power of immune suppression mechanisms in licensing cancer cell proliferation, survival, and metastasis. In terms of immunotherapeutic responses, it seems increasingly clear that in order to "push on the gas" of immune activation, it will be necessary to "get off the brakes" of immune suppression—an idea that cancer geneticists may recognize as analogous to the concept in their field that oncogenes can drive neoplastic cell proliferation only when the blockades imposed by tumor suppressor genes are relieved.

III. THE CHALLENGE OF CANCER

Clearly, the goal of cancer therapy is to kill residual tumor that cannot be excised surgically. However, the inherent nature of the cancer cell limits the full effectiveness of therapies that have been developed, or that arguably can be developed. Being of host origin, cancer cells share features of the host that make effective treatment difficult, due to side effects that limit the therapeutic window. Moreover, the plastic nature of tumors makes them remarkably resilient in rebounding from clinical regimens of radiotherapy and chemotherapy that are traditionally used. For example, even when the vast majority of cancer cells are killed by a cytotoxic chemotherapeutic drug, a small number of residual cells that are resistant to the agent can be sufficient to seed the regrowth of a tumor. Making matters worse, the regrown tumor may no longer respond to the previously successful therapy, due to the capacity of tumor cells to evolve resistance under selective pressures applied by cytotoxic agents. Indeed, the concept of selection is integral to understanding this disease: development and progression in cancer is driven by the selection of cells that survive conditions that are normally lethal. Resistance to any normally lethal pressure can be selected by evolution in a cancer cell population because of the genetic plasticity, an important characteristic of cancer cells. As demonstrated in the treatment of other diseases caused by a highly mutable entity, e.g., HIV, successful targeting of tumor cells may require the application of multiple agents that target different survival mechanisms. However, compared to HIV, the genetic space available for the evolution of a cancer cell is far larger, due to the far greater size of the cancer cell genome. Thus, effective eradication of tumors has proven —and may continue to prove to be—quite challenging, even using multiple agents in combination, because of the diversity of options that the cancer genome can realize to evolve mechanisms of survival in response to multiple selection pressures these agents apply. Our best chance is to identify as many of these mechanisms as possible, and to discover approaches that synergize to inhibit these many mechanisms.

Two general solutions to this dismal situation may be to redirect the focus of attack from the tumor cell itself to the environment that sustains its growth and survival or to engage the immune system in ways that allows it to eradicate tumor cells like an infection. The former strategy is essentially passive in nature insofar as cancer cells are killed by an indirect route. For example, by depriving tumors of a blood supply anti-angiogenic therapies can indirectly kill cancer cells. Resistance to such therapies should be difficult to evolve, as the argument goes, because stromal cells in the tumor environment are not genetically plastic. However, due to their passive nature such therapies are still prone to circumvention through tumor cell evolution (e.g., vascular mimicry in the case of anti-angiogenesis therapies [5]). In contrast, active strategies to engage or "awaken" active immunity in the cancer patient has many appeals,

3

the chief of which is its capability to "dodge and weave" with tumor heterogeneity, the inherent outcome of the response of tumor cells to selection pressures. In this regard, the immune system may be particularly well suited to clear the small numbers of residual tumor cells, particular dormant cells or cancer stem cells, that may be poorly eradicated by radiotherapy and chemotherapy and which could help lengthen remission periods. Indeed, even treatments that did not cure but rather converted cancer to a long-term subclinical condition, by analogy to HIV infections, would represent a resounding success. Therefore, the key question becomes how a tumor can outrun an activated immune system, given that precisely this event has occurred during tumorigenesis, so that the balance might be tipped back in favor of the immune system.

IV. PARTS OF THE BOOK

The second edition of this book provides a significant expansion upon the first edition, reflecting rapid developments in cancer immunology and the new field of immunochemotherapy. The book encompasses two general parts, which are subdivided into three sections each. The first part of the book introduces key concepts, with Sections I—III to introduce basic principles of immunology, cancer immunobiology and cancer therapeutics. The second part of the book introduces strategies to stimulate or heighten (and measure) immunotherapeutic responses, with Sections IV—VI devoted to passive and active immunotherapy, potential improvements with existing tools, and emerging strategies to target mechanisms of tumoral immunosuppression that are being discovered along with novel experimental tools to do so.

Section I introduces basic principles in immunology for the large number of individuals working or interested in cancer research who remain relatively unschooled in this discipline. This section does not delve into every topic but offers rudiments relevant to key directions in the field. Fundamental components of the immune system are introduced in Chapter 2 spanning both innate and adaptive immunity. The following chapters focus more deeply on the adaptive immune system, which tumors must ultimately erect powerful barricades against, with Chapter 3 addressing B cells and antibodies and Chapter 4 addressing T cells and cytokines. Chapter 5 introduces antigen processing and presentation to the adaptive immune system as carried out by dendritic cells, a class of myeloid cells specifically dedicated to antigen presentation. This chapter addresses an important area of cancer immunobiology and therapy at present, insofar as it encompasses the first active immunotherapy to be approved in the U.S. for cancer treatment. Chapter 6 introduces mucosal immunity, an area of rapidly expanding influence due in part to a growing appreciation of how the aerodigestive tracts not only shape tolerance to environmental antigens but also to how the gut microbiome programs immunity overall [6].

Section II moves specifically into the general principles of cancer immunobiology, a seminal area that is renewing its historical impact on cancer research after the divorce of immunology from the mainstream of the field with the molecular genetics revolution of the 1980s. Key chapters highlight the significance of tumor immunoediting and immune suppression mechanisms in progression. Two fundamental ideas here are that subclinical (occult) cancers may arise commonly during aging and that clinical cancer may represent only those rare lesions that have achieved immune escape. In cancer research, models of oncogenesis have exerted the most influence on cancer cell-centric concepts, whereas models of immunoediting have assumed a major influence on cancer microenvironment concepts. Chapter 7 introduces cancer immunoediting as a fundamental process with three parts, namely immunosurveillance, immune equilibrium and immune escape, which lead respectively to control, stasis, or outgrowth of a malignancy. Immunoediting starts with the immune recognition and destruction of cells that have acquired genetic and epigenetic alterations characteristic of tumor cells, but at the same time, the selective pressure produced by immunoediting drives tumor evolution and progression. In this process, the cell-intrinsic traits of cancer (immortalization, growth deregulation, apoptotic resistance, and tumor suppressor inactivation) lead to the development of subclinical or occult lesions that are not clinically important until cell-extrinsic traits (invasion, angiogenesis, metastasis, and immune escape) have been achieved. The complex roles for inflammatory cells and altered immunity in the development of cell-extrinsic traits represent an increasingly important area for investigation. Chapter 8 discusses key aspects of immunosurveillance, including the production of "danger signals" and the generation of innate and adaptive immune responses to tumor cells. Chapter 9 discusses immune "sculpting" processes that occur in the tumor as a result of the evolution of the battle between immune cells and tumor cells, focusing on key roles played in the inflammatory tumor microenvironment by natural killer cells (NK cells). Chapters 10 and 11 discuss immune escape. A timely focus on rapid developments in studies of Th17 helper cell-based immuno-suppression are addressed in Chapter 10, with a broader overview of immunosuppressive networks presented in Chapter 11. With the evolution of immunosuppressive networks by tumors, immunoediting eventually culminates in an escape from immune control, initially locally to permit tumor growth but ultimately to invasive and metastatic states that can challenge or defeat clinical management.

Section III provides an introductory overview to cancer therapeutics and strategies of development, including perspectives on pharmacology and safety assessment, cancer vaccines and immunoguiding tactics. Chapter 12 introduces cytotoxic chemotherapeutics, which continue to provide the major part of the armamentarium employed by medical oncologists. Chapter 13 offers an overview of cancer pharmacology and safety assessment for both "classical" types of cytotoxic drugs as well as modern molecular targeted therapeutics, where the central goal is learning whether "hitting the target" in the tumor cell (pharmacodynamics) can be achieved in a relatively safe and effective manner. Strategies for passive immunotherapy with monoclonal antibodies are reviewed in Chapter 14. Although it took two decades to fully mature, this area of immunotherapy has achieved considerable success yet may see still greater influence in cancer treatment, particularly in targeting T-cell negative co-regulatory pathways with the recent U.S. approval of anti-CTLA4 therapy (ipilumimab or Yervoy®), which is the focus of a later chapter. Chapter 15 introduces strategies for active immunotherapy with a focus on cancer vaccines. While pursued for many years to generally frustrating ends, cancer vaccine strategies appear poised to break through to significant clinical impacts with the combination of targeted strategies that can attenuate tumoral immunosuppression (as introduced in Sections V and VI). Chapter 16 introduces concepts in immunoguiding—that is, the development of tactics to guide the use of immunotherapy based on changes in the quality or quantity of immune metrics in treated subjects. This area encompasses the general area of immunopharmacology, which will be critical for the successful development of tailored or personalized treatments in different disease settings and patients.

Section IV opens the second half of the book, which addresses how to improve survival outcomes using immunotherapeutic strategies. This section offers examples of how different passive or active immune strategies are yielding knowledge into how to harness the immune system to attack tumors, with a focus on cellular therapies, vaccines and immune checkpoint antibodies. These approaches may all benefit considerably from combinations with one or more strategies for reversing tumoral immune suppression introduced in the last section of the book, with the potential to reduce or even relieve needs for traditional chemotherapy, which might ultimately be unseated as a standard of care. In Chapter 17, the field of adoptive T-cell therapy is discussed, focusing on how efforts in engineering T-cell receptors have greatly leveraged therapeutic impact. Chapters 18 and 19 offer lessons gained from study of the first active and passive immunotherapies to be approved by the U.S. FDA for patient treatment, namely, the autologous dendritic cell vaccine sipuleucel-T (Provenge®) and the anti-CTLA4 antibody ipilumimab (Yervoy®). In seeking to promote more effective tumor antigen presentation, Provenge® offers the first of many strategies that will no doubt be developed to improve the activity of dendritic cells in cancer patients. In contrast, Yervoy® offers the first of many strategies that will no doubt be developed to block negative coregulatory signals (immune checkpoint signals) which stanch immune activation by tumor antigens. Chapter 20 describes lessons gained from development of one of the more thoroughly studied tumor antigen vaccines, PSA-TRICOM, which like Provenge® was developed for prostate cancer. As an illustration of the development of the cancer vaccine field, this project has yielded significant information over the years. Lastly, Chapter 21 addresses adjuvant strategies for vaccines. The introduction of appropriate adjuvants to vaccinations against infectious diseases in the 1950s had an enormous impact on efficacy, and similar factors may also affect the impact of cancer vaccines despite interest in their use for treatment as well as prophylaxis.

Section V addresses how to improve clinical responses using combinations of agents that constitute immunochemotherapy (see Figure 1.1). Cancer pharmacology and cancer immunology are each very well-developed fields, but efforts to investigate combinatorial regimens at this interface at either the preclinical or clinical level remain little developed. Conceptual barriers between fields that were created by historical developments are now fading [3], but the lack of cross-communication and cross-fertilization still represent impediments to the development of immunochemotherapy even with existing tools. This section of the book highlights areas where there are some strong arguments for multidisciplinary investigations and clinical trials. Chapter 22 examines the use of small molecule inhibitors of histone deacetylase (HDAC) as an illustration of how epigenetic modification may be important in the immune microenvironment of cancer, as well as cancer cells themselves (where epigenetic studies have

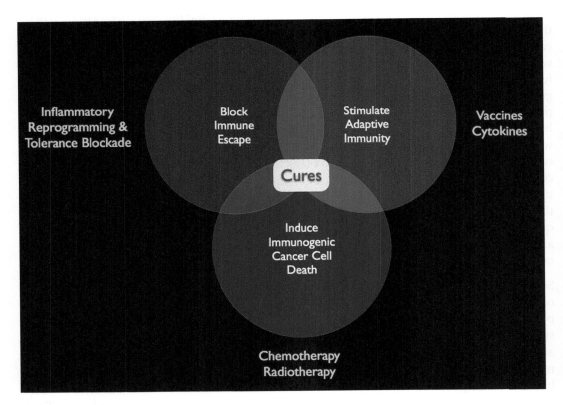

FIGURE 1.1

Immunochemotherapy of the future. The new synthesis of immunological thought with the mainstream of cancer research is stimulating the creation and evaluation of new combinations of therapies that can stimulate the immune system, relieve the immune blockades erected by tumor cells, and trigger pro-immunogenic tumor cell deaths. Immune blockades erected by tumors are associated with altered inflammatory "flavors" of their microenvironment, switching its character from antagonistic to supportive for tumor outgrowth. Thus, agents that can reprogram the inflammatory microenvironment or block tolerance—these may be genetically synonymous [8]—may further leverage the efficacy of immunochemotherapies that are comprised of existing strategies to stimulate immunity and kill cancer cells.

focused to date). Chapter 23 discusses tools to profile immunotherapeutic resistance including such epigenetic changes that affect gene expression. Chapter 24 discusses how traditional cytotoxic chemotherapy not only stimulates immune activity but in doing so improves efficacy. While some of this information has existed for some time, it has not been widely appreciated, and only recently have mechanisms emerged that can begin to explain the basis for immunostimulatory effects of traditional chemotherapy. In closing this section, Chapter 25 discusses how harnessing these effects may represent a golden opportunity in combinations with active immunotherapy. Such ideas have been heterodox until recently, with the bias that chemotherapy could only damage the immune system and thereby hinder the desired effects of immunotherapy. It is now becoming clear this widely held view is incorrect. Indeed, with an emerging appreciation of how traditional cytotoxic chemotherapies engage the immune system—and perhaps must engage it—it may be possible to define immunochemotherapy combinations that improve durable clinical responses and long-term survival in patients.

Section VI introduces the exciting and rapidly growing knowledge base concerning the molecular nature of immunosuppressive barriers erected by tumors. Targeting those barriers now becomes possible with these advances as rational strategies to degrade or defeat immune escape. One common thread in this chapter is the presentation of different perspectives on myeloid cells derived from the innate immune system that help shape the inflammatory state(s) that support invasive cancer and metastatic progression. Tumor stroma include a large number of these cells. Indeed, emerging work tends to support the concept [8] that mechanisms of immune escape overlap genetically with mechanisms of cancer-associated inflammation, perhaps principally involving myeloid cells, such that corrective approaches to immune escape might be viewed as synonymous with inflammatory reprogramming of the tumor microenvironment.

Section VI discusses a variety of cellular and molecular principles along with tractable therapeutic approaches for clinical evaluation. Chapter 26 discusses the area of JAK/STAT signaling, where one of the first clinically approved inhibitors for exploration in the oncology clinic has emerged, with a focus on myeloid cells. Chapters 27 and 28 focus on two myeloid cell subsets of great interest, the tumor-associated macrophages (TAM) and the myeloid-derived suppressor cells (MDSC), each of which contribute strongly to procancerous inflammatory programming in the tissue microenvironment of cancer cells. Chapter 29 introduces Hyper-Acute vaccines, a provocative new class of nonautologous whole tumor cell vaccines engineered to harness the hyperacute xenotransplantation rejection response as a general strategy to reprogram inflammation in the context of tumor antigen presentation. Early clinical trials suggest the HyperAcute approach may broadly degrade suppression mechanisms against tumor antigens in a manner associated with eosinophil recruitment. The remaining chapters shift from cellular to molecular principles of immunosuppression. Chapter 30 discusses the exploding work on tumor-associated exosomes, comprised of small vesicles secreted from cells which convey hormone-like messages in tissues (proteins, microRNAs and other components). Exosomes may tolerize dendritic cells to antigens and mediate critical inflammatory and immune regulatory signals in the tumor microenvironment, with major prognostic and therapeutic import. Chapters 31—34 focus on molecular principles of immunomodulation by galectins, indoleamine 2,3-dioxygenase (IDO), arginase and nitric oxide (NOS). This area encompasses the fascinating new field of tumor immunometabolism. Together, there is growing evidence that these cellular and molecular actors may be broadly involved in cancer immunosuppression, prompting great interest in clinical study of inhibitors that can degrade the metabolic barricades they erect to help tumors evade immune control. Strategies for therapeutic inactivation of these mechanisms, which are now largely well justified from work in preclinical models, are moving forward presently in early clinical trials.

Together, the areas discussed in this section of the book provide an overview of different types of immunotherapeutic approaches being taken to capture different elements of the immune system to more effectively attack and eradicate tumor cells. In the present culture, cancer immunologists tend to be oriented to biological therapies and to have limited knowledge of cancer pharmacology or genetics. Conversely, cancer geneticists and pharmacologists tend to be oriented toward small molecule therapies and to have limited understanding of cancer immunology or immune-based therapies (other than perhaps passive immune therapies, e.g., antibodies). It is hoped that this book can reveal why interactions between these two still relatively disparate groups will be both intellectually and clinically rewarding as the exciting new field of immunochemotherapy unfolds this decade. With the end of a long separation between cancer biologists and cancer immunologists [7], this new conceptual synthesis in cancer research may represent the opening stage of an all-out war on cancer with better hopes of obliterating this terrible disease.

ACKNOWLEDGMENTS

Work in the authors' laboratories has been supported by NIH grants CA109542, CA159337 and CA159315, New Link Genetics Corporation, Sharpe-Strumia Research Foundation, Lankenau Hospital Foundation and the Main Line Health System (G.C.P.) and by NIH grants R01CA122081, P50CA062924, and P50CA088843 (E.M.J.). Dr. Jaffee is the first recipient of the Dana and Albert "Cubby" Broccoli Professorship in Oncology and the co-director of the Skip Viragh Pancreatic Cancer Center at Johns Hopkins University. G.C.P. declares competing interests as a scientific advisor, grant recipient and stockholder in New Link Genetics Corporation, which is developing HyperAcute vaccines and which has licensed patented technology from the author's institution to develop small molecule inhibitors of IDO and the IDO pathway for the treatment of cancer and other diseases. E.M.J. declares competing interests based upon licensing of patented vaccines from the author's institution to BioSante Pharmaceuticals and Aduro BioTech Inc. The inventions from both authors have the potential to generate future royalties.

8

References

[1] Hanahan D, Weinberg RA. The hallmarks of cancer. Cell 2000;100:57—70.

[2] Hanahan D, Weinberg RA. Hallmarks of cancer: the next generation. Cell 2011;144:646—74.

[3] Prendergast. Immunological thought in the mainstream of cancer research: past divorce, recent remarriage and elective affinities of the future. OncoImmunology 2012;1:1—5.

[4] Dunn GP, Old LJ, Schreiber RD. The three Es of cancer immunoediting. Ann Rev Immunol 2004;22:329—60.

[5] Folberg R, Hendrix MJ, Maniotis AJ. Vasculogenic mimicry and tumor angiogenesis. Am J Pathol 2000;156:361—81.

[6] Cho I, Blaser MJ. The human microbiome: at the interface of health and disease. Nat Rev Genet 2012;13:260—70.

[7] Prendergast GC, Jaffee EM. Cancer immunologists and cancer biologists: why we didn't talk then but need to now. Cancer Res 2007;67:3500—4.

[8] Prendergast GC, Metz R, Muller AJ. Towards a genetic definition of cancer-associated inflammation: role of the IDO pathway. Am J Pathol 2010;176:2082—7.

Principles of Basic Immunology

CHAPTER 2

Components of the Immune System

Amanda Norvell
Department of Biology, The College of New Jersey, Ewing NJ USA

I. OVERVIEW

The immune system, which is comprised of a diverse collection of cells, molecules and organs, does an astonishing job of protecting individuals from dangers as varied as foreign pathogens and cancerous cells. When functioning appropriately, the work of the immune system goes unnoticed but in cases of immune dysfunction severe consequences result in the form of autoimmunity or immunodeficiency. Orchestrating appropriate and protective immune responses requires a high degree of coordination and communication between multiple cells. This chapter will present a general overview of the human immune system, describing the general organization of the immune system and introducing the major cell types and responses, thus providing a conceptual framework upon which the future chapters will build.

In the simplest terms, the immune system identifies and eliminates dangerous elements. To do so requires two critical activities: *recognition*, identification of the harmful agent, the "antigen," by specific receptors expressed on the surface of immune system cells, followed by *effector responses*, the cellular behaviors that confer protection. A protective immune response that eliminates or neutralizes the antigen involves the synchronized activity of multiple cell types and a variety of cellular responses. Communication between the cells occurs through both cell–cell contact-mediated signaling, as well as through chemical signals that are secreted from one cell and received by others. Many of the cells, such as macrophages and dendritic cells, that participate in an immune response do so by recognizing foreign cells and then responding through a variety of activities that both promote their destruction or clearance and help to alert other cells of the immune system to the danger. Other specialized cells, called lymphocytes, circulate and patrol the body looking for foreign substances. Each lymphocyte is capable of recognizing only a single antigen, so protection for the organism is achieved by having a veritable army of diverse lymphocytes circulating at any given time. Once a particular lymphocyte encounters an antigen it responds by proliferating and differentiating to form cells with specific functional activities, such as cytotoxic T lymphocytes (CTLs) that are capable of direct killing of target cells, and long-lived memory cells that remain in the body, poised to respond to the antigen if it is encountered again. While the molecular events that occur in individual cells are critical and have been the subject of extensive investigation, the details of how many cells and cellular responses are coordinated to offer robust protection against varied dangers, or how the immune response is deregulated in cases of autoimmunity or immuno-deficiency, are areas of active research.

The study of the immune system grew from concern about human health and the understanding that microbes can cause disease. Immunology as a field of study emerged as scientists of the 19th century, such as Louis Pasteur and Robert Koch, began work on the germ theory of infection.

Cancer Immunotherapy. http://dx.doi.org/10.1016/B978-0-12-394296-8.00002-6

Once establishing that microbes can cause illness, the next natural step was to understand how to protect people from infectious diseases. The historic observation, dating as far back as ancient Greece, that those that had been sick and recovered were naturally resistant to future illness led to the systematic study of how exposure to microbes leads to protection from disease. This characteristic, called memory, is one of the most remarkable features of the immune system. Not only does the immune system remember what foreign agents it has seen, but upon subsequent encounter with the same agent, the "secondary immune response" is greatly enhanced; it occurs more rapidly and with much more effective force. Immune memory is the basis for vaccination and current efforts are focused on understanding how to promote protective, long-lived immunity to particular pathogens or to cancers.

II. PRINCIPAL TISSUES AND ORGANS

The immune system is formed by a varied collection of interconnected cells and tissues distributed throughout the body. The major cell types that comprise the immune system are described briefly below, but for the most part many of these cells are circulatory or migratory. The lymphoid organs, including the primary lymphoid organs (bone marrow and thymus) and the secondary lymphoid organs (including regional lymph nodes and spleen), are connected to one another through two separate circulatory systems, the blood system and the lymphatic system. The primary lymphoid organs are the sites of white blood cell production and differentiation, while the secondary lymphoid organs and the circulatory systems outside of the primary lymphoid organs are collectively referred to as the "periphery." The lymph nodes and spleen serve to filter and trap foreign molecules and cells that are delivered from the tissues via the lymph fluid or the blood. In addition, the secondary lymphoid organs also provide an organized tissue in which the white blood cells can both encounter foreign antigen molecules and can physically interact with other white blood cells to initiate an appropriate immune response. Generally, all secondary lymphoid organs have a similar overall structure, with most having a kidney-bean shape that is covered by a thick capsule [1]. Within the lymphoid organs, subdomains such as the cortex, paracortex and medulla can also be distinguished morphologically because different populations of cells are enriched in specific regions of the organs. Blood and lymph fluid are delivered and drained to and from the lymphoid organs by the afferent and efferent vessels respectively. Additionally, highly specialized subregions of the spleen called germinal centers, which are required for the formation of memory B cells, form during the course of an immune response [2,3].

III. CELLS OF THE IMMUNE SYSTEM

The major cells of the immune system are an assortment of blood cells that can be grouped into three general categories, the *lymphocytes*, including T cells, B cells and Natural Killer (NK cells); the *myeloid cells*, which include the antigen presenting cells, the macrophages, and dendritic cells (DCs); and finally the *granulocytic cells*, such as neutrophils, basophils, and eosinophils. For the most part all of these cells are derived from a common stem cell (Figure 2.1). In adult human blood cell production, a process called hematopoesis takes place in the bone marrow. This microenvironment, which contains multiple support cells in the form of epithelial cells and stromal cells, promotes the division and differentiation of developing blood cells. Throughout human ontogeny the site of hematopoesis shifts: during fetal stages blood cells are initially derived in the fetal liver, then their development shifts to the neonatal spleen, and finally around birth hematopoesis moves to the bone marrow. All blood cells, including red blood cells and the white blood cells of the immune system, develop from hematopoietic stem cells that divide to both self-renew and to produce pluripotent progenitor cells [4]. These progenitors differentiate down one of two major pathways, as either lymphoid cells, which further develop into cells of the B-cell lineage, T-cell lineage or NK-cell lineage, or into granulocyte/monocyte progenitors that can differentiate into specialized

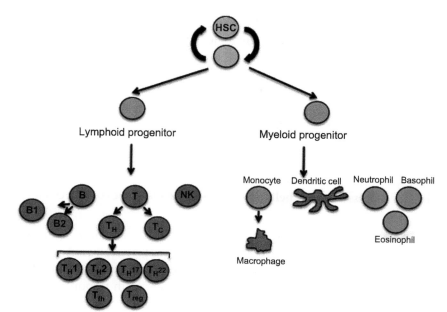

FIGURE 2.1

Schematic diagram of the major cells of the immune system. Blood cells are derived from a common hematopoietic stem cell that gives rise to two lineages of cells: the lymphoid cells and the granulocyte/monocyte lineage. Lymphoid progenitor cells further differentiate into B cells, T cells or Natural Killer cells, while the neutrophils, basophils and eosinophils represent the mature granulocytes and dendritic cells and monocyte/macrophages comprise the mature monocyte lineage.

dendritic cells, macrophages, neutrophils, eosinophils, mast cells, megakaryocytes or red blood cells. With the exception of T cells, which arise within the bone marrow environment but migrate to the thymus where they continue to mature and develop, the remaining blood cells progress through defined steps in their differentiation in the bone marrow and exit to enter the periphery as mature, functional cells. The relatively recent discovery that umbilical cord blood is also a rich source of hematopoietic stem cells has expanded treatment options for individuals requiring bone marrow transplants, and has also facilitated further understanding of stem cell biology as cord blood, which traditionally was discarded at birth, can now provide a non-invasive and relatively non-controversial source of stem cells for study [5]. The external and internal signals that drive the cell fate choices of developing blood cells have not yet been fully elucidated, but unraveling the mysteries of how and why a particular progenitor cell differentiates down a B-cell lineage rather than a T-cell lineage, for example, has important implications for the treatment of human diseases such as various forms of immunodeficiency or in leukemia [6].

A. Lymphocytes

B lymphocytes: B cells, which are named for their site of origin in chickens, the Bursa of Fabricious, are small circulating lymphocytes. All B cells are distinguishable by the surface expression of a B cell specific form of the CD45 protein; this variant is called B220 and it serves as a pan-B cell marker. Two distinct B cell subsets have been described: the B1 B cells and the B2 B cells [7]. B1 cells are a population of long-lived and self-renewing lymphocytes that reside primarily in the peritoneal and pleural cavities. These cells express low levels of B220, and many of them also express the CD5 surface marker. Most B cells, however, fall into the B2 B cell category. These cells are also called "conventional B cells" and are characterized by the expression of high levels of B220. As they are the majority population, discussion of B cells in this chapter will focus on the conventional B2 B cell population exclusively. Finally, all B cells also express a receptor for antigen on the cell surface and, following recognition of antigen, the B cell divides and some of its progeny differentiate into plasma cells that secrete soluble immunoglobulin molecules (also called *antibodies*).

T lymphocytes: T cells are named for the thymus, which is their site of maturation in humans. Early progenitor T cells are derived in tissue of general hematopoesis, for example in the bone marrow of an adult human, and they migrate to the thymus where they continue to

13

develop [8]. Immunocompetent T cells exit the thymus to populate the peripheral circulation. In contrast to B cells, however, which comprise a single major lineage, there are a number of specialized T-cell populations that are phenotypically and functionally distinguished based on the expression of particular surface markers. Just as B220 serves as a marker for all cells of the B lineage, CD3, a complex comprised of multiple surface glycoproteins, is considered a pan-T-cell marker.

Helper T cells: Approximately 60% of mature T cells are said to be helper T cells (Th), which are delineated by surface expression of the CD4 glycoprotein. This category of lymphocytes provides assistance or help to other cells in the immune system through the secretion of soluble chemical signals called cytokines, as well as through cell–cell contact mediated by membrane bound molecules expressed on the helper cell and surface molecules on the cell it is assisting [9,10].

Cytotoxic T cells: The second largest population of T cells in the periphery is the Cytotoxic T cells (CTLs) and these are demarcated by the surface expression of CD8 [11]. These T cells have the ability to recognize and kill virally infected or cancerous cells. Following recognition of the altered-self cells, CTLs kill their targets by inducing a programmed cell death response in the infected or cancerous cell.

Regulatory T cells: Tregs are a small subset of CD4+ T cells that also constitutively expresses CD25 (the alpha chain of the IL-2 receptor). Two distinct Treg populations have been described: those that arise during normal thymic development (natural or nTregs) and those that can be induced in the periphery (induced or iTregs). These populations of T cells fail to develop in individuals carrying mutations in the Foxp3 gene, which encodes a forkhead family transcription factor, and these individuals are susceptible to certain autoimmune syndromes. Thus, Tregs appear to have a major role in preventing autoimmunity [12–14].

Natural Killer cells: NK cells are a third category of lymphocytes and are microscopically distinguished from B and T cells because NK cells are larger and have extensive granules. NK cells are so named because they have the ability to kill target cells through several distinct molecular pathways. NK-cell populations are classified based on the expression of cell surface markers; NK cells do not express CD3 (thus distinguishing them from T cells) but all NK cells are recognized by the expression of both CD16 (an Fc receptor molecule) and CD56 (an adhesion molecule). NK-cell populations can be further divided based on the differential expression of CD56; approximately 90% of circulating NK cells express low levels of CD56, while 10% have high levels of CD56 on the cell surface. At a functional level, NK cells with relatively lower levels of CD56 have increased cytolytic activity, while those with higher CD56 expression appear to secrete large amounts of a variety of cytokines [15–17].

B. Antigen-presenting cells

In order to recognize peptide antigens, T cells must see them in the context of self-MHC molecules, which will be discussed in more detail below, but this fact means that T cells require other cell types in order to do their jobs. With regard to Th-cell function, this group of necessary cells comprises the professional antigen-presenting cells (APCs) and it includes dendritic cells, macrophages and B cells [18–22]. Both macrophages and dendritic cells are of the myeloid lineage; this group is rather heterogeneous with regard to lifespan and phenotypic characteristics. All three populations of APCs, however, can internalize extracellular molecules through the endocytic pathway, and following their breakdown, peptide fragments derived from internalized protein molecules are presented on the surface of the APC in the context of a self molecule called the Major Histocompatibility Complex (MHC) Class II. Macrophages and dendritic cells internalize potential antigens through phagocytosis or by receptor-mediated endocytosis, while B cells can only internalize antigens through receptor-mediated endocytosis.

14

Macrophages: Macrophages, which have phagocytic activity and the ability to produce large amounts of cytokines, differentiate from circulating monocytes in the periphery. Once leaving the bone marrow, monocytes circulate for a short time before they migrate into specific tissues and differentiate into tissue macrophages. Some populations of macrophages remain in specific tissues, becoming what is called "resident macrophages," while others can continue to migrate throughout the body, becoming "infiltrating macrophages." Just as distinct subpopulations of Th cells, which are characterized by patterns of cytokine expression, have been described, it is becoming apparent that there are also subpopulations of macrophages that can be distinguished by their distribution, functional activity and cytokine profiles [19,20].

Dendritic Cells: Dendritic cells were initially named for their morphology; they have long, thin, delicate processes, which look similar to the dendrites on neurons. Two major populations of DCs have been described: myeloid DCs and plasmacytoid DCs that are each derived from distinct progenitor cell types. These major groups of DCs can also be further subdivided based on expression of particular surface proteins and cytokines. Dendritic cells are potent antigen-presenting cells, as they have a large surface area and express high levels of MHC Class II on the surface. DCs play an absolutely critical role in promoting immune responses and, intriguingly, it is now also clear that DCs may also play a direct role in preventing immune responses inappropriately directed against self-molecules [22]. Ralph Steinman was a co-recipient of the 2011 Nobel Prize in Physiology and Medicine for his lifetime of work describing the critical role for DCs in immune responses.

IV. IMMUNE RESPONSES

Simplistically, the immune system can be thought of as having two branches, the innate immune system and the adaptive immune system, although this discrete bifurcation is not truly accurate, as specific cell types and immune responses are found in both branches. Furthermore, it has become more apparent that the signals and cues provided by the innate immune response have a significant effect on the efficiency and strength of the response of the cells of the adaptive branch [23]. Indeed, macrophages and dendritic cells represent critical bridges between both branches and adaptive responses would not be possible without these cell types. While the innate immune system provides immediate, and in some ways a generalized defense against infectious agents, the adaptive immune response takes a bit longer to initiate, but once it is activated it provides exquisitely specific and long-lasting protection. Combined, the power of the two branches of the immune system offers large-scale protection from the world of foreign pathogens, as well as internal dangers such as cancer.

Innate immunity, often described as the more primitive immune system, is found in organisms across phylogeny, including plants and simple multicellular animals. The collection of cells and cellular responses considered to be part of the innate response is quite diverse. Some features of the innate immune system act to prevent microbial colonization through physical or physiological barriers. The skin, for example, is considered a component of the innate branch as it is a first line of defense that must be penetrated, either through cuts or insect bites, for an invading organism to enter a host. Similarly, the pH of the stomach is also inhospitable to many microorganisms and thus serves as an effective physiological barrier. At the cellular level, generally cells of the macrophage/granulocyte lineage, as well as NK cells, are the major players in the innate immune response.

While the role of many of these innate immune system cells in the presentation of antigens to the adaptive branch has been appreciated for some time, the ability of innate system cells to themselves recognize foreign cells and respond appropriately has only been fully understood for a relatively short period. Groundbreaking work from several labs, most notably the work of Bruce A. Beutler and Jules A. Hoffmann which was recognized with the 2011 Nobel Prize in Physiology and Medicine, has offered insight into how microbial cells are recognized by the cells of the innate immune system [24,25]. Microbes, which include bacteria, viruses, fungi and assorted parasites, have conserved motifs that are not found on human cells. For example, lipopolysaccharide (LPS) is a polysaccharide component of the outer cell membrane of gram negative bacteria, while double-stranded RNA is a feature of many viruses, and neither of these features is commonly found in human cells. Collectively, molecular motifs associated with microbes are called Pathogen-Associated Molecular Patterns (PAMPs). These PAMPs are recognized by a broad group of receptors called Pattern Recognition Receptors (PRRs) that are expressed on a wide variety of immune system cells, including those of the innate branch such as NK cells, macrophages and DCs [26]. To date a variety of PRR families have been described, including the retinoic acid-inducible gene I (RIG-I)-like receptor family (RLR) and the C-lectins [27]. The first discovered, and most well-characterized, family of PRRs are the Toll-like Receptors (TLRs), so named for their homology with the *Drosophila* Toll protein [28]. TLRs are transmembrane proteins that are expressed at the cell surface or on internal membranes such as endosomes. To date, 13 different TLR proteins have been identified in humans and these are expressed in a variety of cell types, including cells of the innate branch of the immune system, lymphocytes and on populations of epithelial cells. Ligation of TLRs induces a signaling cascade that ultimately initiates a cellular response of some sort. For example, LPS is recognized by TLR4, and signaling through TLR4 on macrophages and DCs causes them to upregulate expression of pro-inflammatory cytokines, such as Interleukin-6 (IL-6), Interferon-beta (IFN-β) and Tumor Necrosis Factor-alpha (TNF-α). TLR ligation can initiate several different types of responses, including activation of the adaptive branch of the immune system, inflammatory responses or even tissue repair [25]. Understanding the details of how PRRs mediate appropriate responses or how PRRs distinguish pathogenic microbes from harmless microbes, such as those that are found as commensal residents of the intestine, has not yet been fully elucidated.

The adaptive branch of the immune system is comprised predominantly of the lymphocytes of the B-cell and T-cell lineages. The behavior of these cells, with regard to their ability to recognize specific antigens and their responses following antigenic stimulation, gives the adaptive immune response five defining characteristics: **specificity**, **inducibility**, **diversity**, **memory** and **nonresponsiveness to self.** Understanding how these features of the adaptive branch of the immune system are achieved, and how to effectively exploit these characteristics in order to protect from infection or fight disease, has been the focus of intensive research for much of the last century and through today. There are two types of adaptive immune responses: humoral responses and cell-mediated responses, which are directed by the B cells and the T cells, respectively. The humoral response is characterized by the production of soluble immunoglobulins or antibodies. These proteins have a number of specific effector functions that will be described in a bit more detail below, but ultimately they bind to target antigens and mediate either their destruction or clearance from the body, or in the case of molecules like toxins or viruses, antibody binding can render them inactive. Cell-mediated responses are a bit more diverse and include the direct killing of target cells, either virally infected or cancerous cells by specialized T cells or NK cells, as well as the production of cytokines by T cells and the subsequent activation of other cells.

V. LYMPHOCYTE RECOGNITION OF ANTIGEN

The cells of the immune system continually circulate, constantly searching for invading microbes, other dangerous invaders or altered self-cells. Lymphocytes that have entered the periphery and have not yet encountered antigens are said to be naïve, and these cells have a finite lifespan. To initiate an immune response, either humoral or cell-mediated, a specific lymphocyte must be appropriately stimulated by antigenic encounter. This ensures that lymphocytes do not differentiate into effector cells when their target is not present. Thus, the first step of an immune response is specific antigen recognition by a given B or T cell.

One of the key features of both B and T cells is that individual lymphocytes express a single, specific antigen receptor on their surface. In the case of B cells, this antigen receptor is a membrane bound immunoglobulin molecule (surface Ig, or sIg) [29,30], while for T cells it is a membrane bound heterodimeric protein called the T-cell receptor (TCR) [31]. The antigen receptor on each lymphocyte is unique and capable of binding to a single antigenic determinant, which is termed an epitope. Antigen binding, which is mediated by noncovalent interactions between the amino acids of the antigen-binding site of the antigen receptor and the epitope, initiates a biochemical signaling cascade that ultimately leads to the "activation" of the lymphocyte. Importantly, however, sIg and the TCR have short cytoplasmic tails, and thus they cannot transduce an intracellular biochemical signal. To do so, both types of antigen receptors rely on the association with other molecules, the Ig-α and Ig-β proteins on B cells and the proteins of the CD3 complex on T cells. Following appropriate stimulation with foreign antigen, activated B and T cells divide, generating multiple copies of themselves, and these daughter cells go on to differentiate into functional effector cells and long-lived memory cells (Figure 2.2). Importantly, the antigen specificity of the daughter cells, both the effectors and the memory cells, is identical to that of the original lymphocyte. This behavior, the ability of a single cell to recognize foreign antigen and respond by generating multiple effector and memory cells with the same specificity, is termed the *clonal selection theory* and it is a central pillar in our understanding of the immune system [32].

The antigen receptor on B cells is a membrane bound antibody molecule. Antibodies are tetramers comprised of two identical heavy chains and two identical light chains that are held together by covalent bonds to generate a Y-shaped molecule. A functional antibody molecule has two domains: the first is the antigen-binding portion (Fab, for fragment antigen binding), which is formed by the interaction of the heavy and light chains and is located at the membrane-distal portion of the molecule, while the membrane-proximal region of the antibody contains a transmembrane domain that tethers the molecule to the cell surface (Fc portion). A single immunoglobulin molecule is bivalent, containing two identical antigen-binding pockets [33]. Furthermore, the antigen-binding site of an immunoglobulin molecule

17

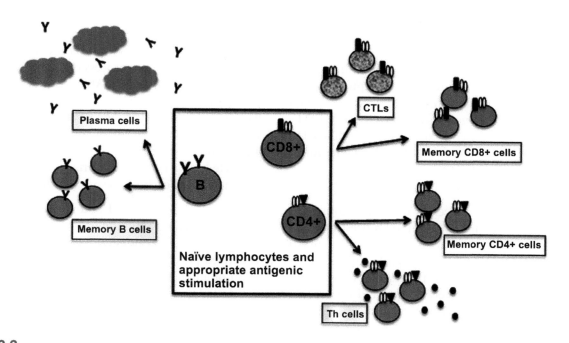

FIGURE 2.2

Following appropriate antigenic stimulation, naïve lymphocytes divide and differentiate into effector and memory populations. Memory lymphocytes retain the same antigenic specificity as the parental cell from which they were derived. Effector B cells, called plasma cells, secrete immunoglobulin molecules, while effector CTLs acquire the ability to lyse target cells, and effector Th populations secrete cytokines.

can recognize antigenic epitopes of nearly any composition, whether protein, nucleic acid, carbohydrate or lipid, or even combinations of macromolecules. The interaction between the antibody and the epitope depends on the three-dimensional shape of the epitope, much as an enzyme-active site recognizes and binds to its substrate. It is important to remember that an antigen is any foreign molecule introduced into the body, while an epitope is the discrete three-dimensional shape that interacts with the Fab portion of the molecule. A complex antigen, such as a polypeptide or an infectious agent, will likely have multiple epitopes capable of activating a number of B-cell clones. An additional feature of the antigens recognized by B cells is that they may be soluble or membrane-bound. Several of these characteristics are in sharp contrast to the characteristics of T-cell antigens, as are described below.

As opposed to the bivalent antigen receptor on B cells, the TCR is monovalent and recognizes a single antigenic epitope [34–36]. Additionally, the TCR comprises two distinct covalently associated polypeptide chains. Greater than 95–99% of circulating T cells express αβTCRs, and a small proportion of T cells express a TCR comprised of γδTCRs. These γδT cells are an unusual population of lymphocytes: they are long-lived cells that appear to be derived mostly during embryonic or early postnatal periods, they express neither CD4 nor CD8, and their mode of antigen recognition is different from that of the αβT cells [37]. For the remainder of this chapter, however, the discussion will be restricted to the majority, traditional αβT-cell population. While the antigen combining site of an antibody molecule can bind a variety of biological macromolecules, the TCR can only recognize peptide antigens, typically peptides 9–15 amino acids in length. Furthermore, the TCR must "see" antigen in the context of a self protein called the Major Histocompatibility Complex (MHC) [38]. MHC molecules are expressed on the surface of cells and they serve to display peptide fragments that have been derived from proteins broken down within the cell. There are two basic types of MHC molecules, MHC Class I and MHC Class II, and these are distinct in several critical ways, but worth noting here is that MHC Class I is expressed on all nucleated cells in the body while MHC II expression is restricted to professional antigen-presenting cells such as macrophages and DCs. Furthermore, the peptides that are presented in the context of MHC Class I are said to be endogenous peptides, that is to say that they are derived from proteins synthesized within the cell. Thus, viral peptides and altered self peptides, such as those that may result in cancer cells, would be displayed by MHC I molecules. In contrast, peptides presented in the context of MHC II are derived from exogenous sources; more specifically they are from proteins that have been internalized and digested through the process of endocytosis. Therefore, MHC II peptides can only be presented by professional APCs, as they are the cells that express MHC II and they are the only cells capable of internalizing and processing exogenous antigens. Finally, CD4+ T cells (Th cells) can only recognize peptides presented in the context of MHC II, while CD8+ T cells (CTLs) are able to interact with peptides in the context of MHC I. In the terminology of immunologists, CD4 T cells are said to be MHC II restricted, while CD8 T cells are MHC I restricted [39]. This has important implications for which type of cell can initiate the effector functions of each of these populations of T cells.

The diversity of antigen combining sites on immunoglobulin and TCR molecules is derived through a unique process of genomic DNA rearrangements in individual B- and T-cell clones [40]. This rearrangement occurs as the lymphocytes are developing in the primary lymphoid organs. Importantly, antigen specificity is derived prior to encounter with antigen and it is a random process. An individual's collection of antigen specificities, or their repertoire, is absolutely unique and it is not shaped or selected by the presence of foreign antigen. Lymphocytes are, however, selected for nonresponsiveness to self antigens [41,42]. This is a complex phenomenon that is achieved through multiple molecular mechanisms. Developing lymphocytes are subjected to rigorous screening, and those that produce an antigen receptor that interacts with a self-molecule are either deleted or rendered non-responsive [43–45]. Potentially autoreactive cells that may escape tolerance induction in the primary lymphoid organs can be held in a nonresponsive state in the periphery through the action of regulatory cells, such as Tregs [46]. Regardless of the mechanism of tolerance induction, however, the end result is a population of lymphocytes that is selected to be nonresponsive to any self antigen. This poses challenges when considering how the immune system recognizes cancerous cells, which may have very few changes relative to their normal counterparts, and thus makes identifying them quite difficult.

Finally, in addition to signals that are generated through their antigen receptors, lymphocytes require co-stimulatory signals to become fully activated and proliferate following antigen encounter. In the case of B cells, co-stimulation comes from ligation of CD40, which is a transmembrane protein constitutively expressed on the surface of mature B lymphocytes. CD40 Ligand, a transmembrane protein expressed on the surface of antigen-activated Th cells, provides the co-stimulatory signal [47]. T-cell activation requires signals sent through CD28, following ligation with its ligands B7.1 (CD80) or B7.2 (CD86) [48,49]. While CD28 expression on T cells is constitutive, B7 family members are expressed on APCs, and their expression patterns are variable. DCs, which are potent APCs, express high levels of B7 at all times, while macrophages and B cells upregulate B7 levels following encounter with antigen. In order to elicit an immune response from lymphocytes multiple signals must be received; the first is stimulation through the antigen receptor, which is always signal one, and the second, the co-stimulatory signal or signal two, is provided by another cell that has also been exposed to antigen (Figure 2.3). This system of checking and double-checking helps to ensure that lymphocytes become fully activated and differentiate into effector cells only after multiple cells have been appropriately stimulated by foreign antigen and thus serves to prevent inappropriate immune responses that could result in autoimmunity.

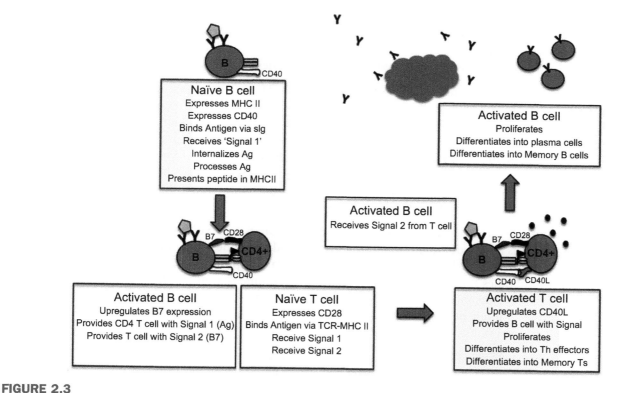

FIGURE 2.3

Full activation, proliferation and differentiation of naïve lymphocytes requires at least two signals; the first is generated through the antigen receptor (signal 1) and the second is a costimulatory signal (signal 2). In this scheme a naïve B cell has interacted with a specific antigen. Following ligation of sIg and internalization and processing of the antigen, the B cell presents a peptide fragment in the context of surface MHC II and upregulates expression of B7. A naïve CD4+ T cell that is specific for that antigen receives signal 1 through the TCR and signal 2, ligation of CD28 by B7 on the B cell, and then upregulates expression of CD40L. This, in turn, provides the B cell with signal 2. Collectively, these signals provide each naïve lymphocyte, the B cell and the T cell, with the two signals they need to differentiate into effector plasma cells and Th cells, respectively.

VI. EFFECTOR FUNCTIONS

Following appropriate stimulation with antigen, lymphocytes proliferate and differentiate into two populations of cells, effector cells and memory cells. The effector cell populations are the cells that actually do the business of eliminating or neutralizing the antigen. In the case of B cells, the effector population is called plasma cells and these cells produce soluble immunoglobulin molecules. T-cell effector populations are much more diverse, but generally T-cell populations can be divided into two major effector types: CD8 Cytotoxic T cells (CTLs) that can kill target cells, and CD4 T helper cells that provide soluble and cell—cell contact mediated help to B lymphocytes and CD8 T cells. As is evidenced by the severe immunodeficiency that eventually occurs following untreated HIV infection, CD4 T cells have a crucial role in both humoral and cell-mediated immunity, and their elimination causes a complete breakdown of both branches of the adaptive immune system.

Ligation of sIg on a mature B cell sends a signal that the cell has seen its antigen. Additionally, antigen that is bound to sIg is internalized by receptor-mediated endocytosis. This allows the B cell to process the antigen and present peptide fragments to Th cells in the context of MHC II, and receive the appropriate help to differentiate into effector plasma cells [18,21]. Plasma cells are essentially factories committed to producing soluble immunoglobulin molecules. The secreted antibody produced by a plasma cell has the same antigenic specificity as the B-cell clone from which it originated. The binding of soluble antibodies to antigens facilitates antigen clearance through several mechanisms. In the case of antigenic epitopes on membrane-bound pathogens, such as bacterial cells or enveloped viruses, antibody binding can cause lysis of the target cell by activating serum complement components (complement fixation). Additionally, antibody-coated antigens can be rapidly cleared by phagocytic cells such as macrophages and DCs through a process called *opsonization*. These APCs have surface receptors for the Fc portion of the antibody molecule and when complexed with antigen, the soluble antibody binds to these Fc receptors and the antibody—antigen complexes are internalized by receptor-mediated endocytosis and degraded.

In humans, there are five major classes of antibody molecules (also called isotypes), IgM, IgD, IgG, IgA and IgE, each of which has unique characteristics. For example, IgM activates complement very well, IgG has a long half-life in serum, and IgA antibodies are secreted across mucous membranes. Following antigenic stimulation, the effector plasma cell population has a finite lifespan, while the memory B cells that are generated do not secrete antibody but survive for much longer periods in circulation. Most plasma cells have a short half-life, on the order of several days to a week; however, recent studies suggest that some long-lived plasma cell populations may exist [50—52].

Primary and secondary humoral immune responses have very different characteristics. While IgM is the predominant immunoglobulin produced following initial antigen encounter, IgGs are the major class secreted during the secondary response. Furthermore, the affinity of the antibodies for the antigen increases in later immune responses. This phenomenon, called *affinity maturation*, is the result of somatic mutation in the DNA that encodes the Fab portion of the antibody molecule and the subsequent selection of B-cell clones that bind the antigen with greater affinity.

Naïve CD8+ T cells circulate in the periphery, performing surveillance on any cell that expresses MHC I molecules. In a healthy individual, most cells display normal self-peptides at the cell surface, and one's T cells should not recognize any of these peptides as foreign. In virally infected cells, or in cancerous cells, however, foreign peptides may be presented in the context of self MHC. If a naïve CD8 T cell recognizes a foreign peptide and receives an appropriate co-stimulatory signal through CD28 and T cell help in the form of the cytokine IL-2, it can proliferate and differentiate into an effector Cytotoxic T cell (CTL). These cells produce granules filled with a small molecule called perforin and a second molecule called

Granzyme B. If and when a CTL effector cell encounters a cell that is displaying the same peptide antigen, it makes contact, called conjugate formation, with the cell through its T-cell receptor and the MHC I on the target. Following conjugate formation, the CTL releases the contents of its granules onto the target. The perforin molecules can insert into the target cell membrane, effectively puncturing the membrane of the target cell and the Granzyme B enzyme enters the target through this breach. Within the target cell cytoplasm, Granzyme B initiates a cascade of events that ultimately leads to apoptosis of the target cell. Importantly, CTLs also induce apoptosis in their targets through a second and unrelated pathway that involves the death receptor protein Fas. Circulating CD8 T cells do not express the Fas Ligand (FasL) on their surface; however, following appropriate stimulation with antigen, activated CTLs upregulate FasL expression. When the CTL forms a conjugate with a target cell, the FasL on the CTL binds to Fas on the target and this initiates a biochemical signaling cascade that induces apoptosis of the target cell. Once a CD8 T clone has been activated by initial antigen encounter, the effector CTLs that are generated become efficient, yet short-lived, assassins that can kill multiple target cells before the CTL clone itself dies [53−55].

T helper populations are absolutely necessary for a functional immune system. Following antigenic stimulation, Th cells provide help through cell−cell contact-dependent signaling and through the production of specific cytokines. CD4+ T-cells can be further categorized into helper cell subsets based predominantly on the spectrum of cytokines they produce. Major Th subsets include the Th1 and Th2 cells which secrete large amounts of IFN-γ or IL-4, respectively [56]. Since the initial recognition that Th cells could be distinguished by the suite of cytokines that they produce, several other CD4+ Th-cell subsets have been described; these include Tregs (regulatory T cells) [12−14], Th17 [57,58], Tfh (follicular helper cells) [59−61] and Th22 cells [62], which are each characterized by the production of a defining set of cytokines. Whether these Th-cell subsets represent distinct Th lineages or whether these distinctions represent more dynamic, transient cellular behaviors, is still an open question [63]. Importantly, however, it is clear that in general, the cytokines produced by a particular Th-cell subset both promote and reinforce that subset's identity and also inhibit the activity or behavior of other Th-cell subsets [64]. Thus, the balance of Th-cell subsets in an individual can have profound effects on the suite of cytokines produced, which in turn can also heavily influence the activity of other Th-cell subsets. How the behavior of Th-cell subsets is maintained during immune responses, and how this balance is perturbed in situations of immune dysfunction, is of great interest.

NK cells are one of the major cell types of the innate branch of the immune system. In addition to secreting cytokines that stimulate multiple cell types and induce a variety of cellular responses, NK cells are somewhat similar to CTLs in that they have cytotoxic activity. NK cells kill their targets through the secretion of perforin and granzymes, as well as the ligation of the death receptors on targets [65,66]. Unlike CTLs, however, NK cells do not require any previous exposure to an antigen in order to differentiate into cytotoxic killers. Activation of their killing activity can be induced through two separate pathways. In the first, target cells coated with antibody molecules can bind to Fc receptors on the NK cells, and this triggers degranulation and killing of the target through a mechanism called antibody-dependent cellular cytotoxicity, or ADCC [67]. The second mechanism involves degranulation induced by the ligation of several classes of receptor proteins on the surface of the NK cell, including adhesion molecules, activating receptors and co-activating receptors [68].

Circulating mature lymphocytes that have not yet encountered antigen are said to be naïve, and these cells have very strict requirements for activation. As described above, in a primary immune response naïve B and T cells must receive two distinct signals, antigen and co-stimulation, in order to proliferate and differentiate into effectors and memory cells. Following this initial stimulation, however, effector populations and memory cell populations have less stringent requirements for activation by antigen. This effectively means that once activated by antigen, the resulting clones of effector and memory cells are easier to trigger following subsequent antigen encounter. When considering CTLs, this means that once a CTL clone has differentiated into a full-fledged killer T cell, it can be triggered to kill antigen-expressing targets more easily than its naïve parental CD8 T-cell clone. How is this achieved? One way in which this can be accomplished is that CTL effectors do not always require co-stimulation to become active, nor do they always require T cell help from CD4 Th clones. This phenomenon, less stringent requirements for antigen activation, is also observed for memory cells, and this helps to ensure that memory responses are magnified as compared to primary responses.

A healthy immune system is capable of responding to an infinite number of foreign or altered-self antigens. Collectively, the responses of the innate and adaptive branches of the immune system provide both a generalized, immediate protection from infectious agents, as well as a long-term specific response to non-self dangers. The ability of the adaptive branch to remember foreign antigens and respond more vigorously and quickly when re-exposed to the same antigen provides opportunities to induce long-lived protection against infectious agents and to altered self. Understanding how the coordinated action of a large number of diverse cells can be harnessed to promote robust and appropriate immune responses remains an ongoing challenge.

References

[1] Ruddle NH, Akirav EM. Secondary lymphoid organs: responding to genetic and environmental cues in ontogeny and the immune response. J Immunol 2009 Aug 15;183(4):2205–12.

[2] Coico RF, Bhogal BS, Thorbecke GJ. Relationship of germinal centers in lymphoid tissue to immunologic memory. VI. Transfer of B cell memory with lymph node cells fractionated according to their receptors for peanut agglutinin. J Immunol 1983 Nov;131(5):2254–7.

[3] Kraal G, Weissman IL, Butcher EC. Memory B cells express a phenotype consistent with migratory competence after secondary but not short-term primary immunization. Cell Immunol 1988 Aug;115(1):78–87.

[4] Seita J, Weissman IL. Hematopoietic stem cell: self-renewal versus differentiation. Wiley Interdiscip Rev Syst Biol Med 2010 Nov-Dec;2(6):640–53.

[5] Alkindi S, Dennison D. Umbilical Cord Blood Banking and Transplantation: A short review. Sultan Qaboos Univ Med J 2011 Nov;11(4):455–61.

[6] Czechowicz A, Weissman IL. Purified hematopoietic stem cell transplantation: the next generation of blood and immune replacement. Immunol Allergy Clin North Am 2010 May;30(2):159–71.

[7] Montecino-Rodriguez E, Dorshkind K. B-1 B cell development in the fetus and adult. Immunity 2012 Jan 27;36(1):13–21.

[8] Thompson PK, Zuniga-Pflucker JC. On becoming a T cell, a convergence of factors kick it up a Notch along the way. Semin Immunol 2011 Oct;23(5):350–9.

[9] Pepper M, Jenkins MK. Origins of CD4(+) effector and central memory T cells. Nat Immunol 2011 Jun;12(6):467–71.

[10] Zhu J, Paul WE. Heterogeneity and plasticity of T helper cells. Cell Res 2010 Jan;20(1):4–12.

[11] Williams MA, Bevan MJ. Effector and memory CTL differentiation. Annu Rev Immunol 2007;25:171–92.

[12] Josefowicz SZ, Rudensky A. Control of regulatory T cell lineage commitment and maintenance. Immunity 2009 May;30(5):616–25.

[13] Sakaguchi S, Yamaguchi T, Nomura T, Ono M. Regulatory T cells and immune tolerance. Cell 2008 May 30;133(5):775–87.

[14] Shevach EM. CD4+ CD25+ suppressor T cells: more questions than answers. Nat Rev Immunol 2002 Jun;2(6):389–400.

[15] Caligiuri MA. Human natural killer cells. Blood 2008 Aug 1;112(3):461–9.

[16] Cooper MA, Fehniger TA, Caligiuri MA. The biology of human natural killer-cell subsets. Trends Immunol 2001 Nov;22(11):633–40.

[17] Fehniger TA, Cooper MA, Nuovo GJ, Cella M, Facchetti F, Colonna M, et al. CD56^{bright} natural killer cells are present in human lymph nodes and are activated by T cell-derived IL-2: a potential new link between adaptive and innate immunity. Blood 2003 Apr 15;101(8):3052–7.

[18] Chen X, Jensen PE. The role of B lymphocytes as antigen-presenting cells. Arch Immunol Ther Exp (Warsz) 2008 Mar-Apr;56(2):77–83.

[19] Geissmann F, Gordon S, Hume DA, Mowat AM, Randolph GJ. Unravelling mononuclear phagocyte heterogeneity. Nat Rev Immunol 2010 Jun;10(6):453–60.

[20] Hume DA. Macrophages as APC and the dendritic cell myth. J Immunol 2008 Nov 1;181(9):5829–35.

[21] Rodriguez-Pinto D. B cells as antigen presenting cells. Cell Immunol 2005 Dec;238(2):67–75.

[22] Steinman RM. Decisions About Dendritic Cells: Past, Present, and Future. Annu Rev Immunol 2011 Oct 13.

[23] Hoebe K, Janssen E, Beutler B. The interface between innate and adaptive immunity. Nat Immunol 2004 Oct;5(10):971–4.

[24] Hoffmann JA. The immune response of Drosophila. Nature 2003 Nov 6;426(6962):33–8.

[25] Moresco EM, LaVine D, Beutler B. Toll-like receptors. Curr Biol 2011 Jul 12;21(13):R488–93.

[26] Janeway Jr CA. Approaching the asymptote? Evolution and revolution in immunology. Cold Spring Harb Symp Quant Biol 1989;54:1–13. Pt 1.

[27] Iwasaki A, Medzhitov R. Regulation of adaptive immunity by the innate immune system. Science 2010 Jan 15;327(5963):291–5.

[28] Medzhitov R, Preston-Hurlburt P, Janeway Jr CA. A human homologue of the Drosophila Toll protein signals activation of adaptive immunity. Nature 1997 Jul 24;388(6640):394–7.

[29] Brezski RJ, Monroe JG. B-cell receptor. Adv Exp Med Biol 2008;640:12–21.

[30] Treanor BB. cell receptor: from resting state to activate. Immunology 2012 Jan 23.

[31] Morris GP, Allen PM. How the TCR balances sensitivity and specificity for the recognition of self and pathogens. Nat Immunol 2012 Feb;13(2):121–8.

[32] Burnet FM. The Clonal Selection Theory of Acquired Immunity. Cambridge, MA: Cambridge University Press; 1959.

[33] Silverton EW, Navia MA, Davies DR. Three-dimensional structure of an intact human immunoglobulin. Proc Natl Acad Sci U S A 1977 Nov;74(11):5140–4.

[34] Garboczi DN, Ghosh P, Utz U, Fan QR, Biddison WE, Wiley DC. Structure of the complex between human T-cell receptor, viral peptide and HLA-A2. Nature 1996 Nov 14;384(6605):134–41.

[35] Garboczi DN, Utz U, Ghosh P, Seth A, Kim J, VanTienhoven EA, et al. Assembly, specific binding, and crystallization of a human TCR-alphabeta with an antigenic Tax peptide from human T lymphotropic virus type 1 and the class I MHC molecule HLA-A2. J Immunol 1996 Dec 15;157(12):5403–10.

[36] Garcia KC, Degano M, Stanfield RL, Brunmark A, Jackson MR, Peterson PA, et al. An alphabeta T cell receptor structure at 2.5 A and its orientation in the TCR-MHC complex. Science 1996 Oct 11;274(5285):209–19.

[37] Hao J, Wu X, Xia S, Li Z, Wen T, Zhao N, et al. Current progress in gammadelta T-cell biology. Cell Mol Immunol 2010 Nov;7(6):409–13.

[38] Zinkernagel RM, Doherty PC. Restriction of in vitro T cell-mediated cytotoxicity in lymphocytic choriomeningitis within a syngeneic or semiallogeneic system. Nature 1974 Apr 19;248(450):701–2.

[39] Braciale TJ, Morrison LA, Sweetser MT, Sambrook J, Gething MJ, Braciale VL. Antigen presentation pathways to class I and class II MHC-restricted T lymphocytes. Immunol Rev 1987 Aug;98:95–114.

[40] Tonegawa S. Somatic generation of antibody diversity. Nature 1983 Apr 14;302(5909):575–81.

[41] Billingham RE, Brent L, Medewar PB. 'Actively acquired tolerance' of foreign cells. Nature 1953;(172):603–6.

[42] Lederberg J. Genes and antibodies: Do antigens bear instructions for antibody specificity or do they select cell lines that arise by mutation? Science 1959;129:1649–53.

[43] Goodnow CC, Crosbie J, Adelstein S, Lavoie TB, Smith-Gill SJ, Brink RA, et al. Altered immunoglobulin expression and functional silencing of self-reactive B lymphocytes in transgenic mice. Nature 1988 Aug 25;334(6184):676–82.

[44] Nemazee DA, Burki K. Clonal deletion of B lymphocytes in a transgenic mouse bearing anti-MHC class I antibody genes. Nature 1989 Feb 9;337(6207):562–6.

[45] von Boehmer H, Kisielow P. Self-nonself discrimination by T cells. Science 1990 Jun 15;248(4961):1369–73.

[46] Bilate AM, Lafaille JJ. Induced CD4(+)Foxp3(+) Regulatory T Cells in Immune Tolerance. Annu Rev Immunol 2011 Mar 24.

[47] Klaus SJ, Pinchuk LM, Ochs HD, Law CL, Fanslow WC, Armitage RJ, et al. Costimulation through CD28 enhances T cell-dependent B cell activation via CD40-CD40L interaction. J Immunol 1994 Jun 15;152(12):5643–52.

[48] Ledbetter JA, Imboden JB, Schieven GL, Grosmaire LS, Rabinovitch PS, Lindsten T, et al. CD28 ligation in T-cell activation: evidence for two signal transduction pathways. Blood 1990 Apr 1;75(7):1531–9.

[49] Turka LA, Ledbetter JA, Lee K, June CH, Thompson CB. CD28 is an inducible T cell surface antigen that transduces a proliferative signal in CD3+ mature thymocytes. J Immunol 1990 Mar 1;144(5):1646–53.

[50] Ahmed R, Gray D. Immunological memory and protective immunity: understanding their relation. Science 1996 Apr 5;272(5258):54–60.

[51] Slifka MK, Ahmed R. Long-lived plasma cells: a mechanism for maintaining persistent antibody production. Curr Opin Immunol 1998 Jun;10(3):252–8.

[52] Good-Jacobson KL, Shlomchik MJ. Plasticity and heterogeneity in the generation of memory B cells and long-lived plasma cells: the influence of germinal center interactions and dynamics. J Immunol 2010 Sep 15;185(6):3117–25.

[53] Berke G. The binding and lysis of target cells by cytotoxic lymphocytes: molecular and cellular aspects. Annu Rev Immunol 1994;12:735–73.

[54] Berke G. The CTL's kiss of death. Cell 1995 Apr 7;81(1):9–12.

[55] Nagata S, Suda T. Fas and Fas ligand: lpr and gld mutations. Immunol Today 1995 Jan;16(1):39–43.

[56] Mosmann TR, Cherwinski H, Bond MW, Giedlin MA, Coffman RL. Two types of murine helper T cell clone. I. Definition according to profiles of lymphokine activities and secreted proteins. J Immunol 1986 Apr 1;136(7):2348–57.

[57] Stockinger B, Veldhoen M, Martin B. Th17 T cells: linking innate and adaptive immunity. Semin Immunol 2007 Dec;19(6):353–61.

[58] Miossec P, Korn T, Kuchroo VK. Interleukin-17 and type 17 helper T cells. N Engl J Med 2009 Aug 27;361(9):888–98.

[59] Zhou L, Chong MM, Littman DR. Plasticity of CD4+ T cell lineage differentiation. Immunity 2009 May;30(5):646–55.

[60] Fazilleau N, Mark L, McHeyzer-Williams LJ, McHeyzer-Williams MG. Follicular helper T cells: lineage and location. Immunity 2009 Mar 20;30(3):324–35.

[61] King C, Tangye SG, Mackay CR. T follicular helper (TFH) cells in normal and dysregulated immune responses. Annu Rev Immunol 2008;26:741–66.

[62] Eyerich S, Eyerich K, Pennino D, Carbone T, Nasorri F, Pallotta S, et al. Th22 cells represent a distinct human T cell subset involved in epidermal immunity and remodeling. J Clin Invest 2009 Dec;119(12):3573–85.

[63] O'Shea JJ, Paul WE. Mechanisms underlying lineage commitment and plasticity of helper CD4+ T cells. Science 2010 Feb 26;327(5969):1098–102.

[64] Knosp CA, Johnston JA. Regulation of CD4+ T-cell polarization by suppressor of cytokine signalling proteins. Immunology 2012 Feb;135(2):101–11.

[65] Arase H, Arase N, Saito T. Fas-mediated cytotoxicity by freshly isolated natural killer cells. J Exp Med 1995 Mar 1;181(3):1235–8.

[66] Bratke K, Kuepper M, Bade B, Virchow Jr JC, Luttmann W. Differential expression of human granzymes A, B, and K in natural killer cells and during CD8+ T cell differentiation in peripheral blood. Eur J Immunol 2005 Sep;35(9):2608–16.

[67] Cooper MA, Fehniger TA, Caligiuri MA. The biology of human natural killer-cell subsets. Trends Immunol 2001;11:633–40.

[68] Bryceson YT, March ME, Ljunggren HG, Long EO. Activation, coactivation, and costimulation of resting human natural killer cells. Immunol Rev 2006 Dec;214:73–91.

CHAPTER 3

Adaptive Immunity: B Cells and Antibodies

Lauren M.F. Merlo, Laura Mandik-Nayak
Lankenau Institute for Medical Research, Wynnewood, PA USA

I. INTRODUCTION TO B CELLS

B cells play many important roles in the immune system, including acting as antigen-presenting cells, cytokine secretion, and setting up the architecture of lymphoid organs, but they are most commonly known as the antibody-producing cells of the adaptive immune system. B cells are capable of producing highly specific antibodies in response to a variety of foreign antigen compounds. In this review, we will describe the stages of B-cell development, the basic processes involved in the generation of B-cell receptors, and the steps in B-cell activation and antibody production (Figure 3.1).

We have only a limited number of genes, yet the immune system may encounter millions of different pathogens or other immune antigens over the lifetime of an organism. Therefore, the immune system must be able to generate an antibody repertoire diverse enough to deal with invading pathogens while avoiding the production of antibodies against "self" and other harmless antigens (e.g., the food we ingest)—and it must do all of this with only a small number of available genes. B cells accomplish this through a unique process of splicing and recombination between different gene segments as well as random nucleotide insertion to introduce further diversity into developing B-cell receptors, which is followed by a selection process to eliminate nonproductive and self-reactive specificities.

The basic stages of B-cell development and maturation can be defined by different steps in the process of B-cell receptor formation. B-cell receptors are formed by 2 heavy chain and 2 light chain molecules (Figure 3.2); these associate to form the mature antigen-recognition molecule—the B-cell receptor (BCR). B cells expressing receptors that are not strongly self-reactive mature and eventually become secreted as antibodies.

B cells and their homologs are important in adaptive immunity in all vertebrates, apparently arising first in jawed fishes during evolution. However, homologs of Ig genes have been found in invertebrates, suggesting that adaptive immunity is derived from ancient immune precursors [1].

II. B-CELL DEVELOPMENT
A. Hematopoietic stem cells

B cells arise in the bone marrow of the long bones of the body and are derived from multipotent hematopoietic stem cells, defined by their ability to self-renew and to produce multiple, more differentiated cell types. These multipotent stem cells differentiate into progenitor cells that produce either lymphoid or myeloid lineages. The lymphoid progenitor produces

25

Cancer Immunotherapy. http://dx.doi.org/10.1016/B978-0-12-394296-8.00003-8

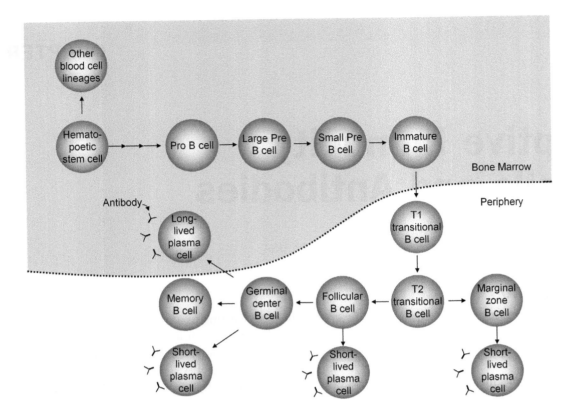

FIGURE 3.1

B-cell development. B cells are derived from hematopoietic stem cells. In the bone marrow VDJ recombination of the heavy chain and VJ recombination of the light chain occur to produce a B-cell receptor. The IgM-expressing immature B-cell can leave the bone marrow and enter the periphery, where it can become activated upon encounter with antigen, generating an initial, short-lived immune response or forming a germinal center where affinity maturation further refines the specificity of the BCR and differentiation of both short- and long-lived plasma cells as well as memory B cells occurs. Plasma cells secrete antibodies that allow for the elimination of pathogens.

T (discussed in Chapter 4), NK (discussed in Chapters 8–9), and B cells. B cells can be differentiated from other blood cell lineages by their cell surface markers (Table 3.1). During hematopoiesis in the bone marrow, blood cell precursors and developing B cells are located in the extravascular spaces between bone marrow medullary vascular sinuses [2].

B. Pro-B cells and heavy chain recombination

The portion of the B-cell receptor (BCR) that recognizes antigens is made up of three disparate genetic regions, termed V, D, and J, that are spliced and recombined at the genetic level in a combinatorial process unique to the immune system. Multiple genes encoding each of these regions exist in the genome and can be joined in different ways to produce a diverse repertoire of receptor molecules. The generation of this diversity is critical; because the body may encounter many more antigens than there are available genes, this process provides a way to produce millions of different combinations of antigen-recognizing receptor molecules.

The rearrangement of the heavy chain (denoted by the subscript H) of the B-cell receptor encompasses the first steps in B-cell development. In early pro-B cells, the short D_H (diversity) and J_H (joining) regions are recombined first, a process dependent on the enzymes RAG1 and RAG2.

Once the D and J regions are recombined, the cell is now considered a "late pro-B" cell (Figure 3.1) and the short DJ region now combines with a longer V_H gene segment. In humans, there are about 50 functional V_H genes located on chromosome 14 [3], along with

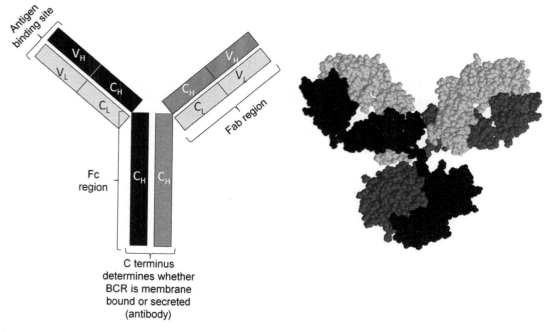

FIGURE 3.2

Antibody structure. The left-hand image shows a schematic of a B-cell receptor/antibody. V_L=variable region of light chain; V_H=variable region of heavy chain; C_L=constant region of light chain; C_H=constant region of heavy chain. The right-hand image is a 3D structure of an IgG antibody [109]. Color-coding between the two images is the same. Light chains=light gray, 1 heavy chain=dark gray, 1 heavy chain=black; note that although colored differently for visualization purposes, the heavy chains are identical.

approximately 25 functional D_H gene segments [4] and 6 J_H segments [5] (in the mouse, approximately 90 V_H, 12 D_H, and 4 J_H genes are located on chromosome 12[6−8]). The VDJ locus itself is highly polymorphic on a population-wide scale, with individuals having different haplotypes with different VDJ genes in varying numbers [9]. The combination of 50 V_H, 25D_H, and 6J_H segments leads to a potential combinatorial diversity of approximately 7500 VDJ heavy chains. The process by which this recombination occurs is highly orchestrated through a RAG-mediated recombination between signal sequences separated by 12 or 23 base pair spacers [10]. This process ensures that only the correct types of genes are recombined, although it does not ensure that the reading frame is preserved, meaning 2/3 of the newly generated VDJ segments will be nonfunctional.

TABLE 3.1 Identifying B Cells by Flow Cytometry—Commonly Used Molecular Markers	
(Surface) Marker	**Use in studying B cells**
B220 (CD45R)	Pan-B cell marker; B-cell development up to but not including plasma cells
CD19	Pan-B cell marker; B-cell development up to but not including plasma cells
CD20	Pan-B cell marker; B-cell development up to but not including plasma cells
IgM	Immature B cells
CD62L (L-selectin)/CD44	Activation markers, together can distinguish naïve from activated B cells
CD69	Early activation marker
MHC Class II	Mature B cells
CD80/CD86	Co-stimulating molecules upregulated on activated B cells
CD138 (syndecan)	Ab secreting cell

At this stage, junctional diversity can be dramatically increased by the addition of N nucleotides in the joints between gene segments. While the addition of nucleotides between joints can also occur during light chain assembly, the enzyme responsible for this addition, terminal deoxytransferase (TdT), is most highly expressed early in B-cell development when the heavy chain is being rearranged [11]. In addition to the N nucleotides added by TdT, a small number of bases, called P bases, can also be added, though these usually represent a smaller contribution to junctional diversity than the N nucleotides [12]. The total number of bases in this region can vary from ~3–25, including the intervening D region, due to the addition of P and N nucleotides and the excision of bases resulting from exonuclease activity [12].

There are, of course, two copies of the VDJ loci in each individual. In general, a B cell produces only a single heavy chain (and, eventually, a single light chain), although rare exceptions have been observed in mouse studies [13]. Recombination at the second locus is inhibited by the process of allelic exclusion, apparently by monoallelic initiation of recombination and feedback inhibition mechanisms, though the molecular details are incompletely understood [14]. It is thought that allelic exclusion reduces the incidence of autoreactivity and autoimmunity [14]. Although the theoretical number of heavy chains that can be generated in the pro-B cell stage between VDJ recombination and junctional diversification is high, the majority of heavy chains will be nonfunctional, often because of an incorrect reading frame generated during splicing. If a Pro-B cell does not produce a heavy chain at the first locus, rearrangement can then proceed at the second locus.

There is a fourth critical component to the heavy chain: the constant (C_H) region. The C region present on heavy chains determines the BCR/antibody class. The initial, immature B cells all express the μ constant region. Constant region genes are located downstream of the recombined VDJ region and the μ constant region is linked with the VDJ region by standard intron splicing processes to produce an IgM molecule.

C. Pre-B cells: Testing of heavy chains and light chain recombination

Once VDJ recombination of the Ig heavy chain is completed, the cell becomes a pre-B cell. First, the newly rearranged heavy chains are tested for reactivity with surrogate light chains [15]. If pairing between the two is successful, a "Pre-B-Cell Receptor" is expressed on the cell surface in association with Igα and Igβ proteins, which are also essential for mature B-cell receptors [16–18], triggering proliferation of the large pre-B cells. At this point, heavy chain rearrangement ceases. The cluster of small pre-B cells generated from the large pre-B cell each has an identical heavy chain but can generate different light chains, further increasing diversity of resultant receptors.

Next, light chain rearrangement occurs. The basic process is the same as for the heavy chain, except that light chains lack a D region. There are two light chain loci in mammals, κ and λ, located on chromosomes 22 and 2 in humans (chromosomes 6 and 16 in mouse), respectively. In an isotype exclusion process, only a single light chain is expressed in each B cell. In humans, the κ chain tends to be rearranged before the λ chain, and the majority of light chains are κ. In mice, this is even more extreme, with κ representing 95% of light chains [19,20]. This ratio is clinically significant, as a distorted κ:λ ratio may indicate a lymphoma. Light chains also have a smaller constant region that does not participate in the Fc region of the BCR/antibody (Figure 3.2). The combination of the VDJ recombined heavy chain and VJ recombined light chain generates a theoretical diversity of $>10^6$ BCRs based on recombination alone, an impressively diverse repertoire from a very limited number of genes.

Light chains are also tested for functionality at this stage. If the initial rearrangement (usually at the κ locus) fails to produce a functional protein, light chains can further rearrange their genes to incorporate an alternative J_L segment located downstream of the original J_L segment. Additionally, rearrangement can occur at the λ locus or at the κ and λ loci on the other chromosome. Light chains also exhibit allelic exclusion, though it is not as complete as in heavy chain rearrangement [14].

D. Immature B cells and B-cell tolerance

Once a light chain is produced that can bind to the existing μ heavy chain, the cell becomes an immature B cell. At this point, the B-cell receptor has formed. These initial, intact IgM molecules are now expressed on the cell surface instead of just intracellularly as in the pre-B cell [21].

Once formed, the IgM molecule is tested for autoreactivity. This central tolerance process is critical for eliminating B cells that have produced receptors that will react with the body's own "self" proteins to avoid development of autoimmune disease. The process is imperfect and cells that are only weakly self-reactive may be allowed to enter the periphery. Effectively, the immune system accepts a small amount of autoreactivity in favor of diversity.

Autoreactive cells can be abolished through one of several processes at this stage. Central tolerance generally alters or eliminates strongly self-reactive B cells either by receptor editing [22–24] or apoptosis through a clonal deletion process [25,26]. It has been estimated that 55–75% of newly arising B cells are autoreactive [27]. If an immature B cell is presented with autoantigen in the bone marrow, it becomes developmentally arrested and reduces expression of B-cell survival factors such as bcl-2 and BAFF [26,28]. For a short period, RAG continues to be expressed, allowing the B cell to rearrange the light chain to alter specificity and potentially reduce autoreactivity [23]. Note that some heavy chain rearrangements are also observed at the pre-B-cell stage [29], but whether the rearrangements are triggered by lack of an in-frame, productive rearrangement or some signal of self-reactivity is not clear [30].

The final tolerance mechanism initiated in the bone marrow is anergy [31–33], whereby a weakly autoreactive cell becomes functionally inactivated and ceases to respond to antigen stimulation. Anergic B cells may leave the bone marrow and enter the periphery. Although it is not a universal phenomenon, anergic cells can be developmentally arrested and may be excluded from the follicle [34] and apoptose within a few days through a process regulated by levels of bcl2 and BIM, with contribution from Fas [28,35,36]. Anergic cells have effectively "tuned down" their antigen receptor signaling and can become activated when presented with large quantities of antigen [37], particularly in cases of restricted antigen repertoire where there is little competition with naïve B cells for survival factors. B cells may also be maintained in an ignorant state whereby, although having the potential for autoreactivity, they do not come into contact with their autoantigen or do not receive T-cell help when encountering autoantigen [38,39].

Tolerance processes occur in the periphery as well as in the bone marrow. A BCR in the periphery may bind to organ-specific proteins not encountered in the bone marrow. In this case, B cells usually do not receive T-cell help, preventing activation of these autoreactive B cells [28,40,41]. Thus, the linked recognition process itself helps dampen autoreactivity. Additionally, autoreactive cells may arise in the periphery as a result of somatic hypermutation in the germinal centers; these cells can be eliminated by apoptosis [42].

These tolerance processes have important implications for human disease. Breakdown in tolerance mechanisms contribute to a variety of autoimmune disorders such as systematic lupus erythematosus (SLE) and rheumatoid arthritis (RA). This also has importance in cancer treatment, as autoimmunity can be a byproduct of cancer therapy, particularly immunotherapies [43].

Cells that are not self-reactive are allowed to leave the bone marrow and enter the periphery. Immature B cells that have migrated to the periphery are often referred to as transitional B cells. These cells can be activated to become mature B cells. In mice, transitional B cells are further subdivided into classes based on surface marker expression and localization, though the transitional B-cell population in humans is less clearly defined [44].

III. MATURE B CELLS
A. Peripheral B cells and lymphoid architecture

Once a B cell develops and becomes mature, these naïve B cells become activated by contact with antigens in peripheral lymphoid tissues, also referred to as secondary lymphoid organs/ tissues (the primary organ being the bone marrow). The chief locations for B-cell activation are the lymph nodes and spleen, with some contribution from other lymphoid tissues such as the tonsils and Peyer's patches. There are multiple classes of mature B cells, but the majority of B cells are the B-2 cells. We will focus on those here, with discussion of the other B-cell subclasses below (see Section III G).

To become activated, a B cell must encounter its antigen either in soluble form or attached to the surface of another cell, generally in the follicles of the spleen and lymph nodes. The structure of these follicles differs somewhat between human and mouse [45]. These areas allow the innate and adaptive immune system to come together to produce a coordinated immune response. B cells spend most of their time in lymphoid tissues; classic studies showed that mature B cells regularly circulate through secondary lymphoid organs, with B cells that have not come into contact with an antigen circulating to another lymphoid organ within 24 hours, spending less than an hour in transit between lymphoid organs [46,47].

The spleen, because it also serves as a blood-filtering organ, tends to "see" systemic, blood-borne pathogens, while the lymph nodes are the primary site for defense against intracellular pathogens and effectively scanning local areas for foreign antigens. Antigens carried to the spleen via the blood enter the lymphoid (white pulp) areas via the marginal sinus. In the lymph nodes, cells enter the cortex, where B cells reside, via high endothelial venules and afferent lymphatic vessels [45]. The conduit systems allowing movement between compartments in the lymph node and spleen appear to differ, allowing for inclusion/exclusion of different sizes and types of particles [45,48]. In both the spleen and lymph nodes, B cells and T cells are segregated into distinct areas called the follicle (B cells) and periarteriolar lymphoid sheaths (T cells), respectively. This segregation (Figure 3.3) is necessary for proper function. Note that B cells themselves are critical for the development of proper lymphoid tissue architecture, especially the splenic marginal zone [49,50].

B. Antigen presentation to B cells

To become activated, first a B cell must come in contact with an antigen. While T cells recognize only short peptide sequences presented in the context of MHC molecules, B cells can recognize large, intact antigens in three dimensions. B cells can recognize some small, soluble

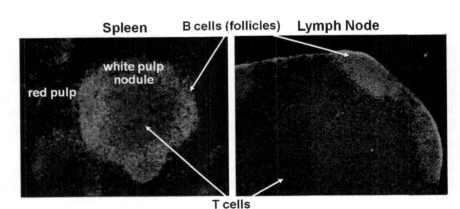

FIGURE 3.3
Murine follicular structure. B- and T-cell areas are separated in secondary lymphoid tissues.

antigens, but more commonly this contact is mediated by antigen-presenting cells of the innate immune system, particularly macrophages and various classes of dendritic cells.

How, exactly, do B cells meet an antigen? Movement of antigen in the lymph node is complex, but recent imaging studies have elucidated a more detailed lymph node structure and allowed for detailed tracking of cell movement [51,52]. Small, soluble antigens appear to pass through poorly defined pores in the subcapsular sinus of the lymph node, where they can enter the follicles directly and encounter naïve B cells. Generally, however, trafficking of antigen in the lymph node is a highly structured process, which improves the odds of a B cell encountering antigen. Presentation of larger, intact antigens such as viruses, bacteria, and immune complexes can be mediated by macrophages located along the subcapsular sinus in lymph nodes, although the exact mechanism by which presentation occurs, whether it be direct presentation of unprocessed antigen or internalization and return to the cell surface is debated [51]. Macrophages may present antigen that can be recognized by the BCR and subsequently internalized and returned to the B-cell surface in the context of MHC to elicit T-cell help [53]. The antigen-presenting properties of dendritic cells are very well studied in relation to T-cell activation, but dendritic cells also can present antigen to B cells. There appears to be a subpopulation of dendritic cells clustered around the high endothelial venules (the entry point of B cells into the lymph node) that can present intact antigen to B cells; the exact molecular mechanisms allowing this intact presentation are under investigation but involve Fc receptors and DC-SIGN [51,54,55].

Follicular dendritic cells (FDCs) are a separate population of dendritic cells that present opsonized antigen to B cells and are likely a key player in antigen presentation. They are present in both the primary follicle, where they present immune complexes to naïve B cells, and in the germinal center during the affinity maturation process [56]. It is not entirely clear how these cells, usually restricted to the follicle, gain access to antigen, but it appears to be through a cell-mediated mechanism, possibly by marginal-zone B cells in the spleen (Section III G) and by follicular B cells themselves [57,58]. FDCs can present antigen through a complement-mediated system and, in germinal centers, by an Fc receptor mechanism [56,59]. FDCs retain antigens for extended periods and can activate cognate B cells for more than one week after antigen administration [52].

Movement of B cells and their antigen in the lymph nodes occurs in response to chemical gradients (e.g., CXCL13 secreted by FDCs) [60] and along a complex network of reticular fibers that can be associated FDC dendritic processes [52]. This highly structured process increases the probability of B cells encountering antigen above what would be expected by a passive diffusion process. Migration of B cells that have internalized antigen via the BCR to the T:B-cell border allows B cells to associate with appropriate helper T cells in a nonrandom manner. Importantly, antigen-specific B cells are effective antigen-presenting cells themselves because they can stimulate T cells under conditions where antigen is limiting, effectively concentrating antigen at the T:B-cell border. These antigen-presentation properties are also critical following this interaction when B cells migrate back to form germinal centers.

B cells that have encountered antigen through one of the mechanisms described above can be activated in a T-cell dependent or independent manner. Although the T-cell dependent mechanism is the more widely studied and thought to be the more important mechanism for providing long-term defense against various pathogens, B cells can become activated without T-cell help when presented with certain types of antigens, particularly bacterial poly-saccharides. Some molecules such as lipopolysaccharide (LPS) can, at high concentrations, produce nonspecific B-cell responses. Other, highly repetitive antigens can stimulate B cells by cross-linking specific B-cell receptors [61]. B cells activated by thymus-independent antigens can undergo class switching and produce short-lived plasma cells, but usually do not undergo affinity maturation or produce memory B cells (but see [62,63]). It is thought that T-cell independent responses are likely important during initial responses to bacterial pathogens.

The more common mechanism is the $CD4^+$ (helper) T-cell dependent activation process, requiring intricate coordination between B and T cells. Once a B-cell receptor recognizes a particular antigen, it internalizes the antigen, degrades it via endocytosis, and subsequently presents peptide pieces on its surface in the context of MHC Class II molecules. MHC Class II molecules are highly polymorphic and are usually expressed only on antigen-presenting cells (B cells, dendritic cells, and macrophages) [64]. CD4+ T cells that recognize the same antigen (though not necessarily the same epitope) as the BCRs initiate a cascade allowing activation of the cognate B cell. In particular, the binding of the CD40 molecule on B cells to the CD40 ligand on T cells and associated release of various cytokines such as IL-4 signals the B cell to divide. At this point, the activated B cells may migrate to the outer portion of the follicle in an EBI-2 mediated process [65] and differentiate quickly into short-lived antibody-producing plasma cells, producing an initial adaptive response to infection. Alternatively, they may migrate into the follicle where they can proliferate and mature further in a germinal center reaction, producing higher-affinity antibody and memory cells but at a slower rate. Whether or not a B cell is directed to the extrafollicular plasma cell formation or a GC reaction may depend on the BCR affinity for the antigen [66].

When B cells respond to T-cell dependent antigen in the follicles in the presence of antigen-retaining FDCs, areas of extensive B-cell proliferation, called germinal centers (GCs), can form within the follicle. Here, B cells undergo clonal expansion, somatic hypermutation, affinity maturation, and class switch recombination (though this also occurs outside GCs), eventually forming antibody-secreting plasma cells. GCs are also the site of memory B-cell formation Section III F). Germinal centers are divided into "dark" and "light" zones based on their characteristic physical appearance. It was long thought that proliferation, class switch recombination, and hypermutation processes generally occurred in the dark zone and T-helper cell interaction at the light zone. It now appears that there may be more B-cell cross-traffic between zones than previously recognized [52,67]. The T-cell subset providing the "help" to B cells in the germinal center, T-follicular helper cells (T_{FH}), has been the subject of extensive recent study [68−70]. T_{FH} cells appear to be the primary T cell responsible for B-cell homing to the follicle and they produce a variety of proteins controlling germinal center formation and plasma and memory cell differentiation, including CD40L, IL-4, and IL-21, which can alter expression of two key regulators of B-cell differentiation, bcl-6 and blimp-1 [68].

C. Class switching

The antibody "class," also referred to as "isotype," is determined by the constant region of the heavy chain. Both short-lived and long-lived antibody-secreting cells can be class switched, and probably receive the signal to switch at the same time as they receive initial T-cell help, with signaling resulting from CD40/CD40L binding [71]. Class switching involves the transfer of the initial µ constant region (IgM) to one of several alternative constant regions, C_γ (IgG), C_ε (IgE), or C_α (IgA). This is accomplished while maintaining the antigen specificity of the variable region at the opposite end of the antibody. The heavy chain class controls the stability of the resultant antibody, and various other proteins can recognize this Fc region of the antibody (Figure 3.2) to help neutralize and clear pathogens. Class switch recombination, like somatic hypermutation (Section III D), is dependent on activation-induced cytidine deaminase (AID) in a well-studied mechanism [72,73]. Briefly, the alternative C regions are arranged in tandem downstream from the initially expressed C_μ region, each with a short "S" (switch) segment upstream. AID deaminates cytosines in the S regions, eventually creating double-stranded breaks which allow for joining of downstream C regions, producing a B-cell receptor with the same VDJ antigen specificity but a new constant region [73]. Humans have 9 C_H regions, arranged C_μ, C_δ, $C_\gamma3$, $C_\gamma1$, $C_\alpha1$, $C_\gamma2$, $C_\gamma4$, C_ε, $C_\alpha2$. The mouse locus and isotypes are different, C_μ, C_δ, $C_\gamma3$, $C_\gamma1$, $C_\gamma2b$, $C_\gamma2a$, C_ε, C_α [74].

32

A fifth immunoglobulin class, IgD, expressed on the surface of transitional B cells, is unusual in that the C_δ region, immediately downstream from the C_μ region, is generally expressed via alternative splicing of a long mRNA transcript encompassing both the C_μ and C_δ, although it may be recombined by class switching in rare instances [75].

We have mentioned that antibodies are secreted B-cell receptors. Each of the C regions can undergo alternative splicing at their C terminus to produce either a membrane-bound B-cell receptor or a secreted receptor (antibody) [75]. The functions of the different immunoglobulin isotypes are discussed more fully in Section IV.

D. Affinity maturation and somatic hypermutation

Affinity maturation is the process by which B cells increase their affinity for a particular antigen. This "fine tuning" of B-cell specificity occurs through a repeated process of somatic hypermutation of B-cell receptors and subsequent clonal selection.

In the GCs, B cells express AID, which initiates somatic hypermutation of the antigen-binding site of B-cell receptors [72]. Both the heavy and light chain Ig genes can be hypermutated, a process of point mutation and repair in the genes encoding the BCR. Hypermutation can occur anywhere along the VDJ region of the Ig gene, beginning with the V region promoter. Generally, AID induces cytosine to uracil deamination, a mismatch that can be repaired by several possible mechanisms including base excision repair and mismatch repair, which recruit error-prone polymerases allowing any base to be incorporated [72]. Most clones generated by somatic hypermutation are likely less specific for the antigen than the original clone. Positive selection for more "fit" clones along with apoptosis of the less fit clones allows for increased affinity. In addition, some of these hypermutated receptors may be autoreactive, so there is likely a tolerance checkpoint associated with this process. Indeed, mice with a deficiency in bcl2-mediated apoptosis develop autoimmunity because autoreactive B cells generated through somatic hypermutation are not eliminated [76,77].

Although the process is not clearly defined, it is thought that the affinity maturation process may be iterative, with positive selection for receptors with the highest antigen affinity and apoptosis of mutated receptors with lower affinity or autoreactivity. Amongst cells with some affinity for the FDC-presented antigen, there may be a subsequent competition step for T-cell help [78]. Ultimately, the germinal center reaction produces two types of cells, memory B cells and antibody secreting plasma cells.

E. Plasma cells

Fully differentiated, antibody-secreting B cells are referred to as plasma cells. While plasma cells are only a small percentage of the total cells in lymphoid tissues, they produce virtually all of the antibody [79]. Plasma cells may be short-lived, providing immediate antibody response to current infection, or long-lived, providing long-term immunity. While short-lived plasma cells can be derived from T-cell dependent or independent processes, long-lived plasma cell formation generally requires T-cell help. Plasma cell differentiation begins with the formation of plasmablasts, mature B cells that have begun to secrete antibody but which still express MHC Class II to elicit T-cell help. These subsequently differentiate into plasma cells, which do not express MHC Class II and are unable to further switch antibody classes. The molecular mechanisms regulating plasma cell differentiation involve upregulation of the transcription factors blimp1 and xbp1 and a concomitant downregulation of bcl6 and pax5 [80]. Short-lived plasma cells may exist in the spleen and lymph nodes, but long-lived plasma cells are generally associated with the bone marrow [81]. Whether the long-lived plasma cells are in fact truly long-lived or are short-lived plasma cells continuously produced from memory B cells has been extensively debated, though it does appear that these cells have an increased longevity associated with the upregulation of anti-apoptotic factors [82] and can persist in the absence of memory B cells [83]. Based on the observation that most of the cells in the bone marrow

33

compartment are class switched and have high affinity for antigen, it is thought that these long-lived plasma cells derive principally from germinal center reactions [84].

F. Immunological memory

Memory cells arise from T-cell dependent reactions in the germinal center and are the critical cell type for immune response to re-challenge from an antigen. Although, like plasma cells, memory B cells differentiate from the GC reaction, they do not secrete antibody and can persist independently of antigen [85]. Following a second challenge with a pathogen, memory B cells present antigen to T_{FH} cells, prompting memory plasma cell formation and possibly secondary germinal center formation [86]. This allows for a rapid, coordinated, T-cell dependent response to rechallenge from a pathogen, a response that, by definition, occurs much more quickly than a primary response [87]. This memory response is also the critical process in providing disease protection via immunization. Many of the factors controlling memory cell formation are similar to those involved in GC formation and plasma cell differentiation, with the exact molecular mechanism still under investigation [86].

G. Types of mature B cells

We have discussed above the general differentiation and maturation process for the most common type of B cells, referred to as B-2 cells, but there are a variety of other mature B-cell types. The cell signaling involved in differentiation or maintenance of these alternative B-cell types is not always clear, especially because these may differ somewhat between mouse and human [88].

Marginal zone (MZ) B cells are a population of B cells found only in the marginal zones between the white and red pulp areas of the spleen. They are thought to be very important in the initial response to a pathogen, as they can respond very rapidly to low amounts of antigen [89]. MZ B cells line the marginal sinus and are involved in T-cell independent responses to bloodborne, bacterial antigens and are also important in T-cell dependent responses. They may serve to elicit T-cell help indirectly by serving as antigen-presenting cells, transferring immune complexes from the marginal sinus to the follicular B cells [90,91], or they may directly activate CD4+ T cells [92]. Marginal zone B cells have also been shown to play a role in autoantibody production in a transgenic rodent model of autoimmunity [93]. The developmental fate decisions involved in MZ B-cell development are still being elucidated, but it appears that they derive mainly from T2 transitional B cells and their development is dependent on BCR signal strength as well as Notch2 and NF-κB signals [90]. MZ B cells usually generate short-lived, IgM-producing plasma cells [94]. The marginal zone B-cell population is much more clearly defined in rodent models than in human systems; in humans, the MZ B cells may undergo some hypermutation and appear to recirculate [95].

B-1 B cells act more like "natural" or "innate" immune cells, as opposed to active components of adaptive immunity. The origin of these cells is debated, although recent evidence suggests that they are developmentally distinct from B-2 cells [96]. B-1 cells in rodents are usually subdivided B-1a and B-1b subtypes, collectively responsible for immune responses in the peritoneal and pleural cavities [94]. B-1 cells are thought to contribute to rapid, initial T-cell independent responses to pathogens, during which they may differentiate into IgM-secreting short-lived plasma cells and may also contribute to IgA responses at mucosal sites [97,98]. Like other B-cell subsets, while existence of B-1 cells in mouse is well characterized, this population is less clear in humans [96].

A class of IL-10 producing B cells has been recently recognized as a regulatory population of B cells, often called B_{regs}. These cells are thought to act at the interface of innate and adaptive immune responses, with IL-10 production triggered by signaling through toll-like receptors, resulting in a decrease in innate inflammatory and dendritic cell functions. These cells, like regulatory T cells, are thought to control immune responses and dysregulation may be associated with autoimmunity. Like T_{regs}, B_{regs} may also be associated with cancer progression by reducing antitumor immunity [99] (Chapter 11), and a possible mechanism for the effect of B-cell depletion cancer therapy is a reduction in B_{reg} populations. B_{regs} are much more clearly defined in mice; human B_{reg} populations have been more difficult to study [100].

IV. ANTIBODY FUNCTION

There are five immunoglobulin isotypes (Section III C), each with unique properties and functions. The different classes respond to different types of antigens and have differing abilities to activate various pathways for neutralizing and clearing pathogens.

IgM, as described previously, is expressed on the cell surface during B-cell development and the secreted form is associated with primary immune responses. While IgMs often have lower affinities for antigens because the variable regions have not undergone somatic hyper-mutation and affinity maturation, the pentameric structure of secreted IgM is highly efficient in coating antigens, targeting them for destruction [75]. IgD tends to be expressed at the membrane with IgM following exit of immature B cells from the bone marrow and is found in very low levels in the serum. The function of IgD is not clear; in B-cell development it seems to be interchangeable with IgM. IgD may be involved in modulating B-cell homeostasis [101]. IgA tends to be found at mucosal surfaces and is thought to protect these surfaces from toxins, viruses, and bacteria by either preventing these antigens from binding to the surface or by direct neutralization [75]. IgA can function as a monomer or dimer. IgE is involved in defense against parasitic infections but is most known for its involvement in allergic reactions. It is considered to be highly potent despite its low serum concentration and short half-life, and appears to function by upregulating expression of an Fc receptor ($Fc\epsilon R$) on various myeloid cells [75].

IgG is the most common antibody isotype, comprising the vast majority of immunoglobulin found in serum, where it is the most stable of all immunoglobulin classes. The four human (three mouse) subclasses are similar in that they are capable of directly neutralizing toxins and viruses. All participate in secondary antibody responses, though they may respond differently to protein vs. polysaccharide antigens. IgG1, 2, and 3 can activate the complement cascade to clear antibody-coated (opsonized) pathogens [75]. IgG molecules generally act in monomeric form.

An antibody can neutralize and/or rid the body of a pathogen using one of several processes. The first, neutralization, occurs when an antibody coats the surface of an invading toxin, virus, or bacteria to prevent the pathogen from functioning. This process has been particularly well studied in viruses, where neutralizing antibodies may block interaction of a viral surface protein and its associated receptor or block the viral components to inhibit assembly [102,103]. The second process, opsonization, is often associated with removal of bacterial pathogens. Here, the variable (Fab) portion of the antibody (Figure 3.2), usually IgG, binds to the cell membrane, forming an immune complex. Phagocytes, particularly monocytes and neutrophils, can recognize the Fc region at the opposite end of the antibody through their activating Fc receptors, allowing for destruction of the pathogen. Once bound to antibody, these activating Fc receptors can increase T-cell responses by promoting antigen presentation on MHC molecules [102]. Components of the complement system are also intricately involved in promoting opsonization and phagocytosis [104]; indeed, activation of the complement system is an important function of antibodies. Antibodies can also clear pathogens via antibody-dependent cell-mediated cytotoxicity (ADCC) in concert with NK cells [102]. NK cells expressing an Fc receptor can recognize antibodies bound to particular types of pathogens, inducing the release of cytokines such as interferon gamma and targeting the cell for apoptosis. There has been considerable recent interest in using this pathway in concert with therapeutic monoclonal antibodies to target cancer cells in cancer immunotherapy [105,106].

35

V. B CELLS AND CANCER

Breakdowns in the B-cell developmental program at a variety of stages can lead to the development of cancers. Of the non-Hodgkin lymphomas diagnosed in the US, approximately 90% are disorders of B cells [107]. Cancers can also arise from more differentiated B cells; uncontrolled growth of plasma cells leads to multiple myeloma. Alternative B-cell subtypes, such as marginal zone B cells, can also contribute to lymphomas [108].

VI. CONCLUSIONS

B cells have been intensively studied for many years, and there are a wide variety of tools available for studying B cells in the lab (Table 3.2). B cells contribute multiple functions critical to the body's adaptive immune response. They not only differentiate into the antibody-producing cells directly responsible for pathogen neutralization and clearance, but are also required for antigen presentation to other cell types and for the development of proper lymphoid architecture.

TABLE 3.2 A Toolbox for Evaluating B Cells

Assay/Tool	Use in studying B cells
Flow Cytometry	Examines surface and intracellular proteins on single cells. Generally, antibodies to proteins of interest are linked to different fluorescent dyes. Multiple markers can be examined simultaneously, dependent on the capability of the flow cytometer. Requires cells to be examined *ex vivo*.
ELISA	Allows for quantitative determination of amount of antibody produced for a given antigen by mature B cells. Antigen is coated on the surface of a plate and then antibody added. The amount of antibody can be quantified by use of a colorimetric assay.
ELISpot	Determines the number of B cells that can bind to a particular antigen of interest. Antigen is bound to a membrane and then cells grown on the surface; the number of spots (representing cells) that secrete the antibody of interest can then be determined. ELISpots are advantageous because they measure secretion by single cells.
B-cell depletion	Some antibodies exist for B-cell depletion in mouse models, especially anti-CD20.
Mouse models (cross to B-cell knockout mice)	A variety of mouse models exist with different mutations in genes regulating B-cell development and maturation. Note that eliminating B cells eliminates more than antibodies, as B cells are required for the development of proper lymphoid structure.
Bone marrow chimeras (mouse models)	Bone marrow, the site of B-cell development, can be transferred from a donor to an irradiated recipient mouse. Differences between donor and recipient can be exploited to allow tracking of the donor B cells *in vivo*.
Immunization	Immune response can be studied in various experimental models by immunization with a novel antigen.
In vitro stimulation	Several different compounds can be added to stimulate *in vitro* cultures of B cells including 1) LPS (Lipopolysaccharide), commonly added to primary B-cell cultures to activate B cells and stimulate antibody production, 2) Anti-IgM, which mimics antigen engagement, and 3) Anti-CD40+IL-4, which mimics T-cell help.

References

[1] Pancer Z, Cooper MD. The evolution of adaptive immunity. Annu Rev Immunol 2006;24:497–518.

[2] Nagasawa T. Microenvironmental niches in the bone marrow required for B-cell development. Nat Rev Immunol 2006;6:107–16.

[3] Tomlinson IM, Cook GP, Walter G, et al. A complete map of the human immunoglobulin VH locus. Ann N Y Acad Sci 1995;764:43–6.

[4] Corbett SJ, Tomlinson IM, Sonnhammer EL, Buck D, Winter G. Sequence of the human immunoglobulin diversity (D) segment locus: a systematic analysis provides no evidence for the use of DIR segments, inverted D segments, 'minor' D segments or D-D recombination. J Mol Biol 1997;270:587–97.

[5] Ravetch JV, Siebenlist U, Korsmeyer S, Waldmann T, Leder P. Structure of the human immunoglobulin mu locus: characterization of embryonic and rearranged J and D genes. Cell 1981;27:583–91.

[6] Wood C, Tonegawa S. Diversity and joining segments of mouse immunoglobulin heavy chain genes are closely linked and in the same orientation: implications for the joining mechanism. Proc Natl Acad Sci USA 1983;80:3030–4.

[7] Kofler R, Geley S, Kofler H, Helmberg A. Mouse variable-region gene families: complexity, polymorphism and use in non-autoimmune responses. Immunol Rev 1992;128:5–21.

[8] de Bono B, Madera M, Chothia C. VH gene segments in the mouse and human genomes. J Mol Biol 2004;342:131–43.

[9] Kidd MJ, Chen Z, Wang Y, et al. The Inference of Phased Haplotypes for the Immunoglobulin H Chain V Region Gene Loci by Analysis of VDJ Gene Rearrangements. J Immunol 2012;188:1333–40.

[10] Schatz DG, Ji Y. Recombination centres and the orchestration of V(D)J recombination. Nat Rev Immunol 2011;11:251–63.

[11] Bentolila LA, Olson S, Marshall A, et al. Extensive junctional diversity in Ig light chain genes from early B cell progenitors of mu MT mice. J Immunol 1999;162:2123–8.

[12] Hofle M, Linthicum DS, Ioerger T. Analysis of diversity of nucleotide and amino acid distributions in the VD and DJ joining regions in Ig heavy chains. Mol Immunol 2000;37:827–35.

[13] Velez M-G, Kane M, Liu S, et al. Ig allotypic inclusion does not prevent B cell development or response. J Immunol 2007;179:1049–57.

[14] Brady BL, Steinel NC, Bassing CH. Antigen receptor allelic exclusion: an update and reappraisal. J Immunol 2010;185:3801–8.

[15] Mårtensson IL, Ceredig R. Review article: role of the surrogate light chain and the pre-B-cell receptor in mouse B-cell development. Immunology 2000;101:435–41.

[16] Sigvardsson M, Clark DR, Fitzsimmons D, et al. Early B-cell factor, E2A, and Pax-5 cooperate to activate the early B cell-specific mb-1 promoter. Mol Cell Biol 2002;22:8539–51.

[17] Herren B, Burrows PD. B cell-restricted human mb-1 gene: expression, function, and lineage infidelity. Immunol Res 2002;26:35–43.

[18] Pelanda R, Braun U, Hobeika E, Nussenzweig MC, Reth M. B cell progenitors are arrested in maturation but have intact VDJ recombination in the absence of Ig-alpha and Ig-beta. J Immunol 2002;169:865–72.

[19] Arakawa H, Shimizu T, Takeda S. Re-evaluation of the probabilities for productive arrangements on the kappa and lambda loci. Int Immunol 1996;8:91–9.

[20] Langman RE, Cohn M. The proportion of B-cell subsets expressing kappa and lambda light chains changes following antigenic selection. Immunol Today 1995;16:141–4.

[21] King LB, Monroe JG. Immunobiology of the immature B cell: plasticity in the B-cell antigen receptor-induced response fine tunes negative selection. Immunol Rev 2000;176:86–104.

[22] Gay D, Saunders T, Camper S, Weigert M. Receptor editing: an approach by autoreactive B cells to escape tolerance. J Exp Med 1993;177:999–1008.

[23] Tiegs SL, Russell DM, Nemazee D. Receptor editing in self-reactive bone marrow B cells. J Exp Med 1993;177:1009–20.

[24] Nemazee D. Receptor editing in lymphocyte development and central tolerance. Nat Rev Immunol 2006;6:728–40.

[25] Hartley SB, Crosbie J, Brink R, Kantor AB, Basten A, Goodnow CC. Elimination from peripheral lymphoid tissues of self-reactive B lymphocytes recognizing membrane-bound antigens. Nature 1991;353:765–9.

[26] Hartley SB, Cooke MP, Fulcher DA, et al. Elimination of self-reactive B lymphocytes proceeds in two stages: arrested development and cell death. Cell 1993;72:325–35.

[27] Wardemann H, Yurasov S, Schaefer A, Young JW, Meffre E, Nussenzweig MC. Predominant autoantibody production by early human B cell precursors. Science 2003;301:1374–7.

[28] Ferry H, Leung JCH, Lewis G, et al. B-cell tolerance. Transplantation 2006;81:308–15.

[29] Zhang Z. VH replacement in mice and humans. Trends Immunol 2007;28:132—7.

[30] Lutz J, Müller W, Jäck H-M. VH replacement rescues progenitor B cells with two nonproductive VDJ alleles. J Immunol 2006;177:7007—14.

[31] Goodnow CC, Crosbie J, Adelstein S, et al. Altered immunoglobulin expression and functional silencing of self-reactive B lymphocytes in transgenic mice. Published online: 25 August 1988, 1988;334:676—82. http://dx.doi.org/10.1038/334676a0.

[32] Goodnow CC, Crosbie J, Jorgensen H, Brink RA, Basten A. Induction of self-tolerance in mature peripheral B lymphocytes. Nature 1989;342:385—91.

[33] Erikson J, Radic MZ, Camper SA, Hardy RR, Carmack C, Weigert M. Expression of anti-DNA immunoglobulin transgenes in non-autoimmune mice. Nature 1991;349:331—4.

[34] Cyster JG, Goodnow CC. Antigen-induced exclusion from follicles and anergy are separate and complementary processes that influence peripheral B cell fate. Immunity 1995;3:691—701.

[35] Yarkoni Y, Getahun A, Cambier JC. Molecular underpinning of B-cell anergy. Immunol Rev 2010;237:249—63.

[36] Fulcher DA, Basten A. Reduced life span of anergic self-reactive B cells in a double-transgenic model. J Exp Med 1994;179:125—34.

[37] Goodnow CC. Balancing immunity and tolerance: deleting and tuning lymphocyte repertoires. Proc Natl Acad Sci USA 1996;93:2264—71.

[38] Shlomchik MJ, Zharhary D, Saunders T, Camper SA, Weigert MG. A rheumatoid factor transgenic mouse model of autoantibody regulation. Int Immunol 1993;5:1329—41.

[39] Shlomchik MJ. Sites and stages of autoreactive B cell activation and regulation. Immunity 2008;28:18—28.

[40] Adelstein S, Pritchard-Briscoe H, Anderson TA, et al. Induction of self-tolerance in T cells but not B cells of transgenic mice expressing little self antigen. Science 1991;251:1223—5.

[41] Fulcher DA, Lyons AB, Korn SL, et al. The fate of self-reactive B cells depends primarily on the degree of antigen receptor engagement and availability of T cell help. J Exp Med 1996;183:2313—28.

[42] Shokat KM, Goodnow CC. Antigen-induced B-cell death and elimination during germinal-centre immune responses. Nature 1995;375:334—8.

[43] Amos SM, Duong CPM, Westwood JA, et al. Autoimmunity associated with immunotherapy of cancer. Blood 2011;118:499—509.

[44] Vossenkämper A, Spencer J. Transitional B cells: how well are the checkpoints for specificity understood? Arch Immunol Ther Exp (Warsz) 2011;59:379—84.

[45] Mebius RE, Kraal G. Structure and function of the spleen. Nat Rev Immunol 2005;5:606—16.

[46] Gowans JL, Knight EJ. The route of re-circulation of lymphocytes in the rat. Proc R Soc Lond B Biol Sci 1964;159:257—82.

[47] von Andrian UH, Mempel TR. Homing and cellular traffic in lymph nodes. Nat Rev Immunol 2003;3:867—78.

[48] Nolte MA, Beliën JAM, Schadee-Eestermans I, et al. A Conduit System Distributes Chemokines and Small Blood-borne Molecules through the Splenic White Pulp. J Exp Med 2003;198:505—12.

[49] Crowley MT, Reilly CR, Lo D. Influence of lymphocytes on the presence and organization of dendritic cell subsets in the spleen. J Immunol 1999;163:4894—900.

[50] Nolte MA, Arens R, Kraus M, et al. B cells are crucial for both development and maintenance of the splenic marginal zone. J Immunol 2004;172:3620—7.

[51] Batista FD, Harwood NE. The who, how and where of antigen presentation to B cells. Nat Rev Immunol 2009;9:15—27.

[52] Gonzalez SF, Degn SE, Pitcher LA, Woodruff M, Heesters BA, Carroll MC. Trafficking of B cell antigen in lymph nodes. Annu Rev Immunol 2011;29:215—33.

[53] Carrasco YR, Batista FD. B cells acquire particulate antigen in a macrophage-rich area at the boundary between the follicle and the subcapsular sinus of the lymph node. Immunity 2007;27:160—71.

[54] Qi H, Egen JG, Huang AYC, Germain RN. Extrafollicular activation of lymph node B cells by antigen-bearing dendritic cells. Science 2006;312:1672—6.

[55] Huang N-N, Han S-B, Hwang I-Y, Kehrl JH. B cells productively engage soluble antigen-pulsed dendritic cells: visualization of live-cell dynamics of B cell-dendritic cell interactions. J Immunol 2005;175:7125—34.

[56] Allen CDC, Cyster JG. Follicular dendritic cell networks of primary follicles and germinal centers: phenotype and function. Semin Immunol 2008;20:14—25.

[57] Cyster JG. B cell follicles and antigen encounters of the third kind. Nat Immunol 2010;11:989—96.

[58] Suzuki K, Grigorova I, Phan TG, Kelly LM, Cyster JG. Visualizing B cell capture of cognate antigen from follicular dendritic cells. J Exp Med 2009;206:1485—93.

[59] Qin D, Wu J, Vora KA, et al. Fc gamma receptor IIB on follicular dendritic cells regulates the B cell recall response. J Immunol 2000;164:6268–75.

[60] Cyster JG, Ansel KM, Reif K, et al. Follicular stromal cells and lymphocyte homing to follicles. Immunol Rev 2000;176:181–93.

[61] Vos Q, Lees A, Wu ZQ, Snapper CM, Mond JJ. B-cell activation by T-cell-independent type 2 antigens as an integral part of the humoral immune response to pathogenic microorganisms. Immunol Rev 2000;176:154–70.

[62] Defrance T, Taillardet M, Genestier L. T cell-independent B cell memory. Curr Opin Immunol 2011;23: 330–6.

[63] Taillardet M, Haffar G, Mondière P, et al. The thymus-independent immunity conferred by a pneumococcal polysaccharide is mediated by long-lived plasma cells. Blood 2009;114:4432–40.

[64] Neefjes J, Jongsma MLM, Paul P, Bakke O. Towards a systems understanding of MHC class I and MHC class II antigen presentation. Nat Rev Immunol 2011;11:823–36.

[65] Pereira JP, Kelly LM, Xu Y, Cyster JG. EBI2 mediates B cell segregation between the outer and centre follicle. Nature 2009;460:1122–6.

[66] Paus D, Phan TG, Chan TD, Gardam S, Basten A, Brink R. Antigen recognition strength regulates the choice between extrafollicular plasma cell and germinal center B cell differentiation. J Exp Med 2006;203:1081–91.

[67] Allen CDC, Okada T, Tang HL, Cyster JG. Imaging of germinal center selection events during affinity maturation. Science 2007;315:528–31.

[68] Crotty S. Follicular helper CD4 T cells (TFH). Annu Rev Immunol 2011;29:621–63.

[69] King C. New insights into the differentiation and function of T follicular helper cells. Nat Rev Immunol 2009;9:757–66.

[70] Nutt SL, Tarlinton DM. Germinal center B and follicular helper T cells: siblings, cousins or just good friends? Nat Immunol 2011;12:472–7.

[71] Basso K, Klein U, Niu H, et al. Tracking CD40 signaling during germinal center development. Blood 2004;104:4088–96.

[72] Peled JU, Kuang FL, Iglesias-Ussel MD, et al. The biochemistry of somatic hypermutation. Annu Rev Immunol 2008;26:481–511.

[73] Stavnezer J, Guikema JEJ, Schrader CE. Mechanism and regulation of class switch recombination. Annu Rev Immunol 2008;26:261–92.

[74] Shimizu A, Takahashi N, Yaoita Y, Honjo T. Organization of the constant-region gene family of the mouse immunoglobulin heavy chain. Cell 1982;28:499–506.

[75] Schroeder Jr HW, Cavacini L. Structure and function of immunoglobulins. J Allergy Clin Immunol 2010;125:S41–52.

[76] Mandik-Nayak L, Nayak S, Sokol C, et al. The origin of anti-nuclear antibodies in bcl-2 transgenic mice. Int Immunol 2000;12:353–64.

[77] Hande S, Notidis E, Manser T. Bcl-2 obstructs negative selection of autoreactive, hypermutated antibody V regions during memory B cell development. Immunity 1998;8:189–98.

[78] Allen CDC, Okada T, Cyster JG. Germinal-center organization and cellular dynamics. Immunity 2007;27:190–202.

[79] Fairfax KA, Kallies A, Nutt SL, Tarlinton DM. Plasma cell development: from B-cell subsets to long-term survival niches. Semin Immunol 2008;20:49–58.

[80] Shapiro-Shelef M, Calame K. Regulation of plasma-cell development. Nat Rev Immunol 2005;5:230–42.

[81] Slifka MK, Matloubian M, Ahmed R. Bone marrow is a major site of long-term antibody production after acute viral infection. J Virol 1995;69:1895–902.

[82] Spets H, Strömberg T, Georgii-Hemming P, Siljason J, Nilsson K, Jernberg-Wiklund H. Expression of the bcl-2 family of pro- and anti-apoptotic genes in multiple myeloma and normal plasma cells: regulation during interleukin-6(IL-6)-induced growth and survival. Eur J Haematol 2002;69:76–89.

[83] Slifka MK, Antia R, Whitmire JK, Ahmed R. Humoral immunity due to long-lived plasma cells. Immunity 1998;8:363–72.

[84] Takahashi Y, Dutta PR, Cerasoli DM, Kelsoe G. In situ studies of the primary immune response to (4-hydroxy-3-nitrophenyl)acetyl. V. Affinity maturation develops in two stages of clonal selection. J Exp Med 1998;187:885–95.

[85] Maruyama M, Lam KP, Rajewsky K. Memory B-cell persistence is independent of persisting immunizing antigen. Nature 2000;407:636–42.

[86] McHeyzer-Williams M, Okitsu S, Wang N, McHeyzer-Williams L. Molecular programming of B cell memory. Nat Rev Immunol 2012;12:24–34.

39

[87] Tangye SG, Avery DT, Deenick EK, Hodgkin PD. Intrinsic differences in the proliferation of naive and memory human B cells as a mechanism for enhanced secondary immune responses. J Immunol 2003;170:686−94.

[88] LeBien TW, Tedder TF. B lymphocytes: how they develop and function. Blood 2008;112:1570−80.

[89] Martin F, Oliver AM, Kearney JF. Marginal zone and B1 B cells unite in the early response against T-independent blood-borne particulate antigens. Immunity 2001;14:617−29.

[90] Pillai S, Cariappa A. The follicular versus marginal zone B lymphocyte cell fate decision. Nat Rev Immunol 2009;9:767−77.

[91] Cinamon G, Zachariah MA, Lam OM, Foss Jr FW, Cyster JG. Follicular shuttling of marginal zone B cells facilitates antigen transport. Nat Immunol 2008;9:54−62.

[92] Attanavanich K, Kearney JF. Marginal zone, but not follicular B cells, are potent activators of naive CD4 T cells. J Immunol 2004;172:803−11.

[93] Mandik-Nayak L, Racz J, Sleckman BP, Allen PM. Autoreactive marginal zone B cells are spontaneously activated but lymph node B cells require T cell help. J Exp Med 2006;203:1985−98.

[94] Allman D, Pillai S. Peripheral B cell subsets. Curr Opin Immunol 2008;20:149−57.

[95] Weill J-C, Weller S, Reynaud C-A. Human marginal zone B cells. Annu Rev Immunol 2009;27:267−85.

[96] Montecino-Rodriguez E, Dorshkind K. B-1 B Cell Development in the Fetus and Adult. Immunity 2012;36:13−21.

[97] Macpherson AJ, Gatto D, Sainsbury E, Harriman GR, Hengartner H, Zinkernagel RM. A primitive T cell-independent mechanism of intestinal mucosal IgA responses to commensal bacteria. Science 2000;288:2222−6.

[98] Suzuki K, Ha S, Tsuji M, Fagarasan S. Intestinal IgA synthesis: a primitive form of adaptive immunity that regulates microbial communities in the gut. Semin Immunol 2007;19:127−35.

[99] Schioppa T, Moore R, Thompson RG, et al. B regulatory cells and the tumor-promoting actions of TNF-α during squamous carcinogenesis. Proc Natl Acad Sci USA 2011;108:10662−7.

[100] Mauri C, Ehrenstein MR. The 'short' history of regulatory B cells. Trends Immunol 2008;29:34−40.

[101] Geisberger R, Lamers M, Achatz G. The riddle of the dual expression of IgM and IgD. Immunology 2006;118:429−37.

[102] Joller N, Weber SS, Oxenius A. Antibody-Fc receptor interactions in protection against intracellular pathogens. Eur J Immunol 2011;41:889−97.

[103] Hangartner L, Zinkernagel RM, Hengartner H. Antiviral antibody responses: the two extremes of a wide spectrum. Nat Rev Immunol 2006;6:231−43.

[104] Dunkelberger JR, Song W-C. Complement and its role in innate and adaptive immune responses. Cell Res 2010;20:34−50.

[105] Houot R, Kohrt HE, Marabelle A, Levy R. Targeting immune effector cells to promote antibody-induced cytotoxicity in cancer immunotherapy. Trends Immunol 2011;32:510−6.

[106] Alderson KL, Sondel PM. Clinical cancer therapy by NK cells via antibody-dependent cell-mediated cytotoxicity. J Biomed Biotechnol 2011;2011:379123.

[107] Morton LM, Turner JJ, Cerhan JR, et al. Proposed classification of lymphoid neoplasms for epidemiologic research from the Pathology Working Group of the International Lymphoma Epidemiology Consortium (InterLymph). Blood 2007;110:695−708.

[108] Sagaert X, Tousseyn T. Marginal zone B-cell lymphomas. Discov Med 2010;10:79−86.

[109] Harris LJ, Skaletsky E, McPherson A. Crystallographic structure of an intact IgG1 monoclonal antibody. J Mol Biol 1998;275:861−72.

CHAPTER 4

Adaptive Immunity: T Cells and Cytokines

Jenni Punt, VMD, PhD
Haverford College, Haverford, PA USA

A successful immune response to a tumor requires strong cytotoxic activity. Natural killer cells and CD8+ cytotoxic T cells are the most potent killers in the cell-mediated immune response arsenal. Once activated, both deliver "the kiss of death" to their target, inducing apoptosis. Unlike NK cells (which are the topic of a subsequent chapter), cytotoxic T cells (CTLs) use antigen-specific T-cell receptors to recognize MHC Class I/peptide combinations expressed by infected cells, allogeneic cells and tumor cells. As you will see below, tumor cells present several challenges to the adaptive immune system that can make them less than ideal targets for CTLs.

In this chapter, we will focus on the regulation of cytotoxic T-cell development and activity. We will first review the fundamental events that initiate the adaptive immune response in general. We will then take a deeper look at the activation and activities of T cells—both the CD8+ killers and the CD4+ helper cells that are required for both cytotoxic T cells and antibody B cells to optimally differentiate. We will also discuss the network of cytokine interactions that regulate CD4+ T-cell differentiation and activity—and ultimately regulate CTL development. Finally, we will discuss the adaptive immune response to tumors, touching briefly on the challenges a T cell faces when trying to generate a successful response to a tumor.

I. AN OVERVIEW OF THE EVENTS THAT INITIATE AN ADAPTIVE IMMUNE RESPONSE

The immune response to invasion by pathogen or tumor depends on the coordinated activities of both the innate immune system and the adaptive immune system. The innate immune system is regulated by cells of the myeloid lineage, including dendritic cells, macrophages and granulocytes. The adaptive immune system is regulated by cells of the lymphoid lineage: T and B lymphocytes.

The adaptive immune system is exquisitely antigen specific and the source of long-term memory cells that participate in immune surveillance for abnormal cells (infected cells and tumor cells). Importantly, it depends entirely on the innate immune system to be activated. When considering the adaptive immune response to tumors, it is therefore important to consider how, and how well, the innate immune system is stimulated. Weak adaptive immune responses to tumors may be caused, in part, by weak innate immune activation.

A. Innate Immune Cells Initiate the Adaptive Immune Response

Cells of the innate immune system (see Chapter 2) express pattern recognition receptors (PRRs) that recognize specific features of broad pathogen categories (gram negative bacteria,

Cancer Immunotherapy. http://dx.doi.org/10.1016/B978-0-12-394296-8.00004-X

gram positive bacteria, RNA viruses, worms, etc.). They can also recognize proteins released by cells that have been damaged. Engagement of pattern recognition receptors generates signals that activate innate immune cells, leading to enhancement of the ability to process and present antigen as well as the release of cytokines and chemokines that induce inflammation and stimulate all immune cells.

Dendritic cells (Chapter 5), which reside in epithelial layers at sites of infection and invasion, are one of the most important innate immune regulators of the adaptive immune response. The most efficient activators of naïve T lymphocytes, they become stimulated after engaging pathogen or encountering proteins generated by cell damage. Once activated, dendritic cells increase their phagocytic activity, engulf and digest pathogens or damaged cells, and present digested peptides on their surface in association with MHC Class I and MHC Class II. They change their migration patterns and travel to secondary lymphoid tissues (lymph nodes, spleen, and mucosal associated lymphoid tissue (MALT)), where they will be scanned by circulating T cells.

B. Adaptive Immune Cells, Lymphocytes, are Activated in Secondary Lymphoid Tissue

At the same time that dendritic cells are circulating through epithelial tissues, the main cell participants in the adaptive immune system, naïve T and B lymphocytes (newly generated cells that have not yet been stimulated), are circulating continually through secondary lymphoid tissue, browsing with their antigen-specific receptors for processed and unprocessed antigen, respectively.

T and B lymphocytes see antigen very differently. B lymphocytes recognize unprocessed proteins via their B-cell receptors (BCRs), which are membrane bound versions of the antibodies that will be secreted. T cells only recognize processed peptides associated with the groove of MHC molecules on the surface of a cell. CD4 T cells, which can develop into helper T lymphocytes, recognize peptide/MHC Class II complexes. CD8 T cells, which can develop into cytotoxic T cells, recognize peptide/MHC Class I complexes.

T and B lymphocytes scan different microenvironments within lymphoid tissue. B cells enter the follicles of a secondary lymphoid organ and browse for unprocessed antigen which decorates the surfaces of follicular dendritic cells. T cells enter T-cell zones (the paracortex of a lymph node or the periarteriolar lymphoid sheath (PALS) of the spleen) where they scan MHC/peptide complexes on surfaces of dendritic cells. Lymphocytes continue browsing for 18 hours or more. If they do not encounter an antigen that they bind with sufficient affinity, they leave the organ and circulate to other secondary lymphoid tissue. If, however, they do recognize antigen with high enough affinity they stop migrating, proliferate, and differentiate into effector cells.

The adaptive immune response includes a humoral arm, which generates antibody (Chapter 3), and a cellular arm, which is responsible for cytotoxic activity. CD4 T-cell activation in secondary lymphoid tissues is critical for optimal development of both arms of the adaptive immune system. When a naïve CD4 T cell recognizes an MHC/peptide combination on the surface of an activated dendritic cell, it will initiate an activation program. Depending on the type of signal the dendritic cell delivers, the CD4 T cell differentiates into one of several types of helper T cells, some of which contribute to the differentiation of B cells, some of which contribute to the differentiation of cytotoxic T cells. Over the next 3−5 days, CD4+ T cells proliferate robustly and differentiate into one of several different effector helper T-cell types that are tailored to the insult that initiated the immune response. Some leave the secondary lymphoid tissue and travel to sites of inflammation, while others stay to enhance the differentiation of B and CD8+ T lymphocytes. Still others differentiate into long-lived memory T cells that protect the body from a second invasion.

C. B-cell Activation Requires CD4+ T-Cell Help

To be fully activated, B cells find and bind to the antigen for which they are specific and must receive the help of a CD4 T cell that shares the same pathogen specificity. This seemingly improbable pair of events is elegantly coordinated in the lymph node. Antigen-specific B cells are directly recognized by antigen-specific, activated CD4+ helper T cells, which scan the follicular boundaries. These helper T cells deliver costimulatory signals and cytokines to B cells that induce their proliferation and differentiation (see Chapter 3).

D. CD8 T-cell Activation Requires CD4+ T-Cell Help

To be fully activated and to generate memory cells, most CD8+ T cells must also receive CD4 T-cell help. Given that CD8 T cells do not express the MHC Class II that is required for recognition by helper CD4 T cells, CD4 T cells cannot deliver help to CD8 T cells as directly as they do to B cells. Instead, a third cell—a dendritic cell—is required to mediate the interaction. This interaction results in the differentiation of CD8 T cells into cytotoxic cells (CTLs) that have the ability to induce apoptosis of their targets.

Once they have differentiated and proliferated, effector B cells and CD8+ cytotoxic T cells leave secondary lymphoid tissue and travel to sites of infection or insult. They are specifically attracted to these sites by chemokine signals generated by the innate immune response, which has been active in this area. Memory cell versions of these antigen specific cells will either stay in secondary lymphoid tissue (e.g., central memory T cells) or will, too, travel to the periphery (e.g., effector memory T cells) to ward off a second attack. For a pictorial summary of the events that occur in a lymph node, see Figure 4.1.

II. T-CELL ACTIVATION: A DEEPER LOOK

In order to fully understand how the most effective antitumor response can be inspired—and why immune responses are not always able to clear tumors—we need to understand in more cellular and molecular detail how the immune system generates helper T cells that stimulate cytotoxic T-cell development (and contributes to the generation of antibodies that can target other killer cells to a tumor).

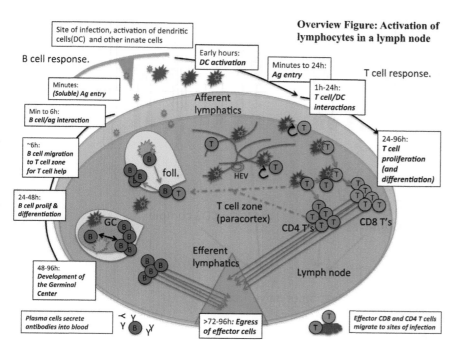

FIGURE 4.1
Overview of adaptive immune system.

A. Naïve T cells are generated in the thymus and recirculate among lymphoid organs

Naïve T cells are continually generated in the thymus, where each cell undergoes DNA rearrangement to generate a unique T-cell receptor and where each cell is screened against autoreactivity and for an affinity ("restriction") for self-MHC (see Chapter 2).

Each naïve T cell recirculates from blood through a lymph node and back to blood every 12 to 24 hours. Because only about 1 in 100,000 naïve T cells is likely to respond to any given antigen, this rapid recirculation increases the chances that a T cell will encounter appropriate antigen.

Naïve T cells enter lymph nodes from the blood via specialized vascular regions called high endothelial venules (HEV). As described above, these cells then browse the dendritic cell networks in the T-cell zone of the lymph node (the paracortex). If a naïve cell does not bind any of the MHC/peptide complexes it encounters, it exits through the efferent lymphatics, which ultimately drain into the thoracic duct and then back into the blood. If a naïve T cell does encounter an antigen-presenting cell that expresses an MHC/peptide to which it can bind, it will initiate an activation program.

B. T-cell activation requires signals from the TCR, co-receptors, and co-stimulatory molecules

Two sets of signals are required to activate naïve T cell: i) a cascade generated by the TCR, a ten membered protein complex composed of an antigen-specific dimer (the TCRαβ dimer), and a signaling multimer known as CD3 (see Figure 4.2) and ii) a cascade generated through the co-stimulatory receptor CD28. A homodimer expressed by most naïve CD4 and CD8 T cells, CD28 binds to two members of the B7 family of proteins, **B7-1** (CD80) and **B7-2** (CD86).

44

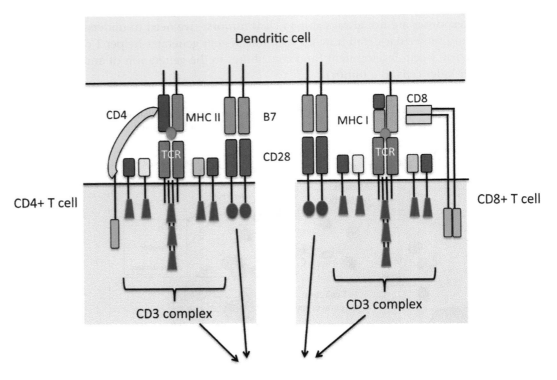

FIGURE 4.2
CD4 and CD8 T-cell recognition of antigen.

These co-stimulatory ligands are only expressed on activated professional antigen-presenting cells (dendritic cells, macrophages and B cells). Dendritic cells express the highest levels of MHC and B7 ligands and are the most potent activators of naïve T cells.

In the absence of CD28 signals, TCR engagement inhibits rather than activates naïve T cells, inducing a state of *anergy* where the cell is unable to respond to subsequent TCR signals—even if CD28 signal are restored.

CD28 is the dominant co-stimulatory receptor on naïve T cells. Another co-stimulatory receptor, ICOS, is structurally related to CD28 but is expressed by memory and effector T cells. Immune cells also express negative co-stimulatory receptors, which turn off, rather than activate, T cells. The negative co-stimulatory molecule CTLA-4 binds the same B7 ligands as CD28, but even more tightly. CTLA-4 is upregulated by T cells only after they have initiated their activation program and helps to control the T-cell response when pathogens are cleared. It also may play a role in inhibiting autoreactive T cells. Clinical scientists have taken advantage of our knowledge of the inhibitory role of CTLA-4 and have designed monoclonal antibodies that block its activity. These reagents (e.g., *ipilimumab* and *tremelimumab*) prolong and enhance the T-cell response to tumors (Chapter 19).

C. T cells become intimately associated with dendritic cells during activation

A key feature of the initiation phase of TCR signaling is the formation of a supramolecular structure known as the *immunological synapse*, or IS. The IS develops over the first few hours of contact between the T cell and dendritic cell, and, in its most organized state, forms two concentric clusters of surface and intracellular proteins.

The center of the most highly organized structures is called the cSMAC (central Supramolecular Aggregative Clusters) and is enriched with TCR/CD3 complexes, the co-receptors CD4 and CD8, which stabilize the interaction by binding MHC Class II and MHC Class I, respectively, as well as associated intracellular signaling proteins. The outer ring, the peripheral (p)SMAC, is enriched for adhesion molecules such as LFA-1, which secure the T cell/APC connection. Interestingly, some potentially inhibitory receptors such as the large transmembrane phosphatase CD45, are absent from these rings, and may be forced out of the central region when the IS is formed. Although the formation of an IS is not absolutely required for the initiation of TCR signaling, it facilitates the long-term interactions that are required for optimal T-cell activation.

D. Cytokines are also involved in T-cell activation

Cytokines contribute an important third signal to T-cell activation. They bind and activate surface cytokine receptors, inducing intracellular signals that enhance proliferation and survival, and influence the effector function that a T cell acquires.

IL-2 is an important cytokine for naïve T-cell activation, particularly when antigen and/or co-stimulatory ligands are limiting. Produced by T cells, themselves, in response to TCR/CD28 co-engagement, IL-2 binds receptors (IL-2R) on the surfaces of activated T cells, maintaining cells in cycle. As we will see below, a network of other cytokines produced by dendritic cells, T cells, NK cells, and other immune cells defines the functional fate of CD4 T cells.

E. T-cell Receptor Signaling Initiates A Cascade of Intracellular Events

TCR/CD28 co-engagement initiates a cascade of biochemical events that 1) enhance T-cell survival, 2) induce cell cycle entry, and 3) induce differentiation into a variety of distinct memory cell and/or effector cell subtypes. The network of events triggered by TCR signaling is dauntingly complex; however, some useful generalizations and themes apply to virtually all growth factor receptors, of which the TCR (and BCR) are specific examples.

- Signal transduction begins with the interaction between a ligand and its receptor and typically results in the aggregation ("cross-linking") of multiple receptors and co-receptors. *For the T cell, this interaction is initiated by TCR/MHC/peptide binding. The co-receptors CD4 or CD8 and co-stimulatory molecules (CD28) are also involved in this initiating engagement aggregation.*
- Receptor aggregation leads to changes of activities of protein phosphatases and tyrosine kinases that in turn can lead to an amplifying cascade of enzymatic activity. *In T cells, CD45 is a key regulatory phosphatases and the initiating tyrosine kinases include lck and ZAP-70.*
- Intracellular signaling cascades are organized in space and time by adaptor proteins that assemble enzymes and their substrates. *Adaptor molecules specific to T cells include SLP-76 and LAT.*
- Enzymes organized by adaptor proteins can set off signal cascades by serine threonine kinases (e.g., **MAPKs** like ERK and JNK) and lipid kinases (e.g., **Phospholipase C**).
- Signal transduction also leads to the generation of intracellular "second messengers," molecules or ions that can diffuse to other sites in the cell and trigger other signaling cascades. **Ca++** is a common and potent second messenger, as is **cAMP**. These second messengers also initiate cascades that change gene expression and intracellular protein locale and activity.

These signaling cascades lead to transcription of new genes, as well as post-translational modifications of enzymes that enhance or inhibit their activities and regulate cell function and fate.

III. THE DIFFERENTIATION OF NAÏVE T CELLS INTO EFFECTOR T CELLS

Successful T cell/dendritic engagement in a lymphoid organ leads to the expression of the pro-survival molecule bcl-x_L, the pro-proliferative cytokine IL-2, and its high affinity receptor chain, CD25. Within 48 hours, a naïve T cell enlarges into a blast cell and undergoes repeated rounds of cell division. Over the next four to five days they divide at least ten times and generate progeny that differentiate into memory or effector T-cell populations.

An effector T cell has acquired unique functional abilities that can have a direct impact on the immune response to pathogen. CD8+ effector T cells bind and kill infected cells and CD4+ effector T cells secrete cytokines that activate or inactivate other cell types. CD4+ helper T cells can adopt different effector fates, which are distinguished by the array of cytokines they produce.

A. CD4+ T cells develop into several different helper cell subtypes

Activated CD4+ T helper (T_H) cells can differentiate ("be polarized to") into at least five distinct effector subpopulations known as T_H1, T_H2, T_H17, T_{FH}, and iT_{REG} cells.

Each of these major CD4+ T helper cell subsets are characterized by 1) a distinct set of *polarizing cytokines* that induce the expression of 2) a set of *master gene regulators* that define the genotype of the effector subset, and define 3) a signature set of *effector cytokines* the T-cell population produces once it is fully differentiated. Each plays a distinct functional role in an immune response. See Table 4.1 for a summary of the factors that define T-helper-cell subsets.

1. T_H1 CELLS

T_H1 cells are known for their ability to enhance the immune response to intracellular pathogens (*cell-mediated immunity*). **IL-12**, which is produced by activated dendritic cells, is the key

TABLE 4.1 Table of Polarizing and Effector Cytokines for CD4 Helper Cells

Helper subtype	Polarizing cytokine	Master transcriptional regulator	Effector cytokines	Function: Physiologic and pathologic
T_H1	IL-12	T-bet	IFN-γ	Protection against intracellular pathogens (helping CD8 T cells); contributes to autoimmune symptoms
T_H17	TGFβ, IL-6, IL-21, IL-23	RORγ	IL-17A, IL-17F, IL-21	Protection against fungi(?) contributes to autoimmune symptoms
iT_{REG}	TGFβ	FoxP3	IL-10	Inhibits immune responses; protects from autoimmunity
T_H2	IL-4	GATA-3	IL-4, IL-5, IL-10, IL-13	Provides protection against extracellular pathogens; Enhances B-cell differentiation, particularly IgE responses; Contributes to allergy
T_{FH}	IL-6, IL-1β, TNFα, IL-21	Bcl-6	IL-21, IFN-γ	Provides protection against extracellular pathogens; Provides help for B cells in follicle and germinal center; Contributes to autoantibody production

polarizing cytokine for differentiation to the T_H1 lineage and induces the expression of the master transcriptional regulator, **T-bet**. Two other cytokines, IFN-γ and IL-18 also contribute to T_H1 polarization. IFN-γ (produced by activated T_H1 cells and NK cells) enhances IL-12 production by dendritic cells and upregulates the IL-12 receptor on activated T cells. IL-18 (produced by NK cells) enhances proliferation and stimulates even more IFN-γ production.

The defining cytokine secreted by the T_H1 subset, **IFN-γ**, activates macrophages and induces antibody class switching to IgG classes (such as IgG2a in the mouse) that support phagocytosis and fixation of complement. Together with IL-2, IFN-γ also promotes CTL differentiation (providing help for the differentiation of CD8 T cells). These cytokine effects, together, make the T_H1 subset particularly suited to respond to viral infections and intracellular pathogens.

This subset can also promote excessive inflammation and tissue injury that is associated with some autoimmune disease, although T_H17 cells may also share this responsibility.

2. T_H2 CELLS

T_H2 cells are known for their ability to promote *humoral* (*antibody mediated*) *immunity*, and are particularly important in the control of helminth infections. They are also involved in allergy. Differentiation to the T_H2 subset depends on **IL-4**, its signature polarizing cytokine. Exposing naïve helper cells to IL-4 at the beginning of an immune response induces expression of **GATA-3**, the master transcriptional regulator that induces differentiation into the T_H2 lineage. Interestingly, T_H2 development is greatly favored over T_H1 development: even in the presence of IFN-γ and IL-12, T cells will differentiate into T_H2 effectors if IL-4 is present.

Several cytokines are produced by the T_H2 subset, including IL-4, itself, IL-5, IL-10, and IL-13. **IL-4**, the signature cytokine secreted by this subset, promotes B-cell activation and class switching to IgE. IgE antibodies engage Fcε receptors on basophils, mast cells and eosinophils, and, when bound to pathogen, trigger the release of proteins that cause serious damage to parasites. IL-5 promotes the production of IgG1 isotypes and IL-13 activities overlap largely with those of IL-4. IL-4 and IL-10 both act to suppress the expansion of T_H1-cell populations.

i. Cross-regulation of T_H1 and T_H2 cells

T_H1 and T_H2 differentiation are tightly co-regulated. Cytokines and transcription factors that promote T_H1 differentiation inhibit T_H2 differentiation, and vice versa. T_H1 and T_H2 polarizing cytokines also have opposing effects on target cells other than T_H subsets. For example, IFN-γ secreted by the T_H1 subset promotes IgG2a production by B cells but inhibits IgG1 and IgE production. On the other hand, IL-4 secreted by the T_H2 subset promotes production of IgG1 and IgE and suppresses production of IgG2a. The phenomenon of cross-regulation explains the observation that there is often an inverse relationship between the production of certain antibodies and cell-mediated immunity; that is, when IgG1 antibody production is high, cell-mediated immunity is low and vice versa.

ii. T_H1/T_H2 balance determines disease outcomes

Studies in both mice and humans show that the balance of activity among T-cell subsets *in vivo* can significantly influence the outcome of the immune response. For example, individuals who suffer from the more severe form of leprosy exhibit more T_H2 activity than T_H1 activity. The progression of HIV infection to AIDS may also be enhanced by a shift from T_H1 to T_H2 response, which is less effective at controlling intracellular infections.

Some pathogens appear to "purposely" influence the activity of the T_H subsets. The Epstein-Barr virus, for example, produces a homolog ("mimic") of human IL-10 called viral (v) IL-10. Like cellular IL-10, vIL-10 suppresses T_H1 activity, thus compromising the immune response to the virus.

3. T_H17 CELLS

Like T_H1 cells, T_H17 cells are involved in cell-mediated immunity (see Chapter 10). They are generated when naïve CD4 T cells are activated in the presence of **IL-6** and **TGFβ**. Together with **IL-23** these polarizing cytokines induce expression of the master TH17 regulator, **RORγ**.

T_H17 cells are so named because they produce IL-17A, a cytokine associated with chronic immune and autoimmune responses, including inflammatory bowel disease, arthritis, and multiple sclerosis. In fact, T_H17 cells appear to be the dominant inflammatory cell type in chronic autoimmune disorders. They also produce IL-17F, IL-21 and IL-22—all cytokines associated with tissue inflammation. We have only begun to understand the true physiological function of T_H17, which in healthy humans have been found in the gut and may play a role in warding off infection by fungus and some bacteria.

4. INDUCED REGULATORY T CELLS (iT_{REG}s)

The fourth major CD4$^+$ T-cell subset, induced T_{REG} cells, is similar in function to the natural T_{REG}s cells that originate from the thymus. These cells negatively regulate T-cell responses and play a critically important role in limiting autoimmune T-cell activity.

Induced T_{REG}s arise from naïve T cells that are activated in the presence of **TGFβ**, the key polarizing cytokine for T_{REG} differentiation. TGFβ induces expression of **FoxP3**, the master transcriptional regulator responsible for T_{REG} commitment.

T_{REG} cells can exert their suppressive function indirectly by secreting the cytokines IL-10 and TGF-β, which inhibit the ability of antigen-presenting cells to stimulate T cells. They can also act more directly on T-cell targets, inducing apoptosis.

i. Cross-regulation between T_H17 and T_{REG} subsets

Like T_H1 and T_H2 cells, iT_{REG} and T_H17 cross-regulate each other. TGFβ induces T_{REG} differentiation; however, when accompanied by IL-6, TGFβ induces T_H17 differentiation. The T_H17 versus iT_{REG} relationship may be very adaptive. A healthy state favors the development of the anti-inflammatory iT_{REG} population, which would be reinforced by iT_{REG} cell's own production of TGFβ. An inflammatory state, where acute response proteins like IL-6 are produced, would induce a shift away from T_{REG} development toward the pro-inflammatory T_H17 lineage, so a proper defense could be mounted.

5. T_{FH} CELLS

Like T_H2 cells, T_{FH} cells regulate humoral responses and antibody production. In fact, they were discovered because of their abundance in B-cell follicles—and appear to play a key role in mediating B-cell help in the germinal center.

IL-6, IL-1β, TNFα and **IL-21** have all been implicated as polarizing cytokines for T_{FH} differentiation, and induce the expression of **bcl-6**, T_{FH}'s "master" transcriptional regulator. Cross-regulation is also a feature of T_{FH} function; bcl-6 expression inhibits T-Bet, GATA-3, and RORγ expression, thus inhibiting T_H1, T_H2, and T_H17 differentiation.

T_{FH} cells secrete both IFN-γ and IL-4 (cytokines typically associated with T_H1 and T_H2 subsets, respectively), but are perhaps best characterized by their secretion of **IL-21** (which is also secreted by T_H17 cells). T_{FH} cells are distinguished from T_H2 cells by their expression of ICOS versus CD28, as well as their expression of surface receptors that localize them in the follicles and germinal centers. How T_{FH} cells divide responsibilities for B-cell help with T_H2 cells remains unclear.

B. T-cell subset plasticity

Investigations now suggest that the relationship among T_H cell subpopulations may be more plastic than previously suspected: at early stages in differentiation, helper cells may be able to shift their commitment and produce another. For example, when exposed to IL-12, young T_H2 cells can be induced to express the signature T_H1 cell cytokine, IFN-γ. Young T_H1 cells can also be induced to express the signature T_H2 cytokine, IL-4, under T_H2 polarizing conditions. T_H1 and T_H2 cells do not seem able to adopt T_H17 or T_{REG} characteristics. On the other hand, T_H17 and T_{REG} cells can adopt the cytokine expression profiles of other subsets, including T_H1 and T_H2. The plasticity of T-cell subsets confounds efforts to categorize them. In fact, novel subpopulations of helper T cells may simply be variants of T_H1, T_H2, T_H17, T_{FH} and T_{REG} cells that have been exposed to other polarizing environments.

IV. THE SIGNIFICANCE OF POLARIZING CYTOKINES

Polarizing cytokines allow the immune system to customize the immune response to the type of insult or infection that has occurred. Which cytokines are made depends on the innate immune interactions that initiated the immune response. For example, some viruses interact with TLR3 expressed by dendritic cells and induce release of IL-12. Parasitic worms interact with pattern recognition receptors on innate immune cells, stimulating production of IL-4.

49

We take advantage of the influence of innate immune responses on T-helper-cell polarization with vaccine *adjuvants*. Adjuvants have been added to vaccine preparations to enhance the immune response long before we understood precisely what they did. We now know that they work in large part by activating the innate immune system and directing the production of specific sets of polarizing cytokines. Although only a few adjuvants (e.g., alum) are approved for human use, investigators are actively working on developing others that can tailor the immune response to a vaccine antigen.

V. CD8+ T CELLS DEVELOP INTO CYTOTOXIC LYMPHOCYTES

Cytotoxic T lymphocytes (CTLs) induce apoptosis of targets, which include pathogen-infected cells, cells from allogeneic tissue grafts, and tumor cells. Although there are exceptions, CTLs are predominantly $CD8^+$ and, therefore, class I MHC restricted. Since virtually all nucleated cells in the body express class I MHC molecules, a CTL can recognize and eliminate almost any cell in the body that displays the MHC Class I/peptide complex to which it is specific.

A. How effector CTLs are generated from naïve CD8 T cells

Naïve CD8+ T cells do not have the molecular equipment to kill targets, but gain this capacity during activation in secondary lymphoid tissue. Two sets of signals are required for optimal differentiation of a CD8+ T cell into a killer. Like their CD4+ counterparts, naïve CD8+ T cells are activated in the paracortex of secondary lymphoid tissues by dendritic cells, and must receive signals through their TCR and CD28. However, they also need the help of an effector CD4+ T helper cell.

T_H1 and T_H17 cells both appear capable of giving this help and observations in living lymph nodes indicate that help is delivered via an interaction among three cells: a CD4+ T_H cell, an activated antigen-presenting cell, and a CD8+ T cell. The antigen-presenting cell acts as a bridge, presenting MHC Class II/peptide complexes to the CD4 T cell and MHC Class I/peptide complexes to the CD8 T cell. Some of the "help" generated by T_H cells is due to their engaging CD40 on the surface of the APC, enhancing its ability to activate CD8+ T cells. T_H cells can also deliver help more directly by binding CD40 on the CD8 T cells and by producing large amounts of the pro-proliferative cytokine, IL-2.

Interestingly, T-cell help is not absolutely required for CD8+ T-cell activation. Some activated antigen-presenting cells can provide signals that induce proliferation and differentiation. Importantly, however, CD4 T cell help is absolutely required for the development of memory CD8 T cells.

CD8 T cells appear to differentiate into two cytotoxic T-cell subtypes. Specifically, 1L-12 induces differentiation to the T_C1 CD8 T-cell subset, which secretes IFN-γ. IL-4 induces differentiation to the T_C2 CD8 T-cell subset, which secretes IL-4.

VI. THE ACTIVITIES OF EFFECTOR AND MEMORY T CELLS IN TISSUES

A. Effector and memory cells alter their activation requirements and migration behavior

Once activated, antigen-experienced effector T cells (both cytotoxic and helper variants) respond more efficiently to antigen receptor stimulation and gain the capacity to traffic to multiple tissues in the body. The reasons for this are several-fold:

> *Effector cells are less dependent on co-stimulatory signals.* Unlike naïve T cells, antigen-experienced effector cells and memory cells can be activated in the absence of

co-stimulation. This allows CTLs, for instance, to interact with, and kill, infected cells in tissue, which are unlikely to express B7 ligands.

Effector cells express a different CD45 isoform. CD45, a transmembrane phosphatase that enhances TCR signaling, exists as several different isoforms. Unlike naïve T cells, which express the CD45RA isoform, effector T cells express a more efficient isoform, CD45RO. Thus they are more sensitive to TCR stimulation.

Effector T cells express higher levels of adhesion molecules than their naïve counterparts. The levels of expression of adhesion molecules CD2 and LFA-1 are two- to four-fold higher on effector T cells than on naïve T cells. This enables effector T cells to bind more effectively to target cells, many of which express low levels of adhesion molecule ligands.

Effector cells express different homing and chemokine receptors. Unlike naïve T cells, effector T cells no longer express L-selectin (CD62L) and CCR7, which regulates homing to the T-cell zones of secondary lymphoid tissue. They now are free to travel to other tissues. Where effector T cells go depends on the chemokine receptors they upregulate during their activation and differentiation. Some upregulate chemokine receptors that direct them to general sites of inflammation. Others upregulate chemokine receptors that target them to specific tissues such as the gut and the skin.

B. CTLs kill cells in two ways

Once they have migrated from secondary lymphoid organs to sites of infection, CTLs scan cell surfaces for the MHC/peptide complex for which they are specific. If they find the combination, they establish an immunological synapse with their target and deliver signals that induce apoptosis (the "kiss of death" (see Figure 4.3)). Their target will die within a few hours, long after the CTL has dissociated and found other targets to kill.

CTLs can kill in one of two ways. First, they can empty the contents of "death" granules which contain granzyme and perforin. After being endocytosed by the target cell, perforin develops pores in the vesicle that allow granzyme to enter the cytoplasm. Granzyme activates caspases, which induce apoptosis. CTLs also express the ligand (FasL) for the death receptor Fas. Engagement of Fas, which is expressed by multiple cells, also activates caspases and induces apoptosis.

51

C. Helper T cells are active in both secondary lymphoid tissue and in the periphery

Some helper T cells remain in the lymph node and continue to regulate the differentiation of B cells and CD8 T cells. Others travel to sites of infection to enhance activation of innate immune cells and/or to quell T-cell responses.

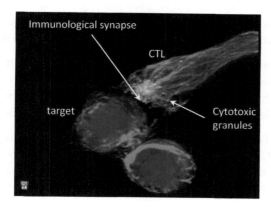

FIGURE 4.3

The kiss of death. A cytotoxic T-cell (CTL) engages a target cell. Cytotoxic granules containing perforin (stained green) and granzyme B are delivered via microtubules (stained red) to the point of contact where an immunological synapse is formed. (Nuclei are stained blue.)

VII. TWO MAJOR TYPES OF MEMORY T CELLS REMAIN AFTER ANTIGEN IS CLEARED

T-cell activation results in a proliferative burst, effector cell generation, and then a dramatic contraction of cell number. At least 90% of effector cells die by apoptosis after pathogen is cleared, leaving behind an all-important population of antigen-specific memory T cells. These cells are long-lived and quiescent, but respond with heightened reactivity to a subsequent challenge with the same antigen, generating a signature secondary response.

Two broad subsets of memory T cells that differ by function and location have been identified: **central memory cells (T_{CM})** and **effector memory cells (T_{EM})**. Central memory cells (T_{CM}) express the activation marker CD44, the adhesion molecule CD62L, and the chemokine receptor that regulates homing to lymphoid tissue, CCR7. They reside in secondary lymphoid organs and retain the ability to self-renew. Once activated, T_{CM} can differentiate into effector T cells. Effector memory cells (T_{EM}) express CD44, but do not express CCR7—allowing them to circulate among non-lymphoid tissues. Many (but not all) T_{EM} also express low levels of CD62L. T_{EM} reside in peripheral tissues (including lung, liver and intestines) and, once activated, quickly express the effector functions that they exhibited during the primary response. T_{EM} appear to be a very important first line of defense during a successful secondary response.

VIII. THE CHALLENGES FACED BY THE ADAPTIVE IMMUNE SYSTEM WHEN RESPONDING TO TUMORS

Tumors offer several challenges to the adaptive immune system. Below we broadly describe what may happen during an immune response to a solid tumor. We also highlight possible reasons that the immune response to tumors is not always optimal.

If a tumor results in tissue damage, innate immune cells will be activated (e.g., via DAMPs, see Chapter 2). Activated antigen-presenting cells increase their phagocytic activity and may engulf damaged tumor cells, process and present tumor peptides, and circulate to secondary lymphoid tissue. However, if a tumor does not damage tissue it may not elicit an all-important innate immune response.

Even if dendritic cells successfully process tumor proteins and travel to T-cell zones of lymphoid organs, they may not engage the thousands of naïve T cells that scan their surfaces. Why not? Recall that naïve T cells have been screened in the thymus against autoreactivity. Tumor cells are often only slightly modified versions of self. Therefore, circulating T cells are likely to be tolerant to many of the peptides that could be generated from tumor proteins. Fortunately, some tumors do express unique proteins (e.g., mutant versions of a normal protein or proteins that were expressed very early in development and are no longer seen by T cells), which can be recognized by and induce activation of some naïve T cells.

In order to be effective against a tumor, an activated T cell needs to differentiate into an effector cell that enhances cell-mediated immunity (e.g., T_H1, T_H17). Whether a dendritic cell that responded to DAMPs at the site of the tumor is capable of polarizing the T cell in this direction depends on other variables, many of which we still do not completely understand.

If naïve tumor specific CD8+ T cells are provided with the appropriate T-cell help, they will develop into functional CTLs, and leave the lymph node. Their ability to return to the site of the tumor, an important next step, depends on cues generated by innate immune cells at the tumor site (e.g., chemokines). Tumors may not inspire the production of these cues as effectively as a pathogen does.

If CTLs form and successfully find their way to a tumor, they also need to be able to engage the MHC Class I/peptide complex that originally stimulated them in secondary lymphoid organs. Recent studies suggest that even when active and eager CTLs find their way to tumors, they do not effectively induce cytolysis. This seems to be due to problems in the tumor cells' own ability to present the antigen.

Solid tumors present even more difficulties. Even if tumor-specific CTLs do find their antigen on the surface of tumor cells, they may have difficulty penetrating the tumor to kill all cell targets.

Although these challenges are real and daunting, understanding them in cellular and molecular detail can inspire specific therapeutic strategies for overcoming them.

Further Reading

[1] Ahmed R, Bevan M, Reiner S, Fearon D. The precursors of memory: models and controversies. Nat Rev Immunol 2009;9:662−8.

[2] Bevan MJ. Helping the CD8(+) T-cell response. Nat Rev Immunol 2004;4:595−602.

[3] Bourgeois C, Tanchot C. Mini-review CD4 T cells are required for CD8 T cell memory generation. Eur J Immunol 2003;33:3225−31.

[4] Jenkins MR, Griffiths GM. The synapse and cytolytic machinery of cytotoxic T cells. Curr Opin Immunol 2010;22:308−13.

[5] Kaiko GE, Horvat JC, Beagley KW, Hansbro PM. Immunological decision making: how does the immune system decide to mount a helper T-cell response? Immunol 2007;123:326−38.

[6] Kapsenberg ML. Dendritic cell control of pathogen-driven T-cell polarization. Nature Reviews Immunol 2003;3:984−93.

[7] Khoury S, Sayegh M. The roles of the new negative T cell costimulatory pathways in regulating autoimmunity. Immunity 2004;20:529−38.

[8] King C. New insights into the differentiation and function of T follicular helper cells. Nat Rev Immunol 2009;9:757−66.

[9] Korn T, Bettelli E, Oukka M, Kuchroo V. IL-17 and Th17 Cells. Annu Rev Immunol 2009;27:485−517.

[10] Owen J, Punt J, Strafford. S, editors. Kuby Immunology. 7th ed. W.H. Freeman and Co; 2013.

[11] Linsley P, Nadler S. The clinical utility of inhibiting CD28-mediated costimulation. Immunol Rev 2009;229:307−21.

[12] Pepper M, Jenkins MK. Origins of CD4+ effector and memory T cells. Nature Immunol 2011;12:467−71.

[13] Reiner S. Inducing the T cell fates required for immunity. Immunol Res 2008;42:160−5.

[14] Sharpe A. Mechanisms of costimulation. Immunol Rev 2009;229:5−11.

[15] Smith-Garvin J, Koretzky G, Jordan M. T cell activation. Annu Rev Immunol 2009;27:591−619.

[16] Trambas CM, Griffiths GM. Delivering the kiss of death. Nat Immunol 2003;4:399−403.

[17] Zhu J, Paul W. Heterogeneity and plasticity of T helper cells. Cell Res 2010;20:4−12.

[18] Zhou L, Chong M, Littman D. Plasticity of CD4+ T cell lineage differentiation. Immunity 2009;30:646−55.

CHAPTER 5

Dendritic Cells: Antigen Processing and Presentation

Nancy Luckashenak, Laurence C. Eisenlohr
Department of Microbiology and Immunology, Kimmel Cancer Center, Thomas Jefferson University, Philadelphia, PA USA

I. DENDRITIC CELLS: INTRODUCTION

Dendritic cells (DCs) are the most potent professional antigen-presenting cells (APCs) *in vivo*, capable of both tolerance induction and the initiation of primary T-cell responses. A number of DC subsets have been described in both men and mice with unique functional attributes ascribed to a few. However, in general, constitutive expression of Major Histocompatibility Complex (MHC) class II and the high migratory capacity exhibited by a number of DC subsets contribute to the high stimulatory capacity of this cell type [1−3]. Under resting conditions, DCs are considered "immature" and have been shown to induce peripheral tolerance by causing T-cell anergy, directing T-cell deletion or by inducing the generation of regulatory T cells (T_{reg}) [4−6]. At the onset of an inflammatory response, DCs undergo a process of "maturation" that includes cytoskeletal rearrangement forming the long dendritic processes that give this cell type its name, an upregulation of cell surface MHC and co-stimulatory molecules, redistribution of proteins involved in antigen processing, and secretion of a number of cytokines such as IL-12 which collectively induce the activation of naïve T cells [1]. These extraordinary properties have placed DCs at the center of many efforts at immune modulation, including cancer immunotherapy (see Chapter 18).

II. ANTIGEN PROCESSING AND PRESENTATION

DCs exert their influence on the immune response by presenting antigen in the context of MHC class I and class II molecules to $CD8^+$ and $CD4^+$ T cells, respectively. For the classical MHC molecules, antigen is presented in the form of peptides (epitopes) derived from proteins originating both within and outside the cell. The result is a considerable expansion of antigen-specific T cells in central lymphoid compartments and their eventual migration, in states of activation, to sites of antigen load, where they carry out a variety of effector and regulating functions that are elaborated upon by other authors in this volume.

III. MHC CLASS I

$CD8^+$ T cells, or cytotoxic T lymphocytes (CTLs), recognize peptides typically 8−10 amino acids (aa) in length presented on MHC class I molecules. MHC class I is composed of two polypeptide chains that are noncovalently associated, a polymorphic α-chain and the nonpolymorphic β2-microglobulin. Peptides displayed on MHC class I molecules are typically

55

derived from intracellular self or viral proteins that are degraded by the proteasome. The system is strikingly inefficient as only ~0.1% of potential MHC class I peptides survive the catabolic processes within the cytosol and endoplasmic reticulum (ER) [7]. The properties of proteins that target them to MHC class I processing are still a matter of debate. Several nonmutually exclusive mechanisms have been proposed, including: 1) defectiveness acquired during transcription, translation or folding resulting in rejection by the quality control machinery [8]; 2) degradation of pioneer translation products that are produced by a specialized ribosome which checks the integrity of nascent mRNA species [9,10]; 3) failure of the cellular folding machinery to intercept a fraction of the nascent polypeptide pool [11]; 4) standard turnover of senescent protein may also contribute. Although this mechanism may be minimally relevant to clearance of acute viral infections (virion assembly usually taking less time than mature protein turnover), it could be a factor in recognition of foreign cells, tumor cells and persistently infected cells. In many cases, cellular proteins are targeted for destruction by the multicatalytic 26S proteasome complex via polyubiquitinylation and this process has been implicated in class I-restricted antigen processing [12]. The multi-subunit proteasome consists of a 20S core and two 19S caps on either end. The 20S core is composed of seven α and seven β nonidentical subunits forming two inner β-rings and two outer α-rings. The inner β-rings contain the active hydrolyzing sites each with a different specificity. However, on the whole, the proteasome tends to cleave at the C-terminus after basic or hydrophobic residues, thereby generating a peptide with a potential anchor residue for the MHC class I binding pocket. In the presence of IFN-γ the β1, β2 and β5 core catalytic β-subunits are replaced with subunits of different specific proteolytic activity and enhanced cleavage rates [7,13–15]. These subunits β1i (LMP2), β2i (MECL-1) and β5i (LMP7) assemble with the noncatalytic subunits of the 20S core proteasome to form the "immunoproteasome" whose peptide products are partially distinct from those of constitutive proteasome. The contribution of the "immuno-proteasome" to particular CTL responses is varied but a number of studies have shown that it is required for the production of specific tumor-derived CTL epitopes [13]. In addition, recent data suggest a role for the "immunoproteasome" in the elimination of proteins that become oxidized during inflammatory responses [16].

The 20S proteasome can also be capped by the PA28 regulatory subunit which has been shown to be both constitutive, IFN-γ-independent and IFN-γ-inducible in most tissues [17]. 19S accessory caps that can associate with both the constitutive proteasome and "immuno-proteasome" bind polyubiquitinated proteins, mediating the subsequent steps of deubiqui-tination, unfolding and guiding of the substrates into the catalytic chamber of the 20S core. PA28 association opens the channel to the catalytic chamber, allowing for catabolism of non-ubiquitinated substrates thereby increasing the breadth of MHC class I peptide species produced by the proteasome [13,18,19]. In addition, there is mounting evidence for ubiquitin-independent processing by uncapped 20S proteasome [20,21], a pathway that may be skewed toward cytosolic vs. ER-targeted proteins [21].

The cytosol also contains several aminopeptidases that are highly destructive to most peptides [22]. The few peptides that survive the hostile environment of the cytosol are candidates for transport into the ER by the TAP (transporter associated with antigen processing) complex. TAP is a member of the ATP-binding cassette transporter family and is localized to the ER membrane but has also been detected on post-ER compartments (Figure 5.1) [23]. TAP preferentially binds peptides whose C-termini favor class I binding [24] thereby ensuring delivery of only relevant species to the ER. Although a number of TAP-independent MHC class I peptides have been described, MHC class I-mediated antigen presentation in the absence of TAP is severely compromised [25]. TAP is a component of the peptide loading complex (PLC) that includes calreticulin, an empty MHC class I molecule and a tapasin-ERp57 conjugate [26]. Calreticulin is a molecular chaperone that binds MHC class I, thereby recruiting it into the PLC and allowing for stabilization and peptide loading by ERp57 and tapasin. Together, ERp57 and tapasin are believed to alter the conformation or stability of MHC class I in a manner that

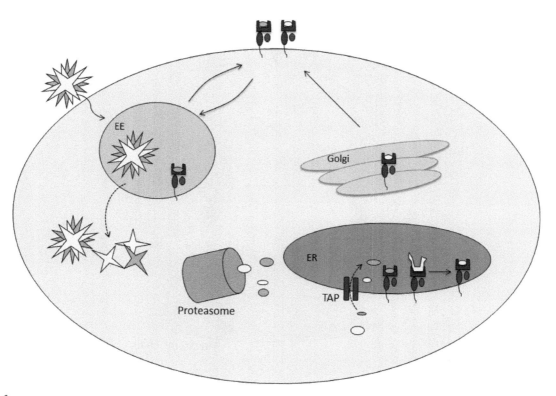

FIGURE 5.1

Processing and presentation of antigen for MHC Class I. Antigen enters the cytosol, via the early endosomes (EE) ("cross presentation") or via direct cytosolic synthesis ("direct presentation"). Proteins may then be processed by the proteasome into peptide fragments that are transported into the endoplasmic reticulum (ER) via the TAP transporter where they bind to nascent MHC Class I. Stable peptide: MHC Class I complexes are then shuttled to the cell surface for inspection by CD8+ T cells. (A variation of crosspresentation, in which antigen is confined to the endosomal compartment, is described in the text.)

allows for the preferential binding of high affinity peptides [7,27−29]. Peptides located in the ER as a result of either TAP-dependent or -independent translocation may be subject to further N-terminal trimming by the ER aminopeptidase associated with antigen processing (ERAAP in mice or ERAP1 and 2 in humans) before or during binding to MHC class I [7,30−33]. Studies in ERAAP deficient mice showed that ERAAP is necessary for the generation of CD8+ T-cell responses to a number of epitopes while other epitopes are apparently ERAAP independent [34]. In humans, a polymorphism in the gene that encodes ERAP1 was correlated with susceptibility to ankylosing spondylitis highlighting the importance of peptide trimming in the ER under certain circumstances [35]. Once fully processed, high affinity peptides are loaded onto MHC class I molecules that passage through the Golgi to reach the cell surface for display to CD8+ T cells.

IV. MHC CLASS II

CD4+ T cells recognize peptide epitopes displayed on APCs in the context of MHC class II molecules. MHC class II is a heterodimer consisting of polymorphic α- and β-chains, each with a transmembrane region. According to the classical paradigm of MHC class II presentation, and distinct from the conventional class I processing pathway, antigen is derived from an extracellular source and enters the cell via phagocytosis/endocytosis and delivery to the endocytic (endosomal/lysosomal) compartment (Figure 5.2) [36]. Antigen is passaged through compartments of increasing acidity and proteolytic activity until reaching the late endosome where loading onto nascent MHC class II occurs. The amount of processing required for epitope presentation is highly variable. Since the peptide-binding groove of class

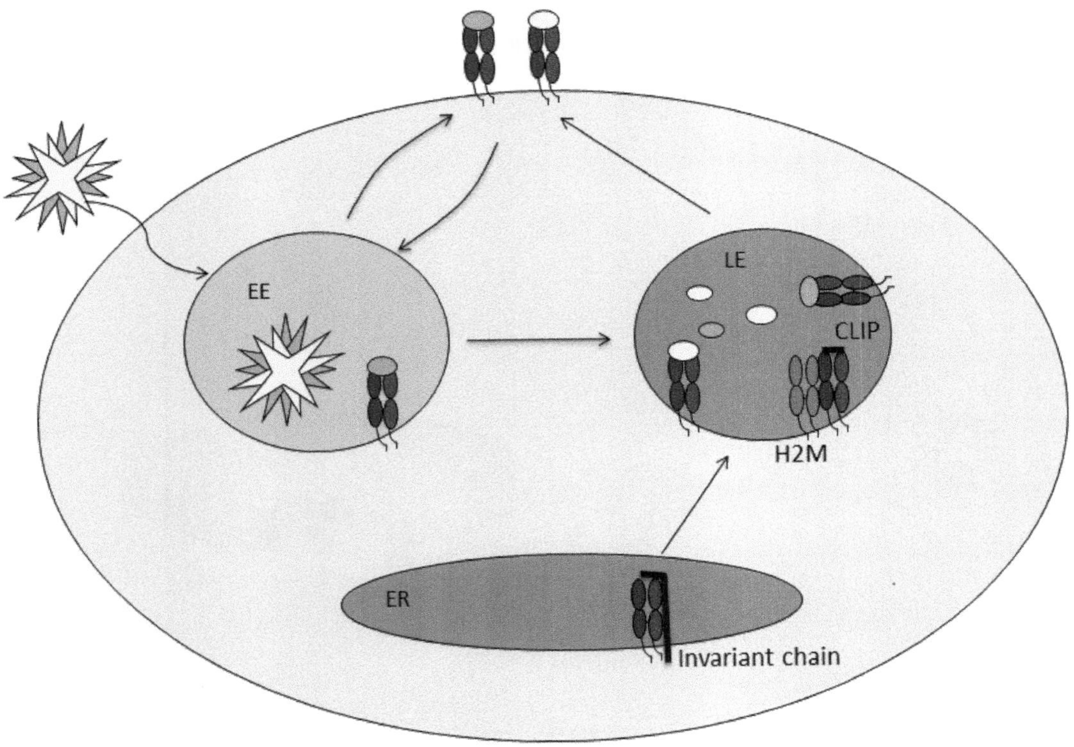

FIGURE 5.2

Classical processing and presentation of antigen for MHC Class II. Antigen gains access to the cell via the early endosome (EE). From there antigen progresses through compartments of increasing acidity and proteolytic activity, undergoing unfolding and fragmentation, until it reaches the late endosome (LE) for loading onto MHC Class II. MHC Class II is synthesized in the ER, bound by the chaperone invariant chain and is targeted to the LE by a dileucine motif in the tail of invariant chain. Following proteolysis, invariant chain is degraded to a form termed "CLIP" that occupies the peptide-binding cleft of MHC Class II. Exchange of CLIP for peptide is facilitated by H-2M (HLA-DM in humans). Stable peptide: MHC II complexes are then transported to the cell surface for presentation to CD4$^+$ T cells. Depending upon the state of maturation of the antigen-presenting cell, surface peptide: MHC Class II complexes may be internalized and degraded internally or recycled back to the cell surface.

II is open at both ends, unfolding of the antigen is ostensibly the only requirement for processing [37]. Indeed, some proteins naturally unfold with acidification and appear to require minimal proteolysis for presentation [38]. Other proteins are highly resistant to unfolding, requiring participation of covalent bond breakers such as gamma-interferon lysosomal thiol reductase (GILT) [39], asparaginyl endopeptidase (AEP) [40] and/or endosomal cathepsins.

MHC class II molecules are initially translated in the ER where three dimers are immediately bound by a trimer of the chaperone molecule invariant chain (Ii) [41]. Ii binds to the peptide-binding cleft of MHC class II preventing premature binding of other peptides and targets MHC class II to endosomes via a dileucine motif within the cytoplasmic tail [42]. The MHC class II/Ii complex reaches the endosomes either directly from the ER or following internalization of complexes that initially traffic to the plasma membrane [43]. Once in the harsh environment of the late endosome, Ii is reduced via a systematic series of proteolytic steps [44] to the small fragment termed CLIP (class II-associated invariant chain peptide) that occupies the peptide-binding groove. Exchange of processed antigen for CLIP occurs with the assistance of the chaperone HLA-DM (H2-M in mice) that prevents aggregation of empty MHC class II molecules and ensures binding of peptides with high affinity [43,45]. Peptide-loaded MHC class II molecules are shuttled to the cell surface of APCs, a process that is highly regulated. When an APC is in an "immature" state, MHC class II molecules are ubiquitinated on a specific lysine residue of the β-chain by the MARCH-1 E3 ubiquitin ligase and perhaps other E3 ligases as well [46]. This signal induces the rapid internalization and transport of MHC class II to endosomes. Once in the endosome, MHC class II molecules are either recycled to the cell surface or targeted for lysosomal degradation. Inflammatory signals that induce DC "maturation" halt ubiquitination of MHC class II molecules and result in an accumulation of MHC class II molecules on the cell surface [46].

V. ALTERNATE PATHWAYS OF ANTIGEN PRESENTATION
A. MHC class I: crosspresentation

Crosspresentation typically refers to MHC class I-restricted presentation of antigen derived from an exogenous source and facilitates presentation by a professional APC in cases where the antigen cannot be acquired directly [47]. Crosspresentation would be required for viruses that do not naturally infect APCs [48] and also for tumor- or tissue-specific antigens expressed by tumor cells, which are unlikely to be potent APCs [49]. In addition, many viruses and tumors develop strategies for thwarting direct antigen processing [50,51], and crosspresentation provides an effective way of separating antigen from these inhibitory processes. Indeed, for these reasons and perhaps others as well, crosspresentation appears to be critical in most cases for an optimal $CD8^+$ T-cell response [52]. Two overarching aspects of crosspresentation remain unelucidated. The first concerns the form of antigen that is actually crosspresented. Although purified, soluble protein can be crosspresented in an *in vitro* setting; this appears to be of limited significance *in vivo* since immunization with purified proteins does not typically induce a $CD8^+$ T-cell response. Rather, evidence suggests that antigen associated with heat shock proteins [53] and/or apoptotic bodies [54] is the transferred material. Either form would result from the cellular stresses associated with infection or tumor burden. The expression by DCs of receptors for both heat shock proteins [55,56] and apoptotic bodies [57] facilitates selective uptake and processing of relevant, "danger"-associated material.

The second major question concerns the intracellular pathways that are involved in crosspresentation. From the perspective of conventional class I antigen processing (reviewed above), crosspresentation is difficult to envision since antigen must reach the cytosol from the extracellular space and this capability is limited in most cells. However, certain DC and macrophage subsets possess this capability [58]. Thus, the general outline is transfer of antigen from an endocytic compartment to the cytosol followed by conventional proteasome- and TAP-dependent processing. Many aspects of this cytosolic crosspresentation pathway remain unclear, including where and how antigen is delivered to the cytosol, and where processed peptide is loaded onto class I molecules. With respect to the latter, the ER is the presumed location but TAP has also been located on endosomal membranes of DCs, particularly in the activated state [59].

In addition to TAP-dependent crosspresentation, there is now convincing evidence for cytosol-free crosspresentation in which antigen processing and peptide loading are confined to the endocytic compartment [52,60]. Findings that implicate this unconventional scheme are: 1) the identification of key components of the class I peptide-loading complex (class I, β-2 microglobulin, calreticulin and calnexin) within endosomes, 2) reduction of crosspresentation by inhibitors of endosomal proteases, and 3) the identification of the insulin-regulated aminopeptidase (IRAP) as the endosomal equivalent of ERAP [61]. Like the more conventional TAP-dependent pathway, many pressing questions remain. For example, is class I delivered directly to the endocytic compartment following synthesis or is it internalized from the cell surface? There is support for both [62,63]. Taking one step back, which of the several crosspresentation schemes that have been reported plays the most prominent role during natural *in vivo* responses? As suggested in a recent review, this is likely to vary depending upon the type of antigen (viral, bacterial, or self-derived proteins), the APC types involved, and the route of internalization [52]. Likewise, the simultaneous operation of several pathways would maximize the probability of successful crosspresentation.

B. MHC class II: endogenous presentation

The classical pathway of MHC class II processing and presentation was developed mainly through the use of purified proteins that initially gained widespread use due to their availability, stability, and ability to stimulate delayed-type hypersensitivity responses. Such proteins focus the action on the endosomal compartment of the cell, particularly when DCs are not utilized as APCs. When viral proteins, tumor antigens, or autoantigens are studied, several additional processing pathways come to light. Most notable are three "endogenous" processing pathways that convert proteins expressed within the APC to MHC class II-bound peptides without an extracellular phase (Figure 5.3). The first route is macroautophagy [64], which typically involves the envelopment of cytosol-resident insoluble protein aggregates and cellular organelles in double membrane vesicles. These vesicles are then fused to lysosomes via a well-coordinated series of protein interactions. Macroautophagy has been implicated in the endogenous MHC class II processing of several viral and self proteins [65]. Second is chaperone-mediated autophagy [66] in which cytosolic proteins bearing a relatively degenerate "KFERQ" sequence are targeted to the lysosome via a specific transport complex. Up to 30% of cytosolic proteins have been estimated to contain this motif. To date, chaperone-mediated autophagy has been implicated in the processing of two autoantigens, glutamate decarboxylase and a mutated version of human immunoglobulin kappa light chain [67]. Thus, a broader role has yet to be identified. Finally, a class I-like pathway involving both the proteasome and TAP has been ascribed to the generation of epitopes from the two glycoproteins of influenza [68]. Proteasome- and TAP-dependence have been individually observed in other systems as well [69,70]. Since these processing pathways are nonredundant (do not produce the same epitopes from the same parent protein) [38,68,71], as with cross-presentation, multiple pathways would serve to broaden the array of presented epitopes.

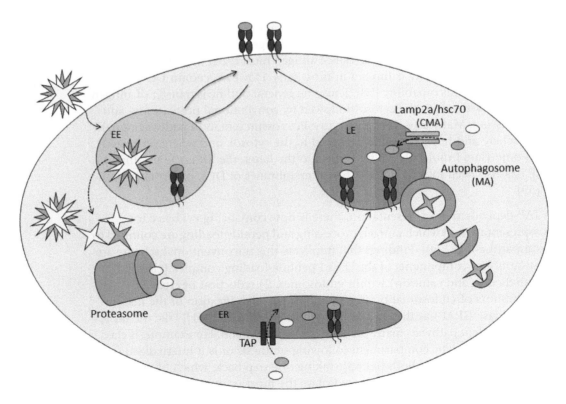

FIGURE 5.3

Endogenous processing and presentation on MHC Class II. Antigen delivered to the cytosol via biosynthesis or delivery from endosomal compartments is targeted to pathways involving 1) macroautophagy (MA), 2) chaperone-mediated autophagy (CMA) or 3) the proteasome dependent and/or TAP. Additional details regarding these pathways remain to be identified.

This appears to be critically important in some cases, such as hepatitis C virus (HCV) where resolution of the infection correlates with a broad CD4$^+$ T-cell response, and transition to chronic carrier state correlates with a narrower CD4$^+$ T-cell response [72,73]. Breadth is also likely to be important for tumor immunity where potential targets are much more limiting.

VI. DENDRITIC CELL SUBSETS AND SPECIALIZED FUNCTIONS

A number of DC subsets have been described to date in mouse and man and more likely remain unidentified. The DC subsets are defined mostly based on the expression of particular cell surface markers, anatomic location and ontogeny, but unique functional attributes have been assigned to a few subsets. In general, when DCs are in an immature or resting state, they express low levels of MHC class I, MHC class II, co-stimulatory molecules such as CD40 and CD86 and low levels of chemokine receptors that promote migration to lymphoid tissues (e.g., CCR7) [74]. Signals that trigger the DC maturation cascade are usually received via the family of toll-like receptors (TLRs) but other signals are also able to induce DC maturation such as those received via cytokine receptors and non-TLR receptors that also recognize viral components such as dsRNA [75]. It must be kept in mind, however, that not all signals that induce some level of DC maturation induce immunogenic DCs. For example, the disruption of E-cadherin-mediated DC–DC adhesion induces a morphological and phenotypic maturation of DCs but these cells do not produce proinflammatory cytokines [76,77]. Additionally, not all fully mature DCs are functionally equivalent, a point that will be addressed in the following description of individual DC subsets.

A. Mouse DC subsets

1. cDCs

Fully differentiated mouse DCs express the integrin CD11c and can be divided into three broad categories: lymphoid tissue resident DCs (LT-DCs), migratory DCs (mDCs) and inflammatory DCs (infDCs) [78]. The LT-DC category contains the conventional DCs (cDCs) and plasmacytoid-like DCs (pDCs). cDCs express high levels of CD11c and intermediate levels of MHC class II. They are typically found in the spleen, lymph nodes and thymus, and may be further classified as CD8$^+$CD11b$^-$ CD207$^{+/-}$ (Langerin), CD4$^+$CD11b$^+$ or CD11b$^+$CD4$^-$CD8$^-$. The CD8$^-$ cDCs subsets reside in the marginal zone of the spleen and migrate into T-cell rich areas only upon stimulation while the CD8$^+$ cDCs are constitutively present in T-cell areas of the spleen. The exact role of CD8$^-$ cDCs is unclear but studies suggest that in an immature state, the CD4$^-$ population is able to induce T-cell tolerance in a TGF-β-dependent manner. However, this same population is fully capable of producing IL-12 and driving a CTL response following TLR stimulation. In contrast, the CD4$^+$ cDC subset is apparently unable to produce IL-12 and therefore has been implicated in the control of autoimmunity [79–81]. Unlike the other cDC subsets, a clear role for the CD8$^+$ cDC subset in antiviral immunity and crosspresentation of exogenous antigen on MHC class I has been described [82,83]. Although CD8$^+$ cDCs express receptors that allow for efficient phagocytosis of dead cells, the ability of these cells to crosspresent has been attributed to yet unidentified differences in antigen-processing machinery and is not solely the result of differential antigen acquisition capabilities [84]. The CD8$^+$ cDC subset has also been shown to induce tolerance when antigen is targeted to the DEC205 endocytic receptor which is highly expressed on CD8$^+$ cDCs, highlighting the plasticity of this potent mouse DC subset [85,86].

2. pDCs

Murine pDCs and human pDCs are most clearly distinguished by their ability to produce large quantities of IFN, 100–1000-fold more than any other DC subset in response to virus [87,88]. This is an astounding feature as pDCs account for only 0.3–0.5% of the cells found in human peripheral blood or mouse lymphoid organs [89]. In the mouse, pDCs can be identified as

CD11c^{Lo}MHC Class II^{Lo}CD11b$^-$B220/CD45RA$^+$Siglec-H$^+$PDCA-1$^+$ and they express only TLR7 and 9 while other DC subsets express a wider array of TLRs including TLR7 and 9 [90,91]. The exclusive expression of viral DNA and RNA sensing TLRs and the unique ability of pDCs to retain stimulatory nucleic acids in the endocytic compartment where these TLRs are localized have been proposed to drive the potent IFN production [92]. pDCs are also characterized by their round plasma cell-like morphology when immature but take on the more dendritic morphology of cDCs when they are stimulated [89,93]. These cells traffic directly to the T-cell areas of lymphoid organs via the blood, do not migrate to peripheral tissue in the steady-state but can be readily detected in tissues at sites of viral infection and active immunity [94—96]. pDCs are capable of priming and crosspriming a T-cell response but, unlike cDCs, they require stimulation through TLRs to acquire this capacity [97,98]. Another unique feature of this DC subset is their continued ability to synthesize MHC class II following maturation, a mechanism that is believed to facilitate the presentation of endogenous viral proteins [98]. Despite this, a requirement for murine pDCs in a number of viral infection models has proven difficult to demonstrate. Only in the context of mouse hepatitis virus has a striking pDC dependence been demonstrated with depletion of pDCs resulting in increased viral replication in the spleen (~1000-fold), spread of virus to tissues that are normally unaffected and severe liver damage [99]. In other viral infections such as lymphocytic choriomeningitis virus (LCMV), murine pDCs were shown to produce IFN in response to viral infection but were not required for T-cell responses or survival [100—102]. Despite the fact that pDCs can promote potent T-cell responses when stimulated, in the steady-state these cells have been implicated in tolerance induction in a number of disease models such as experimental autoimmune encephalomyelitis (EAE) and oral tolerance induction, but results in other models prohibit a generalization of these cells as tolerogenic in the steady-state [103—105].

3. mDCs

The murine mDC subsets have been intensely studied over the past few years. These include epidermal langerhans cells (LCs) that have dominated the DC field as the prototypic migratory DC until a number of additional mDC populations were recently described. mDCs are found in the skin, lung, intestinal tract, liver and kidney as well as spleen and lymph nodes [106]. However, the most well studied and understood are the mDC populations of the skin and cutaneous lymph nodes, which can be distinguished based on differential expression of CD207 (Langerin), CD11b and the integrin CD103 (αE, β7) that binds E-cadherin expressed by epithelial cells and LCs [107,108]. The epidermis of the skin contains only one mDC population, epidermal LCs that are CD207$^+$CD103$^-$ while the dermis is home to at least five mDC subsets: CD207$^-$CD11b$^+$ dermal DCs (DDCs), CD207$^+$CD103$^+$ DDCs, CD207$^+$CD103$^-$ DDCs, CD207$^-$CD11b$^-$ DDCs, and CD207$^+$CD103$^-$ LCs, the latter in the process of migration to the skin-draining lymph nodes [109]. Numerous studies using transgenic mice and ablation models have provided a wealth of data regarding the specific functions of cutaneous DCs that are somewhat contradictory. For example, LCs were shown by *in vitro* and some *in vivo* models to be capable of crosspresentation, while in ablation models CD103$^+$ dDCs, not LCs, were shown to be the only cutaneous DC able to crosspresent antigen [110—113]. In addition, studies of the cutaneous contact hypersensitivity (CHS) response in ablation models have suggested either no role for LCs in the induction of the immune response or a regulatory role, while yet again CD207$^+$ dDCs were demonstrated to be the key APCs required for a CHS response (thoroughly reviewed in [114]). LCs do migrate from the skin to the cutaneous draining lymph nodes in the steady-state, supporting a role for these cells in the maintenance of peripheral tolerance and perhaps suppression of an active response to a foreign pathogen [76,115]. Despite inconsistencies between all of these studies, two models that describe the function of LCs and CD207$^+$ dDCs as proposed by Kaplan are as follows: 1) LCs capture antigen that is present only in the very outermost regions of the epidermis, or 2) direct priming of a CTL response by LCs is determined by the nature of the antigen and the inflammatory environment. No doubt studies in the near future will shed more light on the exact function of this unique mDC subset.

4. Inf-DCs

Inf-DCs are also known as TNF-iNOS DCs (Tip DC) and can be identified as $CD11c^{Lo}CD11b^{+}Ly6C^{+}$ and produce TNF and iNOS [78,116]. As their name suggests, these DCs arise from monocytes during inflammation and have been detected in inflamed lymphoid and nonlymphoid organs such as the spleen, dermis, liver and lung [117]. The recruitment and differentiation of these monocytes into DCs have been observed in a number of murine infection and disease models such as *Listeria, Leishmania*, herpes simplex virus (HSV) infection and EAE, although the exact contribution of this DCs subset to disease resolution or exacerbation remains to be clearly defined [117].

VII. HUMAN DC SUBSETS

Human DC subsets are typically divided more simply into two major subsets, cDCs and pDCs. The cDC subsets in human blood are the $CD1c^{+}BDCA1^{+}$ and $CD141^{+}BDCA3^{+}$ subsets while the human pDC subset can be identified as $BDCA2^{+}BDCA4$/neutropilin-$1^{+}ILT7^{+}$ (immunoglobulin-like transcript 7) $CD123^{+}$ [118–120]. In human skin, three additional cDC subsets have been identified: $Langerin^{+}CD1a^{+}DCIR^{+}$ (dendritic cell immunoreceptor) LCs in the epidermis, and $CD1c^{+}$ and $CD14^{+}$ DCs in the dermis [121].

A. Human cDCs

The $BDCA1^{+}$ and $BDCA3^{+}$ human DC subsets have been shown to be the equivalent of the $CD8^{-}$ and $CD8^{+}$ murine splenic DCs subsets, respectively [118]. Accordingly, human $BDCA3^{+}$ DCs were reported to be more efficient than $BDCA1^{+}$ DCs at crosspresentation to $CD8^{+}$ T cells *in vitro*; however, this finding awaits quantification *in vivo* [121]. Furthermore, the significance of this enhanced crosspresentation in an *in vivo* setting remains questionable as the $BDCA3^{+}$ subset is ten times less abundant than the $BDCA1^{+}$ subset in human blood [118]. As was observed with mouse $CD8^{+}$ DCs, antigen acquisition capabilities appear not to contribute to the unique crosspresentation phenotype of $BDCA3^{+}$ DCs [118]. Interestingly, recent gene profiling in human and mouse DC subsets and protein expression profiling in mouse DC subsets have revealed unique expression patterns of antigen-presentation machinery between DCs that are highly efficient at crosspresentation and those that are not. For example, murine $CD8^{+}$ DCs, and human $BDCA3^{+}$ and LCs exhibit a higher expression of genes involved in MHC class I presentation such as TAP compared to other DC subsets. Conversely, human $BDCA1^{+}$ and $CD14^{+}$ DCs and murine $CD8^{-}$ DCs express higher levels of lysosomal proteases and the MHC class II chaperone HLA-DM (H2M) which may result in enhanced presentation on MHC class II in these DC subsets [122,123].

As mentioned above, human skin contains three populations of cDCs: epidermal LCs, $CD14^{-}CD1c^{+}$ dermal DCs, and $CD14^{+}$ dermal DCs. Unlike mouse cutaneous DCs, no functional studies of human skin DCs subsets have been conducted. However, *in vitro* studies show that human LCs are more efficient at crosspresentation than $CD14^{+}$ DCs while $CD14^{+}$ DCs may be more specialized to prime a humoral immune response [124]. This is in stark contrast to mouse studies that have shown that $CD103^{+}$ DCs, among the dermal subsets, are most efficient at crosspresentation *in vivo* [113,125].

B. Human pDCs

As in the mouse, human pDCs comprise a very small (0.2–0.8% of human blood) population in human blood but are responsible for the production of over 95% of type I IFNs in response to virus, partly due to their selective expression of TLR7 and TLR9 [119,126]. These cells express no other TLRs and, as seen in mouse pDCs, human pDCs possess the unique ability to retain DNA in early endosomes, which is believed to enhance TLR-signaling and subsequent IFN secretion [127]. Human pDCs are able to prime and crossprime T cells *in vitro* but their *in vivo* function remains much more elusive [126,128–132].

In human viral infections, pDCs have been most extensively studied in the context of HIV and HCV infections but their actual function during these viral infections remains unknown. For example, although pDCs are activated by HCV-infected hepatocytes through TLR7 it is controversial whether or not their activity is suppressed during chronic HCV infection [133,134]. On the other hand, during chronic HCV infection the function of individual pDCs was observed to be normal [135]. pDCs are readily infected with HIV and produce IFN in response to the virus but the total number of pDCs in the blood of HIV-infected individuals progressively decreases [89,136]. Furthermore, it remains unclear whether pDCs and the massive amount of IFN they secrete during the course of HIV infection are beneficial or facilitate the spread of the disease. It has been suggested that IFN secretion by pDCs in the early stages of HIV infection is beneficial in halting the spread of the virus but that a continued high level of secretion by pDCs at later stages, when the virus has escaped antiviral strategies, may lead to T cell hyperactivation and depletion [89,137,138]. Clearly more studies need to be conducted in order to determine how pDCs participate in human viral infections and if they will eventually be potential targets for therapy in these settings.

Given the potent IFN production capacity of pDCs and the fact that elevated IFN levels are a hallmark of a number of autoimmune diseases and a cause of pathogenesis, it is not surprising that these cells have been strongly linked to at least two types of autoimmunity in humans, psoriasis and systemic lupus erythematosus (SLE) [139,140]. Elevated levels of pDCs are found in psoriasis skin lesions and blocking this cell type with anti-BDCA-2 antibody in a mouse xenograft model prevented the development of skin lesions altogether, clearly indicating this cell type is disease progression [141].

VIII. CONCLUSIONS

Multiple intracellular and extracellular routes exist for the generation of MHC-associated peptides that activate T cells. Of the various cell types that perform this function, none appears to be as potent and as versatile as the DC. In reality "DC" refers to a variety of subsets, each apparently with a specific "skill set" with respect to antigen processing, cytokine production and migratory capacity that cover the full spectrum of immune response, from profound tolerance induction to heightened activation. As other chapters will show, DCs have been exploited in many cancer immunotherapy settings with a wide range of outcomes. Their effectiveness will no doubt improve as more is learned about their inner and outer workings.

References

[1] Banchereau J, Steinman RM. Dendritic cells and the control of immunity. Nature 1998;392(6673):245–52.

[2] Kushwah R, Hu J. Complexity of dendritic cell subsets and their function in the host immune system. Immunology 133(4):409–19.

[3] Pulendran B, Tang H, Denning TL. Division of labor, plasticity, and crosstalk between dendritic cell subsets. Curr opin Immunol 2008;20(1):61–7.

[4] Steinman RM, Hawiger D, Liu K, Bonifaz L, Bonnyay D, Mahnke K, et al. Dendritic cell function in vivo during the steady state: a role in peripheral tolerance. Ann N Y Acad Sci 2003;987:15–25.

[5] Maldonado RA, von Andrian UH. How tolerogenic dendritic cells induce regulatory T cells. Adv Immunol 2010;108:111–65.

[6] Hu J, Wan Y. Tolerogenic dendritic cells and their potential applications. Immunology 2011;132(3):307–14.

[7] Saunders PM, van Endert P. Running the gauntlet: from peptide generation to antigen presentation by MHC class I. Tissue Antigens 2011;78(3):161–70.

[8] Yewdell JW, Anton LC, Bennink JR. Defective ribosomal products (DRiPs): a major source of antigenic peptides for MHC class I molecules? J Immunol 1996;157(5):1823–6.

[9] Apcher S, Manoury B, Fahraeus R. The role of mRNA translation in direct MHC class I antigen presentation. Curr opin Immunol 2012;24(1):71–6.

[10] Apcher S, Daskalogianni C, Lejeune F, Manoury B, Imhoos G, Heslop L, et al. Major source of antigenic peptides for the MHC class I pathway is produced during the pioneer round of mRNA translation. Proc Natl Acad Sci U S A 2011;108(28):11572–7.

[11] Eisenlohr LC, Huang L, Golovina TN. Rethinking peptide supply to MHC class I molecules. Nat Rev Immunol 2007;7(5):403–10.

[12] Rock KL, Gramm C, Rothstein L, Clark K, Stein R, Dick L, et al. Inhibitors of the proteasome block the degradation of most cell proteins and the generation of peptides presented on MHC class I molecules. Cell 1994;78(5):761–71.

[13] Sijts EJ, Kloetzel PM. The role of the proteasome in the generation of MHC class I ligands and immune responses. Cell Mol Life Sci 2011;68(9):1491–502.

[14] Groll M, Bajorek M, Kohler A, Moroder L, Rubin DM, Huber R, et al. A gated channel into the proteasome core particle. Nat Struct Biol 2000;7(11):1062–7.

[15] Schmidtke G, Eggers M, Ruppert T, Groettrup M, Koszinowski UH, Kloetzel PM. Inactivation of a defined active site in the mouse 20S proteasome complex enhances major histocompatibility complex class I antigen presentation of a murine cytomegalovirus protein. J Exp Med 1998;187(10):1641–6.

[16] Ebstein F, Kloetzel PM, Kruger E, Seifert U. Emerging roles of immunoproteasomes beyond MHC class I antigen processing. Cell Mol Life Sci 2012.

[17] Strehl B, Seifert U, Kruger E, Heink S, Kuckelkorn U, Kloetzel PM. Interferon-gamma, the functional plasticity of the ubiquitin-proteasome system, and MHC class I antigen processing. Immunol Rev 2005;207:19–30.

[18] Hendil KB, Khan S, Tanaka K. Simultaneous binding of PA28 and PA700 activators to 20 S proteasomes. Biochem J 1998;332(Pt 3):749–54.

[19] Tanahashi N, Murakami Y, Minami Y, Shimbara N, Hendil KB, Tanaka K. Hybrid proteasomes. Induction by interferon-gamma and contribution to ATP-dependent proteolysis. J Biol Chem 2000;275(19):14336–45.

[20] Qian SB, Princiotta MF, Bennink JR, Yewdell JW. Characterization of rapidly degraded polypeptides in mammalian cells reveals a novel layer of nascent protein quality control. J Biol Chem 2006;281(1):392–400.

[21] Huang L, Marvin JM, Tatsis N, Eisenlohr LC. Cutting Edge: Selective role of ubiquitin in MHC class I antigen presentation. J Immunol 2011;186(4):1904–8.

[22] Reits E, Griekspoor A, Neijssen J, Groothuis T, Jalink K, van Veelen P, et al. Peptide diffusion, protection, and degradation in nuclear and cytoplasmic compartments before antigen presentation by MHC class I. Immunity 2003;18(1):97–108.

[23] Ghanem E, Fritzsche S, Al-Balushi M, Hashem J, Ghuneim L, Thomer L, et al. The transporter associated with antigen processing (TAP) is active in a post-ER compartment. J Cell Sci 2010;123(Pt 24):4271–9.

[24] Burgevin A, Saveanu L, Kim Y, Barilleau E, Kotturi M, Sette A, et al. A detailed analysis of the murine TAP transporter substrate specificity. PLoS One 2008;3(6):e2402.

[25] Van Kaer L, Ashton-Rickardt PG, Ploegh HL, Tonegawa S. TAP1 mutant mice are deficient in antigen presentation, surface class I molecules, and CD4-8+ T cells. Cell 1992;71(7):1205–14.

[26] Wearsch PA, Cresswell P. The quality control of MHC class I peptide loading. Curr Opin Cell Biol 2008;20(6):624–31.

[27] Garbi N, Tanaka S, Momburg F, Hammerling GJ. Impaired assembly of the major histocompatibility complex class I peptide-loading complex in mice deficient in the oxidoreductase ERp57. Nat Immunol 2006;7(1):93–102.

[28] Peaper DR, Wearsch PA, Cresswell P. Tapasin and ERp57 form a stable disulfide-linked dimer within the MHC class I peptide-loading complex. EMBO J 2005;24(20):3613–23.

[29] Dong G, Wearsch PA, Peaper DR, Cresswell P, Reinisch KM. Insights into MHC class I peptide loading from the structure of the tapasin-ERp57 thiol oxidoreductase heterodimer. Immunity 2009;30(1):21–32.

[30] Koch J, Guntrum R, Heintke S, Kyritsis C, Tampe R. Functional dissection of the transmembrane domains of the transporter associated with antigen processing (TAP). J Biol Chem 2004;279(11):10142–7.

[31] Saric T, Chang SC, Hattori A, York IA, Markant S, Rock KL, et al. An IFN-gamma-induced aminopeptidase in the ER, ERAP1, trims precursors to MHC class I-presented peptides. Nat Immunol 2002;3(12):1169–76.

[32] Saveanu L, Carroll O, Lindo V, Del Val M, Lopez D, Lepelletier Y, et al. Concerted peptide trimming by human ERAP1 and ERAP2 aminopeptidase complexes in the endoplasmic reticulum. Nat Immunol 2005;6(7):689–97.

[33] Serwold T, Gonzalez F, Kim J, Jacob R, Shastri N. ERAAP customizes peptides for MHC class I molecules in the endoplasmic reticulum. Nature 2002;419(6906):480–3.

[34] Hammer GE, Gonzalez F, Champsaur M, Cado D, Shastri N. The aminopeptidase ERAAP shapes the peptide repertoire displayed by major histocompatibility complex class I molecules. Nat Immunol 2006;7(1):103–12.

[35] Burton PR, Clayton DG, Cardon LR, Craddock N, Deloukas P, Duncanson A, et al. Association scan of 14,500 nonsynonymous SNPs in four diseases identifies autoimmunity variants. Nat Genet 2007;39(11):1329–37.

[36] Trombetta ES, Mellman I. Cell biology of antigen processing in vitro and in vivo. Annu Rev Immunol 2005;23:975–1028.

[37] Sercarz EE, Maverakis E. Mhc-guided processing: binding of large antigen fragments. Nat Rev Immunol 2003;3(8):621–9.

[38] Sinnathamby G, Eisenlohr LC. Presentation by recycling MHC class II molecules of an influenza hemagglutinin-derived epitope that is revealed in the early endosome by acidification. J Immunol 2003;170(7):3504–13.

[39] Maric M, Arunachalam B, Phan UT, Dong C, Garrett WS, Cannon KS, et al. Defective antigen processing in GILT-free mice. Science 2001;294(5545):1361–5.

[40] Watts C, Matthews SP, Mazzeo D, Manoury B, Moss CX. Asparaginyl endopeptidase: case history of a class II MHC compartment protease. Immunol Rev 2005;207:218–28.

[41] Roche PA, Marks MS, Cresswell P. Formation of a nine-subunit complex by HLA class II glycoproteins and the invariant chain. Nature 1991;354(6352):392–4.

[42] Bakke O, Dobberstein B. MHC class II-associated invariant chain contains a sorting signal for endosomal compartments. Cell 1990;63(4):707–16.

[43] Rocha N, Neefjes J. MHC class II molecules on the move for successful antigen presentation. EMBO J 2008;27(1):1–5.

[44] Bryant PW, Lennon-Dumenil AM, Fiebiger E, Lagaudriere-Gesbert C, Ploegh HL. Proteolysis and antigen presentation by MHC class II molecules. Adv Immunol 2002;80:71–114.

[45] Kropshofer H, Arndt SO, Moldenhauer G, Hammerling GJ, Vogt AB. HLA-DM acts as a molecular chaperone and rescues empty HLA-DR molecules at lysosomal pH. Immunity 1997;6(3):293–302.

[46] Ishido S, Matsuki Y, Goto E, Kajikawa M. Ohmura-Hoshino M. MARCH-I: a new regulator of dendritic cell function. Mol Cells 2010;29(3):229–32.

[47] Lin ML, Zhan Y, Villadangos JA, Lew AM. The cell biology of cross-presentation and the role of dendritic cell subsets. Immunol Cell Biol 2008;86(4):353–62.

[48] Sigal LJ, Crotty S, Andino R, Rock KL. Cytotoxic T-cell immunity to virus-infected non-haematopoietic cells requires presentation of exogenous antigen. Nature 1999;398(6722):77–80.

[49] Huang AY, Bruce AT, Pardoll DM, Levitsky HI. In vivo cross-priming of MHC class I-restricted antigens requires the TAP transporter. Immunity 1996;4(4):349–55.

[50] Horst D, Verweij MC, Davison AJ, Ressing ME, Wiertz EJ. Viral evasion of T cell immunity: ancient mechanisms offering new applications. Curr Opin Immunol 2011;23(1):96–103.

[51] Chang CC, Ferrone S. Immune selective pressure and HLA class I antigen defects in malignant lesions. Cancer Immunol Immunother 2007;56(2):227–36.

[52] Segura E, Villadangos JA. A modular and combinatorial view of the antigen cross-presentation pathway in dendritic cells. Traffic 2011;12(12):1677–85.

[53] Srivastava P. Interaction of heat shock proteins with peptides and antigen presenting cells: chaperoning of the innate and adaptive immune responses. Annu Rev Immunol 2002;20:395–425.

[54] Arina A, Tirapu I, Alfaro C, Rodriguez-Calvillo M, Mazzolini G, Inoges S, et al. Clinical implications of antigen transfer mechanisms from malignant to dendritic cells. exploiting cross-priming. Exp Hematol 2002;30(12):1355–64.

[55] Kuppner MC, Gastpar R, Gelwer S, Nossner E, Ochmann O, Scharner A, et al. The role of heat shock protein (hsp70) in dendritic cell maturation: hsp70 induces the maturation of immature dendritic cells but reduces DC differentiation from monocyte precursors. Eur J Immunol 2001;31(5):1602–9.

[56] Singh-Jasuja H, Hilf N, Scherer HU, Arnold-Schild D, Rammensee HG, Toes RE, et al. The heat shock protein gp96: a receptor-targeted cross-priming carrier and activator of dendritic cells. Cell Stress Chaperones 2000;5(5):462–70.

[57] Delneste Y, Magistrelli G, Gauchat J, Haeuw J, Aubry J, Nakamura K, et al. Involvement of LOX-1 in dendritic cell-mediated antigen cross-presentation. Immunity 2002;17(3):353–62.

[58] Rock KL, Shen L. Cross-presentation: underlying mechanisms and role in immune surveillance. Immunol Rev 2005;207:166–83.

[59] Burgdorf S, Scholz C, Kautz A, Tampe R, Kurts C. Spatial and mechanistic separation of cross-presentation and endogenous antigen presentation. Nat Immunol 2008;9(5):558–66.

[60] Jutras I, Desjardins M. Phagocytosis: at the crossroads of innate and adaptive immunity. Annu Rev Cell Dev Biol 2005;21:511–27.

[61] Saveanu L, Carroll O, Weimershaus M, Guermonprez P, Firat E, Lindo V, et al. IRAP identifies an endosomal compartment required for MHC class I cross-presentation. Science 2009;325(5937):213–7.

[62] Di Pucchio T, Chatterjee B, Smed-Sorensen A, Clayton S, Palazzo A, Montes M, et al. Direct proteasome-independent cross-presentation of viral antigen by plasmacytoid dendritic cells on major histocompatibility complex class I. Nat Immunol 2008;9(5):551–7.

[63] Basha G, Omilusik K, Chavez-Steenbock A, Reinicke AT, Lack N, Choi KB, et al. A CD74-dependent MHC class I endolysosomal cross-presentation pathway. Nat Immunol 2012;13(3):237–45.

[64] Menzies FM, Moreau K, Rubinsztein DC. Protein misfolding disorders and macroautophagy. Curr Opin Cell Biol 2011;23(2):190–7.

[65] Gannage M, Munz C. Autophagy in MHC class II presentation of endogenous antigens. Curr Top Microbiol Immunol 2009;335:123–40.

[66] Arias E, Cuervo AM. Chaperone-mediated autophagy in protein quality control. Curr Opin Cell Biol 2011;23(2):184–9.

[67] Crotzer VL, Blum JS. Cytosol to lysosome transport of intracellular antigens during immune surveillance. Traffic 2008;9(1):10–6.

[68] Tewari MK, Sinnathamby G, Rajagopal D, Eisenlohr LC. A cytosolic pathway for MHC class II-restricted antigen processing that is proteasome and TAP dependent. Nat Immunol 2005;6(3):287–94.

[69] van Luijn MM, Chamuleau ME, Ressing ME, Wiertz EJ, Ostrand-Rosenberg S, Souwer Y, et al. Alternative Ii-independent antigen-processing pathway in leukemic blasts involves TAP-dependent peptide loading of HLA class II complexes. Cancer Immunol Immunother 2010;59(12):1825–38.

[70] Dani A, Chaudhry A, Mukherjee P, Rajagopal D, Bhatia S, George A, et al. The pathway for MHCII-mediated presentation of endogenous proteins involves peptide transport to the endo-lysosomal compartment. J Cell Sci 2004;117(Pt 18):4219–30.

[71] Sinnathamby G, Maric M, Cresswell P, Eisenlohr LC. Differential requirements for endosomal reduction in the presentation of two H2-E(d)-restricted epitopes from influenza hemagglutinin. J Immunol 2004;172(11):6607–14.

[72] Lechner F, Wong DK, Dunbar PR, Chapman R, Chung RT, Dohrenwend P, et al. Analysis of successful immune responses in persons infected with hepatitis C virus. J Exp Med 2000;191(9):1499–512.

[73] Shoukry NH, Cawthon AG, Walker CM. Cell-mediated immunity and the outcome of hepatitis C virus infection. Annu Rev Microbiol 2004;58:391–424.

[74] Palucka K, Banchereau J, Mellman I. Designing vaccines based on biology of human dendritic cell subsets. Immunity 2010;33(4):464–78.

[75] Granucci F, Foti M, Ricciardi-Castagnoli P. Dendritic cell biology. Adv Immunol 2005;88:193–233.

[76] Jiang A, Bloom O, Ono S, Cui W, Unternaehrer J, Jiang S, et al. Disruption of E-cadherin-mediated adhesion induces a functionally distinct pathway of dendritic cell maturation. Immunity 2007;27(4):610–24.

[77] Manicassamy S, Pulendran B. Dendritic cell control of tolerogenic responses. Immunol Rev 241(1):206–27.

[78] Crozat K, Guiton R, Guilliams M, Henri S, Baranek T, Schwartz-Cornil I, et al. Comparative genomics as a tool to reveal functional equivalences between human and mouse dendritic cell subsets. Immunol Rev 2010;234(1):177–98.

[79] Edwards AD, Chaussabel D, Tomlinson S, Schulz O, Sher A. Reis e Sousa C. Relationships among murine CD11c(high) dendritic cell subsets as revealed by baseline gene expression patterns. J Immunol 2003;171(1):47–60.

[80] Gordon JR, Li F, Nayyar A, Xiang J, Zhang X. CD8 alpha+, but not CD8 alpha-, dendritic cells tolerize Th2 responses via contact-dependent and -independent mechanisms, and reverse airway hyper-responsiveness, Th2, and eosinophil responses in a mouse model of asthma. J Immunol 2005;175(3):1516–22.

[81] Legge KL, Gregg RK, Maldonado-Lopez R, Li L, Caprio JC, Moser M, et al. On the role of dendritic cells in peripheral T cell tolerance and modulation of autoimmunity. J Exp Med 2002;196(2):217–27.

[82] Shortman K, Heath WR. The CD8+ dendritic cell subset. Immunol Rev 2010;234(1):18–31.

[83] den Haan JM, Lehar SM, Bevan MJ. CD8(+) but not CD8(−) dendritic cells cross-prime cytotoxic T cells in vivo. J Exp Med 2000;192(12):1685–96.

[84] Schnorrer P, Behrens GM, Wilson NS, Pooley JL, Smith CM, El-Sukkari D, et al. The dominant role of CD8+ dendritic cells in cross-presentation is not dictated by antigen capture. Proc Natl Acad Sci U S A 2006;103(28):10729–34.

[85] Shrimpton RE, Butler M, Morel AS, Eren E, Hue SS, Ritter MA. CD205 (DEC-205): a recognition receptor for apoptotic and necrotic self. Mol Immunol 2009;46(6):1229–39.

[86] Bonifaz L, Bonnyay D, Mahnke K, Rivera M, Nussenzweig MC, Steinman RM. Efficient targeting of protein antigen to the dendritic cell receptor DEC-205 in the steady state leads to antigen presentation on major histocompatibility complex class I products and peripheral CD8+ T cell tolerance. J Exp Med 2002;196(12):1627–38.

67

[87] Siegal FP, Kadowaki N, Shodell M, Fitzgerald-Bocarsly PA, Shah K, Ho S, et al. The nature of the principal type 1 interferon-producing cells in human blood. Science 1999;284(5421):1835—7.

[88] Liu YJ. IPC: professional type 1 interferon-producing cells and plasmacytoid dendritic cell precursors. Annu Rev Immunol 2005;23:275—306.

[89] Reizis B, Bunin A, Ghosh HS, Lewis KL, Sisirak V. Plasmacytoid dendritic cells: recent progress and open questions. Annu Rev Immunol 2011;29:163—83.

[90] Jarrossay D, Napolitani G, Colonna M, Sallusto F, Lanzavecchia A. Specialization and complementarity in microbial molecule recognition by human myeloid and plasmacytoid dendritic cells. European journal of immunology 2001;31(11):3388—93.

[91] Kadowaki N, Ho S, Antonenko S, Malefyt RW, Kastelein RA, Bazan F, et al. Subsets of human dendritic cell precursors express different toll-like receptors and respond to different microbial antigens. J Exp Med 2001;194(6):863—9.

[92] Honda K, Ohba Y, Yanai H, Negishi H, Mizutani T, Takaoka A, et al. Spatiotemporal regulation of MyD88-IRF-7 signalling for robust type-I interferon induction. Nature 2005;434(7036):1035—40.

[93] Lande R, Gilliet M. Plasmacytoid dendritic cells: key players in the initiation and regulation of immune responses. Ann N Y Acad Sci 2010;1183:89—103.

[94] GeurtsvanKessel CH, Willart MA, van Rijt LS, Muskens F, Kool M, Baas C, et al. Clearance of influenza virus from the lung depends on migratory langerin+CD11b— but not plasmacytoid dendritic cells. J Exp Med 2008;205(7):1621—34.

[95] Smit JJ, Rudd BD, Lukacs NW. Plasmacytoid dendritic cells inhibit pulmonary immunopathology and promote clearance of respiratory syncytial virus. J Exp Med 2006;203(5):1153—9.

[96] Lund JM, Linehan MM, Iijima N, Iwasaki A. Cutting Edge: Plasmacytoid dendritic cells provide innate immune protection against mucosal viral infection in situ. J Immunol 2006;177(11):7510—4.

[97] Mouries J, Moron G, Schlecht G, Escriou N, Dadaglio G, Leclerc C. Plasmacytoid dendritic cells efficiently cross-prime naive T cells in vivo after TLR activation. Blood 2008;112(9):3713—22.

[98] Young LJ, Wilson NS, Schnorrer P, Proietto A, ten Broeke T, Matsuki Y, et al. Differential MHC class II synthesis and ubiquitination confers distinct antigen-presenting properties on conventional and plasmacytoid dendritic cells. Nat Immunol 2008;9(11):1244—52.

[99] Cervantes-Barragan L, Zust R, Weber F, Spiegel M, Lang KS, Akira S, et al. Control of coronavirus infection through plasmacytoid dendritic-cell-derived type I interferon. Blood 2007;109(3):1131—7.

[100] Swiecki M, Colonna M. Unraveling the functions of plasmacytoid dendritic cells during viral infections, autoimmunity, and tolerance. Immunol Rev 2010;234(1):142—62.

[101] Krug A, French AR, Barchet W, Fischer JA, Dzionek A, Pingel JT, et al. TLR9-dependent recognition of MCMV by IPC and DC generates coordinated cytokine responses that activate antiviral NK cell function. Immunity 2004;21(1):107—19.

[102] Dalod M, Salazar-Mather TP, Malmgaard L, Lewis C, Asselin-Paturel C, Briere F, et al. Interferon alpha/beta and interleukin 12 responses to viral infections: pathways regulating dendritic cell cytokine expression in vivo. J Exp Med 2002;195(4):517—28.

[103] Irla M, Kupfer N, Suter T, Lissilaa R, Benkhoucha M, Skupsky J, et al. MHC class II-restricted antigen presentation by plasmacytoid dendritic cells inhibits T cell-mediated autoimmunity. J Exp Med 2010;207(9):1891—905.

[104] Goubier A, Dubois B, Gheit H, Joubert G, Villard-Truc F, Asselin-Paturel C, et al. Plasmacytoid dendritic cells mediate oral tolerance. Immunity 2008;29(3):464—75.

[105] Koyama M, Hashimoto D, Aoyama K, Matsuoka K, Karube K, Niiro H, et al. Plasmacytoid dendritic cells prime alloreactive T cells to mediate graft-versus-host disease as antigen-presenting cells. Blood 2009;113(9):2088—95.

[106] Kushwah R, Hu J. Complexity of dendritic cell subsets and their function in the host immune system. Immunology 2011;133(4):409—19.

[107] Jakob T, Brown MJ, Udey MC. Characterization of E-cadherin-containing junctions involving skin-derived dendritic cells. J Invest Dermatol 1999;112(1):102—8.

[108] Tang A, Amagai M, Granger LG, Stanley JR, Udey MC. Adhesion of epidermal Langerhans cells to keratinocytes mediated by E-cadherin. Nature 1993;361(6407):82—5.

[109] Guilliams M, Henri S, Tamoutounour S, Ardouin L, Schwartz-Cornil I, Dalod M, et al. From skin dendritic cells to a simplified classification of human and mouse dendritic cell subsets. Eur J Immunol 40(8):2089—94.

[110] Stoitzner P, Tripp CH, Eberhart A, Price KM, Jung JY, Bursch L, et al. Langerhans cells cross-present antigen derived from skin. Proc Natl Acad Sci U S A 2006;103(20):7783—8.

[111] Waithman J, Allan RS, Kosaka H, Azukizawa H, Shortman K, Lutz MB, et al. Skin-derived dendritic cells can mediate deletional tolerance of class I-restricted self-reactive T cells. J Immunol 2007;179(7):4535—41.

[112] Wang L, Bursch LS, Kissenpfennig A, Malissen B, Jameson SC, Hogquist KA. Langerin expressing cells promote skin immune responses under defined conditions. J Immunol 2008;180(7):4722–7.

[113] Bedoui S, Whitney PG, Waithman J, Eidsmo L, Wakim L, Caminschi I, et al. Cross-presentation of viral and self antigens by skin-derived CD103+ dendritic cells. Nat Immunol 2009;10(5):488–95.

[114] Kaplan DH. In vivo function of Langerhans cells and dermal dendritic cells. Trends Immunol 31(12): 446–51.

[115] Steinman RM, Nussenzweig MC. Avoiding horror autotoxicus: the importance of dendritic cells in peripheral T cell tolerance. Proc Natl Acad Sci U S A 2002;99(1):351–8.

[116] Hashimoto D, Miller J, Merad M. Dendritic cell and macrophage heterogeneity in vivo. Immunity 2011;35(3):323–35.

[117] Dominguez PM, Ardavin C. Differentiation and function of mouse monocyte-derived dendritic cells in steady state and inflammation. Immunol Rev 2010;234(1):90–104.

[118] Delamarre L, Mellman I. Harnessing dendritic cells for immunotherapy. Semin Immunol 23(1): 2–11.

[119] Lande R, Gilliet M. Plasmacytoid dendritic cells: key players in the initiation and regulation of immune responses. Ann N Y Acad Sci 1183: 89–103.

[120] Novak N, Gros E, Bieber T, Allam JP. Human skin and oral mucosal dendritic cells as 'good guys' and 'bad guys' in allergic immune responses. Clin Exp Immunol 2010;161(1):28–33.

[121] Ueno H, Klechevsky E, Schmitt N, Ni L, Flamar AL, Zurawski S, et al. Targeting human dendritic cell subsets for improved vaccines. Semin Immunol 2011;23(1):21–7.

[122] Robbins SH, Walzer T, Dembele D, Thibault C, Defays A, Bessou G, et al. Novel insights into the relationships between dendritic cell subsets in human and mouse revealed by genome-wide expression profiling. Genome Biol 2008;9(1):R17.

[123] Klechevsky E, Liu M, Morita R, Banchereau R, Thompson-Snipes L, Palucka AK, et al. Understanding human myeloid dendritic cell subsets for the rational design of novel vaccines. Hum Immunol 2009;70(5):281–8.

[124] Klechevsky E, Morita R, Liu M, Cao Y, Coquery S, Thompson-Snipes L, et al. Functional specializations of human epidermal Langerhans cells and CD14+ dermal dendritic cells. Immunity 2008;29(3):497–510.

[125] Heath WR, Carbone FR. Dendritic cell subsets in primary and secondary T cell responses at body surfaces. Nat Immunol 2009;10(12):1237–44.

[126] Tel J, van der Leun AM, Figdor CG, Torensma R, de Vries IJ. Harnessing human plasmacytoid dendritic cells as professional APCs. Cancer Immunol Immunother 2012.

[127] Guiducci C, Ott G, Chan JH, Damon E, Calacsan C, Matray T, et al. Properties regulating the nature of the plasmacytoid dendritic cell response to Toll-like receptor 9 activation. J Exp Med 2006;203(8): 1999–2008.

[128] Mittelbrunn M, Martinez del Hoyo G, Lopez-Bravo M, Martin-Cofreces NB, Scholer A, Hugues S, et al. Imaging of plasmacytoid dendritic cell interactions with T cells. Blood 2009;113(1):75–84.

[129] Fonteneau JF, Gilliet M, Larsson M, Dasilva I, Munz C, Liu YJ, et al. Activation of influenza virus-specific CD4+ and CD8+ T cells: a new role for plasmacytoid dendritic cells in adaptive immunity. Blood 2003;101(9):3520–6.

[130] Kawamura K, Kadowaki N, Kitawaki T, Uchiyama T. Virus-stimulated plasmacytoid dendritic cells induce CD4+ cytotoxic regulatory T cells. Blood 2006;107(3):1031–8.

[131] Cella M, Facchetti F, Lanzavecchia A, Colonna M. Plasmacytoid dendritic cells activated by influenza virus and CD40L drive a potent TH1 polarization. Nat Immunol 2000;1(4):305–10.

[132] Hoeffel G, Ripoche AC, Matheoud D, Nascimbeni M, Escriou N, Lebon P, et al. Antigen crosspresentation by human plasmacytoid dendritic cells. Immunity 2007;27(3):481–92.

[133] Takahashi K, Asabe S, Wieland S, Garaigorta U, Gastaminza P, Isogawa M, et al. Plasmacytoid dendritic cells sense hepatitis C virus-infected cells, produce interferon, and inhibit infection. Proc Natl Acad Sci U S A 2010;107(16):7431–6.

[134] Yonkers NL, Rodriguez B, Milkovich KA, Asaad R, Lederman MM, Heeger PS, et al. TLR ligand-dependent activation of naive CD4 T cells by plasmacytoid dendritic cells is impaired in hepatitis C virus infection. J Immunol 2007;178(7):4436–44.

[135] Decalf J, Fernandes S, Longman R, Ahloulay M, Audat F, Lefrerre F, et al. Plasmacytoid dendritic cells initiate a complex chemokine and cytokine network and are a viable drug target in chronic HCV patients. J Exp Med 2007;204(10):2423–37.

[136] Fitzgerald-Bocarsly P, Jacobs ES. Plasmacytoid dendritic cells in HIV infection: striking a delicate balance. J Leukoc Biol 2010;87(4):609–20.

[137] Meier A, Chang JJ, Chan ES, Pollard RB, Sidhu HK, Kulkarni S, et al. Sex differences in the Toll-like receptor-mediated response of plasmacytoid dendritic cells to HIV-1. Nat Med 2009;15(8):955–9.

[138] Mandl JN, Barry AP, Vanderford TH, Kozyr N, Chavan R, Klucking S, et al. Divergent TLR7 and TLR9 signaling and type I interferon production distinguish pathogenic and nonpathogenic AIDS virus infections. Nat Med 2008;14(10):1077−87.

[139] Gilliet M, Cao W, Liu YJ. Plasmacytoid dendritic cells: sensing nucleic acids in viral infection and autoimmune diseases. Nat Rev Immunol 2008;8(8):594−606.

[140] Ronnblom L, Alm GV, Eloranta ML. Type I interferon and lupus. Curr Opin Rheumatol 2009;21(5):471−7.

[141] Nestle FO, Conrad C, Tun-Kyi A, Homey B, Gombert M, Boyman O, et al. Plasmacytoid predendritic cells initiate psoriasis through interferon-alpha production. J Exp Med 2005;202(1):135−43.

CHAPTER 6

Mucosal Immunity

Cathryn Nagler, Taylor Feehley
Committee on Immunology, Department of Pathology, The University of Chicago, Chicago, IL USA

I. OVERVIEW

Unique structural and functional adaptations are required at the mucosal surfaces that form the interface between the external environment and the rest of the body. The anatomy of these barriers, their specialized mechanisms of protection, and their contribution to immune homeostasis will be discussed in this chapter.

II. MUCOSAL SURFACES ARE THE MAJOR PORTALS OF ENTRY FOR ANTIGEN

The mucus-covered epithelia of the body, namely the respiratory, digestive, and urogenital tracts, cover an enormous surface area and form the boundary between the external environment and the underlying tissue. Mucosal surfaces are therefore major routes of antigen entry and are protected by a wide variety of mechanisms, both mechanical and immunological [1]. The antigens that enter through mucosal sites are numerous and varied, including airborne antigens such as fungal spores, pollen, and dust and ingested antigens such as food and bacteria. The responses mounted at mucosal surfaces depend on the antigens themselves as well as the environment in which these antigens are sensed. These different responses can be broadly divided into tolerogenic or inflammatory responses; maintaining a balance between tolerance and immunity is vital for the health of the host.

Although some antigens are processed and presented within the mucosal immune system, others cross the epithelial barrier and traffic throughout the body. In the gut, many antigens gain access through organized lymphoid structures, known as Peyer's patches, which are located in the small intestine (Figure 6.1). Mucosal surfaces are connected by the lymph and/or blood to lymphoid organs such as lymph nodes. The mesenteric and mediastinal lymph nodes drain the gut and airways respectively via afferent lymphatics (Figure 6.1) [1]. The ability of antigen that enters at the mucosa to reach distal sites allows for cross talk between the mucosal and systemic immune systems and the establishment of systemic responses.

Throughout this chapter, emphasis will be placed on the mucosal surfaces of the intestine and on the responses mounted in the gut associated lymphoid tissue (GALT). However, many of the principles to be discussed can be applied to other mucosal sites as well.

III. EPITHELIAL BARRIER

The epithelial barrier at mucosal surfaces typically consists of a single-cell layered columnar epithelium (with a few notable exceptions, e.g., the squamous epithelium of the esophagus) [2]. This seemingly simple barrier is reinforced by a number of specialized protective adaptations, each of which will be discussed below. These include (1) intercellular *tight junctions* that restrict

71

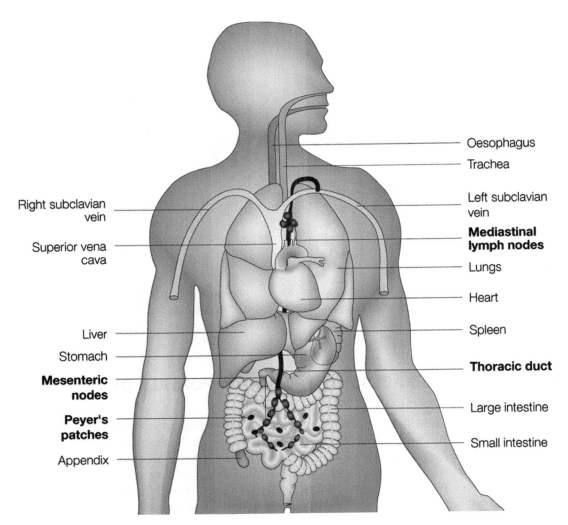

FIGURE 6.1

Antigens enter through mucosal surfaces. Most antigens are either inhaled or ingested and enter the body through the mucosal surfaces of the respiratory and gastrointestinal tracts. In the gut, many antigens gain access through **Peyer's patches**, aggregations of lymphoid follicles found primarily in the distal ileum of the small intestine. Afferent lymphatics transport antigens from the intestinal mucosa to the draining **mesenteric lymph nodes** for presentation to naïve T cells (inhaled antigens are presented in the **mediastinal lymph nodes** that drain the airways). Antigen sensitized T cells migrate out of the draining node through efferent lymphatics and ultimately enter the systemic circulation through the **thoracic duct**. *(From ref. 1, with permission).*

the passage of even small molecules between the cells of the epithelium, (2) *secretory IgA*, a mucosa-associated, structurally stabilized form of immunoglobulin which coats all mucosal surfaces, (3) *defensins*, antimicrobial peptides secreted by epithelial Paneth cells which act as natural antibiotics, and (4) the *mucus* layer itself.

The selectively permeable epithelial barrier is regulated by both tight junctions and adherens junctions located at the apical intercellular space (Figure 6.2) [2]. Tight junctions are formed through cell–cell interactions of proteins, such as occludin and members of the claudin family. Adherens junctions confer stability to the epithelial barrier and are found just basal to the tight junctions. The molecules that make up the tight and adherens junctions interact with actin and myosin rings adjacent to the junctions, allowing them to regulate contraction, tightening or relaxing the contact between neighboring cells and serve to provide a selectively permeable barrier that can regulate the passage of solutes based on both size and charge [2,4]. These junctions ensure that cell–cell contact, and thus barrier integrity, are maintained under

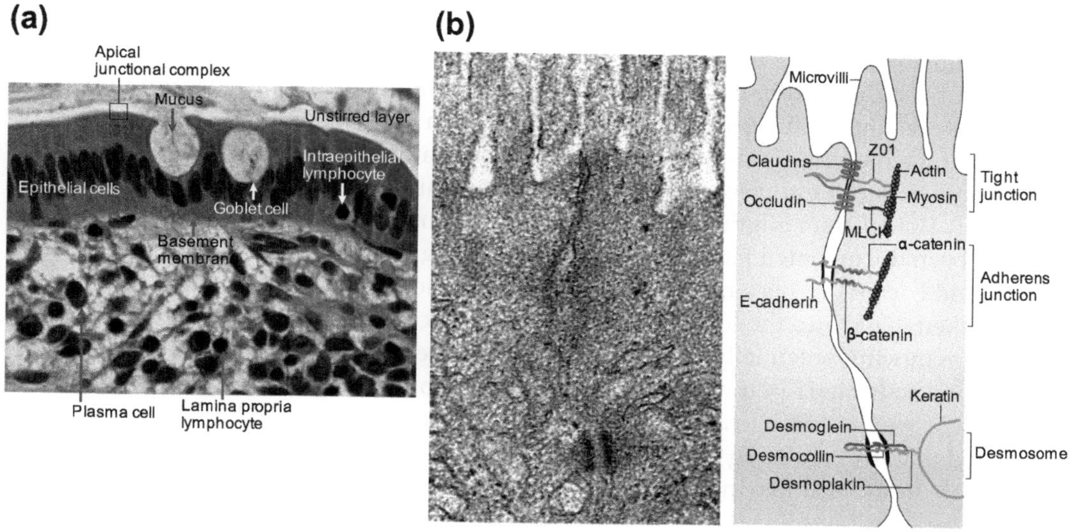

FIGURE 6.2

The epithelial barrier. a. The intestinal mucosa is lined by single cell layered columnar epithelium. **Goblet cells**, which synthesize and release mucin, as well as other specialized cell types, are contained within the epithelial layer. The **tight junction**, a component of the apical junctional complex, seals the paracellular space between epithelial cells. **Intraepithelial lymphocytes** reside above the basement membrane, subjacent to the tight junction. Lymphocytes are readily detectable in the lamina propria. **b.** An electron micrograph, and the corresponding line drawing, of the junctional complex of an intestinal epithelial cell. Just below the base of the microvilli the plasma membranes of adjacent cells seem to fuse at the tight junction, where claudins, zonula occludens 1(ZO1), occludin and F-actin interact. E-cadherin, α-catenin, β-catenin, cateninδ1 and F-actin interact to form the adherens junction *(Adapted from ref. 2, with permission)*.

homeostatic conditions. Two kinds of transport across the epithelial barrier have been described: paracellular and transcellular [2,5]. Paracellular transport is passive and involves the passage of ions through the space between epithelial cells while transcellular transport is active and harnesses the energy of electrochemical gradients across the epithelium into the lamina propria for transport of other nutrients across the barrier. Passive, paracellular transport allows proteins or polysaccharides to pass through the barrier between cells down their concentration gradients. Due to the size and charge selectivity of the epithelial barrier, however, nothing as large as a bacterium or whole cell can pass freely into the lamina propria. Certain stimuli, including infectious pathogens and environmental toxins may, however, disrupt the barrier allowing foreign antigens to enter the lamina propria. For example, proinflammatory cytokines such as TNFα [6] and IFNγ [7] can alter the conformation of the tight junctions to induce barrier dysfunction and increase permeability [2].

Another protective mechanism at mucosal surfaces is the production of secretory IgA [8–10]. IgA exists in both a monomeric and dimeric form; the monomeric form is found predominantly in serum while dimeric IgA is found at epithelial barriers, particularly in the gut. Dimeric IgA is held together by J (joining) chain, a small protein that links the Fc portions of the two immunoglobulin molecules to form a dimer. The production of the J chain seems to be limited to mucosal surfaces, making the dimeric form of IgA a unique feature of these sites. Secretory IgA is produced at the phenomenal rate of 40–60 mg/kg body weight/day [1]. Its secretion into the lumen is regulated by the polymeric Ig receptor (pIgR). This receptor allows dimeric IgA to traffic from the basolateral to the luminal surface, against what might be considered the normal flow of transport across the epithelium. The pIgR is a transmembrane protein that binds to the J chain. Upon binding to the pIgR, IgA traffics in endosomes from the basolateral surface to the apical surface where it is released into the lumen. Release requires the cleavage of pIgR from the membrane, leaving only a small peptide bound to the J chain called the secretory component (SC). In the lumen SC prevents proteolytic degradation of IgA.

IgA's utility at mucosal surfaces is largely related to its ability to neutralize and sequester antigen. Some of the IgA produced under homeostatic conditions is generated by T-cell-independent responses from B1 B cells; this IgA is low affinity because it does not undergo somatic hypermutation in a germinal center [9,10]. Much of this T-independent IgA response is thought to be bacteria specific and broadly reactive against the microbiome because its production is induced upon colonization of germ free mice with intestinal commensal bacteria [10,11,12]. High affinity, T-dependent IgA responses to the commensal microbiota have also been documented [10]. In addition to guarding the epithelium from antigen entry, IgA can bind bacteria or bacterial antigens that do gain access to the lamina propria and transport them back into the lumen. In this role IgA functions as an antigen "sump pump," constantly removing potentially damaging stimuli and helping to control inflammation. IgA can also bind to bacteria in the lumen; this may be important to limit overgrowth of the microbiota as well as block invasion by pathogenic microbes. Indeed, it has recently been appreciated that, by regulating the composition of gut bacterial communities, IgA plays a critical role in the maintenance of immune homeostasis [12].

A third specialized adaptation for the protection of the epithelial barrier is the production of antimicrobial peptides [13,14]. Specialized epithelial cells called Paneth cells, which are located in the crypts of the intestinal villi, secrete these peptides. Antimicrobial peptide production is constitutive, and its mode of action is antigen nonspecific, allowing for broad-spectrum antibacterial protection. Paneth cell-secreted peptides provide an extra layer of protection that prevents bacteria from invading the crypts, thereby guarding the site of epithelial cell regeneration. There are several types of antimicrobial peptides, including defensins, trefoil peptides, C-type lectins, and phospholipases [15]. Given their varied modes of action, these peptides serve as an important first line of defense against certain intestinal pathogens and can limit aberrant expansion of the microbiota.

The goblet cell is another specialized epithelial cell type; these very large cells are distributed throughout the epithelium and are responsible for secreting mucus (see Figure 6.2). Mucus covers the apical face of epithelial cells and is a complex polysaccharide matrix that forms a protective barrier between the epithelial surface and the gut lumen [2]. The mucus layer is particularly important in separating the microbiota from the epithelium, effectively partitioning microbial communities [16]. Although certain bacteria can be associated with enterocytes, most remain embedded in mucus or free in the lumen, limiting their ability to interact directly with the epithelium and trigger inflammatory responses.

Secretory IgA, antimicrobial peptides and mucus are specialized adaptations of the mucosa that provide reinforcement to the physical barrier of the epithelium itself. The combined effect of these defense mechanisms is a well-maintained divide between the lumen and the lamina propria that is not often breached under conditions of health and homeostasis.

IV. INDUCTIVE AND EFFECTOR SITES IN THE MUCOSA-ASSOCIATED LYMPHOID TISSUE

Unique structural features of the intestine contribute to its role as an immunological "organ." The intestinal epithelium has a distinct organization and forms folds called villi; these villi act to increase the surface area of the intestine to aid in the absorption of water and nutrients. Intestinal villi contain primarily columnar epithelial cells, also called enterocytes, which have finger-like protrusions on their apical/luminal side called microvilli. The microvilli further increase the surface area (and corresponding absorptive capacity) of each enterocyte. At the ends of these microvilli are glycoproteins that form a brush border which, along with the mucus layer, creates a thick glycocalyx. Within the small intestine, however, there are cells that have a different morphology and are interspersed between enterocytes, typically as part of organized mucosal lymphoid structures. These cells, called M cells, lack the brush border glycocalyx and are specialized to acquire and transcytose antigen from the gut lumen to the lamina propria of the intestine [17,18]. M cells facilitate transport of antigen or material that is larger than that which passes by paracellular or transcellular transport, including whole microbes [17]. Thus, these specialized cells regulate the amount of antigen that gains access to the mucosa and provide a controlled route for antigen trafficking.

Antigen-presenting cells (APCs) of the lamina propria often reside below the M cells where they have access to newly imported antigens [19]. The population of cells in the lamina propria that can phagocytose and present antigen is highly heterogeneous. Some of these APC are migratory dendritic cells (DC) and can carry antigen to the mesenteric lymph node for presentation to naïve T cells at that site. The migratory DC subset is often identified by its expression of the surface markers CD11c and CD103 [20]. Other DCs are tissue-resident and sample antigen directly from the intestinal lumen by extending dendritic processes between epithelial cells [21,22]. These DCs are identified by their expression of CD11c and CX_3CR_1, a chemokine receptor, on their cell surface. A third class of APC that is present in the intestinal lamina propria is a population of nonmigratory, $CX_3CR_1^+$ macrophages. These macrophages, although partially defined by the same surface receptor as the DCs, are also CD11b$^+$ and F4/80$^+$, do not extend processes and are hypothesized to be potent producers of IL-10, an immunosuppressive cytokine important for limiting inflammation and maintaining regulatory T-cell populations [23]. They do not seem to present antigen effectively to naïve T cells but process antigen efficiently, suggesting a predominant role in the clonal expansion of effector cells that home back to the lamina propria [19].

In addition to epithelial cells (which are derived from the stromal compartment) and APCs, mucosal surfaces are associated with a wide range of other hematopoietic cells. There are more antibody-producing B cells in mucosal tissues than in the spleen and lymph nodes combined [2]! One abundant and unique population of cells is the intestinal intraepithelial lymphocytes (IEL). These atypical and nonmigratory T cells reside between enterocytes, above the basement membrane. Expression of a CD8αα homodimer (rather than the CD8αβ heterodimer expressed by CD8$^+$ T cells at other sites) correlates with the activated/memory phenotype of IEL. Indeed many IEL are constitutively cytolytic directly *ex vivo* [24,25]. The IEL population consists largely of γδ T cells (referring to the structure of their T-cell receptor, TCR), but there are also αβ TCR$^+$ IELs. IELs act as sentinels to detect and repair damaged epithelium [26]. They have also been implicated in protection against colitis as well as intestinal infections [26].

The intestine has gut-associated lymphoid tissue (GALT), the lungs have bronchus-associated lymphoid tissue (BALT), and the nasal passages have nasal-associated lymphoid tissue (NALT). Within these dedicated lymphoid tissues, there are both inductive sites and effector sites. Antigen-specific responses are initiated at inductive sites. Effector sites are populated with memory effector T and B cells which man the barriers, poised to respond quickly and effectively to subsequent antigen challenge [1]. Trafficking between inductive and effector sites is regulated by highly specific homing receptors. Each mucosal tissue has a zip code-like address of chemokine and adhesion/addressin molecules that direct lymphocytes back to these sites upon infection or stimulation. For the gut, homing is directed by CCR9/CCL25 and $\alpha_4\beta_7$/MADCAM1 engagement, while in the lung homing is dependent on CCR10/CCL28 and $\alpha_4\beta_1$/VCAM1 receptor/ligand interactions [27,28]. Given these distinct molecular signatures imparted on lymphocytes as part of their education, cells can migrate from inductive to effector sites and from systemic circulation back to a mucosal surface. Another factor that directs lymphocyte trafficking and education at mucosal surfaces is the presence of vitamins and their metabolites. This is of particular importance in the gut. Dietary vitamin A can be converted to retinoic acid (RA) by DCs that possess the retinaldehyde dehydrogenase (RALDH) enzyme; when these DCs interact with cognate T cells in the presence of RA, the T cells are induced to upregulate gut homing receptors [29]. A similar pathway operates in the skin; DCs convert sunlight-induced vitamin D3 to its active form $1,25(OH)_2D_3$, which induces the expression of CCR10 on activated T cells, allowing their migration into the epidermis [30].

Using the gut as a model mucosal surface again, inductive sites include the mesenteric lymph node, which drains the lymph and trafficking lymphocytes from the lamina propria, and two kinds of tertiary lymphoid organs, the Peyer's patches (Figure 6.3) and the isolated lymphoid follicles (ILFs) [1]. Peyer's patches and ILFs are clusters of lymphocytes in the lamina propria that can support antigen presentation to T cells and the formation of germinal centers for generation of high affinity antibodies [9,10]. All three of these sites contain antigen-loaded APCs that encounter naïve T cells [10]. When these T cells interact with APC loaded with their cognate antigen, their TCR is engaged and they differentiate into an effector T cell (Teff) or a regulatory T cell (Treg). This fate decision is dictated by signals from the APC and the cytokine environment of the inductive site. Cytokines that are of particular relevance for this fate decision are TGFβ, RA, and IL-6. The presence of TGF-β and RA supports the differentiation of Tregs by upregulating expression of the transcription factor

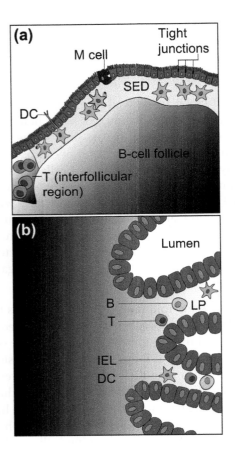

FIGURE 6.3

The gut associated lymphoid tissue. The gut associated lymphoid tissue contains inductive (Peyer's patch) and effector (lamina propria) sites. **a.** The **Peyer's patch** contains B-cell follicles similar to those found in lymph nodes. A follicle-associated epithelium (**FAE**) lines the dome of the Peyer's patch. Antigen is transported across the epithelial barrier by specialized epithelial cells called **M cells** and by dendritic cells (DCs) that reach into the intestinal lumen. **Tight junctions** at the apical surface of epithelial cells maintain barrier integrity. The abundance of DCs and macrophages present in the subepithelial dome (**SED**) of the Peyer's patch facilitates the uptake, processing and presentation of antigen transported across the epithelium. **b.** The intestinal villus epithelium contains an unusual population of intraepithelial lymphocytes (IEL), which reside above the epithelial basement membrane. The lamina propria of the intestinal villi is richly populated with both lymphoid effector cells (e.g., memory T cells and IgA secreting B cells) and antigen-presenting cells (DC and macrophages). *(Adapted from ref. 1, with permission).*

Foxp3 [29,31,32]. By contrast when TGF-β and IL-6 dominate the cytokine milieu, T cells upregulate another transcription factor, RORγt, which drives the proinflammatory Th17 effector program [33—35]. The balance between these lineages, as well as the other effector T-cell subsets (Th1, Th2), is important for the maintenance of homeostasis at mucosal surfaces [36] and TGF-β plays a particularly critical role. In addition to regulating the differentiation of Tregs, TGF-β governs class switching to the IgA isotype [8—10]. Naïve B cells in inductive sites can acquire and present antigen and interact with antigen-experienced T cells in B-cell follicles. When B and T cells that recognize the same antigen interact, the B cell undergoes T-dependent class-switch recombination and somatic hypermutation to produce high affinity antibodies. The choice of antibody isotype produced by these B cells is controlled by cytokines. In the TGF-β rich microenvironment of the GALT, IgA is preferentially produced. T-dependent IgA is antigen specific, meaning it undergoes somatic hypermutation that results ultimately in high affinity antibodies; this is distinctly different from the barrier-protective, low affinity secretory IgA discussed earlier. Other cytokines drive switching to different isotypes (e.g., IL-4 for IgG1 switching), creating a varied repertoire of high affinity antibodies with different functions. Once antigen-specific T and B lymphocytes have clonally expanded, they can traffic back to the lamina propria and villus epithelium, which are the effector sites for the gut. When these cells are reintroduced to their cognate antigen at this effector site, they are engaged again, and can rapidly mount an appropriate immune response.

V. THE MICROBIOME AND MUCOSAL SURFACES

One major challenge to maintaining homeostasis at mucosal surfaces is the presence of the microbiome. The microbiome is defined as the community of bacteria, the commensal microbiota, that colonize all mucosal sites in the body; there are trillions of individual bacteria representing up to 1000 unique bacterial species [37]. Although at least 28 bacterial phyla have been described, in a healthy individual the commensal microbiota is dominated by bacteria from only two of these phyla: Bacteroidetes and Firmicutes [38]. On a species level, the composition of the microbiota varies from site to site and individual to individual. It can also be affected by the environment, age of the host and genetics. The commensal microbiota is essential for the health of the host, providing energy, nutrients, and metabolites that the host is unable to produce itself, including short chain fatty acids such as acetate and butyrate [39].

The microbiome, however, also presents a major conundrum for the immune system. How does the host tolerate and promote homeostasis with the microbiota while mounting the necessary response in the presence of invading intestinal pathogens? Innate immune sensors including Toll-like receptors (TLRs), Nod-like receptors (NLRs), and C-type lectin receptors (CLRs) detect bacterial surface molecules or nucleic acids [40]. Many bacterial pathogen associated molecular patterns (PAMPS), including lipopolysaccharide (LPS), peptidoglycan, and flagellin, are common to both pathogens and members of the microbiota. Responses to the same PAMPS, which trigger inflammation and an adaptive immune response, must be downregulated to avoid a response to the commensals that inhabit mucosal surfaces. Yet, clearance of pathogens often necessitates an inflammatory response. Different classes of pathogens elicit different effector responses at mucosal sites; intracellular bacteria primarily drive Th1 responses, helminth infection drives Th2 responses, and acute bacterial infections drive Th17 responses.

VI. TOLERANCE TO DIETARY ANTIGEN AND THE MICROBIOME

Although pathogens typically evoke host protective effector responses, the commensal microbiome does not. The exact mechanism for maintaining nonresponsiveness to the microbiome has not been fully elucidated. Several mechanisms have been proposed, however, including reduced mucosal responsiveness to major PAMPs such as LPS and alterations in the structure of PAMPs on commensals that change the signaling pathways they induce [41].

There is also compelling new evidence for induction of bacteria-specific Foxp3$^+$Tregs [42]. These regulatory cells are potent producers of the immunoregulatory cytokines IL-10 and TGF-β, which can both prevent the induction of effector responses or limit their duration.

A final hypothesis is that it is not the mere presence of the microbiota or individual isolated species, but the composition of the community, the microbiome, that allows the host to tolerate their presence. The host adaptive immune system, having co-evolved with an enteric microbiome, requires stimuli from the microbiota in order to promote the generation of a balanced lymphocyte compartment with both Teff and Tregs [37]. Recent work has demonstrated that individual species or defined microbial cocktails can have potent immunomodulatory effects such as the induction of Tregs or the induction of pro-inflammatory Th1 and Th17 cells. Single species have even been shown to do one or more of these things under different conditions, and have thus been deemed "pathobionts," referring both to their presence as normal members of the microbiome and their potential to become pathogenic under conditions of dysbiosis or excessive external stress. Dysbiosis refers to the state in which the homeostatic balance of the microbiome is lost; it can be caused by a variety of environmental factors such as diet, antibiotic use, and pathogen exposure and is also influenced by host genetics. Prolonged dysbiosis often leads to increased inflammatory responses and may drive the development of various diseases. This suggests that the homeostasis of the mucosal immune system is regulated by a balance of activating and inhibitory signals provided by both the bacteria themselves and the lymphocytes present to regulate them. Given this model of microbial-immune cross talk, it follows that changes in the microbiota can influence general health and homeostasis.

Along with the microbiome, there is another major class of antigens to which the immune system must become tolerant: food antigens. Mucosal and systemic nonresponsiveness to food is called oral tolerance. The mechanisms regulating tolerance to dietary antigen are likely to have both similarities and differences to those regulating tolerance to the microbiome. The induction of oral tolerance has been the focus of extensive research and has recently been found to be more complicated than originally appreciated. Briefly, food antigen is taken up by APCs in the intestine and presented to naïve T cells, which then are educated not to respond to this antigen on reexposure [43]. Since these food antigens are acquired in an environment that favors anti-inflammatory responses, T cells may undergo anergy or deletion if they are reactive to food antigens, in a mechanism similar to central tolerance. A second mechanism of tolerance is also employed in the intestine, namely the induction of Tregs. The fate of these food antigen-specific T cells was initially hypothesized to depend on the dose of food antigen present; high doses of antigen-induced anergy or deletion while frequent, low-dose exposure favored the induction of Tregs [43]. This theory about antigen dose has recently fallen out of favor among many investigators in light of more compelling models [19]. The actual subsets of APCs that are required for this tolerance, the location of APC/T cell interaction, and the cytokine environment required to promote oral tolerance are still incompletely understood. Recent work promotes a two-step model of oral tolerance where induction of Tregs is the primary mechanism for preventing food-specific effector responses [44,45]. In the first step, antigen can be taken up through a variety of methods, including transcytosis through M cells or enterocytes and diffusion between epithelial cells. Once antigen reaches the lamina propria, it is phagocytosed by the CD103$^+$ subset of migratory DC. This DC population then processes this antigen and traffics to the MLN, where antigen-loaded DCs present their antigen to naïve T cells. Because these DCs can metabolize retinoic acid and TGF-β, they have been shown to be particularly good at inducing Foxp3$^+$ Treg differentiation in food antigen-specific T cells [29]. It has been shown that after feeding/intragastric gavage with soluble antigen, the frequency of antigen-specific CD4$^+$Foxp3$^+$ Tregs increases markedly [44]. It is thought that the environment of the MLN also promotes/supports the induction of Tregs. These induced Tregs, instead of being deleted or becoming nonresponsive to antigenic stimulation, become highly effective producers of IL-10 and can help to suppress effector responses by other cells that may escape tolerization [46,47]. When naïve T cells are stimulated by antigen presented by these DCs, they upregulate key gut homing receptors such as $\alpha_4\beta_7$ and CCR9, allowing them to traffic back to the lamina propria, the second step required for the induction of tolerance in this model [44,45]. Once in the lamina propria, Tregs expand markedly and form the predominant population of lymphocytes at this site [46]. This expanded Treg population contributes to the anti-inflammatory environment in which APCs see antigen, further limiting the chance of generating an effector response to food antigens. While it is not completely known what drives this expansion, there is evidence that it is dependent on the $CX_3CR_1^+$ macrophage population that is resident in the LP [44]. Oral tolerance is impaired in mice deficient in this macrophage population [47]. Significantly fewer Tregs are detectable in the lamina propria of mice lacking $CX_3CR_1^+$ macrophages; bacterial translocation and proinflammatory cytokines are increased [47].

Other cells have also been implicated in oral tolerance, albeit with less clearly defined roles or strict necessity. Antigen-presenting cells in the liver have been proposed to be important for promoting the systemic nonresponsiveness that is characteristic of, and necessary for, successful oral tolerance [19,48]. Plasmacytoid DCs, in particular, have been implicated in inducing anergy in antigen-specific T cells after oral antigen administration [49,50]. Of note, the $CX_3CR_1^+$ DC subset is related to plasmacytoid DCs based on gene-expression profiles [51]. Overall, oral tolerance is a classical process of education of the immune system that takes place uniquely at mucosal sites. When oral tolerance breaks down, multiple pathologies can occur that have both local (mucosal) and systemic effects.

The mucosal surfaces of the body are important sites for the regulation of immune responses. The epithelium and its various protective mechanisms form a physical barrier between the external and internal environments and contain and control responses to the commensal microbiota. Mucosal immune responses regulate the choice between tolerogenic or inflammatory responses to luminal antigen. When all of these specialized mechanisms work in concert, the health and homeostasis of the host is maintained.

References

[1] Nagler-Anderson C. Man the barrier! Strategic defenses in the intestinal mucosa. Nat Rev Immunol 2001;1:59—67.

[2] Turner JR. Intestinal mucosal barrier function in health and disease. Nat Rev Immunol 2009;9:799—809.

[3] Round JL, Mazmanian SK. The gut microbiota shapes intestinal immune responses during health and disease. Nat Rev Immunol 2009;9:313—23.

[4] Van Itallie CM, Anderson JM. Claudins and epithelial paracellular transport. Annu Rev Physiol 2006;68:403—29.

[5] Madara JL. Regulation of movement of solutes across tight junctions. Ann Rev Physiol 1998;60:143—59.

[6] Clayburgh DR, Musch MW, Leitges M, Fu Y-X, Turner JR. Coordinated epithelial NHE3 inhibition and barrier dysfunction are required for TNF-mediated diarrhea in vivo. J Clin Invest 2006;116:2682—94.

[7] Watson CJ, Hoare CJ, Garrod DR, Carlson GL, Warhurst G. Interferon-γ selectively increases epithelial permeability to large molecules by activating different populations of paracellular pores. J Cell Sci 2005;118:5221—30.

[8] Fagarasan S, Honjo T. Regulation of IgA synthesis at mucosal surfaces. Curr Opin Immunol 2004;16: 277—83.

[9] Cerutti A. The regulation of IgA class switching. Nat Rev Immunol 2008;8:421—34.

[10] Fagarasan S, Honjo T. Intestinal IgA synthesis: regulation of front-line body defences. Nat Rev Immunol 2003;3:63—72.

[11] Macpherson AJ, et al. A primitive T cell-independent mechanism of intestinal mucosal IgA responses to commensal bacteria. Science 2000;288:2222—6.

[12] Fagarasan S, et al. Critical Roles of Activation-Induced Cytidine Deaminase in the Homeostasis of Gut Flora. Science 2002;298:1424—7.

[13] Salzman NH, Underwood MA, Bevins CL. Paneth cells, defensins, and the commensal microbiota: a hypothesis on intimate interplay at the intestinal mucosa. Semin Immunol 2007;19:70—83.

[14] Salzman NH, et al. Enteric defensins are essential regulators of intestinal microbial ecology. Nat Immunol 2010;11:76—83.

[15] Gill N, Wlodarska M, Finlay BB. Roadblocks in the gut: barriers to enteric infection. Cell Microbiol 2011;13:660—9.

[16] Sonnenburg JL, Angenent LT, Gordon JI. Getting a grip on things: how do communities of bacterial symbionts become established in our intestine? Nat Immunol 2004;5:569—73.

[17] Neutra MR. Current concepts in mucosal immunity. V. Role of M cells in transepithelial transport of antigens and pathogens to the mucosal immune system. Amer J Physiol 1998;274:G785—791.

[18] Corr SC, Gahan CCGM, Hill C. M-cells: origin, morphology and role in mucosal immunity and microbial pathogenesis. FEMS Immunology & Medical Microbiology 2008;52:2—12.

[19] Pabst O, Mowat AM. Oral tolerance to food protein. Mucosal Immunol 2012.

[20] Schulz O, et al. Intestinal CD103+, but not CX3CR1+, antigen sampling cells migrate in lymph and serve classical dendritic cell functions. J Exp Med 2009;206:3101—14.

[21] Niess JH, et al. CX3CR1-Mediated Dendritic Cell Access to the Intestinal Lumen and Bacterial Clearance. Science 2005;307:254—8.

[22] Chieppa M, Rescigno M, Huang AY, Germain RN. Dynamic imaging of dendritic cell extension into the small bowel lumen in response to epithelial cell TLR engagement. J Exp Med 2006;203:2841—52.

[23] Murai M, et al. Interleukin 10 acts on regulatory T cells to maintain expression of the transcription factor Foxp3 and suppressive function in mice with colitis. Nat Immunol 2009;10:1178—84.

[24] Cheroutre H. IELs: enforcing law and order in the court of the intestinal epithelium. Immunol Rev 2005;206:114—31.

[25] Cheroutre H, Madakamutil L. Acquired and natural memory T cells join forces at the mucosal front line. Nat Rev Immunol 2004;4:290—300.

[26] Cheroutre H, Lambolez F, Mucida D. The light and dark sides of intestinal intraepithelial lymphocytes. Nat Rev Immunol 2011;11:445—56.

[27] Johansson-Lindbom B, Agace WW. Generation of gut-homing T cells and their localization to the small intestinal mucosa. Immunol Rev 2007;215:226—42.

[28] Kunkel EJ, et al. CCR10 expression is a common feature of circulating and mucosal epithelial tissue IgA Ab-secreting cells. J Clin Invest 2003;111:1001—10.

[29] Sun CM, et al. Small intestine lamina propria dendritic cells promote de novo generation of Foxp3 T reg cells via retinoic acid. J Exp Med 2007:1775—85.

[30] Sigmundsdottir H, et al. DCs metabolize sunlight-induced vitamin D3 to 'program' T cell attraction to the epidermal chemokine CCL27. Nat Immunol 2007;8:285—93.

[31] Benson MJ, Pino-Lagos K, Rosemblatt M, Noelle RJ. All-trans retinoic acid mediates enhanced T reg cell growth, differentiation, and gut homing in the face of high levels of co-stimulation. J Exp Med 2007:1765—74.

[32] Kang SG, Lim HW, Andrisani OM, Broxmeyer HE, Kim CH. Vitamin A metabolites induce gut-homing FoxP3+ regulatory T cells. J Immunol 2007;179:3724—33.

[33] Bettelli E, Korn T, Kuchroo VK. Th17: the third member of the effector T cell trilogy. Curr Opin Immunol 2007;19:652—7.

[34] Bettelli E, et al. Reciprocal developmental pathways for the generation of pathogenic effector TH17 and regulatory T cells. Nature 2006;441:235—8.

[35] Veldhoen M, Stockinger B. TGFbeta1, a "Jack of all trades": the link with pro-inflammatory IL-17-producing T cells. Trends Immunol 2006;27:358—61.

[36] Coombes JL, Robinson NJ, Maloy KJ, Uhlig HH, Powrie F. Regulatory T cells and intestinal homeostasis. Immunol Rev 2005;204:184—94.

[37] Lee YK, Mazmanian SK. Has the microbiota played a critical role in the evolution of the adaptive immune system? Science 2010;330:1768—73.

[38] Backhed F, Ley RE, Sonnenburg JL, Peterson DA, Gordon JI. Host-bacterial mutualism in the human intestine. Science 2005;307:1915—20.

[39] Eberl G. A new vision of immunity: homeostasis of the superorganism. Mucosal Immunol 2010;3:450—60.

[40] Delbridge LM, O'Riordan MX. Innate recognition of intracellular bacteria. Curr Opin Immunol 2007;19:10—6.

[41] Sansonetti PJ. To be or not to be a pathogen: that is the mucosally relevant question. Mucosal Immunol 2011;4:8—14.

[42] Lathrop SK, et al. Peripheral education of the immune system by colonic commensal microbiota. Nature 2011;478:250—4.

[43] Weiner HL, da Cunha AP, Quintana F, Wu H. Oral tolerance. Immunol Rev 2011;241:241—59.

[44] Hadis U, et al. Intestinal tolerance requires gut homing and expansion of FoxP3+ regulatory T cells in the lamina propria. Immunity 2011;34:237–46.

[45] Cassani B, et al. Gut-Tropic T Cells That Express Integrin alpha4beta7 and CCR9 Are Required for Induction of Oral Immune Tolerance in Mice. Gastroenterology 2011;141:2109–18.

[46] Rubtsov YP, et al. Regulatory T cell-derived interleukin-10 limits inflammation at environmental interfaces. Immunity 2008;28:546–58.

[47] Medina-Contreras O, et al. CX3CR1 regulates intestinal macrophage homeostasis, bacterial translocation, and colitogenic Th17 responses in mice. J Clin Invest 2011.

[48] Crispe IN. The Liver as a Lymphoid Organ. Annu Rev Immunol 2009;27:147–63.

[49] Goubier A, et al. Plasmacytoid Dendritic Cells Mediate Oral Tolerance. Immunity 2008;29:464–75.

[50] Dubois B, et al. Sequential Role of Plasmacytoid Dendritic Cells and Regulatory T Cells in Oral Tolerance. Gastroenterology 2009;137:1019–28.

[51] Bar-On L, et al. CX3CR1+ CD8α+ dendritic cells are a steady-state population related to plasmacytoid dendritic cells. Proc Natl Acad Sci 2010;107:14745–50.

Principles of Cancer Immunobiology

CHAPTER 7

Cancer Immunoediting: From Surveillance to Escape

Michele W.L. Teng[1,2], Michael H. Kershaw[1,2], Mark J. Smyth[1,2]
[1]Cancer Immunology Program, Peter MacCallum Cancer Centre, East Melbourne, Victoria, Australia
[2]Sir Peter MacCallum Department of Oncology, University of Melbourne, Victoria, Australia

I. INTRODUCTION

The development of human tumors is a multistep process traditionally thought to require the acquisition of six biological capabilities. They are: i) sustaining proliferative signaling, ii) evading growth suppressors, iii) resisting cell death, iv) enabling replicative immortality, v) inducing angiogenesis, and vi) activating invasion and metastasis. Collectively these capabilities are acquired by cancer cells in a temporal manner and allow their survival, proliferation, and metastasis. They are defined as the hallmarks of cancer as originally published in the landmark review by Hanahan and Weinberg [1].

Over the past decade, significant progress in cancer research has strengthened and broadened this concept, revealing that tumor biology cannot be understood simply by characterizing the features of the cancer cells, but rather must include the contributions of the tumor microenvironment to tumorigenesis [2]. Furthermore, a number of observations have raised questions and highlighted new mechanistic concepts that were not fundamental in the original synthesis of the six hallmark traits. Consequently, the hallmarks of cancer have undergone recent revision [2]. Certain characteristics aid in the ability of cancer cells to acquire their hallmarks. The two enabling characteristics that do so are genomic instability and mutation and tumor promoting inflammation. Two new hallmarks have been proposed to be functionally important for the development of cancer. The first involves deregulating cellular energetics whereby cancer cells rewire their ability to metabolize energy so as to fuel cell growth and proliferation. The second is the active evasion of destruction by the immune system which paradoxically can also promote cancer initiation, promotion, and progression.

In this book chapter, we discuss the role of the immune system in the prevention of tumor development, covering a brief history of cancer immunity and summarizing the concept of cancer immunoediting, including its three phases: elimination, equilibrium and escape. We then discuss the mouse models of cancer that have been used to establish this concept. Finally, the latter part of this chapter focuses specifically on the evidence for cancer immunoediting in humans.

85

Cancer Immunotherapy. http://dx.doi.org/10.1016/B978-0-12-394296-8.00007-5

II. HISTORY OF CANCER IMMUNE SURVEILLANCE AND CANCER IMMUNOEDITING

Although the importance of the immune system in protecting the host from microbial pathogens is well accepted, the notion that the immune system can also control cancer has been wrought with controversy for over a century. This is due in part to the lack of appropriate immunodeficient mouse models on pure genetic backgrounds (reviewed in detail in reference [3]). However, interest in this area of tumor immunology was rekindled just over a decade ago when a series of seminal works collectively verified the role of immunity in cancer control.

First, the demonstration that IFN-γ plays a critical function in cancer immunosurveillance, whereby neutralizing antibody to IFN-γ in tumor-bearing mice resulted in accelerated tumor growth compared to control antibody treated wild-type mice [4]. Second, mice unresponsive to IFN-γ were found to be more susceptible to carcinogen-induced and spontaneous primary tumor formation compared to age matched wild-type mice [5,6]. Third, the observation that mice lacking perforin ($pfp^{-/-}$) had an increased incidence of spontaneous B-cell lymphomas compared with wild-type mice [7,8]. Lastly, the demonstration that host tumor necrosis factor related apoptosis-inducing ligand (TRAIL) could suppress tumor formation in various mouse models of cancer [9–12]. Collectively, this work formally demonstrated the importance of lymphocyte cytokine and cytotoxicity pathways in preventing tumorigenesis.

Shanakaran and colleagues described the increased incidence of adenocarcinomas in mice lacking lymphocytes and response to interferons [6]. However, this study also highlighted the comparatively greater immunogenicity of tumors derived from immune compromised mice compared to those derived from wild-type immune competent controls. The finding that the immune system controls not only tumor quantity, but also tumor quality (immunogenicity) [3,6], prompted a significant revision of the cancer immunosurveillance hypothesis. Based on these above-mentioned data, Robert Schreiber and his colleagues then published a series of beautiful reviews outlining the cancer immunoediting concept [3,13,14]. The concept that the immune system shapes tumor immunogenicity was the basis of the cancer immunoediting hypothesis, which stressed the dual host-protective and tumor-promoting actions of immunity on developing tumors.

Cancer immunoediting consists of three phases: elimination, equilibrium, and escape, and as such are termed the "three Es of cancer immunoediting" [3,13,15,16] (Figure 7.1). In their simplest form, tumors sequentially proceed through each of these phases, although it is possible that transit between these phases could occur in a bidirectional manner. External factors such as environmental stress and deterioration of an aging immune system potentially might influence the process.

Elimination. The elimination phase corresponds to the original concept of cancer immunosurveillance in which cells of the immune system recognize cancer cells and successfully eliminate them before they become clinically apparent, thus returning tissues back to their normal state of homeostasis. Many studies have demonstrated the critical requirement for cells from both the innate and adaptive immune system in executing this phase (reviewed in Chapter 8 [13,14,17]). Importantly, while certain effector cell subsets and molecules have been shown to be involved in cancer elimination in general, these studies have also revealed that elimination of any given tumor is regulated by the specific characteristics of the tumor—for example, how the tumor originated (spontaneous versus carcinogen-induced), the anatomical location of the tumor, and the tumor's rate of growth.

Equilibrium. Tumor cells not eradicated in the elimination phase enter into the equilibrium phase whereby the immune system halts tumor growth but is unable to completely eliminate the tumor. Currently, this phase is perceived to be the longest in duration—potentially extending throughout the host's lifespan. As such this phase may represent a second fixed

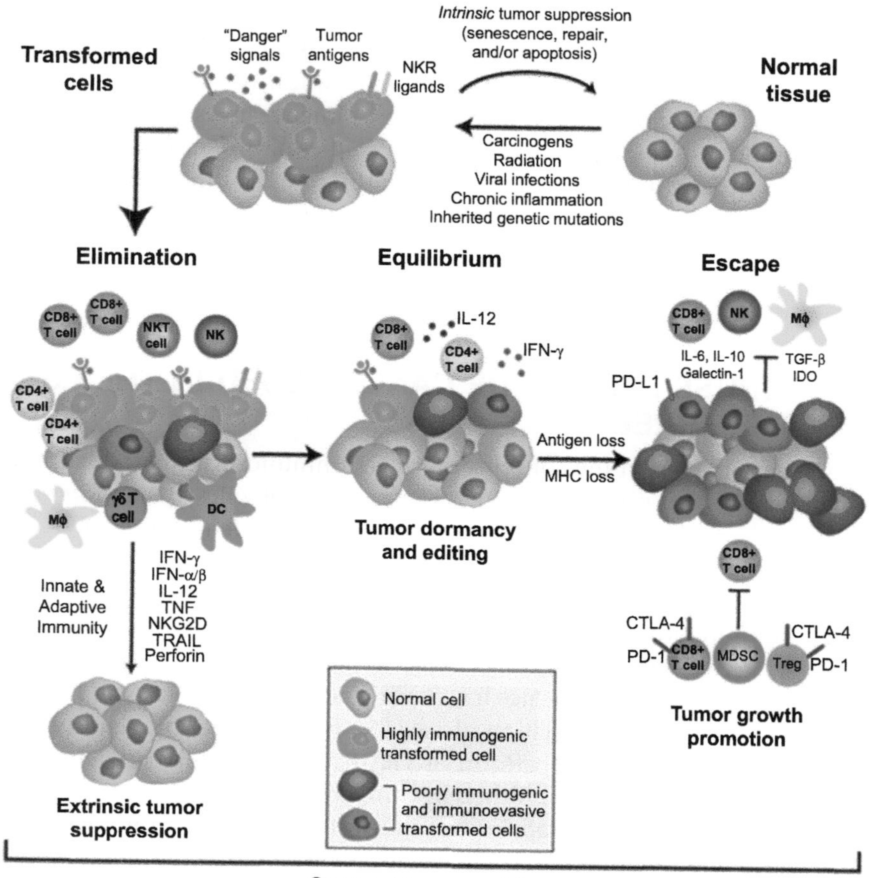

FIGURE 7.1

The cancer immunoediting process. Cancer immunoediting is an extrinsic tumor suppressor mechanism that engages only after cellular transformation has occurred and intrinsic tumor suppressor mechanisms have failed. In its most complex form, cancer immunoediting consists of three sequential phases: elimination, equilibrium, and escape. In the elimination phase, innate and adaptive immunity work together to destroy developing tumors long before they become clinically apparent. Many of the immune molecules and cells that participate in the elimination phase have been characterized, but future work is required to determine their exact sequence of action. If this phase goes to completion, the host remains tumor free, and elimination thus represents the full extent of the process. However, if a rare cancer cell variant is not destroyed in the elimination phase, it may then enter the equilibrium phase, in which its outgrowth is prevented by immunologic mechanisms. T cells, IL-12, and IFN-γ are required to maintain tumor cells in a state of immune-mediated dormancy, whereas NK cells and molecules that participate in the recognition or effector function of cells of innate immunity are not required. This suggests that equilibrium is a function of adaptive immunity only. Editing of tumor immunogenicity occurs in the equilibrium phase. Equilibrium may also represent an end stage of the cancer immunoediting process and may restrain outgrowth of occult cancers for the lifetime of the host. However, as a consequence of constant immune selection pressure placed on genetically unstable tumor cells held in equilibrium, tumor cell variants may emerge that (i) are no longer recognized by adaptive immunity (antigen loss variants or tumor cells that develop defects in antigen processing or presentation), (ii) become insensitive to immune effector mechanisms, or (iii) induce an immunosuppressive state within the tumor microenvironment. These tumor cells may then enter the escape phase, in which their outgrowth is no longer blocked by immunity. These tumor cells emerge to cause clinically apparent disease (this figure was reproduced from [16]).

endpoint of cancer immunoediting. Two possible outcomes are anticipated from the equilibrium phase. The first involves the eventual elimination of all tumor cells by the immune system, resulting in a return to normal tissue homeostasis similar to the elimination phase. In contrast, over a long period of time, the continuous interaction between the immune system with genetically unstable tumors sculpts or "edits" the phenotype of tumor. This prolonged pressure selects for tumor cells that have acquired the most immunoevasive mutations resulting in their outgrowth. Interestingly, unlike the elimination phase, adaptive immunity, but not innate immunity, has been shown to maintain tumor cells in equilibrium. Specifically, interleukin-12 (IL-12), IFN-γ, CD4$^+$, and CD8$^+$ T cells were found to be required [18–21].

Escape. Tumors that cannot be recognized and eradicated by the immune system in the elimination or equilibrium phases progress into the escape phase. These tumors grow progressively to become visible tumors and clinical symptoms are thought to manifest at this stage. The escape phase has been an area of intense investigation in the field of tumor immunology over the past decades. Many studies have demonstrated that tumors in the escape phase avoid the immune system through direct and/or indirect mechanisms to aid in their growth and metastases (reviewed in Chapters 10—11 [15—16]). Focused work is now being undertaken to devise strategies that can target these mechanisms of escape, since they represent means to treat tumors using novel cancer immunotherapies [22—25].

III. MOUSE MODELS OF CANCER USED IN THE ESTABLISHMENT OF THE THREE Es

Evidence to support the concepts of cancer immunosurveillance and immunoediting has historically been obtained through the exposure of wild-type and immunodeficient mice to carcinogens and comparing their relative tumor incidences and latency. The two common carcinogen-induced models of cancer used to study cancer immunoediting are soft tissue fibrosarcomas induced using 3'Methylchloranthene A (3'-MCA) and skin papillomas induced by a combination of 7,12-di-methylbenz[a]-anthracene (DMBA) and 12-O-tetradecanoyl-phorbol-13-acetate (TPA). Collectively, results from exposing a range of mouse strains deficient in various immune genes have clearly demonstrated a central role for innate lymphocyte responses in tumor elimination phase [15]. In particular, mice lacking IFNAR1, IFN-γ, TNF, T cells, NKT cells, NK cells, perforin or TRAIL displayed an increase in MCA-induced sarcomas [6—7,9,12,26—27,28—30]. Although compelling, questions have been raised about the validity of extrapolating conclusions drawn from carcinogen-induced models of cancer to oncogene-induced cancer [2]. Chemical carcinogens used to induce such tumors are prone to generate cancer cells that are highly mutated and especially immunogenic, whereas oncogene-driven cancers appear less immunogenic and from a genetic standpoint better characterized, more simple, and designed to represent human cancers containing the same mutations [2,31,32]. A recent study by Matshushita et al. has elegantly addressed some of these issues [33]. In this study, primary sarcomas derived from immunodeficient Rag2$^{-/-}$ mice, which phenotypically resemble nascent primary tumor cells, had cancer-causing mutations in Kras and Trp53 also frequently observed in *de novo* human and mouse cancers. Using a genomic exome profiling approach, the authors demonstrated that mouse MCA-induced sarcomas had qualitative and quantitative genomic similarities to carcinogen-induced human cancers. Furthermore, transfer of these sarcomas into wildtype mice resulted in a proportion of tumors escaping, where it was demonstrated that T-cell-dependent selection pressure on these tumors caused tumors to lose their highly immunogenic antigens as one mechanism of tumor escape. Complementary to this study, DuPage et al. utilized an oncogene-induced model of primary sarcoma engineered to express a strong model antigen and reported similar findings whereby immunoediting of these tumors by T cells resulted in the loss of the model antigen and subsequent tumor outgrowth [34].

In addition to these recent studies, a higher frequency of hematological malignances and solid tumors have been observed in various immunodeficient mice compared to age matched wild-type mice in aging experiments [6,7,27,35]. Furthermore, immunodeficiency was found to also increase the frequency of cancer in several transgenic mouse models of cancer (e.g., Trp53$^{-/-}$, Her2/neu) [5,7—9,35—37]. Collectively, data across these three different mouse models of cancer have specifically defined the importance of IFN-γ, perforin and TRAIL effector molecules in tumor elimination [15]. By contrast, the requirement for other effector cells and molecules has generally only been validated in some carcinogen-induced tumor models to date. Thus, it will be important to confirm their general role in tumor elimination in genetically defined spontaneous models of cancer. Furthermore, these *de novo* models of cancer are also important for the study of the equilibrium phase, which cannot be studied using transplantable tumor models. The use of both carcinogen-induced and genetic mouse models of cancer will also be required to test whether tumors arising in these two basic model systems display all the 3 Es or whether a fraction of tumors generated *de novo* are never recognized by the immune system. For example, in some settings where mouse mammary cancer has been assessed on a lymphocyte-deficient background, it does not appear that the adaptive immune system plays a critical role in cancer prevention [38]. In our studies of regulatory T-cell depleted mice using the MCA carcinogen-induced fibrosarcoma model, we always noted a proportion of tumors whose growth appeared unaffected by regulatory T-cell depletion [39]. This is despite the fact that a large proportion of tumors were suppressed for growth or rejected under identical experimental conditions. These observations and advanced tumor profiling may now be used to try to answer why certain types of tumors do not appear to be affected by the immune system and whether there are strategies that can unmask them for recognition.

Although genetically engineered mice may more faithfully model the multistage pathogenesis of human cancer and the microenvironmental interplay between emerging neoplastic cells and tissue elements, tumor formation in the transgenic mice is, by its nature, biologically variable and latent compared with tumor transplantation. Experiments simply take considerably longer and at greater cost. Moreover, the continuous expression of transforming genes might actually restrict the ability of the host to eradicate all malignant cells and thus perpetuate inflammatory responses [31]. Lastly, mice still have significant limitations in modeling human cancer, including species—species differences and inaccurate recapitulation of *de novo* human tumor development [32]. Thus, it is very important to try to validate that cancer immunoediting occurs in humans.

IV. CANCER IMMUNOEDITING IN HUMANS

Unlike experimental inbred mice living in well-controlled environments, humans are very polymorphic and live in comparatively uncontrolled environments. Nevertheless, convincing correlative clinical data from human patients have provided unequivocal evidence that cells of both the innate and adaptive immune system are required for the prevention of cancer and also shape tumor immunogenicity. For the rest of this chapter, we review data that support the existence of cancer immunoediting in humans. The mechanisms of tumor escape in humans will not be discussed here given that they greatly overlap with those observed in mice and have been extensively reviewed elsewhere [3,13,14,40—42].

A. Tumor immune infiltrates as a prognostic indicator

Extensive data amassed from large annotated cohorts of human cancers supports the hypothesis that the immune system influences the development of cancer [43]. Indeed, all immune cell types can be found in a tumor and they can be located in the core (center) of the tumor (CT), in the invasive margin (IM) or in the adjacent tertiary lymphoid structures (TLS) [43]. Importantly, different immune contextures, classified as the number, type and location of immune infiltrates in tumor have been linked with either beneficial or deleterious outcomes for cancer patients and these were first demonstrated in colorectal cancer [44]. In a number of key studies using a large number of colorectal samples, Galon, Pages and colleagues analyzed the immune components in the tumor microenvironment using a combination of high-throughput genotypic (microarrays) and phenotypic (immunohistochemistry, flow cytometry) analyses and evaluated their possible influence on tumor dissemination [44—46]. Collectively, the immune contexture correlating with good prognosis in colorectal patients required the presence of $CD3^+CD8^+$ cytotoxic T cells and $CD45RO^+$ memory T cells, in high numbers in both the center of the tumor and invasive margin. Importantly, this particular immune contexture and its correlation with disease-free status and overall survival of cancer patients has now been demonstrated for tumors originating from different organs and of various cancer cell types, such as melanoma [47], head and neck [48], bladder [49], breast [50], ovarian [51,52], oesophageal [53] and prostatic [54,55]. In addition, it has also now been demonstrated that together with cytotoxic and memory T cells, the presence of Th1 polarization signature in the tumor immune infiltrates maximally correlates to a positive clinical outcome for all tumor types [56]. This Th1 immune signature has been demonstrated to consist of Th1 associated factors (IFN-γ, IL-12, T-bet, and interferon regulatory factor 1), cytotoxic factors (granzymes, perforin and granulysin) and chemokines (CX3CL1, CXCL9, CXCL10, CCL5 and CCL2). Collectively, the results of these studies provide strong evidence for cancer immunoediting in humans.

In contrast to Th1 cells, the role of other $CD4^+$ T-cell types such as Th2, Th17 or Tregs correlating with either a positive or negative clinical outcome has been mired in controversy. A striking example is that of regulatory T cells (Tregs) where conflicting data has resulted in difficulties in interpreting their role in cancer immunoediting and surveillance. Tregs can be divided into different subpopulations such as natural Tregs and induced Tregs. However, natural Tregs, which are best defined and generated from the thymus, have been demonstrated to negatively modulate antitumor immunity in numerous mouse and human studies (reviewed in Chapter 33 [57]). Tregs are generally defined as $CD4^+CD25^{hi}FOXP3^+$, although CD25 and FOXP3 are also expressed by activated effector T cells, albeit only transiently for FOXP3 [58]. In addition, there are also FOXP3- suppressor cells [59,60] as well as $CD8^+$ T cells expressing FOXP3 [61,62]. Nevertheless, a landmark study by Curiel et al. demonstrated that regulatory T cells were specifically recruited into ovarian carcinoma and correlated with reduced survival [63]. The correlation of Treg numbers and poor clinical outcome has also been reported for several other malignancies including breast cancer [64,65], lung cancer [66–68], melanoma [69,70], pancreatic cancer [71,72], hepatocellular carcinoma [73–76], and gastric cancer [77,78]. However, other studies have reported no impact of Treg cell infiltration on survival in some of the malignancies mentioned above [79–82]. Interestingly, intratumor Treg numbers have been reported to inversely correlate with improved survival in patients with head and neck cancer [48,83], bladder cancer [84], colorectal cancer [85–88], gastric cancer [89], ovarian cancer [90], follicular lymphoma and Hodgkin's lymphoma [91]. The reasons for these different outcomes are not clear but may be related to the difference in the technical assays used, the stringency in defining Tregs (FOXP3 staining alone versus CD4 FOXP3 CD25 co-staining), the histological and molecular type of malignancy involved and their associated tumor microenvironment. In addition, whether the $FOXP3^+$ cells are truly suppressive in all studies is not clear. Furthermore, given that chronic inflammation promotes carcinogenesis [92–95] and Tregs are key in suppressing inflammation, it is envisioned that the presence of Tregs may be beneficial in such settings.

Likewise, conflicting data have also been reported for Th17 and Th2 cells. Th17 cells have been reported to correlate with poor prognosis in colorectal cancer [85], gastric cancer [96], lung cancer [97] and hepatocellular carcinoma [98], but correlated with better survival in patients with ovarian cancer [99], esophageal cancer [100], and gastric cancer [101]. Association of Th2 cells with poor prognosis in ovarian cancer [102], pancreatic cancer, [103,104] and gastric cancer [105] has been described, while conversely, they correlate with good prognosis in breast cancer [106], Hodgkin's lymphoma [107], and melanoma [108]. In addition, a role for Th17 or Th2 cells in promoting or suppressing antitumor immunity is reported even for the same cancer types. Similar to Tregs, the assays used to define Th17 and Th2 cells may differ between studies. For example in some studies, IL-17 rather than $CD4^+$ $IL-17^+$ cells were quantified [96,97,100,101], which may affect the analyses given that other immune cells such as NK cells and lymphoid tissue inducer-like cells can also produce IL-17 [109]. Furthermore, while nonresolving inflammation is tumor promoting, certain forms in inflammation can promote antitumor immunity [110], and thus it is possible that the conflicting data seen with Th17 cells reflect the differences in inflammatory tumor microenvironment. Most likely, it is the sum total of the ratios of different cytokines and cell types which dictates clinical outcomes. Hence, to be able to categorically define whether certain immune subsets, receptors, chemokines and cytokines are associated with outcomes in different cancer types, there needs to be a uniform approach to assaying tumor immune infiltrates to allow cross comparison of studies. Galon and colleagues have now initiated a taskforce to standardize immunohistochemistry assays used in quantification of immune infiltrates [56]. This quantification allows the establishment of an immune score which can be utilized to predict clinical outcomes in patients where there is no cancer-associated prognostic marker. Remarkably, the use of immune scoring for the classification of colorectal patients for disease free and overall survival has been demonstrated to be superior compared to previous pathological criteria of tumor staging [111,112], underscoring the need for clinical pathologists to consider infiltrating immune cells when determining a patient's prognosis [43].

B. Spontaneous immune responses to cancer

Further data supporting the process of cancer immunosurveillance in humans is the spontaneous recognition of tumors by cells of the adaptive immune system. Even in the early 1970s, screening cancer cell lines with autologous patient serum led to the identification of spontaneous antibody responses to autologous cancers in a subset of patients [113,114]. Spontaneous T-cell responses against autologous tumors have also been reported [115]. These responses, observed in the absence of specific immunotherapy, support the ability of immune system cells to respond spontaneously to antigens on tumors. Antibody responses in patient serum have been reported for over 100 tumor-associated antigens (TAAs), although most reports were isolated and multiple reports were only available for eight antigens, suggesting that for each individual cancer, the immunogenic mutations might be unique (reviewed in [116]). Among these were antibody responses against cancer-testis antigen, NY-ESO-1, the first antigen identified from serum reactivity for an autologous esophageal squamous cell carcinoma [117]. Spontaneous antibody responses specific for NY-ESO-1 have been observed in approximately 8% of patients with liver or breast tumors, and in up to 18% of lung cancer patients. Yet when patients are separated into those whose tumors express NY-ESO-1, frequencies of up to 83% serum responses have been observed [118]. These events are much higher than those found in healthy populations, where serum reactivity to NY-ESO-1 has been found in approximately 0.6% of individuals.

Similarly, quite high spontaneous antibody responses have been reported against p53, mutant forms of which can often be overexpressed in malignancy. Levels vary with tumor types, ranging from 10%—12% for cancers of the lung, breast and liver, up to 30%—40% for esophageal and ovarian cancers. Again, frequencies of antibody responses in healthy individuals to p53 are much less (approximately 2%). Of course, spontaneous responses against self antigens can occur in other circumstances, which can then lead to autoimmunity. For example, antinuclear antibodies are associated with systemic lupus erythmatosis [119], and antibodies reactive with glutamic acid decarboxylase are associated with diabetes [120]. However, the high frequency of antibodies specific for tumor-associated antigens in cancer patients compared to healthy individuals suggests that immunity has been induced in response to malignancy.

Some of the strongest evidence supporting the elimination phase of cancer immunoediting in humans rests with the phenomenon of spontaneously regressing melanoma lesions accompanied by the clonal expansion of T cells [115,121,122]. The observation that such response could occur in the absence of specific immunotherapy supports the ability of the immune system to spontaneously recognize antigens on/in tumors. In addition, it has been reported that specific CD4$^+$ and CD8$^+$ T-cell activity can occur spontaneously against TAAs, including NY-ESO-1 [123,124]. While it is rare for spontaneous T-cell responses specific for some TAAs to develop, such as the MAGE family [125], T-cell responses specific for the melanocyte

91

differentiation antigen MART-1/Melan-A have been found in a relatively high percentage (>50%) of healthy individuals [126]. Overall, there exists a strong correlation between spontaneous T-cell responses and some TAAs, but not others. However, it is unclear if the presence of TAA-specific T cells in healthy individuals reflects past exposure to transformed cells expressing the antigen. Future work is required to isolate TAAs and TSAs in a range of tumors to determine the relative abundance and uniqueness of tumor antigens.

Spontaneous immune responses against malignant cells have also been demonstrated in patients with paraneoplastic autoimmune disorders (PND). These rare disorders that cause neurologic symptoms arise due to high titers of antibodies cross reacting with neuronal antigens that are also expressed on tumor cells [127]. In addition, tumor-specific T cells have also been identified in patients with PND [128]. Despite the presence of humoral and cellular immunity to TAA, nearly all patients with PND succumb to disease, with about half dying from cancer and the rest from neurologic disease. However, the few surviving patients undergo complete tumor remission in response to therapy and no longer display any neurological impairment. These striking clinical cases illustrate that tumor antigens are the drivers of both beneficial immune responses against neoplastic tissues and pathological immune responses against normal tissues (i.e., neurons). Notably, the symptoms of PND can precede tumor diagnosis by several years [129], suggesting that antitumor responses might be primed by undetectable, microscopic tumors early in their development. Yet to be determined is whether the antitumor immune response substantially delays tumor growth in PND patients, and such analysis may be confounded by the lethality of the neurologic complications. Regardless, antineuronal antibodies have been reported to correlate with improved prognosis for some neurological malignancies [130], and there exist case reports of spontaneous complete remission in the absence of specific treatment [131].

More potential evidence, though controversial, can be found in spontaneous regression of cancer in patients. Although rare, estimated at 1 in 80,000 [132], complete regression of tumors has been observed [133]. These observations were made using compiled data prior to 1960 on patients in the absence of therapy or following noncurative measures. There are a number of possible reasons for spontaneous regressions including surgical disruption of tumor vasculature, unusual sensitivity to inadequate treatment or acute infection, but an immune contribution, or what used to be referred to as an "allergic reaction," remains a possible cause for some regressions. It is more difficult to interpret more recent unexpected regressions of tumors since most patients receive intensive therapy. Nevertheless, there are recent isolated reports of spontaneous regression of tumors in patients refusing treatment. In the case study of a 71 year old patient with non small cell lung cancer (NSCLC), spontaneous regression was intriguingly associated with a high titer of antibodies specific for NY-ESO-1 [134]. However, the low rate of spontaneous rejections suggests that either the immune response is absent or the tumor has evolved to escape the immune response in the majority of cases.

C. Other indicators of immune surveillance

While the above observations present strong evidence for immune surveillance of cancer in humans, it is interesting to consider other intriguing observations that may support a role for immunity in tumor control. For example, approximately 5–10% of malignant disease can be classified as of unknown primary [135]. In a proportion of these cases metastases of known histology are found in distant organs in the absence of a primary tumor, suggesting that the primary tumor had regressed spontaneously. Of course, there are many factors that may contribute to regression of individual tumors, but it is interesting to consider a potential contribution from immunity eliminating the primary, while metastases, perhaps after evolving to escape immune attention, continued to progress. Interestingly, improved prognosis of patients with advanced melanoma has been observed for those in whom a primary tumor site could not be identified [136].

Further evidence for immune surveillance can be derived from the range of immune inhibitory measures taken by tumors. After all, why should tumors express such specific molecules unless there is some selection advantage in doing so? Spontaneous immune interaction with tumors can be inferred from associations of poorer prognosis with expression of immune inhibitory molecules within tumor tissue. For example, programmed death-1 ligand can suppress T-cell immunity, and its presence in tumors has been shown to be associated with poorer outcome in several tumor types [137,138]. Similarly, the presence of the immune suppressive enzyme, indoleamine 2,3-deoxygenase, correlates with disease progression in some cancers [139,140]. Tumors can also inhibit innate immune cells including NK cells and γ/δ T cells through the production of soluble MICA/B that can inhibit the activity of the activation receptor NKG2D expressed on these innate immune cell types (Chapter 9) [141−143]. This suggests that tumors can be subject to scrutiny by innate immunity, and it is to the advantage of tumors to employ means of avoiding this process.

D. Summary of human cancer immunoediting

In summary, there is considerable support for the process of immunosurveillance in humans despite the difficulties associated with working with a genetically and immunologically diverse population. In addition to the discussion above, other evidence that supports the existence of cancer immunoediting comes from observations that severely immunodeficient humans such as those who have acquired immunodeficiencies (AIDs), or those on immunosuppressive drugs following organ transplantation have an increased frequency of malignancies. These studies are not discussed here as they have recently been reviewed [15]. The reasons why spontaneous immune responses occur in only a proportion of individuals are not clear, and the complexity of immune interactions make a definitive answer to this question difficult. However, possible reasons included the genetic driver mutations specific to that tumor, the differences in antigenicity and antigen processing in different individuals, and the polymorphisms in the immune repertoire of the host. Tumors also vary with respect to their capacity to inhibit immunity in various individuals. Future advances in gene expression and proteomics of tumors and increasing knowledge of tumor antigens will provide greater insight into immunosurveillance in humans, and may be useful in determining which patients may benefit from particular treatments.

93

ACKNOWLEDGMENTS

The authors wish to thank members of the Smyth and Schreiber laboratories for their collaboration and discussion. This work was supported by the National Health and Medical Research Council of Australia (NH&MRC) Program Grant (454569), and The Association for International Cancer Research. MWLT was supported by a NH&MRC CDF1 award. MJS (Australia) and MHK (SRF) received fellowship support from the NH&MRC.

References

[1] Hanahan D, Weinberg RA. The hallmarks of cancer. Cell 2000 Jan 7;100(1):57−70.

[2] Hanahan D, Weinberg Robert A. Hallmarks of Cancer: The Next Generation Cell 2011;144(5):646−74.

[3] Dunn GP, Bruce AT, Ikeda H, Old LJ, Schreiber RD. Cancer immunoediting: from immunosurveillance to tumor escape. Nat Immunol 2002 Nov;3(11):991−8.

[4] Dighe AS, Richards E, Old LJ, Schreiber RD. Enhanced in vivo growth and resistance to rejection of tumor cells expressing dominant negative IFN gamma receptors. Immunity 1994 Sep;1(6):447−56.

[5] Kaplan DH, Shankaran V, Dighe AS, Stockert E, Aguet M, Old LJ, et al. Demonstration of an interferon gamma-dependent tumor surveillance system in immunocompetent mice. Proc Natl Acad Sci U S A 1998 Jun 23;95(13):7556−61.

[6] Shankaran V. IFNγ and lymphocytes prevent primary tumour development and shape tumour immunogenicity. Nature 2001;410:1107−11.

[7] Smyth MJ, Thia KY, Street SE, MacGregor D, Godfrey DI, Trapani JA. Perforin-mediated cytotoxicity is critical for surveillance of spontaneous lymphoma. J Exp Med 2000 Sep 4;192(5):755–60.

[8] Bolitho P, Street SE, Westwood JA, Edelmann W, Macgregor D, Waring P, et al. Perforin-mediated suppression of B-cell lymphoma. Proc Natl Acad Sci U S A 2009 Feb 24;106(8):2723–8.

[9] Takeda K, Smyth MJ, Cretney E, Hayakawa Y, Kayagaki N, Yagita H, et al. Critical role for tumor necrosis factor-related apoptosis-inducing ligand in immune surveillance against tumor development. J Exp Med 2002 Jan 21;195(2):161–9.

[10] Takeda K, Hayakawa Y, Smyth MJ, Kayagaki N, Yamaguchi N, Kakuta S, et al. Involvement of tumor necrosis factor-related apoptosis-inducing ligand in surveillance of tumor metastasis by liver natural killer cells. Nat Med 2001 Jan;7(1):94–100.

[11] Smyth MJ, Cretney E, Takeda K, Wiltrout RH, Sedger LM, Kayagaki N, et al. Tumor necrosis factor-related apoptosis-inducing ligand (TRAIL) contributes to interferon gamma-dependent natural killer cell protection from tumor metastasis. J Exp Med 2001 Mar 19;193(6):661–70.

[12] Cretney E, Takeda K, Yagita H, Glaccum M, Peschon JJ, Smyth MJ. Increased susceptibility to tumor initiation and metastasis in TNF-related apoptosis-inducing ligand-deficient mice. J Immunol 2002 Feb 1;168(3):1356–61.

[13] Dunn GP, Old LJ, Schreiber RD. The three Es of cancer immunoediting. Annu Rev Immunol 2004;22:329–60.

[14] Dunn GP, Old LJ, Schreiber RD. The immunobiology of cancer immunosurveillance and immunoediting. Immunity 2004 Aug;21(2):137–48.

[15] Vesely MD, Kershaw MH, Schreiber RD, Smyth MJ. Natural innate and adaptive immunity to cancer. Annu Rev Immunol 2011 Apr 23;29:235–71.

[16] Schreiber RD, Old LJ, Smyth MJ. Cancer immunoediting: integrating immunity's roles in cancer suppression and promotion. Science 2011 Mar 25;331(6024):1565–70.

[17] Swann JB, Smyth MJ. Immune surveillance of tumors. J Clin Invest 2007 May;117(5):1137–46.

[18] Koebel CM, Vermi W, Swann JB, Zerafa N, Rodig SJ, Old LJ, et al. Adaptive immunity maintains occult cancer in an equilibrium state. Nature 2007 Dec 6;450(7171):903–7.

[19] Eyles J, Puaux AL, Wang X, Toh B, Prakash C, Hong M, et al. Tumor cells disseminate early, but immuno-surveillance limits metastatic outgrowth, in a mouse model of melanoma. J Clin Invest 2010 Jun;120(6):2030–9.

[20] Loeser S, Loser K, Bijker MS, Rangachari M, van der Burg SH, Wada T, et al. Spontaneous tumor rejection by cbl-b-deficient CD8+ T cells. J Exp Med 2007 Apr 16;204(4):879–91.

[21] Teng MW, Swann JB, Koebel CM, Schreiber RD, Smyth MJ. Immune-mediated dormancy: an equilibrium with cancer. J Leukoc Biol 2008 Oct;84(4):988–93.

[22] Mellman I, Coukos G, Dranoff G. Cancer immunotherapy comes of age. Nature 2011 Dec 22;480(7378):480–9.

[23] Ogino S, Galon J, Fuchs CS, Dranoff G. Cancer immunology—analysis of host and tumor factors for personalized medicine. Nat Rev Clin Oncol 2011;8(12):711–9.

[24] Sharma P, Wagner K, Wolchok JD, Allison JP. Novel cancer immunotherapy agents with survival benefit: recent successes and next steps. Nat Rev Cancer 2011 Nov;11(11):805–12.

[25] Quezada SA, Peggs KS, Simpson TR, Allison JP. Shifting the equilibrium in cancer immunoediting: from tumor tolerance to eradication. Immunol Rev 2011 May;241(1):104–18.

[26] Smyth MJ, Thia KY, Street SE, Cretney E, Trapani JA, Taniguchi M, et al. Differential tumor surveillance by natural killer (NK) and NKT cells. J Exp Med 2000 Feb 21;191(4):661–8.

[27] Street SE, Trapani JA, MacGregor D, Smyth MJ. Suppression of lymphoma and epithelial malignancies effected by interferon gamma. J Exp Med 2002 Jul 1;196(1):129–34.

[28] Swann JB, Uldrich AP, van Dommelen S, Sharkey J, Murray WK, Godfrey DI, et al. Type I natural killer T cells suppress tumors caused by p53 loss in mice. Blood 2009 Jun 18;113(25):6382–5.

[29] Dunn GP, Bruce AT, Sheehan KC, Shankaran V, Uppaluri R, Bui JD, et al. A critical function for type I interferons in cancer immunoediting. Nat Immunol 2005 Jul;6(7):722–9.

[30] Swann JB, Vesely MD, Silva A, Sharkey J, Akira S, Schreiber RD, et al. Demonstration of inflammation-induced cancer and cancer immunoediting during primary tumorigenesis. Proc Natl Acad Sci U S A 2008 Jan 15;105(2):652–6.

[31] Dranoff G. Experimental mouse tumour models: what can be learnt about human cancer immunology? Nat Rev Immunol 2012 Jan;12(1):61–6.

[32] Cheon DJ, Orsulic S. Mouse models of cancer. Annu Rev Pathol 2011;6:95–119.

[33] Matsushita H, Vesely MD, Koboldt DC, Rickert CG, Uppaluri R, Magrini VJ, et al. Cancer exome analysis reveals a T-cell-dependent mechanism of cancer immunoediting. Nature 2012 Feb 16;482(7385):400–4.

[34] DuPage M, Mazumdar C, Schmidt LM, Cheung AF, Jacks T. Expression of tumour-specific antigens underlies cancer immunoediting. Nature 2012 Feb 16;482(7385):405−9.

[35] Zerafa N, Westwood JA, Cretney E, Mitchell S, Waring P, Iezzi M, et al. Cutting edge: TRAIL deficiency accelerates hematological malignancies. J Immunol 2005 Nov 1;175(9):5586−90.

[36] Street SE, Zerafa N, Iezzi M, Westwood JA, Stagg J, Musiani P, et al. Host perforin reduces tumor number but does not increase survival in oncogene-driven mammary adenocarcinoma. Cancer Res 2007 Jun 1;67(11):5454−60.

[37] Finnberg N, Klein-Szanto AJ, El-Deiry WS. TRAIL-R deficiency in mice promotes susceptibility to chronic inflammation and tumorigenesis. J Clin Invest 2008 Jan;118(1):111−23.

[38] Ciampricotti M, Hau C-S, Doornebal CW, Jonkers J, de Visser KE. Chemotherapy response of spontaneous mammary tumors is independent of the adaptive immune system. Nat Med 2012;18(3):344−6.

[39] Teng MW, Ngiow SF, von Scheidt B, McLaughlin N, Sparwasser T, Smyth MJ. Conditional regulatory T-cell depletion releases adaptive immunity preventing carcinogenesis and suppressing established tumor growth. Cancer Res 2010 Oct 15;70(20):7800−9.

[40] Zitvogel L, Tesniere A, Kroemer G. Cancer despite immunosurveillance: immunoselection and immuno-subversion. Nat Rev Immunol 2006;6:715−27.

[41] Smyth MJ, Dunn GP, Schreiber RD. Cancer immunosurveillance and immunoediting: the roles of immunity in suppressing tumor development and shaping tumor immunogenicity. Adv Immunol 2006;90:1−50.

[42] Khong HT, Restifo NP. Natural selection of tumor variants in the generation of "tumor escape" phenotypes. Nat Immunol 2002 Nov;3(11):999−1005.

[43] Fridman WH, Pages F, Sautes-Fridman C, Galon J. The immune contexture in human tumours: impact on clinical outcome. Nat Rev Cancer 2012 Mar 15.

[44] Galon J, Costes A, Sanchez-Cabo F, Kirilovsky A, Mlecnik B, Lagorce-Pages C, et al. Type, density, and location of immune cells within human colorectal tumors predict clinical outcome. Science 2006 Sep 29;313(5795):1960−4.

[45] Pages F. Effector memory T cells, early metastasis, and survival in colorectal cancer. N Engl J Med 2005;353:2654−66.

[46] Pages F. In situ cytotoxic and memory T cells predict outcome in patients with early-stage colorectal cancer. J Clin Oncol 2009;27:5944−51.

[47] Taylor RC, Patel A, Panageas KS, Busam KJ, Brady MS. Tumor-infiltrating lymphocytes predict sentinel lymph node positivity in patients with cutaneous melanoma. J Clin Oncol 2007 Mar 1;25(7):869−75.

[48] Badoual C. Prognostic value of tumor-infiltrating CD4+ T-cell subpopulations in head and neck cancers. Clin Cancer Res 2006;12:465−72.

[49] Sharma P, Shen Y, Wen S, Yamada S, Jungbluth AA, Gnjatic S. CD8 tumor-infiltrating lymphocytes are predictive of survival in muscle-invasive urothelial carcinoma. Proc Natl Acad Sci U S A 2007;104:3967−72.

[50] Menegaz RA, Michelin MA, Etchebehere RM, Fernandes PC, Murta EF. Peri- and intratumoral T and B lymphocytic infiltration in breast cancer. Eur J Gynaecol Oncol 2008;29:321−6.

[51] Shah W, Yan X, Jing L, Zhou Y, Chen H, Wang Y. A reversed CD4/CD8 ratio of tumor-infiltrating lymphocytes and a high percentage of CD4(+)FOXP3(+) regulatory T cells are significantly associated with clinical outcome in squamous cell carcinoma of the cervix. Cell Mol Immunol 2011 Jan;8(1):59−66.

[52] Sato E, Olson SH, Ahn J, Bundy B, Nishikawa H, Qian F. Intraepithelial CD8+ tumor-infiltrating lymphocytes and a high CD8+/regulatory T cell ratio are associated with favorable prognosis in ovarian cancer. Proc Natl Acad Sci U S A 2005;102:18538−43.

[53] Cho Y, Miyamoto M, Kato K, Fukunaga A, Shichinohe T, Kawarada Y. CD4+ and CD8+ T cells cooperate to improve prognosis of patients with esophageal squamous cell carcinoma. Cancer Res 2003;63:1555−9.

[54] Richardsen E, Uglehus RD, Due J, Busch C, Busund LT. The prognostic impact of M-CSF, CSF-1 receptor, CD68 and CD3 in prostatic carcinoma. Histopathology 2008;53:30−8.

[55] Karja V, Aaltomaa S, Lipponen P, Isotalo T, Talja M, Mokka R. Tumour-infiltrating lymphocytes: a prognostic factor of PSA-free survival in patients with local prostate carcinoma treated by radical prostatectomy. Anticancer Res 2005;25:4435−8.

[56] Galon J, Pages F, Marincola FM, Thurin M, Trinchieri G, Fox BA, et al. The immune score as a new possible approach for the classification of cancer. J Transl Med 2012;10:1.

[57] Teng MW, Ritchie DS, Neeson P, Smyth MJ. Biology and clinical observations of regulatory T cells in cancer immunology. Curr Top Microbiol Immunol 2011;344:61−95.

[58] Wang J, Ioan-Facsinay A, van der Voort EI, Huizinga TW, Toes RE. Transient expression of FOXP3 in human activated nonregulatory CD4+ T cells. Eur J Immunol 2007 Jan;37(1):129−38.

[59] Naji A, Le Rond S, Durrbach A, Krawice-Radanne I, Creput C, Daouya M, et al. CD3+CD4low and CD3+CD8low are induced by HLA-G: novel human peripheral blood suppressor T-cell subsets involved in transplant acceptance. Blood 2007 Dec 1;110(12):3936−48.

[60] Elrefaei M, Burke CM, Baker CA, Jones NG, Bousheri S, Bangsberg DR, et al. TGF-beta and IL-10 production by HIV-specific CD8+ T cells is regulated by CTLA-4 signaling on CD4+ T cells. PLoS ONE 2009; 4(12):e8194.

[61] Kiniwa Y, Miyahara Y, Wang HY, Peng W, Peng G, Wheeler TM, et al. CD8+ Foxp3+ regulatory T cells mediate immunosuppression in prostate cancer. Clin Cancer Res 2007 Dec 1;13(23):6947—58.

[62] Dinesh RK, Skaggs BJ, La Cava A, Hahn BH, Singh RP. CD8+ Tregs in lupus, autoimmunity, and beyond. Autoimmun Rev 2010 Jun;9(8):560—8.

[63] Curiel TJ, Coukos G, Zou L, Alvarez X, Cheng P, Mottram P, et al. Specific recruitment of regulatory T cells in ovarian carcinoma fosters immune privilege and predicts reduced survival. Nat Med 2004 Sep;10(9):942—9.

[64] Bates GJ. Quantification of regulatory T cells enables the identification of high-risk breast cancer patients and those at risk of late relapse. J Clin Oncol 2006;24:5373—80.

[65] Gobert M. Regulatory T cells recruited through CCL22/CCR4 are selectively activated in lymphoid infiltrates surrounding primary breast tumors and lead to an adverse clinical outcome. Cancer Res 2009;69:2000—9.

[66] Petersen RP. Tumor infiltrating Foxp3+ regulatory T-cells are associated with recurrence in pathologic stage I NSCLC patients. Cancer 2006;107:2866—72.

[67] Shimizu K. Tumor-infiltrating Foxp3+ regulatory T cells are correlated with cyclooxygenase-2 expression and are associated with recurrence in resected non-small cell lung cancer. J Thorac Oncol 2010;5:585—90.

[68] Tao H, Mimura Y, Aoe K, Kobayashi S, Yamamoto H, Matsuda E, et al. Prognostic potential of FOXP3 expression in non-small cell lung cancer cells combined with tumor-infiltrating regulatory T cells. Lung Cancer 2012 Jan;75(1):95—101.

[69] Miracco C, Mourmouras V, Biagioli M, Rubegni P, Mannucci S, Monciatti I, et al. Utility of tumour-infiltrating CD25+FOXP3+ regulatory T cell evaluation in predicting local recurrence in vertical growth phase cutaneous melanoma. Oncol Rep 2007 Nov;18(5):1115—22.

[70] Mougiakakos D, Johansson CC, Trocme E, All-Ericsson C, Economou MA, Larsson O, et al. Intratumoral forkhead box P3-positive regulatory T cells predict poor survival in cyclooxygenase-2-positive uveal melanoma. Cancer 2010 May 1;116(9):2224—33.

[71] Hiraoka K, Miyamoto M, Cho Y, Suzuoki M, Oshikiri T, Nakakubo Y. Concurrent infiltration by CD8+ T cells and CD4+ T cells is a favourable prognostic factor in non-small-cell lung carcinoma. Br J Cancer 2006;94:275—80.

[72] Kobayashi N, Kubota K, Kato S, Watanabe S, Shimamura T, Kirikoshi H, et al. FOXP3+ regulatory T cells and tumoral indoleamine 2,3-dioxygenase expression predicts the carcinogenesis of intraductal papillary mucinous neoplasms of the pancreas. Pancreatology 2010;10(5):631—40.

[73] Fu J, Xu D, Liu Z, Shi M, Zhao P, Fu B. Increased regulatory T cells correlate with CD8 T-cell impairment and poor survival in hepatocellular carcinoma patients. Gastroenterology 2007;132:2328—39.

[74] Gao Q. Intratumoral balance of regulatory and cytotoxic T cells is associated with prognosis of hepatocellular carcinoma after resection. J Clin Oncol 2007;25:2586—93.

[75] Kobayashi N, Hiraoka N, Yamagami W, Ojima H, Kanai Y, Kosuge T, et al. FOXP3+ regulatory T cells affect the development and progression of hepatocarcinogenesis. Clin Cancer Res 2007 Feb 1;13(3):902—11.

[76] Zhou J, Ding T, Pan W, Zhu LY, Li L, Zheng L. Increased intratumoral regulatory T cells are related to intratumoral macrophages and poor prognosis in hepatocellular carcinoma patients. Int J Cancer 2009 Oct 1;125(7):1640—8.

[77] Kim HI, Kim H, Cho HW, Kim SY, Song KJ, Hyung WJ, et al. The ratio of intra-tumoral regulatory T cells (Foxp3+)/helper T cells (CD4+) is a prognostic factor and associated with recurrence pattern in gastric cardia cancer. J Surg Oncol 2011 Dec;104(7):728—33.

[78] Shen Z, Zhou S, Wang Y, Li RL, Zhong C, Liang C, et al. Higher intratumoral infiltrated Foxp3+ Treg numbers and Foxp3+/CD8+ ratio are associated with adverse prognosis in resectable gastric cancer. J Cancer Res Clin Oncol 2010 Oct;136(10):1585—95.

[79] Hillen F. Leukocyte infiltration and tumor cell plasticity are parameters of aggressiveness in primary cutaneous melanoma. Cancer Immunol Immunother 2008;57:97—106.

[80] Ladanyi A. FOXP3+ cell density in primary tumor has no prognostic impact in patients with cutaneous malignant melanoma. Pathol Oncol Res 2010;16:303—9.

[81] Mahmoud SM. An evaluation of the clinical significance of FOXP3+ infiltrating cells in human breast cancer. Breast Cancer Res Treat 2011;127:99—108.

[82] Mizukami Y. Localisation pattern of Foxp3+ regulatory T cells is associated with clinical behaviour in gastric cancer. Br J Cancer 2008;98:148—53.

[83] Zhang YL. Different subsets of tumor infiltrating lymphocytes correlate with NPC progression in different ways. Mol Cancer 2010;9:4.

[84] Winerdal ME. FOXP3 and survival in urinary bladder cancer. BJU Int 2011;108:1672—8.

[85] Tosolini M. Clinical impact of different classes of infiltrating T cytotoxic and helper cells (Th1, th2, treg, th17) in patients with colorectal cancer. Cancer Res 2011;71:1263–71.

[86] Salama P. Tumor-infiltrating FOXP3+ T regulatory cells show strong prognostic significance in colorectal cancer. J Clin Oncol 2009;27:186–92.

[87] Frey DM. High frequency of tumor-infiltrating FOXP3+ regulatory T cells predicts improved survival in mismatch repair-proficient colorectal cancer patients. Int J Cancer 2010;126:2635–43.

[88] Michel S, Benner A, Tariverdian M, Wentzensen N, Hoefler P, Pommerencke T. High density of FOXP3-positive T cells infiltrating colorectal cancers with microsatellite instability. Br J Cancer 2008;99:1867–73.

[89] Wang B, Xu D, Yu X, Ding T, Rao H, Zhan Y, et al. Association of intra-tumoral infiltrating macrophages and regulatory T cells is an independent prognostic factor in gastric cancer after radical resection. Ann Surg Oncol 2011 Sep;18(9):2585–93.

[90] Leffers N, Gooden MJ, de Jong RA, Hoogeboom BN, ten Hoor KA, Hollema H, et al. Prognostic significance of tumor-infiltrating T-lymphocytes in primary and metastatic lesions of advanced stage ovarian cancer. Cancer Immunol Immunother 2009 Mar;58(3):449–59.

[91] Tzankov A, Meier C, Hirschmann P, Went P, Pileri SA, Dirnhofer S. Correlation of high numbers of intra-tumoral FOXP3+ regulatory T cells with improved survival in germinal center-like diffuse large B-cell lymphoma, follicular lymphoma and classical Hodgkin's lymphoma. Haematologica 2008;93:193–200.

[92] DeNardo DG, Andreu P, Coussens LM. Interactions between lymphocytes and myeloid cells regulate pro- versus anti-tumor immunity. Cancer Metastasis Rev 2010 Jun;29(2):309–16.

[93] Grivennikov SI, Greten FR, Karin M. Immunity, inflammation, and cancer. Cell 2010 Mar 19;140(6):883–99.

[94] Qian BZ, Pollard JW. Macrophage diversity enhances tumor progression and metastasis. Cell 2010 Apr 2;141(1):39–51.

[95] Colotta F, Allavena P, Sica A, Garlanda C, Mantovani A. Cancer-related inflammation, the seventh hallmark of cancer: links to genetic instability. Carcinogenesis 2009 Jul;30(7):1073–81.

[96] Maruyama T, Kono K, Mizukami Y, Kawaguchi Y, Mimura K, Watanabe M, et al. Distribution of Th17 cells and FoxP3(+) regulatory T cells in tumor-infiltrating lymphocytes, tumor-draining lymph nodes and peripheral blood lymphocytes in patients with gastric cancer. Cancer Sci 2010 Sep;101(9):1947–54.

[97] Chen X, Wan J, Liu J, Xie W, Diao X, Xu J, et al. Increased IL-17-producing cells correlate with poor survival and lymphangiogenesis in NSCLC patients. Lung Cancer 2010 Sep;69(3):348–54.

[98] Kuang DM, Peng C, Zhao Q, Wu Y, Chen MS, Zheng L. Activated monocytes in peritumoral stroma of hepatocellular carcinoma promote expansion of memory T helper 17 cells. Hepatology 2010 Jan;51(1):154–64.

[99] Kryczek I. Phenotype, distribution, generation, and functional and clinical relevance of Th17 cells in the human tumor environments. Blood 2009;114:1141–9.

[100] Lv L, Pan K, Li X-d, She K-l, Zhao J-j, Wang W, et al. The Accumulation and Prognosis Value of Tumor Infiltrating IL-17 Producing Cells in Esophageal Squamous Cell Carcinoma. PLoS ONE 2011;6(3):e18219.

[101] Chen JG. Intratumoral expression of IL-17 and its prognostic role in gastric adenocarcinoma patients. Int J Biol Sci 2011;7:53–60.

[102] Kusuda T. Relative expression levels of Th1 and Th2 cytokine mRNA are independent prognostic factors in patients with ovarian cancer. Oncol Rep 2005;13:1153–8.

[103] De Monte L. Intratumor T helper type 2 cell infiltrate correlates with cancer-associated fibroblast thymic stromal lymphopoietin production and reduced survival in pancreatic cancer. J Exp Med 2011;208:469–78.

[104] Tassi E. Carcinoembryonic antigen-specific but not antiviral CD4+ T cell immunity is impaired in pancreatic carcinoma patients. J Immunol 2008;181:6595–603.

[105] Ubukata H, Motohashi G, Tabuchi T, Nagata H, Konishi S. Evaluations of interferon-γ/interleukin-4 ratio and neutrophil/lymphocyte ratio as prognostic indicators in gastric cancer patients. J Surg Oncol 2010;102:742–7.

[106] Yoon NK. Higher levels of GATA3 predict better survival in women with breast cancer. Hum Pathol 2010;41:1794–801.

[107] Schreck S. Prognostic impact of tumour-infiltrating Th2 and regulatory T cells in classical Hodgkin lymphoma. Hematol Oncol 2009;27:31–9.

[108] Ladanyi A, Kiss J, Mohos A, Somlai B, Liszkay G, Gilde K, et al. Prognostic impact of B-cell density in cutaneous melanoma. Cancer Immunol Immunother 2011 Dec;60(12):1729–38.

[109] Takatori H, Kanno Y, Watford WT, Tato CM, Weiss G, Ivanov II, et al. Lymphoid tissue inducer-like cells are an innate source of IL-17 and IL-22. J Exp Med 2009 Jan 16;206(1):35–41.

[110] Mantovani A, Sica A. Macrophages, innate immunity and cancer: balance, tolerance, and diversity. Curr Opin Immunol 2010 Apr;22(2):231–7.

[111] Broussard EK, Disis ML. TNM staging in colorectal cancer: T is for T cell and M is for memory. J Clin Oncol 2011;29:601–3.

97

[112] Mlecnik B. Histopathologic-based prognostic factors of colorectal cancers are associated with the state of the local immune reaction. J Clin Oncol 2011;29:610−8.

[113] Carey TE, Takahashi T, Resnick LA, Oettgen HF, Old LJ. Cell surface antigens of human malignant melanoma: mixed hemadsorption assays for humoral immunity to cultured autologous melanoma cells. Proc Natl Acad Sci U S A 1976 Sep;73(9):3278−82.

[114] Ueda R, Shiku H, Pfreundschuh M, Takahashi T, Li LT, Whitmore WF, et al. Cell surface antigens of human renal cancer defined by autologous typing. J Exp Med 1979 Sep 19;150(3):564−79.

[115] Knuth A, Danowski B, Oettgen HF, Old LJ. T-cell-mediated cytotoxicity against autologous malignant melanoma: analysis with interleukin 2-dependent T-cell cultures. Proc Natl Acad Sci U S A 1984 Jun;81(11):3511−5.

[116] Reuschenbach M, von Knebel Doeberitz M, Wentzensen N. A systematic review of humoral immune responses against tumor antigens. Cancer Immunol Immunother 2009 Oct;58(10):1535−44.

[117] Chen YT, Scanlan MJ, Sahin U, Tureci O, Gure AO, Tsang S, et al. A testicular antigen aberrantly expressed in human cancers detected by autologous antibody screening. Proc Natl Acad Sci U S A 1997 Mar 4;94(5):1914−8.

[118] Jager E, Stockert E, Zidianakis Z, Chen YT, Karbach J, Jager D, et al. Humoral immune responses of cancer patients against "Cancer-Testis" antigen NY-ESO-1: correlation with clinical events. Int J Cancer 1999 Oct 22;84(5):506−10.

[119] Rothfield NF, Stollar BD. The relation of immunoglobulin class, pattern of anti-nuclear antibody, and complement-fixing antibodies to DNA in sera from patients with systemic lupus erythematosus. J Clin Invest 1967 Nov;46(11):1785−94.

[120] Myers MA, Rabin DU, Rowley MJ. Pancreatic islet cell cytoplasmic antibody in diabetes is represented by antibodies to islet cell antigen 512 and glutamic acid decarboxylase. Diabetes 1995 Nov;44(11):1290−5.

[121] Ferradini L, Mackensen A, Genevee C, Bosq J, Duvillard P, Avril MF, et al. Analysis of T cell receptor variability in tumor-infiltrating lymphocytes from a human regressive melanoma. Evidence for in situ T cell clonal expansion. J Clin Invest 1993 Mar;91(3):1183−90.

[122] Zorn E, Hercend T. A MAGE-6-encoded peptide is recognized by expanded lymphocytes infiltrating a spontaneously regressing human primary melanoma lesion. Eur J Immunol 1999 Feb;29(2):602−7.

[123] Gnjatic S, Atanackovic D, Jager E, Matsuo M, Selvakumar A, Altorki NK, et al. Survey of naturally occurring CD4+ T cell responses against NY-ESO-1 in cancer patients: correlation with antibody responses. Proc Natl Acad Sci U S A 2003 Jul 22;100(15):8862−7.

[124] Jager E, Nagata Y, Gnjatic S, Wada H, Stockert E, Karbach J, et al. Monitoring CD8 T cell responses to NY-ESO-1: correlation of humoral and cellular immune responses. Proc Natl Acad Sci U S A 2000 Apr 25;97(9):4760−5.

[125] Griffioen M, Borghi M, Schrier PI, Osanto S. Detection and quantification of CD8(+) T cells specific for HLA-A*0201-binding melanoma and viral peptides by the IFN-gamma-ELISPOT assay. Int J Cancer 2001 Aug 15;93(4):549−55.

[126] Pittet MJ, Valmori D, Dunbar PR, Speiser DE, Lienard D, Lejeune F, et al. High frequencies of naive Melan-A/MART-1-specific CD8(+) T cells in a large proportion of human histocompatibility leukocyte antigen (HLA)-A2 individuals. J Exp Med 1999 Sep 6;190(5):705−15.

[127] Albert ML, Darnell RB. Paraneoplastic neurological degenerations: keys to tumour immunity. Nat Rev Cancer 2004 Jan;4(1):36−44.

[128] Albert ML, Darnell JC, Bender A, Francisco LM, Bhardwaj N, Darnell RB. Tumor-specific killer cells in paraneoplastic cerebellar degeneration. Nat Med 1998 Nov;4(11):1321−4.

[129] Mathew RM, Cohen AB, Galetta SL, Alavi A, Dalmau J. Paraneoplastic cerebellar degeneration: Yo-expressing tumor revealed after a 5-year follow-up with FDG-PET. J Neurol Sci 2006 Dec 1;250(1-2):153−5.

[130] Darnell RB, DeAngelis LM. Regression of small-cell lung carcinoma in patients with paraneoplastic neuronal antibodies. Lancet 1993 Jan 2;341(8836):21−2.

[131] Horino T, Takao T, Yamamoto M, Geshi T, Hashimoto K. Spontaneous remission of small cell lung cancer: a case report and review in the literature. Lung Cancer 2006 Aug;53(2):249−52.

[132] Boyers LM. Letter to the Editor. J A M A 1953;152:986.

[133] Cole WH, Everson TC. Spontaneous regression of cancer: preliminary report. Ann Surg 1956 Sep;144(3):366−83.

[134] Nakamura Y, Noguchi Y, Satoh E, Uenaka A, Sato S, Kitazaki T, et al. Spontaneous remission of a non-small cell lung cancer possibly caused by anti-NY-ESO-1 immunity. Lung Cancer 2009 Jul;65(1):119−22.

[135] van de Wouw AJ, Janssen-Heijnen ML, Coebergh JW, Hillen HF. Epidemiology of unknown primary tumours; incidence and population-based survival of 1285 patients in Southeast Netherlands, 1984-1992. Eur J Cancer 2002 Feb;38(3):409−13.

[136] Lee CC, Faries MB, Wanek LA, Morton DL. Improved survival for stage IV melanoma from an unknown primary site. J Clin Oncol 2009 Jul 20;27(21):3489–95.

[137] Gao Q, Wang XY, Qiu SJ, Yamato I, Sho M, Nakajima Y, et al. Overexpression of PD-L1 significantly associates with tumor aggressiveness and postoperative recurrence in human hepatocellular carcinoma. Clin Cancer Res 2009 Feb 1;15(3):971–9.

[138] Ohigashi Y, Sho M, Yamada Y, Tsurui Y, Hamada K, Ikeda N, et al. Clinical significance of programmed death-1 ligand-1 and programmed death-1 ligand-2 expression in human esophageal cancer. Clin Cancer Res 2005 Apr 15;11(8):2947–53.

[139] Brandacher G, Perathoner A, Ladurner R, Schneeberger S, Obrist P, Winkler C, et al. Prognostic value of indoleamine 2,3-dioxygenase expression in colorectal cancer: effect on tumor-infiltrating T cells. Clin Cancer Res 2006 Feb 15;12(4):1144–51.

[140] Schallreuter KU, Tobin DJ, Panske A. Decreased photodamage and low incidence of non-melanoma skin cancer in 136 sun-exposed caucasian patients with vitiligo. Dermatology 2002;204(3):194–201.

[141] Pietra G, Manzini C, Rivara S, Vitale M, Cantoni C, Petretto A, et al. Melanoma cells inhibit natural killer cell function by modulating the expression of activating receptors and cytolytic activity. Cancer Res 2012 Mar 15;72(6):1407–15.

[142] Salih HR, Rammensee HG, Steinle A. Cutting edge: down-regulation of MICA on human tumors by proteolytic shedding. J Immunol 2002 Oct 15;169(8):4098–102.

[143] Marten A, von Lilienfeld-Toal M, Buchler MW, Schmidt J. Soluble MIC is elevated in the serum of patients with pancreatic carcinoma diminishing gammadelta T cell cytotoxicity. Int J Cancer 2006 Nov 15;119(10):2359–65.

CHAPTER 8

Immunosurveillance: Innate and Adaptive Antitumor Immunity

Kenneth F. May, Jr. [1], Masahisa Jinushi[2], Glenn Dranoff[1]
[1]Department of Medical Oncology and Cancer Vaccine Center, Dana-Farber Cancer Institute and Department of Medicine, Brigham and Women's Hospital and Harvard Medical School, Boston, MA USA
[2]Research Center for Infection-Associated Cancer, Institute for Genetic Medicine, Hokkaido University, Sapporo, Japan

I. INTRODUCTION

The immune response to cancer can be broadly divided into innate and adaptive components. The cellular elements of innate immunity include granulocytes, macrophages, mast cells, dendritic cells, and natural killer (NK) cells. Innate immunity serves as a first line of defense against cancer, as germ-line encoded pattern recognition receptors rapidly detect infected or stressed cells, thereby triggering potent effector mechanisms aimed at tumor containment. In contrast, adaptive immunity, composed of B cells secreting antibodies, $CD4^+$ and $CD8^+$ T cells, evolves over the course of several days, reflecting the requirement for activation and expansion of rare tumor-associated antigen-specific lymphocytes harboring somatically rearranged immunoglobulin or T-cell receptors. NKT cells and $\gamma\delta$ T cells function at the interface of innate and adaptive immunity (Figure 8.1).

The interplay of tumor cells and endogenous immunity is increasingly recognized to play a decisive role throughout the multiple stages of carcinogenesis [1]. Clinico-pathologic studies demonstrate that dense intratumoral lymphocyte infiltrates, especially those enriched in cytotoxic $CD8^+$ T cells, are associated with reduced frequencies of disease recurrence and prolonged survival in several types of cancer [2,3,4,5]. Nonetheless, in the setting of unresolved inflammation, tumor cells and stromal elements subvert host immunity to promote disease progression. These divergent outcomes illustrate the complexity of the host–tumor interaction. In this review, we discuss the mechanisms whereby innate and adaptive antitumor immunity mediate these dual roles during tumor development and the ways by which the tumor microenvironment helps sculpt these responses.

II. INNATE ANTITUMOR RESPONSES

Normal cells are endowed with an intricate machinery that protects against genotoxic stress induced by cell intrinsic and extrinsic insults, including DNA replication errors, oxidative damage, microbial infection, and inflammation. The failure of the DNA damage

101

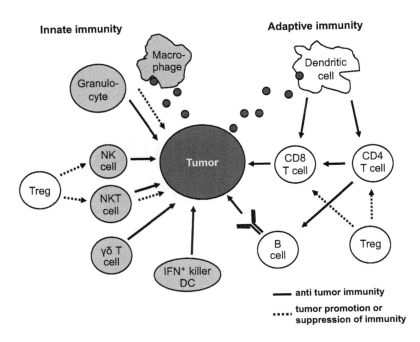

FIGURE 8.1

The complex interplay of innate and adaptive immunity with the tumor determines the intensity and outcome of the endogenous anticancer response. Immune cells mediate both antitumor activity as well as tumor promotion depending on the context. Suppression of antitumor immunity can be mediated directly by the tumor or by certain immune cells such as regulatory T cells. Interactions depicted are greatly simplified, and elements of the innate and adaptive arms of the immune system function as a complex intertwining network.

response to resolve single-stranded or double-stranded DNA breaks poses a significant risk for malignant transformation. In this context, the innate immune system functions as an extrinsic surveillance mechanism for genotoxic injury. NKG2D ligands, which include the MHC class I-related molecules MICA and MICB and six UL16 binding proteins in humans and the retinoic acid-early inducible gene products (RAE) and H60 in rodents, are induced by DNA damage through a pathway involving ATM, ATR, Chk-1, and Chk-2 [6]. The surface expression of these ligands on stressed cells triggers NKG2D-dependent activation of NK, NKT, and $\gamma\delta$ T cells (as well as CD8 T cells), which inhibit tumor growth through cytotoxicity and IFN-γ production (also discussed in Chapter 9). Additionally, the release of cytoplasmic stress-response molecules, such as heat-shock protein 70 (HSP-70), HMGB1 and uric acid, activates macrophages and dendritic cells in part through toll-like receptor (TLR) engagement, resulting in IL-12 production and the transition to adaptive immunity [7].

While these innate responses may contribute to tumor suppression, their aberrant activation may also prove deleterious when normal tissues are perturbed, as during autoimmunity or chronic inflammation. In these settings, the sustained expression of NKG2D ligands leads to downregulation of NKG2D surface expression through increased endocytosis and the consequent suppression of protective responses [8]. Tumor cells and stromal cells in the tumor-microenvironment have been demonstrated to cleave NKG2D ligands from their surface via the isomerase ERp5 and ADAM metalloproteinases, which can further fuel this immune suppression [9,10]. Direct suppression by cytokines such as TGF-β secreted from the stroma may further contribute to suppression. Smoldering inflammation may ensue as well, which may function in tumor promotion. Stress ligand expression may thus either trigger cytotoxic antitumor reactions or facilitate immune escape.

III. INNATE IMMUNE CELLS*

A. NK cells

NK cells are a key participant in innate antitumor responses and employ several effector mechanisms, including perforin, death receptor ligands, and interferon-gamma (IFN-γ) production. NK cells were initially characterized by their ability to lyse MHC class I deficient tumor cells without prior stimulation. In the tumor microenvironment, NK-cell function is regulated through a combination of inhibitory and activating receptors, cytokines such as IL-2 and IL-15, and co-stimulatory molecules including CD80, CD86, CD40, CD70, and ICOS. The NK-cell contribution to tumor defense is highlighted by the increased susceptibility of mice rendered NK-cell deficient, through the administration of antibodies against the membrane proteins NK1.1 or asialo-GM1, to methylcholanthrene-induced tumors [11].

NK cells express several families of inhibitory receptors that deliver negative regulatory signals following engagement with target cell MHC class I molecules. These proteins include the killer cell immunoglobulin-like receptors (KIRs) (primates), the Ly49 lectin-like homodimers (rodents), and the C-type lectin-like molecules (CD94 and NKG2A/E) (primates and rodents). Individual NK cells display varying patterns of inhibitory receptors, yielding an increased ability of the population as a whole to detect losses of individual MHC class I alleles.

NK cells are endowed with several families of activating receptors including the natural cytotoxicity receptors (NKp46, NKp44, NKp30 and NKp80), additional Ly49 proteins, and NKG2D. The natural cytotoxicity receptors have been shown to play a variety of possible roles in tumor cell recognition and killing, and metastasis prevention [12,13]. Interestingly, the activating receptor NKp44 may also have inhibitory properties for tumor immunity depending on which ligand it engages [14]. However, the relative importance of these receptors in overall tumor immunity is not yet clear.

In contrast to the natural cytotoxicity receptors, a major role for the NKG2D pathway in NK-cell tumor recognition has been delineated [15]. NKG2D ligands are frequently expressed in transformed cells as part of the DNA damage response, raising the possibility that NKG2D-triggered responses are a critical link between target cell genotoxic stress and immune-mediated destruction. Illustrating the important role of NKG2D in immunosurveillance, mice deficient in NK2GD develop increased numbers and earlier development of tumors in several spontaneous cancer models [16]. Moreover, chemically induced tumors in wild type mice frequently fail to express NKG2D ligands, underscoring a selective pressure for escape from NKG2D surveillance during chemical carcinogenesis. The administration of blocking antibodies to NKG2D increases the susceptibility of mice to chemically induced tumors, further highlighting the potent NKG2D-dependent mechanism of tumor suppression [17]. These antitumor activities primarily involve perforin, whereas the production of IFN-γ and tumor necrosis factor-related death inducing ligand (TRAIL) are more important for NK-cell tumor suppression in other contexts. Consistent with these findings, chemically induced sarcomas arising in perforin-deficient mice express the NKG2D ligand Rae-1 and are rejected upon transplantation into wild type mice.

Though classically thought to be part of innate immunity, recent studies in animal models provide evidence for the existence of antigen-specific memory-like NK-cell responses to a variety of antigens (viral, haptens) [18,19,20], as well as following cytokine stimulation with IL-12, IL-15, and IL-18 [21]. It is yet unclear whether these NK-cell responses are present in humans, and the role of such responses in tumor immunity await further studies.

103

*Also discussed in Chapter 2.

B. NKT cells

NKT cells express an invariant T-cell receptor alpha chain (Vα14-Jα18 in mice and Vα24-Jα18 in humans) and particular NK-cell markers such as CD161 or NKR-P1 [22]. The invariant T-cell receptors are specific for glycolipid antigens presented by CD1d, an MHC class I-related molecule expressed on antigen-presenting cells and some cancers. A role for NKT cells in tumor suppression was revealed by the increased susceptibility of Jα18 deficient mice, which lack invariant NKT cells, to chemically induced tumors and experimentally induced metastases [23]. Correspondingly, the administration of α-galactosylceramide (α-GalCer), a natural lipid isolated from marine sponges that activates NKT cells through efficient CD1d binding, augments antitumor immunity in multiple model systems. NKT-cell-mediated tumor destruction involves IFN-γ production, which contributes to NK and CD8$^+$ T-cell activation, and cytotoxicity. NKT cells are also required for the therapeutic effects of GM-CSF and IL-12-based cytokine strategies [24,25].

NKT cells produce both Th1 and Th2 cytokines, depending on their mode of activation, underscoring key regulatory roles for the cytokine milieu and glycolipid antigen repertoire present in the tumor microenvironment. Indeed, NKT cells can undermine tumor rejection in some tumor models through a mechanism that involves TGF-β production by Gr-1$^+$ myeloid suppressor cells [26]. CD4$^-$ NKT cells effectuate tumor rejection in the MCA-induced fibrosarcoma and B16F10 melanoma models, whereas CD4$^+$ NKT cells contribute to the pathogenesis of inflammatory diseases such as asthma by the secretion of IL-4, IL-5, and IL-13 [27,28]. NKT cells likely play a role in the immunosurveillance of human cancer as well, with NKT cell defects both in cell number and function being observed in a variety of solid tumor and hematologic settings. However, inconsistent characterization of NKT-cell subsets and heterogeneity of patient populations studied makes a generalized conclusion of the NKT cell role in human cancer challenging [29]. A deeper understanding of the factors determining the induction of NKT-cell subsets during tumor development is an important goal of further investigation.

C. γδ T cells*

γδ cells are a small population of T lymphocytes that integrate features of innate and adaptive immunity. While these cells undergo VDJ recombination during thymic development, their TCR diversity is relatively limited compared to conventional αβ T cells, and they function more in pattern recognition [30]. γδ T cells constitute a significant proportion of intraepithelial lymphocytes (IEL) in the skin and gastrointestinal and genitourinary tract mucosa. Their importance for tumor surveillance has been increasingly recognized, particularly in their ability to recognize unique ligands expressed by tumors that are not recognized by αβ T cells [31]. One example is the increased incidence of chemically induced fibrosarcomas and spindle cell carcinomas in γδ T-cell deficient mice [32]. Vδ1 T cells are enriched in various tumors, where they may be activated through TCR signaling evoked by CD1-presented lipid antigens or NKG2D signaling triggered by MIC or ULBPs. Vδ2 T cells recognize phosphoantigens that can be expressed by tumors. Interestingly, these phosphoantigens are upregulated in tumor cells by bisphosphonate administration, a standard therapy for clinical management of bone metastases, which can enhance killing by Vδ2 T cells [33,34]. γδ T cells serve as a major early source of IFN-γ during disease development and also mediate direct antitumor cytotoxicity. Additionally, these cells might function in antigen presentation, as activated Vγ2δ2 T cells have been shown to prime conventional αβ T cells against soluble antigens following migration to regional lymph nodes [35]. Another subset of IL-17-secreting γδ T cells (Vδ4/Vδ6) demonstrated early trafficking to tumors following chemotherapy administration, and were essential for the recruitment and therapeutic efficacy of traditional cytotoxic T cells in several

---

*Also see Chapter 4

different mouse tumor models [36]. Collectively, these studies illustrate how γδ T cells may serve as first-line defense against a variety of tumors.

D. MACROPHAGES

Macrophages are a prominent component of the cellular response to tumors, where they mediate diverse functions. The release of stress-induced molecules such as HSP-70 or HMGB1 from necrotic tumor cells may trigger TLR-dependent macrophage activation, resulting in the production of cytotoxic reactive oxygen and nitrogen species and the secretion of inflammatory cytokines. Indeed, a spontaneous mutation that developed in SR/CR mice, which manifest a natural resistance to tumor growth, results in striking macrophage activation and cytotoxicity towards multiple tumor cell lines [37]. Macrophages may further contribute to tumor protection by stimulating antitumor T cells while suppressing $CD4^+CD25^+$ regulatory T cells (Tregs) through IL-6 release.

In contrast to these beneficial activities, tumor-associated macrophages also play major roles in promoting tumor progression (discussed in more detail in Chapters 27–28). In the context of unresolved inflammation, tumor cells exploit macrophage activities that are critical for wound healing, including the secretion of angiogeneic molecules, growth factors, and matrix metalloproteinases [38]. Together, these products foster the breakdown of basement membranes and the establishment of a robust vascular network, thereby driving tumor cell invasion, expansion, and metastasis. The key factors that determine whether macrophages mediate tumor protection or promotion remain to be elucidated.

E. GRANULOCYTES

Granulocytes also have complex interactions with tumors. In one role, granulocytes may contribute to tumor destruction through the release of toxic moieties packaged in granules, the generation of reactive oxygen species, and inflammatory cytokine secretion. Experimental tumors engineered to secrete granulocyte-colony stimulating factor were rejected through a pathway requiring neutrophils; moreover, this reaction stimulated the generation of adaptive T-cell responses that mediated eradication of subsequent tumor challenges [39]. Neutrophils were similarly required for the antitumor effects of Her-2/neu-based DNA vaccinations in a transgenic breast cancer model [40]. Alternatively, neutrophils may also enhance tumor progression by secretion of metalloproteinases that promote angiogenesis and tumor cell dissemination [41] or by secretion of elastases that promote tumor cell growth [42]. The specific roles of granulocytes in antitumor immunity versus tumor promotion through tissue remodeling and angiogenesis stimulation remain to be explored.

F. IFN-PRODUCING KILLER DENDRITIC CELLS

IFN-producing killer dendritic cells (IKDC) are a newer subset of dendritic cells that express some NK-cell markers, produce type I interferons, and are cytotoxic [43,44]. The phenotype of these cells is distinct from NK cells and plasmacytoid dendritic cells. IKDCs may be activated with NKG2D ligands and lyse tumor targets through TRAIL, but following migration to draining lymph nodes these cells display antigen-presenting cell features, such as upregulation of MHC and co-stimulatory molecules, and stimulation of T-cell responses. Additional studies are required to clarify the role of IKDC in endogenous and therapeutic tumor immunity and their precise developmental origins.

IV. ADAPTIVE ANTITUMOR RESPONSES

The adaptive antitumor response is typically initiated by dendritic cells, which capture dying tumor cells, process the antigenic cargo for MHC class I and II presentation, migrate to draining lymph nodes, and stimulate antigen-specific T and B lymphocytes. In the tumor microenvironment, dendritic cells may be activated by "danger" signals released from stressed or necrotic tumor cells, thereby triggering a maturation program that includes expression of multiple co-stimulatory molecules and cytokines that result in effector T-cell responses [45]. Alternatively, the production of immunosuppressive cytokines such as TGF-β, IL-10, and VEGF in the microenvironment may inhibit dendritic cell function, instead yielding decreased T-cell effector responses and augmented regulatory T-cell function [46].

Productive antitumor CD4[+] T-cell responses promote potent and long-lasting CD8[+] T-cell responses and contribute to further dendritic cell maturation [47]. CD4[+] T cell CD40 ligand expression may trigger CD40 signaling on dendritic cells, resulting in enhanced IL-12 production and the differentiation of IFN-γ secreting Th1 cells and cytotoxic T lymphocytes. CD4[+] T cells also stimulate B-cell production of antitumor antibodies. These antibodies can have a variety of functions including blocking growth or survival pathways dependent on cell surface receptors, such as Her2/Neu. Antibodies may also target innate immune components to the tumor microenvironment, where specific cytolytic mechanisms may be unleashed, such as complement fixation and antibody-dependent cellular cytotoxicity. Antibodies might also opsonize tumor cells for dendritic cell Fc receptor mediated cross-presentation of tumor antigens, leading to the induction of additional CD4[+] and CD8[+] T-cell responses [48]. Differences in the affinities of IgG subclasses to bind the array of activating and inhibitory Fcγ receptors expressed on dendritic cells influences the balance of effector versus tolerizing function [49]. These findings should advance the development of therapeutic monoclonal antibodies and provide a framework for clarifying the roles of endogenously produced antitumor antibodies.

V. ADAPTIVE IMMUNITY IN IMMUNOSURVEILLANCE

The importance of adaptive immunity for tumor immunosurveillance was first established through studies of mice harboring targeted mutations of the recombinase activating gene-2 (RAG-2), which lack all B lymphocytes, αβ and γδ T cells, and NKT cells [50]. These mice manifested an increased susceptibility to chemically induced tumors, and the fibrosarcomas arising in these animals were frequently rejected upon transplant to wild type animals. Subsequent studies of mice deficient in αβ or γδ T cells alone revealed a similar enhanced susceptibility to chemical carcinogens, highlighting the key roles of T lymphocytes in tumor protection. Consistent with these findings, the development of intra-tumoral T cell infiltrates in multiple cancers is correlated with the absence of early metastasis and prolonged disease-free survival. The adaptive immune system, however, may also promote carcinogenesis within the background of chronic inflammation. In transgenic models of hepatitis B-induced liver cancer, smoldering CD4[+] and CD8[+] T-cell responses are required for progression of hepatocellular carcinoma [51]. Similarly, CD4[+] T cells activated by normal cutaneous bacterial flora promote the evolution of squamous cell carcinoma in a human papilloma virus transgenic model [52].

FoxP3 expressing Tregs may play an important role in modulating the dual roles of adaptive immunity in tumor protection and promotion [53]. Substantial evidence in multiple tumor models indicates that Tregs present a major impediment to cytotoxic T-cell mediated tumor rejection, particularly in the context of therapy-induced responses (discussed in more detail in Chapter 31). Indeed, the presence of FoxP3 expressing Tregs in ovarian cancer patients is tightly linked to inferior clinical outcomes [54]. On the other hand, Tregs function to maintain immune homeostasis, and their disruption leads to severe autoimmune disease and chronic inflammation. These functions may underlie the striking ability of Tregs to effectuate tumor destruction in murine models of inflammation-induced cancer [55]. Moreover, the presence of Tregs in the cellular infiltrates of Hodgkin's lymphomas has been linked to improved survival, perhaps reflecting a dependence of Reed-Sternberg cells on particular components of the host response.

B lymphocytes similarly play dual roles in tumor immunosurveillance. While antibodies may promote tumor destruction through the mechanisms discussed earlier, in the HPV transgenic model of cutaneous squamous cell carcinoma, antibodies were required for disease development [56]. In this setting, antibodies promoted the recruitment of innate immune cells to the tumor microenvironment, where persistent inflammation promoted carcinogenesis. Additional investigations are required to delineate what factors determine whether adaptive immune responses will inhibit or accelerate tumor development.

VI. TARGETS OF ANTITUMOR T-CELL RESPONSES

The principal mechanism involved in the priming of antitumor T cells appears to be cross-presentation of tumor-associated antigens by professional antigen-presenting cells, particularly dendritic cells. This pathway allows processing of exogenously acquired tumor antigens into the MHC class I pathway, whereas proteins captured through endocytosis or autophagy are typically processed for MHC class II-restricted presentation. Tumor-associated antigens can be broadly divided into several categories, including cancer/testis antigens, which show restricted expression in adult germ cells but frequent upregulation in cancers, mutated proteins, differentiation antigens, and pathogen-encoded sequences, such as Epstein-Barr virus in some B-cell lymphomas [57]. However, most of the gene products that stimulate endogenous responses in tumor-bearing hosts are nonmutated and expressed in some normal tissues. In these cases, the tumor-reactive T cells are of low affinity, as thymic deletion has purged the repertoire of high affinity T cells with potential autoreactivity. Overexpressed self-antigens may also stimulate $CD4^+CD25^+$ regulatory T cells, such as the heat shock protein J-like 2 and the cancer/testis antigen LAGE-1 [58,59]. Together, these mechanisms result in intrinsic and extrinsic modes of T cell-tolerance, which limit the overall potency of the antitumor T-cell response. A high priority for further investigation is the identification of recurrent mutations or novel epitopes arising from protein splicing, which could be incorporated into therapeutic strategies to augment antitumor T-cell responses.

VII. ANTITUMOR EFFECTOR MECHANISMS: CYTOKINES*
A. Interferons

IFN-γ classically plays a key role in tumor suppression [60]. NK, NKT and $\gamma\delta$ T cells are major sources of IFN-γ early during tumor development, whereas $CD4^+$ and $CD8^+$ T cells may become additional sources as adaptive immunity evolves. IFN-γ contributes to tumor protection in multiple ways, including inhibition of angiogenesis, the induction of phagocyte cytotoxicity, and the stimulation of dendritic cell IL-12 production, which in turn promote Th1 and cytotoxic T-cell responses. Mice with targeted mutations of IFN-γ or downstream signaling components established a major role for this cytokine in protection from chemically induced and spontaneous tumors. Moreover, IFN-γ functions as a master regulator of tumor cell immunogenicity. Whereas methycholanthrene-induced tumors that arose in RAG-2 deficient mice were efficiently rejected upon transplantation into wild type mice, tumors that developed in mice doubly deficient for RAG-2 and the IFN-γ receptor manifested robust growth after transplant into wild type mice. The immunogenicity of these tumors was enhanced through the restoration of MHC class I presentation, identifying $CD8^+$ T cells as a major component of IFN-γ-stimulated tumor suppression.

More recently, IFN-γ has been implicated in playing a role in the promotion of carcinogenesis. In a neonatal mouse model of melanomagenesis, irradiation of neonatal skin with ultraviolet-B induced a pro-melanoma inflammatory cascade during remodeling that only occurred in the presence of IFN-γ. The proposed mechanism involves the release of

107

* Discussed in detail in Chapter 4

chemokines from damaged skin which attracts IFN-γ-secreting macrophages, that in turn activate melanocytes [61]. In the same study, human melanoma specimens were also demonstrated to contain significant numbers of IFN-γ-secreting macrophages.

A requirement for type I interferons (IFN-α/β) in tumor suppression has also been defined [62]. Mice with targeted mutations of the type I interferon receptors or wild type animals administered neutralizing antibodies to type I interferons manifested enhanced susceptibility to chemical carcinogenesis and tumor transplantation. Protection in these systems involved host immunity and p53 tumor suppressor function in cancer cells [63]. Indeed, impaired interferon signaling and subsequent activation has been demonstrated in peripheral blood lymphocytes from cancer patients [64]. Clinically, exogenous IFN-α administration has shown benefit (albeit with significant side effects) in several types of cancers, including hematologic malignancies and melanoma. Thus, IFN-γ and IFN-α/β mediate critical though distinct functions in tumor immunosurveillance.

B. IL-2, IL-15, and IL-21

IL-2 potently activates the antitumor effector functions of both innate and adaptive cytotoxic cells. The systemic infusion of high doses of recombinant IL-2 or the adoptive transfer of NK cell or CD8$^+$ T lymphocytes stimulated *ex vivo* with IL-2 can evoke durable tumor regressions in a minority of patients with advanced melanoma and renal cell carcinoma [65]. IL-2 induced tumor immunity involves both NKG2D-dependent pathways and perforin mediated killing. Additionally, IL-2 is critical for immune homeostasis, as mice deficient in the cytokine or signaling components succumb to chronic inflammatory disease due to defects in the maintenance of FoxP3 expressing regulatory T cells. Thus, IL-2 may also contribute to tumor protection through the control of inflammation-driven carcinogenesis.

The closely related cytokine IL-15 is critical for NK cell and memory CD8$^+$ T cell homeostasis. The ability of IL-15 to amplify proximal TCR signaling in memory CD8+ T cells overcomes tolerance in a TCR transgenic model of tumor-induced anergy [66]. Constitutive IL-15 expression, however, may contribute to tumor promotion, as IL-15 transgenic mice succumbed to growth-factor-induced NKT-cell leukemias [67].

The IL-21 receptor shares the common gamma-chain subunit employed for IL-2 and IL-15 signaling. IL-21 affects many immune cell types, including the promotion of proliferation and cytotoxic activity of NK cells, NKT cells, and CD8 T cells [68]. Interestingly, endogenous and exogenous IL-21 may have differing functions in antitumor immunity. Endogenous IL-21 can limit CD8 T-cell expansion and tumor rejection, and is not required for NK, NKT, or CD8 T-cell mediated tumor immunity [69]. However, the therapeutic administration of IL-21 has shown efficacy in a variety of animal models, and is being tested clinically as a treatment for human cancers. Collectively, IL-2, IL-15, and IL-21 play complementary roles in tumor surveillance.

C. IL-12 and IL-18

Upon activation, phagocytes secrete IL-12 and IL-18, which in turn stimulate innate and adaptive cells to produce IFN-γ and thereby contribute to tumor suppression. Mice deficient in p40, a subunit shared by IL-12 and IL-23, manifest an increased susceptibility to chemical carcinogens. IL-12 enhances NK and NKT cell antitumor activities through NKG2D and perforin dependent pathways [70]. IL-12 may also stimulate a unique subset of innate immune cells (NKp46+ lymphoid tissue-inducer cells) that can promote leukocyte trafficking into B16 melanoma to enhance rejection [71]. In contrast, IL-18 augments NK cell cytotoxicity in a NKG2D independent fashion that involves Fas ligand mediated killing. However, in some settings, IL-18 may contribute to suppression of tumor immunity. For example, low levels of exogenously administered or tumor-secreted IL-18 cause upregulation of PD-1 expression on NK cells, leading to their suppression [72].

D. IL-23 and IL-17

The roles of IL-23 and IL-17 in tumor immunity and promotion have not yet been clearly defined. IL-23 is a heterodimeric cytokine composed of a p40 subunit, which is shared with IL-12, and a unique p19 subunit. While activated macrophages and dendritic cells produce both IL-12 and IL-23, these cytokines trigger distinct downstream effector pathways. IL-12 promotes the development of IFN-γ-secreting Th1 cells, whereas IL-23 supports the expansion and activation of Th17 cells, a CD4$^+$ T subset that is critical for tissue inflammation. IL-23 stimulates increased expression of IL-17, which may promote tumor cell growth and invasion through upregulation of MMP9, COX-2, and angiogenesis, whereas IL-23 deficiency attenuated tumor formation through a reduction in inflammation [73]. IL-23 also restrains protective immunity through inhibiting the intra-tumoral localization of Th1 cells and cytotoxic CD8+ lymphocytes. In some systems, though, IL-23 might also evoke protective antitumor responses, in part mediated by activated granulocytes, which as discussed earlier can trigger tumor cytotoxicity. Similarly, differences in model system reveal differing functions of Th17 cells and IL-17. In some settings, IL-17 has been demonstrated to promote tumor growth by binding IL-17 receptors both on tumor cells and on stromal cells in the tumor microenvironment, activating the IL-6/Stat3 signaling pathway [74]. Additionally, IL-17 produced by tumor-infiltrating γδ T cells may promote tumor progression by stimulating angiogenesis [75]. However, in other contexts, Th17 cells and endogenous IL-17 seem to play a role in promoting IFN-γ+ effector T cells and NK cells in the tumor environment, leading to enhanced tumor immunity [76,77]. Further investigations are required to understand the multiple roles of IL-23 and IL-17 in tumor surveillance.

E. GM-CSF

Granulocyte-macrophage colony-stimulating factor (GM-CSF) stimulates the production, proliferation, maturation, and activation of granulocytes, macrophages, and dendritic cells. Vaccination with irradiated tumor cells engineered to secrete GM-CSF enhances tumor immunity in mice and patients through enhanced tumor antigen presentation. CD1d-restricted NKT cells, CD4 and CD8+ T cells, and antibodies are required for tumor protection [78]. Whereas GM-CSF deficient mice manifest pulmonary alveolar proteinosis, autoimmune disease, and loss of some protective immune responses, they do not manifest increased spontaneous cancers. In contrast, mice doubly deficient in GM-CSF and IFN-γ develop at high frequency diverse hematological and solid tumors within the background of chronic inflammation and infection [79]. This points to a critical role for GM-CSF in immune homeostasis, balancing the promotion of phagocytosis of apoptotic tumor cells to facilitate antigen presentation to effector lymphocytes with the induction of regulatory T cells and myeloid suppressor cells. GM-CSF has been administered in a variety of clinical settings as an immune adjuvant for cancer vaccines. It has become increasingly clear that dosing, schedule of administration and delivery method are critical for determination of immune stimulatory versus suppressive effects of this cytokine.

VIII. ANTITUMOR EFFECTOR MECHANISMS: CYTOTOXIC MECHANISMS

A. Perforin

Cytotoxicity triggered through the perforin—granzyme pathways is critical to tumor suppression [80]. Perforin-deficient mice display an enhanced susceptibility to chemical carcinogenesis and spontaneously develop lymphomas, which are rejected upon transplantation to wild type animals through a CD8$^+$ T-cell dependent mechanism. Perforin deficiency also compromises NK cell cytotoxicity against MHC class I deficient tumor cells, which may be primarily NKG2D dependent. Together, these findings underscore the importance of the perforin—granzyme pathway for innate and adaptive antitumor cytotoxicity.

B. TNF family members

Death receptors belonging to the tumor necrosis factor (TNF) superfamily constitute the second major mechanism of cellular cytotoxicity. TNF-related apoptosis-inducing ligand (TRAIL) is a type II transmembrane protein that binds to five receptors in humans and one in mice. Among these, DR4 (TRAIL-R1) and DR5 (TRAIL-R2) transduce death signals through caspase-8, FADD and Bax, while the remaining receptors (TRAIL-R3, TRAIL-R4 and osteoprotegrin) may attenuate killing as nonsignaling receptor decoys. TRAIL is upregulated in various innate and adaptive lymphocytes through interferons, IL-2 and IL-15. The IFN-γ-dependent induction of TRAIL on NK cells is critical for the antitumor effects of IL-12 and α-GalCer, whereas TRAIL deficiency augments the development of liver metastasis in perforin, but not IFN-γ-deficient hosts. TRAIL-deficient mice manifest an increased susceptibility to methycholanthrene-induced and hematologic tumors, and when crossed with p53 deficient mice show accelerated tumor formation [81,82]. A number of preclinical studies have shown the therapeutic potential of recombinant TRAIL or anti-TRAIL receptor antibodies, particularly in combination with chemotherapies, and testing in humans is ongoing [83].

The interaction of Fas and Fas ligand similarly triggers antitumor cytotoxicity. Mice deficient in this pathway manifest an increased incidence of spontaneous plasmacytoid lymphomas [84]. In transplantation models, Fas/Fas ligand interactions contribute to control of metastases. Thus, tumor growth may select for escape from this pathway.

LIGHT is another TNF member that participates in tumor suppression by functioning as a co-stimulatory molecule [85]. The engineered expression of LIGHT triggers an antitumor T-cell response that mediates destruction of established tumors, illustrating that appropriate manipulation of the tumor microenvironment may be therapeutic.

110

IX. THE INTERPLAY OF INNATE AND ADAPTIVE ANTITUMOR IMMUNITY

Innate immunity functions not only to exert direct antitumor effects, but also to stimulate the generation of adaptive immune responses through the presentation of tumor antigens by dendritic cells. The types of stimuli present in the tumor microenvironment dictate the program of dendritic cell activation, thereby directing adaptive responses toward either protective immunity or tolerance. The detection of "danger signals" elicited by stress or cell death and interactions with other innate cells appears to be important for triggering dendritic cell activation. Thus, NK cells that recognize NKG2D ligand-positive, MHC class I-deficient tumors, NKT cells that detect CD1d-presented lipids, and γδ T cells that recognize stress antigens can all interact productively with dendritic cells. In this cross-talk, cytokines, B7 family members, and CD40 play critical roles.

X. CONCLUSION

Recent investigations of endogenous antitumor responses have unveiled a previously unappreciated complexity of interaction among tumor cells, stroma, and immune elements. Innate immune activation by stress-inducible signals on tumor cells triggers a response aimed at controlling disease development. Effective responses may transition to adaptive immunity that manifests further specificity and memory. However, persistent immune activation may also result in an interplay of innate and adaptive elements that supports tumor cell proliferation, survival, invasion, angiogenesis, and metastasis. A more detailed understanding of the mechanisms regulating the development of tumor protective or tumor promoting host responses is critical to the crafting of immunotherapeutic strategies.

References

[1] Dranoff G. Cytokines in cancer pathogenesis and cancer therapy. Nat Rev Cancer 2004;4:11—22.

[2] Clark Jr WH, Elder DE, Guerry 4th D, et al. Model predicting survival in stage I melanoma based on tumor progression. J Natl Cancer Inst 1989;81:1893—904.

[3] Galon J, Costes A, Sanchez-Cabo F, et al. Type, density, and location of immune cells within human colorectal tumors predict clinical outcome. Science 2006;313:1960—4.

[4] Pages F, Berger A, Camus M, et al. Effector memory T cells, early metastasis, and survival in colorectal cancer. N Engl J Med 2005;353:2654—66.

[5] Zhang L, Conejo-Garcia JR, Katsaros D, et al. Intratumoral T cells, recurrence, and survival in epithelial ovarian cancer. N Eng J Med 2003;348:203—13.

[6] Gasser S, Orsulic S, Brown EJ, Raulet DH. The DNA damage pathway regulates innate immune system ligands of the NKG2D receptor. Nature 2005;436:1186—90.

[7] Medzhitov R. Toll-like receptors and innate immunity. Nat Rev Immunol 2001;1:135—45.

[8] Oppenheim DE, Roberts SJ, Clarke SL, et al. Sustained localized expression of ligand for the activating NKG2D receptor impairs natural cytotoxicity in vivo and reduces tumor immunosurveillance. Nat Immunol 2005;6:928—37.

[9] Waldhauer I, Goehlsdorf D, Gieseke F, et al. Tumor-associated MICA is shed by ADAM proteases. Cancer Res 2008;68:6368—76.

[10] Zocchi MR, Catellani S, Canevali P, et al. High ERp5/ADAM10 expression in lymph node microenvironment and impaired NKG2D ligands recognition in Hodgkin lymphoma. Blood 2012;119:1479—89.

[11] Smyth MJ, Cretney E, Takeda K, et al. Tumor necrosis factor-related apoptosis-inducing ligand (TRAIL) contributes to interferon gamma-dependent natural killer cell protection from tumor metastasis. J Exp Med 2001;193:661—70.

[12] Brandt CS, Baratin M, Yi EC, et al. The B7 family member B7-H6 is a tumor cell ligand for the activating natural killer cell receptor NKp30 in humans. J Exp Med 2009;206:1495—503.

[13] Glasner A, Ghadially H, Gur C, et al. Recognition and prevention of tumor metastasis by the NK receptor NKp46/NCR1. J Immunol 2012;188:2509—15.

[14] Rosental B, Brusilovsky M, Hadad U, et al. Proliferating cell nuclear antigen is a novel inhibitory ligand for the natural cytotoxicity receptor NKp44. J Immunol 2011;187:5693—702.

[15] Raulet DH. Roles of the NKG2D immunoreceptor and its ligands. Nat Rev Immunol 2003;3:781—90.

[16] Guerra N, Tan YX, Joncker NT, et al. NKG2D-deficient mice are defective in tumor surveillance in models of spontaneous malignancy. Immunity 2008;28:571—80.

[17] Smyth MJ, Swann J, Cretney E, Zerafa N, Yokoyama WM, Hayakawa Y. NKG2D function protects the host from tumor initiation. J Exp Med 2005;202:583—8.

[18] O'Leary JG, Goodarzi M, Drayton DL, von Andrian UH. T cell- and B cell-independent adaptive immunity mediated by natural killer cells. Nat Immunol 2006;7:507—16.

[19] Sun JC, Beilke JN, Lanier LL. Adaptive immune features of natural killer cells. Nature 2009;457:557—61.

[20] Paust S, Gill HS, Wang BZ, et al. Critical role for the chemokine receptor CXCR6 in NK cell-mediated antigen-specific memory of haptens and viruses. Nat Immunol 2010;11:1127—35.

[21] Cooper MA, Elliott JM, Keyel PA, et al. Cytokine-induced memory-like natural killer cells. Proc Natl Acad Sci U S A 2009;106:1915—9.

[22] Taniguchi M, Harada M, Kojo S, Nakayama T, Wakao H. The regulatory role of Valpha14 NKT cells in innate and acquired immune response. Annu Rev Immunol 2003;21:483—513.

[23] Smyth MJ, Thia KY, Street SE, et al. Differential tumor surveillance by natural killer (NK) and NKT cells. J Exp Med 2000;191:661—8.

[24] Cui J, Shin T, Kawano T, et al. Requirement for Vα14 NKT cells in IL-12-mediated rejection of tumors. Science 1997;278:1623—6.

[25] Gillessen S, Naumov YN, Nieuwenhuis EE, et al. CD1d-restricted T cells regulate dendritic cell function and antitumor immunity in a granulocyte-macrophage colony-stimulating factor-dependent fashion. Proc Natl Acad Sci USA 2003;100:8874—9.

[26] Terabe M, Matsui S, Park JM, et al. Transforming growth factor-beta production and myeloid cells are an effector mechanism through which CD1d-restricted T cells block cytotoxic T lymphocyte-mediated tumor immunosurveillance: abrogation prevents tumor recurrence. J Exp Med 2003;198:1741—52.

[27] Akbari O, Faul JL, Hoyte EG, et al. CD4+ invariant T-cell-receptor+ natural killer T cells in bronchial asthma. N Engl J Med 2006;354:1117—29.

[28] Crowe NY, Coquet JM, Berzins SP, et al. Differential antitumor immunity mediated by NKT cell subsets in vivo. J Exp Med 2005;202:1279—88.

[29] Berzins SP, Smyth MJ, Baxter AG. Presumed guilty: natural killer T cell defects and human disease. Nat Rev Immunol 2011;11:131–42.

[30] Hayday AC. γδ cells: a right time and a right place for a conserved third way of protection. Annu Rev Immunol 2000;18:975–1026.

[31] Kabelitz D, Wesch D, He W. Perspectives of γδ T cells in tumor immunology. Cancer Res 2007;67:5–8.

[32] Girardi M, Glusac E, Filler RB, et al. The distinct contributions of murine T cell receptor (TCR)gammadelta+ and TCRalphabeta+ T cells to different stages of chemically induced skin cancer. J Exp Med 2003;198:747–55.

[33] D'Asaro M, La Mendola C, Di Liberto D, et al. Vγ9 Vδ2 T lymphocytes efficiently recognize and kill zolendronate-sensitized, imatinib-sensitive and imatinib-resistant chronic myelogenous leukemia cells. J Immunol 2010;184:3260–8.

[34] Benzaid I, Monkkonen H, Stresing V, et al. High phosphoantigen levels in bisphosphonate-treated human breast tumors promote Vγ9 Vδ2 T-cell chemotaxis and cytotoxicity in vivo. Cancer Res 2011;71:4562–72.

[35] Brandes M, Willimann K, Moser B. Professional antigen-presentation function by human gammadelta T Cells. Science 2005;309:264–8.

[36] Ma Y, Aymeric L, Locher L, et al. Contribution of IL-17-producing γδ T cells to the efficacy of anticancer chemotherapy. J Exp Med 2011;208:491–503.

[37] Hicks AM, Riedlinger G, Willingham MC, et al. Transferable anticancer innate immunity in spontaneous regression/complete resistance mice. Proc Natl Acad Sci U S A 2006;103:7753–8.

[38] Condeelis J, Pollard JW. Macrophages: obligate partners for tumor cell migration, invasion, and metastasis. Cell 2006;124:263–6.

[39] Colombo MP, Ferrari G, Stoppacciaro A, et al. Granulocyte-colony stimulating factor gene suppresses tumorigenicity of a murine adenocarcinoma in vivo. J Exp Med 1991;173:889–97.

[40] Curcio C, Di Carlo E, Clynes R, et al. Nonredundant roles of antibody, cytokines, and perforin in the eradication of established Her-2/neu carcinomas. J Clin Invest 2003;111:1161–70.

[41] Bekes EM, Schweighofer B, Kupriyanova TA, et al. Tumor-recruited neutrophils and neutrophil TIMP-free MMP-9 regulate coordinately the levels of tumor angiogenesis and efficiency of malignant cell intravasation. Am J Pathol 2011;179:1455–70.

[42] Houghton AM, Rzymkiewicz DM, Ji H, et al. Neutrophil elastase-mediated degradation of IRS-1 accelerates lung tumor growth. Nat Med 2010;16:219–23.

[43] Chan CW, Crafton E, Fan HN, et al. Interferon-producing killer dendritic cells provide a link between innate and adaptive immunity. Nat Med 2006;12:207–13.

[44] Taieb J, Chaput N, Menard C, et al. A novel dendritic cell subset involved in tumor immunosurveillance. Nat Med 2006;12:214–9.

[45] Matzinger P. The danger model: a renewed sense of self. Science 2002;296:301–5.

[46] Gabrilovich D. Mechanisms and functional significance of tumour-induced dendritic-cell defects. Nat Rev Immunol 2004;4:941–52.

[47] Hung K, Hayashi R, Lafond-Walker A, Lowenstein C, Pardoll D, Levitsky H. The central role of CD4[+] T cells in the antitumor immune response. J Exp Med 1998;188:2357–68.

[48] Dhodapkar KM, Krasovsky J, Williamson B, Dhodapkar MV. Antitumor monoclonal antibodies enhance cross-presentation of cellular antigens and the generation of myeloma-specific killer T cells by dendritic cells. J Exp Med 2002;195:125–33.

[49] Nimmerjahn F, Ravetch JV. Divergent immunoglobulin g subclass activity through selective Fc receptor binding. Science 2005;310:1510–2.

[50] Shankaran V, Ikeda H, Bruce AT, et al. IFNg and lymphocytes prevent primary tumour development and shape tumour immunogenicity. Nature 2001;410:1107–11.

[51] Nakamoto Y, Guidotti LG, Kuhlen CV, Fowler P, Chisari FV. Immune pathogenesis of hepatocellular carcinoma. J Exp Med 1998;188:341–50.

[52] Daniel D, Meyer-Morse N, Bergsland EK, Dehne K, Coussens LM, Hanahan D. Immune enhancement of skin carcinogenesis by CD4+ T cells. J Exp Med 2003;197:1017–28.

[53] Dranoff G. The therapeutic implications of intratumoral regulatory T cells. Clin Cancer Res 2005;11:8226–9.

[54] Curiel TJ, Coukos G, Zou L, et al. Specific recruitment of regulatory T cells in ovarian carcinoma fosters immune privilege and predicts reduced survival. Nat Med 2004;10:942–9.

[55] Erdman SE, Sohn JJ, Rao VP, et al. CD4+CD25+ regulatory lymphocytes induce regression of intestinal tumors in ApcMin/+ mice. Cancer Res 2005;65:3998–4004.

[56] de Visser KE, Korets LV, Coussens LM. De novo carcinogenesis promoted by chronic inflammation is B lymphocyte dependent. Cancer Cell 2005;7:411–23.

[57] Boon T, van der Bruggen P. Human tumor antigens recognized by T lymphocytes. J Exp Med 1996;183:725–9.

[58] Nishikawa H, Kato T, Tawara I, et al. Definition of target antigens for naturally occurring CD4(+) CD25(+) regulatory T cells. J Exp Med 2005;201:681–6.

[59] Wang HY, Lee DA, Peng G, et al. Tumor-specific human CD4+ regulatory T cells and their ligands: implications for immunotherapy. Immunity 2004;20:107–18.

[60] Dunn GP, Old LJ, Schreiber RD. The immunobiology of cancer immunosurveillance and immunoediting. Immunity 2004;21:137–48.

[61] Zaidi MR, Davis S, Noonan FP, et al. Interferon-γ links ultraviolet radiation to melanomagenesis in mice. Nature 2011;469:548–53.

[62] Dunn GP, Bruce AT, Sheehan KC, et al. A critical function for type I interferons in cancer immunoediting. Nat Immunol 2005;6:722–9.

[63] Takaoka A, Hayakawa S, Yanai H, et al. Integration of interferon-alpha/beta signalling to p53 responses in tumour suppression and antiviral defence. Nature 2003;424:516–23.

[64] Critchley-Thorne RJ, Simons DL, Yan N, et al. Impaired interferon signaling is a common immune defect in human cancer. Proc Natl Acad Sci U S A 2009;106:9010–5.

[65] Rosenberg SA. Progress in human tumour immunology and immunotherapy. Nature 2001;411:380–4.

[66] Teague RM, Sather BD, Sacks JA, et al. Interleukin-15 rescues tolerant CD8+ T cells for use in adoptive immunotherapy of established tumors. Nat Med 2006;12:335–41.

[67] Fehniger TA, Suzuki K, Ponnappan A, et al. Fatal leukemia in interleukin 15 transgenic mice follows early expansions in natural killer and memory phenotype CD8+ T cells. J Exp Med 2001;193:219–31.

[68] Spolski R, Leonard WJ. Interleukin-21: basic biology and implications for cancer and autoimmunity. Annu Rev Immunol 2008;26:57–79.

[69] Sondergaard H, Coquet JM, Uldrich AP, et al. Endogenous IL-21 restricts CD8+ T cell expansion and is not required for tumor immunity. J Immunol 2009;183:7326–36.

[70] Smyth MJ, Swann J, Cretney E, Zerafa N, Yokoyama WM, Hayakawa Y. NKG2D function protects the host from tumor initiation. J Exp Med 2005;202:583–8.

[71] Eisenring M, vom Berg J, Kristiansen G, Saller E, Becher B. IL-12 initiates tumor rejection via lymphoid tissue-inducer cells bearing the natural cytotoxicity receptor NKp46. Nat Immunol 2010;11:1030–8.

[72] Terme M, Ullrich E, Aymeric L, et al. IL-18 induces PD-1-dependent immunosuppression in cancer. Cancer Res 2011;71:5393–9.

[73] Langowski JL, Zhang X, Wu L, et al. IL-23 promotes tumour incidence and growth. Nature 2006;442:461–5.

[74] Wang L, Yi T, Kortylewski M, Pardoll DM, Zeng D, Yu H. IL-17 can promote tumor growth through an IL-6-Stat3 signaling pathway. J Exp Med 2009;206:1457–64.

[75] Wakita D, Sumida K, Iwakura Y, et al. Tumor-infiltrating IL-17-producing γδ T cells support the progression of tumor by promoting angiogenesis. Eur J Immunol 2010;40:1927–37.

[76] Kryczek I, Wei S, Szeliga W, et al. Endogenous IL-17 contributes to reduced tumor growth and metastasis. Blood 2009;114:357–9.

[77] Kryczek I, Banerjee M, Cheng P, et al. Phenotype, distribution, generation, and functional and clinical relevance of Th17 cells in the human tumor environments. Blood 2009;114:1141–9.

[78] Hodi FS, Dranoff G. Combinatorial cancer immunotherapy. Adv Immunol 2006;90:337–60.

[79] Enzler T, Gillessen S, Manis JP, et al. Deficiencies of GM-CSF and interferon-gamma link inflammation and cancer. J Exp Med 2003;197:1213–9.

[80] Smyth MJ, Thia KY, Street SE, MacGregor D, Godfrey DI, Trapani JA. Perforin-mediated cytotoxicity is critical for surveillance of spontaneous lymphoma. J Exp Med 2000;192:755–60.

[81] Takeda K, Smyth MJ, Cretney E, et al. Critical role for tumor necrosis factor-related apoptosis-inducing ligand in immune surveillance against tumor development. J Exp Med 2002;195:161–9.

[82] Zerafa N, Westwood JA, Cretney E, et al. Cutting edge: TRAIL deficiency accelerates hematological malignancies. J Immunol 2005;175:5586–90.

[83] Johnstone RW, Frew AJ, Smyth MJ. The TRAIL apoptotic pathway in cancer onset, progression, and therapy. Nat Rev Cancer 2008;8:782–98.

[84] Davidson WF, Giese T, Fredrickson TN. Spontaneous development of plasmacytoid tumors in mice with defective Fas-Fas ligand interactions. J Exp Med 1998;187:1825–38.

[85] Yu P, Lee Y, Liu W, et al. Priming of naive T cells inside tumors leads to eradication of established tumors. Nat Immunol 2004;5:141–9.

113

CHAPTER 9

Immunological Sculpting: Natural Killer-Cell Receptors and Ligands

Sarah S. Donatelli, Julie Y. Djeu
H. Lee Moffitt Cancer Center, Tampa, FL USA

I. INTRODUCTION

The innate immune system is a crucial component of host defense against both foreign pathogenic invaders and aberrant self cells, such as tissues that have undergone malignant transformation. Natural Killer (NK) cells are integral members of the innate arm of immunity, and cancer patients who are deficient in NK cell number or function exhibit a weakened antitumoral response and ultimately poor prognosis. NK cells are among the first to recognize and kill virally or bacterially infected and cancerous, or "stressed," cells.

NK cells differentiate healthy from stressed cells through a vast array of germline-encoded receptors that confer either activating or inhibitory signals. NK-cell receptors differ from T-cell receptors in that they are recombinase activating gene (RAG) independent; that is, they do not somatically rearrange variable diversity or joining (VDJ) gene segments to form endless combinations of antigen-specific receptors. Rather, NK cells express genes for a finite number of receptors that recognize self antigens, and these ligands provide the basis of the NK cell's reaction to the target cell. Distinct NK clones that exhibit varied combinations of both inhibitory and activating receptors result from the stochastic, or probabilistically determined, expression of the receptors.

The expressed receptors potentiate either stimulatory "kill" or inhibitory "no kill" signals upon contact with ligands provided by the target cell. Major histocompatibility class I (MHC I) molecules constitutively expressed by healthy tissues provide ligands for receptors that transmit inhibitory "no kill" signals to the NK cell. Consequently, a lack of MHC I fails to provide the NK cell with inhibitory signals and thus indirectly potentiates an activation signal. On the other hand, stress-induced proteins normally absent on healthy cells emerge as ligands for receptors that provide the NK cell with an activating "kill" signal. During a given target interaction, the NK-cell's receptors will associate with a combination of MHC I molecules and stress-induced ligands. The balance of signals that emanates from these interactions dictates the NK-cell's response to the stressed cell. This chapter introduces the concepts of NK-cell receptor acquisition and signaling, and reviews current knowledge of individual receptors and their ligands.

II. NK EDUCATION, LICENSING, AND PRIMING

NK cells acquire the capacity to recognize and kill stressed cells through distinct receptor-ligand interactions deemed education and licensing [1]. Before NK cells develop into potent

Cancer Immunotherapy. http://dx.doi.org/10.1016/B978-0-12-394296-8.00009-9

effectors that kill damaged cells, they must first become tolerant to healthy tissues through interaction with and recognition of self MHC I molecules to prevent the occurrence of autoimmunity [2]. In mice, this education occurs through *cis* interactions; that is, through the association of an MHC I molecule with an MHC I-specific receptor expressed on the surface of the NK cell itself [3]. This interaction requires phosphorylation of the tyrosine in the immunotyrosine-based inhibitory motif (ITIM) located within the cytoplasmic tail of the MHC I-binding receptor [4]. NK cells that do not express at least one MHC I-specific receptor or NK cells that cannot engage at least one MHC I molecule in such *cis* interactions do not acquire the ability to kill stressed cells and thus remain "unlicensed" [3,4]. Therefore, it is only after the NK cell is tolerant to self MHC that it can be licensed to kill.

The mechanism by which NK cells are licensed remains incompletely described; however, the prevailing theory, or the "arming" of NK cells, has been experimentally supported. The basis for the arming theory is that a positive signal is conferred through the inhibitory ITIM, as ablation of the ITIM abrogates NK functionality [1,4]. This postulation seemed counterintuitive until recent experiments in mice revealed MHC I-specific receptor variants that exclusively bind MHC I in *cis* (on the surface of the NK cell itself) are utilized for licensing. Association of these variants with *cis* MHC I results in sequestration of the inhibitory receptors, allowing for a physical separation between the activating and inhibitory receptors. The activating receptors then have the freedom to contact their ligands and transmit the resulting positive signals required for the mobilization of lytic granules. Therefore, such spatial segregation positively regulates NK-cell cytolysis, suggesting that physical distance from inhibitory molecules may be required for effective function of activating receptors [3]. This requirement may apply to both MHC I-specific and non-MHC I-specific activating receptors, as their signaling pathways are shared and conserved, with the tyrosine phosphatases recruited by ITIM signaling dephosphorylating kinases crucial early in the lytic cascade. These experiments resolved the seemingly counterintuitive fact that positive regulation can ultimately be conferred by inhibitory ITIM signaling.

NK-cell licensing can occur in both the bone marrow during development, and in peripheral, mature NK cells. Importantly, the capacity to kill can be revoked in the absence of MHC I, suggesting that NK development is a constant and malleable process [5]. The licensing signal varies with respect to the diversity of the host MHC haplotype, the number of MHC I specific receptors per NK cell interacting with host MHC, and the affinity of said receptors for their cognate MHC molecule [1]. Importantly, licensing is a steady-state process involved in NK cell maintenance, and under inflammatory conditions, unlicensed NK cells can kill stressed cells, as cytokine stimulation overrides MHC I-dependent licensing in both mice [1] and humans [6].

During steady-state maintenance as well as inflammatory siege, the killing capacity of NK cells is enhanced by cytokines in the immune milieu. Cytokines particularly important to NK-cell development and function are interleukin (IL) IL-2, IL-15, IL-12, IL-18, IL-21, and type I interferons (IFN). Most of these cytokines are produced by other members of the immune system, such as T cells, activated macrophages, and dendritic cells. IL-2 and IL-15, produced by T cells and dendritic cells respectively, promote NK survival, proliferation, cytokine production, and cytotoxicity [7–12], likely by increase of activating surface killing receptors [13]. Similarly, IL-12 and IL-21, sourced from activated macrophages and T cells respectively, promote proliferation [14,15], cytokine production [16], and cytotoxicity [17,18], while macrophage and dendritic cell-derived IL-18 promotes survival [19]. IL-6 produced by T cells and macrophages increases IFNγ and IL-17 production and cytotoxicity [20,21]. Virally induced type I interferons α/β also induce potent cytokine production and cytotoxicity [22,23]. Therefore, interplay of NK cells with other members of the immune system, as well as with their putative targets, is essential for a healthy NK-mediated host defense.

III. HOW RECEPTOR: LIGAND INTERACTIONS TRIGGER CELL LYSIS
A. Cell-to-cell interactions

NK-cell receptors interact with a combination of stimulating and repressive ligands when they investigate unfamiliar cells, and the balance of signals resulting from these interactions determines the fate of the target. If the activation signals overcome the inhibitory signals, the NK cell will lyse the target cell. Inhibitory signals emanate primarily from MHC I ligands, although there are also non-MHC-related inhibitory ligands [24]. All healthy cells (with the exception of erythrocytes and platelets) express MHC I and thus, will only engage the MHC I-specific inhibitory receptor present on all functionally competent NK cells, signaling the NK cell to spare the cell. Stressed cells, on the other hand, often downregulate MHC I, thus preventing transduction of the inhibitory signal, allowing for triggering of NK-cell activation. The process of NK-mediated rejection of MHC I-deficient targets is known as "missing self." In addition to MHC I dysregulation, stressed cells can also display non-MHC I-related activating ligands, such as stress proteins induced by viral infections or malignant transformation, that will trigger NK-cell-mediated cytolysis through their activating receptors. The specific receptors and their ligands are discussed in detail in the following sections. There is evidence that a stronger signal (determined by either the strength or quantity of the receptor-ligand interactions) is required for cytotoxicity of the target, whereas a weaker signal may only elicit inflammatory cytokines such as IFNγ that will recruit members of the adaptive immune response for a closer investigation of the putative invader. As mentioned earlier, in mice, MHC I-specific receptors can associate with MHC I molecules in *cis*, that is, MHC I molecules expressed on the NK cell's own plasma membrane. These *cis* interactions enhance NK-mediated cytolytic activity of target cells by reducing the necessity for *trans* binding, or NK-expressed MHC I-specific inhibitory receptor binding to target cell MHC I, and lowering the threshold for activation through triggering receptors [25,26]. This caveat suggests that the NK-cell-intrinsic MHC repertoire can contribute to determination of the signal strength required to kill the target cell, and NK cells diverse in MHC alleles may be more innately "active" than NK cells that do not exhibit MHC diversity.

B. Signaling

When an NK cell encounters a potential target, intracellular signals reverberate via the surface receptors. The major stimulatory or inhibitory signaling pathways are conserved among respective receptors (Figure 9.1). Activating receptors have short cytoplasmic tails that lack any capacity for signaling. Therefore, activating receptors generally associate with immunotyrosine-based activation motif (ITAM)-containing adaptor molecules that can be phosphorylated to activate downstream signals that end in lytic granule and/or cytokine secretion. ITAM-containing adaptor proteins associate with the short cytoplasmic tails by binding to charged transmembrane amino acids.

The most frequently used adaptor molecules are dynax activating protein 12kD (DAP12), CD3ζ, FcRγ, and DAP10. DAP12 is associated with NK activating receptors through charged residues in the transmembrane region of the receptor's cytoplasmic tail, and upon receptor-ligand interaction, Src family kinases such as lymphocyte-specific protein tyrosine kinase (Lck) and Fyn phosphorylate the tyrosine in the adaptor's ITAM. Spleen tyrosine kinase (Syk) [27] or zeta-chain-associated protein kinase 70 (Zap70)[28] is recruited by binding to the phosphotyrosine in the ITAM and activating phosphoinositide-3 kinase (PI3K) that leads to sequential Rac1, PAK1, and MAPK/ERK activation to mobilize lytic granules that kill the target cell [29,30]. Recently, protein kinase C-Θ (PKC-Θ) has emerged as a requirement for IFNγ release, but not cytolysis, during sustained ITAM signaling [31]. Other adaptors, such as CD3ζ and FcRγ, function in the same manner as DAP12, as they contain the same ITAM (Figure 9.1). DAP10, on the other hand, does not express an ITAM but contains a PI3K-binding domain. The Fyn/Lck phosphorylation of this tyrosine-containing domain recruits PI3K which results

117

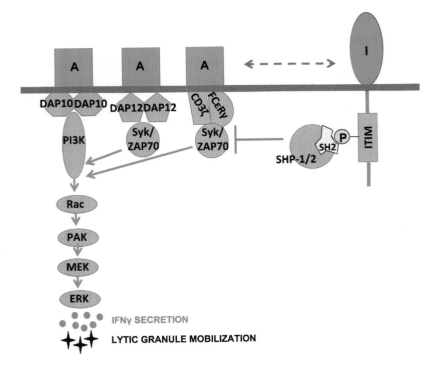

FIGURE 9.1

Conserved signaling pathways of NK receptors.
Activating receptor ligation leads to association of ITAM-containing adaptor proteins and subsequent entry into the PI3K signaling pathway, ultimately leading to IFNγ and lytic granule secretion. Inhibitory receptor ligation leads to activating/inhibitory receptor colocalization, ITIM phosphorylation and subsequent recruitment of SHP-1 and SHP-2 to the SH2 domain, which dephosphorylates critical signaling proteins at the activating receptor/adaptor protein complex. Activating receptors are depicted in green, while inhibitory receptors are depicted as red. Signaling proteins are blue. Green arrows depict sequential activation by phosphorylation of the previous signaling protein.

in mobilization of granules via the same pathway as DAP12 (Figure 9.1)[32]. In addition, antibody-dependent cell cytotoxicity by NK cells can occur via this pathway through FcγRIII (CD16), which couples to CD3ζ, or FcεRγ. Overall, a multitude of ligands can trigger NK cells and the initial signaling molecules activated may vary depending on the receptor, but they merge downstream into a conserved common cascade ending in ERK activation and subsequent lytic granule mobilization.

In contrast, inhibitory receptors have long cytoplasmic tails that contain one or more immunotyrosine inhibitory motifs (ITIM). Upon receptor-ligand interaction, these ITIMs are phosphorylated by Lck and Fyn (Figure 9.1). Src homology-2 domain containing phosphatase 1 and 2 (SHP-1 and SHP-2) then bind to the phosphotyrosine in the ITIM through their SH2 domains [33,34]. SHP-1 and SHP-2 then function to disrupt the lytic cascade by specific dephosphorylation of Syk and Zap70, crucial early signaling proteins necessary for NK activation tyrosines [35].

IV. RECEPTORS FOR MHC I AND MHC I-RELATED MOLECULES
A. Killer immunoglobulin-like receptors (KIR)

MHC I molecules provide the most robust and abundant signals to NK cells. It is through MHC molecules that NK cells can sample the health of the environment. These interactions are crucial to NK function, providing both inhibitory and activating signals. The largest family of molecules expressed in human NK cells that recognize MHC I on target cells are the killer immunoglobulin-like receptors (KIR) and can be inherited as two haplotypes, A and B (Figure 9.2). All KIR contain either two (KIR2D) or three (KIR3D) extracellular immuno-globulin (Ig)-like domains and may exhibit either short (KIR2/3DS) or ITIM-containing long (KIR2/3DL) cytoplasmic tails that play activating or inhibitory roles in NK cell target signaling, respectively (Figure 9.3). For simplicity, in this review, all stimulatory KIR gene products are referred to as "aKIR," and all inhibitory KIR gene products are referred to as "iKIR."

As stated earlier, aKIR provide stimulatory signals to NK cells when they contact their target ligands, causing lytic granule mobilization that induces target cell lysis or cytokine secretion to

HAPLOTYPE A

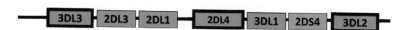

HAPLOTYPE B

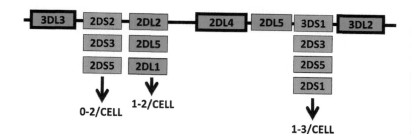

FIGURE 9.2

KIR haplotypes. Schematic depiction of the KIR genotypes of haplotypes A and B. The A haplotype is fixed in gene content, while the B haplotype varies extensively in gene content. The boxes on and below the line are KIRs all variably expressed in a given B haplotype. Framework genes present on all haplotypes are outlined in bold black line, activating KIR are depicted in green and inhibitory KIR in red. The numbers below the series of boxes in haploype B represent the various KIR combinations that can be expressed in a given B haplotype.

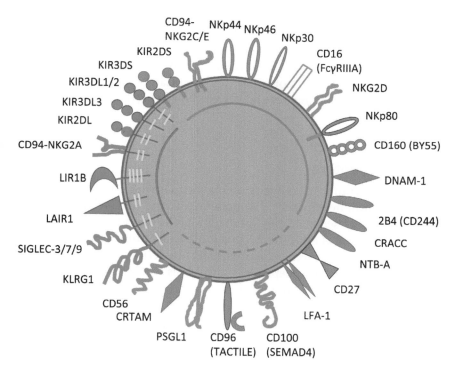

119

FIGURE 9.3

NK-cell surface receptors. Receptors contributing to NK activation are green and grouped with a solid green line, while receptors contributing to NK inhibition are red and grouped with a solid red line. Activating co-receptors are grouped with a dashed, color-coded line. ITIMs are depicted as yellow slashes in the red cytoplasmic tails. Abbreviated receptor names are displayed proximal to the receptor depiction.

amplify the immune response. They contain no intrinsic signaling capacity in their short cytoplasmic tails, but they do contain a charged lysine or arginine that facilitates association with DAP12. Six aKIR that contain two extracellular domains exhibiting different MHC I allelic preferences have been identified. Like their homologous inhibitory relatives, KIR2DS1, KIR2DS2, and KIR2DS3 bind human leukocyte antigen (HLA)-C, MHC I, alleles. This caveat implies that when an NK cell sees a target expressing HLA-C, it can receive both inhibitory and activating signals from the same ligand and adds to the complexity of the ensuing reaction. Furthermore, it suggests that the surface ratio of activating-to-inhibitory KIR may be a determining factor in the fate of the target cell. KIR2DS4 is exceptional in that it is the only KIR expressed in Haplotype A individuals. Furthermore, proteins other than MHC molecules have been identified as ligands. In addition to HLA-C1, -C2, and -A11 [36], KIR2DS4 is triggered by unidentified melanoma proteins [37], and unknown proteins expressed by chronic lymphocytic leukemia (CLL) cells [38], suggesting that this aKIR may play a distinct role in antitumoral defense. Ligands for KIR2DS5 and KIR2DS3 remain unidentified.

In contrast to aKIR, iKIR provide negative intracellular signals by recruiting SHP-1 and SHP-2 to the ITIMs in their long cytoplasmic tails upon ligand binding. Eight iKIR that exhibit different MHC allelic preferences have been identified. KIR2DL1, KIR2DL2, and KIR2DL3 bind HLA-C alleles [39], KIR3DL1 binds HLA-B alleles [40,41], and KIR3DL2 binds HLA-A3 and A11 [42]. The ligand for KIR2DL5 remains unidentified. KIR2DL4 is distinct in that it is expressed in all humans, and it has been experimentally shown to exhibit both activating and inhibitory signals. Furthermore, KIR2DL4 recognizes soluble HLA-G, which is expressed in the placenta, where classical HLA molecules are absent, and functions during pregnancy to prevent spontaneous abortion of the fetus.

It has been documented that KIR expression is controlled epigenetically by DNA methylation of cytosines in CpG dinucleotides rather than by genetic sequence differences in promoters [43]. These DNA methylation patterns are maintained over numerous cell divisions, and contribute to the diversity of gene expression in individual NK clones and their progeny [44]. KIRs are expressed stochastically leading to a repertoire of NK clones that express different combinations of activating and inhibitory KIRs. Genotyping and epidemiological studies have yielded two predominant patterns of KIR expression (Figure 9.2). Haplotype A individuals exhibit a relatively fixed gene content consisting of five iKIRs along with one aKIR, KIR2DS4, and KIR2DL4, which can exhibit both inhibitory and activating functions. Conversely, Haplotype B individuals express variable gene content consisting of multiple aKIR and iKIR combinations [45]. The frequencies of these haplotypes vary significantly with ethnicity; furthermore, correlations between KIR haplotypes and susceptibility to certain cancers and infections are beginning to emerge.

B. Natural cytotoxicity receptors

Apart from MHC-dependent interactions, NK cells rely on interactions with non-MHC-related proteins to distinguish stressed from healthy cells. The presence of non-MHC-related ligands was first noted when NK cells readily lysed MHC I-deficient tumor cells. We now know that this feature is a function due both to a lack of MHC I-mediated inhibition ("missing self") as well as engagement of activating receptors that recognize non-MHC I molecules. The receptors discovered to play a large role in this MHC-independent target lysis were termed the natural cytotoxicity receptors (NCR) (Figure 9.3). Deletion of even one NCR reduces the ability of NK cells to kill tumor targets *in vivo* [46]; this weakness is important because tumor-produced transforming growth factor β-1 (TGFβ) downregulates NCR family members to evade NK cytolysis [47]. Additionally, NCRs can potentiate interactions with antigen-presenting cells, such as dendritic cells, that can aid in cellular maturation for recruitment of the adaptive arm of immunity [48].

The NCR consist of NKp30, NKp44, NKp46, and NKp80 [49−51] and are named for their respective molecular weights. NKp30, NKp46, and Nkp80 are expressed on activated and resting NK cells while NKp44 is upregulated by IL-2. NKp46 ligands include hemagglutinin and hemagglutinin-neuraminidase of influenza and parainfluenza [52], as well as heparin sulfate proteoglycans, which also bind NKp30 [53]. Other ligands for NKp30 are nuclear factor HLA-B-associated transcript 3, a factor released from tumor cells [54], B7-H6 [55], CMV pp65, and BAT3 [56].

Of the NCRs, only NKp44 associates with and signals through DAP12 (Figure 9.1)[49]. NKp30 and NK46 couple to CD3ζ and FcεRγ adaptor molecules, which form heterotrimeric adaptor complexes [50,51]. NKp80 is an activating receptor that binds to the genetically linked activation-induced C-type lectin (AICL) and stimulates NK cytotoxicity against malignant myeloid cells [57]. NKp80 does not require an adaptor protein; rather, it signals through a hemi-ITAM in its cytoplasmic tail through recruitment of Syk [58] and likely progression through the PI3K activation pathway.

C. CD94/NKG2 and NKG2D

The NKG2 family is similar to KIR in that it contains both inhibitory and activating receptors; however, either MHC I or non-MHC I molecules can function as ligands. Furthermore, some family members, NKG2A, NKG2C, and NKG2E, heterodimerize with CD94, while NKG2D associates with itself to form a homodimer (Figure 9.3).

NKG2D is distantly related to the other NKG2 family members and does not dimerize with CD94, but rather forms homodimers that associate with DAP10 to yield an activation signal. In humans, NKG2D complexes bind stress-inducible MHC class I chain-related gene A and B (MICA/ MICB), whose steady-state distribution is restricted to intestinal epithelia, but is upregulated in many epithelial tumors [59,60]. Additional NKG2D ligands are UL16-binding proteins (ULBP) 1/2/3/4 which are induced by cytomegalovirus infection [61–63] and in mice, NKG2D recognizes the retinoic acid-inducible early gene-1 (Rae-1)-like proteins [62] and H-60, a minor MHC derived antigen. NKG2D mediates direct tumor target killing as well as induction of antitumoral T-cell responses [64], and is therefore a crucial component of the NK defense. However, tumors have demonstrated evasion of NKG2D-mediated killing by secretion of TGFβ, which downregulates NKG2D on NK cells [65], and NKG2D ligands on tumor cells [66]. Additionally, tumors shed soluble MICA/B, which functions as a decoy receptor [67].

The other three NKG2 family members, NKG2A, NKG2C, and NKG2E, form heterodimeric complexes with CD94, another lectin-like protein. These complexes recognize the nonclassical MHC molecule, HLA-E. HLA-E is deemed nonclassical in part because it presents only peptides derived from classical MHC I molecules. This feature allows NK cells to indirectly explore the MHC I environment of the putative target [68]. NKG2A contains an ITIM; thus upon binding to HLA-E it elicits an inhibitory signal. Interestingly, NKG2C/E-CD94 also binds HLA-E, yet it does not contain an ITIM. Rather, it associates with DAP12, transmitting an activation signal.

D. CD160 (BY55)

CD160 is an activating receptor expressed in the $CD56^{dim}CD16^+$ cytotoxic NK subset that constitutes the major NK fraction in circulating human NK cells (Figure 9.3)[69,70]. Engagement of CD160 recruits PI3K to activate the lytic cascade [71]. Both glycosylphosphatidylinositol (GPI)-anchored and transmembrane isoforms are found on NK cells. The major GPI-anchored form exhibits homology to KIR2DL4; however, its signaling constituents have not yet been elucidated. On the other hand, the transmembrane isoform, which is transiently expressed on cytokine-activated NK cells, contains a transmembrane region that activates Erk1/2 [72]. CD160 is a promiscuous receptor that binds a variety of ligands including MHC class 1a and 1b molecules HLA-C [69], soluble HLA-G [73], HLA-A2, HLA-B7, and HLA-E [69], as well as the herpesvirus entry mediator protein [74].

E. SLAM family receptors

In vivo, NK cells not only contact tissue cells, they also contact other NK cells. To prevent unmitigated self killing, NK express signaling lymphocyte activation molecule (SLAM)-related receptors. SLAM-family receptors expressed on human NK cells are NTB-A and CRACC, as well as 2B4 (CD244) (Figure 9.3). NTB-A and CRACC serve as self-ligands during homotypic interactions between NK cells, while the 2B4 ligand is CD48, a glycophosphatidylinositol (GPI)-linked member of the CD2 family of receptors expressed on hematopoietic cells [75]. Engagement of 2B4, NTB-A and CRACC on MHC I-negative targets (i.e., stressed cells) activates NK-cell cytotoxicity, while 2B4, NTB-A, or CRACC-expressing, MHC I-positive cells (i.e., neighboring NK cells) are spared [76].

Signaling of SLAM-family members is distinct from that of other NK-cell receptors as they do not recruit traditional ITAM-containing adaptor proteins such as DAP10 or DAP12. Rather, the

121

cytoplasmic domains contain tyrosine-based motifs that undergo phosphorylation to recruit SH2-domain containing SLAM-associated protein (SAP) or Ewing's sarcoma-activated transcripts-2 (EAT-2). In mice, the SLAM-family receptors can exhibit either activating or inhibitory functions, depending on the adaptor that they recruit; however, in humans, SLAM-family receptors have only been shown to be stimulatory [77].

F. Additional NK receptors

In addition to directly lysing target cells, NK also work in concert with B lymphocytes to mediate antibody-dependent cellular cytotoxicity (ADCC) [78]. NK express CD16 which binds IgG-opsonized cells (Figure 9.3). The activating CD16 then associates with ITAM-containing CD3ζ and FCRγ to bind Syk and proceed through the NK activation pathway to ultimately lyse the target cell [79].

NK cells also express an array of receptors that promote the formation of NK-cell–target cell conjugates and therefore act as coreceptors for the lytic granule inducing receptors. Some of these receptors have signaling capacity that promotes activation and cytotoxicity in addition to enhancing adhesion. Others primarily function to form and maintain the contacts between the NK cell and the target cell. Typically, these receptors recognize adhesion molecules present on the target cells. The primary adhesion receptor that is required for stable conjugate formation is leukocyte function associated antigen 1 (LFA-1) (Figure 9.3)[80], an integrin that binds to intercellular adhesion molecule 1 (ICAM-1). The binding of LFA-1 to ICAM-1 results in actin polymerization for enhanced adhesion to the target cell [81]. LFA-1 has been demonstrated as a co-activator during NCR-mediated stromal cell killing and NKG2D-mediated killing of dendritic cells [82]. Another important activating receptor is DNAX accessory molecule-1 (DNAM-1), which also potentiates adhesion and cytotoxicity (Figure 9.3) [31,83] and may have a role in NK-cell migration [84]. The ligands for DNAM-1 in humans are CD155 (polio virus receptor (PVR) or Nectin-5), and CD112 (Nectin-2), both of which are upregulated on tumor cells [85], suggesting a role for the receptor in tumor cell lysis [86]. DNAM-1 signaling is dependent upon Fyn [83], and downstream signaling is dependent upon association with LFA-1 [87]. Two additional receptors that recognize Nectins are class I-restricted T-cell-associated molecule (CRTAM) which binds Necl-2 and enhances NK activation, and CD96 (Tactile), which recognizes Necl-5 and primarily promotes adhesion, but not activation (Figure 9.3). Another molecule that promotes NK-cell–target cell interactions is CD100 (or Semaphorin 4D (SEMA4D)) (Figure 9.3), which potentiates enhanced cytotoxicity and cytokine production upon CD72 ligation by enhancing the adhesion between NK cells and their targets [88]. CD72 is primarily expressed on B cells [89], implicating this interaction in NK-mediated killing of stressed B cells.

In addition to receptors that bind adhesion molecules on target cells and thus promote NK-target cell cytotoxicity, NK cells also exhibit receptors that recognize adhesion molecules, yet are inhibitory. KLRG1 is an ITIM-containing inhibitory receptor that recognizes the classical cadherins, E-, N-, and R-cadherin (Figure 9.3)[90]. Reduced levels of E-cadherin in malignant epithelial tumors correlate with tumor metastasis, suggesting a potential role for NK detection of malignant epithelia [91]. LAIR-1 recognizes a common collagen motif and contains a single extracellular Ig-like domain and two cytoplasmic tyrosine-based inhibitory motifs (ITIMs) (Figure 9.3)[92]. Cross-linking of LAIR-1 on NK cells delivers a potent inhibitory signal that is capable of inhibiting target cell lysis mediated by resting and activated NK cells [92,93] and B cells [94].

Other receptors can help to differentiate subsets of NK cells. While some have known signaling functions, others have only been identified as developmental markers. A major marker for NK subsets is CD56 (Figure 9.3); CD56^{lo} cells constitute the majority of circulating NK cells and exhibit high cytotoxicity capacity to target cells. Conversely, CD56^{hi} cells constitute approximately 10% of circulating NK cells and produce IFNγ but have low cytolytic capacity. In addition, CD27 is expressed on the CD56[hi] subset of NK and binds CD70 (Figure 9.3)[95], and this interaction promotes NK-mediated cytotoxicity and primes CD8+ T-cell responses [96]. Moreover, NK-cell differentiation is accompanied by expression of a post-translation modification of P-selectin glycoprotein ligand-1 (PSGL-1), deemed the PEN5 epitope, that allows for binding to the integrin L-selectin, suggesting that PEN5/PSGL-1 potentially serves as a NK-homing/trafficking receptor [97]. Of note, NK cells also express non-KIR MHC I-specific inhibitory receptors. For example, Lilr1b (ILT2/CD85j /LIR-1), which is a potent MHC I-binding inhibitory receptor, possesses four ITIMs in its cytoplasmic tail (Figure 9.3)[98].

Aberrantly expressed glycoproteins and glycolipids have recently been characterized as tumor markers and can be engaged by sialic acid-binding immunoglobulin (Ig)-like lectins (Siglecs) which are broadly expressed on hematopoietic cells. Of the receptors, Siglec 3 (CD33) is expressed on activated NK cells and contains two ITIMs that negatively regulate NK-cell activation (Figure 9.3)[99,100]. Siglec-7 (p70/AIRM) and Siglec-9 are CD33-related Siglecs that are also expressed on NK cells (Figure 9.3) [101] and have been implicated in clinical pathogenesis. Decreased Siglec-7 expression is an early marker of NK dysfunction and high viral load in HIV infections [102]. Furthermore, Siglec-7 expressed on NK preferentially binds internally branched $\alpha2,6$-linked disialic gangliosides such as disialosyl globopentaosylcer-amide (DSGb5), a ganglioside upregulated on renal cell carcinoma that contributes to metastases [103]. Siglec-9's ligand is MUC-16 [104], which is overexpressed in cancer [105] and functions to inhibit NK-cell-mediated antitumor responses [106] by acting as an anti-adhesive molecule and preventing the formation of the immunological synapse between target cells and NK cells [107].

V. CONCLUSION

NK cells are a crucial part of the first line immune response, particularly in the context of cancer. In contrast to T cells, which are negatively selected and clonally deleted in the thymus if they exhibit self-reactivity, NK cells are genetically primed to tolerate self MHC and yet recognize and kill malignant tissue through detection of aberrantly expressed self-proteins. Through an array of receptors, NK cells can differentiate stressed cancerous cells from healthy tissue, and the balance of inhibitory and activating signals that result from the interactions determines the fate of the putative malignancy (Figure 9.3). Unfortunately, tumors can evade NK-cell-mediated destruction by secretion of immunosuppressive molecules and/or shedding soluble variants of activating receptor ligands. Therefore, in the tumor microenvironment, NK-cell function is compromised. Identifying mechanisms that maintain the expression of stimulatory receptors may provide therapeutic benefit by shifting the intratumoral NK cell towards an aggressive and active phenotype that is ready to detect and destroy invading malignancies.

123

References

[1] Elliott JM, Yokoyama WM. Unifying concepts of MHC-dependent natural killer cell education. Trends Immunol 2011 Aug;32(8):364—72.

[2] Anfossi N, Andre P, Guia S, Falk CS, Roetynck S, Stewart CA, et al. Human NK cell education by inhibitory receptors for MHC class I. Immunity 2006 Aug;25(2):331—42.

[3] Chalifour A, Scarpellino L, Back J, Brodin P, Devevre E, Gros F, et al. A Role for cis Interaction between the Inhibitory Ly49A receptor and MHC class I for natural killer cell education. Immunity 2009 Mar 20;30(3):337—47.

[4] Kim S, Poursine-Laurent J, Truscott SM, Lybarger L, Song YJ, Yang L, et al. Licensing of natural killer cells by host major histocompatibility complex class I molecules. Nature 2005 Aug 4;436(7051):709—13.

[5] Joncker NT, Shifrin N, Delebecque F, Raulet DH. Mature natural killer cells reset their responsiveness when exposed to an altered MHC environment. J Exp Med 2010 Sep 27;207(10):2065—72.

[6] Juelke K, Killig M, Thiel A, Dong J, Romagnani C. Education of hyporesponsive NK cells by cytokines. Eur J Immunol 2009 Sep;39(9):2548—55.

[7] Fehniger TA, Bluman EM, Porter MM, Mrozek E, Cooper MA, VanDeusen JB, et al. Potential mechanisms of human natural killer cell expansion in vivo during low-dose IL-2 therapy. J Clin Invest 2000 Jul;106(1):117–24.

[8] Warren HS, Kinnear BF, Kastelein RL, Lanier LL. Analysis of the costimulatory role of IL-2 and IL-15 in initiating proliferation of resting (CD56dim) human NK cells. J Immunol 1996 May 1;156(9):3254–9.

[9] Lotzova E, Savary CA, Herberman RB. Induction of NK cell activity against fresh human leukemia in culture with interleukin 2. J Immunol 1987 Apr 15;138(8):2718–27.

[10] Brilot F, Strowig T, Roberts SM, Arrey F, Munz C. NK cell survival mediated through the regulatory synapse with human DCs requires IL-15Ralpha. J Clin Invest 2007 Nov;117(11):3316–29.

[11] Carson WE, Giri JG, Lindemann MJ, Linett ML, Ahdieh M, Paxton R, et al. Interleukin (IL) 15 is a novel cytokine that activates human natural killer cells via components of the IL-2 receptor. J Exp Med 1994 Oct 1;180(4):1395–403.

[12] Ferlazzo G, Pack M, Thomas D, Paludan C, Schmid D, Strowig T, et al. Distinct roles of IL-12 and IL-15 in human natural killer cell activation by dendritic cells from secondary lymphoid organs. Proc Natl Acad Sci U S A 2004 Nov 23;101(47):16606–11.

[13] Ferlazzo G, Thomas D, Lin SL, Goodman K, Morandi B, Muller WA, et al. The abundant NK cells in human secondary lymphoid tissues require activation to express killer cell Ig-like receptors and become cytolytic. J Immunol 2004 Feb 1;172(3):1455–62.

[14] Loza MJ, Perussia B. The IL-12 signature: NK cell terminal CD56+high stage and effector functions. J Immunol 2004 Jan 1;172(1):88–96.

[15] Wendt K, Wilk E, Buyny S, Schmidt RE, Jacobs R. Interleukin-21 differentially affects human natural killer cell subsets. Immunology 2007 Dec;122(4):486–95.

[16] Girart MV, Fuertes MB, Domaica CI, Rossi LE, Zwirner NW. Engagement of TLR3, TLR7, and NKG2D regulate IFN-gamma secretion but not NKG2D-mediated cytotoxicity by human NK cells stimulated with suboptimal doses of IL-12. J Immunol 2007 Sep 15;179(6):3472–9.

[17] Wu CY, Gadina M, Wang K, O'Shea J, Seder RA. Cytokine regulation of IL-12 receptor beta2 expression: differential effects on human T and NK cells. Eur J Immunol 2000 May;30(5):1364–74.

[18] Skak K, Frederiksen KS, Lundsgaard D. Interleukin-21 activates human natural killer cells and modulates their surface receptor expression. Immunology 2008 Apr;123(4):575–83.

[19] Hodge DL, Subleski JJ, Reynolds DA, Buschman MD, Schill WB, Burkett MW, et al. The proinflammatory cytokine interleukin-18 alters multiple signaling pathways to inhibit natural killer cell death. J Interferon Cytokine Res 2006 Oct;26(10):706–18.

[20] Malejczyk J, Malejczyk M, Urbanski A, Kock A, Jablonska S, Orth G, et al. Constitutive release of IL6 by human papillomavirus type 16 (HPV16)-harboring keratinocytes: a mechanism augmenting the NK-cell-mediated lysis of HPV-bearing neoplastic cells. Cell Immunol 1991 Aug;136(1):155–64.

[21] Passos ST, Silver JS, O'Hara AC, Sehy D, Stumhofer JS, Hunter CA. IL-6 promotes NK cell production of IL-17 during toxoplasmosis. J Immunol 2010 Feb 15;184(4):1776–83.

[22] Nguyen KB, Salazar-Mather TP, Dalod MY, Van Deusen JB, Wei XQ, Liew FY, et al. Coordinated and distinct roles for IFN-alpha beta, IL-12, and IL-15 regulation of NK cell responses to viral infection. J Immunol 2002 Oct 15;169(8):4279–87.

[23] Sato K, Hida S, Takayanagi H, Yokochi T, Kayagaki N, Takeda K, et al. Antiviral response by natural killer cells through TRAIL gene induction by IFN-alpha/beta. Eur J Immunol 2001 Nov;31(11):3138–46.

[24] Lanier LL. DAP10- and DAP12-associated receptors in innate immunity. Immunol Rev 2009 Jan;227(1):150–60.

[25] Doucey MA, Scarpellino L, Zimmer J, Guillaume P, Luescher IF, Bron C, et al. Cis association of Ly49A with MHC class I restricts natural killer cell inhibition. Nat Immunol 2004 Mar;5(3):328–36.

[26] Scarpellino L, Oeschger F, Guillaume P, Coudert JD, Levy F, Leclercq G, et al. Interactions of Ly49 family receptors with MHC class I ligands in trans and cis. J Immunol 2007 Feb 1;178(3):1277–84.

[27] Jiang K, Zhong B, Gilvary DL, Corliss BC, Vivier E, Hong-Geller E, et al. Syk regulation of phosphoinositide 3-kinase-dependent NK cell function. J Immunol 2002 Apr 1;168(7):3155–64.

[28] Lanier LL, Corliss BC, Wu J, Leong C, Phillips JH. Immunoreceptor DAP12 bearing a tyrosine-based activation motif is involved in activating NK cells. Nature 1998 Feb 12;391(6668):703–7.

[29] Jiang K, Zhong B, Gilvary DL, Corliss BC, Hong-Geller E, Wei S, et al. Pivotal role of phosphoinositide-3 kinase in regulation of cytotoxicity in natural killer cells. Nat Immunol 2000 Nov;1(5):419–25.

[30] Djeu JY, Jiang K, Wei S. A view to a kill: signals triggering cytotoxicity. Clin Cancer Res 2002 Mar;8(3):636–40.

[31] Tassi I, Cella M, Presti R, Colucci A, Gilfillan S, Littman DR, et al. NK cell-activating receptors require PKC-theta for sustained signaling, transcriptional activation, and IFN-gamma secretion. Blood 2008 Nov 15;112(10):4109–16.

[32] Sutherland CL, Chalupny NJ, Schooley K, VandenBos T, Kubin M, Cosman D. UL16-binding proteins, novel MHC class I-related proteins, bind to NKG2D and activate multiple signaling pathways in primary NK cells. J Immunol 2002 Jan 15;168(2):671–9.

[33] Binstadt BA, Brumbaugh KM, Dick CJ, Scharenberg AM, Williams BL, Colonna M, et al. Sequential involvement of Lck and SHP-1 with MHC-recognizing receptors on NK cells inhibits FcR-initiated tyrosine kinase activation. Immunity 1996 Dec;5(6):629—38.

[34] Burshtyn DN, Scharenberg AM, Wagtmann N, Rajagopalan S, Berrada K, Yi T, et al. Recruitment of tyrosine phosphatase HCP by the killer cell inhibitor receptor. Immunity 1996 Jan;4(1):77—85.

[35] McVicar DW, Burshtyn DN. Intracellular signaling by the killer immunoglobulin-like receptors and Ly49. Sci STKE 2001 Mar 27;2001(75): re1.

[36] Graef T, Moesta AK, Norman PJ, Abi-Rached L, Vago L, Older Aguilar AM, et al. KIR2DS4 is a product of gene conversion with KIR3DL2 that introduced specificity for HLA-A*11 while diminishing avidity for HLA-C. J Exp Med 2009 Oct 26;206(11):2557—72.

[37] Katz G, Gazit R, Arnon TI, Gonen-Gross T, Tarcic G, Markel G, et al. MHC class I-independent recognition of NK-activating receptor KIR2DS4. J Immunol 2004 Aug 1;173(3):1819—25.

[38] Giebel S, Nowak I, Wojnar J, Krawczyk-Kulis M, Holowiecki J, Kyrcz-Krzemien S, et al. Association of KIR2DS4 and its variant KIR1D with leukemia. Leukemia 2008 Nov;22(11):2129—30, discussion 30—1.

[39] Winter CC, Long EO. A single amino acid in the p58 killer cell inhibitory receptor controls the ability of natural killer cells to discriminate between the two groups of HLA-C allotypes. J Immunol 1997 May 1;158(9):4026—8.

[40] Cella M, Longo A, Ferrara GB, Strominger JL, Colonna M. NK3-specific natural killer cells are selectively inhibited by Bw4-positive HLA alleles with isoleucine 80. J Exp Med 1994 Oct 1;180(4):1235—42.

[41] Carr WH, Pando MJ, Parham P. KIR3DL1 polymorphisms that affect NK cell inhibition by HLA-Bw4 ligand. J Immunol 2005 Oct 15;175(8):5222—9.

[42] Dohring C, Scheidegger D, Samaridis J, Cella M, Colonna M. A human killer inhibitory receptor specific for HLA-A1,2. J Immunol 1996 May 1;156(9):3098—101.

[43] Santourlidis S, Trompeter HI, Weinhold S, Eisermann B, Meyer KL, Wernet P, et al. Crucial role of DNA methylation in determination of clonally distributed killer cell Ig-like receptor expression patterns in NK cells. J Immunol 2002 Oct 15;169(8):4253—61.

[44] Moretta L, Moretta A. Killer immunoglobulin-like receptors. Curr Opin Immunol 2004 Oct;16(5):626—33.

[45] Kulkarni S, Martin MP, Carrington M. The Yin and Yang of HLA and KIR in human disease. Semin Immunol 2008 Dec;20(6):343—52.

[46] Sivori S, Pende D, Bottino C, Marcenaro E, Pessino A, Biassoni R, et al. NKp46 is the major triggering receptor involved in the natural cytotoxicity of fresh or cultured human NK cells. Correlation between surface density of NKp46 and natural cytotoxicity against autologous, allogeneic or xenogeneic target cells. Eur J Immunol 1999 May;29(5):1656—66.

[47] Ghio M, Contini P, Negrini S, Boero S, Musso A, Poggi A. Soluble HLA-I-mediated secretion of TGF-beta1 by human NK cells and consequent down-regulation of anti-tumor cytolytic activity. Eur J Immunol 2009 Dec;39(12):3459—68.

[48] Moretta A. Natural killer cells and dendritic cells: rendezvous in abused tissues. Nat Rev Immunol 2002 Dec;2(12):957—64.

[49] Cantoni C, Bottino C, Vitale M, Pessino A, Augugliaro R, Malaspina A, et al. NKp44, a triggering receptor involved in tumor cell lysis by activated human natural killer cells, is a novel member of the immunoglobulin superfamily. J Exp Med 1999 Mar 1;189(5):787—96.

[50] Pessino A, Sivori S, Bottino C, Malaspina A, Morelli L, Moretta L, et al. Molecular cloning of NKp46: a novel member of the immunoglobulin superfamily involved in triggering of natural cytotoxicity. J Exp Med 1998 Sep 7;188(5):953—60.

[51] Pende D, Parolini S, Pessino A, Sivori S, Augugliaro R, Morelli L, et al. Identification and molecular characterization of NKp30, a novel triggering receptor involved in natural cytotoxicity mediated by human natural killer cells. J Exp Med 1999 Nov 15;190(10):1505—16.

[52] Mandelboim O, Lieberman N, Lev M, Paul L, Arnon TI, Bushkin Y, et al. Recognition of haemagglutinins on virus-infected cells by NKp46 activates lysis by human NK cells. Nature 2001 Feb 22;409(6823):1055—60.

[53] Bloushtain N, Qimron U, Bar-Ilan A, Hershkovitz O, Gazit R, Fima E, et al. Membrane-associated heparan sulfate proteoglycans are involved in the recognition of cellular targets by NKp30 and NKp46. J Immunol 2004 Aug 15;173(4):2392—401.

[54] Pogge von Strandmann E, Simhadri VR, von Tresckow B, Sasse S, Reiners KS, Hansen HP, et al. Human leukocyte antigen-B-associated transcript 3 is released from tumor cells and engages the NKp30 receptor on natural killer cells. Immunity 2007 Dec;27(6):965—74.

[55] Brandt CS, Baratin M, Yi EC, Kennedy J, Gao Z, Fox B, et al. The B7 family member B7-H6 is a tumor cell ligand for the activating natural killer cell receptor NKp30 in humans. J Exp Med 2009 Jul 6;206(7):1495—503.

[56] Arnon TI, Achdout H, Levi O, Markel G, Saleh N, Katz G, et al. Inhibition of the NKp30 activating receptor by pp65 of human cytomegalovirus. Nat Immunol 2005 May;6(5):515—23.

[57] Tomlinson MG, Lin J, Weiss A. Lymphocytes with a complex: adapter proteins in antigen receptor signaling. Immunol Today 2000 Nov;21(11):584–91.

[58] Dennehy KM, Klimosch SN, Steinle A. Cutting edge: NKp80 uses an atypical hemi-ITAM to trigger NK cytotoxicity. J Immunol 2011 Jan 15;186(2):657–61.

[59] Groh V, Bahram S, Bauer S, Herman A, Beauchamp M, Spies T. Cell stress-regulated human major histocompatibility complex class I gene expressed in gastrointestinal epithelium. Proc Natl Acad Sci U S A 1996 Oct 29;93(22):12445–50.

[60] Groh V, Rhinehart R, Secrist H, Bauer S, Grabstein KH, Spies T. Broad tumor-associated expression and recognition by tumor-derived gamma delta T cells of MICA and MICB. Proc Natl Acad Sci U S A 1999 Jun 8;96(12):6879–84.

[61] Bauer S, Groh V, Wu J, Steinle A, Phillips JH, Lanier LL, et al. Activation of NK cells and T cells by NKG2D, a receptor for stress-inducible MICA. Science 1999 Jul 30;285(5428):727–9.

[62] Steinle A, Li P, Morris DL, Groh V, Lanier LL, Strong RK, et al. Interactions of human NKG2D with its ligands MICA, MICB, and homologs of the mouse RAE-1 protein family. Immunogenetics 2001 May-Jun;53(4):279–87.

[63] Cosman D, Mullberg J, Sutherland CL, Chin W, Armitage R, Fanslow W, et al. ULBPs, novel MHC class I-related molecules, bind to CMV glycoprotein UL16 and stimulate NK cytotoxicity through the NKG2D receptor. Immunity 2001 Feb;14(2):123–33.

[64] Westwood JA, Kelly JM, Tanner JE, Kershaw MH, Smyth MJ, Hayakawa Y. Cutting edge: novel priming of tumor-specific immunity by NKG2D-triggered NK cell-mediated tumor rejection and Th1-independent CD4+ T cell pathway. J Immunol 2004 Jan 15;172(2):757–61.

[65] Castriconi R, Cantoni C, Della Chiesa M, Vitale M, Marcenaro E, Conte R, et al. Transforming growth factor beta 1 inhibits expression of NKp30 and NKG2D receptors: consequences for the NK-mediated killing of dendritic cells. Proc Natl Acad Sci U S A 2003 Apr 1;100(7):4120–5.

[66] Eisele G, Wischhusen J, Mittelbronn M, Meyermann R, Waldhauer I, Steinle A, et al. TGF-beta and metalloproteinases differentially suppress NKG2D ligand surface expression on malignant glioma cells. Brain 2006 Sep;129(Pt 9):2416–25.

[67] Groh V, Wu J, Yee C, Spies T. Tumour-derived soluble MIC ligands impair expression of NKG2D and T-cell activation. Nature 2002 Oct 17;419(6908):734–8.

[68] Borrego F, Ulbrecht M, Weiss EH, Coligan JE, Brooks AG. Recognition of human histocompatibility leukocyte antigen (HLA)-E complexed with HLA class I signal sequence-derived peptides by CD94/NKG2 confers protection from natural killer cell-mediated lysis. J Exp Med 1998 Mar 2;187(5):813–8.

[69] Barakonyi A, Rabot M, Marie-Cardine A, Aguerre-Girr M, Polgar B, Schiavon V, et al. Cutting edge: engagement of CD160 by its HLA-C physiological ligand triggers a unique cytokine profile secretion in the cytotoxic peripheral blood NK cell subset. J Immunol 2004 Nov 1;173(9):5349–54.

[70] Le Bouteiller P, Tabiasco J, Polgar B, Kozma N, Giustiniani J, Siewiera J, et al. CD160: a unique activating NK cell receptor. Immunol Lett 2011 Aug 30;138(2):93–6.

[71] Rabot M, El Costa H, Polgar B, Marie-Cardine A, Aguerre-Girr M, Barakonyi A, et al. CD160-activating NK cell effector functions depend on the phosphatidylinositol 3-kinase recruitment. Int Immunol 2007 Apr;19(4):401–9.

[72] Giustiniani J, Bensussan A, Marie-Cardine A. Identification and characterization of a transmembrane isoform of CD160 (CD160-TM), a unique activating receptor selectively expressed upon human NK cell activation. J Immunol 2009 Jan 1;182(1):63–71.

[73] Fons P, Chabot S, Cartwright JE, Lenfant F, L'Faqihi F, Giustiniani J, et al. Soluble HLA-G1 inhibits angiogenesis through an apoptotic pathway and by direct binding to CD160 receptor expressed by endothelial cells. Blood 2006 Oct 15;108(8):2608–15.

[74] Cai G, Freeman GJ. The CD160, BTLA, LIGHT/HVEM pathway: a bidirectional switch regulating T-cell activation. Immunol Rev 2009 May;229(1):244–58.

[75] Latchman Y, Reiser H. Enhanced murine CD4+ T cell responses induced by the CD2 ligand CD48. Eur J Immunol 1998 Dec;28(12):4325–31.

[76] Stark S, Watzl C. 2B4 (CD244), NTB-A and CRACC (CS1) stimulate cytotoxicity but no proliferation in human NK cells. Int Immunol 2006 Feb;18(2):241–7.

[77] Veillette A, Dong Z, Latour S. Consequence of the SLAM-SAP signaling pathway in innate-like and conventional lymphocytes. Immunity 2007 Nov;27(5):698–710.

[78] Leibson PJ. Signal transduction during natural killer cell activation: inside the mind of a killer. Immunity 1997 Jun;6(6):655–61.

[79] Lanier LL, Yu G, Phillips JH. Analysis of Fc gamma RIII (CD16) membrane expression and association with CD3 zeta and Fc epsilon RI-gamma by site-directed mutation. J Immunol 1991 Mar 1;146(5):1571–6.

[80] Fuchs A, Colonna M. The role of NK cell recognition of nectin and nectin-like proteins in tumor immunosurveillance. Semin Cancer Biol 2006 Oct;16(5):359–66.

[81] Mace EM, Zhang J, Siminovitch KA, Takei F. Elucidation of the integrin LFA-1-mediated signaling pathway of actin polarization in natural killer cells. Blood 2010 Aug 26;116(8):1272–9.

[82] Poggi A, Zocchi MR. Antigen presenting cells and stromal cells trigger human natural killer lymphocytes to autoreactivity: evidence for the involvement of natural cytotoxicity receptors (NCR) and NKG2D. Clin Dev Immunol 2006 Jun-Dec;13(2-4):325–36.

[83] Shibuya A, Campbell D, Hannum C, Yssel H, Franz-Bacon K, McClanahan T, et al. DNAM-1, a novel adhesion molecule involved in the cytolytic function of T lymphocytes. Immunity 1996 Jun;4(6):573–81.

[84] Reymond N, Imbert AM, Devilard E, Fabre S, Chabannon C, Xerri L, et al. DNAM-1 and PVR regulate monocyte migration through endothelial junctions. J Exp Med 2004 May 17;199(10):1331–41.

[85] Soriani A, Zingoni A, Cerboni C, Iannitto ML, Ricciardi MR, Di Gialleonardo V, et al. ATM-ATR-dependent up-regulation of DNAM-1 and NKG2D ligands on multiple myeloma cells by therapeutic agents results in enhanced NK-cell susceptibility and is associated with a senescent phenotype. Blood 2009 Apr 9;113(15):3503–11.

[86] Gilfillan S, Chan CJ, Cella M, Haynes NM, Rapaport AS, Boles KS, et al. DNAM-1 promotes activation of cytotoxic lymphocytes by nonprofessional antigen-presenting cells and tumors. J Exp Med 2008 Dec 22;205(13):2965–73.

[87] Shibuya K, Lanier LL, Phillips JH, Ochs HD, Shimizu K, Nakayama E, et al. Physical and functional association of LFA-1 with DNAM-1 adhesion molecule. Immunity 1999 Nov;11(5):615–23.

[88] Mizrahi S, Markel G, Porgador A, Bushkin Y, Mandelboim O. CD100 on NK cells enhance IFNgamma secretion and killing of target cells expressing CD72. PLoS One 2007;2(9):e818.

[89] Kumanogoh A, Watanabe C, Lee I, Wang X, Shi W, Araki H, et al. Identification of CD72 as a lymphocyte receptor for the class IV semaphorin CD100: a novel mechanism for regulating B cell signaling. Immunity 2000 Nov;13(5):621–31.

[90] Ito M, Maruyama T, Saito N, Koganei S, Yamamoto K, Matsumoto N. Killer cell lectin-like receptor G1 binds three members of the classical cadherin family to inhibit NK cell cytotoxicity. J Exp Med 2006 Feb 20;203(2):289–95.

[91] Colonna M. Cytolytic responses: cadherins put out the fire. J Exp Med 2006 Feb 20;203(2):261–4.

[92] Meyaard L. The inhibitory collagen receptor LAIR-1 (CD305). J Leukoc Biol 2008 Apr;83(4):799–803.

[93] Meyaard L, Adema GJ, Chang C, Woollatt E, Sutherland GR, Lanier LL, et al. LAIR-1, a novel inhibitory receptor expressed on human mononuclear leukocytes. Immunity 1997 Aug;7(2):283–90.

[94] Merlo A, Tenca C, Fais F, Battini L, Ciccone E, Grossi CE, et al. Inhibitory receptors CD85j, LAIR-1, and CD152 down-regulate immunoglobulin and cytokine production by human B lymphocytes. Clin Diagn Lab Immunol 2005 Jun;12(6):705–12.

[95] Vossen MT, Matmati M, Hertoghs KM, Baars PA, Gent MR, Leclercq G, et al. CD27 defines phenotypically and functionally different human NK cell subsets. J Immunol 2008 Mar 15;180(6):3739–45.

[96] Kelly JM, Darcy PK, Markby JL, Godfrey DI, Takeda K, Yagita H, et al. Induction of tumor-specific T cell memory by NK cell-mediated tumor rejection. Nat Immunol 2002 Jan;3(1):83–90.

[97] Andre P, Spertini O, Guia S, Rihet P, Dignat-George F, Brailly H, et al. Modification of P-selectin glycoprotein ligand-1 with a natural killer cell-restricted sulfated lactosamine creates an alternate ligand for L-selectin. Proc Natl Acad Sci U S A 2000 Mar 28;97(7):3400–5.

[98] Cosman D, Fanger N, Borges L, Kubin M, Chin W, Peterson L, et al. A novel immunoglobulin superfamily receptor for cellular and viral MHC class I molecules. Immunity 1997 Aug;7(2):273–82.

[99] Vivier E, Daeron M. Immunoreceptor tyrosine-based inhibition motifs. Immunol Today 1997 Jun;18(6):286–91.

[100] Ulyanova T, Blasioli J, Woodford-Thomas TA, Thomas ML. The sialoadhesin CD33 is a myeloid-specific inhibitory receptor. Eur J Immunol 1999 Nov;29(11):3440–9.

[101] Ikehara Y, Ikehara SK, Paulson JC. Negative regulation of T cell receptor signaling by Siglec-7 (p70/AIRM) and Siglec-9. J Biol Chem 2004 Oct 8;279(41):43117–25.

[102] Brunetta E, Fogli M, Varchetta S, Bozzo L, Hudspeth KL, Marcenaro E, et al. The decreased expression of Siglec-7 represents an early marker of dysfunctional natural killer-cell subsets associated with high levels of HIV-1 viremia. Blood 2009 Oct 29;114(18):3822–30.

[103] Kawasaki Y, Ito A, Withers DA, Taima T, Kakoi N, Saito S, et al. Ganglioside DSGb5, preferred ligand for Siglec-7, inhibits NK cell cytotoxicity against renal cell carcinoma cells. Glycobiology 2010 Nov;20(11):1373–9.

[104] Belisle JA, Horibata S, Jennifer GA, Petrie S, Kapur A, Andre S, et al. Identification of Siglec-9 as the receptor for MUC16 on human NK cells, B cells, and monocytes. Mol Cancer 2010;9:118.

[105] Niloff JM, Knapp RC, Schaetzl E, Reynolds C, Bast Jr RC. CA125 antigen levels in obstetric and gynecologic patients. Obstet Gynecol 1984 Nov;64(5):703–7.

[106] Patankar MS, Jing Y, Morrison JC, Belisle JA, Lattanzio FA, Deng Y, et al. Potent suppression of natural killer cell response mediated by the ovarian tumor marker CA125. Gynecol Oncol 2005 Dec;99(3):704–13.

[107] Gubbels JA, Felder M, Horibata S, Belisle JA, Kapur A, Holden H, et al. MUC16 provides immune protection by inhibiting synapse formation between NK and ovarian tumor cells. Mol Cancer 2010;9:11.

CHAPTER 10

Th17 Cells in Cancer

Ende Zhao[1,2], Lin Wang[2], Shuang Wei[1], Ilona Kryczek[1], Weiping Zou[1,3,4]
[1]Department of Surgery, University of Michigan School of Medicine, Ann Arbor, MI USA
[2]Central Laboratory, Union Hospital, Tongji Medical College, Huazhong University of Science and Technology, Wuhan, China
[3]Graduate Program in Immunology and Cancer Biology, University of Michigan School of Medicine, Ann Arbor, MI USA
[4]University of Michigan Comprehensive Cancer Center, University of Michigan School of Medicine, Ann Arbor, MI USA

I. Th17 DEFINITION

CD4[+] T helper cells (Th) are important mediators in immune response, inflammatory diseases and cancer. Antigen-specific effector CD4[+] T helper cells have been specialized into traditional Th1 and Th2 subsets based on the cytokine profiles and immune function under distinct cytokine and genetic regulation after they are activated by antigen-presenting cells (APC) [1,2]. Th1 cells regulate cellular immunity by producing interferon (IFN)-γ and Th2 cells mediate humoral immunity by secreting interleukin-4 (IL-4), IL-5 and IL-13 [2]. Among CD4[+] T helper cells, there is a subset which secretes the cytokine IL-17 (also known as IL-17A) and plays a crucial role in regulating inflammatory responses [3–5]. These IL-17-secreting CD4[+] T cells have been defined as T helper 17 (Th17) cells since 2005 [5]. Th17 cells are composed of approximately 1% of CD4[+] T cells in peripheral blood in healthy donors [6]. Th17 cells have been proposed to play important roles in many human diseases including inflammation, autoimmune diseases and cancer [7].

II. GENERATION, CYTOKINE PROFILE AND GENETIC CONTROL OF Th17 CELLS
A. Generation

The development of Th17 cells is distinct from that of other traditional T-cell subsets, such as Th1, Th2 and regulatory T (Treg) cells, and is characterized by unique transcriptional factors and cytokine requirements [7–10]. It has been shown that IL-2 reduces Th17-cell development and IL-6 and transforming growth factor beta (TGF-β) mediate the differentiation of Th17 cells [6,11]. IL-6 and TGF-β are considered as the priming cytokines of Th17 lineage [8]. Our group has demonstrated that IL-1 plays a predominant role in inducing Th17-cell production and completely subverts IL-2-mediated suppression on Th17-cell development [12]. We also provided evidence showing that IL-6 is an important but not indispensible factor for Th17 differentiation [6]. IL-23 has been reported to be a crucial regulator of IL-17 expression and a selective inducer of Th17 population [13], and maintains Th17-cells survival and expansion [11]. Furthermore, Th17 differentiation can be antagonized by Th1 and Th2-related cytokines [4,5,14]. However, our group has demonstrated evidence which challenges the dogma of the effect of IFN-γ on Th1 and Th17-cell development by showing that IFN-γ induces memory Th17-cells expansion through triggering IL-1 and IL-23 production of APCs in a B7-H1-independent manner [15–17]. And IFN-γ

129

Cancer Immunotherapy. http://dx.doi.org/10.1016/B978-0-12-394296-8.00010-5

stimulates the migration of Th17 cells by inducing the production of CC chemokine ligand 20 (CCL20, also known as MIP3α) by APCs [16].

Th17 cells share TGF-β with Treg cells during their development, but in the presence of IL-6, naïve CD4$^+$ T cells prefer the commitment to Th17 development. TGF-β is considered an essential regulator for Treg-cells differentiation [11]. However, the involvement of IL-6 and TGF-β in human Th17 development remains controversial because limited numbers of Th17 cells are detected compared with those of Treg and other T-cell subsets in tumor microenvironment which contains high amounts of IL-6 and TGF-β [18,19]. Moreover, our group has reported the induction of Th17 cells by myeloid APCs isolated from ovarian cancer patients is inhibited by blocking IL-1β, but not IL-6 or TGF-β [12]. Therefore, it indicates IL-1β, but not IL-1α, IL-6, IL-23 or TGF-β, is crucial for the induction of Th17 cells by tumor-associated myeloid APCs in human [7,12]. It is worth stressing that the development of Th17 cells largely depends on the context of the ongoing immune response and the components of the cytokine milieu, which can be influenced by disease progression [20].

B. Cytokine profile

IL-17 is the lineage characteristic cytokine of Th17 cells and the founding member of the IL-17 cytokine family (IL-17A-F) (Table 10.1) [7,21]. Human IL-17 is initially found to be derived from activated human CD4$^+$ T cells [3]. IL-17 has an essential proinflammatory activity by inducing the production of IL-6 and granulocyte colony-stimulating factor (G-CSF) [22,23]. IL-17-deficient mice are shown to be resistant to distinct autoimmune diseases [24,25]. There are contradictory observations on the effect of IL-17 on tumor biology by showing that IL-17 has either antitumor or protumor activity [7,26,27]. Details will be provided later. IL-17 is not exclusively produced by Th17 cells, and it has been reported to be expressed by a variety of other innate and adaptive immune cells, including CD8 (Tc17 cells) and Treg cells (Table 10.1) [20,28–33].

As another member of the IL-17 family cytokines, IL-17F is reported to be produced by Th17 cells [11,13,34] and it has a significantly weaker effect compared to IL-17 and can induce the expression of various cytokines, chemokines and adhesion molecules [35–37]. IL-17F can form a heterodimer with IL-17 which signals through the IL-17RA/IL-17RC receptor complex [38]. Several other cytokines are shown to be expressed by Th17 cells. Th17 cells are reported to produce high levels of IL-21 which is induced by IL-6 in a STAT3-dependent manner [39–41]. IL-21 is shown to regulate Th17-cell differentiation in an autocrine manner [8,40,41]. IL-22 is a member of the IL-10 family and is reported to be produced by Th17 cells [42–44]. Interestingly, IL-22 was reported to synergize IL-17 to promote an inflammatory response by regulating β-defensin-2 expression [8,43]. Moreover, IL-26, which is another member of IL-10 family, is also reported to be expressed by Th17 cells in human [45].

In addition to the hallmark cytokine IL-17, tumor infiltrating Th17 cells also express other functionally relevant cytokines in the tumor microenvironment. It is reported that Th17 cells express the anti-inflammatory cytokine IL-10 in mice [46]. Our group demonstrated that human tumor-infiltrating Th17 cells produce minimal levels of IL-10 in ovary cancer patients [12]. And recently, we showed that endogenous IL-10 constrains Th17-cell development through restricting the IL-1 production by dendritic cells (DCs) in patients with inflammatory bowel disease. And DCs from IL-10$^{-/-}$ mice produce more IL-1β and promote Th17 development in an IL-1-dependent manner [47]. On the other hand, Th17 cells from the ovarian cancer microenvironment express high levels of polyfunctional effector cytokines, including IL-2, IFN-γ, TNF-α and granulocyte-macrophage colony-stimulation factor (GM-CSF) [7,12]. The data indicate that tumor-associated Th17 cells exhibit an effector T-cells cytokine profile similar to the cytokine profile of effector T cells in infectious disease [48,49]. The ability of secreting effector cytokines endows Th17 cells potential protective antitumor immunity in tumor immunopathology [7].

TABLE 10.1 IL-17 Family Members

Name	Alias	Receptor	Source	Effect	References
IL-17A	IL-17, CTLA-8	IL-17RA, IL-17RC	Th17, Tc17, $\gamma\delta$T cell, Treg, invariant NKT cell, Lymphoid-tissue inducer (LTi)-like cell, Neutrophil, Eosinophil, Monocyte, Mast cell, Myeloid cells, Paneth cell	Proinflammation; antitumor effect; protumor effect; inducing cytokine, chemokine and adhesion molecule; promoting neutrophila; recruiting neutrophil; protection against infection	[7,8,20,28,133,134]
IL-17B	CX1, NERF	IL-17RB	Chondrocyte, Neuron	Inducing proinflammatory cytokines; recruiting neutrophil	[133,135]
IL-17C	CX2	IL-17RE	Th17, DC, Macrophage, Keratinocyte	Inducing proinflammatory cytokines; activating NF-κB; recruiting neutrophil	[133,136]
IL-17D	IL-27, IL-27A	Unknown	Th17, B cell	Inducing proinflammatory cytokines; inhibiting hematopoietic progenitor colony formation	[133,137,138]
IL-17E	IL-25	IL-17RA, IL-17RB	Th17, Tc17, Th2 cell, DC, Macrophage, Mast cell, Eosinophil, Basophil, Epithelial cell, Paneth cell	Promoting Th2 immune response; promoting Th9 activation; suppressing Th1 and Th17 response; promoting eosinophila; antitumor effect; antiinflammation; protection against infection; promoting allergic lung disease	[133,139−143]
IL-17F	ML-1	IL-17RA, IL-17RC	Th17, Tc17, NKT cell, LTi-like cell, Neutrophil, Basophil, Monocyte, Mast cell, Epithelial cell, Paneth cell	Proinflammation; inducing cytokine; promoting neutrophila; recruiting neutrophil; protection against infection	[8,133,143−146]

Apart from cytokines, Th17 cells also express several chemokines. Th17 cells can be induced to express CCL20 following stimulation by IFN-γ [16]. Interestingly, tumor-infiltrating Th17 cells express high levels of CC chemokine receptor 6 (CCR6), the receptor for CCL20, indicating that Th17 cells might be recruited to inflammatory tissue and tumor microenvironment via CCR6/CCL20 pathway through a paracrine mechanism [8,12]. CXC chemokine receptor 4 (CXCR4) is also reported to be expressed by tumor-infiltrating Th17 cells, which might be associated with the migration and retention of Th17 cells in tumor [12]. Furthermore, Th17 cells can stimulate the production of CXCL9 and CXCL10 to recruit effector T cells to the tumor microenvironment through synergistic effect of IL-17 and IFN-γ [12].

C. Genetic control

STAT family members play an important role during the helper T-cell differentiation at least in part through the induction of lineage-specific transcription factors [8,50]. The genetic control for Th17 cells is distinct from those for Th1, Th2 and Treg cells, which further confirms that Th17 cells are a distinct lineage of Th cells [8]. STAT3 is reported to be an essential mediator of Th17 development, and it is proposed as an upstream mediator of Th17 cells due to detection of a binding site for STAT3 localized on the promoter of the IL-17 gene [8,51,52]. Moreover, $STAT3^{-/-}$ T cells are observed to be defective in Th17 differentiation and the production of their associated cytokines, resulting in protection against EAE, and T cells with overexpression of STAT3 are found to have potentiated differentiation of Th17 cells [53,54]. Interestingly, the expression of retinoic acid receptor-related orphan receptor (ROR)γt and RORα is significantly reduced in $STAT3^{-/-}$ T cells [53,55]. Therefore, all the data indicates STAT3 has an important role in the global regulation of the gene-expression program of Th17 cells [8].

The commitment of helper T cells is mediated by lineage-specific transcription factors. RORγt is identified to be a crucial regulator in orchestrating the differentiation of Th17 cells by showing that overexpression of RORγt promotes Th17 differentiation with subsequent blockade of Th1 and Th2 differentiation and deficiency of RORγt expression results in defective Th17 differentiation and attenuated EAE [41,56–58]. Overexpression of RORα promotes Th17 differentiation with inhibited Th1 and Th2 differentiation in a RORγt-independent manner. Furthermore, overexpression of both RORγt and RORα is demonstrated to have a synergistic effect in promoting Th17 differentiation and compound mutations in both factors result in complete inhibition of Th17 differentiation both *in vitro* and *in vivo* [8,55]. Altogether, it indicates that RORγt is a key transcription factor that orchestrates Th17-cell differentiation and RORγt and RORα have similar and redundant functions [8].

In addition, other transcription factors are reported to be involved in the genetic control of Th17 lineage. Th17 differentiation is reported to be positively regulated through Smad2 which can be phosphorylated by TGF-β [50,59–61]. Furthermore, Smad2 is reported to synergize with RORγt to mediate Th17 differentiation [60], indicating Smad2 might serve as a co-factor for RORγt [50]. Interferon-regulatory factor 4 (IRF4) is reported to be another mediator of Th17 differentiation [62]. However, IRF4 might not be a specific mediator for Th17 cells as it has been reported to be essential for the development of Th2 cells [63,64]. Furthermore, Aryl hydrocarbon receptor (AHR) activation is reported to result in enhanced expression of IL-17, IL-17F and IL-22 [65,66]. Batf is also reported to be a crucial mediator for Th17 differentiation [67]. IκBζ is a member of IκB family, is demonstrated to be required for Th17 differentiation, and has a synergistic effect with RORγt or RORα [50,68]. Taken together, it indicates that the differentiation of Th17 cells might be mediated under distinct transcription factors following different mechanisms under different conditions.

III. Th17-CELL PLASTICITY

The concept of plasticity of T helper cells represents the transition from one committed Th lineage to other Th lineages with distinct characteristic cytokines and function. Although Th17 cells constitute a distinct T helper lineage, more and more evidence indicates that Th17 cells exhibit plasticity under certain conditions and the cytokine profile of Th17 cells may be altered in tissues [28].

It is generally acknowledged that Th1 and Th17 lineages are not only distinct but also mutually antagonistic through cytokines and transcription factors [4,53,69–71]. However, IFN-γ contributes to induced expansion of Th17 cells by promoting the production of IL-1 and IL-23

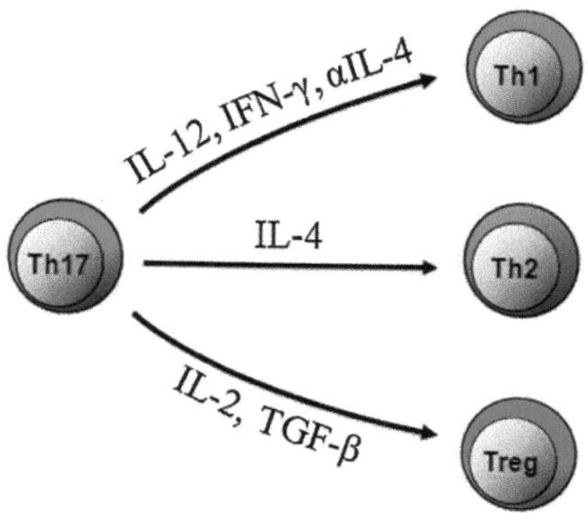

FIGURE 10.1

The plasticity of Th17 cells. Th17 cells may give rise to Th1 cells under the Th1-polarizing condition with IL-12, IFN-γ and anti-IL-4. In the presence of IL-4, Th17 cells may be converted to Th2 cells. In the presence of IL-2 and TGF-β, Th17 cells may be converted into Treg cells.

by APCs [15], and the expression of T-bet can be elevated in Th17 cells in the presence of IL-12 [72,73]. Furthermore, *in vitro* generated Th17 cells are found to be instable in maintaining cytokines expression and they can be converted into Th1 cells in lymphopenic environments [50,73,74]. Recently, we reported that primary Th17 cells can be induced to give rise to Th1 cells under the Th1-polarizing condition, and CD4$^+$ T cells with IFN-γ$^+$IL-17$^+$ phenotype can be detected in human pathological environments (Figure 10.1) [75]. In support of our observations, similar results are shown in mice that indicate that the antitumor effect of Th17 cells requires IFN-γ expression [76]. IFN-γ and IL-12 signaling are reported to be synergic in converting *ex vivo* isolated Th17 cells into Th1 cells [77].

The shared requirement of TGF-β for the development of both Th17 cells and Treg cells indicates that Th17 cells might be developmentally related to Treg cells [78]. High concentrations of TGF-β favor Treg differentiation, while low levels of TGF-β mediate Th17 induction together with proinflammatory cytokines [79]. Although Foxp3 can inhibit the function of RORγt and Treg cells can suppress Th17-cells development, a population of Foxp3$^+$RORγt$^+$CD4$^+$ naïve T cells is detected both *in vitro* and *in vivo* [12,18,79]. In addition, we have shown that primary Th17 cells can be converted into Treg cells under polarization and we observed Foxp3$^+$IL-17$^+$CD4$^+$ T cells in human cancers and further proved that these T cells are functional Treg cells (Figure 10.1) [33,75].

In the presence of IL-4, memory Th17 cells can be converted into Th2 cells (Figure 10.1) [80] and a small population of IL-4$^+$IL-17$^+$ T cells are detected in peripheral blood from healthy donors, but the number of these double positive T cells increases in patients with asthma [80,81]. Therefore, Th17 cells are conferred with flexible plasticity to generate other helper T-cell subsets under biological and pathological circumstances, which might contribute to the function of Th17 cells under both homeostatic and pathological conditions (Figure 10.1).

IV. Th17-CELL STEMNESS

In the immune system, one of the most effective populations that provide antitumor immunity is memory T cells, which are defined as long-lived T cells with heightened capacity to fight against invasion with the experienced pathogens. Th17 cells in human tumor environment are characterized with CD45RO$^+$CD62L$^-$CCR7$^-$ phenotype and enriched in the population expressing CD49 and CCR6 [12,16]. These Th17 cells are confined to memory T-cell compartments. We have reported Th17 cells express higher levels of CD28 and CD127 compared with Th0 and Th1 counterparts and primary Th17 cells express high levels of IL-2

133

and TNF-α and a moderate amount of IFN-γ in blood and disease microenvironment. Furthermore, Th17 cells express high levels of CD95 (Fas receptor, FasR) and low levels of CD27 in human, making them phenotypically resemble terminally differentiated memory T cells [75]. Similar results were reported recently in mice, which confirm that Th17 cells possess a phenotype of terminally differentiated memory T cells [76]. Terminally differentiated memory T cells are considered to be short-lived and have limited antitumor activity as they exhibit senescent and exhausted phenotype. Thus, mouse Th17 cells are assumed to be short-lived T cells based on their phenotype [82]. However, there is no expression of PD-1, KLRG1, CD57, FoxP3 and IL-10 on Th17 cells, indicating that Th17 cells are not functionally exhausted PD-1[+] T cells or senescent CD28[−]CD57[+]KLRG1[+] T cells or suppressive Foxp3[+] or IL-10[+] T cells [75,76]. Moreover, Th17 cells have superior antitumor activity following adoptive transfer [75,83,84]. These findings seem to be contrary to the concept that Th17 cells are short lived because cell persistence in tumor environment is critical to complete eradication of tumor [76,85,86]. Actually, we have shown that adoptively transferred Th17 cells have better persistence *in vivo* compared with Th1 and Th2 cells [75], which is confirmed by showing Th17 cells have better recovery in mice [76]. Although Th17 cells express a high level of CD95, they are resistant to apoptosis through expressing a high amount of Bcl-2 and Bcl-xl in both human and mouse [75,76]. Therefore, Th17 cells are long-lived memory cells and mediate long-term antitumor immunity (Figure 10.2).

Stem cells are defined as a small population with the property of self-renewal, expansion and multilineage developmental potential. Since individual effector cells have a limited lifespan and thymus function reduces in adults, stem cells are needed to maintain the effector memory T-cell pool with their capacity to continuously generate effector memory T cell, which help maintain a constant repertoire of memory T cells for a lifetime [87−89]. We have reported that Th17 cells have increased the capacity of proliferation as they express high levels of Ki67 and efficiently expand both *in vitro* and *in vivo*. Although Th17 cells express high amounts of CD95, they are resistant to apoptosis after CD95 engagement [75]. Interestingly, CD95 is reported to be a stem cell-associated gene [90]. Importantly, we have demonstrated that primary Th17 cells can be induced to give rise to Th1 and Treg-cell subsets respectively under their polarizing

134

FIGURE 10.2
Th17 stemness is controlled by HIF/Notch/Bcl-2 signaling. Human Th17 cells express high levels of HIF-1α, Notch signaling molecules and Bcl-2, and multiple stem cell core genes. HIF/Notch/Bcl-2 signaling pathway controls Th17-cell survival, and promote Th17 cell-mediated T-cell immunity. Th17 cells are polyfunctional and highly plastic in the chronic inflammatory environment, and would be converted into regulatory T cell-type and Th-1 type effector cells. This indicates that Th17 cells have high plasticity and stem cell-like features.

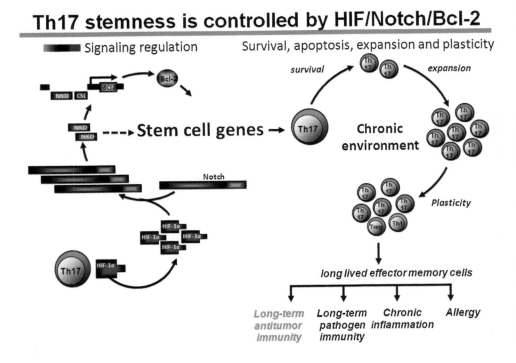

conditions *in vitro* and further confirmed the findings *in vivo* in cancer patients [75]. Supporting this notion, a similar result was gained in mice by showing Th17-polarized cells evolve into Th1 cell-like subset *in vivo* [76]. Moreover, Th17 cells can be converted to Th1 cells under lymphopenic condition in mouse models [72,74,91]. It is well-known that cells are usually under hypoxic condition in inflammatory and tumor tissues [92,93]. It has been proposed that hypoxic environment is required for cancer stem cell function and hypoxia inducible factor 1 (HIF-1) is important for maintaining an active niche for long-term hematopoietic stem cells (HSC) [94]. Our group has reported Th17 cells express large amounts of HIF-1α in human tissues [75]. Furthermore, we have also determined that HIF-1α/Notch/Bcl-2 is a key signaling pathway controlling the survival and apoptosis pattern of Th17 cells [75]. This notion is supported by a recent mouse study showing HIF-1α signaling pathway is crucial for controlling Th17-cell biology [95]. It has been shown cyclin-dependent kinase (CDK) inhibitors are responsible for cellular senescence and exhaustion; therefore, it is essential for HSC self-renewal by suppression of p16^{Ink4A} (CDKN2A) and p19^{Arf} [96]. We found several cyclins are highly expressed in Th17 cells with reduced expression of CDK inhibitors [75]. Our group has also demonstrated that Th17 cells express higher levels of stem cell core genes, such as Nanog, Sox2 and OCT3/4, compared with autologous IL-17$^-$ control cells [75]. In addition, we found the expression of multiple stem cell-associated genes is higher in Th17 cells, including genes encoding Notch signaling pathway (Notch2, Notch3, CHERP, HEY1 and HEY2) and Wnt/β-catenin signaling pathway (LEF-1 and TCF7) and genes for Bcl-2, FOXO3, Myc and PIM2 [75]. A similar study was performed in mice by showing Th17 cells express higher amounts of Wnt/β-catenin signaling-related genes compared with Th1 cells [76]. Altogether, our results indicate that Th17 cells possess stem cell-like properties with the capacity of self-renewal, development potential to other Th subsets, better persistence *in vivo*, better resistance to apoptosis, faster expansion and superior antitumor activity (Figure 10.2).

V. Th17 CANCER IMMUNITY

It is well-known that Th17 cells contribute to inflammation, immune defense and autoimmune diseases [2,8,28]. Recently, more and more investigators focus on the role of Th17 cells in various cancer types, which helps deepen our understanding about the importance of Th17 cells in cancer. Th17 cells are found to be more prevalent in tumor microenvironment even though they represent a minor population in the peripheral blood and tumor draining lymph nodes of cancer patients, which is similar to that reported in the peripheral blood of healthy donors [7]. There are more Th17 cells present in the tumor tissue, regardless of the lower frequencies compared with other T-cell subsets [18]. The cumulative higher levels of Th17 cells in tumor microenvironment might be due to direct induction at the tumor site and/or recruitment from other places [12,18]. Tumor-infiltrating Th17 cells highly express CCR6, CXCR4, c-type lectin receptor CD161 (also known as KLRB1) and multiple isoforms of CD49 integrin (CD49c, CD49d and Cd49e), which might serve as the homing molecules and contribute to the migration and retention of Th17 cells in the tumor microenvironment as it contains high levels of CCL20 and CXCL12 [12,16,83,93,97]. Interestingly, we found Th17 cells can be induced to express CCL20 by the stimulation of IFN-γ, suggesting Th17 cells might mediate their own trafficking to tumor via CCR6/CCL20 pathway [16]. However, there is no expression of CD62L, CCR2, CCR5 or CCR7 on Th17 cells, which might explain their low prevalence in tumor draining lymph nodes [12]. It has been reported Th17 cells express negligible levels of CD25, HLA-DR and granzyme B, which are activation markers for conventional effector T cells, indicating they might not mediate effector functions through granzyme B pathway [7,12]. Furthermore, tumor-infiltrating Th17 cells produce high levels of effector cytokines in both human and mice, including IL-2, IFN-γ, TNF-α and GM-CSF, indicating Th17 cells might promote antitumor immunity in tumor immunopathology [7,12,98].

In the tumor microenvironment, Th17 cells interact with several other immune cells, such as APCs, Th1 cells and Treg cells [7,99]. It has been shown that tumor-associated macrophages and myeloid DCs can stimulate IL-17 production from memory T cells by secreting IL-1β, and they are proven to be more efficient than macrophages from healthy donors [12,15,16]. On the other hand, Th17 cells promote the trafficking of APCs into tumor draining lymph nodes and microenvironment through CCR6/CCL20 pathway [7,12]. It has been proposed that Th17 and Th1 cells might be phenotypically, developmentally and functionally linked in tumor microenvironment [7,84]. There is evidence showing tumor-associated Th17 cells express the typical Th1-lineage cytokine, IFN-γ, in both human and mice [12,27], and IFN-γ$^+$IL-17$^+$CD4$^+$ T cells are observed in human ovarian cancer and colon cancer [75]. Furthermore, we have shown Th17 cells can be induced to Th1 cells under the polarizing condition with IL-12 and anti-IL-4 [75]. Consistent with the human study, mouse Th17 cells have been demonstrated to redifferentiate into Th1 cells under lymphopenic conditions [72,74,91]. It has been shown there is an inverse correlation between the numbers of Th17 and Treg cells in tumor. Tumor-associated Treg cells express high amounts of an ectonucleotidase CD39 (NTPDase 1) and therefore suppress Th17 development via an adenosinergic pathway [12,18]. In addition, human Th17 cells can be converted into Treg cells through *in vitro* polarization [75], and Foxp3$^+$IL-17$^+$CD4$^+$ T cells are found in human tumors [75,100,101]. Interestingly, mouse peripheral mature Treg cells can be converted to Th17 cells which are favored by inflammation and IL-6 production [10,98,102,103]. Therefore, Th17 cells interact with distinct immune cells in the tumor microenvironment and might have a protective role against tumor.

As we already mentioned, human Th17 cells are functional effector T cells with potent antitumor activity as they express high levels of several effector cytokines. Consistent with this hypothesis, we have reported that both Th17 frequency in tumor and IL-17 concentration within ascites predict improved survival in patients with advanced ovarian cancer [12], and Th17 differentiation is inversely correlated with tumor progression in prostate cancer patients [104]. The patients with increased accumulation of Th17 cells in malignant pleural effusion have longer survival with lung cancer (Table 10.2) [105]. Moreover, Th17 increases with specific CTLA4 blockade in patients with metastatic melanoma [106] and the IL-17 level detected in tumor-associated ascites is positively correlated with patient survival (Tables 10.2, 10.3). In support of the findings in human, polarized Th17 transgenic T cells with IL-6 and TGF-β result in tumor eradication in mice [27,83,107]. IL-17 deficiency in mice contributes to accelerated tumor progression and lung metastasis, but overexpression of IL-17 by tumor cells suppresses tumor growth (Table 10.3) [26,108,109]. In addition, it has been shown Th17 cells are conferred with advanced antitumor immunity following immunotherapies which can enhance the activity of Th17 cells [98,110,111]. In IL-6-transduced pancreatic tumor-bearing mice, the number of Th17 cells in tumor is increased, which correlates with slower tumor growth and longer overall median survival [112]. Mechanistically, it has been suggested that Th17 cells may not mediate direct cytotoxic antitumor activity since they do not produce granzyme B or perforin and have no direct effects on the proliferation and apoptosis of tumor cells [12,113]. However, it is possible that Th17 cells might mediate the trafficking of effector T cells into tumor microenvironment to promote antitumor immunity indirectly by inducing the production of Th1-type chemokines CXCL9 and CXCL10 [12,114–116]. Supporting this concept, we found the levels of CXCL9 and CXLC10 are positively correlated with the number of CD8$^+$ T cells and NK cells in tumor microenvironment and the level of IL-17 is positively correlated with the amount of tumor-infiltrating IFN-γ$^+$ effector T cells [12]. In conclusion, it suggests that Th17 cells have an active but indirect role in promoting antitumor immunity by inducing the migration and retention of effector T cells and NK cells in the tumor microenvironment [7]. Therefore, manipulating Th17 cells based on their biology might be therapeutically beneficial for treating patients with cancer (Tables 10.2, 10.3).

TABLE 10.2 Th17 Cells and Tumor

Organism	Tumor type	Tumor initiation	Effect	References
Human	Ovarian cancer	spontaneous	Tumor-infiltrating Th17 cells exhibit a polyfunctional effector T-cell phenotype and synergize with IFN-γ to recruit effector T cells to the tumor microenvironment by stimulating CXCL9 and CXCL10. Th17 levels positively predicts patient outcome.	[12]
Human	Prostate cancer	spontaneous	Th17 differentiation is inversely correlated with tumor progression.	[104]
Human	Lung cancer	spontaneous	Increased accumulation of Th17 cells in malignant pleural effusion predicts longer survival.	[105]
Human	Melanoma	spontaneous	Specific blockade of CTLA4 contributes to increased Th17 cells.	[106]
Human	Head and Neck cancer	spontaneous	Proliferation and angiogenesis of head and neck squamous cell carcinoma are impaired in the presence of Th17 cells.	[147]
Mouse	Melanoma	subcutaneous injection	Polarized tumor-specific Th17 cells have better antitumor effect which is IFN-γ dependent than Th1-polarized cells	[27,76]
Mouse	Pancreatic cancer	subcutaneous injection	Increased Th17 cells in mice bearing IL-6-secreting pancreatic tumor cells contribute to delayed tumor growth and better survival.	[112]
Mouse	Melanoma	subcutaneous injection	Polarized Tc17 cells convert to IFN-γ-producing cells and mediate tumor regression.	[107]
Mouse	Prostate cancer	subcutaneous injection	Hsp70-mediated Th17 autoimmunity induces rejection of established tumor.	[111]
Mouse	Melanoma	subcutaneous injection	Treatment of anti-IDO[a] and antitumor vaccine converts Tregs to the Th17 cells with activation of CD8+ T cells, leading to antitumor efficacy.	[98]
Human	Prostate cancer	spontaneous	Frequency of Th17 pretreatment inversely correlated with time to disease progression in hormone-resistant patients.	[118]
Mouse	Hepatocellular carcinoma	subcutaneous injection	Th17 cells promote HCC progression by fostering angiogenesis. Decreased Th17 infiltration results in decreased tumor growth.	[119]
Mouse	Ovarian cancer	intraperitoneal injection	Th17-derived IL-17 recruits myeloid cells and promotes tumor growth.	[148]
Mouse	Colon cancer	bacteria-induced	Bacterial infection induces Th17 response and results in colonic tumor. Blockade of IL-17 and IL-23R inhibits tumor formation.	[120]

Red, Antitumor effect; Black, Protumor effect.
[a]IDO, Indoleamine 2,3-dioxygenase.

137

TABLE 10.3 Th17-Associated Cytokines and Tumor

Cytokine	Organism	Tumor type	Tumor initiation	Effect	References
IL-17	Mouse	Colon cancer	subcutaneous or intravenous injection	IL-17 deficiency contributes to enhanced tumor growth and metastasis associated with decreased IFN-γ^+ NK cell and tumor-specific IFN-γ^+ T cells.	[26]
IL-17	Mouse	Lung melanoma	intravenous injection	IL-17 deficiency leads to enhanced tumor growth. Tumor-specific Th17 cells activate tumor-specific CD8$^+$ T cells and exhibit stronger antitumor effect than Th1 cells. Th17 cells promote CCL20 production by tumor.	[83]
IL-17	Mouse	Fibrosarcoma	subcutaneous injection	IL-17-transfected Meth-A cells induce tumor-specific antitumor immunity.	[108]
IL-17	Mouse	Plasmocytoma, mastocytoma	subcutaneous injection	Growth of IL-17-producing tumor cells is inhibited in immunocompetent mice, but no difference in nude mice.	[109]
IL-17E	Mouse	Melanoma, Lung cancer, Pancreatic cancer, colon cancer, breast cancer	subcutaneous injection	Repeated administration of IL-17E leads to antitumor activity and B cells are necessary. Combination of IL-17E with chemotherapy or immunotherapy exhibits enhanced antitumor efficacy.	[142]
IL-17F	Mouse	Hepatocellular carcinoma	subcutaneous injection	IL-17F inhibits tumor angiogenesis and contributes to retarded tumor growth in nude mice.	[149]

TABLE 10.3 Th17-Associated Cytokines and Tumor—continued

Cytokine	Organism	Tumor type	Tumor initiation	Effect	References
IL-23	Mouse	Glioma	stereotactic implantation	Injection of IL-23-transduced DC induces antitumor immunity. Treatment with IL-23-expressing cells improves mice survival.	[150,151]
IL-23	Mouse	Melanoma	subcutaneous injection	IL-23 increases vaccine-induced $CD8^+$ T cells and maintains antitumor activity. IL-23-tranfected B16 cells exhibit inhibited tumor growth.	[152,153]
IL-17	Human	Gastric cancer	spontaneous	IL-17 promotes tumor progression. The number of vascular endothelial cells and infiltrating neutrophils positively correlated with IL-17 expression in tumor.	[154]
IL-17	Human	Multiple myeloma	spontaneous	IL-17 inhibits production of Th1-type cytokines with IL-22 and promotes myeloma cell growth.	[155]
IL-17	Human	Lung cancer	spontaneous	Higher level of IL-17 predicts poor patient survival.	[121]
IL-17	Human	Hepatocelluar carcinoma	spontaneous	Level of intratumoral IL-17 inversely correlated with patient survival.	[122]
IL-17	Mouse	Melanoma, Bladder cancer	subcutaneous injection	IL-17 deficiency results in reduced tumor growth. IL-17 induces tumor growth through IL-6/STAT3 pathway.	[125]
IL-17	Mouse	Fibrosarcoma, Colon cancer, Lung cancer	subcutaneous injection	IL-17-expressing tumor cells exhibit faster proliferation. IL-17 promotes CXCR2-dependent angiogenesis.	[123,124]

139

Continued

TABLE 10.3 Th17-Associated Cytokines and Tumor—continued

Cytokine	Organism	Tumor type	Tumor initiation	Effect	References
IL-17	Mouse	Lymphoma, Prostate cancer, Melanoma	subcutaneous injection	IL-17 recruits MDSC and inhibits CD8$^+$ T cells in tumor microenvironment and promotes tumor growth. L-17R deficiency leads to decreased tumor progression.	[126]
IL-23	Mouse	Squamous cancer, Melanoma, Lung cancer, Breast cancer, Colon cancer	Chemical-induced, subcutaneous injection, intradermal injection	IL-23 promotes angiogenesis and inhibit CD8$^+$ T cell infiltration. Inhibition of IL-23 leads to protection against chemical-induced tumor. IL-23R deficiency results in decreased tumor growth.	[132]

Red, Antitumor effect; Black, Protumor effect.

VI. Th17 ASSOCIATED CYTOKINES AND CARCINOGENESIS

The effect of Th17 cells in tumor immunopathology remains controversial. Recently, one group reported that the number of tumor-infiltrating Th17 cells is not correlated with the clinicopathological characteristics or survival of patients with nasopharyngeal carcinoma [117]. It has been reported that Th17 cells even promote tumor development. The pretreatment frequency of circulating Th17 cells has been shown to be inversely correlated with the time to disease progression in patients with hormone-resistant prostate cancer (Table 10.2) [118]. In a mouse study, the decreased level of tumor-infiltrating Th17 cells is associated with reduced tumor growth in hepatocellular carcinoma (HCC) treated with gadolinium chloride [119]. Therefore, these findings seem to be contrary to the observations showing antitumor activity of Th17 cells. However, it is worth pointing out that the elevated level of Th17 cells usually indicates an underlying infection or active inflammatory state, which can promote tumor initiation and development [28,120]. Thus, it is possible that the protumor effect is due to the inflammatory status associated with Th17 cells rather than direct effect of Th17 cells [28]. Consistent with this possibility, high levels of Th17 cells together with IL-17$^+$ Treg cells are detected in patients with ulcerative colitis and associated colon cancer [28,75]. Moreover, it has been reported that the production of several inflammatory cytokines, including IL-1, IL-8 and TNFα, is induced by IL-17$^+$ cells and these cytokines further promote the trafficking of neutrophils to the inflammation site [33]. It is well-known that inflammation can facilitate tumor initiation and progression, suggesting that the tumorigenetic activity of Th17 cells might be due to their proinflammatory role and the accompanied accelerated DNA damage, which enhances tumor angiogenesis and tumorigenesis in the local environment [28].

Furthermore, it is necessary to mention that the Th17 subsets are not synonymous with the cytokine IL-17, and the biological activities of IL-17 should not be equated with those of Th17 cells (Table 10.4) [7,20]. As already described, IL-17 is not exclusively produced by Th17 cells although it is the lineage-signature cytokine of Th17 cells. It has been shown that a higher

TABLE 10.4 Inequalities in Evaluating Th17 and Tumor

Controversial?

Th17 ≠ IL-17$^+$ cell
Th17 ≠ IL-17
Th17 ≠ IL-23
Exogenous IL-17 ≠ Endogenous IL-17
Mouse ≠ Human
Immunodeficient ≠ Immune Competent
Early Cancer Stage ≠ Advanced Cancer Stage
Chemical Carcinogen-induced Cancer ≠
Chronic Infection-associated Cancer ≠
Spontaneous Cancer

amount of IL-17 in tumor microenvironment is correlated with higher blood vessel density and predicts shorter survival in patients with non-small-cell lung cancer and HCC (Table 10.3) [121,122]. Both endogenous and exogenous IL-17 has been reported to promote tumor formation and growth in mouse models [120,123–125]. Several groups have reported slower tumor growth in both IL-17$^{-/-}$ and IL-17R$^{-/-}$ mice [125,126]. In addition, neutralizing IL-17 results in decelerated tumor growth [126]. Furthermore, forced expression of IL-17 in murine tumors leads to faster tumor progression (Table 10.3) [123]. It has been proposed that the protumor activity of IL-17 is due to its proangiogenic property of surrounding endothelial cells and fibroblasts [127]. IL-17 can induce the expression of vascular endothelial growth factor (VEGF), which in turn promotes tumor angiogenesis [128]. TGF-β is also reported to serve as an angiogenic factor and enhance VEGF-mediated angiogenesis by increasing the expression of VEGF receptor on endothelial cells [129]. IL-17 is also shown to induce the expression of IL-6, IL-8, prostaglandin E2 (PGE2) and intracellular adhension molecule 1 (ICAM-1, also known as CD54), which can promote angiogenesis and tumor invasion [33,127]. In support of this notion, the expression level of IL-8 is found to be correlated with the angiogenesis, tumorigenicity and metastasis of distinct tumor models [127,130]. Furthermore, it has been shown that the expression of several angiogenic chemokines by tumor cells and epithelial cells can be selectively induced by IL-17, including CXCL1, CXCL5, CXCL6 and CXCL8 [124,131]. Accordingly, IL-17 can suppress the secretion of angiostatic chemokines by fibroblast [124], indicating IL-17 might contribute to tumor angiogenesis by regulating the balance between angiogenic and angiostatic chemokines [127]. In addition, STAT3 is an important mediator of Th17 differentiation and it is also an oncogenic transcription factor which can upregulate prosurvival and proangiogenic genes. Interestingly, IL-17 can induce the production of IL-6 by tumor cells and tumor-associated stromal cells [125]. It indicates that the protumor activity of IL-17 might be mediated, at least partially, by the IL-6/STAT3 signaling pathway. Furthermore, IL-23 has been proposed to be a possible candidate contributing to Th17 cells-associated carcinogenesis. In a mouse tumor model, IL-23-deficient mice are found to be resistant to tumorigenesis induced by chemical, which is correlated with reduced expression of matrix metalloproteinase 9 (MMP9) and angiogenic markers and increased infiltration of CD8$^+$ T cells [132]. Therefore, the controversial tumorigenic activity of Th17 cells seems to be highly associated with Th17-related cytokines and chemokines rather than Th17 cells themselves (Tables 10.3, 10.4).

VII. CONCLUSION

Th17 cells have been shown to be an important component of the immune system and are involved in various immune events. Th17 cells exhibit an abundant cytokine profile and their generation is mediated under the control of different transcription factors and cytokine milieu.

Recently, Th17 cells have been demonstrated to possess stem cell-like properties and plasticity to give rise to other Th subsets. Their stemness and plasticity may be important factors determining the biological activities of Th17 cells. Furthermore, it will help us better understand the role of Th17 cells in tumor immunopathology by separating Th17 cells and their associated cytokines and analyzing different conditions under a distinct research context. Finally, as experimental and clinical studies have demonstrated meaningful benefits by targeting Th17-cell signaling pathway and/or the related cytokines/receptors to treat patients with inflammation, autoimmune diseases and tumors, it is predictable that manipulation of Th17-cell biology would be a promising therapeutic modality to treat Th17-affected diseases in the years to come.

References

[1] Mosmann TR, Coffman RL. TH1 and TH2 cells: different patterns of lymphokine secretion lead to different functional properties. Annu Rev Immunol 1989;7:145–73.

[2] Dong C. Diversification of T-helper-cell lineages: finding the family root of IL-17-producing cells. Nat Rev Immunol 2006;6(4):329–33.

[3] Yao Z, Painter SL, Fanslow WC, et al. Human IL-17: a novel cytokine derived from T cells. J Immunol 1995;155(12):5483–6.

[4] Park H, Li Z, Yang XO, et al. A distinct lineage of CD4 T cells regulates tissue inflammation by producing interleukin 17. Nat Immunol 2005;6(11):1133–41.

[5] Harrington LE, Hatton RD, Mangan PR, et al. Interleukin 17-producing CD4+ effector T cells develop via a lineage distinct from the T helper type 1 and 2 lineages. Nat Immunol 2005;6(11):1123–32.

[6] Kryczek I, Wei S, Vatan L, et al. Cutting Edge: Opposite Effects of IL-1 and IL-2 on the Regulation of IL-17+ T Cell Pool IL-1 Subverts IL-2-Mediated Suppression. J Immunol 2007;179(3):1423–6.

[7] Zou W, Restifo NP. T(H)17 cells in tumour immunity and immunotherapy. Nat Rev Immunol 2010;10(4):248–56.

[8] Dong C. TH17 cells in development: an updated view of their molecular identity and genetic programming. Nat Rev Immunol 2008;8(5):337–48.

[9] Bettelli E, Korn T, Oukka M, Kuchroo VK. Induction and effector functions of T(H)17 cells. Nature 2008;453(7198):1051–7.

[10] Weaver CT, Hatton RD. Interplay between the TH17 and TReg cell lineages: a (co-)evolutionary perspective. Nat Rev Immunol 2009;9(12):883–9.

[11] Veldhoen M, Hocking RJ, Atkins CJ, Locksley RM, Stockinger B. TGFbeta in the context of an inflammatory cytokine milieu supports de novo differentiation of IL-17-producing T cells. Immunity 2006;24(2):179–89.

[12] Kryczek I, Banerjee M, Cheng P, et al. Phenotype, distribution, generation, and functional and clinical relevance of Th17 cells in the human tumor environments. Blood 2009;114(6):1141–9.

[13] Langrish CL, Chen Y, Blumenschein WM, et al. IL-23 drives a pathogenic T cell population that induces autoimmune inflammation. J Exp Med 2005;201(2):233–40.

[14] Weaver CT, Harrington LE, Mangan PR, Gavrieli M, Murphy KM. Th17: an effector CD4 T cell lineage with regulatory T cell ties. Immunity 2006;24(6):677–88.

[15] Kryczek I, Wei S, Gong W, et al. Cutting edge: IFN-gamma enables APC to promote memory Th17 and abate Th1 cell development. J Immunol 2008;181(9):5842–6.

[16] Kryczek I, Bruce AT, Gudjonsson JE, et al. Induction of IL-17+ T cell trafficking and development by IFN-gamma: mechanism and pathological relevance in psoriasis. J Immunol 2008;181(7):4733–41.

[17] Zou W, Chen L. Inhibitory B7-family molecules in the tumour microenvironment. Nat Rev Immunol 2008;8(6):467–77.

[18] Kryczek I, Wei S, Zou L, et al. Cutting Edge: Th17 and Regulatory T Cell Dynamics and the Regulation by IL-2 in the Tumor Microenvironment. J Immunol 2007;178(11):6730–3.

[19] Zou W. Immunosuppressive networks in the tumour environment and their therapeutic relevance. Nat Rev Cancer 2005;5(4):263–74.

[20] Wilke CM, Kryczek I, Wei S, et al. Th17 cells in cancer: help or hindrance? Carcinogenesis 2011;32(5):643–9.

[21] Zhao E, Xu H, Wang L, et al. Bone marrow and the control of immunity. Cell Mol Immunol 2012;9(1):11–9.

[22] Aggarwal S, Gurney AL. IL-17: prototype member of an emerging cytokine family. J Leukoc Biol 2002;71(1):1–8.

[23] Kolls JK, Linden A. Interleukin-17 family members and inflammation. Immunity 2004;21(4):467–76.

[24] Nakae S, Nambu A, Sudo K, Iwakura Y. Suppression of immune induction of collagen-induced arthritis in IL-17-deficient mice. J Immunol 2003;171(11):6173−7.

[25] Komiyama Y, Nakae S, Matsuki T, et al. IL-17 plays an important role in the development of experimental autoimmune encephalomyelitis. J Immunol 2006;177(1):566−73.

[26] Kryczek I, Wei S, Szeliga W, Vatan L, Zou W. Endogenous IL-17 contributes to reduced tumor growth and metastasis. Blood 2009;114(2):357−9.

[27] Muranski P, Boni A, Antony PA, et al. Tumor-specific Th17-polarized cells eradicate large established melanoma. Blood 2008;112(2):362−73.

[28] Wilke CM, Bishop K, Fox D, Zou W. Deciphering the role of Th17 cells in human disease. Trends Immunol 2011;32(12):603−11.

[29] Stark MA, Huo Y, Burcin TL, Morris MA, Olson TS, Ley K. Phagocytosis of apoptotic neutrophils regulates granulopoiesis via IL-23 and IL-17. Immunity 2005;22(3):285−94.

[30] Ferretti S, Bonneau O, Dubois GR, Jones CE, Trifilieff A. IL-17, produced by lymphocytes and neutrophils, is necessary for lipopolysaccharide-induced airway neutrophilia: IL-15 as a possible trigger. J Immunol 2003;170(4):2106−12.

[31] Michel ML, Keller AC, Paget C, et al. Identification of an IL-17-producing NK1.1(neg) iNKT cell population involved in airway neutrophilia. J Exp Med 2007;204(5):995−1001.

[32] Cua DJ, Tato CM. Innate IL-17-producing cells: the sentinels of the immune system. Nat Rev Immunol 2010;10(7):479−89.

[33] Kryczek I, Wu K, Zhao E, et al. IL-17+ regulatory T cells in the microenvironments of chronic inflammation and cancer. J Immunol 2011;186(7):4388−95.

[34] Harrington LE, Mangan PR, Weaver CT. Expanding the effector CD4 T-cell repertoire: the Th17 lineage. Curr Opin Immunol 2006;18(3):349−56.

[35] Hizawa N, Kawaguchi M, Huang SK, Nishimura M. Role of interleukin-17F in chronic inflammatory and allergic lung disease. Clin Exp Allergy 2006;36(9):1109−14.

[36] Chang SH, Dong C. A novel heterodimeric cytokine consisting of IL-17 and IL-17F regulates inflammatory responses. Cell Res 2007;17(5):435−40.

[37] Wright JF, Guo Y, Quazi A, et al. Identification of an interleukin 17F/17A heterodimer in activated human CD4+ T cells. J Biol Chem 2007;282(18):13447−55.

[38] Wright JF, Bennett F, Li B, et al. The human IL-17F/IL-17A heterodimeric cytokine signals through the IL-17RA/IL-17RC receptor complex. J Immunol 2008;181(4):2799−805.

[39] Wei L, Laurence A, Elias KM, O'Shea JJ. IL-21 is produced by Th17 cells and drives IL-17 production in a STAT3-dependent manner. J Biol Chem 2007;282(48):34605−10.

[40] Korn T, Bettelli E, Gao W, et al. IL-21 initiates an alternative pathway to induce proinflammatory T(H)17 cells. Nature 2007;448(7152):484−7.

[41] Zhou L, Ivanov II , Spolski R, et al. IL-6 programs T(H)-17 cell differentiation by promoting sequential engagement of the IL-21 and IL-23 pathways. Nat Immunol 2007;8(9):967−74.

[42] Chung Y, Yang X, Chang SH, Ma L, Tian Q, Dong C. Expression and regulation of IL-22 in the IL-17-producing CD4+ T lymphocytes. Cell Res 2006;16(11):902−7.

[43] Liang SC, Tan XY, Luxenberg DP, et al. Interleukin (IL)-22 and IL-17 are coexpressed by Th17 cells and cooperatively enhance expression of antimicrobial peptides. J Exp Med 2006;203(10):2271−9.

[44] Wolk K, Kunz S, Witte E, Friedrich M, Asadullah K, Sabat R. IL-22 increases the innate immunity of tissues. Immunity 2004;21(2):241−54.

[45] Wilson NJ, Boniface K, Chan JR, et al. Development, cytokine profile and function of human interleukin 17-producing helper T cells. Nat Immunol 2007;8(9):950−7.

[46] McGeachy MJ, Bak-Jensen KS, Chen Y, et al. TGF-beta and IL-6 drive the production of IL-17 and IL-10 by T cells and restrain T(H)-17 cell-mediated pathology. Nat Immunol 2007;8(12):1390−7.

[47] Wilke CM, Wang L, Wei S, et al. Endogenous interleukin-10 constrains Th17 cells in patients with inflammatory bowel disease. J Transl Med 2011;9:217.

[48] Precopio ML, Betts MR, Parrino J, et al. Immunization with vaccinia virus induces polyfunctional and phenotypically distinctive CD8(+) T cell responses. J Exp Med 2007;204(6):1405−16.

[49] Almeida JR, Price DA, Papagno L, et al. Superior control of HIV-1 replication by CD8+ T cells is reflected by their avidity, polyfunctionality, and clonal turnover. J Exp Med 2007;204(10):2473−85.

[50] Dong C. Genetic controls of Th17 cell differentiation and plasticity. Exp Mol Med 2011;43(1):1−6.

[51] Chen Z, Laurence A, Kanno Y, et al. Selective regulatory function of Socs3 in the formation of IL-17-secreting T cells. Proc Natl Acad Sci U S A 2006;103(21):8137−42.

[52] Mathur AN, Chang HC, Zisoulis DG, et al. Stat3 and Stat4 direct development of IL-17-secreting Th cells. J Immunol 2007;178(8):4901–7.

[53] Yang XO, Panopoulos AD, Nurieva R, et al. STAT3 regulates cytokine-mediated generation of inflammatory helper T cells. J Biol Chem 2007;282(13):9358–63.

[54] Harris TJ, Grosso JF, Yen HR, et al. Cutting edge: An in vivo requirement for STAT3 signaling in TH17 development and TH17-dependent autoimmunity. J Immunol 2007;179(7):4313–7.

[55] Yang XO, Pappu BP, Nurieva R, et al. T helper 17 lineage differentiation is programmed by orphan nuclear receptors ROR alpha and ROR gamma. Immunity 2008;28(1):29–39.

[56] Nurieva R, Yang XO, Martinez G, et al. Essential autocrine regulation by IL-21 in the generation of inflammatory T cells. Nature 2007;448(7152):480–3.

[57] Ivanov II , McKenzie BS, Zhou L, et al. The orphan nuclear receptor RORgammat directs the differentiation program of proinflammatory IL-17+ T helper cells. Cell 2006;126(6):1121–33.

[58] Eberl G, Littman DR. The role of the nuclear hormone receptor RORgammat in the development of lymph nodes and Peyer's patches. Immunol Rev 2003;195:81–90.

[59] Malhotra N, Robertson E, Kang J. SMAD2 is essential for TGF beta-mediated Th17 cell generation. J Biol Chem 2010;285(38):29044–8.

[60] Martinez GJ, Zhang Z, Reynolds JM, et al. Smad2 positively regulates the generation of Th17 cells. J Biol Chem 2010;285(38):29039–43.

[61] Feng XH, Derynck R. Specificity and versatility in tgf-beta signaling through Smads. Annu Rev Cell Dev Biol 2005;21:659–93.

[62] Brustle A, Heink S, Huber M, et al. The development of inflammatory T(H)-17 cells requires interferon-regulatory factor 4. Nat Immunol 2007;8(9):958–66.

[63] Hu CM, Jang SY, Fanzo JC, Pernis AB. Modulation of T cell cytokine production by interferon regulatory factor-4. J Biol Chem 2002;277(51):49238–46.

[64] Rengarajan J, Mowen KA, McBride KD, Smith ED, Singh H, Glimcher LH. Interferon regulatory factor 4 (IRF4) interacts with NFATc2 to modulate interleukin 4 gene expression. J Exp Med 2002;195(8):1003–12.

[65] Quintana FJ, Basso AS, Iglesias AH, et al. Control of T(reg) and T(H)17 cell differentiation by the aryl hydrocarbon receptor. Nature 2008;453(7191):65–71.

[66] Veldhoen M, Hirota K, Westendorf AM, et al. The aryl hydrocarbon receptor links TH17-cell-mediated autoimmunity to environmental toxins. Nature 2008;453(7191):106–9.

[67] Schraml BU, Hildner K, Ise W, et al. The AP-1 transcription factor Batf controls T(H)17 differentiation. Nature 2009;460(7253):405–9.

[68] Okamoto K, Iwai Y, Oh-Hora M, et al. IkappaBzeta regulates T(H)17 development by cooperating with ROR nuclear receptors. Nature 2010;464(7293):1381–5.

[69] Nishihara M, Ogura H, Ueda N, et al. IL-6-gp130-STAT3 in T cells directs the development of IL-17+ Th with a minimum effect on that of Treg in the steady state. Int Immunol 2007;19(6):695–702.

[70] Tanaka K, Ichiyama K, Hashimoto M, et al. Loss of suppressor of cytokine signaling 1 in helper T cells leads to defective Th17 differentiation by enhancing antagonistic effects of IFN-gamma on STAT3 and Smads. J Immunol 2008;180(6):3746–56.

[71] Lazarevic V, Chen X, Shim JH, et al. T-bet represses T(H)17 differentiation by preventing Runx1-mediated activation of the gene encoding RORgammat. Nat Immunol 2010;12(1):96–104.

[72] Nurieva R, Yang XO, Chung Y, Dong C. Cutting edge: in vitro generated Th17 cells maintain their cytokine expression program in normal but not lymphopenic hosts. J Immunol 2009;182(5):2565–8.

[73] Lee YK, Turner H, Maynard CL, et al. Late developmental plasticity in the T helper 17 lineage. Immunity 2009;30(1):92–107.

[74] Martin-Orozco N, Chung Y, Chang SH, Wang YH, Dong C. Th17 cells promote pancreatic inflammation but only induce diabetes efficiently in lymphopenic hosts after conversion into Th1 cells. Eur J Immunol 2009;39(1):216–24.

[75] Kryczek I, Zhao E, Liu Y, et al. Human TH17 Cells Are Long-Lived Effector Memory Cells. Sci Transl Med 2011;3(104):104ra0.

[76] Muranski P, Borman ZA, Kerkar SP, et al. Th17 cells are long lived and retain a stem cell-like molecular signature. Immunity 2011;35(6):972–85.

[77] Lexberg MH, Taubner A, Albrecht I, et al. IFN-gamma and IL-12 synergize to convert in vivo generated Th17 into Th1/Th17 cells. Eur J Immunol 2010;40(11):3017–27.

[78] Peck A, Mellins ED. Plasticity of T-cell phenotype and function: the T helper type 17 example. Immunology 2009;129(2):147–53.

[79] Zhou L, Lopes JE, Chong MM, et al. TGF-beta-induced Foxp3 inhibits T(H)17 cell differentiation by antagonizing RORgammat function. Nature 2008;453(7192):236–40.

[80] Cosmi L, Maggi L, Santarlasci V, et al. Identification of a novel subset of human circulating memory CD4(+) T cells that produce both IL-17A and IL-4. J Allergy Clin Immunol 2010;125(1):222−30 e1−4.

[81] Wang YH, Voo KS, Liu B, et al. A novel subset of CD4(+) T(H)2 memory/effector cells that produce inflammatory IL-17 cytokine and promote the exacerbation of chronic allergic asthma. J Exp Med 2010;207(11):2479−91.

[82] Pepper M, Linehan JL, Pagan AJ, et al. Different routes of bacterial infection induce long-lived TH1 memory cells and short-lived TH17 cells. Nat Immunol 2010;11(1):83−9.

[83] Martin-Orozco N, Muranski P, Chung Y, et al. T helper 17 cells promote cytotoxic T cell activation in tumor immunity. Immunity 2009;31(5):787−98.

[84] Muranski P, Restifo NP. Adoptive immunotherapy of cancer using CD4(+) T cells. Curr Opin Immunol 2009;21(2):200−8.

[85] Zhou J, Shen X, Huang J, Hodes RJ, Rosenberg SA, Robbins PF. Telomere length of transferred lymphocytes correlates with in vivo persistence and tumor regression in melanoma patients receiving cell transfer therapy. J Immunol 2005;175(10):7046−52.

[86] Shen X, Zhou J, Hathcock KS, et al. Persistence of tumor infiltrating lymphocytes in adoptive immunotherapy correlates with telomere length. J Immunother 2007;30(1):123−9.

[87] Fearon DT, Manders P, Wagner SD. Arrested differentiation, the self-renewing memory lymphocyte, and vaccination. Science 2001;293(5528):248−50.

[88] Chang JT, Palanivel VR, Kinjyo I, et al. Asymmetric T lymphocyte division in the initiation of adaptive immune responses. Science 2007;315(5819):1687−91.

[89] Wei S, Zhao E, Kryczek I, Zou W. Th17 cells have stem cell-like features and promote long-term immunity. OncoImmunology 2012;1(4):516−9.

[90] Corsini NS, Sancho-Martinez I, Laudenklos S, et al. The death receptor CD95 activates adult neural stem cells for working memory formation and brain repair. Cell Stem Cell 2009;5(2):178−90.

[91] Bending D, De la Pena H, Veldhoen M, et al. Highly purified Th17 cells from BDC2.5NOD mice convert into Th1-like cells in NOD/SCID recipient mice. J Clin Invest 2009;119(3):565−72.

[92] Semenza GL. Targeting HIF-1 for cancer therapy. Nat Rev Cancer 2003;3(10):721−32.

[93] Kryczek I, Lange A, Mottram P, et al. CXCL12 and vascular endothelial growth factor synergistically induce neoangiogenesis in human ovarian cancers. Cancer Res 2005;65(2):465−72.

[94] Takubo K, Goda N, Yamada W, et al. Regulation of the HIF-1alpha level is essential for hematopoietic stem cells. Cell Stem Cell 2010;7(3):391−402.

[95] Dang EV, Barbi J, Yang HY, et al. Control of T(H)17/T(reg) balance by hypoxia-inducible factor 1. Cell 2011;146(5):772−84.

[96] Bracken AP, Kleine-Kohlbrecher D, Dietrich N, et al. The Polycomb group proteins bind throughout the INK4A-ARF locus and are disassociated in senescent cells. Genes Dev 2007;21(5):525−30.

[97] Zou W, Machelon V, Coulomb-L'Hermin A, et al. Stromal-derived factor-1 in human tumors recruits and alters the function of plasmacytoid precursor dendritic cells. Nat Med 2001;7(12):1339−46.

[98] Sharma MD, Hou DY, Liu Y, et al. Indoleamine 2,3-dioxygenase controls conversion of Foxp3+ Tregs to TH17-like cells in tumor-draining lymph nodes. Blood 2009;113(24):6102−11.

[99] Zou W. Regulatory T cells, tumour immunity and immunotherapy. Nat Rev Immunol 2006;6(4): 295−307.

[100] Beriou G, Costantino CM, Ashley CW, et al. IL-17-producing human peripheral regulatory T cells retain suppressive function. Blood 2009;113(18):4240−9.

[101] Voo KS, Wang YH, Santori FR, et al. Identification of IL-17-producing FOXP3+ regulatory T cells in humans. Proc Natl Acad Sci U S A 2009;106(12):4793−8.

[102] Mucida D, Park Y, Kim G, et al. Reciprocal TH17 and regulatory T cell differentiation mediated by retinoic acid. Science 2007;317(5835):256−60.

[103] Bettelli E, Carrier Y, Gao W, et al. Reciprocal developmental pathways for the generation of pathogenic effector TH17 and regulatory T cells. Nature 2006;441(7090):235−8.

[104] Sfanos KS, Bruno TC, Maris CH, et al. Phenotypic analysis of prostate-infiltrating lymphocytes reveals TH17 and Treg skewing. Clin Cancer Res 2008;14(11):3254−61.

[105] Ye ZJ, Zhou Q, Gu YY, et al. Generation and differentiation of IL-17-producing CD4+ T cells in malignant pleural effusion. J Immunol 2010;185(10):6348−54.

[106] von Euw E, Chodon T, Attar N, et al. CTLA4 blockade increases Th17 cells in patients with metastatic melanoma. J Transl Med 2009;7:35.

[107] Hinrichs CS, Kaiser A, Paulos CM, et al. Type 17 CD8+ T cells display enhanced antitumor immunity. Blood 2009;114(3):596−9.

[108] Hirahara N, Nio Y, Sasaki S, et al. Inoculation of human interleukin-17 gene-transfected Meth-A fibrosarcoma cells induces T cell-dependent tumor-specific immunity in mice. Oncology 2001;61(1):79–89.

[109] Benchetrit F, Ciree A, Vives V, et al. Interleukin-17 inhibits tumor cell growth by means of a T-cell-dependent mechanism. Blood 2002;99(6):2114–21.

[110] Pellegrini M, Calzascia T, Elford AR, et al. Adjuvant IL-7 antagonizes multiple cellular and molecular inhibitory networks to enhance immunotherapies. Nat Med 2009;15(5):528–36.

[111] Kottke T, Sanchez-Perez L, Diaz RM, et al. Induction of hsp70-mediated Th17 autoimmunity can be exploited as immunotherapy for metastatic prostate cancer. Cancer Res 2007;67(24):11970–9.

[112] Gnerlich JL, Mitchem JB, Weir JS, et al. Induction of Th17 cells in the tumor microenvironment improves survival in a murine model of pancreatic cancer. J Immunol 2010;185(7):4063–71.

[113] Yen HR, Harris TJ, Wada S, et al. Tc17 CD8 T cells: functional plasticity and subset diversity. J Immunol 2009;183(11):7161–8.

[114] Galon J, Costes A, Sanchez-Cabo F, et al. Type, density, and location of immune cells within human colorectal tumors predict clinical outcome. Science 2006;313(5795):1960–4.

[115] Zhang L, Conejo-Garcia JR, Katsaros D, et al. Intratumoral T cells, recurrence, and survival in epithelial ovarian cancer. N Engl J Med 2003;348(3):203–13.

[116] Sato E, Olson SH, Ahn J, et al. Intraepithelial CD8+ tumor-infiltrating lymphocytes and a high CD8+/ regulatory T cell ratio are associated with favorable prognosis in ovarian cancer. Proc Natl Acad Sci U S A 2005;102(51):18538–43.

[117] Zhang YL, Li J, Mo HY, et al. Different subsets of tumor infiltrating lymphocytes correlate with NPC progression in different ways. Mol Cancer 2010;9:4.

[118] Derhovanessian E, Adams V, Hahnel K, et al. Pretreatment frequency of circulating IL-17+ CD4+ T-cells, but not Tregs, correlates with clinical response to whole-cell vaccination in prostate cancer patients. Int J Cancer 2009;125(6):1372–9.

[119] Kuang DM, Peng C, Zhao Q, Wu Y, Chen MS, Zheng L. Activated monocytes in peritumoral stroma of hepatocellular carcinoma promote expansion of memory T helper 17 cells. Hepatology 2010;51(1):154–64.

[120] Wu S, Rhee KJ, Albesiano E, et al. A human colonic commensal promotes colon tumorigenesis via activation of T helper type 17 T cell responses. Nat Med 2009;15(9):1016–22.

[121] Chen X, Wan J, Liu J, et al. Increased IL-17-producing cells correlate with poor survival and lymphangiogenesis in NSCLC patients. Lung Cancer 2009;69(3):348–54.

[122] Zhang JP, Yan J, Xu J, et al. Increased intratumoral IL-17-producing cells correlate with poor survival in hepatocellular carcinoma patients. J Hepatol 2009;50(5):980–9.

[123] Numasaki M, Fukushi J, Ono M, et al. Interleukin-17 promotes angiogenesis and tumor growth. Blood 2003;101(7):2620–7.

[124] Numasaki M, Watanabe M, Suzuki T, et al. IL-17 enhances the net angiogenic activity and in vivo growth of human non-small cell lung cancer in SCID mice through promoting CXCR-2-dependent angiogenesis. J Immunol 2005;175(9):6177–89.

[125] Wang L, Yi T, Kortylewski M, Pardoll DM, Zeng D, Yu H. IL-17 can promote tumor growth through an IL-6-Stat3 signaling pathway. J Exp Med 2009;206(7):1457–64.

[126] He D, Li H, Yusuf N, et al. IL-17 promotes tumor development through the induction of tumor promoting microenvironments at tumor sites and myeloid-derived suppressor cells. J Immunol 2010;184(5):2281–8.

[127] Murugaiyan G, Saha B. Protumor vs antitumor functions of IL-17. J Immunol 2009;183(7):4169–75.

[128] Honorati MC, Neri S, Cattini L, Facchini A. Interleukin-17, a regulator of angiogenic factor release by synovial fibroblasts. Osteoarthritis Cartilage 2006;14(4):345–52.

[129] Huang X, Lee C. Regulation of stromal proliferation, growth arrest, differentiation and apoptosis in benign prostatic hyperplasia by TGF-beta. Front Biosci 2003;8:s740–9.

[130] Waugh DJ, Wilson C. The interleukin-8 pathway in cancer. Clin Cancer Res 2008;14(21):6735–41.

[131] Lee JW, Wang P, Kattah MG, et al. Differential regulation of chemokines by IL-17 in colonic epithelial cells. J Immunol 2008;181(9):6536–45.

[132] Langowski JL, Zhang X, Wu L, et al. IL-23 promotes tumour incidence and growth. Nature 2006;442(7101):461–5.

[133] Iwakura Y, Ishigame H, Saijo S, Nakae S. Functional specialization of interleukin-17 family members. Immunity 2011;34(2):149–62.

[134] Kawaguchi M, Adachi M, Oda N, Kokubu F, Huang SK. IL-17 cytokine family. J Allergy Clin Immunol 2004;114(6):1265–73. quiz 74.

[135] Moseley TA, Haudenschild DR, Rose L, Reddi AH. Interleukin-17 family and IL-17 receptors. Cytokine Growth Factor Rev 2003;14(2):155–74.

[136] Gaffen SL. Structure and signalling in the IL-17 receptor family. Nat Rev Immunol 2009;9(8):556—67.

[137] Starnes T, Broxmeyer HE, Robertson MJ, Hromas R. Cutting edge: IL-17D, a novel member of the IL-17 family, stimulates cytokine production and inhibits hemopoiesis. J Immunol 2002;169(2):642—6.

[138] Broxmeyer HE, Starnes T, Ramsey H, et al. The IL-17 cytokine family members are inhibitors of human hematopoietic progenitor proliferation. Blood 2006;108(2):770.

[139] Angkasekwinai P, Park H, Wang YH, et al. Interleukin 25 promotes the initiation of proallergic type 2 responses. J Exp Med 2007;204(7):1509—17.

[140] Ikeda K, Nakajima H, Suzuki K, et al. Mast cells produce interleukin-25 upon Fc epsilon RI-mediated activation. Blood 2003;101(9):3594—6.

[141] Pappu R, Ramirez-Carrozzi V, Ota N, Ouyang W, Hu Y. The IL-17 family cytokines in immunity and disease. J Clin Immunol 2010;30(2):185—95.

[142] Benatar T, Cao MY, Lee Y, et al. IL-17E, a proinflammatory cytokine, has antitumor efficacy against several tumor types in vivo. Cancer Immunol Immunother 2010;59(6):805—17.

[143] Reynolds JM, Angkasekwinai P, Dong C. IL-17 family member cytokines: regulation and function in innate immunity. Cytokine Growth Factor Rev 2010;21(6):413—23.

[144] Kawaguchi M, Onuchic LF, Li XD, et al. Identification of a novel cytokine, ML-1, and its expression in subjects with asthma. J Immunol 2001;167(8):4430—5.

[145] Hymowitz SG, Filvaroff EH, Yin JP, et al. IL-17s adopt a cystine knot fold: structure and activity of a novel cytokine, IL-17F, and implications for receptor binding. EMBO J 2001;20(19):5332—41.

[146] Starnes T, Robertson MJ, Sledge G, et al. Cutting edge: IL-17F, a novel cytokine selectively expressed in activated T cells and monocytes, regulates angiogenesis and endothelial cell cytokine production. J Immunol 2001;167(8):4137—40.

[147] Kesselring R, Thiel A, Pries R, Trenkle T, Wollenberg B. Human Th17 cells can be induced through head and neck cancer and have a functional impact on HNSCC development. Br J Cancer 2010;103(8):1245—54.

[148] Charles KA, Kulbe H, Soper R, et al. The tumor-promoting actions of TNF-alpha involve TNFR1 and IL-17 in ovarian cancer in mice and humans. J Clin Invest 2009;119(10):3011—23.

[149] Xie Y, Sheng W, Xiang J, Ye Z, Yang J. Interleukin-17F suppresses hepatocarcinoma cell growth via inhibition of tumor angiogenesis. Cancer Invest 2010;28(6):598—607.

[150] Hu J, Yuan X, Belladonna ML, et al. Induction of potent antitumor immunity by intratumoral injection of interleukin 23-transduced dendritic cells. Cancer Res 2006;66(17):8887—96.

[151] Yuan X, Hu J, Belladonna ML, Black KL, Yu JS. Interleukin-23-expressing bone marrow-derived neural stem-like cells exhibit antitumor activity against intracranial glioma. Cancer Res 2006;66(5):2630—8.

[152] Overwijk WW, de Visser KE, Tirion FH, et al. Immunological and antitumor effects of IL-23 as a cancer vaccine adjuvant. J Immunol 2006;176(9):5213—22.

[153] Oniki S, Nagai H, Horikawa T, et al. Interleukin-23 and interleukin-27 exert quite different antitumor and vaccine effects on poorly immunogenic melanoma. Cancer Res 2006;66(12):6395—404.

[154] Iida T, Iwahashi M, Katsuda M, et al. Tumor-infiltrating CD4+ Th17 cells produce IL-17 in tumor microenvironment and promote tumor progression in human gastric cancer. Oncol Rep 2011;25(5):1271—7.

[155] Prabhala RH, Pelluru D, Fulciniti M, et al. Elevated IL-17 produced by TH17 cells promotes myeloma cell growth and inhibits immune function in multiple myeloma. Blood 2010;115(26):5385—92.

CHAPTER 11

Immune Escape: Immunosuppressive Networks

Sandra Demaria
Department of Pathology, New York University School of Medicine, and NYU Langone Medical Center, New York, NY USA

I. INTRODUCTION

The mechanisms of immune escape by tumors have been the focus of intense investigations for several years, and much has been learned. When unable to eliminate transformed cells, the immunological pressure results in selection of poorly immunogenic tumor cells that are difficult to kill, recognize, or locate by immune effectors [1,2]. Increased resistance to killing by T cells or natural killer (NK) cells can be due to upregulation of anti-apoptotic molecules, or mutation in death receptors such as Fas/CD95 [3]. Loss or alterations in expression of genes encoding one or more of the molecules required for the generation and assembly of major histocompatibility complex (MHC) class I/antigenic peptide complexes leads to decreased recognition by T cells [4]. Finally, the lack of endothelial signals and altered chemokine gradients impair homing and infiltration of tumors by antitumor T cells [5,6]. In addition to escaping from antitumor effector T cells that have developed, the tumor microenvironment actively prevents immune-mediated rejection by exploiting the immunosuppressive networks that have evolved to maintain tolerance to self during tissue inflammation in infectious diseases. In fact, there are several parallels between the immunological alterations that develop in chronic infectious diseases and cancer. In both conditions, imbalances in stimulatory and inhibitory pathways lead to a dysfunctional immune system unable to eliminate the pathogen.

The three critical imbalances that develop in the tumor microenvironment, between mature and immature dendritic cells (DC), stimulatory and inhibitory B7 family molecules, and regulatory and conventional T cells, have been discussed in detail in the first edition of this book. This chapter will focus on the mechanisms of T-cell dysfunction, with emphasis on the more recent findings that highlight potentially targetable pathways to improve the effects of cancer treatment. Here, the definition of "T-cell dysfunction" will be applied in a broad sense to mean not only the development of T cells that are unable to perform the effector functions intrinsic to their type of functional differentiation, but also the development of T cells that have differentiated towards the erroneous functional program, one that instead of inhibiting the tumor fosters its progression (Figure 11.1).

II. DYSFUNCTIONAL T-CELL DIFFERENTIATION

Functional differentiation, also termed "polarization," of T cells is regulated by signals present in the environment at the time of initial antigen recognition and activation [7]. Several types

Cancer Immunotherapy. http://dx.doi.org/10.1016/B978-0-12-394296-8.00011-7

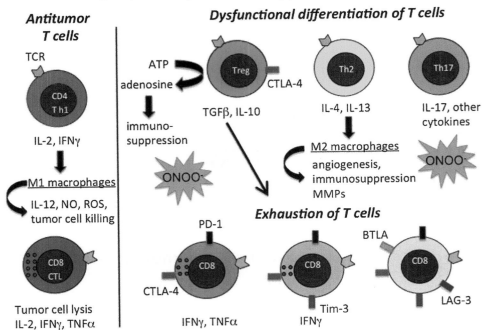

Immune escape: immunosuppressive networks

FIGURE 11.1

Immunosuppressive networks. Left, tumor rejection requires the coordinated action of Th1 CD4$^+$ T cells, M1 macrophages and CTLs, capable of performing several effector functions, including secretion of IFNγ and TNFα and tumor cell killing. Right, immune escape is characterized by dysfunctional differentiation of CD4$^+$ T cells into cells that promote tumor growth and prevent rejection. Treg cells convert ATP into immunosuppressive adenosine and secrete TGFβ and IL-10, cytokines that contribute to CD8$^+$ T-cell exhaustion, a process of progressive loss of effector functions by CD8$^+$ T cells and acquisition of multiple checkpoint/inhibitory receptors (CTLA-4, PD-1, Tim-3, LAG-3, BTLA). IL-4 produced by Th2 CD4$^+$ T cells induces the polarization of macrophages towards M2 phenotype, cells that produce pro-angiogenic and immunosuppressive cytokines and, together with myeloid derived suppressor cells, generate peroxynitrites (ONOO$^-$), highly reactive oxidizing agents that modify tyrosines and other amino acids, altering antigenic peptides, chemokines and other molecules required for T-cells infiltration and recognition of tumor cells.

of functional programs exist, the best defined being T helper (Th)1, Th2, Th17, and regulatory T-cells (Treg) differentiation [8]. Although multiple factors, including the strength of T-cell receptor (TCR)-mediated signals have been shown to influence naïve CD4$^+$ T-cell differentiation [9], cytokines are the key drivers [8]. Th1 differentiation requires the presence of interferon (IFN)-γ produced by NK cells, CD8$^+$ or other Th1 CD4$^+$ T cells, and is sustained by interleukin (IL)-12 produced by innate immune cells. Th2 differentiation is driven by IL-4 produced, at least in some cases, by basophils [10], and is mutually exclusive in that induction of the Th2 transcription factor GATA-3 suppresses expression of the Th1 transcription factor T-bet, and vice versa [11]. Th17 differentiation is dependent on the presence of both (Chapter 10) transforming growth factor β (TGF-β) and IL-6 and is mutually exclusive with adaptive or induced Treg (iTreg) differentiation, which requires TGF-β and IL-2, although some plasticity between these programs seems to exist [12,13].

Experimental evidence has shown that tumor rejection requires T cells that have functionally differentiated to become CD4$^+$ Th1 and CD8$^+$ cytotoxic T cells (CTL) [14]. Th1 cells produce IFN-γ, promote and sustain the development of CTLs, and the polarization of macrophages towards a M1 phenotype, characterized by production of IL-12, reactive oxygen species and nitric oxide (NO), and tumorigenic activity [15]. This functional program, which developed to fight intracellular pathogens such as viruses, is also increasingly recognized as the critical antitumor immune response program in human patients since presence of a dominant Th1 signature in the tumor is associated with better prognosis [16–19]. Conversely, a dominant Th2 polarization of the antitumor immune response has been associated with disease progression and worse outcome in several malignancies [20–23]. Th2 functional differentiation is characterized by production of cytokines that promote humoral immunity required to fight extracellular pathogens, including IL-4, IL-5, IL-10, and IL-13 [8]. In the context of cancer, Th2 skewing can be detrimental in several ways. Because differentiation of naïve CD4$^+$ T cells towards a Th2 program is mutually exclusive with differentiation towards a Th1 program, conditions that favor the first will prevent the latter, thus hindering development of effective antitumor immunity. But more importantly, the cytokines produced by Th2 cells promote the polarization of macrophages towards a M2 phenotype, which is characterized by pro-angiogenic, immunosuppressive and tissue-remodeling activities that promote tumor growth [24]. Recent evidence in a mouse model of mammary carcinogenesis highlights a key role of Th2 CD4$^+$ T cells in promoting metastases mediated by IL-4, which enhanced the protumor activities of macrophages, including the production of epidermal growth factor [25]. Another Th2 cytokine, IL-13, was shown to promote breast cancer development by binding and signaling to the cancer cells themselves [26].

Given the impact of Th2 T cell polarization on tumor progression, it is important to understand which factors drive this dysfunctional differentiation of CD4$^+$ T cells in the tumor microenvironment. Since naïve CD4$^+$ T cells must be exposed to IL-4 during the early stages of activation to undergo Th2 differentiation [27], presumably antigen recognition must occur in a tumor environment rich in IL-4. Two questions that have been puzzling investigators for some time concern the nature of the antigen(s) recognized by CD4$^+$ T cells and the source of IL-4. A superantigen encoded by an endogenous retrovirus was shown to be responsible for activation of protumorigenic Th2 T cells in a mouse lymphoma model [28], but a similar phenomenon has not been reported in humans and may be a rare occurrence. Some epithelial tumor cells have been shown to produce IL-4 and use it as an autocrine survival factor, but their ability to induce Th2 responses was not investigated [29]. Nonetheless, a recent report by Godefroy and colleagues provides some insights into both of the above questions [30]. While studying in melanoma patients CD4$^+$ T-cells specific for matrix metalloproteinase-2 (MMP-2), a proteolytic enzyme that is overexpressed by many tumors, they found that these cells were functionally differentiated towards a Th2 phenotype, and identified the mechanisms responsible for this polarization. Active MMP-2 acted not only as a source of antigen, but also as the endogenous Th2 conditioner, by inducing the expression of OX40L and by degrading type I IFN receptor on DC, thus leading to reduced signal transducer and activator of transcription (STAT)1 phosphorylation and loss of IL-12 production [30]. Importantly, while both signaling via OX40L and inhibition of IL-12 production were required for polarization of MMP-2-specific CD4$^+$ T cells, IL-4 was not required. Additionally, Godefroy et al. showed that DC conditioned by MMP-2 were able to induce Th2 polarization of CD4$^+$ T cells specific for other melanoma-associated antigens, suggesting that this may be a major pathway mediating the dysfunctional differentiation of T cells towards the Th2 program in tumors rich in MMP-2 [30]. This data demonstrates a novel link between a factor involved in tumor invasion, angiogenesis and metastasis [31] and induction of dysfunctional differentiation of antitumor T cells, further supporting the concept that immune escape is intimately connected to the mechanisms of tumor progression.

Among the other two main functional programs, Th17 CD4$^+$ T cells have a strong pro-inflammatory function. Their role in cancer is still under debate [32] and will be discussed in detail in another chapter (see Chapter 10, "Th17 Cells in Cancer"). Treg cells play a critical role in controlling homeostasis of the immune system and preventing excessive inflammation and autoimmunity [33]. Tumor immunity is also, for the most part, a reaction against self antigens and, therefore, the fact that Treg cells protect tumors from immune rejection is a deviation of their physiological function [34]. Expression of the Forkhead Box Protein P3 (FoxP3) transcription factor is necessary for the development and function of Treg cells in mice and humans [35,36], and has been used as a marker for this T-cell subset in tumors. Infiltration of most tumor types by Treg cells correlates with a worse prognosis [37–41], and increased numbers of Treg cells in tumor-draining lymph nodes have been associated with tumor progression [42,43]. However, in some lymphoid malignancies Treg cells may have a beneficial effect, perhaps because of their ability to inhibit neoplastic B cells [44,45]. Likewise, in colorectal cancer Treg cells have a positive prognostic value, something that may be explained by the unique inflammatory environment of the colon [46]. Tregs cells that are present in tumors include natural Treg (nTreg), which differentiate into Treg cells in the thymus, and iTreg, which differentiate or "convert" into regulatory cells because of signals present in the microenvironment at the time of activation [47]. The relative contribution of each Treg type to suppression of the antitumor response remains controversial and may depend on the experimental model [48]. Conversion of conventional CD4$^+$ T cells into iTreg cells is not unique to tumors, and occurs physiologically in seemingly opposite tolerogenic, noninflammatory conditions, as well as serving as a feedback mechanism to prevent uncontrolled immune activation in inflammatory conditions [49]. However, in tumors the conversion of CD4$^+$ T cells into iTregs can become dominant and contribute to pathology, representing a type of dysfunctional differentiation of T cells. This occurs because the tumor microenvironment is rich in TGFβ, the key cytokine promoting Treg differentiation, which is produced by neoplastic cells as well as immature myeloid DC [50,51]. Expression of programmed death 1 ligand (PD-L1) by DC, and the interaction between cytotoxic T-lymphocyte antigen-4 (CTLA-4) and CD80 can also contribute to the generation of iTreg cells [52,53], indicating that the phenotype of DC, which is altered in tumors, modulates the generation of iTreg cells. Reciprocally, Treg cells exert their suppressive function, in part, by direct interaction with DC, leading to downregulation of co-stimulatory molecules and upregulation of indoleamine 2,3-dioxygenase (IDO) by DC [54,55], although the role of this mechanism in mediating Treg suppression *in vivo* remains unclear [56]. Overall, although multiple pathways and mediators of the immunosuppressive activity of Treg cells have been described [56], suppression by tumor-infiltrating iTreg cells is likely mediated predominantly by secretion of IL-10 and TGFβ [57], while nTreg cells act by cell-contact dependent cytotoxicity, a possibility that is supported by recent data comparing gene expression profiles of *in vivo* generated Treg cells [58].

III. T-CELL EXHAUSTION IN CANCER

Tumor escape from immune control can happen due to development of the "wrong" type of T cells, as discussed above, but T cells functionally differentiated towards a Th1 and CTL program that are unable to perform their functions have also been detected in tumors [59]. The loss of effector functions by CD8$^+$ T cells in the context of cancer has many similarities with a process first described in chronic viral infections as T-cell exhaustion [60,61]. The model of T-cell exhaustion that is emerging for CD8$^+$ T cells in chronic infectious diseases is a progressive, hierarchical loss of functions that is accompanied by the increase in the expression and diversity of inhibitory receptors [62]. First, T cells lose the ability to produce IL-2, proliferate and kill, as measured *ex vivo*. Next, the ability to produce tumor necrosis factor (TNF)α is lost, followed by loss of IFNγ production and, finally, physical deletion of the T-cell clone reactive to a given antigen. The degree of exhaustion of CD8$^+$ T cells has been shown to be modulated by several factors that are relevant also to the situation of cancer patients, including the loss of CD4$^+$ T cell help [63,64] and the antigenic load [65], consistent with the observation that increased tumor burden is associated with more severe exhaustion [66].

Inhibitory or immune checkpoint receptors that are expressed on the surface of exhausted T cells are part of a larger group of receptors that regulate immune responses. Most inhibitory receptors dampen the signals downstream to the TCR, often by recruiting the tyrosine phosphatases SHP-1 and SHP-2 to phosphorylated immunoreceptor tyrosine-based inhibition motifs (ITIMs) in the receptor cytoplasmic tail [67]. They are important in maintenance of tolerance and are often transiently upregulated during T-cell activation. However, in exhausted T-cells inhibitory receptors are expressed permanently and at high levels [68]. In addition, co-expression of multiple inhibitory receptors has been reported on exhausted CD8$^+$ T cells, with up to seven receptors being expressed in the most exhausted T cells during viral infections

[69]. Importantly, inhibitory receptors are not simply markers of T-cell dysfunction, but actively control T-cell exhaustion, as demonstrated by the fact that therapeutics blocking these pathways can restore, at least to some degree, T-cell function [70,71].

Among checkpoint receptors, CTLA-4 plays a fundamental role in regulating the activation and proliferation of T cells, and in its absence mice develop a fatal lymphoproliferative disease at a young age that is driven by CD4$^+$ T cells [72]. Although regulation by CTLA-4 impacts predominantly CD4$^+$ T cells, it also affects CD8$^+$ T cells, mostly at the level of secondary responses [73]. In conditions of chronic antigenic stimulation that lead to T-cell exhaustion CTLA-4 is persistently upregulated, impairing T-cell activation. CTLA-4 inhibitory effects are mediated by multiple cell intrinsic and extrinsic mechanisms, including the competition with the activating co-receptor CD28 for binding to co-stimulatory molecules B7-1 and B7-2, triggering of negative signaling pathways that inhibit cytokines production, and reverse signaling mediated by the interaction of CTLA-4 expressed on Treg cells with B7 molecules on DC [70]. The critical role of CTLA-4 in maintenance of immune tolerance to tumors has been unequivocally demonstrated by the therapeutic success of antibodies blocking this checkpoint receptor [74], as will be discussed in more detail in Chapter 19, "Antibodies to Stimulate Host Immunity: Lessons from Ipilimumab."

Programmed death (PD)-1 is another important regulator of T-cell activation that physiologically functions to limit collateral damage to normal tissue during an inflammatory response [71]. PD-1 binds to B7-H1/PD-L1, a broadly expressed ligand that is upregulated in response to pro-inflammatory cytokines [75]. A second ligand, B7-DC/PD-L2, has a more restricted pattern of expression, mainly DC and macrophages, and is also induced by proinflammatory cytokines [76]. Mice deficient in PD-1 show increased severity of auto-immune diseases suggesting that PD-1 is a context-dependent modulator of immune reactivity [77]. In tumors, upregulation of B7-H1/PD-L1 is common [78] and may be driven by IFN-γ that is produced by antitumor T cells, leading to the hypothesis that it is required for cancer cells to escape the antitumor immune response [71]. On the other hand, PD-1 is a major checkpoint receptor expressed by exhausted CD8$^+$ T cells in chronic infections as well as cancer and it is often found on tumor-infiltrating lymphocytes [62,79]. Expression of PD-1 on CD4$^+$ T cells has also been linked to decreased production of Th1 cytokines, and to the conversion of CD4$^+$ T cells into iTreg cells [80]. Therefore, PD-1 plays a central role in T-cell dysfunction in cancer, and its role is nonredundant with CTLA-4, a concept that is supported by the improved antitumor response obtained with concomitant blockade of both receptors [79]. Clinical testing of antibodies that block the PD-1/PD-L1 pathways in cancer patients is still in the early stage, but has shown promising results [81].

T-cell immunoglobulin-3 (Tim-3) is another member of the checkpoint receptors family but it has a more restricted expression compared to CTLA-4 and PD-1, and is specifically expressed on CD4$^+$ Th1 and CD8$^+$ CTL cells that produce IFN-γ [82]. The ligand for Tim-3 is galectin-9, a member of a family of lectins that bind N-acetyllactosamine-containing glycans and perform important immunoregulatory functions [83]. Binding of galectin-9 to Tim-3 leads to T-cell death thus specifically switching off Th1 immune responses [84]. Expression of Tim-3 on tumor-infiltrating lymphocytes has been recently reported in melanoma metastases [85]. In preclinical models, tumor-infiltrating lymphocytes that co-express Tim-3 in addition to PD-1 have been shown to have a more exhausted phenotype [86], and similar findings were reported in cancer patients [87]. In both cases, concomitant blockade of PD-1 and Tim-3 was required to restore T-cell functionality. These data support the clinical development of strategies to block Tim-3 in cancer patients. Additional work is needed, however, to clarify the role of Tim-3 expressed on other cells, including innate immune cells, endothelium, and leukemia stem cells [82].

Lymphocyte activation gene-3 (LAG-3) is an inhibitory receptor structurally similar to CD4 molecule that binds to MHC class II molecules with higher affinity than CD4 [88]. LAG-3 is upregulated in both CD4$^+$ and CD8$^+$ T cells upon activation and can be induced by IL-10 and

IL-6 [89]. In CD4$^+$ T cells signaling via LAG-3 reduces TCR-mediated activation, production of Th1 cytokines, and expansion of activated T cells, thus serving to control the size of the memory T-cell pool [90]. LAG-3 has also been detected on iTreg and activated nTreg cells, and data suggest that it is required for optimal suppressive activity of these cells [91]. In CD8$^+$ T cells LAG-3 is among the inhibitory receptors expressed by exhausted cells [89]. In a model of chronic viral infection LAG-3 blockade did not rescue CD8$^+$ T-cell function [92]. However, recent data have defined the existence of a synergy between PD-1 and LAG-3 expressed by exhausted T cells in mouse models of cancer [93]. Concomitant blockade of both LAG-3 and PD-1 was required to obtain tumor rejection while blockade of a single receptor was not effective. This synergy is further supported by the development of serious autoimmune pathology in mice deficient in both LAG-3 and PD-1, despite the minimal immune dysregulation seen in single knockout mice [93].

B and T-lymphocyte attenuator (BTLA) is an inhibitory receptor expressed by B and T cells and DC [94]. BTLA is increased upon CD4$^+$ T-cell activation and is preferentially expressed on cells with Th1 type of functional differentiation [95]. Studies of BTLA-deficient mice have identified an important role of BTLA in negative regulation of CD8$^+$ T-cell homeostasis and memory generation [96]. The ligand for BTLA, herpes virus entry mediator (HVEM) is expressed on many immune cells as well as some cancer cells [97]. In addition to BTLA, HVEM interacts with other ligands, including CD160, an inhibitory receptor expressed on exhausted CD8$^+$ T cells [69,98], and two co-stimulatory receptors, lymphotoxin-like, inducible expression, compete with herpes simplex virus glycoprotein D for HVEM (LIGHT) and lymphotoxin α (LTα3) and plays a positive or negative role in immunoregulation depending on the context [94]. Persistent high expression of BTLA in tumor antigen-specific CD8$^+$ T cells of melanoma patients was recently reported in two studies [97,99], establishing an important role for BTLA in maintenance of immune tolerance to the tumor. Importantly, Fourcade et al. [99] showed a hierarchy of T-cell exhaustion in NY-ESO-1-specific CD8$^+$ T cells with progressively increasing degree of dysfunction in PD-1$^+$ BTLA$^-$ Tim-3$^-$, PD-1$^+$ BTLA$^+$ Tim-3$^-$, and PD-1$^+$ BTLA$^+$ Tim-3$^+$ T cells. *In vitro*, BTLA blockade enhanced the proliferation and expansion of cytokine-producing NY-ESO-1-specific CD8$^+$ T cells in response to cognate peptide, and showed additive effects in combination with PD-1 but not Tim-3 blockade. However, blockade of BTLA in combination with PD-1 and Tim-3 further enhanced the recovery of T-cell function [99], suggesting that multiple checkpoints receptors need to be targeted to fully recover T-cell function in cancer patients.

Overall, recent data in mouse models and cancer patients are defining the network of inhibitory receptors and their ligands that control T-cell dysfunction in cancer. The picture that is emerging is complex with many similarities to the process of T-cell exhaustion in chronic viral infections, but some possible differences too. For instance, BTLA upregulation has been linked to T-cell anergy [100], and was not seen in exhausted T cells in chronic infections [69]. This may be an important difference with therapeutic implications since, in addition to chronic stimulation by antigens, T cells in cancer patients also face suboptimal stimulation that leads to anergy. In fact, Derré et al. [97] showed that vaccination in the presence of a strong immune activator, the Toll-like receptor (TLR)9 agonist CpG, downregulated BTLA expression and enhanced activation and function of tumor-specific T cells in patients. Although more data are required to understand the mechanisms involved, the possibility that TLR stimulation could contribute to correct T-cell dysfunction should be considered in exploring novel combination treatments [101].

IV. BALANCE OF EXTRACELLULAR ADENOSINE AND ATP IN THE TUMOR: A FUNDAMENTAL REGULATOR OF IMMUNE REACTIVITY

Inhibition of the effector functions of T cells in the tumor microenvironment can also be mediated by imbalances in the levels of extracellular purines [102]. The purinergic receptors and their ligands are part of a network of microenvironmental signals that regulate intercellular communication not only in the nervous system but also in the immune system

[103,104]. Purinergic receptors include three major groups: P2X receptors responsive only to ATP function as ATP-gated ion channels, P2Y receptors which are G protein-coupled receptors (GPCR) and bind to ATP and other nucleotides such as ADP, UDP and UTP, and P1 receptors which are GPCR and bind adenosine. Importantly, ectonucleotidases play a key role in this signaling network by hydrolyzing ATP to ADP, AMP and adenosine, thus regulating the balance between activating and immunosuppressive signals.

ATP is released in a controlled manner by innate and adaptive immune cells and serves, usually as an autocrine signal, in regulation of their activation and effector functions. Release of ATP can occur by vesicular transport, as in neurons, but pannexin 1 hemichannels are a major mechanism of ATP release in T cells and human neutrophils [105–107]. In neutrophils and macrophages autocrine ATP signaling, mediated predominantly by P2Y2 receptors, is involved in regulation of chemotaxis [107,108]. In T cells ATP release is triggered by TCR stimulation [105]. Woehrle et al. [106] have recently shown a key role of the interaction between ATP released by pannexin 1 hemichannels with P2X1 and P2X4 receptors at the immunological synapse for Ca(2+) entry, activation of nuclear factors of activated T cells (NFAT), and IL-2 production, suggesting that purinergic signaling may be a mechanism of amplification to assure T-cell activation to rare antigenic peptides [104]. While ATP is released by healthy immune cells in a defined spatiotemporal way that prevents bystander effects, ATP released by stressed and dying cells in the extracellular environment serves as a signal to attract phagocytic cells to the site of tissue damage, as well as a proinflammatory signal that co-activates the inflammasome [104]. In the absence of microbial pathogens, the presence of damage-associated molecular patterns (DAMPS) molecules released by dying cells together with ATP will determine whether the cell death is perceived as silent and tolerogenic or inflammatory [109–111]. The NLR family, pyrin domain-containing 3 (NLRP3, also known as NAL3) inflammasome is activated by concomitant stimulation of TLRs by DAMP molecules and P2X7 receptor by ATP, and leads to activation of caspase-1 and processing of IL-1β and IL-18 [112]. Importantly, activation of P2X7 receptor by ATP released by dying tumor cells following chemotherapy was recently shown to be required for efficient cross presentation of tumor-associated antigens by DC to T cells, and development of antitumor immunity [111]. Overall, data indicate that extracellular ATP, for the most part, promotes inflammation and activation of the immune response.

In marked contrast adenosine has a fundamental immunosuppressive role, highlighted by the phenotype of the genetic disease due to absence of adenosine deaminase (ADA), which results in severe combined immunodeficiency (SCID), characterized by accumulation of adenosine and defects in B- and T-cell development and activation [113]. P1 A2A adenosine receptor is expressed by most innate and adaptive immune cells, binds with high affinity to adenosine and inhibits immune cell functions [114]. In macrophages, adenosine inhibits phagocytosis and production of superoxide, nitric oxide, TNFα and IL-12 [115]. In addition, recent evidence indicates that adenosine promotes the functional differentiation of protumorigenic M2 macrophages via A2A and A2B receptors [116]. Adenosine skews natural killer T (NKT) cells towards the production of Th2 polarizing IL-4 and immunosuppressive IL-10 and TGFβ cytokines [117]. Adenosine also skews the differentiation of DC into cells that produce pro-angiogenic and immunosuppressive factors and promote tumor growth [118]. Recent data also implicated adenosine in the accumulation of myeloid derived suppressor cells (MDSC) in tumors [119]. Upregulation of A2A receptors occurs upon T-cell activation and, if adenosine is present, signaling via A2A will cause significant inhibition of cytotoxicity and cytokine production by T cells [120]. Adenosine also promotes T-cell anergy and differentiation of CD4$^+$ T cells into iTreg cells [121]. Therefore, extracellular adenosine levels, which have been shown to be elevated in tumors compared to normal tissue [102,122] maintain immuno-suppression and foster immune escape in multiple ways.

The balance of extracellular ATP and its derivatives, including adenosine, is regulated in tissues by ectonuclotidases, enzymes broadly expressed on the surface of mammalian cells [123].

155

Among them, CD39 is the prototypic member of the family of ecto-nucleoside triphosphate diphospho-hydrolases (ENTPDase), which metabolize ATP to ADP and AMP [123]. CD39 is expressed on endothelial cells, where it is involved in regulation of thrombus formation, and on some subsets of immune cells. In T cells, CD39 is expressed by Treg cells and is required for their suppressive function as shown by the impaired suppressive activity of Treg cells from Cd39-null mice [124]. CD73 is an ecto5'-nucleotidase, which generates adenosine from AMP [125]. CD73 plays a role in many physiological processes that are regulated by adenosine, including the control of inflammation and the adaptation to hypoxia, and is upregulated by hypoxia-inducible factor-1 (HIF-1)α in different cell types, including epithelia [125]. Studies using CD73-deficient mice have revealed additional ways in which CD73 expression regulates inflammation and have shown that adenosine generated by CD73 expressed on high endothelial venules in lymph nodes limits lymphocyte migration in response to an inflammatory stimulus [126]. Importantly, Treg cells express high levels of both CD39 and CD73, which work in tandem to convert ATP into adenosine [124], and can be activated by ATP to up-regulate CD73 [127].

In the tumor microenvironment infiltrating Treg cells play an important role in regulating the levels of adenosine, and CD73 expression on Treg cells has been shown to be critical for their protumorigenic effect [128]. In addition, CD73 is frequently upregulated in tumor cells, including human carcinomas of the colon, lung, ovary and pancreas, and has been associated with worse outcome in breast cancer [129]. Data in an experimental mouse breast cancer model demonstrated that CD73 expressed by cancer cells promoted immune escape and metastases [130]. CD73 expressed by tumor cells was also shown to impair tumor rejection by adoptively transferred antitumor CD8[+] T cells [131].

Using CD73-deficient mice and a bone marrow chimera, Stagg et al. [128] showed that CD73 expression on both hematopoietic and nonhematopoietic cells contributed to promoting tumor growth. Importantly, metastases of a CD73-negative mouse melanoma were enhanced by expression of CD73 in nonhematopoietic cells independently from the antitumor immune response, suggesting a role for endothelial CD73 in favoring metastases, and supporting the concept that therapeutic targeting of CD73 could have multiple benefits.

A study analyzing the adenosinergic pathway in suppression by human Treg cells showed that while Treg cells have high levels of CD39 and CD73 and low levels of ADA, the enzyme that breaks down adenosine, the opposite is true for effector T cells [132]. These data suggest that a low ratio of Treg to T effectors cells that has been shown to be a critical determinant of tumor rejection [133], and is associated in human tumors with improved prognosis [41,134], might ultimately reflect a lower concentration of immunosuppressive adenosine.

Overall, canonical pathways that control inflammation are dysregulated in cancer and contribute to immune evasion. Growing evidence indicates that the tumor microenvironment is skewed towards increased levels of adenosine, a pleiotropic immunosuppressive mediator that contributes to impair CTL function, promote the dysfunctional differentiation of CD4[+] T cells into iTreg and Th2 cells and of macrophages towards the M2 phenotype. Physiologically, these effects are meant to promote tissue repair but in the context of cancer they foster tumor growth. Because the ectonucleotidases that generate adenosine can be expressed by multiple cell types, including the neoplastic cells themselves, Treg cells, MDSC [119] and endothelial cells, targeting these enzymes or the A2A and A2B receptors that mediate adenosine effects may prove more effective therapeutically than targeting individual cells that produce adenosine.

V. CHEMICAL BARRIERS FACED BY T CELLS IN THE TUMOR

Hypoxia is a common and critical feature of the tumor microenvironment that shapes many aspects of tumor progression and response to treatment [135]. Recent evidence has provided new insights into the hypoxia-conditioned tumor proteome and its role in immune escape that will be briefly discussed in this section.

While HIF-1α expression is essential for macrophage inflammatory and bactericidal activity in normal tissue during hypoxic conditions found at sites of infection [136], in tumors HIF-1α expression was recently shown to be critical for macrophages immunosuppressive activity [137]. In this study, Doedens et al. [137] showed that arginase I was induced by soluble factors produced by the tumor cells in hypoxic conditions. Arginase I consumes L-arginine limiting the ability of inducible nitric oxide synthase (iNOS) to produce tumoricidal NO, effectively switching the antitumor activity of macrophages into a protumorigenic one. In fact, downstream mediators of L-arginine metabolism can control T-cell function in tumors and are regulated by the coordinated action of iNOS and arginase that are co-expressed by MDSC in the hypoxic tumor environment [138–140]. In addition to polyamines, reactive nitrogen and oxygen species (RNS and ROS) have important immunoregulatory functions, and recent data have uncovered novel molecular mechanisms that explain how RNS alter the tumor proteome to promote tumor escape. In the presence of elevated arginase activity, found in M2 macrophages and MDSC, L-arginine levels are lowered so that iNOS will produce a mixture of NO and O_2^-, which react with each other and form peroxynitrite ($ONOO^-$), a highly reactive oxidizing agent that modifies several amino acids, either directly (cysteine, methionine, tryptophan) or via intermediary secondary species (tyrosine, phenylalanine, histidine) [140,141]. Peroxynitrites have been shown to inhibit protein tyrosine phosphorylation and signal transduction by nitration of tyrosine, and induce T-cell death [142]. In addition to toxic effects, nitration of tyrosines in the TCR/CD8 complex was also shown to impair the ability of T cells to recognize MHC/antigenic peptide thus promoting tolerance [143]. Recent data have identified another mechanisms of tumor cell resistance to CTL mediated by MDSC-produced peroxynitrite, namely the impairment of binding and presentation of antigenic peptides modified by nitrosylation on MHC molecules of tumor cells [144]. Furthermore, Molon et al., [145] demonstrated a novel way in which nitrosylation of proteins in the tumor promotes immune escape by hampering T-cell infiltration. They showed that the nitrosylated chemokine CCL2 was unable to promote chemotaxis of T cells, while still active on myeloid cells that express higher levels of CCL2 receptor CCR2 [145]. This differential activity of modified CCL2 resulted in poor infiltration of T cells in the tumor center, while MDSC, which were largely responsible for peroxynitrite generation were not affected and were fueling the process. Importantly, nitrosylated CCL2 was also detected in human prostate and colon carcinoma, suggesting that it may be a common mechanisms explaining why T cells are seen at the periphery but not center of tumors in many patients [16]. See Chapter 34, "Arginase, Nitric Oxide Synthase, and Novel Inhibitors of L-arginase Metabolism in Immune Modulation" for additional discussions of this pathway.

High levels of nitrotyrosine have been detected in several human cancers, including pancreatic, head and neck, prostate, liver, colon, and breast [146–149]. Given the ability of peroxynitrites to modify multiple amino acids within proteins, they have been considered broad regulator of the proteome in cancer [148]. Protein nitration/nitrosylation is likely to impair T-cell function in the tumor in additional ways, as suggested by downregulation of co-receptors and chemokine receptors in human T cells exposed to RNS [148]. Therefore, this chemical barrier may have a unique place among the immunosuppressive networks that favor immune escape of tumors. Development of new therapeutics to target peroxynitrite production will provide new tools to overcome tumor immune escape [145].

VI. CONCLUSIONS

This chapter summarized recent advances in understanding the bases for T-cell dysfunction in cancer, and the molecules and pathways involved. A high degree of complexity characterizes the immunosuppressive networks that promote tumor escape from immune control. There are multiple, often redundant mechanisms aimed at paralyzing development and function of effector antitumor T cells. The availability of novel and more sophisticated analytical techniques has improved our ability to detect and measure small bioactive molecules and their "footprints" in the tumor microenvironment. The "tumor map" that T cells must navigate to reject an established tumor is getting increasingly more detailed. In addition, we are beginning to appreciate the multiplicity and diversity of checkpoint receptors that fine-tune T-cell activity (Figure 11.1). It is likely that significant advances in cancer treatment will be achieved by strategies that combine the expertise of immunologists in correcting defects in T-cell differentiation and activation with the expertise of biochemists and pharmacologists in designing small molecule inhibitors of RNS and of ectonucleotidases or other immunosuppressive biochemical pathways. Increased understanding of the tumor context, and of the changes caused by treatment is also required for the rational design of combinations of cytocidal agents with immune response modifiers. In fact, both chemotherapy and radiotherapy can induce changes that promote tumor rejection [150–152]. For example, ionizing radiation can act as a modifier of the tumor microenvironment that modulates the antigenic peptide repertoire of tumor cells [153] and induces chemokines that attract T cells [154], while chemotherapy can induce ATP release by tumor cells [155]. Thus, we may already have in our therapeutic armamentarium tools that can disrupt key points in the immunosuppressive networks of tumors. The challenge is to learn how to best use them and combine them with other interventions targeted to the specific characteristics of each individual tumor.

References

[1] Dunn GP, Bruce AT, Ikeda H, Old LJ, Schreiber RD. Cancer immunoediting: from immunosurveillance to tumor escape. Nature Immunol 2002;3:991–8.

[2] Smyth MJ, Dunn GP, Schreiber RD. Cancer immunosurveillance and immunoediting: the roles of immunity in suppressing tumor development and shaping tumor immunogenicity. Adv Immunol 2006;90:1–50.

[3] Takahashi H, Feuerhake F, Kutok JL, Monti S, Dal Cin P, Neuberg D, et al. FAS death domain deletions and cellular FADD-like interleukin 1beta converting enzyme inhibitory protein (long) overexpression: alternative mechanisms for deregulating the extrinsic apoptotic pathway in diffuse large B-cell lymphoma subtypes. Clin Cancer Res 2006;12(11 Pt1):3265–71.

[4] Chang CC, Ferrone S. Immune selective pressure and HLA class I antigen defects in malignant lesions. Cancer Immunol Immunother 2007;56(2):227–36.

[5] Gajewski TF, Meng Y, Blank C, Brown I, Kacha A, Kline J, et al. Immune resistance orchestrated by the tumor microenvironment. Immunol Rev 2006;213:131–45.

[6] Kandalaft LE, Motz GT, Busch J, Coukos G. Angiogenesis and the tumor vasculature as antitumor immune modulators: the role of vascular endothelial growth factor and endothelin. Curr Top Microbiol Immunol 2011;344:129–48.

[7] Guy B. The perfect mix: recent progress in adjuvant research. Nat Rev Microbiol 2007;5(7):505–17.

[8] Wan YY, Flavell RA. How diverse—CD4 effector T cells and their functions. J Mol Cell Biol 2009;1(1):20–36.

[9] Tao X, Constant S, Jorritsma P, Bottomly K. Strength of TCR signal determines the costimulatory requirements for Th1 and Th2 CD4+ T cell differentiation. J Immunol 1997;159(1):5956–63.

[10] Sokol CL, Barton GM, Farr AG, Medzhitov R. A mechanism for the initiation of allergen-induced T helper type 2 responses. Nat Immunol 2008;9(3):310–8.

[11] O'Garra A, Arai N. The molecular basis of T helper 1 and T helper 2 cell differentiation. Trends Cell Biol 2000;10(12):542–50.

[12] Zhou L, Chong MM, Littman DR. Plasticity of CD4+ T cell lineage differentiation. Immunity 2009;30(5):646–55.

[13] Sharma MD, Hou DY, Liu Y, Koni PA, Metz R, Chandler P, et al. Indoleamine 2,3-dioxygenase controls conversion of Foxp3+ Tregs to TH17-like cells in tumor-draining lymph nodes. Blood 2009;113(24):6102–11.

[14] Nishimura T, Nakui M, Sato M, Iwakabe K, Kitamura H, Sekimoto M, et al. The critical role of Th1-dominant immunity in tumor immunology. Cancer Chemother Pharmacol 2000;46(Suppl):S52–61.

[15] Martinez FO, Sica A, Mantovani A, Locati M. Macrophage activation and polarization. Front Biosci 2008;13:453–61.

[16] Galon J, Costes A, Sanchez-Cabo F, Kirilovsky A, Mlecnik B, Lagorce-Pages C, et al. Type, density, and location of immune cells within human colorectal tumors predict clinical outcome. Science 2006;313:1960–4.

[17] Tosolini M, Kirilovsky A, Mlecnik B, Fredriksen T, Mauger S, Bindea G, et al. Clinical impact of different classes of infiltrating T cytotoxic and helper cells (Th1, th2, treg, th17) in patients with colorectal cancer. Cancer Res 2011;71(4):1263–71.

[18] Ascierto ML, De Giorgi V, Liu Q, Bedognetti D, Spivey TL, Murtas D, et al. An immunologic portrait of cancer. J Transl Med 2011;9:146.

[19] Finak G, Bertos N, Pepin F, Sadekova S, Souleimanova M, Zhao H, et al. Stromal gene expression predicts clinical outcome in breast cancer. Nat Med 2008;14:518–27.

[20] Sheu BC, Lin RH, Lien HC, Ho HN, Hsu SM, Huang SC. Predominant Th2/Tc2 polarity of tumor-infiltrating lymphocytes in human cervical cancer. J Immunol 2001;167(5):2972–8.

[21] Lauerova L, Dusek L, Simickova M, Kocák I, Vagundová M, Zaloudík J, et al. Malignant melanoma associates with Th1/Th2 imbalance that coincides with disease progression and immunotherapy response. Neoplasma 2002;49(3):159–66.

[22] Disis ML. Immune regulation of cancer. J Clin Oncol 2010;28(29):4531–8.

[23] Tatsumi T, Kierstead LS, Ranieri E, Gesualdo L, Schena FP, Finke JH, et al. Disease-associated bias in T helper type 1 (Th1)/Th2 CD4(+) T cell responses against MAGE-6 in HLA-DRB10401(+) patients with renal cell carcinoma or melanoma. J Exp Med 2002;196(5):619–28.

[24] Allavena P, Sica A, Garlanda C, Mantovani A. The Yin-Yang of tumor-associated macrophages in neoplastic progression and immune surveillance. Immunol Rev 2008;222:155–61.

[25] DeNardo DG, Barreto JB, Andreu P, Vasquez L, Tawfik D, Kolhatkar N, et al. CD4(+) T cells regulate pulmonary metastasis of mammary carcinomas by enhancing protumor properties of macrophages. Cancer Cell 2009;16(2):91–102.

[26] Aspord C, Pedroza-Gonzalez A, Gallegos M, Tindle S, Burton EC, Su D, et al. Breast cancer instructs dendritic cells to prime interleukin 13-secreting CD4+ T cells that facilitate tumor development. J Exp Med 2007;204:1037–47.

[27] Mowen KA, Glimcher LH. Signaling pathways in Th2 development. Immunol Rev 2004;202:203–22.

[28] Tsiagbe VK, Asakawa J, Miranda A, Sutherland RM, Paterson Y, Thorbecke GJ. Syngeneic response to SJL follicular center B cell lymphoma (reticular cell sarcoma) cells is primarily in V beta 16+ CD4+ T cells. J Immunol 1993;150(12):5519–28.

[29] Todaro M, Lombardo Y, Francipane MG, Alea MP, Cammareri P, Iovino F, et al. Apoptosis resistance in epithelial tumors is mediated by tumor-cell-derived interleukin-4. Cell Death Differ 2008;15(4):762–72.

[30] Godefroy E, Manches O, Dréno B, Hochman T, Rolnitzky L, Labarrière N, et al. Matrix metalloproteinase-2 conditions human dendritic cells to prime inflammatory T(H)2 cells via an IL-12- and OX40L-dependent pathway. Cancer Cell 2011;19(3):333–46.

[31] Kessenbrock K, Plaks V, Werb Z. Matrix metalloproteinases: regulators of the tumor microenvironment. Cell Immunol 2010;141(1):52–67.

[32] Wilke CM, Kryczek I, Wei S, Zhao E, Wu K, Wang G, et al. Th17 cells in cancer: help or hindrance? Carcinogenesis 2011;32(5):643–9.

[33] Wing K, Sakaguchi S. Regulatory T cells exert checks and balances on self tolerance and autoimmunity. Nat Immunol 2010;11(1):7–13.

[34] Nishikawa H, Sakaguchi S. Regulatory T cells in tumor immunity. Int J Cancer 2010;127(4):759–67.

[35] Fontenot JD, Gavin MA, Rudensky AY. Foxp3 programs the development and function of CD4+CD25+ regulatory T cells. Nat Immunol 2003;4(4):330–6.

[36] Hori S, Nomura T, Sakaguchi S. Control of regulatory T cell development by the transcription factor Foxp3. Science 2003;299(5609):1057–61.

[37] Bates GJ, Fox SB, Han C, Leek RD, Garcia JF, Harris AL, et al. Quantification of regulatory T cells enables the identification of high-risk breast cancer patients and those at risk of late relapse. J Clin Oncol 2006;24:5373–80.

[38] Curiel TJ, Coukos G, Zou L, Alvarez X, Cheng P, Mottram P, et al. Specific recruitment of regulatory T cells in ovarian carcinoma fosters immune privilege and predicts reduced survival. Nat Med 2004;10(9):942–9.

[39] Petersen RP, Campa MJ, Sperlazza J, Conlon D, Joshi MB, Harpole DHJ, et al. Tumor infiltrating Foxp3+ regulatory T-cells are associated with recurrence in pathologic stage I NSCLC patients. Cancer 2006;107(12):2866–72.

[40] Kobayashi N, Hiraoka N, Yamagami W, Ojima H, Kanai Y, Kosuge T, et al. FOXP3+ regulatory T cells affect the development and progression of hepatocarcinogenesis. Clin Cancer Res 2007;13(3):902–11.

[41] Gao Q, Qiu SJ, Fan J, Zhou J, Wang XY, Xiao YS, et al. Intratumoral balance of regulatory and cytotoxic T cells is associated with prognosis of hepatocellular carcinoma after resection. J Clin Oncol 2007;25:2586–93.

[42] Gupta R, Babb JS, Singh B, Chiriboga L, Liebes L, Adams S, et al. The Numbers of FoxP3+ Lymphocytes in Sentinel Lymph Nodes of Breast Cancer Patients Correlate With Primary Tumor Size but Not Nodal Status. Cancer Invest 2011;29(6):419–25.

159

[43] Nakamura R, Sakakibara M, Nagashima T, Sangai T, Arai M, Fujimori T, et al. Accumulation of regulatory T cells in sentinel lymph nodes is a prognostic predictor in patients with node-negative breast cancer. Eur J Cancer 2009;45(12):2123–31.

[44] Carreras J, Lopez-Guillermo A, Fox BC, Colomo L, Martinez A, Roncador G, et al. High numbers of tumor-infiltrating FOXP3-positive regulatory T cells are associated with improved overall survival in follicular lymphoma. Blood 2006;108(9):2957–64.

[45] Alvaro T, Lejeune M, Salvadó MT, Bosch R, García JF, Jaén J, et al. Outcome in Hodgkin's lymphoma can be predicted from the presence of accompanying cytotoxic and regulatory T cells. Clin Cancer Res 2005;11(4):1467–73.

[46] Ladoire S, Martin F, Ghiringhelli F. Prognostic role of FOXP3+ regulatory T cells infiltrating human carcinomas: the paradox of colorectal cancer. Cancer Immunol Immunother 2011;60(7):909–18.

[47] Zhou G, Levitsky HI. Natural regulatory T cells and de novo-induced regulatory T cells contribute independently to tumor-specific tolerance. J Immunol 2007;178(4):2155–62.

[48] Bilate AM, Lafaille JJ. Induced CD4(+)Foxp3(+) Regulatory T Cells in Immune Tolerance. Annu Rev Immunol 2012;30:733–58.

[49] Curotto de Lafaille MA, Kutchukhidze N, Shen S, Ding Y, Yee H, Lafaille JJ. Adaptive Foxp3+ regulatory T cell-dependent and -independent control of allergic inflammation. Immunity 2008;29(1):114–26.

[50] Liu VC, Wong LY, Jang T, Shah AH, Park I, Yang X, et al. Tumor evasion of the immune system by converting CD4+CD25- T cells into CD4+CD25+ T regulatory cells: role of tumor-derived TGF-b. J Immunol 2007;178(5):2883–92.

[51] Ghiringhelli F, Puig PE, Roux S, Parcellier A, Schmitt E, Solary E, et al. Tumor cells convert immature myeloid dendritic cells into TGF-beta-secreting cells inducing CD4+CD25+ regulatory T cell proliferation. J Exp Med 2005;202(7):919–29.

[52] Wang L, Pino-Lagos K, de Vries VC, Guleria I, Sayegh MH, Noelle RJ. Programmed death 1 ligand signaling regulates the generation of adaptive Foxp3+CD4+ regulatory T cells. Proc Natl Acad Sci U S A 2008;105(27):9331–6.

[53] Zheng SG, Wang JH, Stohl W, Kim KS, Gray JD, Horwitz DA. TGF-beta requires CTLA-4 early after T cell activation to induce FoxP3 and generate adaptive CD4+CD25+ regulatory cells. J Immunol 2006;176(6):3321–9.

[54] Onishi Y, Fehervari Z, Yamaguchi T, Sakaguchi S. Foxp3+ natural regulatory T cells preferentially form aggregates on dendritic cells in vitro and actively inhibit their maturation. Proc Natl Acad Sci U S A 2008;105(29):10113–8.

[55] Puccetti P, Grohmann U. IDO and regulatory T cells: a role for reverse signalling and non-canonical NF-kappaB activation. Nat Rev Immunol 2007;7(10):817–23.

[56] Tang Q, Bluestone JA. The Foxp3+ regulatory T cell: a jack of all trades, master of regulation. Nat Immunol 2008;9(3):239–44.

[57] Strauss L, Bergmann C, Szczepanski M, Gooding W, Johnson JT, Whiteside TL. A unique subset of CD4+CD25 high Foxp3+ T cells secreting interleukin-10 and transforming growth factor-beta1 mediates suppression in the tumor microenvironment. Clin Cancer Res 2007;13(15 Pt 1):4345–54.

[58] Haribhai D, Williams JB, Jia S, Nickerson D, Schmitt EG, Edwards B, et al. A requisite role for induced regulatory T cells in tolerance based on expanding antigen receptor diversity. Immunity 2011;35(1):109–22.

[59] Frey AB, Monu N. Effector-phase tolerance: another mechanism of how cancer escapes antitumor immune response. J Leukoc Biol 2006;79(4):652–62.

[60] Gallimore A, Glithero A, Godkin A, Tissot AC, Plückthun A, Elliott T, et al. Induction and exhaustion of lymphocytic choriomeningitis virus-specific cytotoxic T lymphocytes visualized using soluble tetrameric major histocompatibility complex class I-peptide complexes. J Exp Med 1998;187(9):1383–93.

[61] Zajac AJ, Blattman JN, Murali-Krishna K, Sourdive DJ, Suresh M, Altman JD, et al. Viral immune evasion due to persistence of activated T cells without effector function. J Exp Med 1998;188(12):2205–13.

[62] Wherry EJ. T cell exhaustion. Nat Immunol 2011;12(6):492–9.

[63] Wherry EJ, Ahmed R. Memory CD8 T-cell differentiation during viral infection. J Virol 2004;78(11):5535–45.

[64] Kmieciak M, Worschech A, Nikizad H, Gowda M, Habibi M, Depcrynski A, et al. CD4+ T cells inhibit the neu-specific CD8+ T-cell exhaustion during the priming phase of immune responses against breast cancer. Breast Cancer Res Treat 2011;126(2):385–94.

[65] Wherry EJ, Blattman JN, Murali-Krishna K, van der Most R, Ahmed R. Viral persistence alters CD8 T-cell immunodominance and tissue distribution and results in distinct stages of functional impairment. J Virol 2003;77(8):4911–27.

[66] Zhou Q, Munger ME, Veenstra RG, Weigel BJ, Hirashima M, Munn DH, et al. Coexpression of Tim-3 and PD-1 identifies a CD8+ T-cell exhaustion phenotype in mice with disseminated acute myelogenous leukemia. Blood 2011;117(17):4501–10.

[67] Vazquez-Cintron EJ, Monu NR, Frey AB. Tumor-induced disruption of proximal TCR-mediated signal transduction in tumor-infiltrating CD8+ lymphocytes inactivates antitumor effector phase. J Immunol 2010;185(12):7133–40.

[68] Virgin HW, Wherry EJ, Ahmed R. Redefining chronic viral infection. Cell 2009;138(1):30–50.

[69] Blackburn SD, Shin H, Haining WN, Zou T, Workman CJ, Polley A, et al. Coregulation of CD8+ T cell exhaustion by multiple inhibitory receptors during chronic viral infection. Nat Immunol 2009;10(1):29–37.

[70] Peggs KS, Quezada SA, Allison JP. Cell intrinsic mechanisms of T-cell inhibition and application to cancer therapy. Immunol Rev 2008;224:141–65.

[71] Topalian SL, Drake CG, Pardoll DM. Targeting the PD-1/B7-H1(PD-L1) pathway to activate anti-tumor immunity. Curr Opin Immunol 2012 Jan 9 [Epub ahead of print].

[72] Chambers CA, Sullivan TJ, Allison JP. Lymphoproliferation in CTLA-4-deficient mice is mediated by costimulation-dependent activation of CD4+ T cells. Immunity 1997;7(6):885–95.

[73] Chambers CA, Sullivan TJ, Truong T, Allison JP. Secondary but not primary T cell responses are enhanced in CTLA-4-deficient CD8+ T cells. Eur J Immunol 1998;28(10):3137–43.

[74] Hodi FS, O'Day SJ, McDermott DF, Weber RW, Sosman JA, Haanen JB, et al. Improved survival with ipilimumab in patients with metastatic melanoma. N Engl J Med 2010;363(8):711–23.

[75] Freeman GJ, Long AJ, Iwai Y, Bourque K, Chernova T, Nishimura H, et al. Engagement of the PD-1 immunoinhibitory receptor by a novel B7 family member leads to negative regulation of lymphocyte activation. J Exp Med 2000;192(7):1027–34.

[76] Latchman Y, Wood CR, Chernova T, Chaudhary D, Borde M, Chernova I, et al. PD-L2 is a second ligand for PD-1 and inhibits T cell activation. Nat Immunol 2001;2(3):261–8.

[77] Okazaki T, Honjo T. The PD-1-PD-L pathway in immunological tolerance. Trends Immunol 2006 Apr;27(4): 195-201 2006;27(4):195–201.

[78] Dong H, Strome SE, Salomao DR, Tamura H, Hirano F, Flies DB, et al. Tumor-associated B7–H1 promotes T-cell apoptosis: a potential mechanism of immune evasion. Nat Med 2002;8(8):793–800.

[79] Curran MA, Montalvo W, Yagita H, Allison JP. PD-1 and CTLA-4 combination blockade expands infiltrating T cells and reduces regulatory T and myeloid cells within B16 melanoma tumors. Proc Natl Acad Sci U S A 2010;107(9):4275–80.

[80] Francisco LM, Salinas VH, Brown KE, Vanguri VK, Freeman GJ, Kuchroo VK, et al. PD-L1 regulates the development, maintenance, and function of induced regulatory T cells. J Exp Med 2009;206(13):3015–29.

[81] Brahmer JR, Drake CG, Wollner I, Powderly JD, Picus J, Sharfman WH, et al. Phase I study of single-agent anti-programmed death-1 (MDX-1106) in refractory solid tumors: safety, clinical activity, pharmacodynamics, and immunologic correlates. J Clin Oncol 2010;28(19):3167–75.

[82] Anderson AC. Tim-3, a negative regulator of anti-tumor immunity. Curr Opin Immunol 2012. In press.

[83] Rabinovich GA, Toscano MA. Turning 'sweet' on immunity: galectin-glycan interactions in immune tolerance and inflammation. Nat Rev Immunol 2009;9(5):338–52.

[84] Zhu C, Anderson AC, Schubart A, Xiong H, Imitola J, Khoury SJ, et al. The Tim-3 ligand galectin-9 negatively regulates T helper type 1 immunity. Nat Immunol 2005;6(12):1245–52.

[85] Baitsch L, Baumgaertner P, Devêvre E, Raghav SK, Legat A, Barba L, et al. Exhaustion of tumor-specific CD8+ T cells in metastases from melanoma patients. J Clin Invest 2011;121(6):2350–60.

[86] Sakuishi K, Apetoh L, Sullivan JM, Blazar BR, Kuchroo VK, Anderson AC. Targeting Tim-3 and PD-1 pathways to reverse T cell exhaustion and restore anti-tumor immunity. J Exp Med 2010;207(10):2187–94.

[87] Fourcade J, Sun Z, Benallaoua M, Guillaume P, Luescher IF, Sander C, et al. Upregulation of Tim-3 and PD-1 expression is associated with tumor antigen-specific CD8+ T cell dysfunction in melanoma patients. J Exp Med 2010;207(10):2175–86.

[88] Sierro S, Romero P, Speiser DE. The CD4-like molecule LAG-3, biology and therapeutic applications. Expert Opin Ther Targets 2011;15(1):91–101.

[89] Matsuzaki J, Gnjatic S, Mhawech-Fauceglia P, Beck A, Miller A, Tsuji T, et al. Tumor-infiltrating NY-ESO-1-specific CD8+ T cells are negatively regulated by LAG-3 and PD-1 in human ovarian cancer. Proc Natl Acad Sci U S A 2010;107(17):7875–80.

[90] Workman CJ, Cauley LS, Kim IJ, Blackman MA, Woodland DL, Vignali DA. Lymphocyte activation gene-3 (CD223) regulates the size of the expanding T cell population following antigen activation in vivo. J Immunol 2004;172(9):5450–5.

[91] Huang CT, Workman CJ, Flies D, Pan X, Marson AL, Zhou G, et al. Role of LAG-3 in regulatory T cells. Immunity 2004;21(4):503–13.

[92] Richter K, Agnellini P, Oxenius A. On the role of the inhibitory receptor LAG-3 in acute and chronic LCMV infection. Int Immunol 2010;22(1):13–23.

[93] Woo SR, Turnis ME, Goldberg MV, Bankoti J, Selby M, Nirschl CJ, et al. Immune inhibitory molecules LAG-3 and PD-1 synergistically regulate T-cell function to promote tumoral immune escape. Cancer Res 2012;72(4):917—27.

[94] Murphy TL, Murphy KM. Slow down and survive: Enigmatic immunoregulation by BTLA and HVEM. Annu Rev Immunol 2010;28:389—411.

[95] Watanabe N, Gavrieli M, Sedy JR, Yang J, Fallarino F, Loftin SK, et al. BTLA is a lymphocyte inhibitory receptor with similarities to CTLA-4 and PD-1. Nat Immunol 2003;4(7):670—9.

[96] Krieg C, Boyman O, Fu YX, Kaye J. B and T lymphocyte attenuator regulates CD8+ T cell-intrinsic homeostasis and memory cell generation. Nat Immunol 2007;8(2):162—71.

[97] Derré L, Rivals JP, Jandus C, Pastor S, Rimoldi D, Romero P, et al. BTLA mediates inhibition of human tumor-specific CD8+ T cells that can be partially reversed by vaccination. J Clin Invest 2010;120(1):157—67.

[98] Cai G, Freeman GJ. The CD160, BTLA, LIGHT/HVEM pathway: a bidirectional switch regulating T-cell activation. Immunol Rev 2009;229(1):244—58.

[99] Fourcade J, Sun Z, Pagliano O, Guillaume P, Luescher IF, Sander C, et al. CD8(+) T cells specific for tumor antigens can be rendered dysfunctional by the tumor microenvironment through upregulation of the inhibitory receptors BTLA and PD-1. Cancer Res 2012;72(4):887—96.

[100] Hurchla MA, Sedy JR, Gavrieli M, Drake CG, Murphy TL, Murphy KM. B and T lymphocyte attenuator exhibits structural and expression polymorphisms and is highly Induced in anergic CD4+ T cells. J Immunol 2005;174(6):3377—85.

[101] Paulos CM, June CH. Putting the brakes on BTLA in T cell-mediated cancer immunotherapy. J Clin Invest 2010;120(1):76—80.

[102] Ohta A, Gorelik E, Prasad SJ, Ronchese F, Lukashev D, Wong MK, et al. A2A adenosine receptor protects tumors from antitumor T cells. Proc Natl Acad Sci U S A 2006;103(35):13132—7.

[103] Bours MJ, Swennen EL, Di Virgilio F, Cronstein BN, Dagnelie PC. Adenosine 5′-triphosphate and adenosine as endogenous signaling molecules in immunity and inflammation. Pharmacol Ther 2006;112(2):358—404.

[104] Junger WG. Immune cell regulation by autocrine purinergic signalling. Nat Rev Immunol 2011;11(3):201—12.

[105] Schenk U, Westendorf AM, Radaelli E, Casati A, Ferro M, Fumagalli M, et al. Purinergic control of T cell activation by ATP released through pannexin-1 hemichannels. Sci Signal 2008;1(39):ra6.

[106] Woehrle T, Yip L, Elkhal A, Sumi Y, Chen Y, Yao Y, et al. Pannexin-1 hemichannel-mediated ATP release together with P2X1 and P2X4 receptors regulate T-cell activation at the immune synapse. Blood 2010;116(18):3475—84.

[107] Chen Y, Yao Y, Sumi Y, Li A, To UK, Elkhal A, et al. Purinergic signaling: a fundamental mechanism in neutrophil activation. Sci Signal 2010;3(125):ra45.

[108] Kronlage M, Song J, Sorokin L, Isfort K, Schwerdtle T, Leipziger J, et al. Autocrine purinergic receptor signaling is essential for macrophage chemotaxis. Sci Signal 2010;3(132):ra55.

[109] Piccini A, Carta S, Tassi S, Lasiglié D, Fossati G, Rubartelli A. ATP is released by monocytes stimulated with pathogen-sensing receptor ligands and induces IL-1beta and IL-18 secretion in an autocrine way. Proc Natl Acad Sci U S A 2008;105(23):8067—72.

[110] Elliott MR, Chekeni FB, Trampont PC, Lazarowski ER, Kadl A, Walk SF, et al. Nucleotides released by apoptotic cells act as a find-me signal to promote phagocytic clearance. Nature 2009;461(7261):282—6.

[111] Ghiringhelli F, Apetoh L, Tesniere A, Aymeric L, Ma Y, Ortiz C, et al. Activation of the NLRP3 inflammasome in dendritic cells induces IL-1beta-dependent adaptive immunity against tumors. Nat Med 2009;15:1170—8.

[112] Di Virgilio F. Liaisons dangereuses: P2X(7) and the inflammasome. Trends Pharmacol Sci 2007;28(9):465—72.

[113] Apasov SG, Blackburn MR, Kellems RE, Smith PT, Sitkovsky MV. Adenosine deaminase deficiency increases thymic apoptosis and causes defective T cell receptor signaling. J Clin Invest 2001;108(1):131—41.

[114] Stagg J, Smyth MJ. Extracellular adenosine triphosphate and adenosine in cancer. Oncogene 2010;29(39):5346—58.

[115] Haskó G, Pacher P. Regulation of macrophage function by adenosine. Arterioscler Thromb Vasc Biol 2012;32(4):865—9.

[116] Csóka B, Selmeczy Z, Koscsó B, Németh ZH, Pacher P, Murray PJ, et al. Adenosine promotes alternative macrophage activation via A2A and A2B receptors. FASEB J 2012;26(1):376—86.

[117] Nowak M, Lynch L, Yue S, Ohta A, Sitkovsky M, Balk SP, et al. The A2aR adenosine receptor controls cytokine production in iNKT cells. Eur J Immunol 2010;40(3):682—7.

[118] Novitskiy SV, Ryzhov S, Zaynagetdinov R, Goldstein AE, Huang Y, Tikhomirov OY, et al. Adenosine receptors in regulation of dendritic cell differentiation and function. Blood 2008;112(5):1822—31.

[119] Ryzhov S, Novitskiy SV, Goldstein AE, Biktasova A, Blackburn MR, Biaggioni I, et al. Adenosinergic regulation of the expansion and immunosuppressive activity of CD11b+Gr1+ cells. J Immunol 2011;187(11):6120—9.

[120] Ohta A, Ohta A, Madasu M, Kini R, Subramanian M, Goel N, et al. A2A adenosine receptor may allow expansion of T cells lacking effector functions in extracellular adenosine-rich microenvironments. J Immunol 2009;183(9):5487–93.

[121] Zarek PE, Huang CT, Lutz ER, Kowalski J, Horton MR, Linden J, et al. A2A receptor signaling promotes peripheral tolerance by inducing T-cell anergy and the generation of adaptive regulatory T cells. Blood 2008;111(1):251–9.

[122] Pellegatti P, Raffaghello L, Bianchi G, Piccardi F, Pistoia V, Di Virgilio F. Increased level of extracellular ATP at tumor sites: in vivo imaging with plasma membrane luciferase. PLoS One 2008;3(7):e2599.

[123] Yegutkin GG. Nucleotide- and nucleoside-converting ectoenzymes: Important modulators of purinergic signalling cascade. Biochim Biophys Acta 2008;1783(5):673–94.

[124] Deaglio S, Dwyer KM, Gao W, Friedman D, Usheva A, Erat A, et al. Adenosine generation catalyzed by CD39 and CD73 expressed on regulatory T cells mediates immune suppression. J Exp Med 2007;204(6):1257–65.

[125] Colgan SP, Eltzschig HK, Eckle T, Thompson LF. Physiological roles for ecto-5'-nucleotidase (CD73). Purinergic Signal 2006;2(2):351–60.

[126] Takedachi M, Qu D, Ebisuno Y, Oohara H, Joachims ML, McGee ST, et al. CD73-generated adenosine restricts lymphocyte migration into draining lymph nodes. J Immunol 2008;180(9):6288–96.

[127] Ring S, Enk AH, Mahnke K. ATP activates regulatory T Cells in vivo during contact hypersensitivity reactions. J Immunol 2010;184(7):3408–16.

[128] Stagg J, Divisekera U, Duret H, Sparwasser T, Teng MW, Darcy PK, et al. CD73-deficient mice have increased antitumor immunity and are resistant to experimental metastasis. Cancer Res 2011;71(8):2892–900.

[129] Zhang B. CD73: a novel target for cancer immunotherapy. Cancer Res 2010;70(16):6407–11.

[130] Stagg J, Divisekera U, McLaughlin N, Sharkey J, Pommey S, Denoyer D, et al. Anti-CD73 antibody therapy inhibits breast tumor growth and metastasis. Proc Natl Acad Sci U S A 2010;107(4):1547–52.

[131] Jin D, Fan J, Wang L, Thompson LF, Liu A, Daniel BJ, et al. CD73 on tumor cells impairs antitumor T-cell responses: a novel mechanism of tumor-induced immune suppression. Cancer Res 2010;70(6):2245–55.

[132] Mandapathil M, Hilldorfer B, Szczepanski MJ, Czystowska M, Szajnik M, Ren J, et al. Generation and accumulation of immunosuppressive adenosine by human CD4+CD25highFOXP3+ regulatory T cells. J Biol Chem 2010;285(10):7176–86.

[133] Quezada SA, Peggs KS, Curran MA, Allison JP. CTLA4 blockade and GM-CSF combination immunotherapy alters the intratumor balance of effector and regulatory T cells. J Clin Invest 2006;116(7):1935–45.

[134] Sato E, Olson SH, Ahn J, Bundy B, Nishikawa H, Qian F, et al. Intraepithelial CD8+ tumor-infiltrating lymphocytes and a high CD8+/regulatory T cell ratio are associated with favorable prognosis in ovarian cancer. Proc Natl Acad Sci U S A 2005;102:18538–43.

[135] Keith B, Johnson RS, Simon MC. HIF1α and HIF2α: sibling rivalry in hypoxic tumour growth and progression. Nat Rev Cancer 2011;12(1):9–22.

[136] Peyssonnaux C, Datta V, Cramer T, Doedens A, Theodorakis EA, Gallo RL, et al. HIF-1alpha expression regulates the bactericidal capacity of phagocytes. J Clin Invest 2005;115(7):1806–15.

[137] Doedens AL, Stockmann C, Rubinstein MP, Liao D, Zhang N, DeNardo DG, et al. Macrophage expression of hypoxia-inducible factor-1 alpha suppresses T-cell function and promotes tumor progression. Cancer Res 2010;70(19):7465–75.

[138] Corzo CA, Condamine T, Lu L, Cotter MJ, Youn JI, Cheng P, et al. HIF-1α regulates function and differentiation of myeloid-derived suppressor cells in the tumor microenvironment. J Exp Med 2010;207(11):2439–53.

[139] Bronte V, Kasic T, Gri G, Gallana K, Borsellino G, Marigo I, et al. Boosting antitumor responses of T lymphocytes infiltrating human prostate cancers. J Exp Med 2005;201(8):1257–68.

[140] Grohmann U, Bronte V. Control of immune response by amino acid metabolism. Immunol Rev 2010;236:243–64.

[141] Abello N, Kerstjens HA, Postma DS, Bischoff R. Protein tyrosine nitration: selectivity, physicochemical and biological consequences, denitration, and proteomics methods for the identification of tyrosine-nitrated proteins. J Proteome Res 2009;8(7):3222–38.

[142] Brito C, Naviliat M, Tiscornia AC, Vuillier F, Gualco G, Dighiero G. Radi RaC, A. M. Peroxynitrite inhibits T lymphocyte activation and proliferation by promoting impairment of tyrosine phosphorylation and peroxynitrite-driven apoptotic death. J Immunol 1999;162:3356–66.

[143] Nagaraj S, Gupta K, Pisarev V, Kinarsky L, Sherman S, Kang L, et al. Altered recognition of antigen is a mechanism of CD8+ T cell tolerance in cancer. Nat Med 2007;13(7):828–35.

[144] Lu T, Ramakrishnan R, Altiok S, Youn JI, Cheng P, Celis E, et al. Tumor-infiltrating myeloid cells induce tumor cell resistance to cytotoxic T cells in mice. J Clin Invest 2011;121(10):4015–29.

163

[145] Molon B, Ugel S, Del Pozzo F, Soldani C, Zilio S, Avella D, et al. Chemokine nitration prevents intratumoral infiltration of antigen-specific T cells. J Exp Med 2011;208(10):1949−62.

[146] Vickers SM, MacMillan-Crow LA, Green M, Ellis C, Thompson JA. Association of increased immunostaining for inducible nitric oxide synthase and nitrotyrosine with fibroblast growth factor transformation in pancreatic cancer. Arch Surg 1999;134(3):245−51.

[147] Bentz BG, GKr Haines, Radosevich JA. Increased protein nitrosylation in head and neck squamous cell carcinogenesis. Head Neck 2000;22(1):64−70.

[148] Kasic T, Colombo P, Soldani C, Wang CM, Miranda E, Roncalli M, et al. Modulation of human T-cell functions by reactive nitrogen species. Eur J Immunol 2011;41(7):1843−9.

[149] Nakamura Y, Yasuoka H, Tsujimoto M, Yoshidome K, Nakahara M, Nakao K, et al. Nitric oxide in breast cancer: induction of vascular endothelial growth factor-C and correlation with metastasis and poor prognosis. Clin Cancer Res 2006;12(4):1201−7.

[150] Demaria S, Formenti SC. Sensors of ionizing radiation effects on the immunological microenvironment of cancer. Int J Radiat Biol 2007;83(11):819−25.

[151] Formenti SC, Demaria S. Systemic effects of local radiotherapy. Lancet Oncol 2009;10(7):718−26.

[152] Ma Y, Kepp O, Ghiringhelli F, Apetoh L, Aymeric L, Locher C, et al. Chemotherapy and radiotherapy: cryptic anticancer vaccines. Semin Immunol 2010;22(3):113−24.

[153] Reits EA, Hodge JW, Herberts CA, Groothuis TA, Chakraborty M, Wansley EK, et al. Radiation modulates the peptide repertoire, enhances MHC class I expression, and induces successful antitumor immunotherapy. J Exp Med 2006;203(5):1259−71.

[154] Matsumura S, Wang B, Kawashima N, Braunstein S, Badura M, Cameron TO, et al. Radiation-induced CXCL16 release by breast cancer cells attracts effector T cells. J Immunol 2008;181:3099−107.

[155] Michaud M, Martins I, Sukkurwala AQ, Adjemian S, Ma Y, Pellegatti P, et al. Autophagy-dependent anticancer immune responses induced by chemotherapeutic agents in mice. Science 2011;334(6062):1573−7.

Introduction to Cancer Therapeutics

CHAPTER 12

Principles of Cytotoxic Chemotherapy

Bradley W. Lash[1], Paul B. Gilman[1,2]
[1]Lankenau Medical Center
[2]Lankenau Institute for Medical Research, Wynnewood, PA USA

I. INTRODUCTION

The year 2006 marked the 60th anniversary of modern chemotherapy [1], during which period tremendous gains were made in the treatment of human cancer. While the use of toxic substances to treat disease, including cancers, dates back thousands of years, the impetus for the modern use of chemotherapy actually stemmed from observations on the effects of chemical warfare in the 20th century. In the aftermath of an accidental spill of nitrogen mustard on troops in Italy, physicians noted the impact of the toxin on normal hematopoiesis and lymph tissue [2]. These observations led a group of physicians to use nitrogen mustard on a patient with refractory non-Hodgkin lymphoma with impressive, but short-lived, results [3]. For the first time it was shown that cancer could be treated with something other than surgery or radiation; thus modern medical oncology was born. Through scientific advances such as animal models of human cancer, genomic sequencing, x-ray crystallography and high-throughput screening, the process of drug development has been streamlined. This process has led to the development of new compounds, both broad spectrum chemotherapy as well as molecularly targeted agents, which have been introduced into the clinic in curative, palliative or adjunctive settings. This chapter offers a broad overview of the principles and use of cytotoxic chemotherapy in modern oncology.

II. CLINICAL USE OF CHEMOTHERAPY

Chemotherapy, now focusing increasingly on the use of targeted therapies that include monoclonal antibodies as well as small molecule agents, provides the core tool for medical oncologists to treat cancer. In general, chemotherapy is used in four main clinical settings:

1. **Primary therapy** for advanced disease or metastatic disease (Table 12.1);
2. **Neoadjuvant therapy before surgery and/or irradiation** is administered for locally advanced disease, to improve the effectiveness of these treatments (Table 12.2);
3. **Combination therapy with radiation** for definitive treatment of localized disease at sites where surgical resection would be too morbid (Table 12.3); and
4. **Adjuvant therapy after cancer has been removed** in efforts to eradicate any remaining micrometastatic disease that could seed relapses (Table 12.4).

Other, albeit less common, uses of chemotherapy include direct instillation of chemotherapy into a sanctuary site (intrathecal therapy) and site-directed therapy, such as liver directed therapy or limb-perfusion therapy. While these modalities are important in several diseases, they are not commonly used in modern clinical oncology and will not be discussed further.

Cancer Immunotherapy. http://dx.doi.org/10.1016/B978-0-12-394296-8.00012-9

TABLE 12.1 Cancers for which Chemotherapy Alone is Potentially Curative

Acute Lymphoblastic Leukemia
Acute Myeloid Leukemia
Hairy Cell Leukemia
Diffuse Large B-Cell Lymphoma

Burkitt's Lymphoma
Wilms' Tumors
Gestational Trophoblastic Tumors

TABLE 12.2 Cancers in which Adjuvant Therapy is Established (Adjuvant Therapy is Given after the Primary Therapy)

Breast Cancer
Ovarian Cancer
Pancreatic Cancer
Osteosarcoma

Colon Cancer
Lung Cancer
Gastric Cancer
Glioblastoma

TABLE 12.3 Diseases in which Neoadjuvant Therapy is Established (Neoadjuvant Therapy is Given before the Primary Therapy)

Disease	Modality
Rectal Cancer	Chemoradiotherapy
Breast Cancer	Chemotherapy
Bladder Cancer	Chemotherapy
Esophageal Cancer	Chemotherapy or chemoradiotherapy
Gastric Cancer	Chemotherapy
Sarcoma	Radiation therapy, chemotherapy, or combination

TABLE 12.4 Cancers in which Therapy is Used to Preserve Organ Function or as an Alternative to Surgery

Head and Neck Cancers
Bladder Cancer
Lung Cancer
Cervical Cancer

Esophageal Squamous Cell Carcinoma
Anal Cancer
Nasopharyngeal Cancer

Primary chemotherapy for advanced/metastatic disease implies the use of chemotherapy as the sole modality of treatment, often with palliative rather than curative intent by the oncologist. However, there are an increasing number of tumors in which chemotherapy alone is curative (Table 12.1). In many diseases, including breast cancer [4], colon cancer [5] and lung cancer [6], chemotherapy has been shown to improve quality of life and there is a suggestion of improved overall survival compared with historical controls [7]. With modern chemotherapies, the overall survival of patients with advanced cancers has increased significantly over the last several years, even in cancers such as lung cancer which has traditionally been viewed as hopeless [8].

Neoadjuvant therapy refers to the administration of chemotherapy and/or chemoradiation to help facilitate a subsequent local therapy [9]. In order for neoadjuvant therapy to be used appropriately, the disease must be surgically curable. The role of chemotherapy in this situation is two-fold, with the intent to shrink or completely eradicate the tumor to allow for complete surgical resection, and to reduce or eliminate micrometastatic disease that may be present afterward in an effort to improve survival. The use of neoadjuvant chemotherapy may allow for less radical surgery, thereby allowing organ preservation, as shown in a number of diseases, most notably sarcoma [10] and rectal cancer [11]. Neoadjuvant chemotherapy has been established by several large Phase III trials as appropriate for breast cancer [12], bladder cancer [13], gastroesophageal cancers [14] and it may be helpful in others as well [15].

A related paradigm of neoadjuvant therapy is in its use as a part of definitive chemoradiotherapy to treat a number of locally advanced diseases, in attempting to allow organ preservation (although in sense this use is not technically neoadjuvant therapy since no further treatment is planned). This strategy has been applied most significantly for treatment of anal cancer [16], a disease that would have resulted previously in a permanent colostomy, but which is now treated routinely with combination chemoradiotherapy. Abdominoperitoneal resection (APR) is saved for cases of refractory disease [17]. Similarly, in head and neck cancer, chemoradiation is now used in an attempt to preserve laryngeal function and improve quality of life [18].

Adjuvant chemotherapy is given to patients after definitive therapy, most commonly surgery [15]. The need for adjuvant chemotherapy stemmed from the observation that even in many patients thought to be cured of their disease by surgery, late/distant relapse remained a major cause of mortality in many diseases. While not definitively established, it was widely thought that the cause of these failures was the persistence of micrometastatic disease that might be eradicated by chemotherapy administered to patients who were cancer-free after surgery. Indeed, chemotherapy in this setting has proved to be beneficial in terms of relapse-free and overall survival in a number of diseases, including, for example, breast cancer [19], colon cancer [20], lung cancer [21] and pancreatic cancer [22].

III. TUMOR GROWTH AND ITS IMPACT ON CHEMOTHERAPY USE

The understanding of human tumor growth and the effects of chemotherapy on tumor growth was worked out in human tumor xenografts generated by transplantation into immuno-compromised mice [23]. One of the earliest models of the effects of chemotherapy on tumor growth was a mouse model of leukemia [24] that provided the first insights into treatment. While this model was by no means ideal—for example, the tumor had a 100% growth fraction (percentage of cells actively dividing) unlike the majority of human tumors—it provided the first characterization of human tumor growth and seeded the core principles of medical oncology still mainly employed today. The critical concept that was developed in these tumor graft models is the concept of log-kill. Log-kill implies that chemotherapy kills a constant percentage of actively dividing cells, not a constant number. Based on this theory, if a tumor grows at an exponential rate and chemotherapy is effective against a percentage of those cells, growth will continue even after chemotherapy is given. Accordingly, this theory holds that tumor burdens exceeding a particular limit cannot be cured by any dose of chemotherapy, i.e., that there exists an inverse relationship between cell number and curability [25]. The theory also supported the concept that higher percentages of cell kill will produce higher survival rates [26].

Initial insights from murine models were recognized as imperfect and in need of more sophisticated refinements. In particular, it was necessary to address the fact that human tumors are not made up of a homogenous population of cells that proliferate at the same rate, but rather than can be viewed as containing varying amounts of three types of cells:

1. Terminally differentiated cells incapable of dividing
2. Actively proliferating cells (tumor growth fraction)
3. Quiescent cells that can be recruited into the growth fraction.

Importantly, the ultimate response to cytotoxic chemotherapies was found to relate to the percentage of cells that were actively dividing [27]. When tumor growth is viewed in this manner, growth becomes more sigmoidal [28], or Gompertzian, as named for the 19th century mathematician who first described the growth curve that is displayed by human breast tumors. This model postulates that the growth fraction is proportional to the size of the tumor. The larger the tumor, the less proliferative the cells are, such that the growth fraction decreases with time. Indeed, studies with human cancer cells have shown that the growth fraction of epithelial tumors may be as low as 10% [29]. This finding is thought to be the reason why, with rare exception (Table 12.1), macroscopic disease is rarely curable with cytotoxic chemotherapy alone.

Given the relative inefficacy of chemotherapy alone against macroscopic tumors, the idea that the growth fraction of human cancer cells varies with size has become paramount to understanding modern medical oncology. Even though the tumor may not be cured when clinically detectable (i.e., palpable or seen on imaging), the same tumor might be curable with chemotherapy in the adjuvant setting. In these settings, when only microscopic disease exists, there is a steep dose-response curve to chemotherapy such that the tumor might be rendered curable [30]. So while the absolute number of cells killed is low, the efficiency with which they are killed is high allowing for possible cure. While this concept and its implications on therapy seem intuitive to the modern oncologist, it led to some poor decisions in early adjuvant trials which probably caused the early negative results of these trials [31]. Early adjuvant trials, recognizing that the growth of cancer cells is proportional to the size of the tumor, employed dose reductions and protracted schedules to minimize systemic toxicity. It was thought that given the low tumor burden and high sensitivity of these tumors to chemotherapy, the medical oncologist could spare toxicity without compromising efficacy, but this was proven to be false [32]. Thus, many of the first trials of chemotherapy were negative and this led to a nihilistic attitude towards adjuvant therapy. While the concept of increased sensitivity and adjusting dosing is important, the early trials were flawed in that the opposite approach should have been taken, i.e. dosing should have been intensified to cure the patient, rather than reduced.

Since that time, dose intensification has been shown in many tumors to improve survival outcomes, most prominently in hematologic malignancies. However, its use in solid tumors, particularly in the adjuvant setting, is still a relatively modern concept. The need for dose intensification lies in findings that, in addition to the varied population of cells in tumors that differ in their growth rate, tumors will inherently differ in their general sensitivity to chemotherapy as well [33]. In essence, even before a tumor is exposed to a cytotoxic agent, there are daughter cells which are resistant to that therapy, so while the chemotherapy may kill sensitive clones the resistant ones can grow. This differential growth pattern and differential sensitivity pattern led to the concepts of sequential therapies and dose-density, both of which have proven critical to increasing cures in the adjuvant setting, most notably in breast cancer [34].

IV. GENERAL PRINCIPLES OF CHEMOTHERAPY USE
A. Overview of combination chemotherapy

The biggest barriers to curative chemotherapy are tumor heterogeneity, toxicity to normal tissues and resistance to chemotherapy. Fundamentally, it is the interplay of these factors that ultimately determines the efficacy of treatment. For example, early studies of chemotherapy in pediatric patients with acute lymphoblastic lymphoma (ALL) showed that while seven different single-agent therapies may induce remission, they were rarely curative as single-agents and relapse was problematic [35]. In fact, single agents at doses which can be delivered safely are almost never curative, whereas rational combinations of different agents and maximization of all dosages later made cure rates of >85% possible in childhood ALL [36]. Unfortunately, not all attempts at combination therapy have been as successful. In general, response rates to combination regimens are considerably lower in solid tumors than in hematologic malignancies [37]. However, while exceptions exist [38], combination chemotherapy is superior to single agents in many cancers, such as, for example, lung cancer [39]. Yet adding chemotherapy agents to diversify a combination regimen is also not always more effective; in essence, more chemotherapy is not better if the dose intensity is not improved. So regimen designs must allow an increased dose intensity without prohibitive toxicities: giving three agents at {1/3} of their known effective dose cannot be better than giving one agent at full dose.

The rational development of combination regimens, for both advanced disease and in the adjuvant settings, has followed a few simple principles outlined in Table 12.5. The idea of using drugs with established efficacy in advanced disease seems clinically obvious; however, it should be noted that just because a drug is effective in the metastatic setting it is not necessarily effective in the adjuvant setting and vice versa [40].

Different classes of cytotoxic drugs have been selected specifically for their additive benefits. The concepts of additive benefit or synergistic benefit are used somewhat interchangeably in the oncology clinic [41], but in general additive is preferred when the agents used in the combination have increased efficacy but nonoverlapping toxicity. Synergism, a rare event in oncology, is reserved for cases when the efficacy of the combination of drugs is greater than what would be predicted from the use of that combination, for example, vincristine and prednisone in ALL. In point of fact, the number of truly synergistic drugs is quite small in medical oncology.

Of course, toxicity to normal tissues is an important consideration in designing combination regimens. While chemotherapeutic agents each have a unique side-effect profile, the most common dose-limiting toxicity is myelosuppression. Dose reductions and delays can compromise efficacy in the curative setting. Use of colony stimulating factors has changed treatment of myelosuppression, allowing for maximal drug delivery while minimizing (but not eliminating) neutropenia [42,43]. Aside from growth factors, there are few agents available to prevent toxicity to normal tissues. Amifostine is a notable example to alleviate mucosal toxicity from chemoradiation in head and neck cancer, although this agent has not received widespread use [44]. In most cases, toxicity from chemotherapy needs to be treated with both supportive care and dose reductions, particularly in metastatic settings where quality of life

TABLE 12.5 Aspects of Rational Design of Combination Chemotherapy

Principle	Rationale
Drugs selected should be active in the metastatic setting	This will maximize response by using the most active agents. If possible those drugs which produce a complete remission should be used
The drugs selected should have differing mechanisms of action	This will help maximize tumor eradication by overcoming resistant clones
The drugs selected should have nonoverlapping toxicities	This will maximize dose intensity and prevent empiric dose reductions which might compromise efficacy
All drugs should be given at full dose and at an optimal schedule	This will maximize efficacy and maintain dose intensity
Dosing interval should be consistent and as short as possible	This will allow for maximizing dose intensity. The interval should be determined by the recovery of normal tissues
Drugs with different resistance mechanisms, when possible, should be used	This will allow for maximal tumor eradication, but decrease the chance of cross-resistance

is of paramount importance. In overcoming this toxicity, medical oncologists must design regimens that, when possible, exert nonoverlapping toxicities to allow for maximal dose intensity. It is clear that scheduling of chemotherapy, for both combination regimens and single agents, is most critical in treating all stages of cancer as it impacts outcomes. Proper scheduling includes consideration of dose, dosing intervals, sequencing of agents and duration of therapy, and a huge number of clinical trials have been devoted to improving efficacy by altering these metrics, often through more empirical than rational processes.

B. Scheduling of chemotherapy

In early studies, scheduling of chemotherapy was determined by empirical considerations based primarily on toxicity, but subsequent randomized trials have shed some greater light on better scheduling. Early models suggested that sequential administration of agents would be superior to alternating cycles, i.e. delivering drug A for three cycles followed by drug B for three cycles would be superior to alternating A and B for six cycles. These models were based primarily on the idea that no two regimens had equal killing potential and no two regimens were truly non-cross resistant [45]. This idea was later grounded in clinical trials, particularly in breast cancer where sequential administration proved superior to alternating cycles, even when dose intensity was controlled [46]. Whether this will hold true with modern chemotherapy regimens has not to be established clearly, and ongoing studies still build mainly on earlier principles to establish proper sequencing of treatments.

Scheduling of cytotoxic chemotherapy depends greatly on the agents used. For example, early studies of the use of the purine analog cytarabine showed that continuous infusion over 5 to 7 days was superior to daily dosing [47]. However, the closely related compound gemcitabine seems to have superior efficacy when given intermittently and without protracted infusions [48]. In addition to the surprisingly large effects that scheduling can have on efficacy, scheduling also dramatically influences drug toxicities. For example, the antimetabolite 5-fluorouracil (5-FU) when given as a bolus injection will produce mainly hematologic toxicity, but when given as a continuous IV infusion diarrhea and mucositis predominate, even though there is no difference in patient survival between the two strategies [49]. Further evidence for the critical importance of scheduling comes from studies of the anthracycline drug doxorubicin. Protracted infusion of doxorubicin may reduce cardiotoxicity compared to standard bolus administration [50]. Similarly, its formulation in a liposomal product providing sustained release also seems to mitigate some cardiotoxicity [51]. Thus, scheduling can greatly affect toxicity in ways that are not readily understood. For the medical oncologist, designing the ideal combination regimen requires a careful consideration of the possible impact of the schedule on individual patients.

The duration of chemotherapy treatment varies widely based on the disease being treated, the goals of the treatment and the stage of the disease. Often the duration is determined by prior clinical trials, and as a general rule chemotherapy would usually be given as administered in trials that showed efficacy. However, this does not mean that clinical trials produced final results that could not be improved upon. For example, in colon cancer, initial trials suggested that 24 months of adjuvant treatment was ideal, but subsequent studies have suggested 6 months is sufficient and early data suggests even three months might be as effective [52]. Thus, the standard of care is continually dynamic and not necessarily clear cut or agreed upon by oncologists in various cases.

In metastatic settings, such questions are even more complicated. Most early clinical trials were designed to give a set number of cycles of chemotherapy at which time responding patients were placed on observation, i.e. they were given a "chemotherapy holiday". Indeed, in some diseases, such as non-small cell lung cancer, longer duration of therapy was not superior to 4–6 cycles but produced higher toxicity [53], while in other diseases, such as breast cancer, data from meta-analyses have suggested that treatment until toxicity or progression occurs might provide a survival advantage [54]. In general, chemotherapy-free intervals are appropriate for most metastatic cancers. Alternatively, using a less toxic single agent may be appropriate after a period of so-called induction chemotherapy with a more toxic combination regimen. Such strategies have been shown to be effective in colon cancer, where giving 5-FU after a period of induction with a combination therapy of 5-FU, leucovorin and oxaliplatin (termed FOLFOX) was found to be as effective as (and better tolerated than) standard treatments with all three agents until progression [55]. In NSCLC, a related paradigm, termed maintenance therapy, is now being used with increasing frequency [56]. Maintenance chemotherapy involves the administration of single agents after completion of induction chemotherapy with a combination regimen. There are two strategies of maintenance therapy that have been used, one "continuation maintenance" where the single agent was part of the induction regimen, and second termed "switch maintenance" where the single agent differs from those used during induction. Continuation maintenance is used most commonly with a biologic agent such as bevacizumab [57] or cetuximab [58], but it can also be used with conventional chemotherapy [59]. Switch maintenance is most commonly done with conventional chemotherapy [60], but occasionally a biologic agent such as erlotinib is used [61]. At present, it remains uncertain whether these treatment designs are superior to treatment to progression, but some data suggests that they might be [62]. Ultimately, the merits of continued chemotherapy versus set-duration therapy are discussed with individual patients, as regardless of the route chosen it is clear that the onset of progressive disease during therapy is a clear signal to change the treatment regimen.

C. Importance of dose in clinical outcomes

Effective and appropriate dosing of cytotoxic chemotherapy, particularly combination chemotherapy, is paramount to the use of chemotherapy whether the goals of treatment are palliative or curative. The ability to cure a cancer with chemotherapy is dependent on many complex interactions, but primarily is impacted by the interplay of the dose given and the tolerance of normal tissues. Further influencing the effective use of chemotherapy is the nonlinear growth of cancer cells as described above and the inherent sensitivity of the cancer cells to the agents given. Nonlinear growth can lead to a false sense of security for the medical oncologist. When tumors are rapidly growing they are more sensitive to chemotherapy, so dose reductions may seem logical to spare normal tissues. This is especially true if clinical responses are seen at lower doses, but there remains risk that dose reductions may influence survival by limiting effective cancer cell kills. The critical importance of dose in oncology is normally expressed in terms of dose-intensity, which is defined as the amount of drug given per unit of time, most widely expressed as milligrams per meter-squared per week ($mg/m^2/week$) [63]. The amount of chemotherapy received by the patient, i.e., the received dose intensity, can be compared to the original planned dose intensity and expressed as a percentage. In the curative setting, the received dose intensity should be maintained greater than 85%. For example, it is estimated that in diffuse large B-cell lymphoma (DLBCL) a dose reduction of as little as 20% might compromise cure by greater than 50%, despite the apparent clinical complete response [64]. Additional studies in adjuvant breast cancer [65] and testicular cancer [66] also illustrate the vast importance of dose. Therefore, arbitrary dose reductions for the elderly or other groups should generally be avoided as it might impact cure.

How dose is used, particularly in combination regimens, has changed during the development of the field. Initially, doses were selected based on either dose-finding studies or based on their efficacy in advanced disease. Work during this earlier period led to another important concept in medical oncology, summation dose intensity (SDI). SDI implies that when chemotherapies are combined in an effort to increase efficacy, they must be given at full therapeutic doses [67]. The importance of this concept has been shown in many clinical trials [59]. The impact of SDI on trial design is relatively simple, in that any effective regimens must include agents with nonoverlapping toxicity to prevent dose reductions and a resultant compromise in efficacy.

173

Given the importance of dose intensity on clinical outcomes, various ways have been designed to maximize chemotherapy administration. Design variations include increasing the amount of each drug given, changing the dosing interval, using modulating agents and changing the schedule of administration. Increasing the dose, while seemingly logical, is rarely practical. The tolerability of normal tissues rarely allows for increasing doses. However, while not often done, there are ways to increase doses based on individual tolerance to the regimen. One such example, in DLBCL, is the use of the dose-adjusted EPOCH (etoposide, prednisone, vincristine, cyclophosphamide and doxorubicin) regimen [68]. This protocol takes a pharmacodynamic approach to dosing, where every patient starts at the standard dose schedule which is then adjusted based on nadir blood counts, either increasing or decreasing the dose based on toxicity; the results of comparative studies of such regimens to standard chemotherapy are still awaited, but the preliminary data appear promising. To date, pharmacodynamic dosing of drugs in this manner has represented a personalized approach to maximize dose-intensity in patients individually.

Changing the dose interval has been shown to be effective in the treatment of a wide variety of cancers in both the adjuvant and metastatic settings. This is most commonly done through the use of a dose-dense schedule, which by definition means giving the same dose of chemotherapy at shorter intervals than normally used. Dose-dense scheduling was first postulated by Norton and Simon in the treatment of breast cancer [69]. The superiority of dose-dense regimens over standard regimens was subsequently shown in adjuvant therapy for breast cancer [70], but to date has yet to be shown as superior to conventional dosing for treatment of metastatic colon cancer [71] or other tumors including lymphoma [72] and lung cancer [73]. So it appears, at least in the adjuvant treatment of breast cancer, that delivering chemotherapy in a dose-dense manner may improve outcomes. Ongoing studies are testing the value of dose-dense regimens in other diseases including in metastatic settings.

One alternative to giving therapy in a dose-dense fashion is to give it in a dose-intensive fashion, not the same dose in a shorter time, but a higher dose in the same period of time. The utility of dose-intensive regimens have been best shown in the use of paclitaxel in breast cancer and ovarian cancer. In breast cancer, paclitaxel administration at a lower dose weekly was found to be superior to giving a higher dose every three weeks [74]. In ovarian cancer, a similar paradigm was shown with weekly paclitaxel being superior as well [75]. Of note, both of these studies were done in the adjuvant setting where, according to the Norton-Simon hypothesis, dose-density (or intensity) would be expected to have the greatest impact. Here it should be noted that the same dosing schedule was not optimal for a related compound, docetaxel, in the breast cancer study noted above [70]. Ultimately, maximizing dose either by altering the dosing interval or increasing the SDI is critical to outcomes, factors that clinicians must remember whether designing trials or seeing patients in the clinic.

One final approach that has improved outcomes in clinical trials has been to modulate the activity of one drug with another compound. This approach has been shown best through the use of leucovorin (LV) to increase the efficacy of 5-FU. In early clinical trials of 5-FU in advanced colon cancer, response rates were disappointing and there was no evidence of efficacy [76]. Adding LV to 5-FU improved response rates significantly [77]. LV is an ideal modulator in that it is relatively nontoxic yet clearly increases efficacy of 5-FU. Even better, leucovorin can modulate toxicity as well, most notably with high-dose methotrexate, where as a result of preserving normal tissues LV use allows for higher doses of MTX to be administered [78]. Regardless of how LV works as a modulator, it improves outcomes because it adheres to the principle of increasing SDI.

In conclusion, regardless of the method chosen to increase SDI, the critical aspect is that the doses of chemotherapy must be maximized to improve response rates and/or curative potential. If a regimen does not increase the SDI either by increasing the number of drugs, the dose, or changing the dosing interval, it is unlikely that it will change survival or other clinical outcomes in any meaningful way.

D. Resistance to cytotoxic chemotherapy

After the challenges of maximizing dose and schedule, the next largest obstacle to treatment of cancer with cytotoxic chemotherapy is resistance to therapy. Resistance to therapy has been known since chemotherapy was first used, in fact in their seminal paper Goodman and Gilman noted resistance with each successive dose of nitrogen mustard [3]. The demonstration of an apparently sensitive tumor becoming less responsive to treatment is an example of acquired resistance to therapy. However, tumors are known to be inherently resistant to therapy, even if there has been no prior exposure to the cytotoxic agent [79]. There are numerous well-documented mechanisms of chemotherapy resistance as outlined in Table 12.6.

To clinically circumvent resistance, proper dosing and scheduling of chemotherapy is imperative to reduce selection for resistant clones, but even with present safeguards resistance will emerge. Aside from the specific checkpoints at which a cell can become resistant, i.e., cellular uptake, drug activation, regulation of drug targets, etc., there appear to be a few critical pathways/proteins in the development of resistance that warrant more focused discussion.

The p53 protein is a critical regulator of G1−S checkpoint in the cell-cycle and a regulator of apoptosis [80]. Mutations in p53 are common in many cancers and may contribute to resistance to therapy. In addition there are many other modulators of p53 activity such as posttranscriptional modulation and accelerated degradation [81] which impact on chemotherapy efficacy. Mutations in p53 may prevent the tumor cell from undergoing apoptosis, may prevent the cell from recognizing the damage to the genome induced by the chemotherapy, or may involve other pathways. Regardless of the mechanism, alterations in p53 expression and function are a critical part of chemotherapy resistance, but are only one mechanism, as not all cancers harboring p53 mutations are resistant to chemotherapy.

Another common molecular mechanism of chemotherapy resistance is the increased expression of anti-apoptotic proteins [82]. With DNA damaging agents, regardless of their mechanism of DNA damage, they invariably trigger apoptosis to exert their cytotoxic effect. Expression of anti-apoptotic proteins such as BCL-2 may play a role in chemotherapy sensitivity [83]. Many tumors are known to harbor or acquire BCL-2 mutations including hematologic cancers, melanoma and lung cancer [84]. In addition to modulation of BCL-2 other alterations in apoptotic pathways, such as modified expression of tumor necrosis factor

175

TABLE 12.6 Mechanisms of Chemotherapy Resistance

Mechanism of Drug Resistance	Prototypical Drug
Decreased drug uptake	Methotrexate
Decreased drug activation	Methotrexate
	Nucleoside analogs
	Cyclophosphamide
Increased drug target	Etoposide
	Anthracyclines
Detoxification	Alkylating agents
Enhanced repair	Alkylating agents
	Platinum compounds
Increased efflux	Anthracyclines
	Taxanes
	Etoposide
Defective DNA repair/p53 alteration	Almost all chemotherapy drugs

super family (TNF) proteins, particularly those with a death domain, can lead to resistance to apoptosis via downstream caspase modification. Furthermore, some tumors, such as myeloma, have an overexpression of nuclear light chain factor kappa beta (NF-kB) which also resists apoptosis and is a target of therapy available in the clinic, the proteosome inhibitor bortezomib [85].

Aside from regulation of the various cellular pathways outlined above, two additional mechanisms of resistance are worth mentioning because they serve as potential targets for therapy: glutathione-S-transferase expression (GST) and multidrug resistance (MDR) protein expression. Glutathione is important for maintaining cellular thiol homeostasis, which is important for the function of many proteins including DNA repair proteins elicited by chemotherapy and radiotherapy. Indeed, GST is induced in response to cytotoxic chemotherapy and it has been implicated in the resistance of tumors to many drugs, most notably the DNA alkylating agents [86]. GST increases levels of reduced glutathione which detoxifies the free-radicals formed by alkylating agents, a pathway that offers a likely target of cancer therapy in the future [87]. Elevation of the MDR glycoprotein gp170 constitutes another important mechanism of resistance, affecting multiple classes of chemotherapy. MDR is normally expressed on most epithelial tissues including many tumors of epithelial origin. MDR expression is increased after treatment of many human tumors [88], acting to decrease intracellular drug concentrations by enhancing drug efflux from cells. Drugs targeting these proteins have been tried with limited clinical success [89].

V. CLASSES OF CHEMOTHERAPIES AND THEIR FUNCTION

Cytotoxic chemotherapy can be divided into several broad categories based on the drug mechanism of action (MOA): alkylating agents, antimetabolites, natural products and microtubule inhibitors [90]. These classes of chemotherapy affect cells in cell-cycle specific or nonspecific fashions. Side effects, effectiveness and dosing vary, based on the disease, the stage and the patient being treated. An overview of the major classes of chemotherapies and their use follows below. In addition, Table 12.7 provides information on key drugs used in oncology.

A. Alkylating agents

The alkylating agents interfere with tumor growth primarily by directly damaging DNA, which ultimately prevents cell replication and initiates apoptosis, although effects on RNA and protein synthesis are also seen. The drugs form covalent bonds with various amino, carboxyl, sulfhydryl and phosphate groups on the molecules, particularly the electron-rich nitrogen at position 7 on guanine. Included in this class of agents are the nitrogen mustards, the nitrosoureas and platinum compounds. They are cell-cycle nonspecific but do require proliferating cells to exert their anticancer effects. The most important mechanisms of resistance appear to be enhanced DNA repair and glutathione reduction [91]. As a class, the dose-limiting side effect is myelosuppression. Most are associated with secondary cancers, particularly leukemias and myelodysplasia (MDS).

Nitrogen mustard is the prototype alkylating agent, but is rarely used in modern oncology. It is highly unstable and rapidly converts to the active metabolite. Notably, it is a potent vesicant and skin infiltration requires immediate medical attention. Infusion of thiosulfate can reverse some of the skin damage [92].

Cyclophosphamide is perhaps the most commonly used alkylating agent, in both solid and liquid tumors. Cyclophosphamide is used as a single agent and in combination regimens. It is inactive until metabolized by the cytochrome P450 system into its active metabolite which then decomposes into chloroacetaldehyde, the active agent, and acrolein, which causes the unique side effect of hemorrhagic cystitis [93]. The drug is well tolerated and while there are a number of rare side effects, myelosuppression is the most common dose-limiting toxicity. Of

TABLE 12.7 Classes, Function and Toxicity of Common Chemotherapies

Drug	Clinical Use	Toxicity	Notes
Nitrogen Mustards			
Chlorambucil	CLL[a] NHL[b] HL[c]	Myelosuppression Secondary AML HL[c] Infertility	No longer commonly used
Cyclophosphamide	Breast Cancer NHL Leukemia Myeloma	Myelosuppression Cystitis	MESNA to prevent bladder toxicity No secondary leukemia risk
Melphalan	Myeloma	Myelosuppression GI toxicity	Stem Cell Toxic Used in high doses for preparation for stem cell transplantation
Ifosfamide	Testicular Sarcoma Lung NHL	Myelosuppression Cystitis CNS toxicity	Methylene blue for CNS toxicity MESNA to prevent bladder toxicity
DTIC	Sarcoma Hodgkin Lymphoma	Myelosuppression Flu-like syndrome Nausea	Oral version: Temozolomide is effective for CNS tumors
Platinum Compounds			
Cisplatin	NHL Lung Ovarian Bladder Testicular HN[d]	Renal Dysfunction Neuropathy Ototoxicity Nausea Myelosuppression	Radiation sensitizer Highly emetogenic
Carboplatin	Lung Cancer NHL Ovarian Gastric	Less renal toxicity Myelosuppressive Nausea	Some suggestion of decreased efficacy compared with cisplatin More myelosuppression than cisplatin Less nausea than cisplatin
Oxaliplatin	Colorectal Pancreas Billiary	Neuropathy Myelosuppression	Two distinct neuropathies: - Acute cold induced - Chronic motor sensory
Antimetabolites			
Folate Analogs			
Methotrexate	NHL CNS Leukemia HN	Mucositis Myelosuppression Pulmonary toxicity	Can be given IT[e] Leucovorin can be used to rescue normal tissues, decrease toxicity Low doses commonly used for nonmalignant conditions
Pemetrexed	Lung Ovarian Mesothelioma	Myelosuppression	Vitamin B12 and folic acid supplementation required
Pyrimidine Analogs			
5-Fluorouracil	Colon Breast HN Biliary Pancreas	Mucositis Myelosuppression Diarrhea	Radiation sensitizer Toxicity varies based on schedule Oral prodrug: capecitabine effective in many of the same situations
Cytarabine	AML ALL NHL	Myelosuppression Nausea CNS toxicity Conjunctivitis	Can be given IT Prolonged infusions appear to improve efficacy

177

Continued

TABLE 12.7 Classes, Function and Toxicity of Common Chemotherapies—continued

Drug	Clinical Use	Toxicity	Notes
Gemcitabine	Biliary Pancreatic NHL Lung Breast Bladder	Myelosuppression Rash	Fixed-rate infusions are proven superior to standard dosing
Purine Analogs			
Fludarabine	CLL NHL	Myelosuppression Infections	Toxic to lymphocytes resulting in increased risk of opportunistic infections Autoimmune Hemolytic Anemia
Cladrabine	HCL[f]	Myelosuppression	
Natural Compounds			
Antitumor Antibiotics			
Bleomycin	HL Testicular	Myelosuppression Pneumonitis	PFT required prior to starting
Anthracyclines			
Doxorubicin	Breast AML ALL NHL Hodgkin Sarcoma	Myelosuppression Nausea Cardiotoxicity Stomatitis Vessicant	Liposomal preparation available
Epirubicin	Breast Sarcoma	Same as above	Equally cardiotoxic in equivalent dosing
Mitoxantrone	NHL Prostate	Same as Doxorubicin	Less cardiotoxicity
Epidophyllotoxin			
Etoposide	Lung Ovarian NHL Testicular	Myelosuppression Nausea Infusion Reactions Allopecia	Available in oral form
Camotothecin Analogs			
Irinotecan	Colon	Diarrhea Myelosuppression	Increased toxicity in liver disease
Microtubule Agents			
Paclitaxe	Breast Lung Ovarian HN	Neuropathy Myelosuppression Myalgias Allergic reactions	Albumin-bound form with decreased neuropathy available
Docetaxel	Breast Lung Prostate HN	Myelosuppression Fatigue Myalgias Neuropathy	
Cabazitaxel	Prostate	Neuropathy Myelosuppression	

178

TABLE 12.7   Classes, Function and Toxicity of Common Chemotherapies—continued

Drug	Clinical Use	Toxicity	Notes
Vinorelbine	Lung	Neuropathy	
	Breast	Constipation	
	NHL	Myelosuppression	
Ixebepilone	Breast	Neuropathy	Also mixed in crème form like
		Myelosuppression	paclitaxel - allergic reactions
Eribulin	Breast	Neuropathy	
		Prolonged QT	
		Myelosuppression	

Abbreviations: a: CLL: chronic lymphocytic leukemia; b: NHL: non-Hodgkin, Lymphoma; c: HL: Hodgkin lymphoma; d: HN: Head and Neck Cancer; e: IT:, intrathecal; f: HCL: Hairy Cell Leukemia

note, this agent is not associated with myelodysplasia or MDS because of the presence of aldehyde dehydrogenase in hematopoietic stem cells, making these cells resistant to cyclophosphamide's leukemogenic effects [94].

The first platinum compound in clinical use was cisplatin which has broad activity against many solid tumors and lymphomas. The drug has significant renal toxicity, is highly emetogenic and neurotoxic, and can generate ototoxicity [95]. The loss toxic cisplatin derivative carboplatin was developed to reduce these side effects, but possibly at the cost of efficacy in certain diseases and also with increased myelosuppression, particularly thrombocytopenia [96]. The newest platinum compound oxaliplatin has even less renal toxicity, but more pronounced neuropathy including a unique cold-induced neuropathy syndrome [97].

B. Antimetabolites

These chemotherapies are either structural analogs of purines and pyrimidines involved in DNA and RNA synthesis, or are inhibitors of key enzymes in nucleotide synthesis. The drugs are either incorporated into DNA or RNA in place of their normal analogs resulting in decreased transcription or translation or the drugs interrupt key metabolic pathways involved in the synthesis of these products. As a class they are cell-cycle specific agents, primarily affecting cells undergoing DNA synthesis in S phase. Their toxicity is variable, but immunosuppression and myelosuppression are most common with the structural analogs (e.g., fludarabine, pentostatin, cytarabine), while mucosal toxicity is more common with the interfering agents (e.g., methotrexate, 5-fluorouracil [5-FU]).

Methotrexate (MTX) is the prototypical agent of this class. MTX inhibits DNA synthesis by inhibiting the enzyme dihydrofolate reductase (DHFR), which is critical for recycling of folic acid needed in DNA synthesis. The drug is cleared by the kidneys and can accumulate in fluid compartments such as pleural effusions, leading to increased toxicity [98]. Myelosuppression and mucositis are the dose-limiting toxicities for MTX, but normal tissues can be salvaged by rescue with LV (a folate analog) [99]. As a newer strategy glucarpidase was recently approved by the FDA for reducing toxic levels of methotrexate in patients receiving high-dose therapy [100].

5-fluorouracil (5-FU) was the first "designer" chemotherapy and arguably the first targeted agent in clinical oncology [101]. This drug was developed from preclinical observations that tumor cells relied upon uracil more than normal tissues. 5-FU is a prodrug which is rapidly metabolized to 5-FdUMP which directly targets thylimidate synthase. A newer, oral version of this drug, capecitabine, is used clinically as well. The toxicity of both agents is primarily gastrointestinal with diarrhea being the most common dose-limiting toxicity.

179

Cytarabine and gemcitabine are two similarly related compounds and are the classic pyrimidine derivatives. These compounds are both cytosine derivatives that upon activation via phosphorylation are incorporated into DNA. Interestingly, their efficacies vary with cytarabine being primarily used in hematologic malignancies and gemcitabine being used in many solid tumors and hematologic malignancies. In addition, cytarabine appears to have the most efficacy when given as a continuous infusion [102], whereas fixed dose-rate infusions of gemcitabine do not appear to offer significant benefit compared with standard infusions [103]. Both drugs are myelosuppressive, but cytarabine has other interesting side effects including a chemical conjunctivitis and acute cerebellar syndrome [104].

Fludarabine is the most commonly used purine analog. This drug is a prodrug that in cells is converted to a phosphorylated form that is incorporated into DNA. The phosphorylated form of fludarabine is resistant to degradation by adenosine deaminase. The drug is profoundly toxic to lymphocytes and is active in many hematologic malignancies. Given its lymphocytotoxic effects, prophylaxis against opportunistic infections is mandatory [105].

C. Natural products

This class of compounds is isolated from plants, bacteria or fungi. They exert a wide range of effects on human cells but most interfere with DNA synthesis. They include the antitumor antibiotics, the anthracyclines, bleomycin and the epipodophyllotoxins. Bleomycin interferes with DNA synthesis by forming reactive oxygen species, whereas the anthracyclines and the epipodophyllotoxins interfere with distinct isomers of DNA topoisomerase. This class of drugs tends to cause myelosuppression and can result in secondary leukemias [106].

The anthracyclines as a class are some of the most active agents used in oncology. The prototypical agent is doxorubicin which exhibits broad activity against many solid and hematologic cancers. This drug directly interferes with topoisomerase II preventing DNA replication. Aside from myelosuppression, it can produce significant cardiac dysfunction in a dose-dependent manner [107]. A newer related compound, mitoxantrone, exerts a similar mechanism of action but with less cardiotoxicity. However, overall results with mitoxantrone have been disappointing to date and its role in oncology as a substitute for traditional anthracyclines is not clear [108]. Interestingly, it appears that continuous infusion of doxorubicin might mitigate some of the cardiotoxicity [109]. This finding has led to a liposomal preparation, which exhibits broad efficacy but with less cardiotoxicity [110].

Etoposide is the classic epipodophyllotoxin, which works by inhibiting DNA topoisomerase II. This drug is active in many solid tumors. Aside from myelosuppression, there is a specific cytogenetic change in chromosome 11q23 that can lead to formation of secondary leukemia that can arise with exposure to this class of drugs [111].

The camptothecin derivatives, of which irinotecan is the only commonly used agent, work by inhibiting topoisomerase I. The drug causes myelosuppression, but diarrhea is the most common side effect [112].

D. Microtubule inhibitors

This class of chemotherapy drugs works by direct binding to tubulin, preventing either its polymerization or disassembly. This class includes the vinca compounds and the taxanes and related compounds. They are effective in a wide range of human cancers and display neuropathy as their main dose-limiting toxicity [113]. Of note, newer compounds including eribulin have been brought to the clinic, with activity even in patients failing taxanes [114].

The vinca alkaloids including vincristine, vinblastine and vinorelbine are used commonly to treat a wide variety of cancers. These agents work by preventing microtubule polymerization. Aside from myelosuppression, neuropathy is the most common complication.

Conversely, the taxanes, which are used ubiquitously in oncology, work not by encouraging microtubule formation but by blocking depolymerization, such that the resultant microtubule is less functional. The two most commonly used agents in this subclass are paclitaxel and docetaxel, which at identical doses are likely equivalent [115].

VI. CONCLUSIONS

In the last 60 years the field of medical oncology has advanced rapidly, largely in part to the development and rational use of chemotherapy. While the use of targeted agents in cancer therapy is increasingly important, they are unlikely anytime soon to widely replace cytotoxic chemotherapy for cancer treatment. Advances in supportive care, along with optimization of dose and scheduling have reduced mortality for a number of cancers in the adjuvant and neoadjuvant settings, and have provided the chance for cures. In addition, the effective use of chemotherapy has allowed for not only survival but also improved quality of life in metastatic disease. The principles discussed in this chapter provide an important starting point to view the development of newer agents, new combinations of targeted agents and classical cytotoxic compounds, and the broader introduction of immunotherapies into the treatment of cancer.

References

[1] Hirsh J. An Anniversary for Cancer Chemotherapy. JAMA 2006;296(12):1518—20.

[2] Krumbhaar EB, Krumbhaar HD. The blood and bone marrow in yellow gas (mustard gas) poisoning. Changes produced in bone marrow in fatal cases. J Med Res 1919;40:497—508.

[3] Goodman LS, Wintrobe MM, Damesheck W, et al. Nitrogen Mustard therapy: use of methyl-bis (B-chloroethyl) amine hydrochloride and tris (B-chloroethyl) amine hydrochloride for Hodgkin's disease, lymphosarcoma, leukemia, and certain allied and miscellaneous disorders. JAMA 1946;132:126—32.

[4] Stockler M, Wilcken NR, Ghersi D, et al. Systematic reviews of chemotherapy and endocrine therapy in metastatic breast cancer. Cancer Treat Rev 2000;26(3):151—68.

[5] Nordic Gastrointestinal Tumor Adjuvant Therapy Group. Expectancy or primary chemotherapy in patients with advanced asymptomatic colorectal cancer: a randomized trial. J Clin Oncol 1992;10(6):904—11.

[6] Spiro SG, Rudd RM, Souhami RL, et al. Chemotherapy versus supportive care in advanced non-small cell lung cancer: improved survival without detriment to quality of life. Thorax 2004;59(10):828—36.

[7] Chia SK, Speers CH, D'yachkova Y, et al. The impact of new chemotherapeutic and hormone agents on survival in a population-based cohort of women with metastatic breast cancer. Cancer 2007;110(5):973—9.

[8] NSCLC Meta-Analyses Collaborative Group. Chemotherapy in addition to supportive care improves survival in advanced non-small-cell lung cancer: a systematic review and meta-analysis of individual patient data from 16 randomized controlled trials. J Clin Oncol 2008;26(28):4617—25.

[9] Goldie JH. The Scientific Basis for adjuvant and primary (neoadjuvant) chemotherapy. Semin Oncol 1987;14:1—7.

[10] LeVay J, O'Sullivan B, Catton C, et al. Outcome and prognostic factors in soft tissue sarcoma in the adult. Int J Radiat Oncol Biol Phys 1993;27(5):1091—8.

[11] Allal AS, Bieri S, Pelloni A, et al. Sphincter-sparing surgery after preoperative radiotherapy for low rectal cancers: feasibility, oncologic results and quality of life outcomes. Br J Cancer 2000;82(6):1131—7.

[12] Rastogi P, Anderson SJ, Bear HD, et al. Preoperative chemotherapy: updates of National Surgical Adjuvant Breast and Bowel Project Protocols B-18 and B-27. J Clin Oncol 2008;26(5):778—85.

[13] Advanced Bladder Cancer Meta-analysis Collaboration. Neoadjuvant chemotherapy in invasive bladder cancer: a systematic review and meta-analysis. Lancet 2003;361(9373):1927—34.

[14] Sjoquist KM, Burmeister BH, Smithers BM, et al. Survival after neoadjuvant chemotherapy or chemo-radiotherapy for resectable oesophageal carcinoma: an updated meta-analysis. Lancet Oncol 2011;12(7):681—92.

[15] Hou JY, Kelly MG, Yu H, et al. Neoadjuvant chemotherapy lessens surgical morbidity in advanced ovarian cancer and leads to improved survival in stage IV disease. Gynecol Oncol 2007;105(1):211—7.

[16] Flam M, John M, Pajak TF, et al. Role of mitomycin in combination with fluorouracil and radiotherapy, and of salvage chemoradiation in the definitive nonsurgical treatment of epidermoid carcinoma of the anal canal: results of a phase III randomized intergroup study. J Clin Oncol 1996;14(9):2527—39.

[17] Eeson G, Foo M, Harrow S, et al. Outcomes of salvage surgery for epidermoid carcinoma of the anus following failed combined modality treatment. Am J Surg 2011 May;201(5):628—33.

[18] Blanchard P, Baujat B, Holostenco V, et al. Meta-analysis of chemotherapy in head and neck cancer (MACH-NC): a comprehensive analysis by tumour site. Radiother Oncol 2011;100(1):33–40.

[19] McArthur HL, Hudis CA. Adjuvant Chemotherapy for early-stage breast cancer. Hematol Oncol Clin North Am. 2997;21:207–222

[20] AndréT Boni C, Mounedji-Boudiaf L, et al. Oxaliplatin, fluorouracil, and leucovorin as adjuvant treatment for colon cancer. N Engl J Med 2004;350(23):2343–51.

[21] Pignon JP, Tribodet H, Scagliotti GV, et al. Lung adjuvant cisplatin evaluation: a pooled analysis by the LACE Collaborative Group. J Clin Oncol 2008;26(21):3552–9.

[22] Neoptolemos JP, Stocken DD, Friess H, et al. A randomized trial of chemoradiotherapy and chemotherapy after resection of pancreatic cancer. N Engl J Med 2004;350(12):1200–10.

[23] Skipper HE, Schabel FM, Mellet LB, et al. Implications of biochemical, cytokinetic, pharmacologic and toxicologic relationships in the design of optimal therapeutic schedules. Cancer Chemother Rep 1950;54:431–50.

[24] Skipper HE. Analysis of multiarmed trials in which animals bearing different burdens of L1210 leukemia cells were treated with two, three, and four drug combinations delivered in different ways with varying dose intensities of each drug and varying average dose intensities. Southern Research Institute Booklet 7 1986;420:87.

[25] Skipper HE. Kinetics of mammary tumor cell growth and implications for therapy. Cancer 1971;28:1479–99.

[26] Norton L. Adjuvant breast cancer therapy: Current Status and future strategies—growth kinetics and the improved drug therapy of breast cancer. Semin Oncol 199;26(suppl 3):1–4

[27] Surbone A, Norton L. Kinetics of breast neoplasms. Minerva Med 1994;85:7–16.

[28] Norton LA. Gompertzain model of human breast cancer growth. Cancer Res 1998;48:7067–71.

[29] Bruce WR, Meeker BE, Valertiote FA. Comparision of the sensitivity of normal and hematopoietic and transplanted lymphoma colony forming cells to chemotherapeutic agents administered in vivo. J Natl Cancer Inst 1966;37:233–45.

[30] Gribben JG. Attainment of a molecular remission: a worthwhile goal? J Clin Oncol 1994;12:1532–4.

[31] DeVita VT, Chu E. Medical Oncology. In: Devita VT, Lawrence TS, Rosenberg SA, editors. Cancer: Principles and Practice of Oncology. 9th ed. Lippincott, Williams and Wilkins; 2011. p. 313.

[32] Hudis C, Norton L. Adjuvant drug therapy for operable breast cancer. Semin Oncol 1996;23:475–93.

[33] Norton L. Theoretical concepts and the Emerging Role of Taxanes in adjuvant therapy. The Oncologist 2001;6(suppl 3):30–5.

[34] Bonadonna G, Zambette M, Valagusa P. Sequential or alternating Doxorubicin and CMF regimens in breast cancer with more than three positive nodes. J Am Med Assoc 1995;273:542–7.

[35] Pui CH, Sandlund JT, Pei D, et al. Improved outcome for children with acute lymphoblastic leukemia: results of Total Therapy Study XIIIB at St Jude Children's Research Hospital. Blood 2004;104(9):2690–969.

[36] Gatta G, Capocaccia R, Stiller C, et al. Childhood cancer survival trends in Europe: a EUROCARE Working Group study. J Clin Oncol 2005;23(16):3742–51.

[37] Frei E, Elias A, Wheeler C, et al. The relationship between high-dose treatment and combination chemotherapy: the concept of summation dose intensity. Clin Cancer Res 1998;4:2027–37.

[38] Huncharek M, Caubet JF, McGarry R. Single-agent DTIC versus combination chemotherapy with or without immunotherapy in metastatic melanoma: meta-analysis of 3273 patients from 20 randomized trials. Melanoma Res 2001;11(1):75–81.

[39] Quoix E, Zalcman G, Oster JP, et al. Carboplatin and weekly paclitaxel doublet chemotherapy compared with monotherapy in elderly patients with advanced lung cancer: IFCT-0501 randomised phase 3 trial. Lancet 2011;378:1079–88.

[40] Ychou M, Raoul JL, Douillard JY, et al. A phase III randomised trial of LV5FU2 + irinotecan versus LV5FU2 alone in adjuvant high-risk colon cancer (FNCLCC Accord02/FFCD9802). Ann Oncol 2009; 20(4):674–80.

[41] Chou TC. Drug combination Studies and Their Synergy Quantification using the Chou-Talalay Method. Cancer Res 2010;70:440–6.

[42] Caggiano V, Weiss RV, Rickert TS, et al. Incidence, cost, and mortality of neutropenia hospitalization associated with chemotherapy. Cancer 2005;103(9):1916–24.

[43] Lyman GH, Michels SL, Reynolds MW, et al. Risk of mortality in patients with cancer who experience febrile neutropenia. Cancer 2010;116(23):5555–63.

[44] Brizel DM, Wasserman TH, Henke M, et al. Phase III randomized trial of amifostine as a radioprotector in head and neck cancer. J Clin Oncol 2000;18(19):3339.

[45] Norton L. Evolving concepts in the systemic treatment of breast cancer. Semin Oncol 1997;25(suppl 10). S10-3–S10–10.

[46] Buzzoni R, Bonnadonna G, Valagussa P, et al. Adjuvant chemotherapy with doxorubicin plus cyclophosphamide and methotrexate in the treatment of resectable breast cancer with more than three positive axillary lymph nodes. J Clin Oncol 1991;9:2134–40.

[47] Volger WR, Cooper LE, Groth DP. Correlation of cytosine arabinoside-induced recruitment in growth fraction of leukemic blasts with clinical response. Cancer 1974;33:603–10.

[48] Poplin E, Feng Y, Berlin J, et al. Phase III, randomized study of gemcitabine and oxaliplatin versus gemcitabine (fixed-dose rate infusion) compared with gemcitabine (30-minute infusion) in patients with pancreatic carcinoma E6201: a trial of the Eastern Cooperative Oncology Group. J Clin Oncol 2009;27(23):3778–85.

[49] Chau I, Norman AR, Cunningham D, et al. A randomised comparison between 6 months of bolus fluoro-uracil/leucovorin and 12 weeks of protracted venous infusion fluorouracil as adjuvant treatment in colorectal cancer. Ann Oncol 2005;16(4):549–57.

[50] Smith LA, Cornelius VR, Plummer CJ, et al. Cardiotoxicity of anthracycline agents for the treatment of cancer: systematic review and meta-analysis of randomised controlled trials. BMC Cancer 2010;10:337.

[51] Andreopoulou E, Gaiotti D, Kim E, et al. Pegylated liposomal doxorubicin HCL (PLD; Caelyx/Doxil): experience with long-term maintenance in responding patients with recurrent epithelial ovarian cancer. Ann Oncol 2007;18(4):716–21.

[52] Wolpin BM, Mayer RJ. Systemic treatment of colorectal cancer. Gastroenterology 2008;134:1296–310.

[53] Soon YY, Stockler MR, Askie LM, et al. Duration of chemotherapy for advanced non-small-cell lung cancer: a systematic review and meta-analysis of randomized trials. J Clin Oncol 2009;27(20):3277–83.

[54] Gennari A, Stockler M, Puntoni M, et al. Duration of chemotherapy for metastatic breast cancer: a systematic review and meta-analysis of randomized clinical trials. J Clin Oncol 2011;29(16):2144–9.

[55] Tournigand C, Cervantes A, Figer A, et al. OPTIMOX1: a randomized of FOLFOX4 or FOLFOX7 with oxaliplatin in a stop and go fashion in advanced colon cancer – a GERCOR study. J Clin Oncol 2006;20:394–400.

[56] Stinchcombe TE, West HL. Maintenance therapy in non-small-cell lung cancer. Lancet 2009;374(9699):1398–400.

[57] Sandler A, Gray R, Perry MC, et al. Paclitaxel-Carboplatin Alone or with Bevacizumab for Non-Small-Cell Lung Cancer. N Engl J Med 2006;355:2542–50.

[58] Pirker R, Pereira JF, Szczesna A, et al. Cetuximab plus chemotherapy in patients with advanced non-small-cell lung cancer (FLEX): an open-label randomised phase III trial. Lancet 2009;373(9674):1525–31.

[59] Paz-Ares L, de Marinis F, Dediu M, et al. Maintenance therapy with pemetrexed plus best supportive care versus placebo plus best supportive care after induction therapy with pemetrexed plus cisplatin for advanced non-squamous non-small-cell lung cancer (PARAMOUNT): a double-blind, phase 3, randomised controlled trial. Lancet Oncol. Early Online Publication February 2012;16(12). http://dx.doi.org/10.1016/S1470–2045. 70063–70063.

[60] Ciuleanu T, Brodowicz T, Zielinski C, et al. Maintenance pemetrexed plus best supportive care versus placebo plus best supportive care for non-small-cell lung cancer: a randomised, double-blind phase 3 study. Lancet 2009;374(9699):1432–40.

[61] Cappuzo F, Ciuleanu T, Stelmakh L, et al. Erlotinib as maintenance treatment in advanced non-small-cell lung cancer: a multicentre, randomized, placebo controlled phase 3 study. Lancet Oncol 2010;11(6):521–9.

[62] Fidias PM, Dakhil SR, Lyss AP, et al. Phase III study of immediate compared with delayed docetaxel after front-line therapy with gemcitabine plus carboplatin in advanced non-small-cell lung cancer. J Clin Oncol 2009;27(4):591–8.

[63] Hryniuk WM. Average relative dose intensity and the impact on design of clinical trials. Semin Oncol 1987;14:65–73.

[64] Kwak LW, Halpern J, Olshen RA, et al. Prognostic significance of actual dose intensity in diffuse large-cell lymphoma: results of a tree-structured survival analysis. J Clin Oncol 1990;8(6):963–77.

[65] Bonadonna G, Valagussa P, Moliterni A, et al. Adjuvant cyclophosphamide, methotrexate, and fluorouracil in node-positive breast cancer: the results of 20 years of follow-up. N Engl J Med 1995;332(14):901–6.

[66] Toner GC, Stockler MR, Boyer MJ, et al. Comparison of two standard chemotherapy regimens for good-prognosis germ-cell tumours: a randomised trial. Australian and New Zealand Germ Cell Trial Group. Lancet 2001;357(9258):739–45.

[67] Hryniuk W, Frei E, Wright FA. A single scale for comparing dose-intensity of all chemotgherapy regimens in breast cancer: summation-dose intensity. J Clin Oncol 1998;16:3137–47.

[68] Wyndam WH, Grossband ML, Pittaluga S, et al. Dose-adjused EPOCH chemotherapy for untreated large B-cell lymphomas: a pharmacodynamic approach with high efficacy. Blood 2002;99:2685–93.

[69] Norton L, Simon R. Tumor Size, sensitivity to therapy and design of treatment protocols. Cancer Treat Rep 1976;61:1307–17.

183

[70] Citron ML, Berry DA, Cirrinocione C, et al. Randomized trial of dose-dense vs conventionally scheduled and sequential vs concurrent combination chemotherapy as post-operative adjuvant treatment of node-positive primary breast cancer: first report of Intergroup Trial C9741/Cancer and Leukemia Group B Trial 9741. J Clin Oncol 2003;21(8):1431–9.

[71] Hurwitz H, Patt YZ, Henry L, et al. Phase III study of standard triweekly vs dose dense biweekly capecitabine (C) + oxaliplatin (O) + bevacizumab (B) as first-line treatment for metastatic colon cancer (mCRC): XELOX-A-DVS (dense versus standard): Interim analysis. J Clin Oncol 2009;27:15 (suppl; abstr 4078).

[72] Watanabe T, Tobinai K, Shibata T, et al. Phase II/III Study of R-CHOP-21 Versus R-CHOP-14 for untreated indolent B-Cell Non-Hodgkin Lymphoma: JCOG 0203 Trial. J Clin Oncol 2011;29(30):3990–8.

[73] Lyman GH, Barron RL, Natoli JL, et al. Systematic Review of efficacy of dose-dense versus non-dose dense chemotherapy in breast cancer, non-Hodgkin lymphoma, and non-small cell lung cancer. Crit Rev Oncol Hematol 2011; May 31 (epub ahead of print).

[74] Sparano JA, Wang M, Martino S, et al. Weekly paclitaxel in the Adjuvant treatment of Breast Cancer. N Engl J Med 2008;358:1663–71.

[75] Kastsumata NYasuda MTakahashi F, et al.Dose-dense paclitaxel once a week in combination with carboplatin every 3 weeks in advanced ovarian cancer: a phase 3, open-label, randomised controlled trial.Lancet 17;374(9698):1331–1338

[76] Doroshow JH, Multhauf P, Leong L, et al. Prospective randomized comparision of fluorouracil versus flourouracil and high-dose continuous infusion leucovorin calcium for the treatment of advanced measurable colorectal cancer in patients previously unexposed to chemotherapy. J Clin Oncol 1990;8:491–501.

[77] O'Connell MJ, Maillard JA, Kahn MJ, et al. Controlled trial of fluorouracil and low-dose leucovorin given for six months as postoperative adjuvant therapy for colon cancer. J Clin Oncol 1997;15:246–50.

[78] Frei E, Blum RH, Pitman SW, et al. High-dose methotrexate with leucovorin rescue. Rationale and spectrum of anti-tumor activity. Am J Med 1980;73:370–6.

[79] Goldie JH, Coldman AJ. A mathematical model for relating the drug sensitivity to the spontancous mutation rate. Cancer Treat Rep 1979;63:1727–33.

[80] El-Diery WS. The role of p53 in chemosensitivity and radiosensitivity. Oncogene 2003;22:7486–95.

[81] Lowe SW, Bodis S, McClatchy A, et al. p53 status and the efficacy of caner therapy in vivo. Science 1994;266:807–10.

[82] Adams JM, Cory S. The BCL-2 apoptotic switch in cancer development and therapy. Oncogene 2007;26:1324–37.

[83] Chanan-Khan A. Bcl-2 antisense therapy in hematologic malignancies. Curr Opin Oncol 2004;16:581–5.

[84] Meng XW, Lee SH, Kaufmann SH. Apoptosis in the treatment of cancer: a promise kept? Curr Opin Cell Biol 2006;18:668–76.

[85] Melisi D, Chiao PJ. NF-kappaB as a target in the treatment for cancer therapy. Expert Opin Ther Targets 2007;11:133–44.

[86] McIwain CC, Townsend DM, Tew KD. Glutathione S-transferase polymorphisms: cancer incidence and therapy. Oncogene 2006;25:1639–48.

[87] Cacciatore I, Caccuri AM, Cocco A, et al. Potent isoenzyme-selective inhibition of human glutathione S-transferase A1-1 by novel glutathione S-conjugate. Amino Acids 2005;29(3):255–61.

[88] Ross DD, Doyle LA. Mining our ABCs: Pharmacogenomic approach for evaluating transporter function in cancer drug resistance. Cancer Cell 2004;6:105.

[89] Zhou SF, Wang LL, Di YM, et al. Substrates and inhibitors of human multidrug resistance associated proteins and the implications in drug development. Curr Med Chem 2008;15(20):1981–2039.

[90] Chabner BA, Longo DL, editors. Cancer Chemotherapy and Biotherapy: Principles and Practice. 4th ed. Philadelphia PA: Lippencott, Williams and Wilkens; 2006.

[91] Hall AG, Tilby MJ. Mechanisms of action of, and modes of resistance to, alkylating agents used in the treatment of haematological malignancies. Blood Rev 1992;6(3):163–73.

[92] Ener RA, Meglathery SB, Styler M. Extravasation of Systemic Hemato-Oncological Therapies. Ann Oncol 2004;15(6):858–62.

[93] Fraiser LH, Kanekal S, Kehrer JP. Cyclophosphamide Toxicity. Characterizing and Avoiding the Problem. Drugs 1991;42(5):781–95.

[94] Brodsky RA, Sensenbrenner LL, Jones RJ. Complete remission in severe aplastic anemia after high-dose cyclophosphamide without bone marrow transplantation. Blood 1996;87(2):491–4.

[95] Higa GM, Wise TC, Crowell EB, "Severe. Disabling Neurologic Toxicity Following Cisplatin Retreatment. Ann Pharmacother 1995;29(2):134–7.

[96] Go RS, Adjei AA. Review of the Comparative Pharmacology and Clinical Activity of Cisplatin and Carboplatin. J Clin Oncol 1999;17(1):409–22.

[97] Cassidy J, Misset JL. Oxaliplatin-Related Side Effects: Characteristics and Management. Semin Oncol 2002;29(5 Suppl 15):11–20.

[98] Jolivet J, Cowan KH, Curt GA, et al. The Pharmacology and Clinical Use of Methotrexate. N Engl J Med 1983;309(18):1094–104.

[99] Treon SP, Chabner BA. Concepts in Use of High-Dose Methotrexate Therapy. Clin Chem 1996;42(8 Pt 2): 1322–9.

[100] Widemann BC, Balis FM, Murphy RF, et al. Carboxypeptidase-G2, Thymidine, and Leucovorin Rescue in Cancer Patients With Methotrexate-Induced Renal Dysfunction. J Clin Oncol 1997;15(5):2125–34.

[101] Kuhn JG. Fluorouracil and the New Oral Fluorinated Pyrimidines. Ann Pharmacother 2001;35(2):217–27.

[102] Löwenberg B, Pabst T, Vellenga E, et al. Cytarabine Dose for Acute Myeloid Leukemia. N Engl J Med 2011; 364(11):1027–36.

[103] Poplin E, Feng Y, Berlin J, et al. Phase III, randomized study of gemcitabine and oxaliplatin versus gemcitabine (fixed-dose rate infusion) compared with gemcitabine (30-minute infusion) in patients with pancreatic carcinoma E6201: a trial of the Eastern Cooperative Oncology Group. J Clin Oncol 2009;27(23):3778–85.

[104] Jolson HM, Bosco L, Bufton MG, et al. Clustering of adverse drug events: analysis of risk factors for cerebellar toxicity with high-dose cytarabine. J Natl Cancer Inst 1992;84(7):500–5.

[105] Keating MJ, O'Brien S, McLaughlin P, et al. Clinical Experience With Fludarabine in Hemato-Oncology. Hematol Cell Ther 1996;38(Suppl 2):3470–83.

[106] Godley LA, Larson RA. Therapy-related myeloid leukemia. Semin Oncol 2008;35(4):418–29.

[107] Floyd JD, Nguyen DT, Lobins RL, et al. Cardiotoxicity of cancer therapy. J Clin Oncol 2005;23(30):7685–96.

[108] Smith LA, Cornelius VR, Plummer CJ, et al. Cardiotoxicity of anthracycline agents for the treatment of cancer: systematic review and meta-analysis of randomised controlled trials. BMC Cancer 2010;10:337.

[109] Casper ES, Gaynor JJ, Hajdu SI, et al. A prospective randomized trial of adjuvant chemotherapy with bolus versus continuous infusion of doxorubicin in patients with high-grade extremity soft tissue sarcoma and an analysis of prognostic factors. Cancer 1991;68(6):1221–9.

[110] Jones RL, Berry GJ, Rubens RD, et al. Clnical and pathological absence of cardiotoxicity after liposomal doxorubicin. Lancet Oncol 2004;5(9):575–7.

[111] Libura J, Slater DJ, Felix CA, et al. Therapy-related acute myeloid leukemia-like MLL rearrangements are induced by etoposide in primary human CD34+ cells and remain stable after clonal expansion. Blood 2005;105(5):2124–31.

[112] Mathijssen RH, van Alphen RJ, Verweij J, et al. Clinical Pharmacokinetics and Metabolism of Irinotecan (CPT-11). Clin Cancer Res 2001;7(8):2182–794.

[113] Perez E. Microtuble inhibitors: Differentiating tubulin-inhibitors based on mechanism of action, clinical efficacy and resistance. Mol Cancer Ther 2009;8:2086–95.

[114] Vahdat LT, Pruitt B, Fabian CJ, et al. Phase II Study of Eribulin Mesylate, a Halichondrin B Analog, in Patients With Metastatic Breast Cancer Previously Treated With an Anthracycline and a Taxane. J Clin Oncol 2009;27(18):2954–61.

[115] Crown J, O'Leary M, Ooi WS. Docetaxel and Paclitaxel in the Treatment of Breast Cancer: A Review of Clinical Experience. Oncol 2004;9(Suppl 2):24–32.

CHAPTER 13

Pharmacokinetics and Safety Assessment

Richard A. Westhouse, Bruce D. Car
Discovery Toxicology, Pharmaceutical Candidate Optimization, Bristol-Myers Squibb Co., Princeton, New Jersey USA

I. INTRODUCTION

In the pharmaceutical industry, the drug discovery process begins with identification of a putative drugable target and culminates with identification of a lead candidate with acceptable pharmaceutical properties for progression to exploratory development. For small molecules, this process involves the selection of a chemical scaffold (or core), followed by optimization within that structural series through serially iterative studies of serial structure-activity relationship (SAR) and/or structure-liability relationship (SLR), so as to increase desirable characteristics and reduce undesirable properties. While initial optimization efforts are usually heavily weighted toward increasing potency and efficacy, they should also build in the optimization of pharmaceutical, pharmacokinetic, and safety properties with the iterative progression of drug candidates towards molecules that can be triage tested in animals, followed by testing in man. Pharmaceutical optimization not only includes identification of formulations to achieve not only efficacy, but also multiples above efficacy so as to enable toxicity studies, demonstration of stability, full characterization of physicochemical profiles, and so forth. Pharmacokinetic optimization usually involves additional investigational iterations, using specific assays in collaboration with the pharmaceutical medicinal chemist, so as to identify SAR and engineer the best molecule. The best pharmacokinetic properties are not always intuitive, and a desired clearance usually balances efficacy and toxicity. Safety optimization includes increased selectivity and specificity. Therefore, to maximize the desired therapeutic window, risk assessment investigations must give perspective to the possibility that a patient will or will not develop a previously identified toxicity in the preclinical animal setting.

The ultimate goal of optimization in drug discovery is to identify the best exploratory drug candidate that provides best-in-class medicinal characteristics, if possible, along with commercial advantages including differentiation from competing agents within the specific market. Given the huge clinical and regulatory expense involved in late stage development of a new drug candidate, commercialization issues cannot be ignored. To improve chances to advance development through late-stage clinical trials, pharmaceutical companies are investing increasingly in discovery optimization so as to reduce later failures due to toxicities identified in rigorous preclinical safety testing, which is required to enable clinical trials but may also predict failures due to clinical safety or lack of efficacy [29].

The discovery and development of nonselective cytotoxic small molecule oncologic agents has adhered to classical regulated paradigms, both requiring and allowing relatively little room for innovation. The regulatory guidelines for these agents have not significantly evolved since their inception. Because the biology and pharmacology underlying cancer immunotherapeutic

Cancer Immunotherapy. http://dx.doi.org/10.1016/B978-0-12-394296-8.00013-0

agents differ fundamentally from cytotoxic oncologics, a markedly different profile of issues is observed in discovery and development. In addition to satisfying proscribed regulatory requirements for oncologic development, sound scientific rationale and innovative thinking must be applied to novel oncologic agents to provide an appropriate risk assessment of those agents entering clinical trials. The typical practice for the testing of oncologic and immuno-oncologic agents has been to identify the maximum tolerated dose (MTD) in patients or healthy volunteers in shorter term studies, and then continue in patients with MTD as the sole dosage selection criterion at those high doses. Additional or progressive safety signals, saturated PK clearance, appearance of undesired, nonselective or toxic metabolites, or exaggerated pharmacology may limit a drug's long-term effectiveness, safety or tolerability at MTD. A detailed knowledge of the level of target engagement associated with efficacy [40] may be needed to allow physicians to limit human dosages to exposures with a potential to be beneficial and thereby to improve long-term success.

Types of agents that would be used in cancer immunotherapy can be categorized as either a small molecule or a biopharmaceutical. Regulatory criteria differ considerably for each class, which are handled by different FDA regulatory agencies. Small molecules or new chemical entities (NCE), in general, have a low molecular weight (<750 kDa); possess physicochemical properties allowing solid dosage formulation and minimal pH-dependent solubility; are chemically synthesized as a single active drug substance that can be efficiently purified; and can be manipulated by a medicinal chemist to change specific activities. In contrast, bio-pharmaceutical agents have a large molecular weight; have complex physicochemical properties; are synthesized by host cell lines (or the entity itself *is* the host cell, as for somatic cell vaccines) or by recombinant bacteria; are not as extensively purified due to the heterogeneous nature of the synthetic mixture; and are less able to be manipulated by a medicinal chemist to alter activities, with the exception of target cytotoxics where small molecule warheads are attached to delivery antibodies.

Classes of biopharmaceutical agents include antibodies (antagonist and activating actions), antibody components, adnectins (fibronectin kringle domains), recombinant proteins (such as cytokines, hormones, growth factors, and enzymes), synthetic oligonucleotides, gene transfer products, vaccines (protein, cellular such as somatic cell therapy), etc., with and without posttranslational modifications such as PEGylation or glycosylation to alter activity and pharmacokinetic properties. The approach of this chapter will be to present concepts in pharmacology and toxicology for targeted small molecule therapeutics for cancer, and contrast to significant differences with specific biopharmaceutical agents. For small molecules, medicinal chemists play a significant role in altering substructures in an effort to alter activities (potency or toxicity), while for biopharmaceutical agents, this approach to improving compound qualities is generally not possible. Resolving issues with biopharmaceutical agents generally requires an intimate understanding of the perturbed biologic process and a clear characterization of biophysical properties.

II. CONCEPTS IN PHARMACOKINETICS (PK)

Pharmacokinetics (PK) is the study of the disposition of a drug when it is delivered to an organism—in short, a study of what "the body does to the drug." The science of metabolism and pharmacokinetics developed from the investigation of the disposition of small molecule chemical entities, either therapeutic or toxic (for further information, see [24,44]). Pharmacokinetic concepts in this section will be presented from the perspective of small molecules; however, significant differences for biotechnology-derived products will be introduced when relevant (for further information, see [38]).

Pharmacokinetic analysis must begin with validated analytical methods to quantify the drug in various *in vivo* and *in vitro* samples. For small molecule agents, this is most commonly, if not exclusively, done chromatographically (GS or LC) in conjunction with single or dual mass spectrometry (MS) [9,16]. Specific bioanalytical methods should be validated for the relevant sample matrix from each species. These methods should also utilize standard curves for the specific analyte as well as relevant internal standards. When stability of the analyte in the matrix is unknown, samples should be analyzed as soon after collection as possible, but it is best to perform stability testing very early in the program. Stability must never be assumed, even in frozen sera. These tests generally involve analyzing samples with concentrations that bracket the relevant concentrations, with re-analysis of samples after processing and storing. Sample handling should always be consistent across studies so as not to add extraneous variables. Some biotechnology-derived agents are quantifiable by chromatography/mass spectrometry, even though these proteins are very complex in nature and often inherently heterogeneous. Peptide and protein drugs are typically quantified by immunoassays (ELISA), protein capture ELISA, bioactivity assays, or other such procedures; however, in some cases MS can also be used [7]. These assays, which often require more extensive development, should undergo the same rigorous qualification as chromatography/mass spectrometry methods. Multiple assays may be required in order to gain a complete assessment of exposure—for example, capture assays for antibodies can bind the active site or the Fc domain, depending on need to quantify specific circulating complexes bound at these and other sites. Various reviews and opinions on more rigorous validation of bioanalytical methods have been published [14] including guidance from the United States Food and Drug Administration Center for Drug Evaluation and Research [9].

Blood or plasma exposure of a drug, while convenient for its easy access, is not always the most relevant parameter to use for correlations with drug-related effects (whether efficacy or toxicity). In practice, the free fraction of drug, that is drug not bound by plasma albumin or rarely other binding proteins, is best correlated with desired pharmacology. As many drugs exhibit a high level of blood-protein binding (<90%), this correction can be extremely important in understanding the pharmacology or toxicity of a drug. Models for investigating pharmacokinetic-pharmacodynamic correlations frequently assume simple passive diffusion of drug from the blood compartment to the site of activity. Transporters, such as multidrug resistance (MDR) transporters and many others, are increasingly being identified in cancer cells. These effectively reduce intracellular exposure of drugs, to the extent of disease refractory to treatment even though plasma exposures may be adequate to confer efficacy in other patients [11,53]. For cancer immunotherapeutics that target molecules on normal patient immune cells, plasma levels are the most relevant parameter for modeling antitumor activity. Similarly, for most toxicologic effects, plasma exposure is most relevant, although brain levels are frequently lower than plasma due to the blood—brain barrier, low free-fraction, and/or transporter activity.

Relative to non-oncologic therapies, small molecule cancer agents generally have much higher unit doses. This factor introduces a host of special issues in toxicity and ADME properties as well as in pharmaceutics. The revelation that idiosyncratic toxicities have rarely or ever been noted for compounds whose daily dose is less than 10 mg [55] unfortunately applies to only a small minority of oncologic agents.

The fundamental ADME properties of absorption, distribution, metabolism and excretion determine blood/plasma exposure of a candidate agent.

A. Absorption

Drug absorption is the process of entry of the drug into the vasculature from the delivery site. Of first concern is the route of delivery. The feasibility of potential routes of delivery are dependent on physicochemical properties of the drug, standard of care, and patient convenience/compliance which is driven by marketing and sometimes the health of the patient (e.g., an unconscious patient is generally administered drugs intravenously). Generally, cytotoxic chemotherapeutics are administered by the intravenous (IV) route because of the necessity to tightly control the exposure, but also often the poor oral bioavailability of many such molecules. Small molecule targeted drugs are generally administered by the oral route, not only because improved safety and physicochemical properties render it feasible but also because commercialization of an oral drug is competitively desirable (e.g., based on the need for daily dosing, chronic usage, or other convenience). Biotechnology-derived peptide and protein drugs must be administered by parenteral routes, such as intralesional/intratumor, subcutaneous, and intramuscular, because of the need to maintain structure, but also the benefit of less frequent administration which allows for better patient compliance.

The intravenous route provides 100% absorption and bioavailability and is the least problematic of routes of administration. When allowed by marketing, patience compliance, pharmacokinetic and biophysical properties (such as solubility in a nonirritant vehicle), the IV route is generally the most desirable. Blood compatibility of both the vehicle and formulated drug should always first be confirmed *ex vivo* in the blood and plasma of the preclinical species and humans. These studies should include osmolality determinations and blood compatibility to rule out risks of hemolysis (red blood cell lysis). Such studies can be conducted *in vitro* with small quantities of different species' blood and drug in vehicle. Although acute tolerability can always be an issue in preclinical toxicity studies, since most are conducted by a slow push of a syringe, these are rarely an issue in clinics where administration occurs slowly via an infusion pump. However, as acute effects are identified preclinically, these must be addressed in registrational applications for first-in-human (FIH) studies or in animal studies with prolonged infusion protocols, so it is best to take steps to avoid this problem altogether.

The oral route of administration is usually more problematic in that it involves passage of drugs through barriers. These barriers include stomach acid, gastroenteric mucus, mucosal epithelial cells, basement membranes, fibrous matrices and capillary endothelia. Drugs can move across cell membranes by simple passive diffusion or carrier-mediated transport (either passive or active). Generally, most drugs penetrate cells by diffusion or passive transport; and as such physicochemical properties are critical for this process. Some physicochemical characteristics that affect absorption through the gastrointestinal tract include solubility, pKa and partition coefficient (log P, lipophilicity). Absorption can also be affected on an individual animal basis by such things as gastric pH and emptying, and intestinal motility.

For small molecule programs seeking oral administration, low aqueous solubility resulting in poor bioavailability is often the biggest challenge. Substructural alterations to a molecule with a very lipophilic core frequently do little to increase bioavailability. More often than not, these modifications also alter the target potency as well. Similarly, heroic efforts on the part of formulations and pharmaceutics (such as milling for nano-sized particles) typically only result in small improvements; however, amorphous forms rather than crystalline forms have recently shown promise [43]. Bioavailability studies with suspensions are necessary to demonstrate proof of concept that solid dosage formulations are feasible for the marketed drug; however, these formulations rarely provide a path forward to generate the supra-efficacious exposures needed for toxicity studies. Pro-drug approaches sometimes prove to be the best alternative to avoiding poor permeability or low biovailability [6], but these approaches can exacerbate problems such as hERG off-target effects by increasing the Cmax to trough ratio.

Bioavailability (F) is a calculated measurement of the extent to which the active drug is absorbed and becomes available at the site of action. Generally, the plasma concentration is considered equivalent to availability at the site of action. Absolute bioavailability is expressed relative to maximum attainable exposure (i.e., by the intravenous route of administration which gives 100% bioavailability):

$$F = \frac{(AUC/dose)oral}{(AUC/dose)_{IV}}$$

where AUC is the area under the drug concentration-time curve for a specific period of time. Dosage levels for the above derivation should be selected to generate relatively similar AUCs, such that similar apparent volumes of distribution and elimination rates are maintained.

B. Distribution

After a drug is absorbed or delivered directly to the blood, it is distributed throughout the body by the systemic circulation. Drug distribution throughout the circulation is rapid, based on the efficiency and effectiveness of the cardiovascular system, and local high concentrations of blood only occur following bolus intravenous injection. Movement of drug from the blood to tissues is relative to concentration in the blood, blood flow, plasma protein binding, penetration and tissue affinity. This movement or translocation of drug molecules from the blood to tissues throughout the body is the more relevant reflection of distribution. The volume of distribution at steady state (Vss) in part reflects how well the drug molecules leave plasma (vascular fluid) and enter interstitial fluid (extravascular extracellular) and intracellular fluid. At some time after dosing, the concentration of drug in the bloodstream reaches equilibrium with the concentration in any given tissue. This is not to imply that the concentrations in these compartments are equal. Although the volume of distribution is relative to circulating concentration, penetration and tissue affinity play significant roles in keeping the drug in the vasculature or concentrating it in specific tissues. Volume of distribution that is equivalent to blood volume indicates no extravascular distribution to tissues. This may be acceptable if the target is circulating in the blood, such as perhaps with immunomodulatory or angiogenic therapy. For small molecules, Vss is generally most dependent on physicochemical properties (charge, lipophilicity, etc.). The distribution of biopharmaceuticals, on the other hand, is usually limited to vascular space and interstitial tissues due to the large size. Some tissues are more difficult to penetrate than others. The brain, for example, has a special barrier called the blood–brain barrier, which maintains an especially clean environment. In certain diseases, however, such as cancer, special barriers are probably compromised to some extent and blood vessels are similarly leaky. Distribution has implications both in efficacy (ability to reach the intended target), metabolism (ability to reach cells that metabolize the drug), and toxicity (ability to reach off-target cells).

Investigation into the distribution of a drug may be necessary when there is a disconnect between expected efficacy (based on *in vitro* or biochemical potency and coverage of that concentration by *in vivo* circulating free fraction) and the actual observed efficacy *in vivo*. Factors that can affect distribution include hemodynamics, protein binding, tissue penetration and affinity. In the case of tumors, poor vascularization can occasionally be problematic. Hemodynamics is rarely a cause for lack of drug distribution, but it is important to recognize that the blood is the main "distributor" of drug throughout the body. Thus, serum protein binding is a common confounding factor that alters the pharmacokinetic profile and biologic activity.

The consequences and implications of protein binding of a drug candidate can differ dramatically for small molecules and biopharmaceutical agents. Small molecule therapeutics that are highly bound to proteins are generally sequestered from pharmacological activity and also clearance. Binding may be irreversible, but far more often it is reversible. Irreversible binding is generally a result of bioactivation of the molecule to a reactive intermediate with covalent binding. Binding of this nature, either to plasma proteins or more frequently to cellular proteins, is usually not of concern regarding sequestering drug from activity, but

191

instead it is of concern from the perspective of toxicological impact. Metabolic bioactivation to a reactive intermediate, such as in the liver, may result in indiscriminate covalent binding. The damage to intracellular proteins and DNA can result in cell dysfunction, cell death or mutagenicity. Binding to blood proteins such as albumin is more frequently reversible and of concern from the perspective of distribution. Hydrogen bonds or van der Waals forces between drugs and plasma proteins effectively hold the drug in the vascular space, because of the impermeability of these large protein-drug complexes to biomembranes. Additionally, even if the target is intravascular, steric hindrance from these types of binding effectively sequesters the drug from activity. High protein binding will not only affect the pharmacokinetic profile and clearance, but also the efficacy and minimum efficacious exposure. Plasma concentrations of small molecule drugs quantified by LC/MS/MS are reported by convention as total drug (i.e., bound and unbound). In most instances, if a drug is 98% protein bound, only 2% of the drug is free for activity (efficacy, toxicity and clearance). Therefore, if biochemical or cellular potency data suggest that efficacy will be achieved at 10 nM and those assays do not contain protein, then the actual efficacious exposure *in vivo* will be 500 nM (corrected for protein binding). Therefore, high protein binding will necessitate larger amounts in circulation than might have been originally expected. Another consequence of protein binding is that the pharmacokinetic profile will generally be prolonged with a longer half-life, for example, due to tight albumin binding affecting drug clearance. This situation makes other factors affecting bioavailability (absorption, metabolism, excretion) all the more important to optimize, because optimization of protein binding is often more difficult to achieve by altering drug structure without affecting pharmacology. Lastly, potential differences in protein binding in preclinical species and humans may account for differences in magnitude of effects.

Albumin is the main component of blood that binds to small molecule drugs. Other circulating proteins that can also bind drugs include alpha acidic glycoprotein, lipoproteins and immunoglobulins. There is wide species variation in these proteins and their ability to bind drugs. Therefore, plasma protein binding should be identified in all relevant animal species and in humans. Plasma protein binding is usually determined by equilibrium dialysis. Drugs can also bind to erythrocytes, mainly to hemoglobin but also potentially to the cell membrane. Blood cell partitioning as reflected by blood-to-plasma concentration in all relevant species should also be investigated. Binding to erythrocytes is not only important from the perspective of affecting distribution, but also because drug—erythrocyte binding can sometimes release haptens resulting in autoimmune hemolysis. Lastly, while direct quantification of drug within a tumor or tissue of interest by bioanalytical methods can confirm distribution, the analytical method needs to be validated for that particular matrix.

There is growing interest in targeted or focused drug distribution to seek to concentrate a drug candidate into a tissue of interest. This strategy concentrates active drug in the target tissue and reduces toxicity in off-target tissues. Two means of targeted delivery have been used successfully, namely, conjugation of a cytotoxic chemotherapeutic agent or radio-isotope to an antibody or to a folate moiety. The rationale of this approach is that conjugation of an active moiety results in an inactive form. The conjugated inactive form circulates rather benignly until interaction with a specific target releases the active parent moiety. This approach has been utilized with antibodies that target tumor-specific antigens and with folate that binds folate receptors (FR) in tumors. For example, antibodies targeted to CD20 on B-cell lymphoid tumors have been conjugated to radio-isotopes (ibritumomab, tositumomab) or a cytotoxic antitumor antibiotic (gentuzumab). The antibodies generally target a tumor-specific antigen with limited expression on normal cells. Upon interaction with the antigen, the active moiety is liberated, resulting in specific delivery of the agent. The absence of the conjugated antibody would allow indiscriminate interaction of the active parent drug with any cell, thereby resulting in widespread off-target effects. Another example is conjugation to folate. Some tumors, such as certain ovarian cancers, overexpress FR. Drugs conjugated to folate, such as BMS-753493, EC145 are concentrated in the cellular milieu of these FR+ tumors, and are also endocytosed by these cells thus creating both extracellular and intracellular high concentrations (Cavallaro, 2006). Another targeted delivery approach involves delivery to the brain. Drug can be concentrated in the endothelium of the blood–brain barrier by utilizing new technology of nano-sized particulate drug carriers differentially adsorbed onto blood proteins, such as apolipoprotein E [41]. As illustrated by these examples, targeted delivery of drugs not only achieves higher local concentrations than would be possible by the free parent drug, but also reduces the potential for adverse effects in other tissues.

Biopharmaceutical agents have a different set of distribution concerns. These agents do not bind to serum proteins extensively, but instead frequently interact with specific endogenous binding proteins that may be involved with transport, clearance, and regulation. A good starting point in understanding the pharmacokinetics and pharmacodynamics of a biopharmaceutical agent is to understand that of the endogenous analog. The distribution and protein interactions of xenobiotic agents will mimic that of the endogenous molecule at least to some extent upon initial dosing. Recombinant cytokine, hormone, and growth factor therapy can be expected to interact with specific binding proteins and/or receptors similar to their endogenous counterpart. These interactions may either potentiate or inhibit activity, but certainly will at least alter the pharmacokinetic profile to some extent. Because of the large size and polarity of therapeutic antibodies, significant extravasation likely does not occur by transcellular diffusion. Recombinant proteins and peptides (cytokines) will diffuse into tissues, but to a lesser extent than small molecule chemical entities. Distribution into tissues is generally thought to occur by convective transport, which involves fluid movement from blood to interstitial spaces driven by hydrostatic pressure, osmotic gradients, pore size, etc. (Flessner et al., 1997). Antibodies and some recombinant proteins enter cells via pinocytosis through a receptor-mediated or fluid-phase endocytosis. Distribution is also affected by the rate of intravenous administration (e.g., bolus versus infusion). The specific interactions that occur should be investigated (or known from the biology of the biopharmaceutical agent) in light of its effect on activity, pharmacokinetics, safety, bioanalytical method and ultimate fate of the complex.

Immunogenicity is a significant factor that will affect the pharmacokinetic profile. Immunogenicity can be a safety concern or a therapeutic strategy, but regardless, the presence of it will generally decrease the half-life and potentially result in significant secondary undesirable effects (discussed in Section IV). Historically, the reduction or elimination of immunogenicity through various techniques has been a major goal in the optimization of antibodies and other recombinant proteins.

C. Metabolism

Drug metabolizing enzymes comprise a system that provides mechanisms for the elimination of xenobiotics and the control of circulating concentrations of endogenous molecules. Generally, small molecule drugs are perceived by the body as undesirable foreign substances and consequently are degraded by metabolism to facilitate their excretion (together referred to as clearance) or are excreted directly when possible, facilitated by drug transporters.

The wide variety of exogenous and endogenous small molecules has necessitated that the metabolic system have great flexibility in place to handle whatever nature or medicinal chemists have to offer. The reactions of drug metabolism have a common goal of generally making products that have greater aqueous solubility than their precursors. Sometimes one reaction is not sufficient to provide the physicochemical characteristics that lead to excretion, and subsequent reactions may be necessary.

Phase I reactions (oxidation, reduction, hydrolysis, hydration) generally provide functional polar groups to molecules for the facilitation of excretion, further metabolism with Phase I reactions or conjugation with Phase II reactions (glucuronidation, sulfation, methylation, acetylation, glutathione conjugation or amino acid conjugation). Oxidation reactions comprise the largest class of Phase I reactions. These occur predominantly at carbon, nitrogen and sulfur and are catalyzed by the cytochrome P-450 linked system. Frequently, if a molecule is metabolized to contain a functional group by Phase I reaction, it can readily be excreted either through the urine or bile. Molecules that are not readily excreted will likely undergo further Phase I metabolism or Phase II conjugation. Phase II reactions require either a high energy cofactor (uridine-diphosphoglucuronic acid, phosphoadenosinephosphosulfate, adenosylmethionine, acetyl coenzyme A, glutathione, or amino acids), or a chemically reactive substrate.

From the perspective of drug discovery of small molecule chemical entities, the medicinal chemist in drug discovery plays a critical role in designing molecules with appropriate metabolic characteristics. It is generally the goal of the chemist to design a drug that is metabolically stable enough to convey efficacy, but not so stable that progressive accumulation would occur with daily dosing. A standard battery of metabolic profiling is recommended. Metabolic stability is routinely evaluated *in vitro* as an indication of clearance from the various relevant species. In the battery of assays that follows, relevant species should include humans and all preclinical species used for efficacy and potentially used for safety studies (rat, mouse, dog, and monkey). While data from human microsomes and hepatocytes is the most relevant, it is important to identify species differences in order to drive a development plan or to make conclusions on species-specific *in vivo* effects. First-tier metabolic stability testing usually involves incubations of compounds in liver microsomes fortified with NADPH as in indication of oxidative metabolism. Samples are analyzed by LC/MS/MS for rate of disappearance of administered compound. This can be done in parallel or sequence with hepatocyte cultures. While microsomes are limited to Phase I reactions, hepatocytes contain a more complete spectrum of Phase II reactions. Second tier metabolic reaction phenotyping uses specific CYP isoforms with cDNA-expressed human CYP enzymes. The list of isoforms should include, but not be limited to: CYP1A1, CYP1A2, CYP1B1, CYP2B6, CYP2A6, CYP2C8, CYP2C9, CYP2C18, CYP2C19, CYP2D6, CYP2E, CYP3A4, and CYP3A5. These assays are used to predict specific major, potentially polymorphic, elimination pathways, and thereby identify the potential for drug–drug interactions. In any of these studies or in subsequent more specific studies, LC/UV/MS can be used to specifically identify metabolite structures. Specific structures can be useful in identifying potentially active metabolites.

The drug discovery profiling panel should also include assays that alert for inhibition or induction of drug metabolizing enzymes. Inhibition and induction of enzymes may have significant implications not only on the metabolic profile of the molecule of interest but also on the metabolism of other drugs that may be co-administered to the patient. Cancer therapeutic regimens usually involve co-administration of multiple drugs either as therapy or palliative treatment, or these patients may be prescribed drugs for other unrelated diseases typical of a certain age or group population. It is extremely important to recognize potential drug–drug interactions, not only for other drugs that are known to be administered for that specific disease, but also for drugs that are typical for the target population of people. CYP inhibition testing can be performed with recombinant human CYPs or in pooled human liver microsomes utilizing specific probe reactions (e.g., testosterone 6β-hydroxylation by CYP 3A4) along with positive controls (e.g., ketoconazole, which is a reversible inhibitor of CYP 3A4). Enzyme inhibition can be further characterized as reversible/irreversible and with regard to dependence on time and/or metabolism.

Metabolic induction will affect a drug's own metabolism, and it can also raise the potential for drug–drug interaction. Because cytochrome P450 3A4 is a major drug metabolizing pathway, induction assays are usually focused on this enzyme. High throughput screening assays usually involve PXR transactivation which correlates with CYP 3A4 induction. More refined assays measure the metabolism of probe reactions (such as midazolam) after incubation with the test article. Alternately, assays may measure mRNA induction of specific CYPs by RT-PCR in human hepatocyte cultures.

D. Excretion

The main routes of excretion for small molecule chemical entities are through the liver and kidney. The biliary system is generally responsible for excretion of larger and less polar molecules. While the hepatic acinus or lobule is the physiologic unit for liver metabolism, the biliary system is the physiologic unit for excretion.

In the urinary system, the nephron is the physiologic unit responsible for excretion. The glomerulus of the nephron is the filtration unit and the combination of high hydrostatic pressure and 8 nm interendothelial pores results in the filtration of molecules with molecular weight greater than 69 kDa. This includes drugs bound to plasma proteins that are too large to be passed through the glomerular filter. Aside from the size and charge of the molecule, the biggest factor affecting the characteristic of the filtrate is glomerular filtration rate or blood flow. Downstream in the nephron, the tubular epithelium is responsible for passive and active reabsorption and excretion of molecules, water and ions and is also active in xenobiotic metabolism. Active secretion of xenobiotics (especially organic acid and bases) may take place in the proximal convoluted tubule through specialized transporters. These transporters act on relevant molecules regardless of protein binding. Additionally, the proximal tubular epithelial cells contain many of the drug-metabolizing enzymes found in the liver. The presence of these enzymes facilitates secretion into the nephron lumen and excretion into the urine, or perhaps into general metabolism for release back into the circulation for further metabolism. In general, small molecules and polar molecules are excreted preferentially through the nephron.

E. Clearance of biopharmaceutical agents

For biopharmaceutical agents, the metabolic processes above generally do not occur and the profiling paradigm in discovery is correspondingly impacted. The ultimate disposition of these agents varies widely according to type of drug and the interventional pathway. As pointed out above, the first consideration is that the molecular make-up of the drug will dictate the disposition to some extent. For instance, proteins and peptides will undergo catabolic processing similar to endogenous or dietary proteins. Peptidases will eventually cleave the molecule to amino acids, which will be recycled. Alternatively, these drugs may interact with endogenous molecules as part of their mechanism of activity, making them unavailable for proteolysis. Antibodies undergo this process, not as they relate to the target, but as they relate to normal turnover of endogenous antibodies. The vast majority of antibodies are eliminated by catabolism at sites that are in rapid equilibrium with the blood plasma. Antibody clearance is generally thought to be associated with receptor- and non-receptor-mediated endocytosis targeted toward the Fc portion of the immunoglobulin. The pharmacokinetics of monoclonal antibodies generated against cellular targets can frequently be impacted by another set of unique factors, specifically, by antigen and antibody concentrations, potentially resulting in nonlinear pharmacokinetics [34]. High antigen concentration relative to antibody could result in a short half-life, due to rapid clearance through antigen—antibody processing, while low antigen concentration relative to antibody could result in a prolonged half-life. Immunogenicity will potentially increase clearance and thereby impact pharmacokinetics, as indicated above.

Although the available options for manipulating a biopharmaceutical agent to optimize its pharmacokinetics are not as numerous as those for small molecule agents, some strategies have proven useful, such as alterations focused around the Fc portion by pegylation [30,39] and glycosylation [17], or by a change in the immunoglobulin subtype. Pegylation and

195

glycosylation have been used for both antibodies and recombinant proteins. Pegylation, which involves the attachment of polyethylene glycol chains, can be used to increase half-life, decrease clearance, lower toxicity, increase stability and solubility, and decrease immunogenicity, but it is accompanied by an increased viscosity that may be problematic for higher dose compounds. Glycosylation, which can be useful for enhancing protein stability, is limited in utility by the fact that it is an endogenous process that is often very species specific. In human cells, altering glycosylation from the norm occasionally increases both activity and immunogenicity, which is generally undesirable.

F. Determination of compound pharmacokinetics: *in vivo* pharmacokinetic studies

Compound pharmacokinetics is determined by collecting blood samples at various times after compound administration and determining plasma concentrations as a function of time. The number of time points and the specific time points used for blood collection are based on the maximum volume that can be collected from the species (as allowed by the Institutional Animal Care and Use Committee) as well as the expected pharmacokinetics. For rodents, composite study designs are generally utilized. In this study design, all data points are not collected from all animals, but the collection of all time points from the various animals gives a composite pharmacokinetic profile. For instance, one-half of the group has collection points at three time points and the other half has collection points at three other time points. This intuitively requires twice the number of animals and the full pharmacokinetic profile cannot be defined for one animal, but the composite is robust because the rodents are genetically inbred and metabolically similar. Collection time points are generally clustered most frequently during the absorption phase of the exposure and bracket the time of maximum plasma concentration (Tmax). For a small molecule chemical entity, this is typically from 0.5 to 4 hours, and for a biologic this can be days to weeks. Good estimations of Tmax will result in more accurate derivations of maximum circulating levels (Cmax). Initially, plasma is analyzed for quantification of the active pharmaceutical agent. For small molecules, liquid chromatography with mass spectrometry (LC/MS/MS) is used and for biologic agents, antibody-based immunoassays (reviewed in [14]) are used. The method or assay should be sensitive enough to detect the molecule at therapeutic levels and at least 10-fold below this level. The method or assay should also be validated to be useful for the specific matrix (plasma, serum, etc.) and species from which the sample is obtained. Sample handling is important when stability of the compound is in question. If little is known about the *ex vivo* stability (storage shelf life), samples should be analyzed as soon as possible after collection. For regulatory purposes, stability must be formally evaluated per GLP protocol and should include collected samples that are processed with aliquots stored for analysis after specific ambient and accelerated storage durations. Stabilizing agents may need to be added to samples. This is especially important for prodrugs which can be metabolized to active drug (parent) *ex vivo*, during sample handling and storage by plasma enzymes. One common stabilizing agent is sodium fluoride. All pro-drugs should be analyzed for the pro-drug and the active (parent) with sufficiently sensitive methods.

Study design for small molecule chemical entities generally includes an intravenous route and a route that is clinically relevant. For this discussion, the oral route will be used as the clinically relevant administration. For nonrodents the same animals are used for both portions of the study (cross-over design), so if a certain animal shows significant variation from the other animals, this can be identified and potentially considered as inter-animal variability. In general, the range of starting doses should be 10 mg/kg PO and 5 mg/kg IV for rats and mice and 5 mg/kg PO and 1 mg/kg IV for dogs and monkeys. Because food effects can impact absorption, overnight fasting of animals is recommended.

Data that are generated by pharmacokinetic studies typically include:

$$\text{AUC}_{(0-Xh)} = \text{Area under the curve for specific time}$$
$$0 \text{ to } X \text{ hours expressed as } \mu M \cdot hr \text{ or } ng \cdot hr/mL$$
$$\text{Cmax} = \text{maximum concentration}$$
$$\text{Tmax} = \text{time of maximum concentration}$$
$$t\tfrac{1}{2} = \text{half-life}$$
$$\text{Vss} = \text{volume of distribution at steady state}$$
$$\text{CL}_{tot} = \text{total clearance in mL/min/kg}$$
$$F = \text{bioavailability of the oral route with respect to intravenous dose as a percent}$$

Concentration measurements are total concentration and include both free and bound fractions.

The pharmacokinetic profile should also be evaluated for linearity with respect to dose. Exposure levels (AUC) should increase in a relatively linear manner with increasing dose, especially over the dose range of efficacy. At some point, increasing oral doses will eventually result in less than proportional or no increase in exposure. This is extremely problematic in the range of efficacy, but can also adversely impact development if exposure limits prohibit the demonstration of toxicity. Nonlinear pharmacokinetics can result from a variety of causes. All too frequently, maximal exposure is attained due to solubility constraints. Sometimes, administration of suspensions may result in, at best, marginal increases in exposure. If there is no promise for identifying chemotypes with better solubility, suspensions of nano-sized particles may offer better exposure; however, these techniques are heroic and frequently prohibitive in terms of cost of goods and risk to carry forward into clinical trials. Some promising strategies to overcome solubility limitations include dosing of spray-dried dispersions which result in amorphous (noncrystalline) formulations, and supersaturated solutions.

Other causes of nonlinear kinetics include: saturation of metabolic pathways or plasma protein binding resulting in higher than expected exposure with increasing dose. These situations offer the converse concern, specifically, escalation of dosing above a certain point will result in significant toxicity at a steeper curve. In other words, above a certain dose, exposure increases at a faster rate, resulting in more difficult titration of dose with respect to control of toxicity. Nonlinear pharmacokinetics are displayed more commonly by biopharmaceutical agents. While inter-animal variability is generally partially responsible for nonlinear kinetics, the exact cause is difficult to completely understand (reviewed in [34,35,36,52]).

Following structural optimization and demonstration of appropriate pharmacologic potency, *in vivo* pharmacokinetic studies are conducted. These data are an important part of predicting human pharmacokinetics. Plasma exposure data is also collected from studies of efficacy (rodent xenograft studies) and toxicity, where the profiling is termed toxicokinetics. The plasma exposure data in efficacy studies is used to determine exposures associated with efficacy, as well as to define suboptimal exposures, and those associated with toxicity. Human dose projection assumes that the exposure (generally as AUC_{0-24h}) which results in efficacy in a rodent xenograft study will equal the therapeutic exposure in patients. The exposure associated with the minimal efficacious dose in rodent xenograft studies is used to rank different compounds and is a frequent starting point for a variety of human dosing projections. In general, the plasma drug available for interacting with the pharmacologic target is the unbound fraction. Highly protein bound drugs (e.g., 99%) frequently require much greater total bound and unbound exposures than drugs for which plasma protein binding is less (e.g., 90%). In general, the best accuracy in projecting activities across species, such as from rat to man, will use as reference the unbound fraction of drug since protein binding may differ substantially between species (as noted above).

Although widely used, the minimum efficacious AUC achieved in animal models for the desired pharmacologic endpoint is a simplistic and potentially flawed tool for comparing drugs. In cancer studies, the most robust parameter used in drawing correlations between efficacy and drug exposure is a minimal time for inhibition of target (receptor or otherwise) during the dosing period (e.g., 16 hr of 100% inhibition within a 24-hr period) that is sufficient to elicit tumor shrinkage or regression. Given the practical difficulty in obtaining such information, the simple AUC is the most relevant because this data considers concentration and time. In some circumstances, Cmax may be more relevant, as in the case where there is very tight binding of the drug candidate to the target, where time is not as critical a factor, or in some cases where there may be a threshold concentration-based toxicity, such as cardiac ion channel liabilities.

G. Optimization of pharmacokinetics in drug discovery

Pharmacokinetic properties are frequently optimized by manipulating the physicochemical properties of a compound understood to be limiting for formulation or permeability. Plasma quantification by bioassay is generally not performed for inactive, nonreplicating vaccines such as protein/peptide-based vaccines or inactive whole cell vaccines. In general, techniques for favorably altering the pharmacokinetics of biotechnology-derived proteins involve either alteration of the structure of the protein to include some non-native aspects that are not readily recognized and cleared through normal means, or conjugation to an agent such as PEG or an Fc fragment that extends clearance and half-life. These modifications are most often driven by the desire to increase exposure time (such as half-life), thereby allowing longer treatment intervals or lower dosages.

III. CONCEPTS IN TOXICOLOGY

198

Toxicology in the pharmaceutical industry begins with hazard identification and should culminate with meaningful risk assessment. Early hazard identification in drug discovery generally utilizes high throughput predictive models (with low concordance to true hazard), while hazard identification in drug development utilizes much more rigorous, robust and validated models. The different strategies are reflective of the different purposes. The purpose of toxicology in drug discovery is to enhance lead candidate selection and/or optimization, while the purpose of toxicology in drug development is to enable first-in-human trials or more extensive later clinical trials. In general, hazards—the undesirable effects of drugs—can be due to either target-related pharmacology or off-target mechanisms.

A. Target validation

Validation of the therapeutic target should take place with similar timing and thoroughness whether from the standpoint of toxicology or disease intervention. This validation can be proactive and performed early in the discovery process, as part of coordinated procedures to document and understand potential undesirable effects, or it can be performed as a reactionary measure over concerns of a particular safety issue that arises later in the discovery/development process. The former is obviously more desirable.

The vast majority of new molecular targets for oncology will most likely play some functional role in normal tissues, as well as in neoplastic cells. Significant toxicities for many marketed drugs usually can be attributed to direct intervention at the drug target (i.e., an on-target liability). For instance, in chronic myelogenous leukemia patients treated with imatinib (a bcr-abl inhibitor), defects in cell-mediated immunity have been reported which may result from a blockade of c-ABL signaling in normal T lymphocytes [58]. In patients treated with epidermal growth factor receptor (EGFR) inhibitors, such as erlotinib [18,31] or cetuximab [42,49], skin rash is the dose-limiting toxicity but it is a useful side effect since it correlates well with efficacy. Lastly, vascular endothelial growth factor (VEGF) inhibitors, such as bevacizumab [20,50] have been associated with peripheral hypertension, which may be also attributed to target-related effects.

Fortunately, target-related effects for oncology drugs can be generally tolerated (relative to the benefit of the drug) or controlled by other pharmaceutical agents. Indeed, as noted above for EGFR inhibitors, some effects can even be exploited as surrogate biomarkers, not only for molecular activity but also for overall efficacy [15,18,31,42,46]. If these effects correlate sufficiently with molecular activity, they can provide very early, inexpensive confirmation of target interaction, reassuring stakeholders of eventual clinical benefit in lieu of tumor response (which might not be fully assessed for years). Thus, targeted-related toxicology can sometimes be framed in the context of strategies to benefit the design or acceleration of a clinical trial. Of course, consideration should be given to abrogate target-related effects, to avoid potential serious side effects. For example, approaches to reduce untoward target-related effects can include pharmaceutical intervention by alternate pathways other than the targeted pathway, dosing regimens that will allow some degree of recovery from a side effect, or targeted delivery of the drug (e.g., by conjugation or pro-drug approaches [8], etc.). For example, the hypertension associated with VEGF inhibition can be managed easily with well-accepted anti-hypertensive drugs [13,20]. Such activities should be proactively investigated in preclinical studies, not only to confirm methods to abrogate any toxic effects but also demonstrate the absence of their potential deleterious effects on efficacy, anticipating actions that could accelerate progression through clinical trials.

Unlike the examples above, validation of novel targets is fraught with a paucity of information to support an indication of the potential for target-related adverse changes. There are a number of ways to model the effects of a specific interaction with a target, and the specific shortcomings for each should be understood at the outset or the results should be interpreted relative to the patient population, kinetics and target affinity of the drug, etc. [1,33,45]. While it is rare that a specific target would not be pursued in oncology based only on preclinical studies suggesting an incompatible or adverse event profile, an early in-depth understanding of the target is nonetheless critical to enable an appropriate strategy for future safety assessment.

B. Off-target effects

The vast majority of work in general toxicology studies of targeted small molecule drugs is related to off-target effects. While biotechnology-derived products are highly selective for their targets, small molecule drugs are usually fraught with at least some degree of non-selectivity, which can result in safety liabilities. For example, small molecule kinase inhibitors are almost exclusively engineered to bind to the ATP binding site of the target kinase, even though the structural features of this site are highly conserved, to the extent that it is counterintuitive that selectivity could even be possible [54]. Improvements in macromolecular crystallography have dramatically improved the art of pharmaceutical chemistry by providing indispensible tools to drive structure-activity investigations [12,19,37]. Through these efforts, many small molecule drugs with exquisite molecular potency for the specific target have been successfully engineered. Unfortunately, it still remains somewhat difficult to engineer a small molecule that selectively interacts only with the intended target (for kinase targets as well as others).

Given their importance in oncology, kinase targets represent a special case of interest. Given the growing sophistication in molecular understanding, most kinase inhibitors developed today would be referred to as multikinase inhibitors. Such inhibitors can be rationally designed to potentially confer improved efficacy and reduced chances of relapse due to acquired resistance (similar to the current polypharmacy being practiced for cancer adjuvant therapy). Nonetheless, these agents frequently present a difficult toxicology challenge. While efficacy will always drive drug discovery for oncology, the potential benefits must always be considered relative to the risks (see below). Thus, preclinical toxicology characterizations should be interpreted in light of the compound's selectivity profile and, as such, it is advantageous to proactively generate this data.

The benefit of a clear understanding of the mechanisms of small molecule off-target liabilities resides in both a higher probability of successfully managing the toxicity and also development of a superior backup drug candidate. If a particular liability can be attributed to a specific molecular entity, then the pharmaceutical chemistry will have sufficient direction to reduce that activity by substructural modifications so as to achieve better selectivity. Unfortunately, more often than not the mechanism of a toxicity is not understood. For this reason, backup candidate efforts are often left to empirical queries based on intuition and *in vivo* toxicity studies.

C. Toxicology in preclinical drug development (clinical trial enabling)

First-in-human (FIH) clinical trial applications are supported by a battery of preclinical studies. In general, these studies provide data that argues the clinical candidate will deliver some clinical benefit to patients that can be administered safely. For FIH studies that utilize cancer patients with late-stage cancer or advanced disease, the investigator should be guided by published regulatory guidance, especially the Note for Guidance on Nonclinical Evaluation for Anticancer Pharmaceuticals [28]. With the aim of the guidance to "facilitate and accelerate the development of anticancer pharmaceuticals and to protect patients from unnecessary adverse effects," this treatise discusses the appropriate design of nonclinical studies for anticancer drugs in the context of risk:benefit to this population. Starting from this unique perspective, the nonclinical package is rather abbreviated (compared to noncancer FIH trials).

FIH studies with anticancer agents using normal healthy volunteers require the much more rigorous safety profiling typical of nononcologic indications [27]. Because this study population does not receive any clinical benefit of the drug, the studies are broader in scope and the drug must be demonstrated to be much safer than it would otherwise need to be for study in cancer patients.

The single most important consideration of the design of *in vivo* toxicity testing to support FIH studies is the selection of the starting dose. This selection is based on the need to identify either a no-effect level (NOEL) if the FIH study is in normal healthy volunteers, or a severely toxic dose to 10% of the animals (STD10) if the FIH study is in cancer patients. These parameters define the starting dose for each specific clinical trial. In the case of a normal healthy volunteer study, the starting dose is scaled off the NOEL, so as to insure the safety of clinical volunteers. In the case of an FIH trial with cancer patients, a starting dose that is closer to that expected to confer clinical benefit to patients is more reasonable; therefore, in this case the starting dose is scaled off the STD10 for the drug candidate.

In addition to determining the starting dose, the other main objective of preclinical toxicology in support of a FIH study in cancer patients is to understand the complete toxicology profile (target-related and off-target). This profile includes information on the reversibility of all drug-related changes. To gain a robust understanding of all the *in vivo* effects of drugs, repeat-dose toxicity studies are usually conducted in two species, including one rodent and one nonrodent species. There are exceptions to this rule for biologics, where a drug is strongly anticipated to interact with the target of a single species. These studies should not only have the typical end-point parameters assessed, but should also include the special assessment of any suspected target-related effects, even when these are nonroutine evaluations. Such evaluations provide the basis for parameters that should be considered for monitoring in future clinical trials. When toxicities are identified that cannot be specifically monitored in clinical trials, due to the lack of a validated biomarker, more robust clinical monitoring should be proposed, or unvalidated biomarkers of toxicity should be investigated. Preclinical data might also suggest that certain populations of patients be excluded from studies, because they pose a higher risk of developing an adverse event. For example, patients to exclude from clinical trials may have concurrent diseases or suboptimal organ functioning that might predispose or exacerbate a toxicity [48].

D. Toxicities of special concern

In general, toxicities of special concern that are always included in FIH application for nononcologic indications, such as safety pharmacology, reproductive toxicology, genotoxicity, carcinogenicity, immunotoxicity, phototoxicity, etc. are of lesser concern for FIH studies in cancer patients.

Safety pharmacology assessments of organ function are usually built in to general toxicology studies, instead of dedicated studies, unless of course there is reason for the sensitivity of a dedicated, more robust study, based on the target or expected effects. Of all safety pharmacology endpoints, drug-related effects on cardiovascular physiology (electrical conduction and hemodynamics) have become increasingly responsible for drug withdrawals from the market (e.g., terfenadine and cisapride) [23,25,57]. Thus, dedicated studies that use conscious telemetrized animals should be considered to deliver the most robust cardiovascular safety assessment. That stated, FIH studies in cancer patients may not need this degree of sensitivity, so assessments of cardiovascular physiology for oncology drug candidates can be conducted as part of a general toxicology study using surface leads and other monitoring devices [28].

Cardiovascular electrical conduction and/or hemodynamic liabilities are mainly a concern for small molecules, rather than biological-derived products. In most cases, the mechanism of action for suspected cardiovascular liabilities involves drug interactions with ion channel currents. While small molecule drug interactions with sodium, potassium, calcium, and chloride channels are well documented, both as intended on-target and off-target effects (see [51] for review), the most problematic channel is the delayed rectifier potassium current IKr, which is expressed by the hERG gene (human ether-a-go-go-related gene). Drug interactions with IKr have generated the most attention as a cause for drug withdrawal from the market, due to an association with fatal tachyarrhythmias (specifically, torsades de pointes) that is always associated with prolonged QT interval on electrocardiograms [2,5]. To screen against interactions with ion channels (and various specific subsets of them), the encoding genes of these channels have been cloned and stably expressed in cell lines for use in ion conductance assays. These assays fairly accurately predict *in vivo* activity and are effectively used in candidate optimization [51].

Clinical trials for late stage or advanced cancers do not require studies of genotoxicity [26]. However, such studies may be useful to differentiate drug candidates within a given class. Nontargeted cytotoxic drugs are generally considered to be genotoxic, but the relative hazard is not considered excessive for the patient population. In contrast, genotoxicity testing is required for FIH studies in normal healthy volunteers. Moreover, it is generally conducted for purposes of environmental exposure safety, for risk evaluation during the drug synthesis process. With increasingly safer cancer therapeutics that are administered more chronically, positive genotoxicity will likely become a recognized liability that negatively impacts physician choice and market share. Thus, an evaluation of the genotoxicity for new therapeutic candidates in oncology should be considered for small molecules. Such testing is considered irrelevant for biotechnology-derived drugs [56], with the possible exception of non-native components in these products that could conceivably intercalate into native macromolecules, like DNA.

The standard battery of genotoxicity assays includes reverse mutation studies (e.g., Ames test in *Salmonella typhimurium* and *E. coli*), *in vitro* assessments of chromosomal damage in mammalian cells (e.g., micronucleus assays or Chinese hamster ovary (CHO) cells), and *in vivo* assessments of chromosomal damage (e.g., micronucleus assay) [26].

E. Biotechnology-derived agents

Biotechnology-derived and biopharmaceutical agents have different safety concerns compared to small molecules. Because the array of products is so vast, the ability to construct specific guidelines that are meaningful to the development of each product is exceedingly difficult, although such efforts have been made by both governmental regulatory agencies [56] and independent authors [4;48]. Since the field continues to rapidly expand, with ever-increasingly novel and creative drug candidates, any guidance with detailed specifics will no doubt have to be frequently updated.

Safety assessment of biotechnology-derived agents should always be designed based on rational scientific decisions that consider the type of agent and expected biology. To this end, tactics that are utilized are increasingly creative.

Selection of the appropriate specie(s) of animal for preclinical safety assessment is probably the most important question. The selection of specie(s) must be decided based upon a number of parameters and their divergence from humans, such as expression level and distribution of the target, affinity of the drug candidate to the target, pharmacokinetics and known or expected effector or downstream functions. Knowledge of the similarities or differences from humans will also be invaluable for interpretation of elicited drug-related effects. Sometimes, for specific types of *in vivo* studies, drug affinity to the endogenous target is nonexistent in preclinical species, so creation of a surrogate drug candidate with affinity to the native target in animals is warranted. This is mainly for the purpose of assessing pharmacodynamic effects of targets that are extremely novel, offering little existing information.

Immunogenicity remains a major safety concern for any biotechnology-derived agent, with implications for both preclinical and clinical development. Novel biologic platforms and various creative modifications to endogenous proteins heighten immunogenicity concerns in particular when optimizing pharmacokinetics, etc. In preclinical development, immunogenicity will obviously impact species selection, pharmacokinetics and pharmacodynamics, study design and endpoints, dosage selection, and so forth. Some immunogenicity in preclinical species might be tolerated, such that adequate safety assessment can still be achieved by creative study design and other novel approaches. Anti-drug antibodies (ADA) can be clearing, neutralizing, neutral or any combination of the above. All of these can individually impact species selection for toxicity testing and give compelling evidence to exclude usage. The presence of clearing antibodies that reduces drug exposure may necessitate adjustment of doses upwards to "dose through" a level of anti-drug antibodies so as to achieve adequate exposures while maintaining the integrity of a toxicity study. Although neutralizing antibodies reduce the pharmacodynamic effect without affecting drug clearance, strategies for resolving these issues are generally similar. There are, however, additional concerns for ADA, such as potential cross-reactivity with other endogenous proteins, immune complex formation with deposit in tissues, and especially anaphylaxis or potent injection site reactions. Making this issue even more complicated, anaphylaxis may be difficult to distinguish from the cytokine release reaction [21]. Nevertheless, immunogenicity in preclinical species should not necessarily impact the viability of a drug candidate, given experience showing that the extrapolation of immunogenicity from animals to humans is poor for all species.

F. Vaccines

In general, the safety issues for cancer vaccines usually relate to the antibody- or T-cell-mediated immune response or the adjuvants/immunomodulators rather than the vaccine antigen itself [3]. These issues are the same whether the vaccine is comprised of inactive protein subunits or a cell therapy. Used in combination with vaccines, traditional adjuvants (where there is considerable knowledge concerning safety) usually do not have to be independently evaluated for safety. However, novel synthetic adjuvants, as well as excipients or preservatives, will likely have to be tested in traditional safety evaluations required by FDA for new chemical entities (NCEs).

Protein-based or biotechnology-derived adjuvants, such as cytokines, should be evaluated for safety based on their mechanism of action similar to these types of products for any indication. One main focus of these tests is to identify the implications of supra-physiologic responses. The selection of a specific animal model should be made based on criteria outlined in Section IIIE, but the selection should also consider the potential expression on normal cells of the tumor-associated antigen that will be targeted. Along with traditional endpoints in safety testing, special attention should be focused on characterizing the nature and duration of the immune response to the vaccine. Regulatory agencies increasingly require studies that demonstrate protection against challenge, not merely studies demonstrating that the vaccine administration results in immunogenicity [10].

IV. CLINICAL CONCERNS FOR PHARMACOLOGY AND SAFETY

The composite nonclinical pharmacology and toxicology package generated in discovery and development supports the justification and enablement of FIH clinical trials. The timely regulatory approval and efficient conduct and progression of a clinical development program of drug candidates is impacted by clear definition of potential efficacy (or benefit to study participants), safe starting dose, and identification of potential toxicities. A discussion of preclinical models for efficacy is beyond the scope of this chapter.

The derivation of a safe starting dose for FIH studies is a main focus for preclinical toxicity testing, and the necessary components are dependent on the clinical plan, specifically the use of normal healthy volunteers or cancer patients with late-stage or advanced disease (see Section IIIC). The most common parameter for overall safety is the therapeutic index (or window), which is a ratio of the exposure at which some relevant toxicity is manifest and the exposure that confers some empirical parameter of efficacy. While preclinical therapeutic indices frequently do not translate into actual clinical safety parameters, because oncology clinicians tend to dose up to a maximum tolerated dose, so as to achieve maximal potential efficacy, a high preclinical therapeutic index does, however, give a degree of confidence that clinical doses can be sufficiently escalated beyond what would have been considered minimal efficacious dose, especially in the event the tumor response is not achieved. Cancer immunotherapies, however, have the promise to potentially be safer than typical targeted-therapeutics and demonstrate a true clinical therapeutic window, and would likely be administered to a maximum pharmacologic activity level, instead of a maximum tolerated dose.

Beyond hazard identification in preclinical toxicology for the purposes of derivation of a safe starting dose, a robust risk assessment for particular significant preclinical toxicities should be performed. This gives additional perspective on the specific toxicities with regard to relevance to humans and it guides the interpretation of the seriousness of the toxicities for human risk. Alternatively, without perspective on toxicities, robust biomarkers should be investigated.

The standard of care for cancer is frequently combination therapy and many FIH studies include arms that investigate combination of the drug candidate with various marketed drugs. While demonstration of clinical benefit from that combination is imperative [28], toxicological concerns can frequently be addressed by a logical paper justification for not doing combination preclinical toxicity studies. This should include not only primary toxicological concerns regarding the potential for synergistic toxicities based on mechanism or target organ, but also pharmacokinetic drug–drug interactions based on metabolizing enzyme inhibitions or inductions. For two therapeutic agents that have common target organs for toxicity, the potential combination effect is generally considered to be additive if the two drug targets are different, such as with the cardiotoxicity associated with the combination of trastuzumab and anthracyclines [47]. The risk of clinical drug—drug interaction is not adequately modeled by preclinical testing [22,32], but it does alert the clinical investigator to proactively include drug—drug interaction studies in the clinical program.

V. CONCLUSIONS

The key elements to initiating and developing clinical plans to test therapeutic oncologics depend on carefully conducted nonclinical pharmacokinetic, pharmacological, and toxicologic studies and on an integrated understanding of the potential liabilities. Within the broader discipline of toxicology, knowledge from traditional cytotoxics and current accumulating practical concepts from targeted cytostatic agents increasingly demonstrate that the approach to the safety assessment for novel cytostatic and biopharmaceutical agents should be based more on scientific soundness than traditional approaches.

References

[1] Bolon B. Genetically engineered animals in drug discovery and development: a maturing resource for toxicologic research. Basic Clin Pharmacol Toxicol 2004;95:154—61.

[2] Brell JM. Prolonged QTc interval in cancer therapeutic drug development: defining arrhythmic risk in malignancy. Prog Cardiovasc Dis 2010;53:164—72.

[3] Brennan FR, Dougan G. Non-clinical safety evaluation of novel vaccines and adjuvants: new products, new strategies. Vaccine 2005;23:3210—22.

[4] Brennan RF, Morton LD, Spindeldreher S, Kiessling A, Altenspach R, Hey A, et al. Safety and immunotoxicity assessment of immunomodulatory monoclonal antibodies. MAbs 2010;2:233—55.

[5] Briasoulis A, Agarwal V, Pierce WJ. QT prolongation and torsade de pointes induced by fluoroquinolones: infrequent side effects from commonly used medications. Cardiology 2011;120:103—10.

[6] Cai ZW, Zhang Y, Borzilleri RM, Qian L, Barbosa S, Wei D, et al. Discovery of brivanib alaninate ((S)-((R)-1-(4-(4-fluoro-2-methyl-1H-indol-5- yloxy)-5-methylpyrrolo[2,1-f][1,2,4]triazin-6-yloxy)propan-2yl) 2-aminopropanoate), a novel prodrug of dual vascular endothelial growth factor receptor-2 and fibroblast growth factor receptor-1 kinase inhibitor (BMS-540215). J Med Chem 2008;51:1976—80.

[7] Campbell FL, Le Blanc JC. Peptide and protein drug analysis by MS: challenges and opportunities from the discovery environment. Bioanalysis 2011;3:645—57.

[8] Cavallara G, Mariano L, Salmoso S, Caliceti P, Gaetano G. Folate-mediated targeting of polymeric conjugates of gemcitabine. Int J Pharm 2006;307:258—69.

[9] Center for Drug Evaluation and Research (CDER) and US Department of Health and Human Services. Food and Drug Administration (FDA), Bioanalytical Method Validation: Guidance for the Industry. Rockville: Maryland; 2001. CDER and FDA.

[10] Center for Proprietary Medicinal Products (CPMP). Notes for Guidance on Preclinical Pharmacological and Toxicological Testing of Vaccines. European Medicines Agency (EMEA) 1997. CPMP/SWP/465/95.

[11] Chen ZA, Tiwari AK. Multidrug resistance proteins (MRPs/ABCCs) in cancer chemotherapy and genetic diseases. FEBS J 2011;278:3226—45.

[12] Cherry M, Williams DH. Recent kinase and kinase inhibitor X-ray structures: mechanisms of inhibition and selectivity insights. Curr Med Chem 2004;11:663—73.

[13] Copur MS, Obermiller A. An algorithm for the management of hypertension in the setting of vascular endothelial growth factor signaling inhibition. Clin Colorectal Cancer 2011;10:151—6.

[14] DeSilva B, Smith W, Weiner R, Kelley M, Smolec J, Lee B, et al. Recommendations for the bioanalytical method validation of ligand-binding assays to support pharmacokinetic assessments of macromolecules. Pharm Res 2003;22:1425—31.

[15] De Stefano A, Carlomagno C, Pepe S, Bianco R, De Placido S. Bevacizumab-related arterial hypertension as a predictive marker in metastatic colorectal cancer patients. Cancer Chemother Pharmacol 2011;68:1207—13.

[16] Evans G. A handbook of Bioanalysis and Drug Metabolism. Boca Raton, Florida: CRC Press; 2004.

[17] Drickamer K, Taylor ME. Evolving views of protein glycosylation. Trends Biochem Sci 1998;23:321—4.

[18] Faehling M, Eckert R, Kuom S, Kamp T, Stoiber KM, Schumann C. Benefit of erlotinib in patients with non-small-cell lung cancer is related to smoking status, gender, skin rash and radiological response but not to histology and treatment line. Oncology 2010;78:249—58.

[19] Fedorov O, Sundstrom M, Marsden B, Knapp S. Insights for the development of specific kinase inhibitors by targeted structural genomics. Drug Discov Today 2007;12:365–72.

[20] Gorgon MS, Cunningham D. Managing patients treated with bevacizumab combination therapy. Oncology 2005;69(Suppl. 3):25–33.

[21] Greenberger PA. Drug allergy. J Allergy Clin Immunol 2006;117(Suppl. 2):S464–70.

[22] Grime KH, Bird J, Ferguson D, Riley RJ. Mechanism-based inhibition of cytochrome P-450 enzymes: an evaluation of early decision making in vitro approaches and drug-drug interaction prediction methods. Eur J Pharm Sci 2009;36:175–91.

[23] Hennessy S, Leonard CE, Newcomb C, Kimmel SE, Bilker WB. Cisapride and ventricular arrhythmia. Br J Clin Pharmacol 2008;66:375–85.

[24] Ho RJY, Gibaldi M. Biotechnology and Biopharmaceuticals: Transferring Proteins and Genes into Drugs. Hoboken, New Jersey: John Wiley & Sons; 2003.

[25] Hondeghem LM, Dugardin K, Hoffmann P, Dumotier B, De Clerck F. Drug-induced QTC prolongation dangerously underestimates proarrhythmic potential: lessons from terfenadine. J Cardiovasc Pharmacol 2011;57:589–607.

[26] International Conference on Harmonization (ICH). Genotoxicity: a standard battery of genotoxicity testing of pharmaceuticals. ICH Topic S2B. European Medicines Agency (EMEA) 1997. EMEA/CHMP/ICH/174/95.

[27] International Conference on Harmonization (ICH). Non-clinical safety studies for the conduct of human clinical trials and marketing authorization of pharmaceuticals. ICH Topic M3. European Medicines Agency (EMEA) 2009. EMEA/CHMP/ICH/286/95.

[28] International Conference on Harmonization (ICH). Nonclinical evaluation for anticancer pharmaceuticals. ICH Topic S9. European Medicines Agency (EMEA) 2008. EMEA/CHMP/ICH/646107/2008.

[29] Kola I. The state of innovation in drug development. Clin Pharmacol Ther 2008;83:227–30.

[30] Kozlowski A, Charles SA, Harris JM. Development of pegylated interferons for the treatment of chronic hepatitis C. BioDrugs 2001;15:419–29.

[31] Lee Y, Shim HS, Park MS, Kim JH, Ha SJ, Kim SH, et al. High EGFR gene copy number and skin rash as predictive markers for EGFR tyrosine kinase inhibitors in patients with advanced squamous cell lung carcinoma. Clin Cancer Res 2012;18:1760–8.

[32] Li AP, Maurel P, Gomez-Lechon MJ, Cheng LC, Jurima-Romet M. Preclinical evaluation of drug-drug-interaction potential: present status of the application of primary human hepatocytes in the evaluation of cytochrome P450 induction. Chem Biol Interact 1997;6:5–16.

[33] Lin JH. Application and limitation of genetically modified mouse models in drug discovery and development. Curr Drug Metab 2008;9:419–38.

[34] Lobo ED, Hansen RJ, Balthasar JP. Antibody pharmacokinetics and pharmacodynamics. J Pharmaceut Sci 2004;93:2645–68.

[35] Mahmood I, Green MD, Fisher JE. Selection of the first-time dose in humans: comparison of different approaches based on interspecies scaling of clearance. J Clin Pharmacol 2003;43:692–7.

[36] Mahmood I. Interspecies scaling of protein drugs: prediction of clearance from animals to humans. J Pharmaceut Sci 2003;93:177–85.

[37] McInnes C, Fischer PM. Strategies for the design of potent and selective kinase inhibitors. Curr Pharm Des 2005;11:1845–63.

[38] Meibohm B, editor. Pharmacokinetics and Pharmacology of Biotech Drugs: Principles and Case Studies in Drug Development. Weinheim, Germany: Wiley-VCH; 2007.

[39] Molineux G. Pegylation: engineering improved biopharmaceutical for oncology. Pharmacotherapy 2004;8(Pt 2):3S–8S.

[40] Morgan P, Van Der Graaf P, Arrowsmith J, Feltner D, Drummond K, Wegner C, et al. Can the flow of medicines be improved? Fundamental pharmacokinetic and pharmacological principles toward improving Phase II survival. Drug Disc Today 2012;17:419–24.

[41] Muller RH, Keck CM. Drug delivery to the brain—realization by novel drug carriers. J Nanosci Nanotechnol 2004;4:471–83.

[42] Orditura M, De Vita F, Galizia G, Lieto E, Vecchione L, Vitiello F, et al. Correlation between efficacy and skin rash occurrence following treatment with the epidermal growth factor receptor inhibitor cetuximab: a single institution retrospective analysis. Oncol Rep 2009;21:1023–8.

[43] Qiu Y, Chen Y, Zhang GGZ. Developing Solid Oral Dosage Forms. Burlington, Massachusetts: Academic Press; 2009.

[44] Rowland M, Tozer T. Clinical Pharmacokinetics: Concepts and Applications. Manchester, UK: Lippincott, Williams, & Wilkins; 1995.

[45] Sacca R, Engle SJ, Qin W, Stock JL, McNeish JD. Genetically engineered mouse models in drug discovery research. Methods Mol Biol 2010;602:37–54.

205

[46] Scartozzi M, Galizia E, Chiorrini S, Giampieri R, Berardi R, Pierantoni C, et al. Arterial hypertension correlates with clinical outcome in colorectal cancer patients treated with first-line bevacizumab. Ann Oncol 2009;20:227–30.

[47] Slamon DJ, Leyland-Jones B, Shak S, Fuchs H, Paton V, Bajamonde A, et al. Use of chemotherapy plus a monoclonal antibody against HER2 for metastatic breast cancer that overexpresses HER2. New Engl J Med 2001;344:783–92.

[48] Snodin DJ, Ryle PR. Understanding and applying regulatory guidance on the nonclinical development of biotechnology-derived pharmaceuticals. Biodrugs 2006;20:25–52.

[49] Su X, Lacouture ME, Jia Y, Wu S. Risk of high-grade skin rash in cancer patients treated with cetuximab—an antibody against epidermal growth factor receptor: systemic review and meta-analysis. Oncology 2009;77:124–33.

[50] Syringos KN, Karapanangiotou E, Boura P, Manegold C, Harrington K. Bevacizumab-induced hypertension: pathogenesis and management. BioDrugs 2011;25:159–69.

[51] Szentandrassy N, Nagy D, Ruzsnavsky F, Harmati G, Banyasz T, Magyar J, et al. Powerful technique to test selectivity of agents acting on cardiac ion channels: the action potential voltage clamp. Curr Med Chem 2011;18:3737–56.

[52] Tang L, Persky AM, Hochhaus G, Meibohm B. Pharmacokinetic aspects of biotechnology products. J Pharmaceut Sci 2004;93:2184–204.

[53] Tiwari AK, Sodani K, Dai CL, Ashby CR, Chen ZS. Revisiting the ABCs of multidrug resistance in cancer chemotherapy. Curr Pharm Biotechnol 2011;12:570–94.

[54] Toledo LM, Lydon NB, Elbaum D. The structure-based design of ATP-site directed protein kinase inhibitors. Curr Med Chem 1999;6:775–805.

[55] Uetrecht J. Immune-mediated adverse drug reactions. Chem Res Toxicol 2009;22:24–34.

[56] Food and Drug Administration. Guidance for Industry: S6 preclinical safety evaluation of biotechnology-derived pharmaceuticals. U.S. Department of Health and Human Services; 1997.

[57] Woosley RL, Chen Y, Freiman JP, Gillis RA. Mechanism of the cardiotoxic actions of terfenadine. JAMA 1993;269:1532–6.

[58] Zipfel PA, Zhang W, Quiroz M, Pendergast AM. Requirement for Abl kinases in T cell receptor signaling. Curr Biol 2004;14:1222–31.

CHAPTER 14

Monoclonal Antibodies for Cancer Therapy and Prevention: Paradigm Studies in Targeting the *neu*/ERBB2/HER2 Oncoprotein

Hongtao Zhang[1], Arabinda Samanta[1], Yasuhiro Nagai[1], Hiromichi Tsuchiya[1], Takuya Ohtani[1], Zheng Cai[1], Zhiqiang Zhu[1], Jing Liu[2], Mark I. Greene[1]

[1]Department of Pathology and Lab Medicine, University of Pennsylvania Perelman School of Medicine, Philadelphia, PA USA

[2]School of Life Sciences, University of Science and Technology of China, Hefei, Anhui China

207

I. INTRODUCTION

A. Original identification of the *neu* oncogene (also known as HER2/ERBB2)

One of the origins of targeted therapy of oncoproteins was built upon early studies of the transforming properties of the middle T antigen of polyoma (PymT antigen) [1]. Subsequent studies by Lathe and colleagues showed that recombinant vaccinia viruses expressing PymT could act as vaccines to immunize against tumors [2]. Molecular studies of polyoma middle T antigen which began in 1978 evolved in 1980 into a collaboration with Robert Weinberg's laboratory at MIT to study nonviral oncogenes in solid tumors. In our laboratory, novel immunization approaches were developed to create monoclonal antibodies against cells transformed by the *neu* oncogene [3].

As reported initially in 1984, our initial work [4] was concerned with isolation of a high molecular weight fragment containing a putative oncogene obtained from B104 neuroblastoma, which arose in the offspring of female rats treated during gestation with the carcinogen ethylnitrosourea. It was from this source that the *neu* oncogene (termed *ERBB2* or more commonly *HER2* in humans) was isolated and named for its original tissue of origin (neuroblastoma). The *neu* oncogene was shown to be responsible for the malignant phenotype of the B104 tumor cells. Immortalized mouse fibroblasts (NIH3T3 cells) were transformed with iterative transfections of high molecular weight neuroblastoma DNA containing the oncogene. Transformants were selected for foci formation, a phenotypic property reflecting neoplastic transformation. The transfection process was repeated several times to enrich the high molecular weight transforming DNA. An NIH3T3 subline transfected with the enriched *neu* oncogene was developed and named B104-1-1, which led to progressive tumors when injected subcutaneously into mice. This isolation method was characteristic of similar approaches taken in the 1980s to discover many oncogenes.

The monoclonal antibodies we developed identified a phosphorylated 185 kDa protein product of the *neu* oncogene (p185) in the neuroblastoma cell lysates [4]. This antibody (7.16.4) bound p185[erbB2/neu] orthologs in both rat and human cells [5] (Real and Greene, unpublished data). Flow cytometry showed that the p185[neu] protein existed on the cell surface, an unexpected finding at the time [3]. Strikingly, cDNA sequencing revealed subsequently that the *neu* oncogene was highly homologous to the Epidermal Growth Factor Receptor (EGFR). Thus, p185[erbB2/neu] belonged to the ErbB family of receptor tyrosine kinases. By comparing the sequence of the proto-oncogene expressed by normal tissues, the *neu* oncogene was found to differ from the normal proto-oncogene by a single base mutation that substituted a valine residue for a glutamic acid residue, adding a negative charge into the transmembrane region of the receptor.

B. The human ortholog of *neu*

Soon after the rat *neu* gene and protein were defined, several laboratories identified the human ortholog *ERBB2*, or *HER2*, and showed it was expressed in human neural tissues developmentally and in adenocarcinomas of the stomach, intestine and lung [6–10]. Other groups found that the *ERBB2/HER2/neu* was overexpressed in breast cancers including Stuart Aaronson's and Martin Cline's groups [11–15]. The Nusse and Slamon laboratories then showed that amplification of this gene correlated to some degree with disease [12,14]. The reasons for the dominant development of adenocarcinomas became obvious through our laboratory's developmental studies in the mouse, which identified expression of the *neu* gene mainly in secretory epithelial cells [16].

C. Expression of *erbB2/neu* in mammalian development

Murine *erbB2/neu* is expressed in secretory epithelial cells of every germ layer. Our studies found that the *erbB2/neu* gene and protein were expressed widely in neural and connective tissues of rats during a short embryonic time frame, but there was persistent expression in specific sites in the skin, lung, intestine, breast and brain into adulthood. Lymphoid tissues did not express *erbB2/neu* or its product at any time point [16]. Therefore normal secretory epithelial cells of all mammals express *erbB2/neu* at detectable levels into adulthood. This pattern of expression of the *erbB2/neu* gene and proteins in the adult led us to examine hyperplasia and early tumor lesions in breast, lung and other tumor sites to determine the pathways of transformation. The development of the transformed cell occurs in distinct stages in which transforming genes promote activation of distinct pathways needed to overcome cellular processes to maintain normal phenotype and which induce mechanisms to limit cell death.

D. ErbB family receptors function as dimers

Our laboratory first showed that the p185[erbB2/neu] oncoprotein assembled as a dimeric complex, with the thermodynamic drive to a dimeric form the consequence of the negatively charged glutamic acid mutation in the transmembrane region. This dimeric complex possessed tyrosine kinase activity that was solely responsible for transformation [17]. We also examined how the p185[c-neu] proto-oncogenic receptors become activated at a biochemical level. The proto-oncogenic receptors could form kinase active homodimers at high expression levels. However, cellular expression of modest amounts of both proto-oncogenic *c-neu* and EGFR enabled the malignant transformation of the cells, while transfecting either of them alone did not [18]. NIH3T3 cells expressing moderate amounts of rat proto-oncogenic p185 receptor or

EGFR alone did not develop progressively growing tumors when implanted into athymic mice, but elevating the levels of p185[erbB2/neu] was sufficient to cause complete transformation.

p185[erbB2/neu] and EGFR proteins formed heterodimers in the absence of EGF ligand but more readily in the presence of ligands [19]. The heterodimer was far more active than EGFR homodimers and could readily transform NIH3T3 cells. These studies suggest that heterodimer formation influences functional properties and may contribute to the diversification of their signaling properties. Two other members of the ErbB receptor family, ErbB3 and ErbB4, were later identified by other laboratories. These receptors also form homomeric and heteromeric associations [20], but p185[erbB2/neu] is the preferred heterodimerization partner for all members [19,21]. Initial molecular modeling [22] and crystallographic studies [23] elucidated some features of the structural basis for dimer formation, although this remains incompletely resolved. Once these receptors are dimerized and become active, they promote proliferative and phenotype-altering cascades by activating the MAP kinase (MAPK) and phosphatidylinositol kinase (PI3K/AKT) pathways. We found that the PI3K/AKT pathway was the most relevant for the transformed phenotype, whereas the MAP kinase pathway was more relevant to proliferative processes. p185[erbB2/neu] activation induces uncontrolled proliferation and disrupts normal epithelial organization in epithelial cells [24]. Aranda and colleagues discovered that p185[erbB2/neu] activation disrupted membrane polarity in kidney epithelial cells [25], leading to the formation of hyper-proliferative, multi-acinar structures with filled lumens in certain mammary epithelial cells. Collectively, these studies identified a dynamic evolution of cellular properties with the acquisition of functionally active homomeric or heteromeric ErbB kinases.

II. *ERBB2/HER2/NEU* IN HUMAN DISEASE

A. *ERBB2/HER2/NEU* expression patterns in early lesions of the breast

Increased p185[erbB2/neu] levels can be readily detected in human breast tissues that show the earliest signs of transformation but are not completely transformed. *erbB2* is expressed at low levels in benign breast lesions. Our work found that atypical ductal hyperplasia was associated with increased p185[erbB2/neu] expression in 10% of samples studied [26]. Pechoux and colleagues have performed perhaps the most detailed analysis of premalignant lesions of the breast, finding significant staining of p185[erbB2/neu] in hyperplastic lesions and proliferating mastosis [27]. Pechoux suggested that these changes occur in a pattern corresponding to malignant phenotypic changes. Other studies have confirmed their findings with (for the most part) similar observations [12,27–31]. In some studies increased levels of p185[erbB2/neu] expression were less obvious in terminal duct lobular units (TDLUs) [32,33], but as mentioned were noted in atypical ductal hyperplasia (ADH) [26,32–34].

p185[erbB2/neu] is more consistently over-expressed in high-grade ductal carcinoma *in situ* (DCIS), particularly of the comedo type, and in high-grade inflammatory breast cancer (IBC) [12,32,35–39]. Further increased expression of p185[erbB2/neu] may thus correspond to events that occur at the transition from hyperplasia to DCIS [26,32,34,38,40,41,27]. These studies support the notion of a gradual increase in expression corresponding to the evolution of a more malignant phenotype.

B. Allelic changes

Incompletely transformed lesions possess some transformed properties, such as a loss of growth control, but they lack the ability to invade and metastasize. Additional allelic or adaptive biological changes may cause some lesions to remain stable and others to progress to invasive tumors. Patients with benign breast lesions with low levels of *ERBB2* gene amplification [42], or elevated levels of p53 protein [30], have an increased relative risk of developing breast cancer. Similarly, women with benign breast biopsies demonstrating both *ERBB2* amplification and a proliferative phenotype may have an increased risk for subsequent

209

invasive breast cancer [42]. While activation of *ERBB2* by overexpression seems to be the principal transformation mechanism in human tumors, and overexpression alone has the same effect as the oncogenic mutations found in the rat gene [43], there is also a correlation between *ERBB2* amplification/overexpression and aneuploidy in clinical breast cancer samples [44−49]. *ERBB2* amplification/overexpression and aneuploidy may represent associated consequences of abnormal p53 or other allelic dysfunctions [50].

Alterations of *ras* are also commonly seen in aneuploid cells where *ERBB2* is overexpressed [51] and the presence of both *ERBB2* and *RAS* abnormalities defines a subset of aggressive high-grade tumors [50]. However, in addition to allelic changes, adaptive processes are also important. It should be noted that while *ERRB2* overexpression is correlated with gene amplification [38,52−54], approximately 20% of malignant tissues, including breast cancers, overexpress *ERBB2* while maintaining diploid copies of the gene [53,55−57]. Therefore allelic changes of *ERBB2* lead to the development and progression of premalignant breast disease with induced proliferation. Subsequent allelic changes contributed by alterations of the *p53* or *RAS* or other genes including mutation or loss of *PTEN* [58] may then lead to the further acquisition of the transformed phenotypic features.

C. Adaptive changes

Adaptive changes in the microenvironment may contribute significantly in the evolution of incompletely transformed cells to fully malignant cells. For example, elevation of interleukin-6 (IL-6) has emerged as an important stromal signal that augments transitions from incomplete to more completely transformed cells in murine models of breast cancer using *neu* as well as in human breast cancer cell [59]. Rokavec and colleagues studied the effects of microRNA-200c and its suppression by IL-6, which was critical for tumorigenesis in the MMTV-*neu* mouse model of breast cancer. IL-6 deficient mice crossed to MMTV-*neu* animals were studied and found to accumulate changes in their breasts consisting of incompletely transformed cells. Notably, loss of IL-6 limited *neu* tumorigenesis. This finding highlighted the concept that inflammatory processes may be important to promote phenotypic transitions stimulated by oncogenic activation of *ERRB2* from early to premalignant cells and later to completely transformed cells.

Furthering this concept, Tan and colleagues found that the proinflammatory RANK ligand (RANKL) secreted by tumor-infiltrating T cells recruited into the tumor microenvironment by cancer-associated fibroblasts promoted the *in vivo* dissemination of *erbB2/neu*-transformed breast cells [60]. RANK signaling in mammary carcinoma cells that overexpress the proto-oncogenic *c-neu* was influential for pulmonary metastasis. RANKL-producing T cells were mainly FoxP3+ and found in close proximity to stromal cells expressing smooth muscle actin in mouse and human breast cancers. Thus, the T-cell dependence of pulmonary metastasis could be induced by exogenous RANKL. In this manner, adaptive processes in the tumor microenvironment contribute to promoting the development of early oncogenic lesions and also inciting movement of transformed cells to distal metastatic sites.

Adaptive and allelic changes may also help drive epithelial to mesenchymal transition (EMT), which is increasingly accepted as a key step in malignant conversion. This phenotypic change represents an evolutionarily conserved developmental process, and it may also represent an important feature of immune escape during malignant progression. Epithelial cells normally display polarity as characterized by well-developed tight junctions and adherens junctions. Mesenchymal cells are not polarized in the same manner and they possess multifunctional roles in tissue repair and wound healing that in the context of oncogenic lesions can engender malignant character. During development, certain differentiated polarized epithelial cells change morphologically to a mesenchymal phenotype. In this transition, epithelial cells develop less adherent cell−cell junctions and polarity, easing the acquisition of migratory properties characteristic of mesenchymal cells that are typically more motile than epithelial cells. In this manner, cancer cells may obtain the capacity to migrate and invade through processes similar to those conferred during development by EMT. Inducers of EMT, such as transforming growth factors (TGF) and Wnt, cause changes of gene expression profiles that lead to upregulation of several transcriptional repressors that coordinately engage EMT during development, including Snail [61], Slug [62], Zeb1 [63], Zeb2/SIP1 [64] and the bHLH transcription factors Twist [65] and E47 [66]. Of note, many of these proteins suppress the transcription and expression of the adherens junction protein E-cadherin, which is a pivotal suppressor of the mesenchymal phenotype.

As a nodal event in the induction of EMT, the reduction in E-cadherin leads to adherens junction breakdown, loss of polarity, and induction of mesenchymal characteristics. Cancer cells that have undergone EMT may acquire the capacity to more readily detach from substratum and survive dissemination away from the primary breast lesion into the blood or lymph vessels. In the mouse, *erbB2/neu* appears to confer this capacity. Upon orthotopic transplant to wild-type mice, mammary glands from *neu* transgenic mice develop disseminated tumor cells and micrometastases in the bone marrow and lungs, and the number of disseminated cancer cells and their karyotypic abnormalities are comparable for both small and large tumors [67]. This process of $p185^{erbB2/neu}$ overexpression and subsequent loss of E-cadherin contributes to mammary tumor dissemination and metastasis [68−70]. One can envision a scenario beginning with atypical ductal hyperplasia, in which elevated levels of $p185^{erbB2/neu}$ promotes processes associated with early dissemination. Extending these results, Podsypanina and colleagues have shown that untransformed mouse mammary cells engineered to express inducible oncogenic transgenes can bypass transformation at the primary site when introduced directly into the systemic circulation of a mouse, illustrating direct formation of metastatic pulmonary lesions upon oncogene induction [71].

This experiment suggests that previously untransformed mammary cells may establish residence in the periphery once they have entered the bloodstream and at distal sites assume malignant growth upon oncogene activation. Indeed, disease-free periods can last from several years up to as long as 20−25 years in breast cancer patients after treatment of the primary disease [72]. Consistent with recent studies [59,60], concepts of immunoediting described in Chapter 7 demonstrate that the microenvironment can favor change in premalignant cell colonies at equilibrium that exist in a latent, dormant phenotype to the malignant manifestations characteristic of escape in disseminated tumor cells [73].

III. ERBB2/NEU AS A THERAPEUTIC TARGET
A. Targeted therapy of established tumors and reversal of the malignant phenotype

We [74,75] discovered that downregulation of cell surface $p185^{neu}$ blocks downstream signaling and reverses the malignant phenotype of *neu*-transformed cells. This discovery was made possible with the use of purified monoclonal antibodies (mAb 7.16.4, IgG2a) capable of cross-linking the $p185^{neu}$ receptor on *neu*-transfected NIH3T3 cells. Antibody treatment led to rapid $p185^{neu}$ downregulation and an increased rate of degradation of the receptor. Overall, this effect reversed the malignant phenotype both *in vitro* and *in vivo*. Anti-$p185^{neu}$ also exerted cytostatic effects on anchorage-independent growth of the *neu*-transformed cell lines. The presence of the antibody was required for conversion in phenotype, because when the antibody was removed, the malignant properties of the cell lines became evident again.

In this manner, our laboratory was the first to show that disabling a protein complex needed for transformation could reverse the malignant properties of tumor cells *in vitro* and *in vivo*. In a murine xenograft model, anti-$p185^{neu}$ monoclonal antibodies inhibited the outgrowth of *neu* transformed cells but tumor growth resumed once antibody treatment ceased. These studies established the principles of targeted therapy and heralded the clinical development of receptor-blocking mAb with overlapping target specificity by commercial entities.

For ERBB2/HER2/NEU-targeted therapy, this new age for solid tumor treatment opened with FDA approval of the targeted mAb trastuzumab (Herceptin®; Genentech Inc., South San Francisco, CA). Trastuzumab has proven to be an effective treatment for the ERBB2/NEU overexpressing metastatic breast cancer, with response rates ranging from 17—35% in the clinic [76]. Currently trastuzumab is being used to treat both breast and stomach cancer patients in regimens that include other traditional chemotherapeutic agents. Trastuzumab is also used in the treatment of operable p185$^{erbB2/neu}$-positive breast cancer in the adjuvant setting [77]. The preclinical studies we conducted anticipated this development and also explain how targeted therapy functions to prevent the emergence of tumors. Additionally, our work found that the mAb 7.16.4 competes with antibodies such as trastuzumab, binding to the same or over-lapping epitopes in the fourth subdomain of the p185$^{erbB2/neu}$ ectodomain that is targeted by the approved commercial agent [5].

B. Downregulation of p185$^{erbB2/neu}$ through internalization and a unique mAb that supports the tetramer model

In addition to dimeric kinase complexes, EGFR and human p185$^{erbB2/neu}$ form homo- and heterotetramers. EGF-induced phosphorylation of the tetramers was less than that of the dimers, indicating that the tetrameric receptor complexes have impaired signaling activity. We also noted that kinase disabled tetramers physiologically assemble at the cell surface naturally. The early appearance of kinase-disabled forms suggests that signal attenuation begins before receptor internalization. Therefore, tetramers likely exist as part of the normal dynamic process of receptor formation, signal attenuation, trafficking and function [78].

Our work established p185$^{erbB2/neu}$ receptor downregulation as a mechanistic principle for how targeted mAb therapy functions [75]. We extended these studies biochemically [78,79] to show that mAb exposure disabled receptor dimerization and promoted formation of kinase inactive receptor tetramers. Thus, mAbs that effectively targeted these receptor kinases appeared to act by promoting tetramer assembly and shifting the equilibrium from active dimeric complexes to impaired tetrameric complexes. This concept was extended by molecular structure studies, by crystallizing a new targeting monoclonal antibody chA21 as a complex with the ERBB2 receptor ectodomain [80] (see Figure 14.1 which also shows the position of two anti-p185$^{erbB2/neu}$ mAbs, pertuzumab and trastuzumab, on the ectodomain).

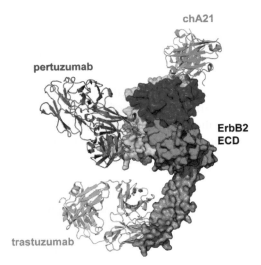

FIGURE 14.1

mAb binding sites on p185$^{erbB2/neu}$. chA21 scFv (*green*) binds to the back and top of the p185$^{erbB2/neu}$ ECD domain, which is distinct to trastuzumab (*cyan*) and pertuzumab (*magenta*). ECD subdomain1: *blue*; subdomain 2: *yellow*; subdomain 3: *red*; subdomain 4: *orange*. The model was constructed using structures in PDB: 1IVO (EGFR), 1N8Z (p185$^{erbB2/neu}$); 3H3B (chA21 scFv).

On the basis of these structural studies, we proposed a model in which chA21 crosslinks two $p185^{erbB2/neu}$ molecules on separate homo- or heterodimers to form a large oligomer on the cell surface [80]. This atomic level model supported the biochemistry, revealing a mechanism by which the targeted mAbs could drive $p185^{erbB2/neu}$ receptors into pathways for internalization or degradation, first as inactive dimeric receptor complexes that could organize into inactive hypophosphorylated tetrameric complexes. In this manner, the mAbs recapitulated normal physiological processes of receptor clearance that occur naturally during receptor downregulation [78].

These studies were a direct extension of a large body of work dealing with targeted therapy of $p185^{erbB2/neu}$ leading to downregulation of the kinase functions and reversal of phenotype. Further studies that deconstructed the binding of mAb to smaller structural elements of the mAb, such as the Fv subdomain or the 3rd CDR, has led to what is now a fairly complete atomic understanding of signals needed to induce downregulation [81,82]. Additionally, this work has revealed that the Fc region of the mAb is dispensable for biological activity, although important for the half-life of the binding elements.

C. Targeted therapies using two intact monoclonals binding distinct epitopes of $p185^{erbB2/neu}$

Perhaps the most convincing feature of mAb-targeted therapy was observed when two antibodies reactive with distinct epitopes of $p185^{erbB2/neu}$ were employed using *in vivo* mouse models of *erbB2/neu*-driven tumor growth [83]. In those studies, the two mAbs synergized to cure 9/17 mice of lethal $p185^{erbB2/neu}$-induced tumors. This strong finding was confirmed with the mAb trastuzumab and pertuzumab approved for human use.

Further studies of how two therapeutic mAb could synergize to produce cures deepened understanding of how receptor kinase activity was disabled in multimer complexes. Specifically, these studies evaluated the effects of the anti-$p185^{c-neu}$ antibody 7.16.4 and a scFv fragment of this mAb. Of note, 7.16.4 binds to rat $p185^{c-neu}$ and to a lesser extent ($\sim$70 times less) to human $p185^{HER2/neu}$. While MAb 7.16.4 could induce disabled tetrameric complexes of human erbB receptors, it is notable that the ScFv of 7.16.4 fragment was unable to induce tetramers to any significant extent [78]. The conclusion of these studies was that formation of ERBB receptor tetramers driven by mAb was a dominant event in impeding receptor kinase activity in complexes.

As noted above, we had demonstrated previously that mixtures of antibodies reactive with two distinct regions on the $p185^{erbB2/neu}$ molecule resulted in synergistic antitumor effects *in vivo* [83]. However, the contribution of tetramerization in cells treated with two mAb had not been studied. To address this issue, we treated SKBR3 human breast cancer cells with cocktails of monoclonal antibodies targeting the ectodomain of $p185^{erbB2/neu}$ receptors (e.g., 4D5 and 2C4, or 4D5 and 1E1), which synergize to enhance formation of phosphorylation-impaired tetrameric receptor complexes [78]. Notably, the tetramers formed after only a brief 15-min treatment with mAb cocktails had significantly diminished kinase activity. Together, the results obtained from these studies strongly rationalized the use of dual antibody therapies for human disease.

D. Targeted therapies arrest the development of preliminary hyperplasia and prevent the progression of premalignant lesions

Since *ERBB2/NEU* plays such an important role in early metastasis, targeted therapies may be critical to prevent premalignant lesions from developing into breast cancer. We found that $p185^{erbB2/neu}$ targeted antibodies not only inhibited growth of already established tumors, but also prevented tumor development in transgenic mice overexpressing the activated *neu* oncogene in mammary epithelial cells [84]. We employed the Jolicoeur stochastic MMTV-*neu*

213

mouse model of breast cancer, in which the rat oncogenic *neu* gene is expressed under the control of the MMTV promoter [85]. Tumors arise stochastically in this model approximately 30 weeks after oncogene induction. The tumor phenotype is completely penetrant with all females developing tumors. In this model, only 50% of the animals treated with the mAb 7.16.4 (10 μg twice weekly) developed breast tumors during the observation period of 70 weeks [84]. When the two distributions of time to tumor development were compared using a log-rank test, the 7.16.4 treatment group clearly displayed longer tumor-free survival than the control group (median time to breast tumors as follows: control, 44 weeks; 7.16.4 treatment, 64.1 weeks, log-rank chi-square (1 df) =13.17, p ≤ 0.001) (personal communication, J. D. Goldberg, New York University School of Medicine).

E. Epithelial hyperplasia can be inhibited by downmodulation of p185 molecules at early times in tumorigenesis, before acquisition of a fully malignant phenotype

One fundamentally interesting cellular event we observed in our studies of the transgenic MMTV-*neu* murine breast tumors was the absence of ductal epithelial hyperplasia in mAb-treated mice. Examining the breast tissue of female mice prior to tumor development, we found that tissues from breasts of these transgenic mice expressed basal levels of p185 kinase and that treated mice had greatly reduced kinase signals. This observation suggested that oncoproteins targeting mAb could act at very early times to inhibit kinase-active receptor function. Very recent studies have suggested a contributory role for erbB3-erbB2 heteromers in some aspects of early breast tumor development [86], where targeting mAb may seem likely to act.

F. Can we prevent invasion of early stage lesions which begin to express active kinase dimers of p185?

In considering possible applications of receptor targeting mAb to prevent progression, we have also evaluated effects on the spread of *erbB2/neu* tumors in the MMTV-*neu* mouse model. We carefully analyzed the normal tissues of 20–25 week old mice to determine whether partially transformed cells may leave the tumor at early stages. The results indicated that $p185^{erbB/neu}$ kinase expressing incompletely transformed tumor cells can leave the breast and move to other locations. Moreover, we found evidence of kinase active $p185^{erbB2/neu}$ derived from the rat *neu* transgene in this model in the spleen, kidney and brain of untreated animals.

In MMTV-*neu* mice that are tumor-free at this early stage, administration of high doses of the anti-$p185^{erbB2/neu}$ mAb 7.16.4 reduced levels of detectable kinase-active $p185^{erbB2/neu}$ compared to controls at 24 weeks of age [84], indicating that breast cells manifest an increased ErbB2/neu receptor kinase activity at times before conversion to frank malignancy. In preliminary studies of the spread of premaligant cells that we had observed, we detected the transgenic rat $p185^{erbB2/neu}$ signal in brain, even in the antibody-treated animals. This observation suggested that the blood–brain barrier prevented the mAb from eradicating partially transformed cells in the brain where they could localize before frank tumor development occurred in the breast tissue of the MMTV-*neu* mice. Thus, mAb treatment as a strategy before early stage tumor cells can depart their site of residence (e.g., as dormant occult cells in immune equilibrium) may comprise the most effective preventive therapy. We also obtained some evidence of $p185^{erbB2/neu}$ activity in mouse splenic cells. The spleen lacks afferent lymphatics, so this observation was important in establishing for the first time that circulating premalignant cells can leave the breast and enter the spleen via the bloodstream. However, in this site, unlike the brain, the access of the targeting mAb would conceivably be effective before or after cell deposition at that site.

Targeted therapy with anti-$p185^{erbB2/neu}$ may prevent emergence of early tumor foci, thereby preventing the rise of metastatic clones. While we found that targeted mAb therapy could prevent or delay the development of primary tumors in the MMTV-*neu* model, we also noted that in female mice where tumors were not prevented completely by mAb treatment only a single small breast tumor would arise, compared to untreated animals where multiple large breast tumors invariably arose. These findings were confirmed and extended by Finkle and colleagues at Genentech using trastuzumab [87]. Additional supportive obserrvations regarding the spread of p185 positive cells were obtained by other groups. In the BALB-NeuT mouse model, where the *neu* transgene is mutated and as a result more active than in the MMTV-*neu* model, Husemann and colleagues reported that p185$^{erbB2/neu}$-positive cells with the cytokeratin marker became detectable in bone marrow as early as 4–9 weeks of age [67]. At this time, only atypical ductal hyperplasia was observed in the mammary gland. Thus, studies in *neu* transgenic mice provide insights into the pattern of cell spreading, at early times before frank primary breast tumor development, and further establish that mAb treatment can downregulate p185$^{erbB2/neu}$ and spread of dormant mutant cells even at times when fully malignant tumors are not present, an idea proposed in our original study of mAb-based cancer prevention [84]. We believe these results remain directly relevant to preventative therapy of early spread of partially or incompletely transformed cells in humans. Consistent with this assertion, a study examining circulating cells derived from benign breast lesions showed that premalignant cells could be identified in individuals with atypical ductal/lobular hyperplasia (ADH or ALH) [88]. At such times, when rank malignancy is not yet present, the administration of receptor targeting mAb might conceivably offer a powerful tool to prevent or reduce the risk of later disease.

G. Interferon and ADCC in mediating the effects of p185$^{erbB/neu}$ mAb therapy

Recent work by several groups [89,90] has defined a role for CD8$^+$ interferon-γ (IFN-γ) secreting cells and natural killer immune cells (NK cells) as contributory elements in 7.16.4 mAb therapy of *neu*-induced murine tumors. Some of these studies were focused on immune elements that cooperated with targeted therapy in a *neu*-tumor implant model, similar to our early work [74]. CD8$^+$ T cells were found to facilitate some aspects of tumor growth reduction mediated by anti-p185$^{erbB2/neu}$ and an important role for IFN-γ was identified in that process. The effects of IFN-γ are complex, as this important cytokine is known to dampen *erbB2/neu* expression at the transcriptional level [91] while increasing the levels of TGFα and EGFR expression [92,93]. IFN-γ elaborated by CD8+ cells may blunt early tumor spread, but later may also contribute to resistance to targeted therapies by formation of heteromers of EGFR with other kinases. If so, IFN-γ may phenotypically alter some aspect of *neu*-transformed cell growth collaboratively with 7.16.4 mAb, specifically with respect to downregulation of p185$^{erbB2/neu}$ during tumorigenesis. In any case, on the basis of the existing information, there seems to be a logical rationale to combine receptor targeting mAbs with IFN-γ to accentuate the antitumor effects of the receptor targeting mAb on ERBB2/NEU-driven breast cancer cell growth.

Our laboratory had suggested a minor role for ADCC [83,89] whereas Clynes found more evidence for ADCC activity with some tumors [94]. However, the mouse model used by Clynes may be less compelling than initially considered [95]. Stagg has now suggested that ADCC lytic activity is not important in the implant model [90] and that the role of NK cells that had been implicated may be to leverage full activation of IFN-γ secretion, by elaborating Type I interferons after MYD88 dependent Toll receptor activation. Therefore, the extent of the role for NK cell dependence in the MMTV-*neu* implant model might be argued to be peripheral and indirect relative to IFN-γ. Furthermore, recent genetic analyses of humans with low or high affinity polymorphisms of their Fc receptors revealed a lack of correlation with clinical outcome, leading some to question the role of ADCC in human responses to mAb therapy [96]. This question will no doubt receive more attention as interest continues to grow in understanding the basis for immune collaboration with passive immunotherapy.

Importantly, in many of these rodent models, tumors emerge despite mAb therapy and the CD8 cell elaborated IFN-γ. That is, over time some of the breast cancer cells appear to **become resistant** despite this combined activity.

H. Resistance to targeted therapies

In many rodent models of cancer, tumors emerge despite mAb therapy and the collaborative immune effects of CD8+ T-cell elaborated IFN-γ. Thus, resistance to mAb therapy can exist before administration or arise after administration, as seen with all cancer therapies developed to date. In human breast cancer, only a small percentage of cases can be rationally targeted with p185 disabling reagents. Unfortunately, many of these patients become resistant to these therapeutics during their therapy. We and others have proposed that resistance to targeted therapy may evolve by allelic events or adaptively by emergence of new heteromeric complexes that arise as either adaptive or genetic changes driven by intrinsic or extrinsic signals (tissue related or immune signals) [97].

As mentioned above, when activated by their ligands the ErbB family receptors EGFR, p185$^{erbB2/neu}$ (HER2), ErbB3 and ErbB4 form homodimeric or heterodimeric complexes that are catalytically active. EGFR is activated by epidermal growth factor (EGF), transforming growth factor alpha (TGFα) and several other ligands. The ErbB3 and ErbB4 receptors are the principal receptors for the neuregulins. Our laboratory established that p185$^{erbB2/neu}$ forms heteromeric associations with EGFR [19]. Multiple homodimeric and heteromeric ErbB receptor complexes exist, together constituting a complex signaling network [98–101]. Notably, p185$^{erbB2/neu}$ is the preferred heterodimerization partner for all of the other ErbB family members [18,19,102–104].

In some ErbB tumors driven by homomeric p185$^{erbB2/neu}$, new heteromers form with EGFR or ErbB3 and may contribute to resistance to p185$^{erbB2/neu}$ targeted therapeutics and metastasis to brain [105]. Elevated levels of heteromers were also observed in tumor cells resistant to the anti-EGFR antibody cetuximab [106]. Engelman has described a role for c-MET in activating ErbB3 and PI3K signaling in resistant breast cancer cells [107]. We suggested that other tyrosine kinases may also complex with ErbB family proteins [108]. More recently Tanizaki and colleagues [109] made the important observation that MET can associate with certain ErbB members, in particular EGFR and ErbB (complexes were identified from cell lysates in this study, but purified proteins were not used to confirm whether direct binding occurred). Our group has found that the Survivin dimeric protein complex is activated and its level of expression enhanced during ErbB-mediated malignant transformation. Disabling Survivin function by targeted disruption of Survivin dimers can limit many malignant properties in cell lines resistant to therapy [110]. However, some cells resist targeting of Survivin and we believe this situation may relate to different modes for activation of Survivin and alterations of Survivin complexes.

I. Phenotypic effects of regulatory T cells on tumors that emerge despite mAb therapy and in the absence of CD8$^+$ or regulatory T cells

Historically, our group was the first to raise the question whether regulatory T cells (Treg) contribute to the escape of tumors from immune surveillance [111]. It is possible that the early spread of receptor kinase-active but incompletely transformed cells is accelerated by effects mediated by FOXP3$^+$ Treg, which are characterized by active FOXP3 transcription factors [112–115]. In addition, it is possible that FOXP3$^+$ Treg promote the emergence of mAb resistant cells by limiting the contributory role of adaptive immune CD8$^+$ T cells. Indeed, we have examined tumor infiltrates in some untreated MMTV-*neu* transgenic animals and noted FOXP3$^+$ T cells amongst the infiltrating cells (M.I.G., M. Katsumata and W. Hancock, unpublished observations). Tan and colleagues have noted that tumor infiltrating T cells, in this case RANKL-producing Treg, could facilitate mammary tumor metastasis [60]. We believe it is possible that therapeutics targeting Treg will find an ancillary role in ErbB-targeted therapies for human tumors. More generally, one clear interest is to develop strategies to target FOXP3 or the enzymes needed to activate it. For example, we expect that modifying enzymes such as TIP60 [116] could limit the function of FOXP3 and relieve Treg-mediated immune suppression seen in malignant disease.

J. Adaptive resistance can be overcome by the dual-antibody therapy

As mentioned above [83] we were able to leverage greater antitumor effects by administering a cocktail of anti-p185$^{erbB2/neu}$ mAbs reactive with distinct p185$^{erbB2/neu}$ epitopes. In support of these preclinical results, results from a Phase II clinical trial presented at the 2008 American Society of Clinical Oncology (ASCO) meeting showed that half of the patients with advanced, trastuzumab-resistant, ERBB2/NEU-positive metastatic breast cancer benefited from a combination of trastuzumab (4D5) and pertuzumab (2C4), an p185$^{erbB2/neu}$ specific mAb which affects ErbB2-ErbB3 dimerization but has only limited effects on EGFR-ErbB2 dimerization [117]. These data supported our earlier contention that two mAbs binding distinct receptor epitopes can overcome adaptive features of trastuzumab resistance in human tumors, by improving p185 clearance from the cell surface. On this basis, we believe the process of inactive tetramer formation can be greatly leveraged by a dual antibody therapy.

IV. CONCLUSIONS

The targeted antibody response to partially or fully transformed cells has provided insight into the evolution of therapies for human cancer. The fact that partially transformed cells leave the breast and enter the circulation is indicative that targeted therapy can be used to prevent the emergence of fully transformed cells. This phenomenon is also indicative of an early genesis of metastases at very early times in tumor formation. Combinations of targeted mAb along with therapeutic supplementation with additional immune adjuvants will likely be helpful in limiting the emergence of resistant tumors *in vivo*, addressing one of the most challenging long-standing problems in oncology.

ACKNOWLEDGMENTS

This work was supported by grants to M.I.G. from the National Institutes of Health (R01 CA055306, R01 CA149425-02 and PO1 AI073489-04), the Breast Cancer Research Foundation, and the Abramson Family Cancer Research Institute. We thank Dr. Aaron Runkle for critical reading and his comments on the manuscript.

217

References

[1] Greene MI, Perry LL, Kinney-Thomas E, Benjamin TL. Specific thymus-derived (T) cell recognition of papova virus-transformed cells. J Immunol 1982;128(2):732–6.

[2] Lathe R, Kieny MP, Gerlinger P, Clertant P, Guizani I, Cuzin F, et al. Tumour prevention and rejection with recombinant vaccinia. Nature 1987;326(6116):878–80.

[3] Drebin JA, Stern DF, Link VC, Weinberg RA, Greene MI. Monoclonal antibodies identify a cell-surface antigen associated with an activated cellular oncogene. Nature 1984;312(5994):545–8.

[4] Schechter AL, Stern DF, Vaidyanathan L, Decker SJ, Drebin JA, Greene MI, et al. The neu oncogene: an erb-B-related gene encoding a 185,000-Mr tumour antigen. Nature 1984;312(5994):513–6.

[5] Zhang H, Wang Q, Montone KT, Peavey JE, Drebin JA, Greene MI, et al. Shared antigenic epitopes and pathobiological functions of anti-p185(her2/neu) monoclonal antibodies. Exp Mol Pathol 1999;67(1):15–25.

[6] Coussens L, Yang-Feng TL, Liao YC, Chen E, Gray A, McGrath J, et al. Tyrosine kinase receptor with extensive homology to EGF receptor shares chromosomal location with neu oncogene. Science 1985;230(4730):1132–9.

[7] Semba K, Kamata N, Toyoshima K, Yamamoto T. A v-erbB-related protooncogene, c-erbB-2, is distinct from the c-erbB-1/epidermal growth factor-receptor gene and is amplified in a human salivary gland adenocarcinoma. Proceedings of the National Academy of Sciences of the United States of America 1985;82(19):6497–501.

[8] Yamamoto T, Ikawa S, Akiyama T, Semba K, Nomura N, Miyajima N, et al. Similarity of protein encoded by the human c-erb-B-2 gene to epidermal growth factor receptor. Nature 1986;319(6050):230–4.

[9] Cohen JA, Weiner DB, More KF, Kokai Y, Williams WV, Maguire Jr HC, et al. Expression pattern of the neu (NGL) gene-encoded growth factor receptor protein (p185neu) in normal and transformed epithelial tissues of the digestive tract. Oncogene 1989;4(1):81–8.

[10] Kern JA, Schwartz DA, Nordberg JE, Weiner DB, Greene MI, Torney L, et al. p185neu expression in human lung adenocarcinomas predicts shortened survival. Cancer Res 1990;50(16):5184–7.

[11] Cline MJ. Oncogenes and the pathogenesis of human cancers. La Ricerca in clinica e in laboratorio 1986;16(4):503–7.

[12] van de Vijver MJ, Peterse JL, Mooi WJ, Wisman P, Lomans J, Dalesio O, et al. Neu-protein overexpression in breast cancer. Association with comedo-type ductal carcinoma in situ and limited prognostic value in stage II breast cancer. N Engl J Med 1988;319(19):1239–45.

[13] King CR, Kraus MH, Aaronson SA. Amplification of a novel v-erbB-related gene in a human mammary carcinoma. Science 1985;229(4717):974–6.

[14] Slamon DJ, Clark GM, Wong SG, Levin WJ, Ullrich A, McGuire WL. Human breast cancer: correlation of relapse and survival with amplification of the HER-2/neu oncogene. Science 1987;235(4785):177–82.

[15] Yokota J, Yamamoto T, Toyoshima K, Terada M, Sugimura T, Battifora H, et al. Amplification of c-erbB-2 oncogene in human adenocarcinomas in vivo. Lancet 1986;1(8484):765–7.

[16] Kokai Y, Cohen JA, Drebin JA, Greene MI. Stage- and tissue-specific expression of the neu oncogene in rat development. Proceedings of the National Academy of Sciences of the United States of America 1987;84(23):8498–501.

[17] Weiner DB, Kokai Y, Wada T, Cohen JA, Williams WV, Greene MI. Linkage of tyrosine kinase activity with transforming ability of the p185neu oncoprotein. Oncogene 1989;4(10):1175–83.

[18] Kokai Y, Myers JN, Wada T, Brown VI, LeVea CM, Davis JG, et al. Synergistic interaction of p185c-neu and the EGF receptor leads to transformation of rodent fibroblasts. Cell 1989;58(2):287–92.

[19] Wada T, Qian XL, Greene MI. Intermolecular association of the p185neu protein and EGF receptor modulates EGF receptor function. Cell 1990;61(7):1339–47.

[20] Sliwkowski MX, Schaefer G, Akita RW, Lofgren JA, Fitzpatrick VD, Nuijens A, et al. Coexpression of erbB2 and erbB3 proteins reconstitutes a high affinity receptor for heregulin. J Biol Chem 1994;269(20):14661–5.

[21] Graus-Porta D, Beerli RR, Daly JM, Hynes NE. ErbB-2, the preferred heterodimerization partner of all ErbB receptors, is a mediator of lateral signaling. Embo J 1997;16(7):1647–55.

[22] Berezov A, Chen J, Liu Q, Zhang HT, Greene MI, Murali R. Disabling receptor ensembles with rationally designed interface peptidomimetics. J Biol Chem 2002;277(31):28330–9.

[23] Garrett TP, McKern NM, Lou M, Elleman TC, Adams TE, Lovrecz GO, et al. The crystal structure of a truncated ErbB2 ectodomain reveals an active conformation, poised to interact with other ErbB receptors. Mol Cell 2003;11(2):495–505.

[24] Muthuswamy SK, Li D, Lelievre S, Bissell MJ, Brugge JS. ErbB2, but not ErbB1, reinitiates proliferation and induces luminal repopulation in epithelial acini. Nat Cell Biol 2001;3(9):785–92.

[25] Aranda V, Haire T, Nolan ME, Calarco JP, Rosenberg AZ, Fawcett JP, et al. Par6-aPKC uncouples ErbB2 induced disruption of polarized epithelial organization from proliferation control. Nat Cell Biol 2006;8(11):1235–45.

[26] Lodato RF, Maguire Jr HC, Greene MI, Weiner DB, LiVolsi VA. Immunohistochemical evaluation of c-erbB-2 oncogene expression in ductal carcinoma in situ and atypical ductal hyperplasia of the breast. Modern pathology: an official journal of the United States and Canadian Academy of Pathology, Inc 1990;3(4):449–54.

[27] Pechoux C, Chardonnet Y, Noel P. Immunohistochemical studies on c-erbB-2 oncoprotein expression in paraffin embedded tissues in invasive and non-invasive human breast lesions. Anticancer Res 1994;14(3B):1343–60.

[28] Borg A, Tandon AK, Sigurdsson H, Clark GM, Ferno M, Fuqua SA, et al. HER-2/neu amplification predicts poor survival in node-positive breast cancer. Cancer Res 1990;50(14):4332–7.

[29] Maguire HC, Greene MI. Neu (c-erbB-2), a tumor marker in carcinoma of the female breast. Pathobiology 1990;58:297.

[30] Rohan TE, Hartwick W, Miller AB, Kandel RA. Immunohistochemical detection of c-erbB-2 and p53 in benign breast disease and breast cancer risk. J Natl Cancer Inst 1998;90(17):1262–9.

[31] Wells CA, McGregor IL, Makunura CN, Yeomans P, Davies JD. Apocrine adenosis: a precursor of aggressive breast cancer? J Clin Pathol 1995;48(8):737–42.

[32] Allred DC, Clark GM, Molina R, Tandon AK, Schnitt SJ, Gilchrist KW, et al. Overexpression of HER-2/neu and its relationship with other prognostic factors change during the progression of in situ to invasive breast cancer. Hum Pathol 1992;23(9):974–9.

[33] De Potter CR, Van Daele S, Van de Vijver MJ, Pauwels C, Maertens G, De Boever J, et al. The expression of the neu oncogene product in breast lesions and in normal fetal and adult human tissues. Histopathology 1989;15(4):351–62.

[34] Gusterson BA, Machin LG, Gullick WJ, Gibbs NM, Powles TJ, Price P, et al. Immunohistochemical distribution of c-erbB-2 in infiltrating and in situ breast cancer. Int J Cancer 1988;42(6):842–5.

[35] Bobrow LG, Happerfield LC, Gregory WM, Springall RD, Millis RR. The classification of ductal carcinoma in situ and its association with biological markers. Semin Diagn Pathol 1994;11(3):199–207.

[36] Claus EB, Chu P, Howe CL, Davison TL, Stern DF, Carter D, et al. Pathobiologic findings in DCIS of the breast: morphologic features, angiogenesis, HER-2/neu and hormone receptors. Exp Mol Pathol 2001;70(3):303–16.

[37] Leal CB, Schmitt FC, Bento MJ, Maia NC, Lopes CS. Ductal carcinoma in situ of the breast. Histologic categorization and its relationship to ploidy and immunohistochemical expression of hormone receptors, p53, and c-erbB-2 protein. Cancer 1995;75(8):2123–31.

[38] Liu E, Thor A, He M, Barcos M, Ljung BM, Benz C. The HER2 (c-erbB-2) oncogene is frequently amplified in situ carcinomas of the breast. Oncogene 1992;7(5):1027–32.

[39] Moreno A, Lloveras B, Figueras A, Escobedo A, Ramon JM, Sierra A, et al. Ductal carcinoma in situ of the breast: correlation between histologic classifications and biologic markers. Mod Pathol 1997;10(11):1088–92.

[40] Coene ED, Schelfhout V, Winkler RA, Schelfhout AM, Van Roy N, Grooteclaes M, et al. Amplification units and translocation at chromosome 17q and c-erbB-2 overexpression in the pathogenesis of breast cancer. Virchows Arch 1997;430(5):365–72.

[41] Parkes HC, Lillycrop K, Howell A, Craig RK. C-erbB2 mRNA expression in human breast tumours: comparison with c-erbB2 DNA amplification and correlation with prognosis. Br J Cancer 1990;61(1):39–45.

[42] Stark A, Hulka BS, Joens S, Novotny D, Thor AD, Wold LE, et al. HER-2/neu amplification in benign breast disease and the risk of subsequent breast cancer. J Clin Oncol 2000;18(2):267–74.

[43] Zhang H, Berezov A, Wang Q, Zhang G, Drebin J, Murali R, et al. ErbB receptors: from oncogenes to targeted cancer therapies. J Clin Invest 2007;117(8):2051–8.

[44] Jimenez RE, Wallis T, Tabasczka P, Visscher DW. Determination of Her-2/Neu status in breast carcinoma: comparative analysis of immunohistochemistry and fluorescent in situ hybridization. Mod Pathol 2000;13(1):37–45.

[45] Kallioniemi OP, Holli K, Visakorpi T, Koivula T, Helin HH, Isola JJ. Association of c-erbB-2 protein overexpression with high rate of cell proliferation, increased risk of visceral metastasis and poor long-term survival in breast cancer. Int J Cancer 1991;49(5):650–5.

[46] Lottner C, Schwarz S, Diermeier S, Hartmann A, Knuechel R, Hofstaedter F, et al. Simultaneous detection of HER2/neu gene amplification and protein overexpression in paraffin-embedded breast cancer. J Pathol 2005;205(5):577–84.

[47] Mrozkowiak A, Olszewski WP, Piascik A, Olszewski WT. HER2 status in breast cancer determined by IHC and FISH: comparison of the results. Pol J Pathol 2004;55(4):165–71.

[48] Smith CA, Pollice AA, Gu LP, Brown KA, Singh SG, Janocko LE, et al. Correlations among p53, Her-2/neu, and ras overexpression and aneuploidy by multiparameter flow cytometry in human breast cancer: evidence for a common phenotypic evolutionary pattern in infiltrating ductal carcinomas. Clin Cancer Res 2000;6(1):112–26.

[49] Wang S, Hossein Saboorian M, Frenkel EP, Haley BB, Siddiqui MT, Gokaslan S, et al. Aneusomy 17 in breast cancer: its role in HER-2/neu protein expression and implication for clinical assessment of HER-2/neu status. Mod Pathol 2002;15(2):137–45.

[50] Shackney SE, Silverman JF. Molecular evolutionary patterns in breast cancer. Adv Anat Pathol 2003;10(5):278–90.

[51] Shackney SE, Pollice AA, Smith CA, Alston L, Singh SG, Janocko LE, et al. The accumulation of multiple genetic abnormalities in individual tumor cells in human breast cancers: clinical prognostic implications. Cancer J Sci Am 1996;2(2):106–13.

[52] Press MF, Pike MC, Chazin VR, Hung G, Udove JA, Markowicz M, et al. Her-2/neu expression in node-negative breast cancer: direct tissue quantitation by computerized image analysis and association of overexpression with increased risk of recurrent disease. Cancer Res 1993;53(20):4960–70.

[53] Robertson KW, Reeves JR, Smith G, Keith WN, Ozanne BW, Cooke TG, et al. Quantitative estimation of epidermal growth factor receptor and c-erbB-2 in human breast cancer. Cancer Res 1996;56(16):3823–30.

219

[54] Venter DJ, Tuzi NL, Kumar S, Gullick WJ. Overexpression of the c-erbB-2 oncoprotein in human breast carcinomas: immunohistological assessment correlates with gene amplification. Lancet 1987;2(8550):69–72.

[55] Friedrichs K, Lohmann D, Hofler H. Detection of HER-2 oncogene amplification in breast cancer by differential polymerase chain reaction from single cryosections. Virchows Arch B Cell Pathol Incl Mol Pathol 1993;64(4):209–12.

[56] Persons DL, Borelli KA, Hsu PH. Quantitation of HER-2/neu and c-myc gene amplification in breast carcinoma using fluorescence in situ hybridization. Mod Pathol 1997;10(7):720–7.

[57] Slamon DJ, Godolphin W, Jones LA, Holt JA, Wong SG, Keith DE, et al. Studies of the HER-2/neu proto-oncogene in human breast and ovarian cancer. Science 1989;244(4905):707–12.

[58] Nagata Y, Lan KH, Zhou X, Tan M, Esteva FJ, Sahin AA, et al. PTEN activation contributes to tumor inhibition by trastuzumab, and loss of PTEN predicts trastuzumab resistance in patients. Cancer Cell 2004;6(2):117–27.

[59] Rokavec M, Wu W, Luo JL. IL6-Mediated Suppression of miR-200c Directs Constitutive Activation of Inflammatory Signaling Circuit Driving Transformation and Tumorigenesis. Mol Cell 2012;45(6):777–89.

[60] Tan W, Zhang W, Strasner A, Grivennikov S, Cheng JQ, Hoffman RM, et al. Tumour-infiltrating regulatory T cells stimulate mammary cancer metastasis through RANKL-RANK signalling. Nature 2011;470(7335):548–53.

[61] Cano A, Perez-Moreno MA, Rodrigo I, Locascio A, Blanco MJ, del Barrio MG, et al. The transcription factor snail controls epithelial-mesenchymal transitions by repressing E-cadherin expression. Nat Cell Biol 2000;2(2):76–83.

[62] Savagner P, Yamada KM, Thiery JP. The zinc-finger protein slug causes desmosome dissociation, an initial and necessary step for growth factor-induced epithelial-mesenchymal transition. J Cell Biol 1997;137(6):1403–19.

[63] Sanchez-Tillo E, Lazaro A, Torrent R, Cuatrecasas M, Vaquero EC, Castells A, et al. ZEB1 represses E-cadherin and induces an EMT by recruiting the SWI/SNF chromatin-remodeling protein BRG1. Oncogene 2010;29(24):3490–500.

[64] Vandewalle C, Comijn J, De Craene B, Vermassen P, Bruyneel E, Andersen H, et al. SIP1/ZEB2 induces EMT by repressing genes of different epithelial cell-cell junctions. Nucleic acids research 2005;33(20):6566–78.

[65] Ansieau S, Bastid J, Doreau A, Morel AP, Bouchet BP, Thomas C, et al. Induction of EMT by twist proteins as a collateral effect of tumor-promoting inactivation of premature senescence. Cancer cell 2008;14(1):79–89.

[66] Lee K, Gjorevski N, Boghaert E, Radisky DC, Nelson CM. Snail1, Snail2, and E47 promote mammary epithelial branching morphogenesis. EMBO J 2011;30(13):2662–74.

[67] Husemann Y, Geigl JB, Schubert F, Musiani P, Meyer M, Burghart E, et al. Systemic spread is an early step in breast cancer. Cancer cell 2008;13(1):58–68.

[68] Cavallaro U, Christofori G. Cell adhesion and signalling by cadherins and Ig-CAMs in cancer. Nat Rev Cancer 2004;4(2):118–32.

[69] Conacci-Sorrell M, Zhurinsky J, Ben-Ze'ev A. The cadherin-catenin adhesion system in signaling and cancer. J Clin Invest 2002;109(8):987–91.

[70] Derksen PW, Liu X, Saridin F, van der Gulden H, Zevenhoven J, Evers B, et al. Somatic inactivation of E-cadherin and p53 in mice leads to metastatic lobular mammary carcinoma through induction of anoikis resistance and angiogenesis. Cancer Cell 2006;10(5):437–49.

[71] Podsypanina K, Du YC, Jechlinger M, Beverly LJ, Hambardzumyan D, Varmus H. Seeding and propagation of untransformed mouse mammary cells in the lung. Science 2008;321(5897):1841–4.

[72] Karrison TG, Ferguson DJ, Meier P. Dormancy of mammary carcinoma after mastectomy. J Nat Cancer Insti 1999;91(1):80–5.

[73] Aguirre-Ghiso JA. Models, mechanisms and clinical evidence for cancer dormancy. Nat Rev Cancer 2007;7(11):834–46.

[74] Drebin JA, Link VC, Stern DF, Weinberg RA, Greene MI. Down-modulation of an oncogene protein product and reversion of the transformed phenotype by monoclonal antibodies. Cell 1985;41(3):697–706.

[75] Drebin JA, Link VC, Weinberg RA, Greene MI. Inhibition of tumor growth by a monoclonal antibody reactive with an oncogene-encoded tumor antigen. Proc Natl Acad Sci U S A 1986;83(23):9129–33.

[76] Vogel CL, Cobleigh MA, Tripathy D, Gutheil JC, Harris LN, Fehrenbacher L, et al. Efficacy and safety of trastuzumab as a single agent in first-line treatment of HER2-overexpressing metastatic breast cancer. J Clin Oncol 2002;20(3):719–26.

[77] Romond EH, Perez EA, Bryant J, Suman VJ, Geyer Jr CE, Davidson NE, et al. Trastuzumab plus adjuvant chemotherapy for operable HER2-positive breast cancer. N Engl J Med 2005;353(16):1673–84.

[78] Furuuchi K, Berezov A, Kumagai T, Greene MI. Targeted antireceptor therapy with monoclonal antibodies leads to the formation of inactivated tetrameric forms of ErbB receptors. J Immunol 2007;178(2):1021–9.

[79] Qian X, LeVea CM, Freeman JK, Dougall WC, Greene MI. Heterodimerization of epidermal growth factor receptor and wild-type or kinase-deficient Neu: a mechanism of interreceptor kinase activation and transphosphorylation. Proceedings of the National Academy of Sciences of the United States of America 1994;91(4):1500−4.

[80] Zhou H, Zha Z, Liu Y, Zhang H, Zhu J, Hu S, et al. Structural insights into the down-regulation of overexpressed p185(her2/neu) protein of transformed cells by the antibody chA21. J Biol Chem 2011; 286(36):31676−83.

[81] Park BW, Zhang HT, Wu C, Berezov A, Zhang X, Dua R, et al. Rationally designed anti-HER2/neu peptide mimetic disables P185HER2/neu tyrosine kinases in vitro and in vivo. Nat Biotechnol 2000;18(2):194−8.

[82] Masuda K, Richter M, Song X, Berezov A, Murali R, Greene MI, et al. AHNP-streptavidin: a tetrameric bacterially produced antibody surrogate fusion protein against p185her2/neu. Oncogene 2006;25(59): 7740−6.

[83] Drebin JA, Link VC, Greene MI. Monoclonal antibodies specific for the neu oncogene product directly mediate anti-tumor effects in vivo. Oncogene 1988;2(4):387−94.

[84] Katsumata M, Okudaira T, Samanta A, Clark DP, Drebin JA, Jolicoeur P, et al. Prevention of breast tumour development in vivo by downregulation of the p185neu receptor. Nat Med 1995;1(7):644−8.

[85] Bouchard L, Lamarre L, Tremblay PJ, Jolicoeur P. Stochastic appearance of mammary tumors in transgenic mice carrying the MMTV/c-neu oncogene. Cell 1989;57(6):931−6.

[86] Vaught DB, Stanford JC, Young C, Hicks DJ, Wheeler F, Rinehart C, et al. HER3 Is Required for HER2-Induced Preneoplastic Changes to the Breast Epithelium and Tumor Formation. Cancer Res 2012;72(10):2672−82.

[87] Finkle D, Quan ZR, Asghari V, Kloss J, Ghaboosi N, Mai E, et al. HER2-targeted therapy reduces incidence and progression of midlife mammary tumors in female murine mammary tumor virus huHER2-transgenic mice. Clin Cancer Res 2004;10(7):2499−511.

[88] Ignatiadis M, Rothe F, Chaboteaux C, Durbecq V, Rouas G, Criscitiello C, et al. HER2-positive circulating tumor cells in breast cancer. PloS one 2011;6(1):e15624.

[89] Park S, Jiang Z, Mortenson ED, Deng L, Radkevich-Brown O, Yang X, et al. The therapeutic effect of anti-HER2/neu antibody depends on both innate and adaptive immunity. Cancer cell 2010;18(2):160−70.

[90] Stagg J, Loi S, Divisekera U, Ngiow SF, Duret H, Yagita H, et al. Anti-ErbB-2 mAb therapy requires type I and II interferons and synergizes with anti-PD-1 or anti-CD137 mAb therapy. Proceedings of the National Academy of Sciences of the United States of America 2011;108(17):7142−7.

[91] Marth C, Widschwendter M, Kaern J, Jorgensen NP, Windbichler G, Zeimet AG, et al. Cisplatin resistance is associated with reduced interferon-gamma-sensitivity and increased HER-2 expression in cultured ovarian carcinoma cells. Br J Cancer 1997;76(10):1328−32.

[92] Hamburger AW, Pinnamaneni GD. Increased epidermal growth factor receptor gene expression by gamma-interferon in a human breast carcinoma cell line. Br J Cancer 1991;64(1):64−8.

[93] Uribe JM, McCole DF, Barrett KE. Interferon-gamma activates EGF receptor and increases TGF-alpha in T84 cells: implications for chloride secretion. Am J Physiol Gastrointest Liver Physiol 2002;283(4):G923−31.

[94] Clynes RA, Towers TL, Presta LG, Ravetch JV. Inhibitory Fc receptors modulate in vivo cytotoxicity against tumor targets. Nat Med 2000;6(4):443−6.

[95] Barnes N, Gavin AL, Tan PS, Mottram P, Koentgen F, Hogarth PM. FcgammaRI-deficient mice show multiple alterations to inflammatory and immune responses. Immunity 2002;16(3):379−89.

[96] Hurvitz SA, Betting DJ, Stern HM, Quinaux E, Stinson J, Seshagiri S, et al. Analysis of Fcgamma Receptor IIIa and IIa Polymorphisms: Lack of Correlation with Outcome in Trastuzumab-Treated Breast Cancer Patients. Clin Cancer Res 2012;18(12):3478−86.

[97] Jardines L, Weiss M, Fowble B, Greene M. neu(c-erbB-2/HER2) and the epidermal growth factor receptor (EGFR) in breast cancer. Pathobiology 1993;61(5-6):268−82.

[98] Alroy I, Yarden Y. The ErbB signaling network in embryogenesis and oncogenesis: signal diversification through combinatorial ligand-receptor interactions. FEBS letters 1997;410(1):83−6.

[99] Dougall WC, Qian X, Peterson NC, Miller MJ, Samanta A, Greene MI. The neu-oncogene: signal transduction pathways, transformation mechanisms and evolving therapies. Oncogene 1994;9(8):2109−23.

[100] Pinkas-Kramarski R, Alroy I, Yarden Y. ErbB receptors and EGF-like ligands: cell lineage determination and oncogenesis through combinatorial signaling. J Mammary Gland Biol Neoplasia 1997;2(2):97−107.

[101] Riese 2nd DJ, Stern DF. Specificity within the EGF family/ErbB receptor family signaling network. Bioessays 1998;20(1):41−8.

[102] Tzahar E, Waterman H, Chen X, Levkovitz G, Karunagaran D, Lavi S, et al. A hierarchical network of interreceptor interactions determines signal transduction by Neu differentiation factor/neuregulin and epidermal growth factor. Mol Cell Biol 1996;16(10):5276−87.

[103] Cai Z, Zhang G, Zhou Z, Bembas K, Drebin JA, Greene MI, et al. Differential binding patterns of monoclonal antibody 2C4 to the ErbB3-p185her2/neu and the EGFR-p185her2/neu complexes. Oncogene 2008;27(27):3870—4.

[104] Cai Z, Zhang H, Liu J, Berezov A, Murali R, Wang Q, et al. Targeting erbB receptors. Semin Cell Dev Biol 2010;21(9):961—6.

[105] Da Silva L, Simpson PT, Smart CE, Cocciardi S, Waddell N, Lane A, et al. HER3 and downstream pathways are involved in colonization of brain metastases from breast cancer. Breast Cancer Res 2010;12(4):R46.

[106] Wheeler DL, Huang S, Kruser TJ, Nechrebecki MM, Armstrong EA, Benavente S, et al. Mechanisms of acquired resistance to cetuximab: role of HER (ErbB) family members. Oncogene 2008;27(28):3944—56.

[107] Engelman JA, Zejnullahu K, Mitsudomi T, Song Y, Hyland C, Park JO, et al. MET amplification leads to gefitinib resistance in lung cancer by activating ERBB3 signaling. Science 2007;316(5827):1039—43.

[108] Wang Q, Greene MI. Mechanisms of resistance to ErbB-targeted cancer therapeutics. J Clin Invest 2008;118(7):2389—92.

[109] Tanizaki J, Okamoto I, Sakai K, Nakagawa K. Differential roles of trans-phosphorylated EGFR, HER2, HER3, and RET as heterodimerisation partners of MET in lung cancer with MET amplification. Br J Cancer 2011;105(6):807—13.

[110] Berezov A, Cai Z, Freudenberg JA, Zhang H, Cheng X, Thompson T, et al. Disabling the mitotic spindle and tumor growth by targeting a cavity-induced allosteric site of survivin. Oncogene 2011.

[111] Greenberg AH, Greene M. Non-adaptive rejection of small tumour inocula as a model of immune surveillance. Nature 1976;264(5584):356—9.

[112] Li B, Greene MI. Special regulatory T-cell review: FOXP3 biochemistry in regulatory T cells—how diverse signals regulate suppression. Immunology 2008;123(1):17—9.

[113] Xiao Y, Li B, Zhou Z, Hancock WW, Zhang H, Greene MI. Histone acetyltransferase mediated regulation of FOXP3 acetylation and Treg function. Curr Opin Immunol 2010;22(5):583—91.

[114] Zhang H, Xiao Y, Zhu Z, Li B, Greene MI. Immune regulation by histone deacetylases: a focus on the alteration of FOXP3 activity. Immunol Cell Biol 2012;90(1):95—100.

[115] Song X, Li B, Xiao Y, Chen C, Wang Q, Liu Y, et al. Structural and Biological Features of FOXP3 Dimerization Relevant to Regulatory T Cell Function. Cell Rep 2012.

[116] Li B, Samanta A, Song X, Iacono KT, Bembas K, Tao R, et al. FOXP3 interactions with histone acetyltransferase and class II histone deacetylases are required for repression. Proc Natl Acad Sci U S A 2007;104(11):4571—6.

[117] Sakai E, Morioka T, Yamada E, Ohkubo H, Higurashi T, Hosono K, et al. Identification of preneoplastic lesions as mucin-depleted foci in patients with sporadic colorectal cancer. Cancer Sci 2012;103(1):144—9.

CHAPTER 15

Genetic Vaccines against Cancer: Design, Testing and Clinical Performance

Freda K Stevenson, Gianfranco di Genova, Christian H Ottensmeier, Natalia Savelyeva
Molecular Immunology Group, Cancer Sciences Unit, University of Southampton Faculty of Medicine, Southampton General Hospital, Southampton, United Kingdom

I. INTRODUCTION

Vaccination against cancer in patients is a lofty ambition, especially when our knowledge of the human immune system is so limited. The success of conventional vaccines against infectious organisms encouraged the hope that we could direct immune attack towards cancer cells. This was perhaps optimistic given that preventative vaccines have succeeded mainly due to induction of protective antibody, in healthy subjects. This success continues, with the recent dramatic demonstration of the effectiveness of antibodies induced by a recombinant vaccine in protecting against human papilloma virus (HPV) [1]. Here there is relevance to cancer since HPV infection is associated with subsequent development of cervical and other cancers. Protection again is antibody-mediated but, since antigen expression changes in infected cells, the vaccine had no significant effect in already infected patients [2]. For HPV *in situ*, for other persistent infections, and for most cancers, it became clear that there was an additional need to activate effector T cells against MHC-bound peptides derived from intracellular antigens. Unfortunately, knowledge of T-cell responses in human subjects has lagged behind that of mice, with, until recently, little systematic analysis, even against conventional vaccines. The need to develop vaccines against human immunodeficiency virus and other emerging infections is now remedying this situation [3]. In parallel, for new vaccines against persistent infections and against cancer, there is a clear requirement to monitor immune responses using agreed and objective criteria.

Another complication for cancer is that the desired durable responses have to be induced in patients with a variably damaged or suppressed immune system. Patients with cancer also tend to be older, raising questions about age-related changes in immune capacity [4]. Clearly such a challenge has demanded new knowledge and technology. It seems obvious to apply all the tools of modern genetics to this challenge. Not only does DNA analysis provide insights into the molecular genetics of pathogens and cancer cells, but gene-based vaccines offer a way to connect this information to immune therapy. In parallel, our knowledge of immune effector mechanisms is increasing so that we can aim to induce specific pathways, or block regulation. The flexibility of construction of genetic vaccines provides unprecedented opportunities for expressing selected genes and should at last help us to solve the difficulties of activating immunity against persistent antigens, a setting common to long-term infection and cancer.

Cancer Immunotherapy. http://dx.doi.org/10.1016/B978-0-12-394296-8.00015-4

II. DNA VACCINES

The two overriding requirements for DNA vaccines are intelligent design and effective delivery. Immunological principles can be incorporated into the design, with inclusion of genes encoding tumor antigens +/− additive molecules to amplify and direct immune outcome. Preclinical models have been essential in testing the ability of a wide range of designs to induce immunity and to suppress tumors [5]. Three components are essential for success: first, the plasmid backbone which acts as a natural adjuvant; second, the tumor antigen, genetically assembled in a form most likely to induce the desired immune effectors; third, an inducer of T-cell help, required for induction of durable immune memory, and to overcome any pre-existing regulation. Optional extras include genes encoding cytokines, chemokines, co-stimulatory molecules or antibodies to target antigen-presenting cells (Figure 15.1) [6,7]. There is also the potential to improve performance of DNA vaccines, possibly by formulation in microparticles or liposomes [8] with a cationic lipid-based adjuvant (Vaxfectin) already in the clinic [9]. Vaccine delivery methods are advancing rapidly, with electroporation (EP) [10] now apparently overcoming previous barriers to effective translation to the clinic [11].

A. Activation of innate immunity

The plasmid backbone was first thought to stimulate innate immunity only via specific CpG dinucleotide repeats, following principles largely gleaned from synthetic oligonucleotides [12]. This pathway involves uptake of CpG-rich DNA via a receptor for advanced glycated end products (RAGE) and signaling through endosomal TLR-9/MyD88 to induce type I IFN. However, DNA vaccines proved effective in TLR9−/− mice [13] and it is now becoming clear, mainly from investigators of the DNA of infectious agents, that there are multiple cytoplasmic pattern recognition receptors which act as sensors for DNA, including DAI (DNA-dependent activator of IFN-regulatory factor), RIG-1 (retinoic acid-inducible protein 1) and helicases DHX9/DH36, which lead to activation of IFN regulatory factors 3/7 and NF-κB, transcription factors that induce expression of interferons and proinflammatory cytokines [14]. In addition, DNA activates AIM-2 (absent in melanoma 2) and its family members, generating active IL-1β and IL-18 by caspase-dependent cleavage. As our understanding of the pathways of activation of innate immunity develops, it offers new opportunities to improve performance of DNA vaccines. Already, DAI has been co-delivered with a DNA melanoma antigen vaccine adding to its effectiveness in preclinical testing [15].

B. Tumor antigens

Tumor antigens can arise from viruses or from mutated, overexpressed or aberrantly expressed normal proteins [16]. There are few tumor-specific antigens, with idiotypic (Id)

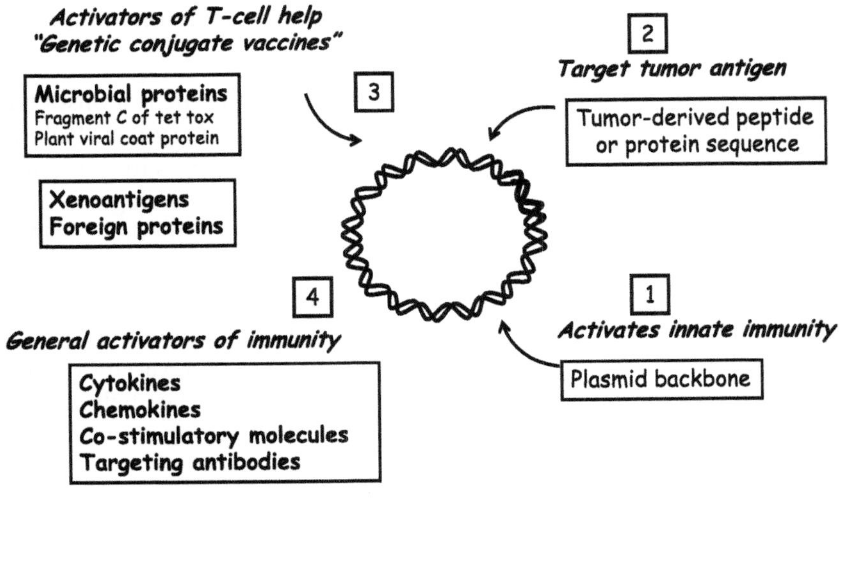

FIGURE 15.1

DNA fusion gene vaccines can provide multiple immune manipulators. (1) The plasmid backbone which activates innate immunity. (2) Tumor antigen sequences encoding full length protein or MHC Class I-binding peptides. (3) Sequences encoding proteins to induce CD4+ T-cell help, derived from microbial sequences or from xenoantigens. (4) Sequences encoding a range of candidate immune activators.

immunoglobulin of B-cell malignancies being a notable exception. Lineage-specific proteins can be useful targets especially when, as in prostate or ovarian cancer, the normal tissue has been removed by surgery. However, for the many tumor antigens also expressed by normal tissue, a successful vaccine has the possibility of inducing autoimmunity. The National Cancer Institute has recently published a priority list of 75 cancer antigens, providing a useful basis for those aiming to test vaccine design and operation against well-documented targets [17]. An important advantage for DNA vaccines, in contrast to recombinant proteins expressed *in vitro*, is that protein is expressed *in vivo*, making it more likely that post-translational modifications mimic those of the host's tumor cells.

C. Activation of T-cell help

CD4+ T-cell help is required for induction of both high affinity antibody and memory CD8+ T cells [18]. Since tumor antigens tend to be similar to normal proteins, they often fail to induce adequate CD4+ T-cell responses. This was the reason for conjugation of tumor-derived idiotypic proteins to foreign proteins such as keyhole limpet hemocyanin [19]. Our strategy was to create "genetic conjugate vaccines" by fusing idiotypic single chain Fv (scFv) sequences to the Fragment C (FrC) sequence of tetanus toxin [20]. This amplified anti-idiotypic antibody levels dramatically, leading to a pilot clinical trial of DNA scFv-FrC fusion vaccines in patients with follicular lymphoma. Although promising results were obtained, with 38% of patients generating anti-Id responses [5], the use of patient-specific vaccines did not allow an overall assessment of vaccine performance. This required a single vaccine applicable to all patients and a translocation sequence characteristic of a subset of acute myeloid leukemia was selected, with amplification of immunity by FrC sequence again demonstrated [21].

Incorporation of FrC into the vaccine draws high levels of T-cell help from an undamaged antimicrobial repertoire. This can also be achieved with other proteins, including plant viral coat proteins, which, possibly because of the self-aggregating quality of the protein, modify the outcome toward a Th1-dominated response, important for attacking cancer cells [22]. It is likely that the same principle applies to DNA-based melanoma vaccines which contain xenogeneic sequences potentially able to induce some level of T-cell help. A DNA vaccine encoding human tyrosinase is now licensed for use in dogs [23] and a DNA vaccine encoding mouse gp100 has been tested in patients [24]. If the goal of vaccination is to induce antibody against a cell surface antigen such as gp100, boosting with viral vectors may be appropriate, although pre-existing or induced antivector antibodies will develop and may inhibit the ability to boost with the same vector [25].

DNA vaccines are ideal vehicles for induction of CD8+ T cells against the wide range of candidate intracellular tumor antigens. However, durable responses again require CD4-T-cell help [18]. This has been illustrated by the failure of exogenous short peptide vaccines to induce memory CD8+ T-cell responses [26]. While it is tempting to use the same genetic conjugate vaccines able to induce antibody, there is a relatively unappreciated problem for T cells. The natural CD8+ T-cell response against even large viruses appears highly focused on only a few MHC Class I-binding peptides, due to the phenomenon of immunodominance [27]. This focus means that delivery of cancer antigens via, for example, pox viral vectors, may fail due to competition from strong viral epitopes [28], as well as from blockade by pre-existing antiviral antibodies. Failure has in fact been demonstrated in a clinical trial of an MVA-delivered melanoma antigen, where T-cell responses apparently directed against vector peptides rather than on the desired tumor peptides were observed [29]. Several other viral delivery systems, including DNA replicon vectors based on alphaviruses, are being investigated, mainly for infectious diseases, with potential application for cancer, provided that immunodominance does not intervene [30].

To avoid this problem, we designed DNA vaccines encoding a single domain (DOM) of FrC which contains no detectable competing MHC Class I (HLA-A2)-binding peptides, and we

225

fused the tumor-derived peptide sequence to the 3'-terminus [31]. This created p.DOM-epitope vaccines able to induce high levels of T-cell help with a tumor peptide placed in an optimal position to generate CD8+ T-cell responses. Efficacy against different target peptides has been demonstrated in a wide range of preclinical models and several are in clinical trials [32]. Importantly, vaccines encoding different tumor-derived peptides can be injected in separate sites without fear of competition [33] and this approach is under formal evaluation in one of our ongoing trials in hematological malignancies.

While the focus is on induction of CD8+ T cells, we are conscious of the fact that antitumor CD4+ T cells will not be induced. This might be a benefit in avoiding expansion of Treg [34]. If required, our DOM-based vaccines can be used with full length tumor antigen sequence, thereby activating CD4+ T cells as well as being applicable to all MHC Class I alleles [35]. However we have found that these are usually less effective at inducing peptide-specific CD8+ T cells than the p.DOM-epitope design [36].

D. Vaccine delivery

The major problem for DNA vaccines has been efficient delivery to large animals. The failure of the first attempts to immediately reproduce the exciting preclinical performance of DNA vaccines in human subjects should perhaps have been no surprise [37], but it has led to an unfortunate view that such vaccines have no place in the clinic. There is still debate about the reasons for failure, but the two key requirements of sufficient levels of transfection and activation of innate immunity were clearly not being met. At least for intramuscular sites, the volume injected, large in mice and impossible to scale up appropriately for patients, was an important factor [38]. Now, several strategies to mimic the effects of the excessive volume for patients have been developed, including electroporation, mainly for muscle sites, and high-pressure injection, dermal patches, tattooing or particle bombardment of DNA on gold particles, mainly for skin [11]. The amount of DNA injected varies with the site, with less required for skin sites than for muscle [11], and EP improving performance for both. In our experience so far, dose escalation between 500–2000 µg +/− EP did not result in a clear increase in immune responses and 1 mg in muscle sites appears adequate (unpublished data).

EP is emerging as a clinically acceptable strategy for DNA vaccination of cancer patients. The procedure is to pass an electric current across the tissue site at the same time as, or immediately after, injection, or very soon after. There is no doubt that this increases transfection levels and therefore antigen expression, but it also creates local inflammation required for attracting antigen-presenting cells [10]. Preclinical models have demonstrated amplification of immune responses by adding EP, especially for antibody and CD8$^+$ T cells [39]. We and others are now studying the effects of EP in clinical trials [40].

III. MESSENGER RNA VACCINES

Although early studies of gene transfer into mouse muscle showed that injection of either DNA or RNA led to protein expression [41], development of RNA-based vaccines has lagged far behind DNA vaccines. The main reason for this is the unstable nature of RNA, which shortened the extracellular half-life due to degradation by RNAses. This made direct injection untenable and largely restricted the approach to RNA-loaded dendritic cells, with some success against a prostate cancer antigen [42]. Progress has been made more recently with a range of stabilization techniques and by injecting into skin or lymph nodes [43]. Advantages of mRNA are that it does not enter the nucleus and is therefore safe. There is also the potential to stimulate the innate immunity via TLR3, TLR7 and TLR8 when delivered to the endosome. Some clinical trials have been carried out in patients with metastatic melanoma but the setting was perhaps not ideal and objective responses were not achieved [44]. A modified approach using mRNA vaccines containing both free and protamine-complexed mRNA shows promise and this is currently in clinical trials [45]. Other trials, reported so far only in abstract form, suggest that mRNA can induce a broad antigen-specific immunity, with antibody, CD4+ and CD8+ T-cell responses detected [46]. Also intradermal delivery of self-adjuvanted mRNA targeting prostate antigens in patients with prostate cancer induced responses against multiple prostate cancer epitopes in 58% of patients [47]. However, it remains to be seen if mRNA vaccines can compete with, or possibly complement, the flexible, stable and easily manipulated DNA vaccines.

IV. VIRUS-LIKE PARTICLE VACCINES

Virus-like particles (VLP) form because of the ability of the viral coat proteins to self-aggregate without the need for other viral components. They therefore mimic the viral structure, displaying antigen in a multimeric form, particularly effective in activating naïve B cells and in eliciting high levels of protective antibody. The successful preventative vaccine against HPV using the L1 coat protein is an example [1]. The VLP from HPV also activates innate immunity via TLR4 expressed by B cells and dendritic cells [48,49]. Performance is increased by adding an adjuvant, either alum (Gardasil, Merck) or alum plus LPS-derived monophosphoryl lipid A (Cervarix, GSK) the latter apparently improving the longevity of antibody responses [50].

The success of the HPV vaccine has led to development of VLP as carriers for weakly immunogenic antigens. One approach is to use the hepatitis B virus (HBV) core antigen (HBcAg), which can self-assemble into VLP [51]. A number of chimeric HBcAg VLP have been developed which express defined epitopes from infectious agents genetically fused to the core protein [52]. Recently this approach has been adopted for cancer vaccines using an epitope from the differentiation antigen claudin 18 isoform 2 (CLDN18.2) expressed in gastroesophageal, pancreatic and other cancers. Fusion to HBcAg led to induction of auto anti-epitope antibodies and partial protection against CLDN18.2 expressing tumor [53].

V. PLANT VIRAL PARTICLES AND THEIR DERIVATIVES AS VACCINES

Plant viruses provide alternative highly immunogenic candidates as carriers for human cancer antigens as they are nonpathogenic, with no pre-existing immunity, and are VLP-like, being assembled from multiple virus coat protein (CP) subunits. An additional advantage is that they encapsulate the ssRNA viral genome. The use of plant virus-based chimeric vaccines expressing defined B-cell epitopes from bacterial and viral pathogens, placed at the termini or in the loops exposed at the viral surface, began ~25 years ago [54]. Genetic linkage to the viral CP leads to display of the peptide on the surface of the plant viral particle, thereby concentrating and aggregating the antigen. These vaccines could be expressed in plants with the yields similar to the wild types and can be purified by methods established for the wild type viruses. Such vaccines have been tested in a number of infectious diseases with induction of good levels of anti-epitope antibodies and provision of protection in rodents [55] and in larger animals [56,57].

One problem, however, is that there is a restriction on the size of the epitope to be included, with larger polypeptides compromising the structural integrity of the viral particle [54]. The use of flexible linkers was helpful for individual larger fragments but could not be adopted as a generic approach [58,59]. Another problem has been the need for exclusion of particular amino acids such as cysteine and tryptophan putting further restriction on the choice of epitopes [60,61,62]. A parallel approach which could potentially avoid this has been to use plant viral coat proteins alone, without including viral RNA. These have been expressed with attached epitopes in several nonplant expression systems including bacteria and yeast [63,64]. Papaya mosaic virus (PapMV) has the ability to assemble into VLP similar to HBcAg without the presence of genomic nucleic acids [64]. These VLP have superior immunogenicity to monomeric proteins and confer long lasting antibody response against the candidate epitope [64]. They have been largely tested for their ability to induce immunity against infectious diseases.

VI. PVX-BASED PLANT VIRAL PARTICLE (PVP) CONJUGATE VACCINES

The goal for vaccines against tumor antigens expressed at the cell surface is to induce high levels of antibody. Although DNA fusion vaccines delivered with EP can achieve this, we have also explored the approach of attaching target antigens to whole virus. We have selected potato virus X (PVX), which comprises CP monomers repeated 1000 times and surrounding the viral ssRNA. Attachment of antigen is nongenetic and does not require individual tailoring for each candidate molecule as is required for chimeric viruses incorporating individual epitopes. There is also a smaller limit on the size of antigen since full-sized antigens or large fragments can be conjugated, ensuring induction of a broadly specific antibody response.

To generate the PVP conjugate vaccine we have initially linked PVX to tumor antigen using streptavidin-biotin. With an Id antigen, this vaccine was superior in induction of antitumor antibody to the DNA fusion vaccine and was able to induce protective antibody without addition of adjuvant (unpublished data). Viral ssRNA clearly has a role in engaging TLR7. Interestingly combination with alum acted synergistically to further increase the antibody levels. Collectively this vaccine design incorporated features important for cancer conjugate vaccines such as multivalency, foreign proteins to activate T-cell help and ssRNA for stimulating innate immunity (Figure 15.2). Targeting TLR7 has particular advantages for induction of antibody responses since it is expressed on plasmacytoid dendritic cells (DC) and on resting B cells in the mouse and also on activated B cells in humans [65,66]. Additionally, in humans, TLR8, another receptor for ssRNA, is expressed on a wider range of DC subsets than TLR7, thereby offering additional advantages to vaccines incorporating ssRNA [67]. The PVP-conjugate vaccine design induces levels of antibody comparable to those induced by KLH

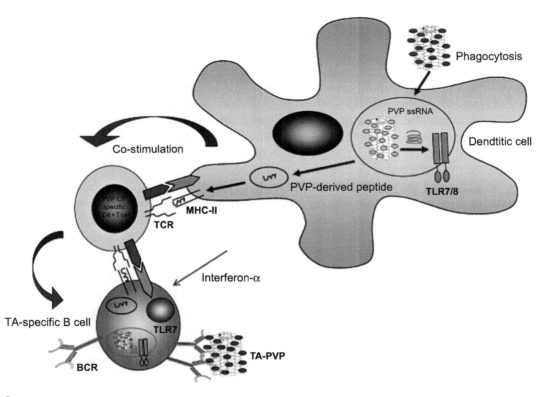

FIGURE 15.2

Mechanism of immune induction for PVP vaccines. Three critical components are important for activation of the immune system, namely, delivery of the antigen aggregated and concentrated on the surface of PVP for efficient activation of B cells, PVP-specific T-cell help for helpless tumor-antigen and activation of dendritic cells by ssRNA through TLR7/8.

conjugates, now ready for clinical trials targeting Id antigen in lymphoma [68]. However, PVP conjugates induce a wider spectrum of antibody isotypes with, in contrast to KLH, prevalence of Th1-driven IgG2 (unpublished data).

Certainly the PVP-conjugate vaccines appear ideal for induction of high levels of Th1-driven antitumor antibody, a desired goal for attacking cancer. Whether these vaccines can also induce antitumor CD8+ T cells is the next question. It may be that one design does not fit all purposes and that specific designs can be selected for optimal immune outcome.

VII. VACCINATION OF HUMAN SUBJECTS

The goal of cancer vaccines is to induce tumor-specific immune responses in patients, which are able to eliminate minimal residual disease and exert long-term surveillance. Although antibodies can attack cell surface molecules, and passive transfer of monoclonal antibodies has clear clinical impact [69], the focus is mainly on induction of tumor-specific cytotoxic lymphocytes (CTL) and, in some cases, CD4+ T cells. The design and testing of DNA vaccines to induce tumor-specific CTL has been discussed in previous sections. For the clinic, we need to consider the setting for vaccination of patients, which is difficult to model, and how to identify and to then monitor the immune responses most relevant for controlling tumor behavior. Assessment in patients is very revealing but is necessarily limited by the restriction of analysis to blood, with few opportunities to investigate events in tissue sites.

Therapeutic efficacy can only be achieved if the primed, tumor-specific CTLs leave the site of injection and the draining lymph nodes, migrate to tumor-bearing tissues and kill tumor cells, despite a likely immunosuppressive tumor microenvironment. Furthermore, long-term protection against tumor recurrence requires successful establishment of tumor-specific memory responses. Now, single cell assays offer a range of surrogate markers useful for estimating vaccine efficacy [70] and systems biology and high throughput analysis can be applied [71].

VIII. QUANTITATIVE AND QUALITATIVE FEATURES OF VACCINE-INDUCED T-CELL RESPONSES

Although quantifying IFN-γ–producing T cells remains a common endpoint assay for cancer vaccines, recent studies in infectious diseases have indicated that qualitative features of T-cell responses are important [72,73]. These include breadth, clonality and functional avidity [70,73]. High avidity allows T cells to recognize peptide expressed at low density on target cells, and to display effector functions and killing activity more promptly [73]. The quality of the T-cell response is also defined by the type and the number of functions that T cells can exert, such as cytokine or chemokine production, cytotoxicity and proliferation. Importantly, the presence of polyfunctional or multifunctional CD8+ and CD4+ T cells has been associated with better control of HIV infection in humans [74,75]. Furthermore, in a mouse model of parasitic infection (*Leishmania major*), it correlates with the degree of vaccine-induced protection [76].

Crucially, long-lasting polyfunctional CD4+ and CD8+ T-cell responses can be induced by DNA vaccination, as found with HIV antigens in nonhuman primates [77] and human subjects [78,79,80]. Interestingly, route and dose of administration appear to influence the quality of the immune response [81]. Immunomonitoring of trials of cancer vaccines needs to be extended to include such assays and to evaluate their relevance for predicting clinical outcomes.

IX. CLINICAL TRIALS OF DNA VACCINES

After initial reservations that DNA vaccines would not be sufficiently potent to deliver immune responses in patients, the field is now changing rapidly. Currently there are 57 trials of DNA vaccination in cancer patients alone that are recruiting patients (www.clinicaltrials.gov, accessed 04 March 2012), illustrating the growing perception in the community of the promise of this approach. A number of DNA vaccines have been licensed, targeting infectious hematopoietic necrosis virus in salmon [82] and rainbow trout. Perhaps more relevant for human application is the protective immunity that is conferred in large mammals, horses, by DNA vaccination against equine encephalitis virus [83]. Furthermore, the first licensed mammalian anti-melanoma vaccine is a DNA vaccine [84], conferring therapeutic benefit in dogs. It is an illustration of the power of this strategy against a cancer antigen [85].

DNA vaccines show an excellent safety in patients with few or no side effects beyond the site of vaccination. Observations in our own trial in prostate cancer [40] confirm data from other groups. Clinically relevant side effects beyond the site of vaccination appear uncommon, using DNA alone or with electroporation [86], even in healthy volunteers [87]. Genomic integration does not appear to be an issue [88,89] and there is no evidence for anti-DNA immune responses or changes in other markers of autoimmunity in nontarget organs [11,90].

With regard to autoantigens as targets, safety data concerning the effects of attacking normal cells may be misleading if immunogenicity is low. Revealing information comes from transfer of autoantigen-specific T cells. Dose limiting toxicity is seen in patients when very high affinity T cells, not induced by vaccination of patients, but expressing a T-cell receptor (TCR) engineered from transgenic mice, are injected [91]. Using T cells with TCR specific for the HLA-A0201*-restricted IMI peptide from carcino-embryonic antigen (CEA) led to diarrhea of such an extent that the study was stopped after three patients, in spite of clinical effects on both CEA levels and on tumor size. Data consistent with this have also been observed in CEA-transgenic mice [92], after transfer of CEA-specific T cells. Our own study in patients with CEA-expressing cancers [93] of a DNA vaccine directed against the CAP1 peptide from CEA [94] showed that low-grade diarrhea was induced, suggesting that vaccination with DNA is able to break tolerance in humans [93]. The data indicate a vaccine-associated effect but formal demonstration that the diarrhea is mediated by bowel-homing T cells was not investigated and will demand a further clinical trial for proof. It will be essential to evaluate over time whether, as vaccine performance improves, immunity against self antigens leads to related adverse events. Similar events have been observed in melanoma patients treated with an immunomodulatory antibody directed against CLTA-4 [95], where removal of regulatory T cells in the gut is the likely mechanism.

X. IMMUNE RESPONSES TO DNA VACCINATION

There is still limited information about the immunogenicity of DNA vaccines in human subjects. It might be anticipated from preclinical studies that DNA vaccines, known to be efficient in induction of cytotoxic T cells, might curtail antigen expression by CTL-mediated removal of the depot cells [96], thus changing the kinetic of antigen expression. There is also the question of boosting to consider, since induced CTL could remove antigen-presenting cells, thereby preventing efficient stimulation [27]. Spacing of booster injections to allow decay of the CTL response would be a way of avoiding this. One difficulty in gaining insight into these questions in patients is the necessarily restricted access to tissue sites, with only blood lymphocytes generally available. Since T cells are likely to be located at tumor sites, this could explain the apparent mismatch between immune responses as measured in the blood and clinical effects.

In our own prostate cancer vaccine trial in men who had failed radical therapy and presented with rising PSA [40] we found strong induction of CD4+ T-cell responses against the DOM helper sequence in 30/31 patients. The majority (60%) of patients additionally developed CD8+ T-cell responses against the vaccine-encoded HLA-A0201*-restricted PSMA27 epitope [5,36,40] detectable by ELISPOT. In contrast to peptide vaccination [26] immune responses to both the DOM helper sequence and the tumor epitope were durable up to the end of follow-up at 18 months.

In our study we also evaluated the delivery of the vaccine by electroporation [40]. We found a highly significant increase of antibody responses when electroporation was used for delivery, but only a trend to improved CD4+ T cell responses. This is in contrast to data following xenogenic (HIV) DNA sequences in healthy volunteers [86], where electroporation increased both the breadth and durability of T cell responses to the DNA vaccine. This apparent contradiction may simply result from the fact that in our study DNA vaccine alone was able to generate strong immunity to the tetanus toxin-derived DOM helper sequence in 30/31 individuals without requiring additional support from electroporation.

Vaccination with DNA encoding full-length PSA has been tested [97] and induces measurable T cell immunity in patients. The overall frequency of responses to the tumor antigen appears to be lower as it was reported [97] that 3/22 patients had measurable CD8$^+$ T cell responses compared to 6/30 patients in our dataset, using *ex vivo* ELISPOT. However vaccine immunogenicity is difficult to compare with small numbers and differences in immune monitoring, highlighting the urgent need for harmonization or standardization of T cell assays to make comparisons possible. Clinically McNeel et al [97]. report significant effects on PSA doubling time in a subgroup of patients.

DNA vaccination against full-length PSMA induced anti-PSMA antibodies in a phase I/II study, but the effect on cellular immunity has not been reported [98]. This approach is also being explored in a prime boost setting where adenoviral PSMA delivery was followed by plasmid DNA vaccination with serological responses in the majority of patients [99]. Studies exploiting xenogeneic sequences following on from the canine vaccine approach, for example using monkey PSA in human subjects [100], are ongoing [101]. A similar approach in melanoma patients has recently been reported, using a DNA encoding mouse gp100 in patients. Immune responses to the human gp100 were detected in 30% of patients [24] with no association of immune responses with outcome and immunogenicity seems comparatively low. Perhaps this is in part related to the complexity of using xenogeneic approaches, which makes it much more difficult to predict and to identify T cell responses in the vaccine recipient. Immunogenicity has also been shown in humans when PSA was delivered as a DNA vaccine into the skin and muscle in a phase I study with GM-CSF and/or IL-2 [102].

In our own trials we have so far focused on targeting single epitopes from the tumor antigen. The reasons for this are immunological, to avoid antigenic competition at the stage of priming and boosting [103] and additionally this approach makes comprehensive immune-monitoring relatively straightforward. Incorporation of full-length antigen sequence into the DNA vaccine seems attractive since it would allow vaccination of all rather than of the 40% of patients who carry the HLA-A2 gene [97]. However, there are cogent reasons for using a peptide-focused vaccine since the inductive power of the repositioned peptide is generally considerably higher than from full length sequence [31,36]. CD8+ T cells specific for a single epitope are clearly capable of suppressing even an acute viral infection [104]. Should escape from focused attack occur, a second vaccine against a different epitope could be used [33] and we are exploring double attack in our current clinical trial against the WT-1 antigen [105] in chronic and acute myeloid leukemia. Although our vaccine design could readily incorporate tumor-derived MHC Class II-binding epitopes, there is no clear evidence that these are required for maintenance of cytotoxic T cells and there is a danger that regulatory T cells might be induced [106,107]. This phenomenon has been described after vaccination with long synthetic peptides in patients with HPV-driven cervical dysplasia [108].

XI. IMMUNOTHERAPY TRIAL ENDPOINTS AND CHOICE OF CLINICAL SETTINGS

A major concern over the interpretation of previous vaccine failures has been voiced, using not only DNA, but other vaccine approaches [109]. The author concluded that the low objective response rate of 3.5% in a large number of vaccinated patients, mostly with metastatic melanoma, made a case for switching to alternative immunotherapy strategies such as adoptive T-cell transfer. With hindsight this conclusion appears to have been premature: since 2009, randomized vaccine trials have demonstrated benefit in a rapidly growing number of indications: melanoma [110], prostate cancer [111], lung cancer [112], colorectal cancer [113] and follicular lymphoma [114]. These observations have led to attempts to not only define better at which stage to vaccinate patients, but also to re-evaluate clinical trials endpoints in vaccine studies.

The most robust outcome for patient benefit in cancer clinical trials remains survival and this is acknowledged in many of the ongoing randomized vaccine studies in Phase III. For example there are five such studies in lung cancer alone which will overall report on >5500 patients in this one condition (reviewed in [115]). For early phase studies, survival is a challenging endpoint and unless end-stage patients are chosen it is simply not feasible to wait for eventual outcomes, which may additionally be affected by subsequent treatments [116]. A frequently used surrogate clinical endpoint in cancer trials is tumor shrinkage using RECIST criteria [117]. However, it has become evident that for immunotherapeutic studies tumor shrinkage may not correlate with survival benefit. An attempt to overcome this has been formulated in the description of immune-related response criteria [118], developed to capture the clinical effects of ipilimumab. Here, not uncommonly, apparent early progression followed by later regression of metastases has been interpreted as a reflection of lymphocytic infiltration into the tumor, causing a net size increase of the lesion but without a true increase in tumor cell number. It is uncertain whether this approach will be relevant to other immunotherapeutic strategies and prospective validation is required.

Confounding factors in the interpretation of the effects of any particular immunotherapeutic strategy are the extent to which the patient's immune system has been damaged by disease or treatment. In terms of treatment, there are clearly agents with long-term deleterious effect on humoral immunity (e.g., anti-CD20 antibodies) or on T-cell immunity (e.g., purine analogues), although there is now considerable controversy as to whether cytotoxic chemotherapy is immunosuppressive or immune-permissive [119,120]. This will require formal evaluation of individual drugs or drug combinations and trials are now testing the addition of vaccines to cytotoxics [121,122], in particular cyclophosphamide [123]. This question is also relevant for new tyrosine kinase inhibitors, which are in wide clinical use. The evidence is mounting that some agents are immune-permissive [124,125], while others are not [125].

In terms of the effects of disease, tumor volume as a predictor of systemic and local immune responses has not been studied systematically [126] and there is little comparative data from within individual trials that compare the immunogenicity of vaccination in patients at different stages of disease. Increasingly, however, there is awareness that early vaccination is preferable, when immunosuppression by the cancer is still limited [127], for example, after resection of primary disease. In our own dataset [93] in patients with advanced solid tumors about 50% mounted cellular responses to the DOM adjuvant sequence and of these about 50% developed CD8+ T-cell responses to the CAP1 epitope. In contrast 11/12 patients without radiologically detectable disease had CD4+ T-cell responses to DOM and 7/12 patients CAP1 responses and it is intriguing how similar these response frequencies are to those in our prostate cancer vaccine study where patients also had a relatively low tumor volume. Evaluation of multiple randomized studies by Gulley et al. [128] based on trial reports on prostate cancer, lung cancer, colorectal and prostate cancer also concludes that vaccinating in early disease is more likely to yield benefit for patients. Overall, we believe that, in common with all cancer vaccines, the potency of nucleic acid vaccines is best evaluated in early disease or in the adjuvant setting, and only when this has been achieved should they be tested in later stage disease.

XII. IMMUNOLOGICAL ASSAY HARMONIZATION

If cancer vaccines mediate their effect through immunological mechanisms, it must be possible to understand and to quantify this effect through immunological assays. A number of such assays have been proposed and are widely used, such as ELISPOT, tetramer analysis or intracellular cytokine measurement. Flow cytometry is developing strongly and *in vitro* cytotoxicity assays remain useful. The major handicap in comparing the evaluations from early phase clinical trials is the variation of assay systems and results in the hands of different groups, making it almost impossible to come to comparative conclusions [129,130]. To overcome the biological and technical variability of these tests for cancer vaccines the CIMT and CIC collaboratives have in recent years undertaken large-scale evaluation of the core assays, identifying key parameters that lead to assay variability and working towards assay harmonization in the community. This has been very successful for ELISPOT [131–133] and tetramer staining [134], with a number of multicenter experiments in the reporting phase for tetramer staining and intracellular staining (http://cimt.eu/workgroups/cip/proficiency-panel-program/). More recently a broad consensus has been reached, which aims to establish a minimal set of information about T-cell assays (www.miataproject.org) in order to overcome the lack of comparability. As we learn more about the most relevant T-cell assays that predict for vaccine outcome, we will be in a good position from this study to validate them for comparative testing between trials.

One problem for evaluation of immune responses in human subjects is the relative lack of knowledge of the normal human immune system. It is extraordinary that while vaccination against infectious disease has been so successful we still know so little about T-cell responses. A new focus on human immunity and the mechanisms of immunological memory is revealing novel features [135], including an unanticipated route of bystander activation for maintenance of CD4+ T-cell memory cells [136]. In contrast to laboratory mice, which are kept in an artificial environment, human subjects are continuously buffeted by infectious organisms. Thus, we need to understand the consequential dynamic nature of immunity and how we can turn it against cancer.

ACKNOWLEDGMENTS

The authors gratefully acknowledge support from the Leukaemia and Lymphoma Research, Tenovus and Cancer Research UK and the Southampton NIHR Experimental Cancer Medicine Centre. We thank Lynsey Block for invaluable help with preparation of the manuscript.

References

[1] Lowy DR, Schiller JT. Prophylactic human papillomavirus vaccines. J Clin Invest 2006;116(5):1167–73.

[2] Schiller JT, Castellsague X, Villa LL, Hildesheim A. An update of prophylactic human papillomavirus L1 virus-like particle vaccine clinical trial results. Vaccine 2008;26(Suppl 10):K53–61.

[3] McMichael AJ. HIV vaccines. Annu Rev Immunol 2006;24:227–55.

[4] Fulop T, Larbi A, Kotb R, de Angelis F, Pawelec G. Aging, immunity, and cancer. Discov Med 2011;11(61):537–50.

[5] Rice J, Ottensmeier CH, Stevenson FK. DNA vaccines: precision tools for activating effective immunity against cancer. Nat Rev Cancer 2008;8(2):108–20.

[6] Abdulhaqq SA, Weiner DB. DNA vaccines: developing new strategies to enhance immune responses. Immunol Res 2008;42(1-3):219–32.

[7] Fredriksen AB, Sandlie I, Bogen B. DNA vaccines increase immunogenicity of idiotypic tumor antigen by targeting novel fusion proteins to antigen-presenting cells. Mol Ther 2006;13(4):776–85.

[8] Kutzler MA, Weiner DB. DNA vaccines: ready for prime time? Nat Rev Genet 2008;9(10):776–88.

[9] Smith LR, Wloch MK, Ye M, Reyes LR, Boutsaboualoy S, Dunne CE, et al. Phase 1 clinical trials of the safety and immunogenicity of adjuvanted plasmid DNA vaccines encoding influenza A virus H5 hemagglutinin. Vaccine 2010;28(13):2565–72.

[10] Ahlen G, Soderholm J, Tjelle T, Kjeken R, Frelin L, Hoglund U, et al. In vivo electroporation enhances the immunogenicity of hepatitis C virus nonstructural 3/4A DNA by increased local DNA uptake, protein expression, inflammation, and infiltration of CD3+ T cells. J Immunol 2007;179(7):4741–53.

[11] Ferraro B, Morrow MP, Hutnick NA, Shin TH, Lucke CE, Weiner DB. Clinical applications of DNA vaccines: current progress. Clin Infect Dis 2011;53(3):296–302.

[12] Krieg AM. CpG motifs in bacterial DNA and their immune effects. Annu Rev Immunol 2002;20:709–60.

[13] Spies B, Hochrein H, Vabulas M, Huster K, Busch DH, Schmitz F, et al. Vaccination with plasmid DNA activates dendritic cells via Toll-like receptor 9 (TLR9) but functions in TLR9-deficient mice. J Immunol 2003;171(11):5908–12.

[14] Kawasaki T, Kawai T, Akira S. Recognition of nucleic acids by pattern-recognition receptors and its relevance in autoimmunity. Immunol Rev 2011;243(1):61–73.

[15] Lladser A, Mougiakakos D, Tufvesson H, Ligtenberg MA, Quest AF, Kiessling R, et al. DAI (DLM-1/ZBP1) as a genetic adjuvant for DNA vaccines that promotes effective antitumor CTL immunity. Mol Ther 2011;19(3):594–601.

[16] Stevenson FK, Rice J, Zhu D. Tumor vaccines. Adv Immunol 2004;82:49–103.

[17] Cheever MA, Allison JP, Ferris AS, Finn OJ, Hastings BM, Hecht TT, et al. The prioritization of cancer antigens: a national cancer institute pilot project for the acceleration of translational research. Clin Cancer Res 2009;15(17):5323–37.

[18] Janssen EM, Lemmens EE, Wolfe T, Christen U, von Herrath MG, Schoenberger SP. CD4+ T cells are required for secondary expansion and memory in CD8+ T lymphocytes. Nature 2003;421(6925):852–6.

[19] Timmerman JM, Levy R. Linkage of foreign carrier protein to a self-tumor antigen enhances the immunogenicity of a pulsed dendritic cell vaccine. J Immunol 2000;164(9):4797–803.

[20] King CA, Spellerberg MB, Zhu D, Rice J, Sahota SS, Thompsett AR, et al. DNA vaccines with single-chain Fv fused to fragment C of tetanus toxin induce protective immunity against lymphoma and myeloma. Nat Med 1998;4(11):1281–6.

[21] Padua RA, Larghero J, Robin M, le Pogam C, Schlageter MH, Muszlak S, et al. PML-RARA-targeted DNA vaccine induces protective immunity in a mouse model of leukemia. Nat Med 2003;9(11):1413–7.

[22] Savelyeva N, Munday R, Spellerberg MB, Lomonossoff GP, Stevenson FK. Plant viral genes in DNA idiotypic vaccines activate linked CD4+ T-cell mediated immunity against B-cell malignancies. Nat Biotechnol 2001;19(8):760–4.

[23] Grosenbaugh DA, Leard AT, Bergman PJ, Klein MK, Meleo K, Susaneck S, et al. Safety and efficacy of a xenogeneic DNA vaccine encoding for human tyrosinase as adjunctive treatment for oral malignant melanoma in dogs following surgical excision of the primary tumor. Am J Vet Res 2011;72(12):1631–8.

[24] Ginsberg BA, Gallardo HF, Rasalan TS, Adamow M, Mu Z, Tandon S, et al. Immunologic response to xenogeneic gp100 DNA in melanoma patients: comparison of particle-mediated epidermal delivery with intramuscular injection. Clin Cancer Res 2010;16(15):4057–65.

[25] Cooney EL, Collier AC, Greenberg PD, Coombs RW, Zarling J, Arditti DE, et al. Safety of and immunological response to a recombinant vaccinia virus vaccine expressing HIV envelope glycoprotein. Lancet 1991;337(8741):567–72.

[26] Rezvani K, Yong AS, Mielke S, Jafarpour B, Savani BN, Le RQ, et al. Repeated PR1 and WT1 peptide vaccination in Montanide-adjuvant fails to induce sustained high-avidity, epitope-specific CD8+ T cells in myeloid malignancies. Haematologica 2011;96(3):432–40.

[27] Yewdell J, Anton LC, Bacik I, Schubert U, Snyder HL, Bennink JR. Generating MHC class I ligands from viral gene products. Immunol Rev 1999;172:97–108.

[28] Yewdell JW. Designing CD8+ T cell vaccines: it's not rocket science (yet). Curr Opin Immunol 2010;22(3):402–10.

[29] Smith CL, Mirza F, Pasquetto V, Tscharke DC, Palmowski MJ, Dunbar PR, et al. Immunodominance of poxviral-specific CTL in a human trial of recombinant-modified vaccinia Ankara. J Immunol 2005;175(12):8431–7.

[30] Tubulekas I, Berglund P, Fleeton M, Liljestrom P. Alphavirus expression vectors and their use as recombinant vaccines: a minireview. Gene 1997;190(1):191–5.

[31] Rice J, Buchan S, Stevenson FK. Critical components of a DNA fusion vaccine able to induce protective cytotoxic T cells against a single epitope of a tumor antigen. J Immunol 2002;169(7):3908–13.

[32] Stevenson FK, Ottensmeier CH, Rice J. DNA vaccines against cancer come of age. Curr Opin Immunol 2010;22(2):264–70.

[33] Liu J, Ewald BA, Lynch DM, Nanda A, Sumida SM, Barouch DH. Modulation of DNA vaccine-elicited CD8+ T-lymphocyte epitope immunodominance hierarchies. J Virol 2006;80(24):11991–7.

[34] Zhou G, Drake CG, Levitsky HI. Amplification of tumor-specific regulatory T cells following therapeutic cancer vaccines. Blood 2006;107(2):628–36.

234

[35] Joseph-Pietras D, Gao Y, Zojer N, Ait-Tahar K, Banham AH, Pulford K, et al. DNA vaccines to target the cancer testis antigen PASD1 in human multiple myeloma. Leukemia 2010;24(11):1951–9.

[36] Vittes GE, Harden EL, Ottensmeier CH, Rice J, Stevenson FK. DNA fusion gene vaccines induce cytotoxic T-cell attack on naturally processed peptides of human prostate-specific membrane antigen. Eur J Immunol 2011;41(8):2447–56.

[37] MacGregor RR, Boyer JD, Ugen KE, Lacy KE, Gluckman SJ, Bagarazzi ML, et al. First human trial of a DNA-based vaccine for treatment of human immunodeficiency virus type 1 infection: safety and host response. J Infect Dis 1998;178(1):92–100.

[38] Buchan S, Gronevik E, Mathiesen I, King CA, Stevenson FK, Rice J. Electroporation as a "prime/boost" strategy for naked DNA vaccination against a tumor antigen. J Immunol 2005;174(10):6292–8.

[39] Tollefsen S, Tjelle T, Schneider J, Harboe M, Wiker H, Hewinson G, et al. Improved cellular and humoral immune responses against Mycobacterium tuberculosis antigens after intramuscular DNA immunisation combined with muscle electroporation. Vaccine 2002;20(27-28):3370–8.

[40] Low L, Mander A, McCann K, Dearnaley D, Tjelle T, Mathiesen I, et al. DNA vaccination with electroporation induces increased antibody responses in patients with prostate cancer. Hum Gene Ther 2009;20(11):1269–78.

[41] Wolff JA, Malone RW, Williams P, Chong W, Acsadi G, Jani A, et al. Direct gene transfer into mouse muscle in vivo. Science 1990;247(4949 Pt 1):1465–8.

[42] Heiser A, Coleman D, Dannull J, Yancey D, Maurice MA, Lallas CD, et al. Autologous dendritic cells transfected with prostate-specific antigen RNA stimulate CTL responses against metastatic prostate tumors. J Clin Invest 2002;109(3):409–17.

[43] Kreiter S, Diken M, Selmi A, Tureci O, Sahin U. Tumor vaccination using messenger RNA: prospects of a future therapy. Curr Opin Immunol 2011;23(3):399–406.

[44] Weide B, Pascolo S, Scheel B, Derhovanessian E, Pflugfelder A, Eigentler TK, et al. Direct injection of protamine-protected mRNA: results of a phase 1/2 vaccination trial in metastatic melanoma patients. J Immunother 2009;32(5):498–507.

[45] Fotin-Mleczek M, Zanzinger K, Heidenreich R, Lorenz C, Thess A, Duchardt KM, et al. Highly potent mRNA based cancer vaccines represent an attractive platform for combination therapies supporting an improved therapeutic effect. J Gene Med 2012.

[46] Sebastian M, von Boehmer L, Zippelius A, Mayer F, Reck M, Atanackovic D, et al. Messenger RNA vaccination in NSCLC: Findings from a phase I/IIa clinical trial. ASCO Meeting Abstracts 2011;29(15_suppl):2584.

[47] Kubler H, Maurer T, Stenzl A, Feyerabend S, Steiner U, Schostak M, et al. Final analysis of a phase I/IIa study with CV9103, an intradermally administered prostate cancer immunotherapy based on self-adjuvanted mRNA. ASCO Meeting Abstracts 2011;29(15_suppl):4535.

[48] Yang R, Murillo FM, Delannoy MJ, Blosser RL, WHt Yutzy, Uematsu S, et al. B lymphocyte activation by human papillomavirus-like particles directly induces Ig class switch recombination via TLR4-MyD88. J Immunol 2005;174(12):7912–9.

[49] Yan M, Peng J, Jabbar IA, Liu X, Filgueira L, Frazer IH, et al. Activation of dendritic cells by human papillomavirus-like particles through TLR4 and NF-kappaB-mediated signalling, moderated by TGF-beta. Immunol Cell Biol 2005;83(1):83–91.

[50] Einstein MH, Baron M, Levin MJ, Chatterjee A, Fox B, Scholar S, et al. Comparative immunogenicity and safety of human papillomavirus (HPV)-16/18 vaccine and HPV-6/11/16/18 vaccine: follow-up from months 12-24 in a Phase III randomized study of healthy women aged 18-45 years. Hum Vaccin 2011;7(12):1343–58.

[51] Pumpens P, Grens E. HBV core particles as a carrier for B cell/T cell epitopes. Intervirology 2001;44(2-3):98–114.

[52] Schodel F, Moriarty AM, Peterson DL, Zheng JA, Hughes JL, Will H, et al. The position of heterologous epitopes inserted in hepatitis B virus core particles determines their immunogenicity. J Virol 1992;66(1):106–14.

[53] Klamp T, Schumacher J, Huber G, Kuhne C, Meissner U, Selmi A, et al. Highly specific auto-antibodies against claudin-18 isoform 2 induced by a chimeric HBcAg virus-like particle vaccine kill tumor cells and inhibit the growth of lung metastases. Cancer Res 2011;71(2):516–27.

[54] Porta C, Lomonossoff GP. Scope for using plant viruses to present epitopes from animal pathogens. Rev Med Virol 1998;8(1):25–41.

[55] Staczek J, Bendahmane M, Gilleland LB, Beachy RN, Gilleland Jr HE. Immunization with a chimeric tobacco mosaic virus containing an epitope of outer membrane protein F of Pseudomonas aeruginosa provides protection against challenge with P. aeruginosa. Vaccine 2000;18(21):2266–74.

[56] Dalsgaard K, Uttenthal A, Jones TD, Xu F, Merryweather A, Hamilton WD, et al. Plant-derived vaccine protects target animals against a viral disease. Nat Biotechnol 1997;15(3):248–52.

[57] Palmer KE, Benko A, Doucette SA, Cameron TI, Foster T, Hanley KM, et al. Protection of rabbits against cutaneous papillomavirus infection using recombinant tobacco mosaic virus containing L2 capsid epitopes. Vaccine 2006;24(26):5516–25.

[58] Cruz SS, Chapman S, Roberts AG, Roberts IM, Prior DA, Oparka KJ. Assembly and movement of a plant virus carrying a green fluorescent protein overcoat. Proc Natl Acad Sci U S A 1996;93(13):6286–90.

[59] Werner S, Marillonnet S, Hause G, Klimyuk V, Gleba Y. Immunoabsorbent nanoparticles based on a tobamovirus displaying protein A. Proc Natl Acad Sci U S A 2006;103(47):17678–83.

[60] Li Q, Jiang L, Li M, Li P, Zhang Q, Song R, et al. Morphology and stability changes of recombinant TMV particles caused by a cysteine residue in the foreign peptide fused to the coat protein. J Virol Methods 2007;140(1-2):212–7.

[61] Lico C, Capuano F, Renzone G, Donini M, Marusic C, Scaloni A, et al. Peptide display on Potato virus X: molecular features of the coat protein-fused peptide affecting cell-to-cell and phloem movement of chimeric virus particles. J Gen Virol 2006;87(Pt 10):3103–12.

[62] Frolova OY, Petrunia IV, Komarova TV, Kosorukov VS, Sheval EV, Gleba YY, et al. Trastuzumab-binding peptide display by Tobacco mosaic virus. Virology 2010;407(1):7–13.

[63] Jagadish MN, Hamilton RC, Fernandez CS, Schoofs P, Davern KM, Kalnins H, et al. High level production of hybrid potyvirus-like particles carrying repetitive copies of foreign antigens in Escherichia coli. Biotechnology (N Y) 1993;11(10):1166–70.

[64] Denis J, Majeau N, Acosta-Ramirez E, Savard C, Bedard MC, Simard S, et al. Immunogenicity of papaya mosaic virus-like particles fused to a hepatitis C virus epitope: evidence for the critical function of multimerization. Virology 2007;363(1):59–68.

[65] Diebold SS. Recognition of viral single-stranded RNA by Toll-like receptors. Adv Drug Deliv Rev 2008;60(7):813–23.

[66] Jarrossay D, Napolitani G, Colonna M, Sallusto F, Lanzavecchia A. Specialization and complementarity in microbial molecule recognition by human myeloid and plasmacytoid dendritic cells. Eur J Immunol 2001;31(11):3388–93.

[67] Heil F, Hemmi H, Hochrein H, Ampenberger F, Kirschning C, Akira S, et al. Species-specific recognition of single-stranded RNA via toll-like receptor 7 and 8. Science 2004;303(5663):1526–9.

[68] Bendandi M, Marillonnet S, Kandzia R, Thieme F, Nickstadt A, Herz S, et al. Rapid, high-yield production in plants of individualized idiotype vaccines for non-Hodgkin's lymphoma. Ann Oncol 2010;21(12):2420–7.

[69] Weiner LM, Surana R, Wang S. Monoclonal antibodies: versatile platforms for cancer immunotherapy. Nat Rev Immunol 2010;10(5):317–27.

[70] Kern F, LiPira G, Gratama JW, Manca F, Roederer M. Measuring Ag-specific immune responses: understanding immunopathogenesis and improving diagnostics in infectious disease, autoimmunity and cancer. Trends Immunol 2005;26(9):477–84.

[71] Nakaya HI, Wrammert J, Lee EK, Racioppi L, Marie-Kunze S, Haining WN, et al. Systems biology of vaccination for seasonal influenza in humans. Nat Immunol 2011;12(8):786–95.

[72] Seder RA, Darrah PA, Roederer M. T-cell quality in memory and protection: implications for vaccine design. Nat Rev Immunol 2008;8(4):247–58.

[73] Appay V, Douek DC, Price DA. CD8+ T cell efficacy in vaccination and disease. Nat Med 2008;14(6):623–8.

[74] Betts MR, Nason MC, West SM, De Rosa SC, Migueles SA, Abraham J, et al. HIV nonprogressors preferentially maintain highly functional HIV-specific CD8+ T cells. Blood 2006;107(12):4781–9.

[75] Kannanganat S, Kapogiannis BG, Ibegbu C, Chennareddi L, Goepfert P, Robinson HL, et al. Human immunodeficiency virus type 1 controllers but not noncontrollers maintain CD4 T cells coexpressing three cytokines. J Virol 2007;81(21):12071–6.

[76] Darrah PA, Patel DT, De Luca PM, Lindsay RW, Davey DF, Flynn BJ, et al. Multifunctional TH1 cells define a correlate of vaccine-mediated protection against Leishmania major. Nat Med 2007;13(7):843–50.

[77] Burgers WA, Chege GK, Muller TL, van Harmelen JH, Khoury G, Shephard EG, et al. Broad, high-magnitude and multifunctional CD4+ and CD8+ T-cell responses elicited by a DNA and modified vaccinia Ankara vaccine containing human immunodeficiency virus type 1 subtype C genes in baboons. J Gen Virol 2009;90(Pt 2):468–80.

[78] Harari A, Bart PA, Stohr W, Tapia G, Garcia M, Medjitna-Rais E, et al. An HIV-1 clade C DNA prime, NYVAC boost vaccine regimen induces reliable, polyfunctional, and long-lasting T cell responses. J Exp Med 2008;205(1):63–77.

[79] Churchyard GJ, Morgan C, Adams E, Hural J, Graham BS, Moodie Z, et al. A phase IIA randomized clinical trial of a multiclade HIV-1 DNA prime followed by a multiclade rAd5 HIV-1 vaccine boost in healthy adults (HVTN204). PLoS One 2011;6(8):e21225.

[80] Goonetilleke N, Moore S, Dally L, Winstone N, Cebere I, Mahmoud A, et al. Induction of multifunctional human immunodeficiency virus type 1 (HIV-1)-specific T cells capable of proliferation in healthy subjects by using a prime-boost regimen of DNA- and modified vaccinia virus Ankara-vectored vaccines expressing HIV-1 Gag coupled to CD8+ T-cell epitopes. J Virol 2006;80(10):4717–28.

[81] Bansal A, Jackson B, West K, Wang S, Lu S, Kennedy JS, et al. Multifunctional T-cell characteristics induced by a polyvalent DNA prime/protein boost human immunodeficiency virus type 1 vaccine regimen given to healthy adults are dependent on the route and dose of administration. J Virol 2008;82(13):6458–69.

[82] Ramstad A, Romstad AB, Knappskog DH, Midtlyng PJ. Field validation of experimental challenge models for IPN vaccines. Journal of fish diseases 2007;30(12):723–31.

[83] Ledgerwood JE, Pierson TC, Hubka SA, Desai N, Rucker S, Gordon IJ, et al. A West Nile virus DNA vaccine utilizing a modified promoter induces neutralizing antibody in younger and older healthy adults in a phase I clinical trial. J Infect Dis 2011;203(10):1396–404.

[84] USDA licenses DNA vaccine for treatment of melanoma in dogs. J Am Vet Med Assoc 2010;236(5):495.

[85] Manley CA, Leibman NF, Wolchok JD, Riviere IC, Bartido S, Craft DM, et al. Xenogeneic murine tyrosinase DNA vaccine for malignant melanoma of the digit of dogs. J Vet Intern Med 2011;25(1):94–9.

[86] Vasan S, Hurley A, Schlesinger SJ, Hannaman D, Gardiner DF, Dugin DP, et al. In vivo electroporation enhances the immunogenicity of an HIV-1 DNA vaccine candidate in healthy volunteers. PLoS ONE 2011;6(5):e19252.

[87] Sardesai NY, Weiner DB. Electroporation delivery of DNA vaccines: prospects for success. Curr Opin Immunol 2011;23(3):421–9.

[88] Dolter KE, Evans CF, Ellefsen B, Song J, Boente-Carrera M, Vittorino R, et al. Immunogenicity, safety, biodistribution and persistence of ADVAX, a prophylactic DNA vaccine for HIV-1, delivered by in vivo electroporation. Vaccine 2011;29(4):795–803.

[89] Ramirez K, Barry EM, Ulmer J, Stout R, Szabo J, Manetz S, et al. Preclinical safety and biodistribution of Sindbis virus measles DNA vaccines administered as a single dose or followed by live attenuated measles vaccine in a heterologous prime-boost regimen. Hum Gene Ther 2008;19(5):522–31.

[90] Fioretti D, Iurescia S, Fazio VM, Rinaldi M. DNA vaccines: developing new strategies against cancer. J Biomed Biotechnol 2010;2010:174378.

[91] Parkhurst MR, Yang JC, Langan RC, Dudley ME, Nathan DA, Feldman SA, et al. T Cells Targeting Carcinoembryonic Antigen Can Mediate Regression of Metastatic Colorectal Cancer but Induce Severe Transient Colitis. Mol Ther 2011.

[92] Bos R, van Duikeren S, Morreau H, Franken K, Schumacher TN, Haanen JB, et al. Balancing between antitumor efficacy and autoimmune pathology in T-cell-mediated targeting of carcinoembryonic antigen. Cancer Res 2008;68(20):8446–55.

[93] Ottensmeier CH, Mander A, McCann K, Low L, Hall E, Bateman A, et al. Clinical and immunological responses to a DNA fusion vaccine in patients with carcinoembryonic antigen-expressing tumors: A Cancer Research UK phase I/II study. ASCO Meeting Abstracts 2010;28(15_suppl):2579.

[94] Tsang KY, Zaremba S, Nieroda CA, Zhu MZ, Hamilton JM, Schlom J. Generation of human cytotoxic T cells specific for human carcinoembryonic antigen epitopes from patients immunized with recombinant vaccinia-CEA vaccine. J Natl Cancer Inst 1995;87(13):982–90.

[95] Hodi FS, O'Day SJ, McDermott DF, Weber RW, Sosman JA, Haanen JB, et al. Improved survival with ipilimumab in patients with metastatic melanoma. N Engl J Med 2010;363(8):711–23.

[96] Davis HL, Millan CL, Watkins SC. Immune-mediated destruction of transfected muscle fibers after direct gene transfer with antigen-expressing plasmid DNA. Gene Ther 1997;4(3):181–8.

[97] McNeel DG, Dunphy EJ, Davies JG, Frye TP, Johnson LE, Staab MJ, et al. Safety and immunological efficacy of a DNA vaccine encoding prostatic acid phosphatase in patients with stage D0 prostate cancer. J Clin Oncol 2009;27(25):4047–54.

[98] Mincheff M, Zoubak S, Makogonenko Y. Immune responses against PSMA after gene-based vaccination for immunotherapy-A: results from immunizations in animals. Cancer gene therapy 2006;13(4):436–44.

[99] Mincheff M, Tchakarov S, Zoubak S, Loukinov D, Botev C, Altankova I, et al. Naked DNA and adenoviral immunizations for immunotherapy of prostate cancer: a phase I/II clinical trial. Eur Urol 2000;38(2):208–17.

[100] Gregor PD, Wolchok JD, Turaga V, Latouche JB, Sadelain M, Bacich D, et al. Induction of autoantibodies to syngeneic prostate-specific membrane antigen by xenogeneic vaccination. Int J Cancer 2005;116(3):415–21.

[101] Doehn C, Bohmer T, Kausch I, Sommerauer M, Jocham D. Prostate cancer vaccines: current status and future potential. BioDrugs 2008;22(2):71–84.

[102] Roos AK, Pavlenko M, Charo J, Egevad L, Pisa P. Induction of PSA-specific CTLs and anti-tumor immunity by a genetic prostate cancer vaccine. Prostate 2005;62(3):217–23.

[103] Galea I, Stasakova J, Dunscombe MS, Ottensmeier CH, Elliott T, Thirdborough SM. CD8(+) T-cell cross-competition is governed by peptide-MHC class I stability. European journal of immunology 2011.

[104] Bartholdy C, Stryhn A, Christensen JP, Thomsen AR. Single-epitope DNA vaccination prevents exhaustion and facilitates a broad antiviral CD8+ T cell response during chronic viral infection. J Immunol 2004;173(10):6284–93.

[105] Chaise C, Buchan SL, Rice J, Marquet J, Rouard H, Kuentz M, et al. DNA vaccination induces WT1-specific T-cell responses with potential clinical relevance. Blood 2008;112(7):2956–64.

[106] Antony PA, Piccirillo CA, Akpinarli A, Finkelstein SE, Speiss PJ, Surman DR, et al. CD8+ T cell immunity against a tumor/self-antigen is augmented by CD4+ T helper cells and hindered by naturally occurring T regulatory cells. J Immunol 2005;174(5):2591−601.

[107] Disis ML. Immune regulation of cancer. Journal of Clinical Oncology 2010;28(29):4531−8.

[108] van der Burg SH, Piersma SJ, de Jong A, van der Hulst JM, Kwappenberg KM, van den Hende M, et al. Association of cervical cancer with the presence of CD4+ regulatory T cells specific for human papillomavirus antigens. Proc Natl Acad Sci U S A 2007;104(29):12087−92.

[109] Rosenberg SA, Yang JC, Restifo NP. Cancer immunotherapy: moving beyond current vaccines. Nat Med 2004;10(9):909−15.

[110] Schwartzentruber DJ, Lawson DH, Richards JM, Conry RM, Miller DM, Treisman J, et al. gp100 peptide vaccine and interleukin-2 in patients with advanced melanoma. The New England journal of medicine 2011;364(22):2119−27.

[111] Kantoff PW, Higano CS, Shore ND, Berger ER, Small EJ, Penson DF, et al. Sipuleucel-T immunotherapy for castration-resistant prostate cancer. N Engl J Med 2011;363(5):411−22.

[112] Quoix E, Ramlau R, Westeel V, Papai Z, Madroszyk A, Riviere A, et al. Therapeutic vaccination with TG4010 and first-line chemotherapy in advanced non-small-cell lung cancer: a controlled phase 2B trial. Lancet Oncol 2011;12(12):1125−33.

[113] Mayer F, Mayer-Mokler A, Nowara E, Torday L, Ludwig J, Kuttruff S, et al. A phase I/II trial of the multipeptide cancer vaccine IMA910 in patients with advanced colorectal cancer (CRC). ASCO Meeting Abstracts 2012;30(4_suppl):555.

[114] Schuster SJ, Neelapu SS, Gause BL, Muggia FM, Gockerman JP, Sotomayor EM, et al. Idiotype vaccine therapy (BiovaxID) in follicular lymphoma in first complete remission: Phase III clinical trial results. ASCO Meeting Abstracts 2009;27(18S):2.

[115] Decoster L, Wauters I, Vansteenkiste JF. Vaccination therapy for non-small-cell lung cancer: review of agents in phase III development. Ann Oncol 2011.

[116] Hoos A, Parmiani G, Hege K, Sznol M, Loibner H, Eggermont A, et al. A clinical development paradigm for cancer vaccines and related biologics. J Immunother 2007;30(1):1−15.

[117] Therasse P, Arbuck SG, Eisenhauer EA, Wanders J, Kaplan RS, Rubinstein L, et al. New guidelines to evaluate the response to treatment in solid tumors. European Organization for Research and Treatment of Cancer, National Cancer Institute of the United States, National Cancer Institute of Canada. J Natl Cancer Inst 2000;92(3):205−16.

[118] Wolchok JD, Hoos A, O'Day S, Weber JS, Hamid O, Lebbe C, et al. Guidelines for the evaluation of immune therapy activity in solid tumors: immune-related response criteria. Clin Cancer Res 2009;15(23):7412−20.

[119] Martins I, Kepp O, Schlemmer F, Adjemian S, Tailler M, Shen S, et al. Restoration of the immunogenicity of cisplatin-induced cancer cell death by endoplasmic reticulum stress. Oncogene 2011;30(10):1147−58.

[120] Tesniere A, Schlemmer F, Boige V, Kepp O, Martins I, Ghiringhelli F, et al. Immunogenic death of colon cancer cells treated with oxaliplatin. Oncogene 2010;29(4):482−91.

[121] Coleman S, Clayton A, Mason MD, Jasani B, Adams M, Tabi Z. Recovery of CD8+ T-cell function during systemic chemotherapy in advanced ovarian cancer. Cancer Res 2005;65(15):7000−6.

[122] Arlen PM, Gulley JL, Parker C, Skarupa L, Pazdur M, Panicali D, et al. A randomized phase II study of concurrent docetaxel plus vaccine versus vaccine alone in metastatic androgen-independent prostate cancer. Clin Cancer Res 2006;12(4):1260−9.

[123] Ghiringhelli F, Menard C, Puig PE, Ladoire S, Roux S, Martin F, et al. Metronomic cyclophosphamide regimen selectively depletes CD4+CD25+ regulatory T cells and restores T and NK effector functions in end stage cancer patients. Cancer Immunol Immunother 2007;56(5):641−8.

[124] Comin-Anduix B, Chodon T, Sazegar H, Matsunaga D, Mock S, Jalil J, et al. The oncogenic BRAF kinase inhibitor PLX4032/RG7204 does not affect the viability or function of human lymphocytes across a wide range of concentrations. Clin Cancer Res 2010;16(24):6040−8.

[125] Hipp MM, Hilf N, Walter S, Werth D, Brauer KM, Radsak MP, et al. Sorafenib, but not sunitinib, affects function of dendritic cells and induction of primary immune responses. Blood 2008;111(12):5610−20.

[126] Mocellin S, Mandruzzato S, Bronte V, Marincola FM. Cancer vaccines: pessimism in check. Nat Med 2004;10(12):1278−9. author reply 9−80.

[127] Gray A, Raff AB, Chiriva-Internati M, Chen SY, Kast WM. A paradigm shift in therapeutic vaccination of cancer patients: the need to apply therapeutic vaccination strategies in the preventive setting. Immunol Rev 2008;222:316−27.

[128] Gulley JL, Madan RA, Schlom J. Impact of tumor volume on the potential efficacy of therapeutic vaccines. Curr Oncol 2011;18(3):e150−7.

[129] van der Burg SH, Kalos M, Gouttefangeas C, Janetzki S, Ottensmeier C, Welters MJ, et al. Harmonization of immune biomarker assays for clinical studies. Sci Transl Med 2011;3(108). 108ps44.

[130] Fox BA, Schendel DJ, Butterfield LH, Aamdal S, Allison JP, Ascierto PA, et al. Defining the Critical Hurdles in Cancer Immunotherapy. J Transl Med 2011;9(1):214.

[131] Mander A, Gouttefangeas C, Ottensmeier C, Welters MJ, Low L, van der Burg SH, et al. Serum is not required for ex vivo IFN-gamma ELISPOT: a collaborative study of different protocols from the European CIMT Immunoguiding Program. Cancer Immunol Immunother 2010;59(4):619–27.

[132] Britten CM, Gouttefangeas C, Welters MJ, Pawelec G, Koch S, Ottensmeier C, et al. The CIMT-monitoring panel: a two-step approach to harmonize the enumeration of antigen-specific CD8(+) T lymphocytes by structural and functional assays. Cancer Immunol Immunother 2008;57(3):289–302.

[133] Britten CM, Gouttefangeas C, Schoenmaekers-Welters MJP, Pawelec G, Koch S, Ottensmeier C, et al. The CIMT monitoring panel: enumeration of antigen-specific CD8(+) T lymphocytes by structural and functional assays. Conference on Strategies for Immune Therapy 2006:406–7. 2006 May 04-05; Mainz, GERMANY.

[134] Moodie Z, Price L, Gouttefangeas C, Mander A, Janetzki S, Lower M, et al. Response definition criteria for ELISPOT assays revisited. Cancer Immunol Immunother 2010;59(10):1489–501.

[135] Zielinski CE, Corti D, Mele F, Pinto D, Lanzavecchia A, Sallusto F. Dissecting the human immunologic memory for pathogens. Immunol Rev 2011;240(1):40–51.

[136] Di Genova G, Roddick J, McNicholl F, Stevenson FK. Vaccination of human subjects expands both specific and bystander memory T cells but antibody production remains vaccine specific. Blood 2006;107(7):2806–13.

CHAPTER 16

Comprehensive Immunomonitoring to Guide the Development of Immunotherapeutic Products for Cancer

Marij J.P. Welters, Sjoerd H. van der Burg
Experimental Cancer Immunology and Therapy Group, Department of Clinical Oncology, Leiden University Medical Center, Leiden, The Netherlands

I. IMMUNOTHERAPY OF CANCER

Immunotherapy is becoming increasingly anchored in treatment of cancer patients. This approach to cancer treatment is based on exploitation of the effector mechanisms of the immune system to prevent or combat cancer. At present, the most commonly applied form of cancer immunotherapy is so-called passive immunotherapy with monoclonal antibodies [1]. One prominent example is the anti-CD20 monoclonal antibody rituximab (trade name MabThera® from Roche and Rituxan® from Genentech/Biogen) for the treatment of non-Hodgkin's lymphoma (NHL) and B-cell leukemia. Rituximab binds to the cell surface of the tumor cells, marking them for destruction by the patient's immune cells [2]. Other monoclonal antibodies are directed against the epidermal growth factor receptor (EGFR), e.g., cetuximab, which is approved to treat head and neck cancer and colon cancer (Erbitux® from ImClone, Merck and Bristol-Myers Squibb) [3,4], and the HER2 receptor-specific antibody trastuzumab for treatment of breast cancer, both of which prevent tumor cell growth signaling through these receptors (Herceptin® from Roche) [5]. Additionally, methods to combat cancer in a more indirect fashion have been developed by blocking the soluble factor vascular endothelial growth factor (VEGF), for example, by using the VEGF-binding monoclonal antibody bevacizumab (Avastin® from Genentech/Hoffmann-LaRoche) [6,7].

More recently, antibodies have been developed that can block feedback control mechanisms in the immune system, which tumors exploit to dampen antitumor responses. Mechanistically, these antibodies prevent exploitation, by blocking negative-acting interactions between antigen-presenting cells (APCs) and T cells. The prototypical example of this approach, now being tested for a variety of immune suppressive co-regulatory T-cell receptors implicated in tumor progression, is the antibody ipilimumab (Yervoy® from Bristol-Myers Squibb) against cytotoxic T lymphocyte-associated antigen 4 (CTLA-4) [8], which releases a break on the patient's spontaneously induced tumor-specific T-cell responses. Ipilumimab was approved in 2011 by the FDA for treatment of advanced melanoma [9,10]. In a related approach, antibodies

Cancer Immunotherapy. http://dx.doi.org/10.1016/B978-0-12-394296-8.00016-6

that block the programmed death receptor 1 (PD-1), another immune suppressive co-regulatory T-cell receptor, is presently in late-stage clinical development. Chronically stimulated T cells express PD-1, which interacts with its ligand PD-L1 expressed on activated APC and some cancer cells. As a result, the function of effector T cells in the tumor milieu is inhibited, favoring tumor outgrowth [11].

In addition, an increasing number of immune-modulating agents have been approved to treat cancer. Interferon-alpha (IFNα-2a [Roferon-A® from Roche]) has been approved to treat hematological cancers (leukemia and lymphomas) and acquired immune deficiency syndrome-related Kaposi's sarcoma, as well as tested for the treatment of melanoma and kidney cancers [12–15]. Agonistic compounds to trigger innate immune responses of cells via their toll-like receptors (TLRs), such as poly-ICLC (Hiltonol® from Oncovir) [16] and poly [I]:poly [C(12)U] (Ampligen® from Hemispherx Biopharma) [17] for TLR3[18], detoxified Lipopolysaccharide (LPS) called monophosphoryl lipid A (MPL® from Corixa) for TLR4 [19,20], imiquimod (Aldara® from 3M Pharma) for TLR7 [21,22] and synthetic oligodeoxynucleotides containing unmethylated CG dinucleotides (CpG) for TLR9 [23,24] have also been studied for the treatment of various cancer types. These agents either are tested as a single treatment agent or in combination with chemotherapy or additional immuno-therapeutic modalities. For instance, CpG has been injected at a single tumor site in combination with low-dose radiotherapy at the same site in 15 patients with low-grade B-cell lymphoma, resulting in one complete regression and three partial responses [25]. In mice, CpG loaded on whole tumor cells adoptively transferred into recipients with large established lymphomas was demonstrated to cure all cases. Currently, the efficacy of this approach is determined in the treatment of mantle-cell lymphoma patients.

More recently, active immunotherapy has been developed to induce and boost adaptive immune responses, particularly T-cell responses, against tumor-associated or tumor-specific antigens. Active forms of immunotherapy are not yet embedded in clinic, but this promises to change with the first FDA approval of a vaccine to advanced prostate cancer termed sipuleucel-T (Provenge® from Dendreon). Following the lead of this agent, many different strategies of active immunotherapy to induce or reinforce tumor-specific T-cell immunity are now being tested in Phase I and II trials. As described in detail in other chapters of this book, these strategies include (i) autologous tumor cell lysate, (ii) whole tumor cell vaccines, (iii) tumor cells engineered to express certain cytokines or chemokines, (iv) dendritic cells (DC) pulsed with antigen or engineered to do so (v) DNA vaccines, (vi) recombinant viral vector vaccines, (vii) recombinant proteins, and (viii) peptide vaccines [26–31]. Additionally, there are trials for adoptive transfer of *ex vivo* expanded autologous tumor-specific T cells that express a tumor-specific receptor or are engineered to do so. In this approach, small numbers of tumor-specific T cells are expanded in the laboratory, free from endogenous inhibitory factors, and then transferred into a patient, who has been manipulated to provide an optimal environment for the transferred cells to exert their tumor-rejecting function [32–36].

We have studied synthetic long peptides (SLP vaccines) as a vaccine strategy. In our own trials in human papillomavirus type 16 (HPV16)-induced cancers, colorectal cancer and ovarian cancer, we have shown that SLP vaccines are highly immunogenic, even in patients with end-stage cancer [37–43]. Clinical success was obtained in patients with high-grade dysplastic vulvar lesions vaccinated with the SLP vaccine directed against the HPV16 oncoproteins E6 and E7. Notably, complete regression of vulvar lesions was correlated with a strong and broad T-cell response to these antigens, whereas failure of the vaccine to induce a clinical response was associated with the increase in HPV16-specific CD4+CD25+Foxp3+ T cells [40,41]. In another strategy to improve T-cell responses, melanoma patients were subjected to lymphodepletion regimens before *ex vivo* expanded tumor-specific T cells were infused, resulting in impressive objective clinical response rates of up to 80% [30,35,44]. More recently, clinical success was reported in the treatment of chronic lymphoid leukemia by adoptively transferring *ex vivo* manipulated T cells, which were genetically engineered to express chimeric antigen receptors (CARs) specific for CD19 and connected to domains that activate these modified T cells [45−47]. The engineered T cells expanded >1000-fold *in vivo*, homed to the bone marrow and expressed the CARs for at least 6 months. A portion of these cells developed into CAR-positive memory T cells which retained their anti-CD19 effector function [47−49]. Now that the use of immune modulating agents is beginning to demonstrate strong benefits in patients, it is high time to better understand and monitor their underlying mechanisms of action. This is the purpose of immunomonitoring, which is rapidly growing in importance with the growing interest and ongoing progress in cancer immunotherapy.

II. IMMUNOMONITORING

Cancer immunotherapy takes an indirect approach to disease management by targeting the patient's immune system. Therefore, the study of the patient's immune response to such treatment is an essential component of immunotherapy trials. This analysis is typically accomplished through various laboratory assays to measure differences in the number and activity of specific immune parameters before, during, and after treatment. If performed adequately, immunological monitoring will lead to the identification of biomarkers serving as surrogate endpoints for clinical efficacy. The type and number of assays are likely to differ between the type of treatment and phase of the trial. They can be focused on measurements of the treatment's expected mechanism of action, but may also comprise broader, more comprehensive biomarker studies that capture as much information about general treatment-related immune modulation and patient-specific data to provide insights about the treatment response [50−52]. In the end, a more comprehensive strategy may allow the identification of immune signatures as measures of biological activity, treatment efficacy or toxicity, thereby playing a role in selecting patient populations and establishing surrogate endpoints for clinical efficacy.

In some cases, immunomonitoring of therapy-induced changes can be quite straightforward and totally focused on the mechanism of action. For instance, the efficacy of rituximab used to treat patients with B-cell lymphoma is readily measured by a decrease in the number of B cells in the blood [2]. It becomes more difficult when the therapy consists of the infusion of antibodies against the epidermal growth factor receptor (EGFR) expressed at the tumor cell surface (e.g., colon or lung cancer). The principal mechanism of action is the inhibition of ligand-induced EGFR activation but some of them (Cetuximab®) are also expected to induce antibody-dependent cell cytotoxicity (ADCC) by recruitment of immune effector cells that become activated via their Fc-gamma receptors (e.g., NK cells) [53]. Here, immunomonitoring would require showing the binding of antibody to the tumor cells of the patient as well as the attraction of these immune effector cells to the tumor [54−56]. In such cases, although it is clear what should be studied, it can prove challenging in practice to obtain samples to do this.

Another example is the treatment of melanoma patients with the CTLA-4 targeting antibody ipilimumab. Mouse models revealed that CTLA-4 is inducibly expressed on activated effector CD4+ and CD8+ T cells as well as constitutively expressed on a subset of regulatory T cells (Tregs). To obtain a maximal antitumor effect, the immune system requires concomitant activation of effector T cells and blockade of Tregs [10]. Based on the expected mechanism of action, one would like to measure the increase in the number and function of the total melanoma-specific T-cell population in the patients treated with such an antibody. Although such analyses can be performed for selected antigens [57], it is quite challenging in view of the many different antigens that form targets for the immune system in melanoma. Whereas new techniques have been developed that in principal allow to measure responses against many different antigens [40,41,58,59], either the amount of blood that can be taken, the limitation in the number of human leukocyte antigen (HLA)-restriction elements that can be analyzed, or both will prohibit scientists from analyzing the full spectrum of T-cell responses that are modulated by treatment and as such the translation of such reactivity into appropriate surrogate biomarkers. Therefore, more general measurements such as an increase in the absolute lymphocyte count or the expression of activation markers by T cells in the blood, in particular that of inducible co-stimulator (ICOS) for recent activation or HLA-DR as a late activation marker, have been found retrospectively as biomarkers in the CTLA-4 antibody early phase clinical trials [10,60]. However, validation of these biomarkers in a prospective randomized trial is still warranted and the next step to be undertaken.

Others have studied the frequency of intratumoral CD8+ T cells and Foxp3+ T cells in pre- and post-treatment tumor biopsies [61,62]. Similar problems will be encountered in monitoring of the full spectrum of tumor-specific T-cell responses during adoptive T-cell transfer therapies based on *ex vivo* expanded tumor-infiltrating lymphocyte (TIL) populations. Here one would like to know the actual number of tumor-specific T cells in the product, their specificities, their functionality and their *in vivo* behavior after infusion. Except for those cases for which an autologous tumor cell line was generated in the laboratory [36], it will be impossible to measure total tumor reactivity either in the infused product or in the blood of patients post-treatment. Notably, a recent large screen of the specificity of TIL populations showed that T-cell reactivity against the majority of known T-cell epitopes was of low frequency and, moreover, that the frequencies of these tumor-specific T cells decreased during the rapid expansion of TILs [58]. Therefore, monitoring of more general surrogate markers such as the percentage of CD8+CD27+ T cells and the telomere length of the T cells was determined in the T-cell product [34,63]. As one would like to know whether these cells survive and expand in the patient as well as whether they are able to migrate into the patient's tumor, a comparison of T-cell receptor clonotypes in the infused TIL population and the blood post-treatment has been performed [34,35]. In the setting that autologous tumor cells are available it is far easier to measure the percentage of tumor-specific T cells in the product or blood of patients by stimulation of peripheral blood mononuclear cells (PBMCs) with these tumor cells and the measurement of activated T cells by flow cytometry [36], albeit that their specificity will remain unknown.

Immunomonitoring of vaccine-based immunotherapeutic approaches should be relatively simple, in particular when well-defined tumor antigens are used. Animal tumor models and studies on the spontaneous local antitumor response revealed that tumor-specific T cells, in particular the T helper type 1 (Th1) cells and the cytotoxic T lymphocytes (CTL), are important in controlling the growth of tumors [64−66]. Therefore, as a first step to determine vaccine efficacy, the response of circulating T cells to the vaccine can be measured [67,68]. The choice of assays is fairly simple, albeit dependent on the vaccine type tested, but it is recommended to use at least two assays in parallel, preferably one structural (i.e., quantitative) and one functional assay [69−72]. Prime examples are the ELISPOT assay [73−75], intracellular cytokine staining (ICS) [76,77], Major Histocompatibility Complex (MHC)-peptide multimer staining [78] and proliferation assays [79]. The immunomonitoring of the T-cell responses induced by vaccines able to trigger both CD4+ and CD8+ T cells to a broad number of epitopes (multi-peptide vaccines, proteins, DNA, recombinant viral vector vaccines, DC vaccines) may require the use of a number of complementary assays and as such relatively high volumes of blood, which sometimes are not available or otherwise precludes its use for other types of measurements. In a large number of cases, the response to one or a few well-known T-cell epitopes has been used as a measurement of vaccine efficacy, but the results never correlated with clinical outcome, partly because in these studies the clinical response rates were low [80−85]. Based on our own studies on the immunotherapy of HPV-induced diseases we recommend a full analysis of the response to all potential epitopes as in our case a strong and broad T-cell response was correlated with clinical success whereas a narrow T-cell response was not [38,41]. Although, this analysis required large numbers of PBMCs in each assay, the near future will bring some relief as the current trend in the field of immunological monitoring is toward micronized assays that allow a more comprehensive analysis of T-cell reactivity per sample. For example, multi-parametric flow cytometry-based approaches enable comprehensive phenotyping and functional assessment of T cells [59,86–91]. Another method to gain as much as possible information about T-cell reactivity constitutes the stimulation of PBMCs with overlapping peptide pools of defined antigens to simultaneously analyze functionally activated CD4+ and CD8+ T cells both by IFNγ ELISPOT assay and by ICS in flow cytometry [39,40,42,43,92–95]. Whilst the protocols used to detect antigen-specific T-cell responses generally involve prestimulation protocols and may not be suitable to simultaneously detect antigen-specific CD4+ and CD8+ T cells directly *ex vivo* in cryopreserved samples, new optimized protocols have started to surface that allow the *ex vivo* detection of low-frequency antigen-specific T cells in cryopreserved PBMCs and can be applied to evaluate clinical trials [96]. An old but still useful method to detect low-frequency tumor-specific T cells *in vivo* are delayed hypersensitivity (DTH) tests, albeit a bit different from the old days [97]. Recently, it was shown that the presence of antigen-specific infiltrating T cells cultured from a biopsy from the DTH site, rather than induration of the DTH site itself—a more classical measurement of DTH—correlated with improved progression-free survival after immunotherapy [98–100]. Similarly, one may use the inflamed vaccine site itself to test for the presence of antigen-specific immune cells [41,101]. However, the promise that immunomonitoring will identify biomarkers, as surrogate endpoints for clinical efficacy in immunotherapeutic trials to restore and reinforce tumor-specific T-cell responses, has yet to be fulfilled. Recent data suggest that clinical reactivity is associated with absolute lymphocyte counts after CTLA-4 antibody treatment [102], elevated levels of IFNγ–responsive cytokines and the expansion of antigen-specific infused cells [47] or vaccine-induced T cells [38,41]. A low clinical efficacy of the tested treatments [26,31,103,104] or the induction of potential T-cell reactions against unknown antigens [34,105] makes it difficult to correlate T-cell reactivity to the clinical outcome in many of the studies. Further explanations for this difficulty are discussed below.

III. MONITORING OF UNWANTED IMMUNE REACTIONS

In the preclinical phase of development, nearly all novel immunotherapeutic regimens are studied in murine models of cancer where the efficacy of the treatment modality is defined typically by growth delay or eradication of the tumor. Depending on the immunotherapeutic compound, different immunological parameters—generally comprising the presence and function of tumor-specific T cells—are measured in blood, lymph nodes and/or tumor biopsies. However, in contrast to what is found in the human setting, responsiveness in mouse models often is correlated with the measured immune response. In the vast majority of these models, tumors are established by injecting relative high numbers of *in vitro* cultured tumor cells, which subsequently need only 1–2 weeks to grow to form a palpable tumor. Thus, the disease period in the models is relatively short and hardly representative of the development of cancers in patients, where detectable tumor masses develop far more slowly. Tumor growth in patients is a long multi-step process in which cells of the innate immune system are attracted to support tumor growth by their production of growth and angiogenic factors. In addition, variable proportions of tumor-promoting and tumor-antagonizing T cells are attracted. During this process the immunogenicity of the tumor evolves in a manner that can promote its escape from the immune system [65,106–108]. In parallel, the immune response also can become altered, due to chronic stimulation leading to exhaustion or to development of an immune-suppressing microenvironmental milieu shaped by the growing tumor. To a significant degree, such alterations may influence the expression of inhibitory receptors on T cells, e.g., programmed death-1 (PD-1), T cell immunoglobulin mucin-3 (TIM-3), B- and T-lymphocyte attenuator (BTLA) [109–112], along with an impaired effector function of these cells, thwarting the Th1/CTL response towards a Th2 response, the attraction and/or induction of Tregs and different types of myeloid cells that can suppress local immunity [113–119]. Nevertheless, such interactions between immune cells along with the interplay with the tumor can also systematically be studied in (transplantable) murine tumor models, which makes them still indispensable for the investigation of immune mechanism [120,121].

In many studies on the interaction between tumors and the immune system, it has been shown that the balance between tumor-promoting immune cells and tumor-antagonizing T cells bears impact on the prognosis of patients [122–127]. Therefore, it is safe to assume that the presence of tumor-promoting immune cells in the tumor and blood may also determine the efficacy of immunotherapeutic approaches. In advanced melanoma, a high frequency of Tregs correlated with general impaired T-cell responsiveness to recall antigens [128], suggesting that these patients are not able to mount effective tumor immunity anymore. Indeed, the ability to respond to an NY-ESO-1 vaccine depended on the frequency of Tregs [129]. Similarly, higher frequencies of Tregs were found to negatively influence the outcome of immunotherapy in renal cell cancer and HPV-induced cancer [130,131]. Furthermore, it turns out that many of the tumor-associated antigens not only form targets for the effector T-cell population but also targets for so-called adaptive Tregs. Different adaptive Tregs have been described so far, some of which do not express Foxp3 [132,133]. Studies in colorectal cancer, melanoma, leukemia, oropharyngeal and cervical cancers have identified a number of cancer-associated antigens that are recognized by adaptive Tregs as well as showed that such Tregs influence T-cell activity in an antigen-selective manner [134–141]. Notably, mouse studies reported that vaccination may enhance the number of tumor-specific Tregs, which then curtail the protective function of vaccine-induced effector cells [142,143]. Also in recent clinical studies, vaccination resulted in the expansion of Tregs [144], some of which were specific to the injected antigen (e.g., MAGE-A3, HPV16 E6 and E7 oncoproteins) [40,41,145]. As the balance between these tumor-promoting Tregs and the tumor-antagonizing effector T cells may bear impact on the clinical outcome of patients, it is clear that monitoring of both components of the immune system will help explain the measured immunological and clinical efficacy of a vaccine.

Our own work on the immune response to HPV-induced diseases clearly illustrates the process of immune response alteration during the development of cancer and its impact on immunotherapy. In healthy individuals, who are protected against HPV-induced disease, over 60% display a broad HPV16-specific T-cell response with a mixed type 1 and 2 cytokine profile [146]. In contrast, less than half of the patients with HPV16-induced cervical cancer displayed HPV16-specific T-cell immunity [147–149]. These responses were weak and poorly polarized toward type 1 immunity as determined by a proliferation assay and cytokine analysis of antigen-stimulated PBMCs. Notably, HPV-induced cancers are preceded by clear premalignant phases of increasing intraepithelial neoplasia that are already associated with decreased immune responsiveness [140,150]. Furthermore, in both the premalignant and cancer phase of HPV-induced disease HPV-specific Tregs could be detected [139,140]. These Tregs specifically inhibited the function of effector T cells when stimulated with cognate antigen [138]. In an attempt to reinforce the immune response to HPV16 in these patients, they were injected with a highly immunogenic HPV16 E6 and E7 synthetic overlapping peptide vaccine. In a small therapeutic vaccination study in cervical cancer patients, the vaccine was able to trigger HPV16-specific effector T cells in all patients. However, in two patients with a recurrence of disease during the trial also an increase in HPV16-specific CD4+ CD25+FoxP3+ T cells was found [40], suggesting a vaccine enhanced response of HPV16-specific Tregs.

The results of our vaccination trial in 20 patients with HPV16-induced high-grade premalignant lesions of the vulva (vulvar intraepithelial neoplasia grade 3, VIN3) were even more instructive in this respect. After vaccination about half of the patients with HPV16+ VIN3 displayed a complete regression of the lesion. The size of the lesion at the start of the trial was correlated with clinical outcome. Relatively smaller lesions completely regressed whereas larger lesions displayed only a partial regression or did not show a clinical response at all [38]. Analyses of the immune response revealed a strong and broad type 1 T-cell response in patients with a relatively smaller lesion. Notably, patients with larger lesions displayed a significantly lower and more restricted type 1 T-cell response. Moreover, patients with larger lesions displayed a significant increase in the frequency of HPV16-specific CD4+CD25+Foxp3+ T cells in their blood. This was not found in the group of patients with relatively smaller lesions [41]. The negative impact of Tregs on the immunotherapy of cancer has been acknowledged in the treatment of melanoma patients, where the use of drugs to deplete or suppress the Tregs is extensively studied in combination with peptide vaccination or DC therapy [151–154]. Importantly, vaccination should result not only in the induction or boosting of a proper tumor antigen-specific T-cell reactivity, i.e., type 1 T-cell immunity, but these vaccine-induced T cells also need to travel from the blood circulation into the tumor and this is certainly not always the case. This is demonstrated clearly in vaccinated melanoma patients where vaccine-induced CD8+ T cells were detected in the blood but not in the tumor [155]. The lack of tumor infiltration may be determined by the status of the tumor microenvironment [156–160]. In our vaccination trial we observed a patient with a partial response in whom a strongly enhanced type 1 and type 2 HPV16-specific CD4+ T-cell response was detected in the blood, whereas only the type 2 cytokine producing HPV16-specific CD4+ T cells were found to be present in the lesion [41], suggesting that the microenvironment of the lesion preferably attracted Th2 cells. Thus, in order to gain a better understanding of both the immunological and clinical outcomes of T-cell based immunotherapeutic modalities in patients one would like to measure the whole population of vaccine-specific T cells in the blood, and when possible also locally at the tumor site in order to determine whether the vaccine-induced T cells migrated into the tumor tissue [161].

Once the T cells have entered the tumor environment they have to overcome the blockades imposed on their function [162]. For instance, other immune cells in the tumor environment may suppress these T cells. In many tumor types, the presence of tumor-associated macrophages (TAMs) is inversely correlated with clinical outcome of the patient [163–166]. TAMs are generally called M2 macrophages, which produce anti-inflammatory cytokines and support the cancer cells in their survival, expansion and metastasis [115,167–171]. M2 macrophages do not support T-cell reactivity but rather hamper it [172–174]. Another example is the myeloid-derived suppressor cell (MDSC), which also hampers the function of effector T cell [117,119,175–177]. However, in some cases M1 macrophages can be present in the tumor tissue and outnumber the counterpart macrophage type M2 [167,168,178,179]. M1 macrophages drive a proinflammatory response by presenting antigen to T cells in a stimulatory context associated with production of IL-12 and other stimulatory cytokines [116,180]. Interestingly, myeloid cells retain their capacity to switch phenotypes. M2 macrophages may switch to M1 macrophages and vice versa [181,182]. M2 macrophages can be redirected into M1 macrophages by stimulation via CD40 and the IFN-γ receptor, such as is delivered upon cognate interaction with CD4+ Th1 cells [114,181].

An immunosuppressive tumor microenvironment was also found to restrain tumor immunity to pancreatic ductal adenocarcinoma (PDA). Injection of an agonist CD40 antibody with gemcitabine resulted in tumor regression in some patients. Reproduction of the treatment in a PDA mouse model revealed that CD40-activated macrophages rapidly infiltrated tumors [183], suggesting that a loss of MDSC through the use of gemcitabine and the activation of tumor-rejecting M1 macrophages mediated tumor regression. Antibody therapy may also be negatively affected by the tumor microenvironment. The combined treatment of patients with colorectal cancer with the anti-EGFR antibody cetuximab, the anti-VEGF antibody bevicizumab and chemotherapy resulted in a poorer disease-free survival than when patients were treated with the anti-VEGF antibody and chemotherapy [184]. The anti-EGFR antibody was expected to block EGFR signaling and activation of NK cells. However, an immunohistochemical staining of tumor sections revealed that tumor-promoting M2 macrophages were abundantly present rather than NK cells. Indeed, in co-cultures of EGFR-positive tumor cells, cetuximab and M2 macrophages, the latter were stimulated to release high levels of the tumor-promoting cytokines IL-10 and VEGF [185], providing an explanation for the unexpectedly worse outcome observed. In summary, immunomonitoring at the local level thus is warranted in order to be able to explain the results of immunotherapeutic approaches for cancer.

IV. HARMONIZATION OF IMMUNE MONITORING

The majority of the clinically tested immunotherapeutics aim to reinforce tumor-specific T-cell immunity to combat tumors. In all these trials, particularly those testing therapeutic vaccines, it is essential to monitor the T-cell response in order to determine the efficacy of the immunotherapeutic agent being tested. Unfortunately, there is an enormous variation in the data produced by different laboratories by various assays measuring different numbers and activity of specific immune parameters before, during and after administration of the immunotherapy. This situation makes it impossible to compare the immunological results obtained with similar therapeutic products among the various testing groups. Moreover, it hampers the identification of specific immune correlates or immune signatures associated with biological activity of the vaccine or other product and even the clinical outcome [68,186,187]. The most commonly used and widely applied T-cell assays are proliferation assays, cytokine analysis, IFNγ-ELISPOT, MHC-peptide multimer staining and ICS. Although each has been optimized over the last decade(s), they still lack an assay standard or reference sample that would render the results more comparable and interpretable. Validation of the assay is only performed in a few cases where the antigen of interest is well defined and the same standard operation procedures (SOPs) are applied in the different laboratories [188–191]. Standardization of biomarker assays enforces the use of identical reagents and/or protocols across laboratories and has been employed successfully in late stage trials. However, the assays often are not validated for general usage, i.e., for different tumor-(associated) antigens. Moreover, the same tumor antigens are not expressed by tumors or targeted in the therapy tested. Further, the lack of a correlation between the T-cell assay outcome and the clinical effect prevents a willingness to validate the assays used, especially as implementation may be prohibitively expensive during early clinical development where biomarker studies are exploratory [192].

An important alternative to assay validation is assay harmonization [68]. Assay harmonization involves the participation of multiple laboratories in an iterative testing process to identify and optimize critical performance variables. One key to this process is proficiency panels in which the same samples are tested by the laboratories using their own protocols, with the results obtained centrally evaluated with respect to the impact of harmonization on the intra- and inter-laboratory assay performance. The outcome of this process is the establishment of harmonization guidelines which are applicable for the larger community. The awareness to validate or harmonize T-cell assays is starting to increase in the field of cancer immunotherapy [186]. In fact, there are now two nonprofit organizations, the European-based Association for Cancer Immunotherapy (CIMT) immunoguiding program (CIP; www.cimt.eu/workgroup/CIP) and the USA-based Cancer Immunotherapy Consortium (CIC; www.cancerresearch.org/consortium), which actively support the harmonization process. Both the CIP and CIC consist of more than 110 laboratories involved in the (>25) international proficiency panels organized by these groups. Outcomes of the proficiency panels used for the ELISPOT [72,193–197] and HLA-peptide multimer staining assay [72,194,198] have resulted in protocols with an increased signal-to-noise ratio of the assay, i.e., improved test performance, along with a decreased variability of the test results among the participating laboratories. The participating laboratories gain a clear benefit from participation in the harmonization process, because they can still use their preferred reagents and potentially an improved protocol, with some modifications according to the guidelines, with the knowledge that they have a performance level equal to their peers. Guidelines for two harmonized T-cell assays are available for the public community that can be found on their websites. Current efforts of both groups focus on the ICS assay.

Harmonization of T-cell assays is an effective way to overcome data variability but the use of the data still can be hampered by inconsistent practices of data reporting. To overcome this issue, the immune monitoring community has come up with a checklist of minimal information about T-cell assays (MIATA) that is essential to properly interpret the reported data of T-cell assay experiments [199,200]. The consequences of fully harmonized assays and reports will be a higher probability of identifying immune biomarkers that identify patient populations benefiting from a given intervention or immune markers associated with success and failure of therapy.

V. IMMUNOGUIDING

Immunoguiding is the systematic use of comprehensive immunomonitoring of biological samples obtained from treated patient groups to understand the strengths, weaknesses and efficacy of the tested immune-modulating compound(s), using these results to steer decisions with respect to developmental aspects of the tested compound [67]. As cancer immunotherapy begins to advance more impactfully, immunoguiding may encourage investigators to move their immunotherapeutic product forward into bigger randomized trials or to go one step back to optimize the vaccine or strategy used. Typically the process starts fairly simply with one or two assays to test if the immune-modulating compound effectively alters the immune response according to the expected mechanism of action (Figure 16.1). It requires a good knowledge of the pharmacokinetics of the compound used in order to determine when and which biological materials should be sampled. The second phase is more intensive as this aims to unravel both wanted and unwanted immune responses that are altered by the compound. Furthermore, it includes the identification and study of immune parameters that may influence the efficacy of the compound to induce the required immune response or the intended clinical response (Figure 16.1). Clearly, this phase requires the use of a set of complementary immune assays with enough power to produce data that allows the generation of hypotheses explaining why the end point was (not) reached. Whether this phase is successful stands or falls by a thorough understanding of the immunological interactions occurring during the natural course of the specific disease for which the compound is developed, as this will help to understand the data coming from large screens or to determine the most logical specific assays

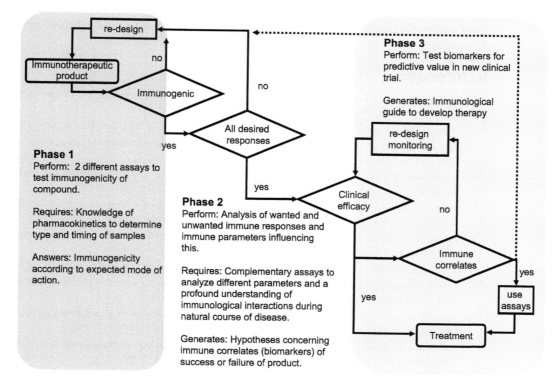

FIGURE 16.1
Phases of the immunoguiding process.

to be performed. These first two phases are not mutually exclusive and may use samples of the same clinical trial. Only if the second phase has successfully identified such biomarkers may the third phase ensue. Here, the identified biomarkers are tested for their predictive value in new trials. If they prove false, the process falls back to phase 2 (Figure 16.1).

Immunoguiding is a highly demanding process for both the clinic and patient. A major challenge the field faces as a whole is how to obtain sufficient amounts of all the biological samples required for the monitoring from the patients participating in clinical trials. While in general sufficient volumes and number of blood samples can be obtained, there is often limited accessibility to (multiple) samples from the tumor and tumor draining lymph nodes. Samples of local tissue, however, will be needed to optimally monitor the results of immunological intervention (e.g., infiltration by tumor-specific T cells, expression of inhibitory molecules) and to assess potential immune suppressive or evasive mechanisms (e.g., Tregs, MDSC, decreased HLA expression) which may block an otherwise successful therapy. For immunoguiding to be carried out successfully, a setting is required where the monitoring laboratory and clinic are in close collaboration and where the underlying reasons for the analysis of the different samples are well understood. Although immunological monitoring as a whole still has not been shown to possess predictive power there are still good reasons to embrace the concept of immunoguiding. Datasets generated may provide a proficient understanding of the effects of a therapy on the patient's immune system, helping explain for each individual patient why a therapy was successful or not and, consequently, pointing out the strengths and weaknesses of the immunotherapeutic strategy tested. In our trials with the HPV16-SLP vaccine, the observation of immunogenic competition between the two co-injected E6 and E7 antigens provided the rationale to separate these antigens in a subsequent trial [37]. Similarly, the association between vaccine failure, large lesions and Tregs in the patients with HPV16-induced VIN3 has prompted further evaluation of patient selection and the treatment strategy [41]. In conclusion, immunoguiding will become increasingly indispensable in understanding the impact of the immunotherapy on the immune response in relation to the clinical outcome, and also advancing most rapidly the most successful immunotherapeutic approaches through more clearly guided optimization strategies.

References

[1] Dienstmann R, Markman B, Tabernero J. Application of Monoclonal Antibodies as Cancer Therapy in Solid Tumors. Curr Clin Pharmacol 2012.

[2] Robak T. Rituximab for chronic lymphocytic leukemia. Expert Opin Biol Ther 2012;12:503—15.

[3] Kabolizadeh P, Kubicek GJ, Heron DE, Ferris RL, Gibson MK. The role of cetuximab in the management of head and neck cancers. Expert Opin Biol Ther 2012;12:517—28.

[4] Van CE, Kohne CH, Hitre E, Zaluski J, Chang Chien CR, Makhson A, et al. Cetuximab and chemotherapy as initial treatment for metastatic colorectal cancer. N Engl J Med 2009;360:1408—17.

[5] Mukohara T. Role of HER2-Targeted Agents in Adjuvant Treatment for Breast Cancer. Chemother Res Pract 2011;2011:730360.

[6] Los M, Roodhart JM, Voest EE. Target practice: lessons from phase III trials with bevacizumab and vatalanib in the treatment of advanced colorectal cancer. Oncologist 2007;12:443—50.

[7] Young RJ, Reed MW. Anti-angiogenic therapy: concept to clinic. Microcirculation 2012;19:115—25.

[8] Loke P, Allison JP. Emerging mechanisms of immune regulation: the extended B7 family and regulatory T cells. Arthritis Res Ther 2004;6:208—14.

[9] Hodi FS, O'Day SJ, McDermott DF, Weber RW, Sosman JA, Haanen JB, et al. Improved survival with ipilimumab in patients with metastatic melanoma. N Engl J Med 2010;363:711—23.

[10] Callahan MK, Wolchok JD, Allison JP. Anti-CTLA-4 antibody therapy: immune monitoring during clinical development of a novel immunotherapy. Semin Oncol 2010;37:473—84.

[11] Flies DB, Sandler BJ, Sznol M, Chen L. Blockade of the B7-H1/PD-1 pathway for cancer immunotherapy. Yale J Biol Med 2011;84:409—21.

[12] Kirkwood J. Cancer immunotherapy: the interferon-alpha experience. Semin Oncol 2002;29:18—26.

[13] Gore ME, Griffin CL, Hancock B, Patel PM, Pyle L, Aitchison M, et al. Interferon alfa-2a versus combination therapy with interferon alfa-2a, interleukin-2, and fluorouracil in patients with untreated metastatic renal cell carcinoma (MRC RE04/EORTC GU 30012): an open-label randomised trial. Lancet 2010;375:641—8.

[14] Lipton JH, Khoroshko N, Golenkov A, Abdulkadyrov K, Nair K, Raghunadharao D, et al. Phase II, randomized, multicenter, comparative study of peginterferon-alpha-2a (40 kD) (Pegasys) versus interferon alpha-2a (Roferon-A) in patients with treatment-naive, chronic-phase chronic myelogenous leukemia. Leuk Lymphoma 2007;48:497—505.

[15] Richtig E, Langmann G. Interferon for melanoma. Ophthalmology 2010;117:1861.

[16] Rosenfeld MR, Chamberlain MC, Grossman SA, Peereboom DM, Lesser GJ, Batchelor TT, et al. A multi-institution phase II study of poly-ICLC and radiotherapy with concurrent and adjuvant temozolomide in adults with newly diagnosed glioblastoma. Neuro Oncol 2010;12:1071—7.

[17] Jasani B, Navabi H, Adams M. Ampligen: a potential toll-like 3 receptor adjuvant for immunotherapy of cancer. Vaccine 2009;27:3401—4.

[18] Salaun B, Zitvogel L, Asselin-Paturel C, Morel Y, Chemin K, Dubois C, et al. TLR3 as a biomarker for the therapeutic efficacy of double-stranded RNA in breast cancer. Cancer Res 2011;71:1607—14.

[19] Cluff CW. Monophosphoryl lipid A (MPL) as an adjuvant for anti-cancer vaccines: clinical results. Adv Exp Med Biol 2010;667:111—23.

[20] Cluff CW. Monophosphoryl lipid A (MPL) as an adjuvant for anti-cancer vaccines: clinical results. Adv Exp Med Biol 2009;667:111—23.

[21] van Seters M, van Beurden M, ten Kate FJ, Beckmann I, Ewing PC, Eijkemans MJ, et al. Treatment of vulvar intraepithelial neoplasia with topical imiquimod. N Engl J Med 2008;358:1465—73.

[22] Gollnick H, Barona CG, Frank RG, Ruzicka T, Megahed M, Maus J, et al. Recurrence rate of superficial basal cell carcinoma following treatment with imiquimod 5% cream: conclusion of a 5-year long-term follow-up study in Europe. Eur J Dermatol 2008;18:677—82.

[23] Krieg AM. Toll-like receptor 9 (TLR9) agonists in the treatment of cancer. Oncogene 2008;27:161—7.

[24] Jahrsdorfer B, Weiner GJ. CpG oligodeoxynucleotides as immunotherapy in cancer. Update Cancer Ther 2008;3:27—32.

[25] Brody JD, Ai WZ, Czerwinski DK, Torchia JA, Levy M, Advani RH, et al. In situ vaccination with a TLR9 agonist induces systemic lymphoma regression: a phase I/II study. J Clin Oncol 2010;28:4324—32.

[26] Mocellin S, Mandruzzato S, Bronte V, Lise M, Nitti D. Part I: Vaccines for solid tumours. Lancet Oncol 2004;5:681—9.

[27] Mellman I, Coukos G, Dranoff G. Cancer immunotherapy comes of age. Nature 2011;480:480—9.

[28] Sharma P, Wagner K, Wolchok JD, Allison JP. Novel cancer immunotherapy agents with survival benefit: recent successes and next steps. Nat Rev Cancer 2011;11:805—12.

[29] Tartour E, Sandoval F, Bonnefoy JY, Fridman WH. [Cancer immunotherapy: recent breakthroughs and perspectives]. Med Sci (Paris) 2011;27:833—41.

[30] Turcotte S, Rosenberg SA. Immunotherapy for metastatic solid cancers. Adv Surg 2011;45:341—60.

[31] Lesterhuis WJ, Haanen JB, Punt CJ. Cancer immunotherapy—revisited. Nat Rev Drug Discov 2011;10:591—600.

[32] Hughes MS, Yu YY, Dudley ME, Zheng Z, Robbins PF, Li Y, et al. Transfer of a TCR gene derived from a patient with a marked antitumor response conveys highly active T-cell effector functions. Hum Gene Ther 2005;16:457—72.

[33] Park TS, Rosenberg SA, Morgan RA. Treating cancer with genetically engineered T cells. Trends Biotechnol 2011;29:550—7.

[34] Rosenberg SA, Dudley ME. Adoptive cell therapy for the treatment of patients with metastatic melanoma. Curr Opin Immunol 2009;21:233—40.

[35] Rosenberg SA, Yang JC, Sherry RM, Kammula US, Hughes MS, Phan GQ, et al. Durable complete responses in heavily pretreated patients with metastatic melanoma using T-cell transfer immunotherapy. Clin Cancer Res 2011;17:4550—7.

[36] Verdegaal EM, Visser M, Ramwadhdoebe TH, van der Minne CE, van Steijn JA, Kapiteijn E, et al. Successful treatment of metastatic melanoma by adoptive transfer of blood-derived polyclonal tumor-specific CD4+ and CD8+ T cells in combination with low-dose interferon-alpha. Cancer Immunol Immunother 2011;60:953—63.

[37] Kenter GG, Welters MJ, Valentijn AR, Lowik MJ, Berends-van der Meer DM, Vloon AP, et al. Phase I immunotherapeutic trial with long peptides spanning the E6 and E7 sequences of high-risk human papillomavirus 16 in end-stage cervical cancer patients shows low toxicity and robust immunogenicity. Clin Cancer Res 2008;14:169—77.

251

[38] Kenter GG, Welters MJ, Valentijn AR, Lowik MJ, Berends-van der Meer DM, Vloon AP, et al. Vaccination against HPV-16 oncoproteins for vulvar intraepithelial neoplasia. N Engl J Med 2009;361:1838–47.

[39] Speetjens FM, Kuppen PJ, Welters MJ, Essahsah F, Voet van den Brink AM, Lantrua MG, et al. Induction of p53-specific immunity by a p53 synthetic long peptide vaccine in patients treated for metastatic colorectal cancer. Clin Cancer Res 2009;15:1086–95.

[40] Welters MJ, Kenter GG, Piersma SJ, Vloon AP, Lowik MJ, Berends-van der Meer DM, et al. Induction of tumor-specific CD4+ and CD8+ T-cell immunity in cervical cancer patients by a human papillomavirus type 16 E6 and E7 long peptides vaccine. Clin Cancer Res 2008;14:178–87.

[41] Welters MJ, Kenter GG, de Vos van Steenwijk PJ, Lowik MJ, Berends-van der Meer DM, Essahsah F, et al. Success or failure of vaccination for HPV16-positive vulvar lesions correlates with kinetics and phenotype of induced T-cell responses. Proc Natl Acad Sci U S A 2010;107:11895–9.

[42] Vermeij R, Leffers N, Hoogeboom BN, Hamming IL, Wolf R, Reyners AK, et al. Potentiation of a p53-SLP vaccine by cyclophosphamide in ovarian cancer: A single-arm phase II study. Int J Cancer 2011.

[43] Leffers N, Lambeck AJ, Gooden MJ, Hoogeboom BN, Wolf R, Hamming IE, et al. Immunization with a P53 synthetic long peptide vaccine induces P53-specific immune responses in ovarian cancer patients, a phase II trial. Int J Cancer 2009;125:2104–13.

[44] Rosenberg SA. Cell transfer immunotherapy for metastatic solid cancer—what clinicians need to know. Nat Rev Clin Oncol 2011;8:577–85.

[45] Porter DL, Levine BL, Kalos M, Bagg A, June CH. Chimeric antigen receptor-modified T cells in chronic lymphoid leukemia. N Engl J Med 2011;365:725–33.

[46] Kalos M. Biomarkers in T cell therapy clinical trials. J Transl Med 2011;9:138.

[47] Kalos M, Levine BL, Porter DL, Katz S, Grupp SA, Bagg A, et al. T cells with chimeric antigen receptors have potent antitumor effects and can establish memory in patients with advanced leukemia. Sci Transl Med 2011;3:95ra73.

[48] Curran KJ, Pegram HJ, Brentjens RJ. Chimeric antigen receptors for T cell immunotherapy: current understanding and future direction. J Gene Med 2012.

[49] Kalos M. Muscle CARs and TcRs: turbo-charged technologies for the (T cell) masses. Cancer Immunol Immunother 2012;61:127–35.

[50] Khleif SN, Doroshow JH, Hait WN. AACR-FDA-NCI Cancer Biomarkers Collaborative consensus report: advancing the use of biomarkers in cancer drug development. Clin Cancer Res 2010;16:3299–318.

[51] Mischak H, Allmaier G, Apweiler R, Attwood T, Baumann M, Benigni A, et al. Recommendations for biomarker identification and qualification in clinical proteomics. Sci Transl Med 2010;2:46ps42.

[52] Davis MM. A prescription for human immunology. Immunity 2008;29:835–8.

[53] Ciardiello F, Tortora G. EGFR antagonists in cancer treatment. N Engl J Med 2008;358:1160–74.

[54] Bae JH, Kim SJ, Kim MJ, Oh SO, Chung JS, Kim SH, et al. Susceptibility to natural killer cell-mediated lysis of colon cancer cells is enhanced by treatment with epidermal growth factor receptor inhibitors through UL16-binding protein-1 induction. Cancer Sci 2012;103:7–16.

[55] Kim H, Kim SH, Kim MJ, Kim SJ, Park SJ, Chung JS, et al. EGFR inhibitors enhanced the susceptibility to NK cell-mediated lysis of lung cancer cells. J Immunother 2011;34:372–81.

[56] Pander J, Gelderblom H, Guchelaar HJ. Pharmacogenetics of EGFR and VEGF inhibition. Drug Discov Today 2007;12:1054–60.

[57] Yuan J, Gnjatic S, Li H, Powel S, Gallardo HF, Ritter E, et al. CTLA-4 blockade enhances polyfunctional NY-ESO-1 specific T cell responses in metastatic melanoma patients with clinical benefit. Proc Natl Acad Sci U S A 2008;105:20410–5.

[58] Andersen RS, Thrue CA, Junker N, Lyngaa R, Donia M, Ellebaek E, et al. Dissection of T cell antigen specificity in human melanoma. Cancer Res 2012;72:1642–50.

[59] Hadrup SR, Bakker AH, Shu CJ, Andersen RS, van VJ, Hombrink P, et al. Parallel detection of antigen-specific T-cell responses by multidimensional encoding of MHC multimers. Nat Methods 2009;6:520–6.

[60] Inman BA, Frigola X, Dong H, Kwon ED. Costimulation, coinhibition and cancer. Curr Cancer Drug Targets 2007;7:15–30.

[61] Hodi FS, Butler M, Oble DA, Seiden MV, Haluska FG, Kruse A, et al. Immunologic and clinical effects of antibody blockade of cytotoxic T lymphocyte-associated antigen 4 in previously vaccinated cancer patients. Proc Natl Acad Sci U S A 2008;105:3005–10.

[62] Hamid O, Schmidt H, Nissan A, Ridolfi L, Aamdal S, Hansson J, et al. A prospective phase II trial exploring the association between tumor microenvironment biomarkers and clinical activity of ipilimumab in advanced melanoma. J Transl Med 2011;9:204.

[63] Shen X, Zhou J, Hathcock KS, Robbins P, Powell Jr DJ, Rosenberg SA, et al. Persistence of tumor infiltrating lymphocytes in adoptive immunotherapy correlates with telomere length. J Immunother 2007;30:123–9.

[64] Ostrand-Rosenberg S. CD4+ T lymphocytes: a critical component of antitumor immunity. Cancer Invest 2005;23:413–9.

[65] Hanahan D, Weinberg RA. Hallmarks of cancer: the next generation. Cell 2011;144:646–74.

[66] Cavallo F, De GC, Nanni P, Forni G, Lollini PL. 2011: the immune hallmarks of cancer. Cancer Immunol Immunother 2011;60:319–26.

[67] van der Burg SH. Therapeutic vaccines in cancer: moving from immunomonitoring to immunoguiding. Expert Rev Vaccines 2008;7:1–5.

[68] van der Burg SH, Kalos M, Gouttefangeas C, Janetzki S, Ottensmeier C, Welters MJ, et al. Harmonization of immune biomarker assays for clinical studies. Sci Transl Med 2011;3:108ps44.

[69] Hoos A, Parmiani G, Hege K, Sznol M, Loibner H, Eggermont A, et al. A clinical development paradigm for cancer vaccines and related biologics. J Immunother 2007;30:1–15.

[70] Keilholz U, Weber J, Finke JH, Gabrilovich DI, Kast WM, Disis ML, et al. Immunologic monitoring of cancer vaccine therapy: results of a workshop sponsored by the Society for Biological Therapy. J Immunother 2002;25:97–138.

[71] Britten CM, Janetzki S, van der Burg SH, Gouttefangeas C, Hoos A. Toward the harmonization of immune monitoring in clinical trials: quo vadis? Cancer Immunol Immunother 2008;57:285–8.

[72] Britten CM, Gouttefangeas C, Welters MJ, Pawelec G, Koch S, Ottensmeier C, et al. The CIMT-monitoring panel: a two-step approach to harmonize the enumeration of antigen-specific CD8+ T lymphocytes by structural and functional assays. Cancer Immunol Immunother 2008;57:289–302.

[73] Czerkinsky C, Andersson G, Ekre HP, Nilsson LA, Klareskog L, Ouchterlony O. Reverse ELISPOT assay for clonal analysis of cytokine production. I. Enumeration of gamma-interferon-secreting cells. J Immunol Methods 1988;110:29–36.

[74] Herr W, Protzer U, Lohse AW, Gerken G. Meyer zum Buschenfelde KH, Wolfel T. Quantification of CD8+ T lymphocytes responsive to human immunodeficiency virus (HIV) peptide antigens in HIV-infected patients and seronegative persons at high risk for recent HIV exposure. J Infect Dis 1998;178:260–5.

[75] van der Burg SH, Ressing ME, Kwappenberg KM, de JA, Straathof K, de JJ, et al. Natural T-helper immunity against human papillomavirus type 16 (HPV16) E7-derived peptide epitopes in patients with HPV16-positive cervical lesions: identification of 3 human leukocyte antigen class II-restricted epitopes. Int J Cancer 2001;91:612–8.

[76] Assenmacher M, Schmitz J, Radbruch A. Flow cytometric determination of cytokines in activated murine T helper lymphocytes: expression of interleukin-10 in interferon-gamma and in interleukin-4-expressing cells. Eur J Immunol 1994;24:1097–101.

[77] Jung T, Schauer U, Heusser C, Neumann C, Rieger C. Detection of intracellular cytokines by flow cytometry. J Immunol Methods 1993;159:197–207.

[78] Altman JD, Moss PA, Goulder PJ, Barouch DH, McHeyzer-Williams MG, Bell JI, et al. Phenotypic analysis of antigen-specific T lymphocytes. Science 1996;274:94–6.

[79] Goodell V, Dela RC, Slota M, MacLeod B, Disis ML. Sensitivity and specificity of tritiated thymidine incorporation and ELISPOT assays in identifying antigen specific T cell immune responses. BMC Immunol 2007;8:21.

[80] Godet Y, Fabre-Guillevin E, Dosset M, Lamuraglia M, Levionnois E, Ravel P, et al. Analysis of spontaneous tumor-specific CD4 T cell immunity in lung cancer using promiscuous HLA-DR telomerase-derived epitopes: potential synergistic effect with chemotherapy response. Clin Cancer Res 2012.

[81] McNeel DG, Dunphy EJ, Davies JG, Frye TP, Johnson LE, Staab MJ, et al. Safety and immunological efficacy of a DNA vaccine encoding prostatic acid phosphatase in patients with stage D0 prostate cancer. J Clin Oncol 2009;27:4047–54.

[82] Ginsberg BA, Gallardo HF, Rasalan TS, Adamow M, Mu Z, Tandon S, et al. Immunologic response to xenogeneic gp100 DNA in melanoma patients: comparison of particle-mediated epidermal delivery with intramuscular injection. Clin Cancer Res 2010;16:4057–65.

[83] Arlen PM, Gulley JL, Parker C, Skarupa L, Pazdur M, Panicali D, et al. A randomized phase II study of concurrent docetaxel plus vaccine versus vaccine alone in metastatic androgen-independent prostate cancer. Clin Cancer Res 2006;12:1260–9.

[84] Amato RJ, Shingler W, Goonewardena M, de BJ, Naylor S, Jac J, et al. Vaccination of renal cell cancer patients with modified vaccinia Ankara delivering the tumor antigen 5T4 (TroVax) alone or administered in combination with interferon-alpha (IFN-alpha): a phase 2 trial. J Immunother 2009;32:765–72.

[85] Bercovici N, Haicheur N, Massicard S, Vernel-Pauillac F, Adotevi O, Landais D, et al. Analysis and characterization of antitumor T-cell response after administration of dendritic cells loaded with allogeneic tumor lysate to metastatic melanoma patients. J Immunother 2008;31:101–12.

[86] Lovelace P, Maecker HT. Multiparameter intracellular cytokine staining. Methods Mol Biol 2011;699:165–78.

[87] Lugli E, Roederer M, Cossarizza A. Data analysis in flow cytometry: the future just started. Cytometry A 2010;77:705–13.

253

[88] Tesfa L, Volk HD, Kern F. A protocol for combining proliferation, tetramer staining and intracellular cytokine detection for the flow-cytometric analysis of antigen specific T-cells. J Biol Regul Homeost Agents 2003;17:366—70.

[89] Newell EW, Klein LO, Yu W, Davis MM. Simultaneous detection of many T-cell specificities using combinatorial tetramer staining. Nat Methods 2009;6:497—9.

[90] Ornatsky O, Bandura D, Baranov V, Nitz M, Winnik MA, Tanner S. Highly multiparametric analysis by mass cytometry. J Immunol Methods 2010;361:1—20.

[91] Maecker HT, Nolan GP, Fathman CG. New technologies for autoimmune disease monitoring. Curr Opin Endocrinol Diabetes Obes 2010;17:322—8.

[92] Tobery TW, Wang S, Wang XM, Neeper MP, Jansen KU, McClements WL, et al. A simple and efficient method for the monitoring of antigen-specific T cell responses using peptide pool arrays in a modified ELISpot assay. J Immunol Methods 2001;254:59—66.

[93] Betts MR, Ambrozak DR, Douek DC, Bonhoeffer S, Brenchley JM, Casazza JP, et al. Analysis of total human immunodeficiency virus (HIV)-specific CD4(+) and CD8(+) T-cell responses: relationship to viral load in untreated HIV infection. J Virol 2001;75:11983—91.

[94] de Jong A, van der Hulst JM, Kenter GG, Drijfhout JW, Franken KL, Vermeij P, et al. Rapid enrichment of human papillomavirus (HPV)-specific polyclonal T cell populations for adoptive immunotherapy of cervical cancer. Int J Cancer 2005;114:274—82.

[95] Karlsson AC, Martin JN, Younger SR, Bredt BM, Epling L, Ronquillo R, et al. Comparison of the ELISPOT and cytokine flow cytometry assays for the enumeration of antigen-specific T cells. J Immunol Methods 2003;283:141—53.

[96] Singh SK, Meyering M, Ramwadhdoebe TH, Stynenbosch LF, Redeker A, Kuppen PJ, et al. The simultaneous ex-vivo detection of low frequency antigen-specific CD4+ and CD8+ T-cell responses using overlapping peptide pools. Cancer Immunol.Immunother 2012. in press.

[97] Hopfl R, Sandbichler M, Sepp N, Heim K, Muller-Holzner E, Wartusch B, et al. Skin test for HPV type 16 proteins in cervical intraepithelial neoplasia. Lancet 1991;337:373—4.

[98] de Vries IJ, Bernsen MR, Lesterhuis WJ, Scharenborg NM, Strijk SP, Gerritsen MJ, et al. Immunomonitoring tumor-specific T cells in delayed-type hypersensitivity skin biopsies after dendritic cell vaccination correlates with clinical outcome. J Clin Oncol 2005;23:5779—87.

[99] de Vries IJ, Bernsen MR, van Geloof WL, Scharenborg NM, Lesterhuis WJ, Rombout PD, et al. In situ detection of antigen-specific T cells in cryo-sections using MHC class I tetramers after dendritic cell vaccination of melanoma patients. Cancer Immunol Immunother 2007;56:1667—76.

[100] Lesterhuis WJ, de Vries IJ, Schuurhuis DH, Boullart AC, Jacobs JF, de Boer AJ, et al. Vaccination of colorectal cancer patients with CEA-loaded dendritic cells: antigen-specific T cell responses in DTH skin tests. Ann Oncol 2006;17:974—80.

[101] van den Hende M, van Poelgeest MI, van der Hulst JM, de JJ, Drijfhout JW, Fleuren GJ, et al. Skin reactions to human papillomavirus (HPV) 16 specific antigens intradermally injected in healthy subjects and patients with cervical neoplasia. Int J Cancer 2008;123:146—52.

[102] Ku GY, Yuan J, Page DB, Schroeder SE, Panageas KS, Carvajal RD, et al. Single-institution experience with ipilimumab in advanced melanoma patients in the compassionate use setting: lymphocyte count after 2 doses correlates with survival. Cancer 2010;116:1767—75.

[103] Restifo NP, Rosenberg SA. Use of standard criteria for assessment of cancer vaccines. Lancet Oncol 2005;6:3—4.

[104] Klebanoff CA, Acquavella N, Yu Z, Restifo NP. Therapeutic cancer vaccines: are we there yet? Immunol Rev 2011;239:27—44.

[105] Hodi FS, Butler M, Oble DA, Seiden MV, Haluska FG, Kruse A, et al. Immunologic and clinical effects of antibody blockade of cytotoxic T lymphocyte-associated antigen 4 in previously vaccinated cancer patients. Proc Natl Acad Sci U S A 2008;105:3005—10.

[106] Schreiber RD, Old LJ, Smyth MJ. Cancer immunoediting: integrating immunity's roles in cancer suppression and promotion. Science 2011;331:1565—70.

[107] Dunn GP, Koebel CM, Schreiber RD. Interferons, immunity and cancer immunoediting. Nat Rev Immunol 2006;6:836—48.

[108] Dunn GP, Old LJ, Schreiber RD. The three Es of cancer immunoediting. Annu Rev Immunol 2004;22:329—60.

[109] Jin HT, Anderson AC, Tan WG, West EE, Ha SJ, Araki K, et al. Cooperation of Tim-3 and PD-1 in CD8 T-cell exhaustion during chronic viral infection. Proc Natl Acad Sci U S A 2010;107:14733—8.

[110] Sakuishi K, Apetoh L, Sullivan JM, Blazar BR, Kuchroo VK, Anderson AC. Targeting Tim-3 and PD-1 pathways to reverse T cell exhaustion and restore anti-tumor immunity. J Exp Med 2010;207:2187—94.

[111] Fourcade J, Sun Z, Pagliano O, Guillaume P, Luescher IF, Sander C, et al. CD8(+) T cells specific for tumor antigens can be rendered dysfunctional by the tumor microenvironment through upregulation of the inhibitory receptors BTLA and PD-1. Cancer Res 2012;72:887—96.

[112] Fourcade J, Sun Z, Benallaoua M, Guillaume P, Luescher IF, Sander C, et al. Upregulation of Tim-3 and PD-1 expression is associated with tumor antigen-specific CD8+ T cell dysfunction in melanoma patients. J Exp Med 2010;207:2175—86.

[113] Harlin H, Kuna TV, Peterson AC, Meng Y, Gajewski TF. Tumor progression despite massive influx of activated CD8(+) T cells in a patient with malignant melanoma ascites. Cancer Immunol Immunother 2006;55:1185—97.

[114] Heusinkveld M, de Vos van Steenwijk PJ, Goedemans R, Ramwadhdoebe TH, Gorter A, Welters MJ, et al. M2 macrophages induced by prostaglandin E2 and IL-6 from cervical carcinoma are switched to activated M1 macrophages by CD4+ Th1 cells. J Immunol 2011;187:1157—65.

[115] Allavena P, Mantovani A. Immunology in the clinic review series; focus on cancer: tumour-associated macrophages: undisputed stars of the inflammatory tumour microenvironment. Clin Exp Immunol 2012;167:195—205.

[116] Porta C, Riboldi E, Totaro MG, Strauss L, Sica A, Mantovani A. Macrophages in cancer and infectious diseases: the 'good' and the 'bad'. Immunotherapy 2011;3:1185—202.

[117] Gabrilovich DI, Nagaraj S. Myeloid-derived suppressor cells as regulators of the immune system. Nat Rev Immunol 2009;9:162—74.

[118] Ostrand-Rosenberg S, Sinha P, Beury DW, Clements VK. Cross-talk between myeloid-derived suppressor cells (MDSC), macrophages, and dendritic cells enhances tumor-induced immune suppression. Semin Cancer Biol 2012.

[119] Chioda M, Peranzoni E, Desantis G, Papalini F, Falisi E, Solito S, et al. Myeloid cell diversification and complexity: an old concept with new turns in oncology. Cancer Metastasis Rev 2011;30:27—43.

[120] Zwaveling S, Ferreira Mota SC, Nouta J, Johnson M, Lipford GB, Offringa R, et al. Established human papillomavirus type 16-expressing tumors are effectively eradicated following vaccination with long peptides. J Immunol 2002;169:350—8.

[121] Welters MJ, Bijker MS, van den Eeden SJ, Franken KL, Melief CJ, Offringa R, et al. Multiple CD4 and CD8 T-cell activation parameters predict vaccine efficacy in vivo mediated by individual DC-activating agonists. Vaccine 2007;25:1379—89.

[122] Fridman WH, Pages F, Sautes-Fridman C, Galon J. The immune contexture in human tumours: impact on clinical outcome. Nat Rev Cancer 2012;12:298—306.

[123] Tosolini M, Kirilovsky A, Mlecnik B, Fredriksen T, Mauger S, Bindea G, et al. Clinical impact of different classes of infiltrating T cytotoxic and helper cells (Th1, th2, treg, th17) in patients with colorectal cancer. Cancer Res 2011;71:1263—71.

[124] Jordanova ES, Gorter A, Ayachi O, Prins F, Durrant LG, Kenter GG, et al. Human leukocyte antigen class I, MHC class I chain-related molecule A, and CD8+/regulatory T-cell ratio: which variable determines survival of cervical cancer patients? Clin Cancer Res 2008;14:2028—35.

[125] DeNardo DG, Barreto JB, Andreu P, Vasquez L, Tawfik D, Kolhatkar N, et al. CD4(+) T cells regulate pulmonary metastasis of mammary carcinomas by enhancing protumor properties of macrophages. Cancer Cell 2009;16:91—102.

[126] Wada H, Sato E, Uenaka A, Isobe M, Kawabata R, Nakamura Y, et al. Analysis of peripheral and local anti-tumor immune response in esophageal cancer patients after NY-ESO-1 protein vaccination. Int J Cancer 2008;123:2362—9.

[127] Badoual C, Sandoval F, Pere H, Hans S, Gey A, Merillon N, et al. Better understanding tumor-host interaction in head and neck cancer to improve the design and development of immunotherapeutic strategies. Head Neck 2010;32:946—58.

[128] Correll A, Tuettenberg A, Becker C, Jonuleit H. Increased regulatory T-cell frequencies in patients with advanced melanoma correlate with a generally impaired T-cell responsiveness and are restored after dendritic cell-based vaccination. Exp Dermatol 2010;19:e213—21.

[129] Nicholaou T, Ebert LM, Davis ID, McArthur GA, Jackson H, Dimopoulos N, et al. Regulatory T-cell-mediated attenuation of T-cell responses to the NY-ESO-1 ISCOMATRIX vaccine in patients with advanced malignant melanoma. Clin Cancer Res 2009;15:2166—73.

[130] Berntsen A, Brimnes MK, Thor SP, Svane IM. Increase of circulating CD4+CD25highFoxp3+ regulatory T cells in patients with metastatic renal cell carcinoma during treatment with dendritic cell vaccination and low-dose interleukin-2. J Immunother 2010;33:425—34.

[131] Daayana S, Elkord E, Winters U, Pawlita M, Roden R, Stern PL, et al. Phase II trial of imiquimod and HPV therapeutic vaccination in patients with vulval intraepithelial neoplasia. Br J Cancer 2010;102:1129—36.

[132] Piersma SJ, Welters MJ, van der Burg SH. Tumor-specific regulatory T cells in cancer patients. Hum Immunol 2008;69:241—9.

[133] Welters MJ, Piersma SJ, van der Burg SH. T-regulatory cells in tumour-specific vaccination strategies. Expert Opin Biol Ther 2008;8:1365—79.

[134] Bonertz A, Weitz J, Pietsch DH, Rahbari NN, Schlude C, Ge Y, et al. Antigen-specific Tregs control T cell responses against a limited repertoire of tumor antigens in patients with colorectal carcinoma. J Clin Invest 2009;119:3311−21.

[135] Wang HY, Lee DA, Peng G, Guo Z, Li Y, Kiniwa Y, et al. Tumor-specific human CD4+ regulatory T cells and their ligands: implications for immunotherapy. Immunity 2004;20:107−18.

[136] Wang HY, Peng G, Guo Z, Shevach EM, Wang RF. Recognition of a new ARTC1 peptide ligand uniquely expressed in tumor cells by antigen-specific CD4+ regulatory T cells. J Immunol 2005;174:2661−70.

[137] Vence L, Palucka AK, Fay JW, Ito T, Liu YJ, Banchereau J, et al. Circulating tumor antigen-specific regulatory T cells in patients with metastatic melanoma. Proc Natl Acad Sci U S A 2007;104:20884−9.

[138] van der Burg SH, Piersma SJ, de JA, van der Hulst JM, Kwappenberg KM, van den Hende M, et al. Association of cervical cancer with the presence of CD4+ regulatory T cells specific for human papillomavirus antigens. Proc Natl Acad Sci U S A 2007;104:12087−92.

[139] Heusinkveld M, Welters MJ, van Poelgeest MI, van der Hulst JM, Melief CJ, Fleuren GJ, et al. The detection of circulating human papillomavirus-specific T cells is associated with improved survival of patients with deeply infiltrating tumors. Int J Cancer 2011;128:379−89.

[140] de Vos van Steenwijk PJ, Piersma SJ, Welters MJ, van der Hulst JM, Fleuren G, Hellebrekers BW, et al. Surgery followed by persistence of high-grade squamous intraepithelial lesions is associated with the induction of a dysfunctional HPV16-specific T-cell response. Clin Cancer Res 2008;14:7188−95.

[141] Lehe C, Ghebeh H, Al-Sulaiman A, Al QG, Al-Hussein K, Almohareb F, et al. The Wilms' tumor antigen is a novel target for human CD4+ regulatory T cells: implications for immunotherapy. Cancer Res 2008;68:6350−9.

[142] Zhou G, Drake CG, Levitsky HI. Amplification of tumor-specific regulatory T cells following therapeutic cancer vaccines. Blood 2006;107:628−36.

[143] Warncke M, Buchner M, Thaller G, Dodero A, Bulashevska A, Pfeifer D, et al. Control of the specificity of T cell-mediated anti-idiotype immunity by natural regulatory T cells. Cancer Immunol Immunother 2011;60:49−60.

[144] Slingluff Jr CL, Petroni GR, Chianese-Bullock KA, Smolkin ME, Ross MI, Haas NB, et al. Randomized multicenter trial of the effects of melanoma-associated helper peptides and cyclophosphamide on the immunogenicity of a multipeptide melanoma vaccine. J Clin Oncol 2011;29:2924−32.

[145] Francois V, Ottaviani S, Renkvist N, Stockis J, Schuler G, Thielemans K, et al. The CD4(+) T-cell response of melanoma patients to a MAGE-A3 peptide vaccine involves potential regulatory T cells. Cancer Res 2009;69:4335−45.

[146] Welters MJ, de JA, van den Eeden SJ, van der Hulst JM, Kwappenberg KM, Hassane S, et al. Frequent display of human papillomavirus type 16 E6-specific memory t-Helper cells in the healthy population as witness of previous viral encounter. Cancer Res 2003;63:636−41.

[147] de Jong A, van Poelgeest MI, van der Hulst JM, Drijfhout JW, Fleuren GJ, Melief CJ, et al. Human papillomavirus type 16-positive cervical cancer is associated with impaired CD4+ T-cell immunity against early antigens E2 and E6. Cancer Res 2004;64:5449−55.

[148] Welters MJ, van der Logt P, van den Eeden SJ, Kwappenberg KM, Drijfhout JW, Fleuren GJ, et al. Detection of human papillomavirus type 18 E6 and E7-specific CD4+ T-helper 1 immunity in relation to health versus disease. Int J Cancer 2006;118:950−6.

[149] Piersma SJ, Welters MJ, van der Hulst JM, Kloth JN, Kwappenberg KM, Trimbos BJ, et al. Human papilloma virus specific T cells infiltrating cervical cancer and draining lymph nodes show remarkably frequent use of HLA-DQ and -DP as a restriction element. Int J Cancer 2008;122:486−94.

[150] van Poelgeest MI, Nijhuis ER, Kwappenberg KM, Hamming IE, Wouter DJ, Fleuren GJ, et al. Distinct regulation and impact of type 1 T-cell immunity against HPV16 L1, E2 and E6 antigens during HPV16-induced cervical infection and neoplasia. Int J Cancer 2006;118:675−83.

[151] Jacobs JF, Punt CJ, Lesterhuis WJ, Sutmuller RP, Brouwer HM, Scharenborg NM, et al. Dendritic cell vaccination in combination with anti-CD25 monoclonal antibody treatment: a phase I/II study in metastatic melanoma patients. Clin Cancer Res 2010;16:5067−78.

[152] Jacobs JF, Nierkens S, Figdor CG, de Vries IJ, Adema GJ. Regulatory T cells in melanoma: the final hurdle towards effective immunotherapy? Lancet Oncol 2012;13:e32−42.

[153] de Vries IJ, Castelli C, Huygens C, Jacobs JF, Stockis J, Schuler-Thurner B, et al. Frequency of circulating Tregs with demethylated FOXP3 intron 1 in melanoma patients receiving tumor vaccines and potentially Treg-depleting agents. Clin Cancer Res 2011;17:841−8.

[154] Appay V, Voelter V, Rufer N, Reynard S, Jandus C, Gasparini D, et al. Combination of transient lymphodepletion with busulfan and fludarabine and peptide vaccination in a phase I clinical trial for patients with advanced melanoma. J Immunother 2007;30:240−50.

[155] Appay V, Jandus C, Voelter V, Reynard S, Coupland SE, Rimoldi D, et al. New generation vaccine induces effective melanoma-specific CD8+ T cells in the circulation but not in the tumor site. J Immunol 2006;177:1670−8.

[156] Davidson EJ, Boswell CM, Sehr P, Pawlita M, Tomlinson AE, McVey RJ, et al. Immunological and clinical responses in women with vulval intraepithelial neoplasia vaccinated with a vaccinia virus encoding human papillomavirus 16/18 oncoproteins. Cancer Res 2003;63:6032—41.

[157] Ganss R, Limmer A, Sacher T, Arnold B, Hammerling GJ. Autoaggression and tumor rejection: it takes more than self-specific T-cell activation. Immunol Rev 1999;169:263—72.

[158] Wang E, Miller LD, Ohnmacht GA, Mocellin S, Perez-Diez A, Petersen D, et al. Prospective molecular profiling of melanoma metastases suggests classifiers of immune responsiveness. Cancer Res 2002; 62:3581—6.

[159] Kilinc MO, Aulakh KS, Nair RE, Jones SA, Alard P, Kosiewicz MM, et al. Reversing tumor immune suppression with intratumoral IL-12: activation of tumor-associated T effector/memory cells, induction of T suppressor apoptosis, and infiltration of CD8+ T effectors. J Immunol 2006;177:6962—73.

[160] Wall EM, Milne K, Martin ML, Watson PH, Theiss P, Nelson BH. Spontaneous mammary tumors differ widely in their inherent sensitivity to adoptively transferred T cells. Cancer Res 2007;67:6442—50.

[161] Malyguine AM, Strobl SL, Shurin MR. Immunological monitoring of the tumor immunoenvironment for clinical trials. Cancer Immunol Immunother 2012;61:239—47.

[162] Gajewski TF. Cancer immunotherapy. Mol Oncol 2012.

[163] Bronkhorst IH, Jager MJ. Uveal Melanoma: The Inflammatory Microenvironment. J Innate Immun 2012.

[164] Fujii N, Shomori K, Shiomi T, Nakabayashi M, Takeda C, Ryoke K, et al. Cancer-associated fibroblasts and CD163-positive macrophages in oral squamous cell carcinoma: their clinicopathological and prognostic significance. J Oral Pathol Med 2012.

[165] Cai QC, Liao H, Lin SX, Xia Y, Wang XX, Gao Y, et al. High expression of tumor-infiltrating macrophages correlates with poor prognosis in patients with diffuse large B-cell lymphoma. Med Oncol 2011.

[166] Mahmoud SM, Lee AH, Paish EC, Macmillan RD, Ellis IO, Green AR. Tumour-infiltrating macrophages and clinical outcome in breast cancer. J Clin Pathol 2012;65:159—63.

[167] Heusinkveld M, van der Burg SH. Identification and manipulation of tumor associated macrophages in human cancers. J Transl Med 2011;9:216.

[168] Biswas SK, Mantovani A. Macrophage plasticity and interaction with lymphocyte subsets: cancer as a paradigm. Nat Immunol 2010;11:889—96.

[169] Vasievich EA, Huang L. The suppressive tumor microenvironment: a challenge in cancer immunotherapy. Mol Pharm 2011;8:635—41.

[170] Sica A. Role of tumour-associated macrophages in cancer-related inflammation. Exp Oncol 2010;32:153—8.

[171] van DM, Savage ND, Jordanova ES, Briaire-de Bruijn IH, Walburg KV, Ottenhoff TH, et al. Anti-inflammatory M2 type macrophages characterize metastasized and tyrosine kinase inhibitor-treated gastrointestinal stromal tumors. Int J Cancer 2010;127:899—909.

[172] Lepique AP, Daghastanli KR, Cuccovia IM, Villa LL. HPV16 tumor associated macrophages suppress anti-tumor T cell responses. Clin Cancer Res 2009;15:4391—400.

[173] Wei J, Wu A, Kong LY, Wang Y, Fuller G, Fokt I, et al. Hypoxia potentiates glioma-mediated immunosuppression. PLoS One 2011;6:e16195.

[174] Mantovani A, Germano G, Marchesi F, Locatelli M, Biswas SK. Cancer-promoting tumor-associated macrophages: new vistas and open questions. Eur J Immunol 2011;41:2522—5.

[175] Nagaraj S, Gabrilovich DI. Myeloid-derived suppressor cells in human cancer. Cancer J 2010;16:348—53.

[176] Ostrand-Rosenberg S. Myeloid-derived suppressor cells: more mechanisms for inhibiting antitumor immunity. Cancer Immunol Immunother 2010;59:1593—600.

[177] Ostrand-Rosenberg S, Sinha P. Myeloid-derived suppressor cells: linking inflammation and cancer. J Immunol 2009;182:4499—506.

[178] Erdag G, Schaefer JT, Smolkin ME, Deacon DH, Shea SM, Dengel LT, et al. Immunotype and immunohistologic characteristics of tumor-infiltrating immune cells are associated with clinical outcome in metastatic melanoma. Cancer Res 2012;72:1070—80.

[179] Pages F, Galon J, Dieu-Nosjean MC, Tartour E, Sautes-Fridman C, Fridman WH. Immune infiltration in human tumors: a prognostic factor that should not be ignored. Oncogene 2010;29:1093—102.

[180] Schmieder A, Michel J, Schonhaar K, Goerdt S, Schledzewski K. Differentiation and gene expression profile of tumor-associated macrophages. Semin Cancer Biol 2012.

[181] Sica A, Mantovani A. Macrophage plasticity and polarization: in vivo veritas. J Clin Invest 2012;122:787—95.

[182] Rakhmilevich AL, Baldeshwiler MJ, Van De Voort TJ, Felder MA, Yang RK, Kalogriopoulos NA, et al. Tumor-associated myeloid cells can be activated in vitro and in vivo to mediate antitumor effects. Cancer Immunol Immunother 2012.

[183] Beatty GL, Chiorean EG, Fishman MP, Saboury B, Teitelbaum UR, Sun W, et al. CD40 agonists alter tumor stroma and show efficacy against pancreatic carcinoma in mice and humans. Science 2011;331:1612—6.

[184] de Gramont A, de Gramont A, Chibaudel B, Bachet JB, Larsen AK, Tournigand C, et al. From chemotherapy to targeted therapy in adjuvant treatment for stage III colon cancer. Semin Oncol 2011;38:521—32.

[185] Pander J, Heusinkveld M, van der Straaten T, Jordanova ES, Baak-Pablo R, Gelderblom H, et al. Activation of tumor-promoting type 2 macrophages by EGFR-targeting antibody cetuximab. Clin Cancer Res 2011; 17:5668—73.

[186] Hoos A, Britten CM, Huber C, O'Donnell-Tormey J. A methodological framework to enhance the clinical success of cancer immunotherapy. Nat Biotechnol 2011;29:867—70.

[187] Hoos A, Eggermont AM, Janetzki S, Hodi FS, Ibrahim R, Anderson A, et al. Improved endpoints for cancer immunotherapy trials. J Natl Cancer Inst 2010;102:1388—97.

[188] Maecker HT, Rinfret A, D'Souza P, Darden J, Roig E, Landry C, et al. Standardization of cytokine flow cytometry assays. BMC Immunol 2005;6:13.

[189] Maecker HT, Maino VC. T cell immunity to HIV: defining parameters of protection. Curr HIV Res 2003;1:249—59.

[190] Gill DK, Huang Y, Levine GL, Sambor A, Carter DK, Sato A, et al. Equivalence of ELISpot assays demonstrated between major HIV network laboratories. PLoS One 2010;5:e14330.

[191] Maecker HT, McCoy JP, Nussenblatt R. Standardizing immunophenotyping for the Human Immunology Project. Nat Rev Immunol 2012;12:191—200.

[192] Disis ML. Immunologic biomarkers as correlates of clinical response to cancer immunotherapy. Cancer Immunol Immunother 2011;60:433—42.

[193] Janetzki S, Cox JH, Oden N, Ferrari G. Standardization and validation issues of the ELISPOT assay. Methods Mol Biol 2005;302:51—86.

[194] Britten CM, Janetzki S, Ben-Porat L, Clay TM, Kalos M, Maecker H, et al. Harmonization guidelines for HLA-peptide multimer assays derived from results of a large scale international proficiency panel of the Cancer Vaccine Consortium. Cancer Immunol Immunother 2009;58:1701—13.

[195] Janetzki S, Panageas KS, Ben-Porat L, Boyer J, Britten CM, Clay TM, et al. Results and harmonization guidelines from two large-scale international Elispot proficiency panels conducted by the Cancer Vaccine Consortium (CVC/SVI). Cancer Immunol Immunother 2008;57:303—15.

[196] Moodie Z, Price L, Gouttefangeas C, Mander A, Janetzki S, Lower M, et al. Response definition criteria for ELISPOT assays revisited. Cancer Immunol Immunother 2010;59:1489—501.

[197] Mander A, Gouttefangeas C, Ottensmeier C, Welters MJ, Low L, van der Burg SH, et al. Serum is not required for ex vivo IFN-gamma ELISPOT: a collaborative study of different protocols from the European CIMT Immunoguiding Program. Cancer Immunol Immunother 2010;59:619—27.

[198] Attig S, Price L, Janetzki S, Kalos M, Pride M, McNeil L, et al. A critical assessment for the value of markers to gate-out undesired events in HLA-peptide multimer staining protocols. J Transl Med 2011;9:108.

[199] Janetzki S, Britten CM, Kalos M, Levitsky HI, Maecker HT, Melief CJ, et al. "MIATA"-minimal information about T cell assays. Immunity 2009;31:527—8.

[200] Britten CM, Janetzki S, van der Burg SH, Huber C, Kalos M, Levitsky HI, et al. Minimal information about T cell assays: the process of reaching the community of T cell immunologists in cancer and beyond. Cancer Immunol Immunother 2011;60:15—22.

Strategies of Passive and Active Immunotherapy

CHAPTER 17

Adoptive T-cell Therapy: Engineering T-cell Receptors

Richard A. Morgan
Surgery Branch, National Cancer Institute, National Institutes of Health, Bethesda, MD USA

I. EARLY TRIALS OF ADOPTIVE T-CELL THERAPY

The paradigm for the development of adoptive cell therapy (ACT) for cancer lies in the studies of cell therapy for hematological malignancies and melanoma. While metastatic melanoma is generally resistant to both chemotherapy and radiotherapy, spontaneous regression of melanoma has been observed in some cases suggesting the immunogenic nature of this tumor in comparison with other tumors [1,2]. Melanoma was the first human cancer for which T cells were shown to recognize specific tumor antigens [3]. The subsequent identification of a large number of tumor-associated antigens opened up the possibility of specifically targeting candidate tumor antigens to selectively eliminate tumor cells by immunotherapy [4]. Currently there are two US FDA approved immunological-based therapies for patients with metastatic melanoma, Interleukin-2 and the anti-CLTA-4 antibody ipilimumab, resulting in objective response rates ranging from 5% to 15% [5,6]. The possibility that physicians might be able to use this immunogenicity as a foundation for the development of an adoptive cell therapy has generated significant progress in the use of immunotherapy, particularly for the treatment of melanoma.

Adoptive cellular immunotherapy involves the administration of autologous or allogenic tumor reactive T cells into patients to achieve tumor regression and has been successful in transplant-related malignancies, leukemia and melanoma [7]. In melanoma, this process involves the identification of lymphocytes with high affinity for tumor antigens that can be selected *in vitro* and expanded and administered to patients. When autologous antitumor lymphocyte cultures are administered to patients with high-dose interleukin IL-2 following a lympho-depleting-conditioning regimen, the cells can expand *in vivo*, traffic to tumor, and mediate tumor regression resulting in durable objective clinical responses. The administration of naturally occurring TIL has been shown to have an objective response rate ranging from 49–72% in metastatic melanoma patients; including bulky invasive tumors at multiple sites including liver, lung, soft tissue and brain [8,9,10]. The use of cloned cytotoxic lymphocytes (CTL) has also been shown to mediate tumor regression in melanoma patients, but response rates were <10% [11,12]. To be a candidate for TIL therapy a patient must meet several requirements. Tumor must be accessible for surgical resection or biopsy and viable tumor reactive TIL must be generated from the tumor in adequate numbers. A major limitation to the widespread application of TIL therapy is the difficulty in generating human T cells with antitumor reactivity. It has been reported that approximately only one half of melanomas reproducibly give rise to antitumor TILs [13]. As an alternative approach, TCR genes from

261

Cancer Immunotherapy. http://dx.doi.org/10.1016/B978-0-12-394296-8.00017-8

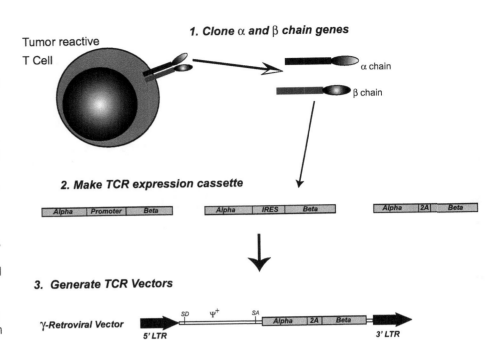

FIGURE 17.1

Production of TCR expression vectors. The first step in the production of a TCR expression vector is to isolate a tumor-reactive T cell and clone the individual TCR alpha and beta chain genes. This can come from a human tumor reactive T-cell clone, it can be a murine T-cell isolate from the immunization of human HLA transgenic mice, or it could come from an alternative source such as bacteriophage or yeast display technology. The second step is the construction of the TCR expression cassette. This has been accomplished by linking the alpha and beta chain genes using an internal promoter, an internal ribosome entry site (IRES), or using a picornavirus 2A peptide. The third and final step is to insert the TCR expression cassette into a gene transfer such as a gamma-retroviral vector shown here.

262

tumor reactive T cells can be isolated and transferred to normal T cells (Figure 17.1). TCR gene transfer would allow the generation of large numbers of defined antigen-specific T cells for therapeutic application. Therefore, TCR based immunotherapy has the advantage that we can administer very large numbers of genetically engineered T cells with high avidity for tumor antigens. Ultimately it may be possible to establish a collection of defined TCR genes that could be used to treat a diverse set of patients' cancer tailored to each patient depending on the tumor antigen expression pattern [4].

II. ISOLATING TCRs FOR GENE TRANSFER

The success of adoptive transfer of T cells as a therapy for the treatment of metastatic melanoma formed a strong foundation for TCR engineered T cells. The first step in TCR gene therapy is to isolate a T-cell clone with high affinity for a defined target antigen. Genes encoding the TCR can be isolated from patients with rare reactive high avidity T-cell clones that recognize and lyse target tumor cells [14]. The TCR α and β chains are identified, isolated and cloned into a gene transfer vector using recombinant DNA techniques. The genetic transfer of TCR α and β chains directed against specific tumor antigens can create generic antigen-specific T cells. The first successful transfer of melanoma reactive TCR to human peripheral blood lymphocytes conferring antitumor reactivity was reported in 1999 [15]. Since then several reports demonstrated that transfer of a tumor antigen-specific TCR into T cells results in an antigen-specific T-cell population [16–18]. This approach bypasses the need to isolate the tumor-specific effector cells from each patient. TCR engineered T cells upon encounter with antigen positive tumor cells secrete immunostimulatory cytokines, exert antigen-specific cytotoxicity and are able to expand in response to the antigen stimulation. It has been shown that the specificity of the TCR-transduced T cells is not altered compared to the parental T-cell clone [17].

The possibility of using HLA-transgenic mice to generate TCR against human tumor antigens offers a valuable strategy to overcome the tolerance of patients to self-tumor antigens and thus allow investigators to generate high avidity TCRs. High affinity TCRs can be obtained by immunization of transgenic mice expressing human HLA with human tumor antigenic peptides. Murine CTL generated by this method are used to isolate murine TCR specific for HLA-restricted human peptides. This strategy has been shown feasible for peptides from the human tumor antigens such as gp100 [19], p53 [20], CEA [21] and MAGE-A3 [22]. Expression of mouse TCRs in human T cells could generate an immune response against the transgene potentially resulting in the rejection of transduced T cells, but we have not observed such an event in humans [23]. In addition to the use of transgenic mice to generate TCRs, technologies such as the use of yeast or phage display have shown the ability to generate very highly avid TCRs [24,25].

Recent advances in gene transfer technology opened up the possibilities of creating large numbers of genetically modified lymphocytes with appropriate therapeutic properties [16,17,26]. High-affinity T-cell receptors can be introduced into normal T cells of cancer patients and the adoptive transfer of these cells into the lymphodepleted patients has been shown to mediate cancer regression [19,26]. TCR engineered T cells complement the clinical success of adoptive cell transfer therapy of TIL by offering the benefit of this therapy to patients who fail to generate TIL.

III. ANTIGEN CHOICE FOR TCR THERAPY

In the past two decades, fundamental advances in immunology and tumor biology combined with the identification of a large number of tumor antigens have led to significant progress in the field of cell-based immunotherapy [27,28]. Many antigens recognized by autologous T lymphocytes have been identified on human melanoma [29]. The first step in TCR-based therapy is the choice of appropriate tumor antigen to target the T cells. The TCR should target a protein that is widely and selectively expressed in tumor cells, and the TCR should have high affinity for its antigen, and be strongly expressed in T cells. The many human tumor associated antigens are nonmutated self-antigens shared between individuals [30] that are normal differentiation antigens, which are overexpressed in tumor cells. Several TCRs have been identified targeting a variety of melanocyte differentiation antigens like gp100 [17], MART-1 [31] and Tyrosinase [32,33].

In addition to targeting differentiation antigens, many investigators have focused on cancer testis antigens. Cancer testis antigens (CTAs) are immunogenic proteins, which are normally expressed in non-MHC expressing germ cells of the testis yet are aberrantly expressed in many tumors. More than 110 CTA genes have been identified that are expressed in multiple tumor types including melanoma, and carcinomas of the bladder, lung and liver [34,35] (many of the CTA are found on the human X chromosome)[36]. The expression pattern of CTA defines three categories of genes: testis-restricted (CTA whose expression is limited to the testis in adults), testis/brain-restricted (CTA whose expression is limited to the testis and brain in adults), and testis-selective (CTA whose expression is limited to the testis and occasionally in various other tissues in adults)[37]. The first human tumor antigen to be described was the CTA gene MAGE-A1. Since the identification of the first human CTA gene (MAGE-A1) in 1991, [3] the number of MAGE family genes has grown to 25 members. MAGE-A is a multigene family consisting of 12 homologous genes MAGE-A1 to MAGE-A12 located at chromosome Xq28. The precise function and biological role of MAGE proteins have not been completely elucidated. The expression of MAGE-A3 has been shown to be higher in more advanced stages of the disease and is associated with poor disease prognosis [38,39]. CTA NY-ESO-1 is also widely expressed in a variety of cancers and has been chosen as the initial target for TCR-based therapy at the NCI Surgery Branch [18,40], and the preliminary results are encouraging (see Section VI). Significant efforts are underway to identify TCRs for a large number of other cancer testis antigens that are expressed in various human cancers. Selection of appropriate target tumor antigen is crucial for ultimate long-term tumor regression and to reduce the severity of associated toxicity to the normal tissue. Targeting T cells against tumor-associated CT antigens might selectively eliminate tumor cells and avoid or reduce toxicity to normal tissue.

Ideally, T-cell-based therapy for cancer would target tumor antigens that are unique to the cancer. In the case of viral-associated malignancies, (e.g., those associated with Epstein-Barr virus or human papillomavirus), targeting this class of antigens can lead to complete eradication of tumors in animal models [7,41,42]. An example of nonviral tumor-specific mutations are those resulting from chromosomal rearrangements. The epidermal growth factor receptor (EGFR) is frequently amplified in glioma and often these amplifications are associated with gene rearrangements. EGFR variant III (EGFRvIII) is the most prevalent of several EGFR mutations found in human glioma, and is expressed in about 30% of glioblastoma [43,44]. The expression of EGFRvIII results from intragene deletion rearrangements that eliminate EGFR exons 2−7, and cause the joining of exons 1 and 8 of the coding sequences. While EGFRvIII drives enhanced tumorigenicity through constitutive and unattenuated activation, its expression has not been detected in any normal tissue examined, thus making this aberrant receptor an ideal target for immunotherapy [45]. Ultimately, it is within possibility, using the current technology of high-throughput DNA sequencing and antigen peptide prediction software, that TCR for patient-specific mutations could be developed [4].

IV. ENGINEERING TO IMPROVE TCR ACTIVITY

TCRs used for engineering T cells for clinical application have to exhibit high affinity for its specific peptide-HLA complex, as the transgenic TCR has to compete for cell-surface expression with the endogenous TCR. Numerous strategies have been developed to generate high-affinity TCR and increase specificity (Figure 17.2). One of the anticipated potential problems in ectopic expression of tumor-specific TCR is the formation of mixed dimmers between endogenous and introduced TCR chains. While toxicity associated with mixed dimmer formation has been observed *in vitro* and in mice models [46], no evidence of toxicity or autoimmunity has been observed in TCR clinical trials [47].

Several strategies have been developed to prevent mixed dimer formation while increasing TCR expression. Development of murine−human hybrid TCRs are reported in which constant region of human receptors are replaced by the murine counterparts. The hybrid TCRs exhibited enhanced expression leading to superior function of the engineered T cells, including high levels

264

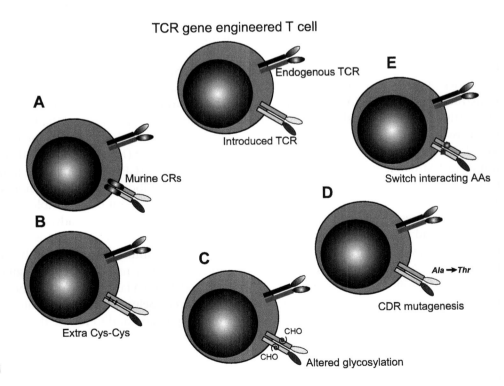

FIGURE 17.2
Protein engineering of TCR genes.
Several protein engineering methodologies have been reported to increase specific TCR chain pairing and/or reactivity. **A.** The introduced TCR can be modified to make a chimeric TCR containing murine constant regions, which has been shown to promote specific chain pairing. **B.** Addition of a second cysteine bridge can be used to increase specific chain pairing. **C.** Alteration of N-linked glycosylation sites has been reported to increase TCR reactivity. **D.** Using site directed mutagenesis, it is possible to make specific amino acid changes within the complementarity determining region (CDR), which can increase antigen reactivity. **E.** The TCR constant regions have a pair of amino acid that interact with each other and these can be flipped to the other chain to facilitate specific chain pairing.

TCR gene engineered T cell

Endogenous TCR
Introduced TCR
Murine CRs
Extra Cys-Cys
CHO CHO Altered glycosylation
Ala → Thr CDR mutagenesis
Switch interacting AAs

of cytokine release and cytolytic activity [48]. In another approach introduction of additional cysteine residues at the constant region of the TCR α and β was used to increase the pairing of TCR chains [49,50]. Single or dual amino acid substitutions in the CDR α or β chains has been shown to provide modest increase in TCR affinity that can enhance the antigen-specific reactivity in T cells [40]. Removal of defined N-glycosylation motifs in the constant domains of TCR-chains resulted in increased functional avidity and enhanced recognition of tumor cells [51]. Some reports described improved expression of TCR on cell surfaces by codon optimization. In this approach, rare codons used by the wild type or murine derived TCR are replaced by those codons most frequently distributed in highly expressed human genes. During the optimization process cis-acting AT or GC rich sequence stretches, cryptic splicing and RNA instability motifs are also removed [52]. A final protein engineering approach uses mutational inversions of the critical interacting amino acids in the TCR α and β chain constant region favors the pairing of the introduced chains and also increases TCR reactivity [53]. As an alternative to protein engineering, it has been reported that small interfering RNA (siRNA) can be used to specifically down-regulate the endogenous TCR, resulting in improved expression and reactivity of the transduced TCR [54,55]. A nonmolecular approach to avoid mispairing is to use γδ T cells for αβ TCR gene engineering; however, the function and persistence of γδ T cells in adoptive cell therapy is not well studied [56]. For a more detailed review of the concepts involved in TCR engineering see these reviews [57,58].

V. TCR DELIVERY

The majority of TCR transfer studies reported have employed murine leukemia virus-based gene delivery systems. These vectors (classified as gamma-retroviral vectors) have been safely used to treat thousands of patients over the past two decades of clinical experimentation. With the rare exception of insertional mutagenesis observed in a few individuals being treated by gene transfer into hematopoietic progenitor cells for treatment of immunodeficiency, there have been no reports of safety issues associated with the gamma-retroviral vector gene transfer system [59]. Although gamma-retroviral vectors are the preferred system for gene delivery to date in the clinical trials, they have limitations. As an alternative, lentiviral vectors are being developed to engineer human T cells with TCR for tumor immunotherapy [60,61]. Lentiviral systems may have the advantage of their ability to transduce the T cells in the absence of TCR mediated activation. This may be useful in keeping the transduced cell population in a less differentiated state that is superior for adoptive immunotherapy [62]. It is also suggested that lentiviral vectors may be less prone to insertional mutagenesis due to their random integration, unlike gamma-retroviral vectors that have preferential integration at the transcription start sites of the genes [63].

Transposons are a relatively new gene transfer system, but provide the advantage of being a nonviral plasmid DNA-based system that is easier to produce and requires less upfront safety testing [64]. Using these methods, genetically engineered T cells have been able to be grown $>1\times10^9$ cells in a short period of time and have shown the ability to expand upon antigenic stimulation, secrete cytokines and exhibit tumor lytic ability [64,65]. Transposon-mediated TCR gene expression has been shown to be comparable to gamma-retroviral vector and lentiviral vector gene transfer systems [66]. Transposon-based nonviral gene delivery systems, such as Sleeping Beauty and PiggyBac, also have random integration profiles with acceptable gene transfer efficiency and are under development for potential clinical application [64,67,68]. Finally, it is reported that electroporation/necleofection could yield good gene transfer with RNA-based expression systems [69]. Although the short half-life of RNA expression post-transfer may limit its clinical application, RNA-based therapy would eliminate the safety concern of gene transfer caused by genome integration [70].

As the TCR is a heterodimer, any gene transfer vector must express both the alpha and beta chains of the TCR. TCR α and β chains have been assembled in different configurations in retroviral vectors either alone or together. Initial bicistronic vectors were generated with dual promoters or linked with IRES sequences [17]. The gene inserted downstream of the IRES is expressed poorly compared to the gene positioned upstream [71]. This might lead to a suboptimal level of expression of the TCR and poor T-cell response. More recent vectors are constructed with the picronavirus derived 2A cleavage peptide elements that allow optimal stoichiometric expression of both α and β chains [19,60,72].

VI. CLINICAL TRIALS

The first human clinical trial of TCR gene therapy was reported in 2006 [26]. In this phase I trial HLA-A2 positive metastatic melanoma patients were treated with retrovirally transduced autologous PBL engineered to expressing a TCR against MART-1. The TCR was cloned from the TIL of a resected melanoma lesion that recognized MART-1: 27—35 epitope. Gene transfer efficiency in this trial was in the range of 21—72% as assessed by the staining for the Vβ12 protein in this TCR. Gene transfer was achieved equally between CD4 and CD8 cells. Gene modified T cells were detected as long as 1 year after adoptive cell transfer. Following T-cell infusion, tumor regression was observed in 2 out of 17 patients. In addition to the initial report, a total of 31 patients were treated in this protocol and 4 patients (13%) experienced an objective regression of metastatic melanoma. Response rate in this first human TCR clinical trial was less than that of the TIL trials that are reported to be in the range of 50—70%. However, this trial provided the first proof of principle for the novel genetic immunotherapy involving TCR modified T cells.

In an effort to improve the efficacy of TCR based therapy, a high avidity TCR that recognized MART-1: 27—35 epitope was generated [19]. It was anticipated that a more highly reactive TCR might yield more effective tumor response in patients. In this second trial objective cancer regression was observed in 30% of patients. However, patients exhibited destruction of normal melanocytes in the skin, eye, and ear. Local steroid administration was employed to treat hearing loss and uveitis. This trial revealed that T cells expressing highly reactive TCRs mediate cancer regression and also target cognate-antigen expressing cells throughout the body. In another trial a highly reactive TCR against human melanocyte differentiation antigen gp100: 154-162 epitope raised by immunizing HLA-A0201 transgenic mice was used to treat melanoma patients [19]. Sixteen melanoma patients were treated in this protocol. Cells expressing murine TCR in this trial persisted at similar levels as the human TCR against MART-1 and mediated tumor regression [19]. An objective clinical response rate of 19% was reported in this trial, and similar on-target/off-tumor toxicity was observed in the skin, ear, and eye.

The transfer of T cells engineered with TCRs directed against melanoma differentiation antigens MART-1 and gp100 resulted in a 13—30% objective response rate, which was lower than the 50—70% rate seen in TIL therapy. Several reasons could be attributed to these lower response rates, including the fact that shared melanoma differentiation proteins may not be the ideal target antigens. Phenotype of the PBL used to engineer TCR may be different from that of the TIL in terms of the expression of homing and other molecules necessary for the efficient trafficking and effector function of the T cells. Alternatively the immune response by the TIL against the tumor may be of polyclonal nature targeting a variety of normal as well as mutated tumor antigens.

The approach to redirect effector cells using genetically modified T cells with tumor-specific T-cell receptors (TCR) has opened the possibility of treating patients with a variety of cancer types other than melanoma. The first clinical trial utilizing lymphocytes transduced with a TCR targeting carcinoembryonic antigen (CEA) to treat metastatic colorectal cancer was reported by Parkhurst et al [73]. CEA is a 180-kDa tumor-associated glycoprotein overexpressed in many epithelial cancers, most notably in colorectal adenocarcinoma. As reported by Parkhurst et al., three patients with metastatic colorectal cancer were treated; all patients experienced a decrease in serum CEA levels (74–99%), and one experienced a measurable response. Severe transient colitis was also observed in the patients presumptively due to targeting CEA, which is also expressed in normal intestinal epithelial cells [73]. This is another example of how targeting self-antigens with a high affinity TCR can mediate cancer regression as well as recognize and destroy normal tissue(s), which may be a limitation to this treatment.

CTA such as NY-ESO-1 are expressed in a wide variety of epithelial cancers including melanoma, and carcinomas of bladder, liver, and lung [34,35] and at a high frequency in synovial cell sarcoma [74]. NY-ESO-1 (gene name $CTAG1\beta$) is a testis-restricted CTA whose expression is restricted in normal adult tissues to the testis, whose cells do not express HLA molecules, and are thus not susceptible to recognition by a TCR. The first clinical trial using adoptive transfer of autologous lymphocytes genetically engineered to express a TCR against CT antigen-NY-ESO-1 has recently been conducted at Surgery Branch, NCI. In this trial reported by Robbins et al., there was a measurable response rate in synovial cell sarcoma patients of 66% (4/6) and in melanoma patients of 45% (5/11) with two melanoma patients being ongoing complete responders [75]. In contrast to the vigorous on-target/off-tumor toxicity seen using TCRs targeting melanoma differentiation antigens, and in the trial targeting CEA, none of the patients who received NY-ESO-1 TCR gene-modified T cells experienced toxicity related to the infused cells. These objective regressions, with the concomitant lack of toxicity observed in this trial, suggest that some CT antigens may be excellent targets for adoptive cell therapy to treat established solid tumors without off-tumor toxicity.

VII. OVERCOMING TUMOR MICROENVIRONMENT INHIBITION OF T-CELL FUNCTION

Recent TCR-based clinical trials have highlighted the promise as well as the challenges facing this therapy. Various factors will contribute towards the clinical efficacy of TCR gene therapy including, the affinity of the transgenic TCR, the maintenance of the TCR gene expression over time, and the *in vivo* persistence of the TCR engineered T cells. Significant progress has been made towards improving the clinical scale transduction and expression of TCR on T cells.

Highly effective T cells can be generated against the desired tumor antigens and yet have no impact at all on tumor growth. Both the T-cell phenotype used for TCR gene modification and the condition these cells encounter at the tumor site can be major determining factors on the outcome of the therapy (Figure 17.3). It has been shown in some cases normal tumor growth proceeds despite having as much as 30% of all circulating CD8 cells with antitumor reactivity [76]. T cells in the tumor microenvironment can be suppressed, whereas similar cells at other sites or peripheral blood can exhibit profound effector function [77]. The mechanism of the local suppression of effector T-cell function at the tumor is not completely understood. Several factors responsible for this phenomenon are proposed, including the local presence of inhibitory cytokines such as IL-10 [78], TGF-β [79], the presence of other cell types capable of actively suppressing immune reactions such as CD4+ regulatory T cells [80] or the stimulation of inhibitory molecules on T cells such as PD-1 [81,82] and CTLA-4 [83].

The programmed death 1 receptor (PD-1) is an inhibitory receptor that is expressed by chronically activated CD4 and CD8 T cells [84,85]. PD-1 is expressed by a larger number of T cells infiltrating metastatic melanoma lesions than T cells in normal tissues and peripheral blood in melanoma patients. The PD-1$^+$ TIL exhibit an exhausted phenotype with impaired effector function compared with PD-1$^-$ TIL and PBL [82]. This observation suggests that the PD-1 pathway has a suppressive role on T-cell effector function. To overcome this suppression, current TCR engineered T cells could be improved by incorporating potential anti-PD-1 strategies like inhibitory RNA to suppress the expression of PD-1 [86]. Similar strategies to prevent the expression of CTLA-4 can potentially enhance the activity of transferred cells *in vivo*. T cells can undergo apoptosis after infusion due to the lack of growth factors or

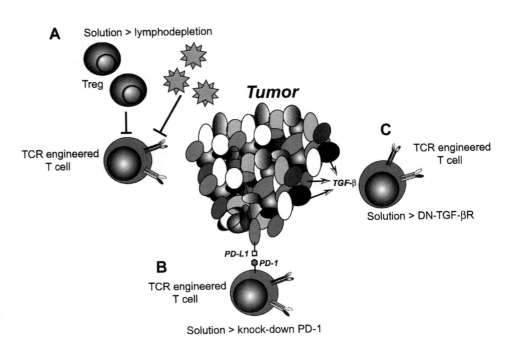

FIGURE 17.3

Overcoming the immunosuppressive tumor environment. The tumor microenvironment is a complex mixture of cells that can actively suppress tumor reactive T cells. **A.** Suppressive cells such as T-regulatory (Treg) cells and myeloid derived suppressor cells (MDSC) can exert a negative effect on antitumor reactive T cells. This can potentially be overcome by lymphodepleting preconditioning. **B.** Several tumor types are known to express the inhibitory ligand PD-L1, which upon binding the T-cells receptor PD-1, inhibits T-cell function. This can potentially be overcome by engineering the T cells with an RNAi-based PD-1 knockdown gene. **C.** Tumors can produce immunosuppressive cytokines such as TGF-b. T cells can be engineered with a dominant negative mutation of the TGF-b receptor (DN-TGF-bR), which can negate the effect of exogenous TGF-b.

co-stimulation. Survival of tumor-specific T cells may be enhanced by engineering them to co-express anti-apoptotic genes like Bcl-2 [87,88]. Finally, to block TGF-β signaling, T cells have been modified to express a dominant-negative TGF-β receptor, which resulted in improvement of TCR transfer therapy in several mouse models [89–91].

Strategies to address some of these issues are already incorporated in the current clinical trials involving TCR modified T cells—for example, lymphodepletion of the host increases the effectiveness of cell transfer therapy by eliminating cellular elements like regulatory T cells and myeloid derived suppressor cells and also by removing the lymphocyte pool in the body that might compete for the available growth factors.

VIII. CONCLUSION

Within a decade of the first demonstration of TCR gene transfer into T cells, significant progress has been made leading to a small number of initial clinical trials. Meaningful clinical responses have been observed using TCR gene-modified T cells in patients with melanoma, colorectal adenocarcinoma, and synovial cell sarcoma, including complete responders. At the same time, these early trials point out the power of TCR engineered T cells to recognize any cell/tissue in the body that expresses the antigen that they are engineered to react with. Thus, the search for appropriate tumor antigens, either tumor specific or those expressed in nonessential organs (e.g., prostate) remains essential for the long-term success of this field. With these encouraging results several efforts are underway to advance this therapy to identify TCRs to treat a variety of cancers. It is likely that progress in this field will evolve rapidly and that TCR gene therapy will become a reality for the treatment of many diverse human malignancies.

References

[1] Chong CA, Gregor RJ, Augsburger JJ, Montana J. Spontaneous regression of choroidal melanoma over 8 years. Retina 1989;9(2):136–8.

[2] King M, Spooner D, Rowlands DC. Spontaneous regression of metastatic malignant melanoma of the parotid gland and neck lymph nodes: a case report and a review of the literature. Clin Oncol (R Coll Radiol) 2001;13(6):466–9.

[3] van der Bruggen P, Traversari C, Chomez P, Lurquin C, De Plaen E, Van den Eynde B, et al. A gene encoding an antigen recognized by cytolytic T lymphocytes on a human melanoma. Science 1991;254(5038):1643–7.

[4] Restifo NP, Dudley ME, Rosenberg SA. Adoptive immunotherapy for cancer: harnessing the T cell response. Nat Rev Immunol 2012;12(4):269–81.

[5] Alexandrescu DT, Ichim TE, Riordan NH, Marincola FM, Di Nardo A, Kabigting FD, et al. Immunotherapy for melanoma: current status and perspectives. J Immunother 2010;33(6):570–90.

[6] Tsao H, Atkins MB, Sober AJ. Management of cutaneous melanoma. N Engl J Med 2004;351(10):998–1012.

[7] Brenner MK, Heslop HE. Adoptive T cell therapy of cancer. Curr Opin Immunol 2010;22(2):251–7.

[8] Rosenberg SA, Yang JC, Sherry RM, Kammula US, Hughes MS, Phan GQ, et al. Durable complete responses in heavily pretreated patients with metastatic melanoma using T-cell transfer immunotherapy. Clin Cancer Res 2011;17(13):4550–7.

[9] Dudley ME, Yang JC, Sherry R, Hughes MS, Royal R, Kammula U, et al. Adoptive cell therapy for patients with metastatic melanoma: evaluation of intensive myeloablative chemoradiation preparative regimens. J Clin Oncol 2008;26(32):5233–9.

[10] Rosenberg SA, Restifo NP, Yang JC, Morgan RA, Dudley ME. Adoptive cell transfer: a clinical path to effective cancer immunotherapy. Nat Rev Cancer 2008;8(4):299–308.

[11] Hunder NN, Wallen H, Cao J, Hendricks DW, Reilly JZ, Rodmyre R, et al. Treatment of metastatic melanoma with autologous CD4+ T cells against NY-ESO-1. N Engl J Med 2008;358(25):2698–703.

[12] Chapuis AG, Thompson JA, Margolin KA, Rodmyre R, Lai IP, Dowdy K, et al. Transferred melanoma-specific CD8+ T cells persist, mediate tumor regression, and acquire central memory phenotype. Proc Natl Acad Sci U S A 2012;109(12):4592–7.

[13] Dudley ME, Wunderlich JR, Shelton TE, Even J, Rosenberg SA. Generation of tumor-infiltrating lymphocyte cultures for use in adoptive transfer therapy for melanoma patients. J Immunother 2003;26(4):332–42.

[14] Johnson LA, Heemskerk B, Powell Jr DJ, Cohen CJ, Morgan RA, Dudley ME, et al. Gene transfer of tumor-reactive TCR confers both high avidity and tumor reactivity to nonreactive peripheral blood mononuclear cells and tumor-infiltrating lymphocytes. J Immunol 2006;177(9):6548–59.

[15] Clay TM, Custer MC, Sachs J, Hwu P, Rosenberg SA, Nishimura MI. Efficient transfer of a tumor antigen-reactive TCR to human peripheral blood lymphocytes confers anti-tumor reactivity. J Immunol 1999;163(1):507–13.

[16] Schaft N, Willemsen RA, de Vries J, Lankiewicz B, Essers BW, Gratama JW, et al. Peptide fine specificity of anti-glycoprotein 100 CTL is preserved following transfer of engineered TCR alpha beta genes into primary human T lymphocytes. J Immunol 2003;170(4):2186–94.

[17] Morgan RA, Dudley ME, Yu YY, Zheng Z, Robbins PF, Theoret MR, et al. High efficiency TCR gene transfer into primary human lymphocytes affords avid recognition of melanoma tumor antigen glycoprotein 100 and does not alter the recognition of autologous melanoma antigens. J Immunol 2003;171(6):3287–95.

[18] Zhao Y, Zheng Z, Robbins PF, Khong HT, Rosenberg SA, Morgan RA. Primary human lymphocytes transduced with NY-ESO-1 antigen-specific TCR genes recognize and kill diverse human tumor cell lines. J Immunol 2005;174(7):4415–23.

[19] Johnson LA, Morgan RA, Dudley ME, Cassard L, Yang JC, Hughes MS, et al. Gene therapy with human and mouse T-cell receptors mediates cancer regression and targets normal tissues expressing cognate antigen. Blood 2009;114(3):535–46.

[20] Cohen CJ, Zheng Z, Bray R, Zhao Y, Sherman LA, Rosenberg SA, et al. Recognition of fresh human tumor by human peripheral blood lymphocytes transduced with a bicistronic retroviral vector encoding a murine anti-p53 TCR. J Immunol 2005;175(9):5799–808.

[21] Parkhurst MR, Joo J, Riley JP, Yu Z, Li Y, Robbins PF, et al. Characterization of genetically modified T-cell receptors that recognize the CEA:691-699 peptide in the context of HLA-A2.1 on human colorectal cancer cells. Clin Cancer Res 2009;15(1):169–80.

[22] Chinnasamy N, Wargo JA, Yu Z, Rao M, Frankel TL, Riley JP, et al. A TCR targeting the HLA-A*0201-restricted epitope of MAGE-A3 recognizes multiple epitopes of the MAGE-A antigen superfamily in several types of cancer. J Immunol 2011;186(2):685–96.

[23] Davis JL, Theoret MR, Zheng Z, Lamers CH, Rosenberg SA, Morgan RA. Development of human anti-murine T-cell receptor antibodies in both responding and nonresponding patients enrolled in TCR gene therapy trials. Clin Cancer Res 2010;16(23):5852–61.

[24] Kieke MC, Sundberg E, Shusta EV, Mariuzza RA, Wittrup KD, Kranz DM. High affinity T cell receptors from yeast display libraries block T cell activation by superantigens. J Mol Biol 2001;307(5):1305–15.

[25] Li Y, Moysey R, Molloy PE, Vuidepot AL, Mahon T, Baston E, et al. Directed evolution of human T-cell receptors with picomolar affinities by phage display. Nat Biotechnol 2005;23(3):349–54.

[26] Morgan RA, Dudley ME, Wunderlich JR, Hughes MS, Yang JC, Sherry RM, et al. Cancer regression in patients after transfer of genetically engineered lymphocytes. Science 2006;314(5796):126–9.

[27] Blattman JN, Greenberg PD. Cancer immunotherapy: a treatment for the masses. Science 2004;305(5681):200–5.

[28] Rosenberg SA. A new era for cancer immunotherapy based on the genes that encode cancer antigens. Immunity 1999;10(3):281–7.

[29] Romero P, Cerottini JC, Speiser DE. The human T cell response to melanoma antigens. Adv Immunol 2006;92:187–224.

[30] Rosenberg SA. Progress in human tumour immunology and immunotherapy. Nature 2001;411(6835): 380–4.

[31] Hughes MS, Yu YY, Dudley ME, Zheng Z, Robbins PF, Li Y, et al. Transfer of a TCR gene derived from a patient with a marked antitumor response conveys highly active T-cell effector functions. Hum Gene Ther 2005;16(4):457–72.

[32] Roszkowski JJ, Lyons GE, Kast WM, Yee C, Van Besien K, Nishimura MI. Simultaneous generation of CD8+ and CD4+ melanoma-reactive T cells by retroviral-mediated transfer of a single T-cell receptor. Cancer Res 2005;65(4):1570–6.

[33] Frankel TL, Burns WR, Peng PD, Yu Z, Chinnasamy D, Wargo JA, et al. Both CD4 and CD8 T cells mediate equally effective in vivo tumor treatment when engineered with a highly avid TCR targeting tyrosinase. J Immunol 2010;184(11):5988–98.

[34] Suri A. Cancer testis antigens—their importance in immunotherapy and in the early detection of cancer. Expert Opin Biol Ther 2006;6(4):379–89.

[35] Simpson AJ, Caballero OL, Jungbluth A, Chen YT, Old LJ. Cancer/testis antigens, gametogenesis and cancer. Nat Rev Cancer 2005;5(8):615–25.

[36] Caballero OL, Chen YT. Cancer/testis (CT) antigens: potential targets for immunotherapy. Cancer Sci 2009;100(11):2014–21.

[37] Hofmann O, Caballero OL, Stevenson BJ, Chen YT, Cohen T, Chua R, et al. Genome-wide analysis of cancer/ testis gene expression. Proc Natl Acad Sci U S A 2008;105(51):20422–7.

[38] Chen YT, Ross DS, Chiu R, Zhou XK, Chen YY, Lee P, et al. Multiple cancer/testis antigens are preferentially expressed in hormone-receptor negative and high-grade breast cancers. PLoS One 2011;6(3):e17876.

[39] Kim J, Reber HA, Hines OJ, Kazanjian KK, Tran A, Ye X, et al. The clinical significance of MAGEA3 expression in pancreatic cancer. Int J Cancer 2006;118(9):2269–75.

[40] Robbins PF, Li YF, El-Gamil M, Zhao Y, Wargo JA, Zheng Z, et al. Single and dual amino acid substitutions in TCR CDRs can enhance antigen-specific T cell functions. J Immunol 2008;180(9):6116–31.

[41] Kenter GG, Welters MJ, Valentijn AR, Lowik MJ, Berends-van der Meer DM, Vloon AP, et al. Vaccination against HPV-16 oncoproteins for vulvar intraepithelial neoplasia. N Engl J Med 2009;361(19):1838–47.

[42] Anders K, Buschow C, Herrmann A, Milojkovic A, Loddenkemper C, Kammertoens T, et al. Oncogene-targeting T cells reject large tumors while oncogene inactivation selects escape variants in mouse models of cancer. Cancer Cell 2011;20(6):755–67.

[43] Gan HK, Kaye AH, Luwor RB. The EGFRvIII variant in glioblastoma multiforme. J Clin Neurosci 2009;16(6):748–54.

[44] Friedman HS, Bigner DD. Glioblastoma multiforme and the epidermal growth factor receptor. The New England journal of medicine 2005;353(19):1997–9.

[45] Johnson LA, Sampson JH. Immunotherapy approaches for malignant glioma from 2007 to 2009. Curr Neurol Neurosci Rep 2010;10(4):259–66.

[46] Bendle GM, Linnemann C, Hooijkaas AI, Bies L, de Witte MA, Jorritsma A, et al. Lethal graft-versus-host disease in mouse models of T cell receptor gene therapy. Nat Med 2010;16(5):565–70. 1p following 70.

[47] Rosenberg SA. Of mice, not men: no evidence for graft-versus-host disease in humans receiving T-cell receptor-transduced autologous T cells. Mol Ther 2010;18(10):1744–5.

[48] Cohen CJ, Zhao Y, Zheng Z, Rosenberg SA, Morgan RA. Enhanced antitumor activity of murine-human hybrid T-cell receptor (TCR) in human lymphocytes is associated with improved pairing and TCR/CD3 stability. Cancer Res 2006;66(17):8878–86.

[49] Cohen CJ, Li YF, El-Gamil M, Robbins PF, Rosenberg SA, Morgan RA. Enhanced antitumor activity of T cells engineered to express T-cell receptors with a second disulfide bond. Cancer Res 2007;67(8):3898–903.

[50] Kuball J, Dossett ML, Wolfl M, Ho WY, Voss RH, Fowler C, et al. Facilitating matched pairing and expression of TCR chains introduced into human T cells. Blood 2007;109(6):2331–8.

[51] Kuball J, Hauptrock B, Malina V, Antunes E, Voss RH, Wolfl M, et al. Increasing functional avidity of TCR-redirected T cells by removing defined N-glycosylation sites in the TCR constant domain. J Exp Med 2009;206(2):463–75.

[52] Scholten KB, Kramer D, Kueter EW, Graf M, Schoedl T, Meijer CJ, et al. Codon modification of T cell receptors allows enhanced functional expression in transgenic human T cells. Clin Immunol 2006;119(2): 135–45.

[53] Voss RH, Willemsen RA, Kuball J, Grabowski M, Engel R, Intan RS, et al. Molecular design of the Calphabeta interface favors specific pairing of introduced TCRalphabeta in human T cells. J Immunol 2008;180(1):391−401.

[54] Okamoto S, Mineno J, Ikeda H, Fujiwara H, Yasukawa M, Shiku H, et al. Improved expression and reactivity of transduced tumor-specific TCRs in human lymphocytes by specific silencing of endogenous TCR. Cancer Res 2009;69(23):9003−11.

[55] Ochi T, Fujiwara H, Okamoto S, An J, Nagai K, Shirakata T, et al. Novel adoptive T-cell immunotherapy using a WT1-specific TCR vector encoding silencers for endogenous TCRs shows marked antileukemia reactivity and safety. Blood 2011;118(6):1495−503.

[56] van der Veken LT, Hagedoorn RS, van Loenen MM, Willemze R, Falkenburg JH, Heemskerk MH. Alphabeta T-cell receptor engineered gammadelta T cells mediate effective antileukemic reactivity. Cancer Res 2006;66(6):3331−7.

[57] Kieback E, Uckert W. Enhanced T cell receptor gene therapy for cancer. Expert Opin Biol Ther 2010;10(5):749−62.

[58] Govers C, Sebestyen Z, Coccoris M, Willemsen RA, Debets R. T cell receptor gene therapy: strategies for optimizing transgenic TCR pairing. Trends Mol Med 2010;16(2):77−87.

[59] Hacein-Bey-Abina S, von Kalle C, Schmidt M, Le Deist F, Wulffraat N, McIntyre E, et al. A serious adverse event after successful gene therapy for X-linked severe combined immunodeficiency. N Engl J Med 2003;348(3):255−6.

[60] Yang S, Cohen CJ, Peng PD, Zhao Y, Cassard L, Yu Z, et al. Development of optimal bicistronic lentiviral vectors facilitates high-level TCR gene expression and robust tumor cell recognition. Gene Ther 2008;15(21):1411−23.

[61] Tsuji T, Yasukawa M, Matsuzaki J, Ohkuri T, Chamoto K, Wakita D, et al. Generation of tumor-specific, HLA class I-restricted human Th1 and Tc1 cells by cell engineering with tumor peptide-specific T-cell receptor genes. Blood 2005;106(2):470−6.

[62] Gattinoni L, Powell Jr DJ, Rosenberg SA, Restifo NP. Adoptive immunotherapy for cancer: building on success. Nat Rev Immunol 2006;6(5):383−93.

[63] Wu X, Li Y, Crise B, Burgess SM. Transcription start regions in the human genome are favored targets for MLV integration. Science 2003;300(5626):1749−51.

[64] Hackett PB, Largaespada DA, Cooper LJ. A transposon and transposase system for human application. Mol Ther 2010;18(4):674−83.

[65] Hackett Jr PB, Aronovich EL, Hunter D, Urness M, Bell JB, Kass SJ, et al. Efficacy and safety of Sleeping Beauty transposon-mediated gene transfer in preclinical animal studies. Curr Gene Ther 2011;11(5):341−9.

[66] Peng PD, Cohen CJ, Yang S, Hsu C, Jones S, Zhao Y, et al. Efficient nonviral Sleeping Beauty transposon-based TCR gene transfer to peripheral blood lymphocytes confers antigen-specific antitumor reactivity. Gene Ther 2009;16(8):1042−9.

[67] Singh H, Manuri PR, Olivares S, Dara N, Dawson MJ, Huls H, et al. Redirecting specificity of T-cell populations for CD19 using the Sleeping Beauty system. Cancer Res 2008;68(8):2961−71.

[68] Nakazawa Y, Huye LE, Salsman VS, Leen AM, Ahmed N, Rollins L, et al. PiggyBac-mediated Cancer Immuno-therapy Using EBV-specific Cytotoxic T-cells Expressing HER2-specific Chimeric Antigen Receptor. Mol Ther 2011.

[69] Zhao Y, Zheng Z, Cohen CJ, Gattinoni L, Palmer DC, Restifo NP, et al. High-efficiency transfection of primary human and mouse T lymphocytes using RNA electroporation. Mol Ther 2006;13(1):151−9.

[70] Zhao Y, Moon E, Carpenito C, Paulos CM, Liu X, Brennan AL, et al. Multiple injections of electroporated autologous T cells expressing a chimeric antigen receptor mediate regression of human disseminated tumor. Cancer Res 2010;70(22):9053−61.

[71] Mizuguchi H, Xu Z, Ishii-Watabe A, Uchida E, Hayakawa T. IRES-dependent second gene expression is significantly lower than cap-dependent first gene expression in a bicistronic vector. Mol Ther 2000;1(4):376−82.

[72] Leisegang M, Engels B, Meyerhuber P, Kieback E, Sommermeyer D, Xue SA, et al. Enhanced functionality of T cell receptor-redirected T cells is defined by the transgene cassette. J Mol Med (Berl) 2008;86(5):573−83.

[73] Parkhurst MR, Yang JC, Langan RC, Dudley ME, Nathan DA, Feldman SA, et al. T cells targeting carcinoem-bryonic antigen can mediate regression of metastatic colorectal cancer but induce severe transient colitis. Mol Ther 2011;19(3):620−6.

[74] Jungbluth AA, Antonescu CR, Busam KJ, Iversen K, Kolb D, Coplan K, et al. Monophasic and biphasic synovial sarcomas abundantly express cancer/testis antigen NY-ESO-1 but not MAGE-A1 or CT7. Int J Cancer 2001;94(2):252−6.

[75] Robbins PF, Morgan RA, Feldman SA, Yang JC, Sherry RM, Dudley ME, et al. Tumor regression in patients with metastatic synovial cell sarcoma and melanoma using genetically engineered lymphocytes reactive with NY-ESO-1. J Clin Oncol 2011;29(7):917−24.

271

[76] Rosenberg SA, Sherry RM, Morton KE, Scharfman WJ, Yang JC, Topalian SL, et al. Tumor progression can occur despite the induction of very high levels of self/tumor antigen-specific CD8+ T cells in patients with melanoma. J Immunol 2005;175(9):6169−76.

[77] Bai A, Higham E, Eisen HN, Wittrup KD, Chen J. Rapid tolerization of virus-activated tumor-specific CD8+ T cells in prostate tumors of TRAMP mice. Proc Natl Acad Sci U S A 2008;105(35):13003−8.

[78] O'Garra A, Barrat FJ, Castro AG, Vicari A, Hawrylowicz C. Strategies for use of IL-10 or its antagonists in human disease. Immunol Rev 2008;223:114−31.

[79] Wrzesinski SH, Wan YY, Flavell RA. Transforming growth factor-beta and the immune response: implications for anticancer therapy. Clin Cancer Res 2007;13(18 Pt 1):5262−70.

[80] Colombo MP, Piconese S. Regulatory-T-cell inhibition versus depletion: the right choice in cancer immuno-therapy. Nat Rev Cancer 2007;7(11):880−7.

[81] Barber DL, Wherry EJ, Masopust D, Zhu B, Allison JP, Sharpe AH, et al. Restoring function in exhausted CD8 T cells during chronic viral infection. Nature 2006;439(7077):682−7.

[82] Ahmadzadeh M, Johnson LA, Heemskerk B, Wunderlich JR, Dudley ME, White DE, et al. Tumor antigen-specific CD8 T cells infiltrating the tumor express high levels of PD-1 and are functionally impaired. Blood 2009.

[83] Sarnaik AA, Weber JS. Recent advances using anti-CTLA-4 for the treatment of melanoma. Cancer J 2009;15(3):169−73.

[84] Sharpe AH, Wherry EJ, Ahmed R, Freeman GJ. The function of programmed cell death 1 and its ligands in regulating autoimmunity and infection. Nat Immunol 2007;8(3):239−45.

[85] Greenwald RJ, Freeman GJ, Sharpe AH. The B7 family revisited. Annu Rev Immunol 2005;23:515−48.

[86] Borkner L, Kaiser A, van de Kasteele W, Andreesen R, Mackensen A, Haanen JB, et al. RNA interference targeting programmed death receptor-1 improves immune functions of tumor-specific T cells. Cancer Immunol Immunother 2010;59(8):1173−83.

[87] Kalbasi A, Shrimali RK, Chinnasamy D, Rosenberg SA. Prevention of interleukin-2 withdrawal-induced apoptosis in lymphocytes retrovirally cotransduced with genes encoding an antitumor T-cell receptor and an antiapoptotic protein. J Immunother 2010;33(7):672−83.

[88] Charo J, Finkelstein SE, Grewal N, Restifo NP, Robbins PF, Rosenberg SA. Bcl-2 overexpression enhances tumor-specific T-cell survival. Cancer Res 2005;65(5):2001−8.

[89] Hu Z, Gerseny H, Zhang Z, Chen YJ, Berg A, Stock S, et al. Oncolytic Adenovirus Expressing Soluble TGFbeta Receptor II-Fc-mediated Inhibition of Established Bone Metastases: A Safe and Effective Systemic Therapeutic Approach for Breast Cancer. Mol Ther 2011.

[90] Yang YA, Dukhanina O, Tang B, Mamura M, Letterio JJ, MacGregor J, et al. Lifetime exposure to a soluble TGF-beta antagonist protects mice against metastasis without adverse side effects. J Clin Invest 2002;109(12):1607−15.

[91] Lacuesta K, Buza E, Hauser H, Granville L, Pule M, Corboy G, et al. Assessing the safety of cytotoxic T lymphocytes transduced with a dominant negative transforming growth factor-beta receptor. J Immunother 2006;29(3):250−60.

272

CHAPTER 18

Dendritic Cell Vaccines: Sipuleucel-T and Other Approaches

Nicholas M. Durham, Charles G. Drake
Department of Oncology, Johns Hopkins University, Baltimore, MD USA

I. GENERATING A CANCER VACCINE

Edward Jenner coined the term "vaccine" to describe his strategy of proactively inoculating patients with cowpox to protect them from contracting the deadly smallpox virus. Since that time, the term vaccine has expanded to include a variety of treatment approaches attempting to harness the immune system to prevent and treat disease. The success of vaccination as a public health measure, notably exemplified by the eradication of polio and smallpox from the Western World, has driven development of well-characterized, reproducible methods of generating a vaccine against a targeted pathogen. The principles of successful vaccination consist of providing the competent immune system with foreign antigen in the context of a "danger" signal (adjuvant). The specific conditions of immunization can be modified based on the strength, type, and location of the response desired. Furthermore, successful vaccines serve as a primary exposure of the immune system to a particular antigen and thus generate immunological memory that protects the host long after the immediate threat has been cleared. Each subsequent exposure generates a faster and more robust antigen-specific response. It is not surprising that this system works so powerfully and reliably given that the immune system has evolved over thousands of years to recognize foreign antigen and generate long-lasting, protective immunity. Generating a vaccine against an established cancer, on the other hand, is much more challenging.

Unlike foreign pathogens, cancer cells are derived from the host. This means that the majority of genes expressed by cancer cells are expressed either transiently or constitutively by normal human cells. Consequently, the multiple layers of protection in place to guard against auto-immunity are commandeered by the tumor to thwart an antitumor immune response. Identifying molecular targets or genes that differentiate a patient's normal cells from tumor cells is an essential first step in designing an effective vaccine against a tumor. This process requires knowledge of two characteristics of a candidate tumor antigen: density and location. If an antigen is more abundant in tumor tissue than in normal tissue, this differential expression can theoretically be used to direct an appropriately titrated immune response that destroys tumor cells while causing minimal damage to normal tissue. Location is also an important consideration, as an antigen expressed even at high levels in nonvital normal tissue might be targeted given the acceptable morbidity associated with autoimmune destruction of this tissue.

At the time of detection, most tumors have been present in an afflicted patient for over a decade [1,2]. During this time, the tumor has been slowly progressing and interacting with

Cancer Immunotherapy. http://dx.doi.org/10.1016/B978-0-12-394296-8.00018-X

18

normal host tissue, including the immune system. There are three possible outcomes for the interaction between a tumor and immune cells. The immune system can either eliminate the cancer cells, maintain equilibrium in which the tumor neither grows nor shrinks, or allow the tumor to escape [3,4]. This failure can be due to the immune system's inability to recognize (ignorance) or remove cancerous cells (tolerance), or simply because the immune system cannot kill faster than the tumor can grow. In order to develop an effective cancer vaccine, ignorance or tolerance must be overcome in order to produce a functional immune response that is capable of selectively killing tumor tissue. It must have a specific target antigen (or antigens). An active, functional response must be generated to this antigen. Responding cells must traffic to the correct anatomical site, and effectively kill tumor cells once there. Dendritic cell vaccines occupy a pivotal position in the immune response, potentially addressing all of these challenges.

II. DENDRITIC CELLS: CRITICAL FOR GENERATING AN IMMUNE RESPONSE*

Immature DCs are found throughout the human body and are constantly sampling the environment for antigens [5,6]. This sampling continues until the DC is activated either upon detection of pathogens by pattern recognition receptors or in response to cytokines secreted by neighboring cells. Activated DCs (Mature DCs) stop sampling the environment, upregulate activation markers, and migrate though the lymphatics to secondary lymphoid organs. In the lymph node, DCs present antigen on both MHC Class I and Class II to CD8 (cytotoxic) and CD4 (helper) cells, respectively. Activation markers, such as B7-1 and B7-2, serve as co-stimulation for T cells to drive differentiation toward the subtypes of functional effector T cells. Nonactivated DCs can also be found in the lymph nodes, presenting antigen without activation markers. In this context, immature DCs drive a tolerogenic immune response via generation of regulatory CD4 T cells (Treg) and/or deletion or anergizing of antigen-specific cells. Depending on the activation state of the DC, the immune system can be skewed toward an anergic, humoral, or cytolytic response. T cells and B cells proliferate, differentiate, and subsequently migrate to the site of DC activation. In this way, DCs serve as central coordinators of the immune response [7,8].

DCs are able to activate many different types of immune cells, but historically it has been shown that CD8 T cells are likely the most important cell type in detecting and lysing tumor cells [9,11]. T cells are able to detect extracellular and intracellular antigens presented by MHC molecules. A CD8 cytolytic response is the preferred immune response based on data developed in many mouse systems as well as data from human CD8 adoptive transfer clinical studies [12]. A robust and long lasting CD8 T-cell response can only be developed with the help of activated CD4 T cells [13,14]. Tumor cells tend to be poor activators of the immune system because they express MHC Class I in the absence of co-stimulatory molecules [15,17]. Consequently, most tumor cells can only stimulate CD8 T cells in a manner that makes them become unresponsive to antigen [18,19]. Dendritic cells, conversely, are the most efficient antigen-presenting cells known and can, therefore, have the potential to activate both types of T-cell response and generate a potent CD8 cytotoxic T lymphocyte (CTL) response.

III. HISTORY AND BASIC BIOLOGY OF DC VACCINES**

The first cancer vaccine trials used autologous tumor lysate, or tumor antigen peptide alone [20—23]. Trials of these peptide vaccines in patients with melanoma reported no survival advantage. Subsequent studies have revealed that peptide vaccines have generally failed at reliably generating immune activation due to their inability to break self-tolerance [24].

---

* Discussed in detail in Chapter 5
** Also see Chapter 5

These early disappointments have driven the development of alternative vaccine strategies, including autologous infusion of DCs. One of the first Phase I clinical trials of a DC-based vaccine used DCs pulsed with two different epitopes of the protein PMSA restricted to the Class I MHC molecule HLA-A0201 in patients with metastatic prostate cancer [25]. The primary endpoints of this study were safety and tolerability. Secondary endpoints were T-cell responses and PSA levels. Prostate cancer is a reasonable setting to test immunotherapy. Since, the prostate gland is molecularly unique, with a number of proteins expressed in a relatively restricted manner. Furthermore, the prostate is a nonvital tissue, reducing the potential impact of autoimmune side effects. In these trials, peripheral blood mononuclear cells (PBMCs) were isolated, plated, and enriched for monocytes. These monocytes were subsequently cultured with GM-CSF and IL-4 to generate monocyte-derived DCs. Patients were then infused with either DC alone, peptide alone, or peptide pulsed DCs. Notably, this trial did not include a specific DC activation step. In general, DC infusion was well-tolerated with few adverse events (AEs). After treatment, patients' PBMCs were isolated for analysis. Prostate membrane specific antigen (PMSA) protein was added to PBMC cultures and proliferation was measured. Only peptide pulsed DCs generated peptide specific lymphocyte proliferation.

This basic paradigm served as a platform for the development of DC vaccines for the next several years. Clinical trials were conducted in renal cell carcinoma, glioblastoma, melanoma, and lymphoma [26—30]. In each of these trials, the same general DC derivation strategy was used: isolate PBMC, select for adherent cells, and culture with IL-4 and GM-CSF. In each case, DC vaccines were found to be safe and well-tolerated, as no significant adverse events were observed. The studies differed in terms of antigen source/loading and activation of DCs.

Antigen loading is specific to the type of antigen under evaluation. To pulse peptides onto DCs, a specific epitope must be known that corresponds with that patient's HLA type. To circumvent this issue, several groups have used tumor lysate directly derived from resected tumor to load DC. For example, Nestle et al. [26] used freeze thaw lysis from biopsies to provide melanoma specific antigens directly from the tumor. In glioma, Yu et al. [29] used acid elution of MHC molecules to provide a peptide library to load DCs. Holtl et al. [28] used enzymatic digestion of tissue removed by nephrectomy to load DCs. These methods are potentially effective because they provide direct access to the antigens that are natively accessible. The drawback is that many of these antigens are not tumor-specific and this process may thus dilute the pool of tumor-specific antigens. In contrast, the identification and synthesis of tumor-specific proteins or peptides can potentially provide a more concentrated source of material with which to load or pulse DC. Other options for DC loading include the use of cDNA libraries isolated from tumor samples as well as overexpression constructs for particular tumor-associated genes [31]. One especially straightforward method for loading DC involves loading of whole protein. This method of DC loading is particularly relevant in hematological malignancies, where the malignant clone is characterized by the production of a monoclonal paraprotein. Reichardt et al. [30] performed a trial in which idiotype (Id) antibodies from multiple myeloma patients were loaded onto DCs after a peripheral blood stem cell transplant. This yielded strong B- and T-cell responses in several patients.

The particular antigen employed in a DC vaccine must be dictated by the disease. For example, in multiple myeloma, the antigen is accessible to B and T cells. Patients who received Id loaded vaccine and produced a T-cell response to the Id loaded vaccine were significantly more likely to become complete responders (75%) than those who received the vaccine but did not mount a Id specific response (4.5%) [32]. Another group tested an antigen loading technique where the Id protein was conjugated directly to GM-CSF [33]. Tao et al. showed that this mechanism allowed for intake and processing of the conjugated antigen without the need for additional adjuvant. While the monoclonal paraprotein serves as a nearly perfect tumor-restricted antigen in patients with multiple myeloma and certain lymphomas, in other diseases tumor antigens are harder to identify and, with the possible exception of melanoma, choice

275

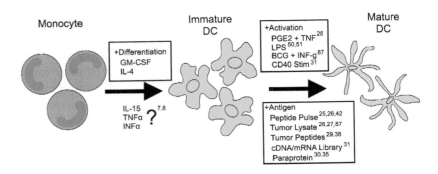

FIGURE 18.1

Generation of DC vaccines. PBMC is isolated from patient blood. Monocytes are differentiated and matured using various methods referenced.

of target antigen becomes increasingly challenging in solid tumors. For a relatively recent review of various tumor antigens in clinical development, see Cheever et al. [34].

The state of the DC defines how well it activates T cells, regardless of the antigen utilized. This principle applies to both the differentiation phase, when monocytes become DCs, as well as the maturation phase, when DCs upregulate co-stimulatory molecules. This is important to consider as differentiation and maturation conditions varied somewhat amongst DC vaccine clinical trials—though most of these DCs were cultured for 4–7 days in the presence of differentiating cytokines. Some trials used no additional activation beyond GM-CSF and IL-4 [25,26,35] while others employed additional cytokines such as TNF-alpha or Prostaglandin E2 to activate and mature DCs [28] (Figure 18.1). These cytokines have been shown to significantly upregulate activation and co-stimulation markers on DCs including CD83, CD86, and MHC-II. Holtl et al. [28] detected lymphocyte proliferation to tumor lysate as well as normal kidney tissue lysate after the addition of TNF-alpha and PGE2. The question of how to optimally activate DCs to generate an antitumor immune response remains an open question in the field [7].

IV. SIPULEUCEL-T: A DENDRITIC CELL VACCINE FOR PROSTATE CANCER

In the late 1980s several groups identified prospective antigens found on prostate tumor samples as well as prostate cancer cell lines, including PSA, PMSA, and PAP [36,37]. The development of Provenge (Sipuleucel-T) began with the discovery of organ-specific autoimmunity (prostatitis) in rats immunized with human Prostatic Acid Phosphatase (PAP)[38]. Rats were immunized with either whole protein in CFA, a vaccinia virus overexpressing humanPAP, or a vaccinia virus expressing ratPAP. Whole human PAP + adjuvant generated a strong humoral response but only vaccinia-PAP was able to generate a CTL response and induce rat prostatitis. Interestingly, rats immunized with ratPAP did not generate a CTL response or subsequent prostatitis, demonstrating that this vaccine strategy did not overcome endogenous tolerance.

In 1999, using PAP as an antigen, Dendreon produced its first vaccine, using a technology that is somewhat different from preceding DC vaccines. To generate this vaccine, patients undergo leukapheresis and large numbers of PBMC are isolated from the blood. PMBCs are enriched for monocytes by gradient density centrifugation. Enriched monocytes are then washed and incubated in serum-free media with a proprietary fusion protein coupling prostatic acid phosphatase (PAP) to GM-CSF (PA2024). No additional cytokines are added to the culture. After approximately 36 hours, the cells are shipped back to an infusion center (without cryopreservation) and are subsequently infused back into the patient [39,40](Figure 18.2). Importantly, DCs are not the only cell type infused into patients as the final product includes significant fractions of T cells, B cells, and NK cells [39].

Two early Phase I trials evaluated the safety and tolerability of Sipuleucel-T in patients with metastatic prostate cancer. The first of these clinical trials administered two DC+PA2024 infusions one month apart followed by three subcutaneous (SQ) injections of the fusion

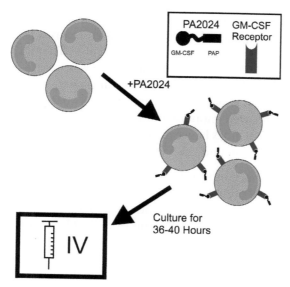

FIGURE 18.2
Generation of Sipuleucel-T. See text for additional details.

protein. Humoral and T-cell responses were followed, as were levels of circulating PAP and PSA. In this trial, 8 of 9 patients developed PA2024 specific T-cell responses, confirming immunological activity. Unfortunately, this response was primarily limited to the GM-CSF portion of the fusion protein, and all patients demonstrated significantly higher proliferation to GM-CSF alone as compared to PAP. This result was perhaps to be expected, given that the fusion protein represents a neo-antigen, whilst mature PAP would be expected to be a self-protein in the majority of patients. After treatment, 2 of the 3 patients whose PSA level dropped after administration of the vaccine also showed T-cell proliferation responses to PAP alone. Antibody responses to either PAP or GM-CSF were detected, but did not correlate with PSA responses.

A second trial administered a total of three IV DC+PA2024 infusions. All patients developed T-cell proliferative responses to PA2024, but only about one-third of the patients developed responses to native PAP. Additionally, this study showed clear evidence of an induced humoral response, with antibody titers to native PAP detectable in over half of the treated patients. While both of these Phase I studies were relatively small, it is interesting to speculate that perhaps the decreased PAP specific responses found by the first group could have been a result of the additional SC injections of PA2024. This notion is supported by preclinical data showing that DC vaccination can break tolerance but only if given after peptide vaccination [41,42]. Considering all patients who received the DC vaccine, there was no observed difference in time to progression with treatment; however, patients who demonstrated a PAP-specific immune response did show a reduction in PSA and PAP. Importantly, both Phase I trials showed Sipuleucel-T to be safe and well tolerated. Fever was the most common adverse event in both trials, along with the development of a mild flu-like syndrome. No adverse events grade III or higher were reported in either trial.

The promising results from these trials led to the initiation of a Phase III trial of the vaccine (Sipuleucel-T) in men with asymptomatic or minimally symptomatic metastatic castrate-resistant prostate cancer [43]. This trial (D9901) enrolled 127 patients and subsequently randomized them 2:1 between Sipuleucel-T and placebo. Patients randomized to active treatment were given 3 infusions of Sipuleucel-T every 2 weeks. Patients in the placebo group underwent leukapheresis and were re-infused with one third of the leukapheresis product. For placebo patients, the remaining {2/3} of the leukapheresis product was cryopreserved, and could later be used to prepare a vaccine product (APC8015F) for salvage therapy. All patients given placebo were unblinded at the time of progression and offered APC8015F in separate salvage treatment protocol. The primary endpoint of this trial was time to progression (TTP), although overall survival (OS) was followed as a planned secondary endpoint. The results of this study showed that patients receiving Sipuleucel-T had a TTP of 11.7 weeks while patients receiving placebo had a TTP of 10 weeks. This difference was not statistically significant; however, patients that received Sipuleucel-T had a median survival of 25.9 months compared to the placebo group's median survival of 21.4 months ($p = 0.01$ HR $= 1.70$). Approximately 39% of the enrolled patients were monitored for immune activation, and while there was an eight-fold higher proliferation index between Sipuleucel-T and placebo patients, no correlative data between immune activation and OS have yet been presented.

In summary, this Phase III trial confirmed the safety and tolerability of Sipuleucel-T, and corroborated previous reports of clinical activity. When these data were reported, a second Phase III trial (D9902) had already enrolled 98 patients. This trial also evaluated TTP as the primary endpoint. In several analyses, the initial 98 patients from D9902A were either analyzed alone, or pooled with the patients from D9901 and analyzed for TTP and OS [44]. The results from these analyses showed an overall survival of 23.2 months in the Sipuleucel-T arm compared with 18.9 months in the placebo group [45] ($p = 0.02$, HR $= 0.77$). This led to an application for a Biologics License Application in November of 2006 (STN125197). As is typical, a scientific advisory panel was convened in March of 2007. The panel voted 17−0 on the issue of Sipuleucel-T safety, and 13−4 on the question of efficacy. In a rare but not unprecedented decision, the FDA did not grant full approval, instead requesting additional data on overall survival. There was significant controversy over the FDA's decision to deny full approval, partially because of the FDA's decision to overturn the advisory panel's recommendations [46]. Ultimately the FDA maintained that if OS is the primary benefit of the agent, it should be the primary endpoint of a larger trial. These events led to the pivotal Phase III trial, D9902B (IMPACT).

This trial was a 512 patient double-blinded study similar in design to D9901 and D9902. The most notable difference between this and the earlier trials was that the primary endpoint was OS. This trial demonstrated a survival advantage, with a median survival of 25.8 months in patients on the active treatment arm, as compared to 21.4 months for those patients treated with placebo [47] (HR $= 0.78$, P $= 0.03$). In this trial (as in the earlier trials) progressors in the placebo group were offered vaccine prepared from cryopreserved cells as part of a salvage protocol. Approximately half of the patients on placebo ultimately received salvage treatment. Thus, this crossover could potentially confound a larger difference in the survival results. It should be noted that, as in earlier trials, the agent was well-tolerated with side effects primarily limited to fever and flu-like syndromes. In April 2010, Sipuleucel-T was approved by the FDA for metastatic castrate resistant prostate cancer [48]. This event was a landmark for cancer immunotherapy in general, and for DC vaccines in particular, marking the first active cancer immunotherapy to demonstrate a survival benefit in a randomized Phase III trial.

V. IMPROVING DC VACCINES

Currently Sipuleucel-T is the only cancer vaccine FDA approved for therapeutic use in humans. As described above, Phase III data showed that this agent provides a significant overall survival advantage of approximately 4 months. Yet neither D9902B (IMPACT) nor D9901 showed a significant difference in time to progression of disease, nor in progression free survival [47]. Since development of this agent began in 1998 a significant amount of research has transpired regarding DC infusion as a vaccine strategy. There are two basic concepts by which these data can be utilized to improve current DC vaccines to treat cancer. First, it is possible to alter the way DCs are generated in order to create a vaccine that generates a stronger, reliable, and more long-lasting immune response. Second, combining currently approved or in trial vaccines with other drugs or treatments may alter the immune system or the tumor to increase the efficacy of both. Since the vast majority of current cancer treatments involve combinatorial therapy, it does not seem unreasonable that combinatorial immunotherapy would be more effective than monotherapy.

The canonical means of generating DCs is to use GM-CSF and IL-4 to drive differentiation of monocytes into DCs. In the case of Sipuleucel-T, only GM-CSF is used. Additionally Sipuleucel-T enriches for monocytes, but leaves reasonable percentages of lymphocytes in culture that end up being re-infused during drug treatment. On average, CD54+ cells make up approximately 5−15% of the total cells [39]. This is important because it has been shown that CD54+ cells are most able to take up PA2024 and present it to T cells [49]. No additional cytokines are added to these DC cultures. We now know that different conditions of DC culture can generate DCs with different phenotypes and functions [7,8]. Monocytes treated with IL-15 with GM-CSF are skewed to a Langerhans-like DC that is a potent activator of CTL responses [50]. After differentiation, DCs cultured with different cytokines, TLR agonists, and/or chemokines will demonstrate differences in activation status, and the expression of co-stimulatory molecules. For example, DCs exposed to IL-1, TNF-alpha, and CD40 significantly upregulate CD54 [51]. Thus, modifying conditions of DC differentiation and activation may generate a more potent inducer of a CD8 CTL response.

VI. IMPROVING DC VACCINES: COMBINATION TREATMENT APPROACHES

A. Androgen deprivation therapy

Although not without controversy, androgen deprivation therapy has been shown to improve the overall survival of high-risk metastatic prostate cancer patients [52]. Physiologically, androgen deprivation therapy (ADT) operates by altering androgen signaling in men. From an endocrine perspective, the androgen signaling axis begins in the brain, where the hypothalamus secretes gonadotropin-releasing hormone (GNRH) which travels down neurosecretory neurons to the anterior portion of the pituitary. This signals the pituitary to secrete FSH and LH which enter the bloodstream. These hormones reach the testes where they bind to high affinity receptors, mediating the secretion of testosterone [53]. Thus ADT can be accomplished in two ways. One method uses a GNRH super-agonist (such as leuprolide acetate) to block release of FSH and LH at the level of the pituitary. Another way to block the androgen axis is with androgen receptor blocking agents, such as bicalutamide, nilutamide or flutamide. These agents bind to androgen receptor in the tissues, rendering physiological levels of androgen nonfunctional.

Perhaps somewhat surprisingly, many cells and organs in the mammalian immune system express androgen receptors (AR), including the thymic epitheilium [54,55]. Thymocytes express the receptor, but there is very little evidence of its presence on mature T cells [56]. Several groups have shown that altering androgens directly affects the thymic epithelium by driving the secretion of thymic regressing factors [57]. Blocking AR signaling by ADT drives thymopoesis and thymic regeneration, even in older mice, rats, and humans [58,59]. This is important because in the case of prostate cancer, both central and peripheral tolerance have most likely depleted the repertoire of self-reactive T cells specific for prostate-restricted antigens. Thymopoesis is thus likely to drive the generation of naïve CD4 and CD8 T cells [59], potentially with novel specificities. This phenomenon has been observed in the B-cell compartment as well after ADT [60,61].

Thus, more T cells are generated in patients on ADT for prostate cancer. In addition, the majority of prostate epithelial cells are dependent on androgen signaling for survival. Thus androgen-deprivation therapy results in rapid apoptotic death of both benign and malignant prostate tissues, which drives recruitment of immune cells to the prostate. Several studies in patients that received ADT have showed dramatic recruitment of T and B cells to the prostate [62,63]. In the first of these studies, Mercader et al [63] administered ADT prior to surgery, and reported a significantly increased population of CD4 T cells and a smaller increase in CD8s in patients that received ADT. These data showed T-cell infiltration to be time-dependent, with a maximal increase noted when androgen-deprivation was initiated two weeks prior to surgery. In more recent work, Gannon et al. [62] further characterized the infiltrating lymphocyte population by staining tissue samples for FoxP3 (Treg); these studies showed that androgen ablation results in an increase in Treg populations. Still, there was a strong increase in immune infiltrate of CD3+ and CD8+ T cells, which may overcome the observed increase in Tregs. To potentially maximize the clinical potential of this ADT-driven increase in T-cell infiltrate, several groups have attempted to combine ADT with immunological treatments to test whether this increased infiltrate corresponds to a break in T-cell tolerance [64,65]. Using an adoptive transfer model in mice where spontaneous prostate tumors overexpress hemagglutinin (HA), we found that adoptively transferred, prostate-specific CD4 and CD8 TCR transgenic cells were rendered tolerant by recognition of tumor-associated antigen. This tolerance was largely mitigated by ADT; we found that castration significantly increased the HA specific CD4 and CD8 T cell's ability to divide and produce INF-gamma. Koh et al [65]. tested combining immunotherapy with ADT in another system, comparing the use of ADT along with a DNA vaccine specific for PSCA. This group found that ADT alone increased the number of DCs found in the prostate draining lymph nodes and that these DCs had an increased expression of DC activation markers CD80, CD83, CD86, CD40, and OX-40L. They then combined DNA vaccination to PSCA followed by ADT (castration) and found a significant increase in the amount of PSCA-specific T cells secreting INF-gamma. Perhaps most significantly, this study also explored the relative timing of ADT with respect to vaccination and found that ADT augments an antitumor immune response optimally when administered after immunization, but not before.

This question is currently being addressed in an ongoing clinical trial, utilizing Sipuleucel-T in men with nonmetastatic, castrate sensitive (biochemically recurrent) prostate cancer. In this trial, 60 patients will be randomized to either ADT prior to Sipuleucel-T or the opposite order. The primary readout will be changes in immune responses to PA2024, which will be assayed by antigen-specific proliferation, antibody production, and INF-gamma production. Secondary endpoints are CD54 upregulation and total CD54+ cell number. This is an important trial, which is likely to influence the initiation and design of future trials exploring ADT/immunotherapy combination treatment.

In 2011, a novel ADT drug, abiraterone acetate, was FDA approved for the treatment of metastatic castrate resistant prostate cancer that has progressed after chemotherapy [66]. Approval of this drug means that more patients will be receiving this treatment earlier in the disease and could be receiving the agent either immediately before or after Sipuleucel-T. Thus, it is clinically important to understand whether abiraterone acetate (with prednisone) can be administered without affecting an antitumor immune response initiated by Sipuleucel-T [67,68]. To evaluate this question clinically, a Phase II trial (NCT01487863) has been initiated. In this trial, men with metastatic castrate resistant prostate cancer will be randomized and treated with abiraterone either concurrent with Sipuleucel-T or immediately following the last infusion of Sipuleucel-T. The primary readout in this study will be upregulation of CD54 in the vaccine product; secondary endpoints will be total CD54+ cell counts and T-cell activation. Taken together these two ongoing trials will determine the optimal sequence with which to combine ADT and Sipuleucel-T, and will also determine whether the novel hormonal therapy abiraterone acetate can be combined with immunotherapy in a straightforward manner.

VII. IMMUNE CHECKPOINT BLOCKADE

In general, DC vaccines are intended to induce antitumor cytotoxic CD8 T-cell responses. DC vaccines do this by increasing the number of antigen-presenting cells that can initiate this type of a response, as well as by increasing the relative concentration of specific antigen(s) being targeted. Based on the co-stimulation that the DC is capable of providing at time of activation, it is possible to change the quality of the initial T-cell response, but after the T cell has migrated to the site of antigen encounter, several factors can alter the ability of the T cell to kill its target. When manufacturing DC vaccines, one notion is to maximize vaccine preparation such that DCs express CD54+, HLA-DR, CD40, CD80, and CD86. These cell surface molecules play a role in providing a strong co-stimulation signal from the DC. T cells that recognize their cognate antigen may also express a number of molecules on the surface such as CTLA-4, PD-1, LAG-3 and BTLA. These molecules serve as checkpoints, controlling the quality and magnitude of a T-cell response [69—71]. In normal circumstances, these checkpoints serve to protect the host from an overactive immune system and autoimmunity. In the case of cancer, antibody blockade therapy of these checkpoints could help break tolerance and could serve as a means to increase the quality of the initial response when primed by a DC vaccine, as well as to help maintain a high quality long-lasting T-cell response. The first T-cell immune checkpoint targeted for antibody blockade was CTLA-4. During the initial stages of activation, CTLA-4 is one of the first inhibitory molecules to be upregulated and transported to the surface. Upon TCR engagement, stored CTLA-4 molecules are transported from intracellular vesicles to the cell surface. The stronger the TCR stimulus, the more CTLA-4 is expressed at the cell surface. CTLA-4 binds CD80 and CD86 with a higher affinity than CD28, thus outcompeting CD28's co-stimulatory role. Mice that have CTLA-4 knocked out show significant and lethal autoimmunity [72—74]. In a pivotal murine study, anti-CTLA inhibited the growth of several tumor cell lines in various mouse models [74]. In other studies, antibody blockade was combined with a GM-CSF secreting tumor vaccine to treat exogenous tumor and compared to no treatment or each monotherapy. Combined blockade with vaccine increased survival, increased tumor regression, and increased secretion of IFN-gamma [75]. This effect was dependent on the presence of CD8+ cells. So, when combined with a DC vaccine, anti-CTLA-4 may help increase the quality of the initial T-cell response and create a T cell that is more sensitive to antigen.

Mouse models led to the engineering of two human anti CTLA-4 antibodies for Phase I clinical trials, tremelimumab (Pfizer, Inc) and Ipilimumab (BMS, Inc). Initial trials alone and with peptide vaccines showed promising results but with significant risks of grade III/IV autoimmune manifestations, mainly colitis [76,77]. After substantial clinical development, anti-CTLA-4 was FDA-approved for the treatment of melanoma [78,79]. There are two early studies currently combining CTLA-4 blockade with DC vaccines in melanoma [80,81]. Both studies use melanoma mRNA to express melanoma-specific antigens. The primary endpoint of these trials is safety and tolerability, but T-cell activation will also be monitored via INF-gamma production and CTL activity. These trials are in early stages but will hopefully clarify whether combining DC vaccines with checkpoint blockade is safe, and whether combination increases either monotherapy's efficacy. It should be noted that the objective response rate to anti-CTLA-4 therapy is in the 10—15% range. This may be because of lack of tumor antigen presentation, or because of other factors that limit immune recognition of tumors. It is thus plausible that DC vaccines can improve antigen exposure to T cells and provide an opportunity for CTLA-4 blockade to directly target tumor reactive T cells.

Several other checkpoint molecules are upregulated after the T-cell/APC interaction is complete. These molecules help limit the T-cell response once the cells begin to migrate to tissue. This is believed to be a means of maintaining peripheral tolerance [69—71]. One of these molecules, Programmed Cell Death-1 (PD-1), is significantly upregulated on T cells present in cancerous tissue in various tumor types, including prostate cancer [82,83]. When PD-1 binds either of its ligands, B7-H1 or B7-DC, cytokine production and total T-cell activation are decreased [84,85]. This mechanism is present to help prevent peripheral autoimmunity. In the case of tumor tolerance, PD-1 antibody blockade may serve as a means to maintain a high level T-cell response post DC vaccine.

A monoclonal antibody blocking PD-1 is currently in clinical development. A Phase I trial tested human anti-PD-1(MDX-1106) in patients with metastatic solid tumors [86]. This dose escalation trial showed a very low incidence of adverse events, with only rare grade III toxicities. A single incidence of grade III colitis was seen. Although these autoimmune adverse events appeared to be significantly less frequent than those noted with CTLA-4 blockade, this small Phase I trial should not be directly compared with the extensive clinical experience accrued using CTLA-4 blockade. In terms of clinical activity, a single complete response and two partial responses were observed. This trial showed PD-1 blockade to be relatively safe and verified that single-agent PD-1 blockade can induce objective antitumor responses in some patients. Since DC vaccines primarily activate T cells and presumably induce them to migrate to the site of immune function, their function is very likely to be limited by the tumor microenvironment, in which B7-H1 is expressed. Thus, combining DC vaccines with PD-1 blockade could lead to a clinical scenario in which activated CD8s are generated, and their functionality later preserved at the tumor site.

VIII. SELECTED DC VACCINES IN CLINICAL DEVELOPMENT

There are two later stage trials employing DC vaccines for treatment of kidney cancer and glioblastoma. Both are promising, and each combines additional treatment with the DC vaccine to maximize its efficacy. AGS-003, a renal cell carcinoma vaccine from Argos Therapeutics, is a patient specific, autologous DC vaccine where the patient's DCs are electroporated with the subjects' tumor mRNA and CD40L mRNA. This is a relatively unique strategy, in which the DC will be able to provide CD40L stimulation without the help of CD4 T cells. This may significantly increase the ability of the DC to generate potent CD8 CTL responses. In a planned Phase III trial, AGS-003 will be administered concurrently with sunitinib, a receptor tyrosine kinase inhibitor. In data from a single-armed Phase III trial, an increase in progression free survival from the addition of AGS-003 to sunitinib was reported [31]. Full data from this trial are not yet available, as median overall survival has not yet been reached,

Northwest Biotherapeutics is currently testing "DCvax", a DC vaccine that is loaded with autologous glioblastoma lysate. Phase I data showed significant extension of time to recurrence from 6.9 months with standard of care (historical controls), to >18 months on DCvax. Overall survival was also increased from SOC of 14.6 months to 33.8 months on DCvax [87]. This was a small nonrandomized Phase I study with only 29 patients, and the comparison group was historical, but the potential clinical activity of DCvax in this challenging disease is intriguing. A larger Phase II study with between 140–240 patients is currently in progress. As is the case for most of the DC-based vaccines discussed here, the side effects of DCvax were minimal, with no grade III/IV adverse events noted. The most frequent AEs were fever, injection site itching, myalgias, and seizures, possibly associated with GBM progression. By comparison, standard of care treatment for GBM involves 60 Gy of radiation over 6 weeks administered with the chemotherapy agent temozolomide. Side effects of that regimen include fatigue, bone marrow suppression, infections, cerebral hemorrhage, and liver irritation [88]. Thus, if the promising clinical data observed in the initial trials of DCvax are supported in a larger, randomized study, this treatment could present an interesting option for patients with GBM.

IX. CONCLUSION

The clinical development of Sipuleucel-T has shown that cancer vaccines can help patients live longer with cancer. Importantly, this immunotherapy is safe, with low rates of adverse events. While technically Sipuleucel-T is quite different from other DC vaccines, it demonstrates the potential of this type of therapy. Despite these encouraging results, it seems likely that the promise of DC vaccines has not yet been fully realized. Progress in this area will likely require a method of consistently activating and maturing DCs in a manner that reliably and reproducibly stimulates T cells. Producing an immune response in the majority of patients that receive a DC vaccine is a viable, short-term goal. Despite these challenges, DC vaccines have shown promise in renal cell carcinoma and glioblastoma, leading to Phase II and III clinical trials (Table 18.1). In the future, DC vaccines combined with other immunotherapies, hormone treatment, or chemotherapy could achieve higher levels of efficacy. The favorable

TABLE 18.1 Selected DC Vaccine Trials

Trial Title	Trial Phase	Clinicaltrials.gov
Study to investigate an anticancer cellular immunotherapeutic, AGS-003, when used in combination with sunitinib in subjects with Renal Cell Carcinoma	Phase II	NCT00678119
A Phase II Clinical Trial Evaluating DCVax®-L, Autologous Dendritic Cells Pulsed With Tumor Lysate Antigen for the Treatment of Glioblastoma Multiforme	Phase II	NCT00045968
IL15 DC Vaccine in Patients with High Risk Melanoma - an Exploratory Phase I/II Study	Phase I/II	NCT01189383
Concurrent versus Sequential Treatment with Sipuleucel-T and Abiraterone in Men with Metastatic Castrate Resistant Prostate Cancer	Phase II	NCT01487863
Sequencing of Sipuleucel-T and ADT in Men with Non-metastatic Prostate Cancer	Phase II	NCT01431391
Autologous TriMix-DC Therapeutic Vaccine in Combination with Ipilimumab in Patients with Previously Treated Unresectable Stage III or IV Melanoma	Phase II	NCT01302496

side effect profile of DC vaccines may prove beneficial in designing combination therapy regimens as compared with other immune therapies.

DISCLAIMER

Dr. Drake has served as a paid consultant for Dendreon and Bristol-Myers Squibb (BMS) and is a co-inventor for a patent licensed to BMS.

ACKNOWLEDGMENTS

This work was supported by the National Institutes of Health R01 CA127153 and 1P50CA58236-15, the Patrick C. Walsh Fund, the OneInSix Foundation, and the Prostate Cancer Foundation.

References

[1] Jones S, et al. Comparative lesion sequencing provides insights into tumor evolution. Proceedings of the National Academy of Sciences of the United States of America 2008;105:4283–8.

[2] Yachida S, et al. Distant metastasis occurs late during the genetic evolution of pancreatic cancer. Nature 2010;467:1114–7.

[3] Dunn GP, Bruce AT, Ikeda H, Old LJ, Schreiber RD. Cancer immunoediting: from immunosurveillance to tumor escape. Nat Immunol 2002;3:991–8.

[4] Koebel CM, et al. Adaptive immunity maintains occult cancer in an equilibrium state. Nature 2007;450:903–7.

[5] Banchereau J, Steinman RM. Dendritic cells and the control of immunity. Nature 1998;392:245–52.

[6] Steinman RM. The dendritic cell system and its role in immunogenicity. Annu Rev Immunol 1991;9:271–96.

[7] Palucka K, Banchereau J. Cancer immunotherapy via dendritic cells. Nat Rev Cancer 2012;12:265–77.

[8] Banchereau J, Palucka AK. Dendritic cells as therapeutic vaccines against cancer. Nat Rev Immunol 2005;5:296–306.

[9] Zinkernagel R, Doherty P. Immunological surveillance against altered self components by sensitised T lymphocytes in lymphocytic choriomeningitis. Nature 1974;251:547–8.

[10] Cerottini J, Nordin A, Brunner K. vitro cytotoxic activity of thymus cells. Nature 1970;227:72–3.

[11] Brunner KT, Mauel J, Cerottini JC, Chapuis B. Quantitative assay of the lytic action of immune lymphoid cells on 51-Cr-labelled allogeneic target cells in vitro; inhibition by isoantibody and by drugs. Immunology 1968;14:181–96.

[12] Yee C, et al. Adoptive T cell therapy using antigen-specific CD8+ T cell clones for the treatment of patients with metastatic melanoma: in vivo persistence, migration, and antitumor effect of transferred T cells. Proceedings of the National Academy of Sciences of the United States of America 2002;99:16168–73.

[13] Ridge JP, Di Rosa F, Matzinger P. A conditioned dendritic cell can be a temporal bridge between a CD4+ T-helper and a T-killer cell. Nature 1998;393:474–8.

[14] Schoenberger S, Toes R, Voort E. van der T-cell help for cytotoxic T lymphocytes is mediated by CD40–CD40L interactions. Nature 1998;393:480–3.

[15] Hirano N, et al. Expression of costimulatory molecules in human leukemias. Leukemia 1996;10:1168–76.

[16] Chong H, Hutchinson G, Hart IR, Vile RG. Expression of co-stimulatory molecules by tumor cells decreases tumorigenicity but may also reduce systemic antitumor immunity. Hum Gene Ther 1996;7:1771–9.

[17] Baskar S. Constitutive Expression of B7 Restores Immunogenicity of Tumor Cells Expressing Truncated Major Histocompatibility Complex Class II Molecules. Proceedings of the National Academy of Sciences 1993;90:5687–90.

[18] Schwartz RH. Costimulation of T lymphocytes: the role of CD28, CTLA-4, and B7/BB1 in interleukin-2 production and immunotherapy. Cell 1992;71:1065–8.

[19] Schwartz R. A cell culture model for T lymphocyte clonal anergy. Science 1990;248:1349–56.

[20] Sondak BVK, et al. Adjuvant Immunotherapy of Resected, Intermediate-Thickness, Node-Negative Melanoma With an Allogeneic Tumor Vaccine: Overall Results of a Randomized Trial of the Southwest Oncology Group. J Clin Oncol 2002;20:2058–66.

[21] Rosenberg SA. Principles and practice of the biologic therapy of cancer. 916. Lippincott Williams & Wilkins. at, <http://books.google.com/books?id=C8ZpQgAACAAJ&pgis=1>; 2000.

[22] Haigh PI, Difronzo LA, Gammon G, Morton DL. Vaccine therapy for patients with melanoma. Oncology (Williston Park, N.Y.) 1999;13:1561–74. discussion 1574 passim.

[23] Rosenberg S a, Yang JC, Restifo NP. Cancer immunotherapy: moving beyond current vaccines. Nat Med 2004;10:909–15.

[24] Diehl L, et al. CD40 activation in vivo overcomes peptide-induced peripheral cytotoxic T-lymphocyte tolerance and augments anti-tumor vaccine efficacy. Nat Med 1999;5:774–9.

[25] Murphy G, Tjoa B, Ragde H, Kenny G, Boynton a. Phase I clinical trial: T-cell therapy for prostate cancer using autologous dendritic cells pulsed with HLA-A0201-specific peptides from prostate-specific membrane antigen. Prostate 1996;29:371–80.

[26] Nestle FO, et al. Vaccination of melanoma patients with peptide- or tumor lysate-pulsed dendritic cells. Nat Med 1998;4:328–32.

[27] Timmerman JM. Idiotype-pulsed dendritic cell vaccination for B-cell lymphoma: clinical and immune responses in 35 patients. Blood 2002;99:1517–26.

[28] Höltl L, et al. Cellular and humoral immune responses in patients with metastatic renal cell carcinoma after vaccination with antigen pulsed dendritic cells. J Urol 1999;161:777–82.

[29] Yu JS, et al. Advances in Brief Vaccination of Malignant Glioma Patients with Peptide-pulsed Dendritic Cells Elicits Systemic Cytotoxicity and Intracranial T-cell Infiltration 1. Methods 2001;10:842–7.

[30] Reichardt VL, et al. Idiotype vaccination using dendritic cells after autologous peripheral blood stem cell transplantation for multiple myeloma—a feasibility study. Blood 1999;93:2411–9.

[31] Healey D, Gamble AH, Amin A, Cohen V, T.L., C.A.N. Immunomonitoring of a phase I/II study of AGS-003, a dendritic cell immunotherapeutic, as first-line treatment for metastatic renal cell carcinoma. JCO (meeting abstracts May; 2010.

[32] Liso A, et al. Idiotype vaccination using dendritic cells after autologous peripheral blood progenitor cell transplantation for multiple myeloma. Biol Blood Marrow Transplant 2000;6:621–7.

[33] Tao M-H, Levy R. Idiotype/granulocyte-macrophage colony-stimulating factor fusion protein as a vaccine for B-cell lymphoma. Nature 1993;362:755–75.

[34] Cheever MA, et al. The prioritization of cancer antigens: a national cancer institute pilot project for the acceleration of translational research. Clin Cancer Res 2009;15:5323–37.

[35] Murphy GP, et al. Phase II prostate cancer vaccine trial: report of a study involving 37 patients with disease recurrence following primary treatment. Prostate 1999;39:54–9.

[36] Solin T, Kontturi M, Pohlmann R, Vihko P. Gene expression and prostate specificity of human prostatic acid phosphatase (PAP): evaluation by RNA blot analyses. Biochimica et biophysica acta 1990;1048:72–7.

[37] Lam KW, et al. Improved immunohistochemical detection of prostatic acid phosphatase by a monoclonal antibody. Prostate 1989;15:13–21.

[38] Fong L, et al. Dendritic cell-based xenoantigen vaccination for prostate cancer immunotherapy. J Immunol (Baltimore, Md. : 1950) 2001;167:7150–6.

284

[39] Small EJ, et al. Immunotherapy of hormone-refractory prostate cancer with antigen-loaded dendritic cells. J Clin Oncol 2000;18:3894—903.

[40] Burch PA, et al. Priming Tissue-specific Cellular Immunity in a Phase I Trial of Autologous Dendritic Cells for Prostate Cancer 1. Clin Cancer Res 2000:2175—82.

[41] Larché M, Wraith DC. Peptide-based therapeutic vaccines for allergic and autoimmune diseases. Nat Med 2005;11:S69—76.

[42] Toes RE, et al. Enhancement of tumor outgrowth through CTL tolerization after peptide vaccination is avoided by peptide presentation on dendritic cells. J Immunol (Baltimore, Md. : 1950) 1998;160:4449—56.

[43] Small EJ, et al. Placebo-controlled phase III trial of immunologic therapy with sipuleucel-T (APC8015) in patients with metastatic, asymptomatic hormone refractory prostate cancer. J Clin Oncol 2006;24:3089—94.

[44] Zhen B-guang A, Gupta G. FDA Statistical review for BLA 125197; 2007.

[45] Higano CS, et al. Integrated data from 2 randomized, double-blind, placebo-controlled, phase 3 trials of active cellular immunotherapy with sipuleucel-T in advanced prostate cancer. Cancer 2009;115:3670—9.

[46] The regulator disapproves. Nat Biotechnol 2008;26:1.

[47] Kantoff PW, et al. Sipuleucel-T immunotherapy for castration-resistant prostate cancer. N Engl J Med 2010;363:411—22.

[48] Higano CS, et al. Sipuleucel-T. Nat Rev Drug Discov 2010;9:513—4.

[49] Sheikh N a, Jones L a. CD54 is a surrogate marker of antigen presenting cell activation. Cancer Immunol Immunother 2008;57:1381—90.

[50] Mohamadzadeh M, et al. Interleukin 15 skews monocyte differentiation into dendritic cells with features of Langerhans cells. J Exp Med 2001;194:1013—20.

[51] Yellin MJ, et al. Functional interactions of T cells with endothelial cells: the role of CD40L-CD40-mediated signals. J Exp Med 1995;182:1857—64.

[52] Sharifi N, Gulley J. Androgen deprivation therapy for prostate cancer. JAMA 2005;294:238—44.

[53] Aragon-Ching J, Williams K, Gulley J. Impact of androgen-deprivation therapy on the immune system: implications for combination therapy of prostate cancer. Front Biosci 2007;12:4957—71.

[54] Kovacs WJ, Olsen NJ. Androgen receptors in human thymocytes. J Immunol 1987;139:490—3.

[55] Viselli SM, Olsen NJ, Shults K, Steizer G, Kovacs WJ. Immunochemical and flow cytometric analysis of androgen receptor expression in thymocytes. Mol Cell Endocrinol 1995;109:19—26.

[56] Benten WP, et al. Functional testosterone receptors in plasma membranes of T cells. FASEB journal ASEB journatestosterone receptors in plasma membranes of T cells. analy analyflow cyto 1999;13:123—33.

[57] Kumar N. Mechanism of androgen-induced thymolysis in rats. Endocrinology 1995;136:4887—93.

[58] Greenstein BD, Fitzpatrick FTA, Kendall MD, Wheeler MJ. Regeneration of the thymus in old male rats treated with a stable analogue of LHRH. J Endocrinol 1987;112. 345—NP.

[59] Sutherland JS, et al. Activation of Thymic Regeneration in Mice and Humans following Androgen Blockade. J Immunol 2005;175:2741—53.

[60] Viselli SM, Stanziale S, Shults K, Kovacs WJ, Olsen NJ. Castration alters peripheral immune function in normal male mice. Immunology 1995;84:337—42.

[61] Wilson C, Mrose S, Thomas D. Enhanced production of B lymphocytes after castration. Blood 1995;85:1535—9.

[62] Gannon PO, et al. Characterization of the intra-prostatic immune cell infiltration in androgen-deprived prostate cancer patients. J Immunol Methods 2009;348:9—17.

[63] Mercader M, et al. T cell infiltration of the prostate induced by androgen withdrawal in patients with prostate cancer. Proceedings of the National Academy of Sciences of the United States of America 2001;98:14565—70.

[64] Drake CG, et al. Androgen ablation mitigates tolerance to a prostate/prostate cancer-restricted antigen. Cancer cell 2005;7:239—49.

[65] Koh YT, Gray A, Higgins SA, Hubby B, Kast WM. Androgen ablation augments prostate cancer vaccine immunogenicity only when applied after immunization. Prostate 2009;69:571—84.

[66] Reid AHM, et al. Significant and sustained antitumor activity in post-docetaxel, castration-resistant prostate cancer with the CYP17 inhibitor abiraterone acetate. J Clin Oncol 2010;28:1489—95.

[67] Dendreon. Sequencing of Sipuleucel-T and ADT in Men With Non-metastatic Prostate Cancer 2012. ClinicalTrials.gov NLM(US), NLM: NCT0143139.

[68] Dendreon. Concurrent Versus Sequential Treatment With Sipuleucel-T and Abiraterone in Men With Metastatic Castrate Resistant Prostate Cancer (mCRPC) 2012. ClinicalTrials.gov NLM(US), NLM: NCT0148786.

[69] Korman AJ, Peggs KS, Allison JP. Checkpoint blockade in cancer immunotherapy. Adv Immunol 2006;90:297—339.

285

[70] Pardoll DM. The blockade of immune checkpoints in cancer immunotherapy. Nat Rev Cancer 2012;12:252—64.

[71] Melero I, Hervas-Stubbs S, Glennie M, Pardoll DM, Chen L. Immunostimulatory monoclonal antibodies for cancer therapy. Nat Rev Cancer 2007;7:95—106.

[72] Tivol EA, et al. Loss of CTLA-4 leads to massive lymphoproliferation and fatal multiorgan tissue destruction, revealing a critical negative regulatory role of CTLA-4. Immunity 1995;3:541—7.

[73] Waterhouse P, et al. Lymphoproliferative disorders with early lethality in mice deficient in Ctla-4. Science (New York, N.Y. 1995;270:985—8.

[74] Leach DR, Krummel MF, Allison JP. Enhancement of Antitumor Immunity by CTLA-4 Blockade. Science 1996;271:1734—6.

[75] Elsas BAV, Hurwitz AA, Allison JP. Combination Immunotherapy of B16 Melanoma Using AntiCytotoxic T Lymphocyteassociated Antigen 4 (CTLA-4) and Granulocyte/Macrophage Colony-Stimulating Factor (GM-CSF)-producing Vaccines Induces Rejection of Subcutaneous and Metastatic Tumors Accompanied by. J Exp Med 1999;190:355—66.

[76] Attia P, et al. Autoimmunity correlates with tumor regression in patients with metastatic melanoma treated with anti-cytotoxic T-lymphocyte antigen-4. J Clin Oncol 2005;23:6043—53.

[77] Phan GQ, et al. Cancer regression and autoimmunity induced by cytotoxic T lymphocyte-associated antigen 4 blockade in patients with metastatic melanoma. Proceedings of the National Academy of Sciences of the United States of America 2003;100:8372—7.

[78] Lipson EJ, et al. Targeted Therapeutics in Melanoma. Curr Clin Oncol 2012:291—306. http://dx.doi.org/10.1007/978-1-61779-407-0.

[79] Lipson EJ, Drake CG. Ipilimumab: an anti-CTLA-4 antibody for metastatic melanoma. Clin Cancer Res 2011;17:6958—62.

[80] Duke University Local Modulation of Immune Receptors to Enhance the Response to Dendritic Cell Vaccination in Metastatic Melanoma. ClinicalTrials.gov at, <http://clinicaltrials.gov/ct2/show/NCT01216436?term=CTLA+and+DC+vaccine&rank=2>.

[81] Neyns B. Autologous TriMix-DC Therapeutic Vaccine in Combination With Ipilimumab in Patients With Previously Treated Unresectable Stage III or IV Melanoma. ClinicalTrials.gov. at, <http://clinicaltrials.gov/ct2/show/NCT01302496?term=CTLA+and+DC+vaccine&rank=1>; 2012.

[82] Ahmadzadeh M, et al. Tumor antigen-specific CD8 T cells infiltrating the tumor express high levels of PD-1 and are functionally impaired. Blood 2009;114:1537—44.

[83] Sfanos KS, et al. Human prostate-infiltrating CD8+ T lymphocytes are oligoclonal and PD-1+. Prostate 2009;69:1694—703.

[84] Shin TT, et al. In vivo costimulatory role of B7-DC in tuning T helper cell 1 and cytotoxic T lymphocyte responses. J Exp Med 2005;201:1531—41.

[85] Butte MJ, Keir ME, Phamduy TB, Sharpe AH, Freeman GJ. Programmed death-1 ligand 1 interacts specifically with the B7-1 costimulatory molecule to inhibit T cell responses. Immunity 2007;27:111—22.

[86] Brahmer JR, et al. Phase I study of single-agent anti-programmed death-1 (MDX-1106) in refractory solid tumors: safety, clinical activity, pharmacodynamics, and immunologic correlates. J Clin Oncol 2010;28:3167—75.

[87] Bosch M, Boynton A, Prins R, Liau L. A phase II clinical trial to test the efficacy of DCVax-brain, autologous dendritic cells pulsed with autologous tumor lysate, for the treatment of patients with glioblastoma multiforme. Neuro Oncol 2007;9:509.

[88] Stupp R, et al. Radiotherapy plus concomitant and adjuvant temozolomide for glioblastoma. N Engl J Med 2005;352:987—96.

CHAPTER 19

Antibodies to Stimulate Host Immunity: Lessons from Ipilimumab

Margaret K. Callahan[1,2], Michael A. Postow[1,2], Jedd D. Wolchok[1,2,3,4]
[1]Department of Medicine, Memorial Sloan-Kettering Cancer Center, New York, NY USA
[2]Weill—Cornell Medical College, New York, NY USA
[3]Ludwig Center for Cancer Immunotherapy, Immunology Program, New York, NY USA
[4]The Ludwig Institute for Cancer Research, New York Branch, New York, NY USA

I. INTRODUCTION

Cytotoxic T-lymphocyte antigen 4 (CTLA-4) is a negative regulator of T-cell function, and antibodies have been developed which block this important immunologic checkpoint. In preclinical studies, CTLA-4 blocking antibodies were able to induce potent antitumor immunity in mice and provided rationale for clinical use. Ipilimumab (Yervoy™, formerly MDX-010, Bristol-Myers Squibb, Princeton, NJ) is a monoclonal antibody against CTLA-4 and was the first drug to demonstrate an overall survival benefit for patients with melanoma in a Phase III trial [1].

In this chapter, we describe the preclinical rationale behind the development of ipilimumab and the key clinical trials leading to its approval by the US Food and Drug Administration (FDA) for the treatment of metastatic melanoma. We examine some of the distinct patterns of response and the side effect profile for this novel immunotherapy. Further, we explore efforts in monitoring immunologic parameters in patients treated with ipilimumab to develop biomarkers that might inform clinical decisions. The clinical development of ipilimumab in malignancies outside of melanoma will be briefly discussed. The chapter concludes with a discussion of efforts to improve upon ipilimumab therapy by combining it with traditional and experimental cancer therapies.

II. PRECLINICAL DEVELOPMENT OF CTLA-4 BLOCKADE

A. The biology of T-cell activation: CTLA-4 as a checkpoint

The clinical development of ipilimumab was built upon a foundation of basic research into the mechanisms that regulate T-cell activation. The "two signal" model of T-cell activation was the product of fundamental studies performed in the 1970s and 1980s. In this model, antigen-specific T-cell activation requires both T-cell receptor (TCR) engagement (signal 1) and a co-stimulatory signal (signal 2) [2—5]. In subsequent decades, this hypothesis has been validated and expanded upon. It is now clear that a diversity of co-stimulatory and co-inhibitory molecules are required to both promote and regulate the complex process of T-cell activation. CTLA-4 plays a fundamental role as an inhibitory receptor, or checkpoint, in the process of T-cell activation.

Cancer Immunotherapy. http://dx.doi.org/10.1016/B978-0-12-394296-8.00019-1

The first co-stimulatory molecule expressed on T cells, CD28, was identified in 1980 [6,7]. Two ligands for CD28 were later identified, B7-1 (CD80) and B7-2 (CD86) [8−11]. B7-1 and B7-2 are expressed on antigen-presenting cells (APCs) and can be induced under inflammatory conditions [11−13]. Ligation of CD28 by B7-1 or B7-2 provides the necessary second signal for naïve T-cell activation resulting in cytokine production, proliferation, and cytotoxic function (Figure 19.1, Panel A) [14,15].

CTLA-4 was cloned in 1987 and its similarity to CD28 was recognized early [16]. Like CD28, CTLA-4 binds to B7-1 and B7-2, albeit with higher affinity [17]. Unlike CD28, engagement of CTLA-4 inhibits T-cell activation [18−20]. Important experiments using crosslinking antibodies to stimulate T cell *in vitro* suggested that CTLA-4 acts as a negative regulator of CD28-mediated co-stimulation [18,21]. CTLA-4 engagement on activated T cells inhibits cytokine synthesis and restricts cell proliferation [18,20,22−24]. Later on, the characterization of CTLA-4 −/− knockout mice established a critical negative regulatory function for CTLA-4 *in vivo*. These mice develop a profound, hyperproliferative lymphocyte expansion which is lethal within 3 weeks after birth [25−27].

B. CTLA-4: Mechanisms of inhibition

CTLA-4 functions as a checkpoint, or "brake," on the activation of T cells through several overlapping mechanisms (depicted in a simplified model in Figure 19.1). First, CTLA-4

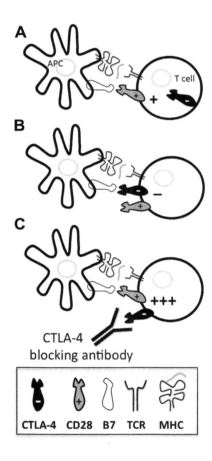

FIGURE 19.1
A. T-cell activation requires two signals. In signal one, the TCR engages a cognate peptide antigen and MHC complex. In signal two, the T cell receives co-stimulation via CD28 interation with B7 (B7-1/CD80 or B7-2/CD86) molecules on the APC. B. Upon T-cell activation, the CTLA-4 molecule is recruited to the cell surface where it competes with CD28 to bind B7 and transmits an inhibitory signal. C. Ipilimumab blocks the engagement of CTLA-4 and prevents engagement of this inhibitory molecule, consequently promoting T-cell activation.

competes with CD28 for binding to its ligands B7-1 and B7-2. CD28 is constituitively expressed on T cells; whereas cell surface expression of CTLA-4 is limited to activated T cells controlled by changes in expression and subcellular trafficking [20,28–33]. CTLA-4 has a higher affinity and out-competes CD28 to bind B7 molecules [32,34,35]. Secondly, CTLA-4 engagement triggers intracellular changes that inhibit T-cell activation. Proposed mechanisms of inhibitory signaling include: (1) association with intracellular phosphatases like Src homology 2 (SH2) domain-containing phosphatase-1 (SHP-1), SHP-2, and protein phosphatase 2A (PP2A), (2) blockade of lipid-raft expression, and (3) disruption of microcluster formation (reviewed by Rudd et al. [15]). Lastly, CTLA-4 transmits suppressive signals via B7 to the APC. This "reverse" signaling results in the induction of indoleamine 2,3-dioxygenase (IDO), an enzyme that degrades tryptophan into byproducts that inhibit T-cell proliferation [36,37].

In vivo, CLTA-4 functions to modulate T-cell activation, employing the cell-intrinsic mechanisms described above [24,27,38–40]. In addition, CTLA-4 expressed on regulatory T cells (Tregs) may play a distinct role in controlling T-cell responses. CTLA-4 is constitutively expressed by natural and inducible Foxp3+ Tregs and engagement of CTLA-4 on Tregs may enhance their regulatory function [41]. Supporting this notion, mice with a conditional deletion of CTLA-4 in the Treg compartment develop a phenotype typified by immune cell hyperactivation similar to, but less severe than, CTLA-4 −/− knockout mice [42].

C. CTLA-4 blockade: A novel approach to stimulate antitumor immunity

Based upon the evidence that CTLA-4 attenuates T-cell activation, it was proposed that blockade of CTLA-4 could enhance antitumor immune responses [43]. This hypothesis was initially validated using transplantable murine tumor lines of colon carcinoma and fibrosarcoma [44–48]. These experiments demonstrated that established tumors could be rejected by administration of a CTLA-4 blocking antibody. This observation has since been expanded to transplantable tumors of many types including prostate carcinoma, breast carcinoma, melanoma, ovarian carcinoma, lymphoma, and others [44–48]. In some poorly immunogenic tumors, such as the B16 melanoma and the SM1 mammary tumor, monotherapy was not effective, but combinations of CTLA-4 blockade with GM-CSF-expressing tumor cells, peptide, or DNA vaccines were active [49–51]. CTLA-4 blockade has since shown activity in combination with conventional cancer therapies including surgery [52], radiation [53,54], chemotherapy [55], cryoablation [56], and radiofrequency ablation [57]. CTLA-4 has also been combined successfully with a diversity of immunotherapies [49–51, 58–66, 67]. Treated mice were resistant to subsequent tumor challenge, confirming the generation of a memory response. Side effects of CTLA-4 blockade in mouse models were minimal, with depigmentation and prostatitis reported in mouse models of melanoma and prostate cancer respectively [49,59,60].

III. CLINICAL DEVELOPMENT OF IPILIMUMAB
A. Development of reagents for human studies

CTLA-4 blocking antibody therapy in humans was developed based on the preclinical activity seen in mouse models. Both ipilimumab and tremelimumab (formerly CP-675, 206 or ticilimumab, Pfizer, New York, NY) are fully human antibodies against CTLA-4 [68–70]. Ipilimumab is an IgG1 antibody with a plasma half-life of 12–14 days. Tremelimumab is an IgG2 antibody with a plasma half-life of approximately 22 days. Both of these agents have been most widely tested in patients with metastatic melanoma, where durable clinical responses have been well documented (Table 19.1). Based on an overall survival benefit in Phase III studies, the US Food and Drug Administration (FDA) approved ipilimumab for the treatment of patients with unresectable or metastatic melanoma in 2011. A Phase III study of tremelimumab was halted after an interim analysis failed to demonstrate a benefit (OS 10.7 versus 11.7 months) [71].

289

TABLE 19.1 Ipilimumab for the Treatment of Advanced Melanoma—Responses in Selected Studies

Reference	Study Population	Dose/Schedule	Treatment Arms	Response Rates	irAEs	Median OS	Survival
Phase III							
Robert et al., 2011	502 patients previously untreated metastatic melanoma	10 mg/kg q3 weeks x 4 doses, then q3 months	Dacarbazine plus ipilimumab	BORR 15.2% DCR 33.2 % 4 CR, 34 PR, 45 SD	Any: 78% Grade III/IV: 42%	11.2 months	47.3% at 1 year 28.5% at 2 years 20.8% at 3 years
			Dacarbazine plus placebo	BORR 10.3% DCR 30.2% 2 CR, 24 PR, 50 SD	Any: 38% Grade III/IV: 6%	9.1 months	36.2% at 1 year 17.9% at 2 years 12.2% at 3 years
Hodi et al., 2010	676 patients previously treated, unresectable stage III or IV melanoma	3 mg/kg q3 weeks x 4 doses option for repeat dosing	Ipilimumab alone	BORR 10.9% DCR 28.5% 2 CR, 13 PR, 24 SD	Any: 61.1% Grade III/IV: 14.5%	10.1 months	45.6% at 1 year 23.5% at 2 years
			Ipilimumab plus gp100 peptide	BORR 5.7% DCR 20.1% 1 CR, 22 PR, 58 SD	Any: 58.2% Grade III/IV: 10.2%	10.0 months	43.6% at 1 year 21.6% at 2 years
			gp100 peptide alone	BORR 1.5% DCR 11.0% 0 CR, 2 PR, 13 SD	Any: 31.8% Grade III/IV: 3%	6.4 months	25.3% at 1 year 13.7% at 2 years
Phase II							
Hersh et al., 2011	72 patients chemotherapy naïve metastatic melanoma	3 mg/kg q3 weeks x 4 doses	Ipilimumab plus dacarbazine	BORR 14.3% DCR 37.1% 2 CR, 3 PR, 8 SD	Any: 65.7% Grade III/IV: 17.1%	14.3 months	62% at 1 year 24% at 2 years 20% at 3 years
			Ipilimumab alone	BORR 5.4% DCR 21.6% 0 CR, 2 PR, 6 SD	Any: 53.8% Grade III/IV: 7.7%	11.4 months	45% at 1 year 21% at 2 years 9% at 3 years

Study	Dosing	Treatment arm	Response	Toxicity	Median OS	Survival
Wolchok et al., 2010	0.3 v. 3 v. 10 mg/kg q3 weeks x 4 doses, then q3 months	Ipilimumab 0.3 mg/kg	BORR 0% DCR 13.7% 0 CR, 0 PR, 10 SD	Any: 26% Grade III/IV: 0%	8.6 months	39.6% at 1 year 18.4% at 2 years
217 patients previously treated metastatic melanoma		Ipilimumab 3 mg/kg	BORR 4.2% DCR 26.4% 0 CR, 3 PR, 16 SD	Any: 65% Grade III/IV: 7%	8.7 months	39.3% at 1 year 24.2% at 2 years
		Ipilimumab 10 mg/kg	BORR 11.1% DCR 29.2% 2 CR, 6 PR, 13 SD	Any: 70% Grade III/IV: 25%	11.4 months	48.6% at 1 year 29.8% at 2 years
Weber et al., 2009	10 mg/kg q3 weeks x 4 doses, then q3 months	Ipilimumab plus budesonide	BORR 12.1% DCR 31% 1 CR, 6 PR, 11 SD	Any: 81% Grade III/IV: 41%	17.7 months	55.9% at 1 year
115 patients previously treated metastatic melanoma		Ipilimumab plus placebo	BORR 15.8% DCR 35% 0 CR, 9 PR, 11 SD	Any: 84% Grade III/IV: 38%	19.3 months	62.4% at 1 year

291

B. Selected phase I and II studies in advanced melanoma

Based upon preclinical evidence, a pilot study was conducted in 17 patients with unresectable melanoma who were treated with a single dose of ipilimumab at 3mg/kg [72]. Two patients in this cohort achieved partial responses (PR). There was no toxicity other than a mild rash. A subsequent pilot study enrolled nine patients who had previously been treated with cancer vaccines (seven patients with melanoma and two patients with ovarian cancer) [73]. Ipilimumab was administered as a single dose at 3mg/kg. After one dose of ipilimumab, tumor necrosis was seen in all three patients with melanoma who were previously treated with an irradiated, autologous granulocyte–macrophage colony-stimulating factor (GM-CSF) secreting tumor cell vaccine. Both ovarian cancer patients had a reduction or stabilization in serum cancer antigen 125 (CA-125), a tumor marker of ovarian cancer. Toxicities were minimal and included one acute hypersensitivity reaction, one grade 3 liver function test abnormality, and rash.

After establishing the safety of single-dose ipilimumab and based upon preclinical evidence suggesting possible benefits of combining CTLA-4 therapy with vaccination [49,51], subsequent early trials evaluated ipilimumab administered in sequential doses and in combination with vaccines. In 2003, Phan et al. published a cohort of 14 patients with metastatic melanoma who received ipilimumab with glycoprotein 100 (gp100) peptide vaccination [68]. At the time the trial was published, three patients achieved objective tumor responses; six patients developed grade 3/4 immune-related adverse events (irAEs), including dermatitis, enterocolitis, and hypophysitis. Ultimately, this trial was expanded to include a total of 56 patients and an overall response (OR) rate of 13% was reported [74].

The question of dosing was further explored in the Phase II setting. Weber et al. treated 88 patients with unresectable Stage III/IV melanoma with ipilimumab over a dose range of 2.8 mg/kg to 20 mg/kg comparing single vs. multiple dose schedules. The overall response rate was 4.5% and an additional 16% of patients had prolonged stable disease (median 194 days) [70]. Downey et al. reported a response rate of 17% for a Phase II trial of 139 patients treated with ipilimumab at doses of 3–9 mg/kg [75]. A dose-response relationship was clearly defined in a double-blind Phase II study comparing ipilimumab at doses of 0.3, 3, and 10 mg/kg every 3 weeks, followed by maintenance doses administered every 12 weeks. The highest dose cohort, 10 mg/kg, had the greatest response rate (11%), followed by 3 mg/kg (4.2%), and 0.3 mg/kg (0%). The irAEs followed a similar pattern [76].

Additional combinations were also tested in the Phase II setting including combinations with chemotherapy or IL-2. Maker et al. tested the combination of ipilimumab with IL-2 in a selected group of 36 patients with advanced melanoma. The dose of ipilimumab was escalated in the Phase I portion of the study, from 0.3 up to 3 mg/kg. In the Phase II portion, the 3 mg/kg cohort was expanded to a total of 24 patients. The study reported a response rate of 22%. Grade 3/4 irAEs were reported in 5 patients (14%). Hersh et al. reported a randomized Phase II study comparing ipilimumab at a dose of 3 mg/kg with or without dacarbazine, with a trend favoring combination therapy [77]. There was a 14.3% response rate for the 35 patients treated with the combination compared with a 5.3% response rate for the 37 patients treated with ipilimumab alone. The combination had only a slightly higher incidence of irAEs (65.7 % vs. 53.8).

C. Phase III trials: Establishing a survival benefit for patients with advanced melanoma

The promising results seen in Phase II studies led to Phase III evaluation. In the first Phase III trial, 676 patients with previously treated advanced melanoma were randomized in a 3:1:1 fashion to receive ipilimumab in combination with the gp100 vaccine, ipilimumab alone, or gp100 vaccine alone [1]. Patients who initially achieved a confirmed partial or complete response or at least stable disease ≥24 weeks were eligible for re-induction within their original treatment arm should they subsequently have developed disease progression.

For the first time ever in melanoma, an overall survival (OS) benefit was demonstrated in a Phase III trial. The median OS for patients who received ipilimumab with gp100 (10.0 months) and ipilimumab alone (10.1 months) was significantly longer than for patients treated with gp100 alone (6.4 months). Based upon the survival benefit demonstrated in this study, ipilimumab was approved by the FDA on March 25th, 2011 for patients with unresectable or metastatic melanoma, marking the first time a drug was approved by the FDA for the treatment of advanced melanoma in over 12 years.

The survival benefit of ipilimumab was confirmed in a subsequent randomized Phase III trial [78]. In this trial, 502 patients with untreated melanoma were randomized 1:1 to receive dacarbazine with ipilimumab (10mg/kg) or dacarbazine with placebo. OS was significantly longer for patients who received dacarbazine with ipilimumab (11.2 months) than patients who received dacarbazine with placebo (9.1 months). Though the overall improvement in median survival of 2.1 months could be interpreted as modest, the number of patients alive at 1 year (47.3% vs. 36.3%), 2 years (28.5% vs. 17.9%), and 3 years (20.8% vs. 12.2%) was also significant for patients receiving dacarbazine with ipilimumab vs. dacarbazine alone, respectively (hazard ratio for death, 0.72; $P<0.001$). Caution should be exercised when comparing OS across different trials, but the three year survival (20.8%) of patients treated with dacarbazine and ipilimumab compares favorably to historical data of patients treated with dacarbazine alone [79].

IV. LESSONS LEARNED DURING THE CLINICAL DEVELOPMENT OF IPILIMUMAB

A. Kinetics of response—immune related response criteria (irRC)

Guidelines for the evaluation of radiographic responses to investigational anticancer agents were developed to standardize evaluations and aid comparisons between clinical trials. The Response Evaluation Criteria in Solid Tumors (RECIST) and modified World Health Organization (mWHO) criteria are used routinely in clinical studies. Responses to ipilimumab were assessed using these criteria in key clinical trials during its development [1]. However, early observations suggested that these criteria may not be optimal for assessing the benefit of ipilimumab. Compared to traditional cytotoxic therapies, ipilimumab was associated with distinct response patterns [80]. First, responses to ipilimumab can develop more slowly than responses to traditional agents. Next, in some patients, an initial period of disease progression may be followed by ultimate disease regression. Lastly, responses to ipilimumab may be heterogeneous with the appearance of new lesions coinciding with regression of larger, index lesions.

293

These patients, not captured using traditional response criteria, all appeared to benefit from therapy. These observations suggested that traditional criteria developed for cytotoxic therapy might not accurately reflect the activity of this novel immunotherapy. To systematically evaluate the novel response kinetics associated with ipilimumab, a pooled retrospective analysis of 487 patients treated across three Phase II studies was undertaken [81]. In this study, improved overall survival was associated with a variety of response patterns, including novel response patterns excluded from traditional criteria. To more accurately reflect the unique patterns of response associated with ipilimumab, the immune-related response criteria (irRC) were proposed. As a modification of the WHO criteria, the irRC takes into account the patient's "total tumor burden" and requires confirmation of suspected disease progression with a repeat radiographic assessment [82]. Studies to prospectively test the irRC are presently underway. This experience has led to an important re-evaluation of the optimal endpoints for measuring the clinical benefit of ipilimumab and may apply to other immunotherapeutic approaches [83].

B. Durability of response

The improvement in OS for patients treated with ipilimumab in two randomized Phase III trials is remarkable. Perhaps most important, however, is the dramatic durable disease control and long-term survival a subset of patients treated with ipilimumab achieve. Prieto et al. evaluated 177 patients treated on some of the earliest clinical trials in ipilimumab's development [68,74,84,85]. In their long-term analysis [86], 15 patients achieved long-term durable complete responses (CR). All CRs, except for one patient, are ongoing with the longest lasting 99+ months (median 83 months). Partial responses (PR) to ipilimumab can also demonstrate remarkable durability. Nine patients who achieved PRs are alive many years after ipilimumab treatment.

C. Unique toxicities—immune-related adverse events

For some patients, the potent ability of CTLA-4 blockade to activate the immune system results in inflammation of normal tissues, characterized as immune-related adverse events (irAEs). The frequency of irAEs depends upon the dose of ipilimumab and may also change when ipilimumab is given in combination with other agents.

1. COLITIS

Inflammation in the gastrointestinal tract can lead to serious complications if left untreated, with colitis progressing to bowel perforation or sepsis. For most patients, typical colitis symptoms are frequent loose or watery nonbloody stools occurring four to eight times daily, rarely associated with abdominal pain, nausea or fever. Endoscopic evaluation is not routinely necessary for diagnosis, but gross endoscopic findings typically show erythema or ulceration consistent with colitis. Histopathologic features of ipilimumab-related colitis may be characterized by a pattern of neutrophilic inflammation, lymphocytic infiltration or mixed infiltration, resembling an autoimmune enteropathy [87]. In one study, colonic biopsy samples were evaluated in patients treated with ipilimumab, and Treg numbers failed to correlate with colitis symptoms [88]. Radiographic findings associated with colitis secondary to ipilimumab have been described [89].

At the 3 mg/kg dose, gastrointestinal irAEs of any grade are reported in ∼30% of patients and Grade 3/4 events are reported in <5% of patients treated with ipilimumab [90]. At the higher dose of 10 mg/kg, these toxicities are more frequent (Table 19.2). In the Hodi study, five deaths (<1%) were attributed to complications from colitis. In the Robert study, there were no deaths related to colitis. With early intervention, colitis symptoms are typically transient and reversible with dose-interruption and steroid treatment; antitumor necrosis factor (TNF) therapy can be helpful in steroid refractory cases [90]. Formal guidelines for the management of ipilimumab-related colitis have been established. Notably, treatment with steroids does not appear to compromise the efficacy of ipilimumab [75]. In a randomized, placebo controlled study, however, prophylactic budesonide failed to reduce rates of ipilimumab-induced colitis [91].

2. DERMATITIS

The most common irAEs reported in studies of ipilimumab are dermatologic and typically include pruritis and/or rash. Rash has been described as beginning with small pink to bright red dome-shaped papules that may coalesce to form thin plaques. The distribution typically includes proximal extensor surfaces of the limbs and may spread to the trunk and the extremities, usually sparing the palms and soles [92]. On histopathologic analysis, epidermal spongiosis and perivascular lymphocytic infiltrate with a predominance of eosinophils and CD4+ T cells have been described [68,92].

Dermatologic toxicity is typically mild and affects approximately half of the patients treated with ipilimumab. Grade 3/4 dermatologic toxicities are rare but have been reported as have vitiligo and alopecia. Topical emollients, antihistamines, or topical steroids are often helpful to minimize dermatologic symptoms. Systemic steroids are rarely required. Severe or desquamating skin reactions are extremely uncommon.

TABLE 19.2 IrAEs in Selected Anti-CTLA-4 Antibody Clinical Trials

Study Reference	Population	Ipilimumab Dose/Schedule	Treatment Arms	Grade	Gastrointestinal*	Skin*	Liver*	irAE	Endocrine
Robert 2011	502 patients previously untreated metastatic melanoma	10 mg/kg q3 weeks x 4 doses, then q3 months	Dacarbazine plus ipilimumab	Any	27% (66/247)	29% (72/247)	33% (81/247)	78%	2% (5/247)
				Grade III/IV	4% (10/247)	3% (7/247)	21% (51/247)	42%	0% (0/247)
			Dacarbazine plus placebo	Any	6% (15/251)	4% (11/251)	16% (40/251)	38%	1% (2/251)
				Grade III/IV	0% (0/251)	0% (0/251)	0% (0/251)	6%	0% (0/251)
Hodi 2010	676 patients previously treated, unresectable stage III or IV melanoma	3 mg/kg q3 weeks x 4 doses, option for repeat dosing	Ipilimumab alone	Any	29% (38/131)	44% (57/131)	4% (5/131)	61%	8% (10/131)
				Grade III/IV	8% (10/131)	2% (2/131)	0% (0/131)	15%	4% (5/131)
			Ipilimumab plus gp100 peptide	Any	32% (122/380)	40% (152/380)	2% (8/380)	58%	4% (15/380)
				Grade III/IV	6% (22/380)	2% (9/380)	1% (4/380)	10%	1% (4/380)
			gp100 peptide alone	Any	14% (19/132)	17% (22/132)	5% (6/132)	32%	2% (2/132)
				Grade III/IV	1% (1/132)	0% (0/132)	2% (3/132)	3%	0% (0/132)
Weber 2009	115 patients previously treated metastatic melanoma	10 mg/kg q3 weeks x 4 doses, then q3 months	Ipilimumab plus budesonide	Any	48% (28/58)	60% (35/58)	16% (9/58)	81%	9% (5/58)
				Grade III/IV	24% (14/58)	5% (3/58)	9% (6/58)	41%	5% (3/58)
			Ipilimumab plus placebo	Any	46% (26/57)	68% (39/57)	14% (8/57)	84%	11% (6/57)
				Grade III/IV	23% (13/57)	0% (0/57)	12% (7/57)	38%	5% (3/57)
Wolchok 2010	217 patients previously treated metastatic melanoma	0.3 v. 3 v. 10 mg/kg q3 weeks x 4 doses, then q3 months	Ipilimumab 0.3 mg/kg	Any	17% (12/72)	0% (0/72)	0% (0/72)	26%	0% (0/72)
				Grade III/IV	0% (0/72)	0% (0/72)	0% (0/72)	0%	0% (0/72)
			Ipilimumab 3 mg/kg	Any	32% (23/71)	45% (32/71)	0% (0/71)	65%	6% (4/71)
				Grade III/IV	3% (2/71)	1% (1/71)	0% (0/71)	7%	3% (2/71)
			Ipilimumab 10 mg/kg	Any	40% (28/71)	46% (33/71)	3% (2/71)	70%	4% (3/71)
				Grade III/IV	15% (11/71)	4% (3/71)	3% (2/71)	25%	1% (1/71)

*For Roberts et al. 2011, the table reports the following irAEs: diarrhea (gastrointestinal), pruritis (skin), and elevation in ALT (liver).

3. HEPATITIS

Inflammation of the liver is a rare complication generally seen in <5% of patients treated with ipilimumab monotherapy (Table 19.2). In combination with dacarbazine, this toxicity appears more frequent. In the Robert et al. study, grade 3/4 elevation in AST were seen in 21% of patients treated on the combination arm compared to 1% of patients treated with dacarbazine alone [78].

Typically, patients present with a transaminitis (elevated AST and ALT) with a minimal change in bilirubin levels. Liver biopsy in one patient with high grade hepatitis showed lymphocytic infiltration into the portal triad and areas of necrosis [68]. Low grade hepatitis may be treated with dose interruption. Grade 3 hepatitis should prompt treatment discontinuation and initiation of high dose steroids. In some high-grade cases, intravenous steroids and mycophenolate mofetil may be necessary. In one case report, aggressive, steroid-resistant hepatitis was successfully treated with antithymocyte globulin [93].

4. ENDOCRINOPATHIES

Endocrinopathies that may develop in patients treated with ipilimumab include hypophysitis (inflammation of the pituitary), thyroiditis, and adrenal insufficiency. Ipilimumab-related hypophysitis has been well described, with an incidence ranging from 0 to 17%, but most typically <5%, depending upon the clinical trial [94,95]. The clinical symptoms, radiographic findings, and laboratory abnormalities in patients with ipilimumab-related hypophysitis appear indistinguishable from autoimmune hypophysitis [95–98]. Patients may be asymptomatic or may present with headache, visual disturbance, fatigue or weakness. Laboratory findings may include one or more of the following: secondary adrenal insufficiency, hypothyroidism, or hypogonadism [99]. Interruption of ipilimumab treatment coupled with high-dose steroids can be effective in reversing acute hypophysitis. However, for many patients, replacement hormones are required long-term, presumably due to irreversible damage to the pituitary. Thyroid dysfunction may develop secondary to hypophysitis or due to isolated thyroiditis. A pattern of ipilimumab-related thyroid dysfunction resembling Graves' disease has been described in a case series [100]. Lastly, cases of primary adrenal insufficiency related to ipilimumab have been reported rarely.

5. RARE irAEs

A diversity of additional irAEs or suspected irAEs have been reported infrequently (1–2% or less) [101–112] (Table 19.3).

TABLE 19.3 Immune-related Adverse Events	
Common	
Colitis	Rash/Pruritis
Infrequent	
Hepatitis	Hypophysitis
Rare	
Pancreatitis	Pneumonitis
Arthritis	Iritis
Uveitis	Myopathy
Nephritis	Neuropathy
Red Blood Cell Aplasia	Thrombocytopenia
Neutropenia	Hemophilia
Meningitis/Encephalopathy	

6. UNDERSTANDING irAEs

The factors that determine which patients develop irAEs and which tissues are affected are uncertain. The identification of patient characteristics or biomarkers that stratify risk for particular irAEs could aid clinical decision-making and is the focus of ongoing research. While the pattern of symptoms for individual irAEs may resemble defined autoimmune diseases, unlike autoimmune disease, irAEs are typically transient and reversible with cessation of CTLA-4 blockade and temporary use of steroids or other immunosuppressants. This may be more consistent with temporary loss of control of pre-existing self-reactive T cells rather than *de novo* development of true autoimmunity. Murine studies have failed to demonstrate that CTLA-4 blockade alone generates symptomatic autoimmunity, although CTLA-4 blockade can exacerbate autoimmune disease in susceptible mouse strains. In preclinical studies, depigmentation and prostatitis were reported in mice treated with CTLA-4 blockade combined with tumor vaccines for melanoma and prostate cancer respectively [49,59,60]. In two studies, mice treated with very high doses of CTLA-4 blocking antibodies developed measurable anti-DNA antibodies, but no detectable organ dysfunction or symptoms. Patients with a history of autoimmune disease have been excluded from clinical trials of ipilimumab thus far.

The overlap between patients who develop irAEs and those who derive clinical benefit from ipilimumab was noticed in early studies. In a Phase I study of 14 patients with metastatic melanoma, Phan et al. reported that 3/3 responding patients (1 CR, 2 PR) had Grade 3/4 toxicities, whereas only 3/11 of nonresponders had similar toxicity [113]. The correlation between Grade 3/4 irAEs and clinical response has since been reported in several larger analyses [70,74,75,103,114,115]. It should be emphasized, however, that high-grade irAEs are not required for clinical response, nor do high-grade irAEs guarantee a clinical response.

D. Potential biomarkers

Despite the OS improvement demonstrated in Phase III trials for patients who receive ipilimumab, unfortunately not all patients derive benefit. Ongoing efforts continue to evaluate biomarkers that correlate with benefit from ipilimumab therapy. A set of putative biomarkers have been reported based upon the results of primarily small, retrospective analyses. Larger, prospective trials are necessary.

The absolute lymphocyte count (ALC) in peripheral blood during treatment with ipilimumab has been correlated positively with clinical outcomes in several retrospective studies. In the largest study, 379 patients with unresectable or metastatic melanoma pooled from three Phase II studies were retrospectively analyzed. Patients who achieved clinical benefit (SD $\geq$24 weeks, PR, CR) had a greater mean rate of ALC increase than did patients without clinical benefit ($P=0.0013$) [116]. No patient with a decline in ALC during treatment achieved clinical benefit. An additional 64 patients were examined prospectively and a similar relationship was found, consistent with reports from earlier studies [68,85].

In a second retrospective study, the ALC of 51 patients treated with ipilimumab (10mg/kg) was associated with a survival benefit. Patients whose ALC was $\geq$1000/μL prior to the third dose of ipilimumab had improved survival compared to patients whose ALC <1000/μL [115]. ALC was also associated with response. No patients with an ALC <1000/μL had achieved stable disease or response by week 24 compared to the 52% of patients with ALC $\geq$ 1000/μL who achieved stable disease or response ($P < 0.01$). Yang et al. identified CD8+ T cells as the pertinent subset in the ALC [117]. In a study of 35 patients, those with clinical benefit were noted to have a statistically significant increase in CD8+ T cells ($P = 0.0294$) but not CD4+ T cells or CD4+CD25+ T cells, compared with patients that did not achieve clinical benefit. Larger prospective studies are necessary to confirm these exploratory findings.

Inducible co-stimulator (ICOS) is a member of the immunoglobulin gene family and is expressed on the cell surface of T cells after activation [118]. ICOS functions as a co-stimulatory

297

molecule and has been associated with effector T-cell expansion and survival [119]. Initial studies suggested ICOS as a pharmacodynamic biomarker of ipilimumab treatment. In a series of six patients with bladder cancer treated with neoadjuvant ipilimumab prior to radical cystoprostatectomy, the frequency of CD4+ T cells which expressed high levels of ICOS (CD4+ICOS^{high}) in both the peripheral blood and bladder tumor increased after treatment [120]. Elevated numbers of CD4+ICOS^{high} cells were also seen in incidentally discovered malignant prostate tissue removed during the operation [121]. In an analysis of 14 patients with melanoma treated with ipilimumab at 10mg/kg, a sustained increase in CD4+ICOS^{high} cells in the peripheral blood over 12 weeks was associated with improved survival [122].

T-helper 17 (Th17) cells represent a unique CD4+ T-cell population and produce interleukin (IL)-17 and IL-22. Th17 cells have previously been described to play a role in the development of autoimmunity and may have a role in antitumor immune responses [123,124]. In a study of 18 patients with metastatic prostate cancer treated with ipilimumab in combination with GVAX, an increase in the frequency of Th17 cells was noted after *in vitro* stimulation for 5 of 18 patients [125]. Three of these five patients achieved a partial response and two achieved stable disease. Th17 cells have also been shown to associate positively with freedom from relapse ($P = 0.049$) in a trial of 75 patients with melanoma treated with ipilimumab alone or in combination with a multipeptide vaccine [126].

Antigen-specific cellular and humoral immune responses to tumor associated antigens have additionally been investigated as potential biomarkers predictive of benefit from ipilimumab. Though antigen-specific responses to MAGE, Melan-A, gp100, tyrosinase, and PSA among others have been evaluated, antigen-specific responses to the cancer-testis antigen, NY-ESO-1 are the most thoroughly described. NY-ESO-1 is expressed in 30–40% of melanomas and is not present in normal adult tissues except testicular germ cells and placenta [127]. In one study of 144 patients with melanoma treated with ipilimumab, 22 patients were found to be seropositive for antibodies to NY-ESO-1 as detected by enzyme-linked immunosorbent assay (ELISA) prior to ipilimumab, and an additional nine patients became seropositive after ipilimumab [128]. Patients who were seropositive had a greater chance of experiencing clinical benefit 24 weeks after ipilimumab initiation ($P = 0.02$). Seropositive patients who additionally had CD8+ T-cell responses to NY-ESO-1 peptide as assessed by intracellular multicytokine staining had increased survival ($P = 0.01$) and more frequent clinical benefit than those who had seropositivity without an additional CD8+ T-cell response. The antigen-specific immune responses to NY-ESO-1 may be a surrogate marker of the broader mechanisms of ipilimumab's antitumor immunity, rather than direct mediators.

A majority of correlative studies have focused on analyzing immunologic changes in peripheral blood; a small number of studies have analyzed the tumor microenvironment. Hamid et al. reported the results of a prospective, double-blind Phase II study exploring candidate biomarkers from the tumor microenvironment [129]. Tissue was collected prior to ipilimumab and after the second dose. Immunohistochemistry and histology on tumor biopsies revealed significant associations between clinical benefit (SD ≥24 weeks, PR, CR) and high baseline expression of FoxP3 ($P = 0.014$) and indoleamine 2,3-dioxygenase ($P = 0.012$). Clinical activity also correlated with the increase in tumor-infiltrating lymphocytes (TILs) from baseline to after the second dose of ipilimumab ($P = 0.005$).

In a study of tumor biopsies collected from 45 patients before and after starting treatment on a Phase II study, Ji et al. report on gene expression patterns in the tumor microenvironment. They observe that expression of inflammatory response genes at baseline predict clinic benefit ($P < 0.01$). A number of immunologically relevant genes are upregulated during treatment and the post-treatment gene expression profile is likewise predictive. In contrast, expression of melanoma-associated and cellular proliferation-related genes was decreased after ipilimumab treatment [130,131].

Several other small case series have described intratumoral changes after treatment with ipilimumab consistent with induction of a productive antitumor immune response. In a series of six patients treated with GVAX and subsequent ipilimumab, therapy-induced tumor necrosis was related to the CD8+ to FoxP3+ ratio in post-treatment biopsies [132]. In a case report of a patient with melanoma who had a complete response to ipilimumab, tumor tissue was infiltrated with CD8+ effector T cells specific for Melan-A [133]. A second case report compared intratumoral infiltrate in two melanoma lesions (one responding, one progressing) in a patient treated with ipilimumab. Tumor response was associated with increased infiltration of activated effector T cells and decreased Tregs [131].

V. CLINICAL TESTING OF IPILIMUMAB IN DISEASES OTHER THAN MELANOMA

Outside of melanoma, the largest clinical trial experience with ipilimumab is in the treatment of metastatic prostate cancer. In a pilot study, 14 patients with castrate-resistant metastatic prostate cancer received a single dose of 3 mg/kg [134]. Two patients had a biochemical response according to consensus criteria (>50% decrease in PSA). An additional eight patients had a decline in PSA that was <50%. A Phase II study expanding to multiple doses of ipilimumab randomized 43 patients with castrate-resistant metastatic prostate cancer to receive ipilimumab 3 mg/kg every four weeks for four doses alone or in combination with a single dose of docetaxel [135]. Six patients, three in each arm, had a decrease in PSA; there were no radiographic responses, and five patients had grade 3/4 irAEs. Several additional studies combining ipilimumab with GM-CSF, radiation, or vaccines have reported promising results [136−140]. A Phase II study comparing hormone therapy with or without ipilimumab in the treatment of advanced prostate cancer has completed accrual (NCT00170157). At present, two Phase III trials of ipilimumab in prostate cancer are ongoing. The first study targets patients who have received prior docetaxel. This study is a randomized, double-blind study comparing ipilimumab with placebo in patients who have received radiotherapy (NCT00861614). A second study includes only patients with castrate-resistant prostate cancer who are chemotherapy naïve randomizing patients to receive ipilimumab or placebo (NCT01057810).

Ipilimumab has also been tested in several additional malignancies including non-small cell lung cancer (NSCLC), renal cell cancer, pancreatic cancer, and hematologic malignancies. The largest of these is a Phase II study combining ipilimumab with chemotherapy in patients with stage IIIb/IV NSCLC. The study accrued 203 patients with chemotherapy-naïve NSCLC who were randomized 1:1:1 to receive either chemotherapy alone or ipilimumab combined with chemotherapy in two different schedules. There was a statistically significant ($P = 0.024$), but very modest (<1 month), improvement in progression-free survival (PFS) for patients receiving ipilimumab in combination with chemotherapy in one arm compared to those receiving chemotherapy alone and a nonsignificant trend toward improved OS for patients who received ipilimumab [141]. Small studies treating patients with non-Hodgkin lymphoma (NHL) who had relapsed after allogeneic bone marrow transplant and RCC have shown some promise [101,108,142]. A Phase II study of 27 patients with metastatic pancreatic cancer demonstrated minimal activity [143,140].

VI. OUTSTANDING QUESTIONS AND FUTURE DIRECTIONS
A. Dosing and schedule

The FDA has approved ipilimumab at a dose of 3 mg/kg to be administered once every three weeks for four doses as "induction" therapy. This dosing and schedule was utilized by Hodi et al. in a Phase III study which reported a response rate of ∼10% and a demonstrated overall survival benefit. However, it is not clear that this regimen reflects the best clinical activity for ipilimumab and several important questions are outstanding. First, what is the most effective dose of ipilimumab? Phase I studies did not identify a maximum tolerated dose. Furthermore, the randomized, double-blinded Phase II study comparing ipilimumab at three dose levels, 0.3, 3, and 10 mg/kg, demonstrated dose-dependent antitumor activity. The improved response rate (0% vs. 4.2% vs. 11.1%) must be balanced against an increased rate of Grade 3/4 irAEs (0% vs. 7% vs. 25%). The activity of ipilimumab at the 10 mg/kg dose will be formally compared to the FDA-approved 3 mg/kg dose in an upcoming randomized, double-blind Phase III study (NCT01515189). Another unanswered question related to dosing is how individual patients differ in their sensitivity to ipilimumab. The idea that the optimal dose of ipilimumab might be personalized was explored in an intrapatient dose-escalation study published by Maker et al [85]. In this study, patients were treated with ipilimumab, starting at a dose of either 3 or 5 mg/kg and were eligible for dose escalation up to 9 mg/kg in the absence of significant toxicities. The overall response (11%) in this population of 46 patients with metastatic melanoma was similar to response rates observed in studies without dose escalation. All responses occurred in patients who escalated to the 9 mg/kg dose. However, the lack of a comparator arm and differences in scheduling make it difficult to draw firm conclusions on dosing from this study.

The FDA-approved schedule for ipilimumab treatment is one dose every three weeks for a total of four doses. Some clinical trials have permitted additional, so-called "maintenance," doses of ipilimumab administered every three months after initial induction therapy. Alternatively, some trials have permitted repeat dosing or "reinduction" therapy using the original four-dose induction schedule. The Hodi study provides some limited evidence that "re-induction" with ipilimumab may help patients who have previously benefitted but then ultimately developed disease progression. In this study, 31 patients with progressive disease were offered re-induction with subsequent evaluation showing 1 CR, 5 PRs, and 15 with SD. The utility of the maintenance dosing schedule has not been tested in a randomized fashion.

B. Ipilimumab in the adjuvant setting

In addition to its thorough evaluation for patients with advanced melanoma, ipilimumab has been evaluated as adjuvant therapy after surgical resection of high risk melanoma. In one Phase I study, 19 patients with resected stage III and IV melanoma were administered ipilimumab in escalating dose cohorts (0.3mg/kg, 1mg/kg, and 3mg/kg) in combination with tumor antigen epitope peptides from gp100, MART-1, and tyrosinase emulsified with the adjuvant Montanide ISA 51 [144]. The primary goal of the study was to assess toxicity of this adjuvant therapeutic approach. Five patients experienced grade 3 gastrointestinal toxicity. Though the overall number of patients was small, there appeared to be an association between the occurrence of irAEs and decreased risk of relapse. Three of eight patients who experienced an irAE relapsed; nine of 11 patients who did not experience an irAE relapsed.

Ipilimumab monotherapy in the adjuvant setting is being evaluated in two ongoing Phase III trials (NCT00636168 and NCT01274338). In NCT00636168, ipilimumab is being compared to placebo after resection of high risk stage III melanoma with recurrence-free survival as the primary endpoint. Accrual has been completed and results are anticipated. Ipilimumab is also being compared to high-dose recombinant interferon-alpha-2b (NCT01274338).

C. Combination therapies

Although ipilimumab is an important new therapy for the treatment of melanoma, its benefit is limited to a subset of patients. Combining ipilimumab with traditional or experimental therapies may represent one avenue to improve upon response rates and expand the durable benefits of ipilimumab. Preclinical evidence from mouse models offers support for combinations with conventional cancer therapies including surgery [52], radiation [53,54], chemotherapy [55] cryoablation [56], and radiofrequency ablation [57]. CTLA-4 has also been combined successfully with a diversity of immunotherapies including tumor vaccines and immunomodulatory antibodies [49–51,58–67]. Lastly, limited evidence supports the combination of CTLA-4 blockade with molecularly targeted agents, an area likely to enjoy increased attention [145].

A number of combination strategies have been explored in clinical trials to date. Combinations of ipilimumab with tumor vaccines have been the most common, including peptide vaccines [1,74,75], cellular vaccines [139], and DNA/RNA vaccines [140]. The combination of ipilimumab with a peptide vaccine against gp100 was tested in a randomized Phase III study but failed to show superior activity to ipilimumab alone [1]. Alternative vaccination strategies may be more successful in combination with ipilimumab but have not yet been tested in larger, randomized studies. A regimen combining ipilimumab and IL-2 was tested in a single arm Phase I/II study [84]. The combination proved tolerable and responses were seen in 22% of patients, but it is unclear if this regimen is superior to monotherapy.

Combinations with chemotherapy have been tested in melanoma and NSCLC [77,78,141]. In an open label, randomized Phase II study, Hersh et al. reported a nonsignificant trend favoring ipilimumab combined with dacarbazine compared to ipilimumab alone, with disease control rates of 37.1% vs. 21.6%, respectively. In the Phase III study reported by Robert et al., ipilimumab alone was not included as a comparator arm, but with a response rate of 15% and over 40% of patients experiencing Grade 3/4 toxicity, it seems unlikely that this combination is superior. The results from a randomized Phase II study combining docetaxel with ipilimumab for hormone-refractory prostate cancer have not yet been reported (NCT00050596). A Phase III randomized, placebo controlled study comparing paclitaxel and carboplatin alone or with ipilimumab for squamous NSCLC is presently open. Studies adding ipilimumab to conventional chemotherapy regimens are also ongoing for small cell lung cancer (NCT01331525) and pancreatic cancer (NCT01473940). In a case report, radiation therapy has been identified as an attractive partner for combination with ipilimumab [146].

On the horizon, combinations of ipilimumab with novel immunotherapies or molecularly targeted therapies are likely to be promising based upon preclinical studies. At present, ipilimumab is being tested in combination with MDX-1106, a PD-1 blocking antibody, in the Phase I setting (NCT01024231). A first in human trial combining ipilimumab with vemurafenib, an inhibitor of BRAF, has recently opened (NCT01400451).

VII. CONCLUSIONS

The development and FDA approval of ipilimumab has been a remarkable advance in the treatment of advanced melanoma. Important lessons about its unusual response pattern, unique side effect profile, and immunologic changes associated with antitumor responses continue to refine our understanding of this promising immunotherapy. Future trials will further explore ipilimumab's activity in treating cancers outside of melanoma and its potential synergy in combination with other promising antitumor agents.

References

[1] Hodi FS, O'Day SJ, McDermott DF, Weber RW, Sosman JA, Haanen JB, et al. Improved survival with ipilimumab in patients with metastatic melanoma. N Engl J Med 2010;363(8):711–23.

[2] Baxter AG, Hodgkin PD. Activation rules: the two-signal theories of immune activation. Nat Rev Immunol 2002;2(6):439–46.

[3] Jenkins MK, Schwartz RH. Antigen presentation by chemically modified splenocytes induces antigen-specific T cell unresponsiveness in vitro and in vivo. J Exp Med 1987;165(2):302–19.

[4] Lafferty KJ, Cunningham AJ. A new analysis of allogeneic interactions. Aust J Exp Biol Med Sci 1975;53(1):27–42.

[5] Bretscher P, Cohn M. A theory of self-nonself discrimination. Science 1970;169(950):1042–9.

[6] Gmunder H, Lesslauer WA. 45-kDa human T-cell membrane glycoprotein functions in the regulation of cell proliferative responses. Eur J Biochem 1984;142(1):153–60.

[7] Hansen JA, Martin PJ, Nowinski RC. Monoclonal antibodies identifying a novel T-Cell antigen and Ia antigens of human lymphocytes. Immunogenetics 1980;11(1):429–39.

[8] Yokochi T, Holly RD, Clark EA. B lymphoblast antigen (BB-1) expressed on Epstein-Barr virus-activated B cell blasts, B lymphoblastoid cell lines, and Burkitt's lymphomas. J Immunol 1982;128(2):823–7.

[9] Azuma M, Ito D, Yagita H, Okumura K, Phillips JH, Lanier LL, et al. B70 antigen is a second ligand for CTLA-4 and CD28. Nature 1993;366(6450):76–9.

[10] Hathcock KS, Laszlo G, Dickler HB, Bradshaw J, Linsley P, Hodes RJ. Identification of an alternative CTLA-4 ligand costimulatory for T cell activation. Science 1993;262(5135):905–7.

[11] Freeman GJ, Gribben JG, Boussiotis VA, Ng JW, Restivo Jr VA, Lombard LA, et al. Cloning of B7–2: a CTLA-4 counter-receptor that costimulates human T cell proliferation. Science 1993;262(5135):909–11.

[12] Hathcock KS, Laszlo G, Pucillo C, Linsley P, Hodes RJ. Comparative analysis of B7-1 and B7-2 costimulatory ligands: expression and function. J Exp Med 1994;180(2):631–40.

[13] Larsen CP, Ritchie SC, Hendrix R, Linsley PS, Hathcock KS, Hodes RJ, et al. Regulation of immunostimulatory function and costimulatory molecule (B7-1 and B7-2) expression on murine dendritic cells. J Immunol 1994;152(11):5208–19.

[14] Lenschow DJ, Walunas TL, Bluestone JA. CD28/B7 system of T cell costimulation. Annu Rev Immunol 1996;14:233–58.

[15] Rudd CE, Taylor A, Schneider H. CD28 and CTLA-4 coreceptor expression and signal transduction. Immunol Rev 2009;229(1):12–26.

[16] Brunet JF, Denizot F, Luciani MF, Roux-Dosseto M, Suzan M, Mattei MG, et al. A new member of the immunoglobulin superfamily—CTLA-4. Nature 1987;328(6127):267–70.

[17] Linsley PS, Brady W, Urnes M, Grosmaire LS, Damle NK, Ledbetter JA. CTLA-4 is a second receptor for the B cell activation antigen B7. J Exp Med 1991;174(3):561–9.

[18] Krummel MF, Allison JP. CD28 and CTLA-4 have opposing effects on the response of T cells to stimulation. J Exp Med 1995;182(2):459–65.

[19] Thompson CB, Allison JP. The emerging role of CTLA-4 as an immune attenuator. Immunity 1997;7(4):445–50.

[20] Walunas TL, Lenschow DJ, Bakker CY, Linsley PS, Freeman GJ, Green JM, et al. CTLA-4 can function as a negative regulator of T cell activation. Immunity 1994;1(5):405–13.

[21] Krummel MF, Allison JP. CTLA-4 engagement inhibits IL-2 accumulation and cell cycle progression upon activation of resting T cells. J Exp Med 1996;183(6):2533–40.

[22] Walunas TL, Bakker CY, Bluestone JA. CTLA-4 ligation blocks CD28-dependent T cell activation. J Exp Med 1996;183(6):2541–50.

[23] Brunner MC, Chambers CA, Chan FK, Hanke J, Winoto A, Allison JP. CTLA-4-Mediated inhibition of early events of T cell proliferation. J Immunol 1999;162(10):5813–20.

[24] Greenwald RJ, Boussiotis VA, Lorsbach RB, Abbas AK, Sharpe AH. CTLA-4 regulates induction of anergy in vivo. Immunity 2001;14(2):145–55.

[25] Waterhouse P, Penninger JM, Timms E, Wakeham A, Shahinian A, Lee KP, et al. Lymphoproliferative disorders with early lethality in mice deficient in Ctla-4. Science 1995;270(5238):985–8.

[26] Tivol EA, Borriello F, Schweitzer AN, Lynch WP, Bluestone JA, Sharpe AH. Loss of CTLA-4 leads to massive lymphoproliferation and fatal multiorgan tissue destruction, revealing a critical negative regulatory role of CTLA-4. Immunity 1995;3(5):541–7.

[27] Chambers CA, Sullivan TJ, Allison JP. Lymphoproliferation in CTLA-4-deficient mice is mediated by costimulation-dependent activation of CD4+ T cells. Immunity 1997;7(6):885–95.

[28] Chuang E, Alegre ML, Duckett CS, Noel PJ, Vander Heiden MG, Thompson CB. Interaction of CTLA-4 with the clathrin-associated protein AP50 results in ligand-independent endocytosis that limits cell surface expression. J Immunol 1997;159(1):144–51.

[29] Shiratori T, Miyatake S, Ohno H, Nakaseko C, Isono K, Bonifacino JS, et al. Tyrosine phosphorylation controls internalization of CTLA-4 by regulating its interaction with clathrin-associated adaptor complex AP-2. Immunity 1997;6(5):583–9.

[30] Egen JG, Kuhns MS, Allison JP. CTLA-4: new insights into its biological function and use in tumor immunotherapy. Nat Immunol 2002;3(7):611–8.

[31] Zhang Y, Allison JP. Interaction of CTLA-4 with AP50, a clathrin-coated pit adaptor protein. Proc Natl Acad Sci U S A 1997;94(17):9273–8.

[32] Pentcheva-Hoang T, Egen JG, Wojnoonski K, Allison JP. B7-1 and B7-2 selectively recruit CTLA-4 and CD28 to the immunological synapse. Immunity 2004;21(3):401–13.

[33] Egen JG, Allison JP. Cytotoxic T lymphocyte antigen-4 accumulation in the immunological synapse is regulated by TCR signal strength. Immunity 2002;16(1):23–35.

[34] Stamper CC, Zhang Y, Tobin JF, Erbe DV, Ikemizu S, Davis SJ, et al. Crystal structure of the B7-1/CTLA-4 complex that inhibits human immune responses. Nature 2001;410(6828):608—11.

[35] Peggs KS, Quezada SA, Allison JP. Cell intrinsic mechanisms of T-cell inhibition and application to cancer therapy. Immunol Rev 2008;224:141—65.

[36] Grohmann U, Orabona C, Fallarino F, Vacca C, Calcinaro F, Falorni A, et al. CTLA-4-Ig regulates tryptophan catabolism in vivo. Nat Immunol 2002;3(11):1097—101.

[37] Munn DH, Sharma MD, Mellor AL. Ligation of B7-1/B7-2 by human CD4+ T cells triggers indoleamine 2,3-dioxygenase activity in dendritic cells. J Immunol 2004;172(7):4100—10.

[38] Chambers CA, Kuhns MS, Allison JP. Cytotoxic T lymphocyte antigen-4 (CTLA-4) regulates primary and secondary peptide-specific CD4(+) T cell responses. Proc Natl Acad Sci U S A 1999;96(15):8603—8.

[39] Greenwald RJ, Oosterwegel MA, van der Woude D, Kubal A, Mandelbrot DA, Boussiotis VA, et al. CTLA-4 regulates cell cycle progression during a primary immune response. Eur J Immunol 2002;32(2):366—73.

[40] McCoy KD, Hermans IF, Fraser JH, Le Gros G, Ronchese F. Cytotoxic T lymphocyte-associated antigen 4 (CTLA-4) can regulate dendritic cell-induced activation and cytotoxicity of CD8(+) T cells independently of CD4(+) T cell help. J Exp Med 1999;189(7):1157—62.

[41] Salomon B, Lenschow DJ, Rhee L, Ashourian N, Singh B, Sharpe A, et al. B7/CD28 costimulation is essential for the homeostasis of the CD4+CD25+ immunoregulatory T cells that control autoimmune diabetes. Immunity 2000;12(4):431—40.

[42] Wing K, Onishi Y, Prieto-Martin P, Yamaguchi T, Miyara M, Fehervari Z, et al. CTLA-4 control over Foxp3+ regulatory T cell function. Science 2008;322(5899):271—5.

[43] Allison JP, Hurwitz AA, Leach DR. Manipulation of costimulatory signals to enhance antitumor T-cell responses. Curr Opin Immunol 1995;7(5):682—6.

[44] Leach DR, Krummel MF, Allison JP. Enhancement of antitumor immunity by CTLA-4 blockade. Science 1996;271(5256):1734—6.

[45] Kwon ED, Hurwitz AA, Foster BA, Madias C, Feldhaus AL, Greenberg NM, et al. Manipulation of T cell costimulatory and inhibitory signals for immunotherapy of prostate cancer. Proc Natl Acad Sci U S A 1997;94(15):8099—103.

[46] Yang YF, Zou JP, Mu J, Wijesuriya R, Ono S, Walunas T, et al. Enhanced induction of antitumor T-cell responses by cytotoxic T lymphocyte-associated molecule-4 blockade: the effect is manifested only at the restricted tumor-bearing stages. Cancer Res 1997;57(18):4036—41.

[47] Shrikant P, Khoruts A, Mescher MF. CTLA-4 blockade reverses CD8+ T cell tolerance to tumor by a CD4+ T cell- and IL-2-dependent mechanism. Immunity 1999;11(4):483—93.

[48] Sotomayor EM, Borrello I, Tubb E, Allison JP, Levitsky HI. In vivo blockade of CTLA-4 enhances the priming of responsive T cells but fails to prevent the induction of tumor antigen-specific tolerance. Proc Natl Acad Sci U S A 1999;96(20):11476—81.

[49] van Elsas A, Hurwitz AA, Allison JP. Combination immunotherapy of B16 melanoma using anti-cytotoxic T lymphocyte-associated antigen 4 (CTLA-4) and granulocyte/macrophage colony-stimulating factor (GM-CSF)-producing vaccines induces rejection of subcutaneous and metastatic tumors accompanied by autoimmune depigmentation. J Exp Med 1999;190(3):355—66.

[50] Davila E, Kennedy R, Celis E. Generation of antitumor immunity by cytotoxic T lymphocyte epitope peptide vaccination, CpG-oligodeoxynucleotide adjuvant, and CTLA-4 blockade. Cancer Res 2003; 63(12):3281—8.

[51] Gregor PD, Wolchok JD, Ferrone CR, Buchinshky H, Guevara-Patino JA, Perales MA, et al. CTLA-4 blockade in combination with xenogeneic DNA vaccines enhances T-cell responses, tumor immunity and autoimmunity to self antigens in animal and cellular model systems. Vaccine 2004;22(13-14):1700—8.

[52] Kwon ED, Foster BA, Hurwitz AA, Madias C, Allison JP, Greenberg NM, et al. Elimination of residual metastatic prostate cancer after surgery and adjunctive cytotoxic T lymphocyte-associated antigen 4 (CTLA-4) blockade immunotherapy. Proc Natl Acad Sci U S A 1999;96(26):15074—9.

[53] Dewan MZ, Galloway AE, Kawashima N, Dewyngaert JK, Babb JS, Formenti SC, et al. Fractionated but not single-dose radiotherapy induces an immune-mediated abscopal effect when combined with anti-CTLA-4 antibody. Clin Cancer Res 2009;15(17):5379—88.

[54] Demaria S, Kawashima N, Yang AM, Devitt ML, Babb JS, Allison JP, et al. Immune-mediated inhibition of metastases after treatment with local radiation and CTLA-4 blockade in a mouse model of breast cancer. Clin Cancer Res 2005;11(2 Pt 1):728—34.

[55] Mokyr MB, Kalinichenko T, Gorelik L, Bluestone JA. Realization of the therapeutic potential of CTLA-4 blockade in low-dose chemotherapy-treated tumor-bearing mice. Cancer Res 1998;58(23): 5301—4.

[56] Waitz R, Solomon SB, Petre EN, Trumble AE, Fasso M, Norton L, et al. Potent Induction of Tumor Immunity by Combining Tumor Cryoablation with Anti-CTLA-4 Therapy. Cancer Res 2012;72(2):430—9.

[57] den Brok MH, Sutmuller RP, Nierkens S, Bennink EJ, Frielink C, Toonen LW, et al. Efficient loading of dendritic cells following cryo and radiofrequency ablation in combination with immune modulation induces anti-tumour immunity. Br J Cancer 2006;95(7):896—905.

[58] Hurwitz AA, Yu TF, Leach DR, Allison JP. CTLA-4 blockade synergizes with tumor-derived granulocyte-macrophage colony-stimulating factor for treatment of an experimental mammary carcinoma. Proc Natl Acad Sci U S A 1998;95(17):10067—71.

[59] van Elsas A, Sutmuller RP, Hurwitz AA, Ziskin J, Villasenor J, Medema JP, et al. Elucidating the autoimmune and antitumor effector mechanisms of a treatment based on cytotoxic T lymphocyte antigen-4 blockade in combination with a B16 melanoma vaccine: comparison of prophylaxis and therapy. J Exp Med 2001;194(4):481—9.

[60] Hurwitz AA, Foster BA, Kwon ED, Truong T, Choi EM, Greenberg NM, et al. Combination immunotherapy of primary prostate cancer in a transgenic mouse model using CTLA-4 blockade. Cancer Res 2000;60(9):2444—8.

[61] Mangsbo SM, Sandin LC, Anger K, Korman AJ, Loskog A, Totterman TH. Enhanced tumor eradication by combining CTLA-4 or PD-1 blockade with CpG therapy. J Immunother 2010;33(3):225—35.

[62] Curran MA, Allison JP. Tumor vaccines expressing flt3 ligand synergize with ctla-4 blockade to reject preimplanted tumors. Cancer Res 2009;69(19):7747—55.

[63] Met O, Wang M, Pedersen AE, Nissen MH, Buus S, Claesson MH. The effect of a therapeutic dendritic cell-based cancer vaccination depends on the blockage of CTLA-4 signaling. Cancer Lett 2006;231(2):247—56.

[64] Daftarian P, Song GY, Ali S, Faynsod M, Longmate J, Diamond DJ, et al. Two distinct pathways of immuno-modulation improve potency of p53 immunization in rejecting established tumors. Cancer Res 2004;64(15):5407—14.

[65] Gao Y, Whitaker-Dowling P, Griffin JA, Barmada MA, Bergman I. Recombinant vesicular stomatitis virus targeted to Her2/neu combined with anti-CTLA4 antibody eliminates implanted mammary tumors. Cancer Gene Ther 2009;16(1):44—52.

[66] Youlin K, Li Z, Xiaodong W, Xiuheng L, Hengchen Z. Combination Immunotherapy with 4-1BBL and CTLA-4 Blockade for the Treatment of Prostate Cancer. Clin Dev Immunol 2012;2012:439235.

[67] Curran MA, Kim M, Montalvo W, Al-Shamkhani A, Allison JP. Combination CTLA-4 blockade and 4-1BB activation enhances tumor rejection by increasing T-cell infiltration, proliferation, and cytokine production. PLoS One 2011;6(4):e19499.

[68] Phan GQ, Yang JC, Sherry RM, Hwu P, Topalian SL, Schwartzentruber DJ, et al. Cancer regression and autoimmunity induced by cytotoxic T lymphocyte-associated antigen 4 blockade in patients with metastatic melanoma. Proc Natl Acad Sci U S A 2003;100(14):8372—7.

[69] Ribas A, Camacho LH, Lopez-Berestein G, Pavlov D, Bulanhagui CA, Millham R, et al. Antitumor activity in melanoma and anti-self responses in a phase I trial with the anti-cytotoxic T lymphocyte-associated antigen 4 monoclonal antibody CP-675,206. J Clin Oncol 2005;23(35):8968—77.

[70] Weber JS, O'Day S, Urba W, Powderly J, Nichol G, Yellin M, et al. Phase I/II study of ipilimumab for patients with metastatic melanoma. J Clin Oncol 2008;26(36):5950—6.

[71] Ribas A, Hauschild A, Kefford R, Punt CJ, Haanen JB, Marmol M, et al. Phase III, open-label, randomized, comparative study of tremelimumab (CP-675,206) and chemotherapy (temozolomide or dacar- bazine) in patients with advanced melanoma [abstract LBA9011]. J Clin Oncol 2008;26 (Suppl.) 2009.

[72] Tchekmedyian S. MDX-010 (human anti-CTLA4): a phase I trial in malignant melanoma. Proc Am Soc Clin Oncol 2002;21(abstr 56).

[73] Hodi FS, Mihm MC, Soiffer RJ, Haluska FG, Butler M, Seiden MV, et al. Biologic activity of cytotoxic T lymphocyte-associated antigen 4 antibody blockade in previously vaccinated metastatic melanoma and ovarian carcinoma patients. Proc Natl Acad Sci U S A 2003;100(8):4712—7.

[74] Attia P, Phan GQ, Maker AV, Robinson MR, Quezado MM, Yang JC, et al. Autoimmunity correlates with tumor regression in patients with metastatic melanoma treated with anti-cytotoxic T-lymphocyte antigen-4. J Clin Oncol 2005;23(25):6043—53.

[75] Downey SG, Klapper JA, Smith FO, Yang JC, Sherry RM, Royal RE, et al. Prognostic factors related to clinical response in patients with metastatic melanoma treated by CTL-associated antigen-4 blockade. Clin Cancer Res 2007;13(22 Pt 1):6681—8.

[76] Wolchok JD, Neyns B, Linette G, Negrier S, Lutzky J, Thomas L, et al. Ipilimumab monotherapy in patients with pretreated advanced melanoma: a randomised, double-blind, multicentre, phase 2, dose-ranging study. Lancet Oncol 2010;11(2):155—64.

[77] Hersh EM, O'Day SJ, Powderly J, Khan KD, Pavlick AC, Cranmer LD, et al. A phase II multicenter study of ipilimumab with or without dacarbazine in chemotherapy-naive patients with advanced melanoma. Invest New Drugs 2010.

[78] Robert C, Thomas L, Bondarenko I, O'Day S, M DJ Garbe C, et al. Ipilimumab plus dacarbazine for previously untreated metastatic melanoma. N Engl J Med 2011;364(26):2517—26.

[79] Chapman PB, Einhorn LH, Meyers ML, Saxman S, Destro AN, Panageas KS, et al. Phase III multicenter randomized trial of the Dartmouth regimen versus dacarbazine in patients with metastatic melanoma. J Am Soc Clin Oncol 1999;17(9):2745–51.

[80] Saenger YM, Wolchok JD. The heterogeneity of the kinetics of response to ipilimumab in metastatic melanoma: patient cases. Cancer Immun 2008;8:1.

[81] Wolchok JD, Hoos A, O'Day S, Weber JS, Hamid O, Lebbe C, et al. Guidelines for the evaluation of immune therapy activity in solid tumors: immune-related response criteria. Clin Cancer Res 2009;15(23):7412–20.

[82] Pennock GK, Waterfield W, Wolchok JD. Patient Responses to Ipilimumab, a Novel Immunopotentiator for Metastatic Melanoma: How Different are these From Conventional Treatment Responses? Am J Clin Oncol 2011.

[83] Kantoff PW, Higano CS, Shore ND, Berger ER, Small EJ, Penson DF, et al. Sipuleucel-T immunotherapy for castration-resistant prostate cancer. New Engl J Med 2010;363(5):411–22.

[84] Maker AV, Phan GQ, Attia P, Yang JC, Sherry RM, Topalian SL, et al. Tumor regression and autoimmunity in patients treated with cytotoxic T lymphocyte-associated antigen 4 blockade and interleukin 2: a phase I/II study. Ann Surg Oncol 2005;12(12):1005–16.

[85] Maker AV, Yang JC, Sherry RM, Topalian SL, Kammula US, Royal RE, et al. Intrapatient dose escalation of anti-CTLA-4 antibody in patients with metastatic melanoma. J Immunother 2006;29(4):455–63.

[86] Prieto PA, Yang JC, Sherry RM, Hughes MS, Kammula US, White DE, et al. CTLA-4 Blockade with Ipilimumab: Long-Term Follow-up of 177 Patients with Metastatic Melanoma. Clin Cancer Res 2012.

[87] Oble DA, Mino-Kenudson M, Goldsmith J, Hodi FS, Seliem RM, Dranoff G, et al. Alpha-CTLA-4 mAb-associated panenteritis: a histologic and immunohistochemical analysis. Am J Surg Pathol 2008;32(8):1130–7.

[88] Lord JD, Hackman RC, Moklebust A, Thompson JA, Higano CS, Chielens D, et al. Refractory colitis following anti-CTLA4 antibody therapy: analysis of mucosal FOXP3+ T cells. Dig Dis Sci 2010;55(5):1396–405.

[89] Bronstein Y, Ng CS, Hwu P, Hwu WJ. Radiologic manifestations of immune-related adverse events in patients with metastatic melanoma undergoing anti-CTLA-4 antibody therapy. AJR Am J Roentgenol 2011;197(6): W992–W1000.

[90] Di Giacomo AM, Biagioli M, Maio M. The Emerging Toxicity Profiles of Anti-CTLA-4 Antibodies Across Clinical Indications. Semin Oncol 2010;37(5):499–507.

[91] Weber J, Thompson JA, Hamid O, Minor D, Amin A, Ron I, et al. A randomized, double-blind, placebo-controlled, phase II study comparing the tolerability and efficacy of ipilimumab administered with or without prophylactic budesonide in patients with unresectable stage III or IV melanoma. Clin Cancer Res 2009;15(17):5591–8.

[92] Jaber SH, Cowen EW, Haworth LR, Booher SL, Berman DM, Rosenberg SA, et al. Skin reactions in a subset of patients with stage IV melanoma treated with anti-cytotoxic T-lymphocyte antigen 4 monoclonal antibody as a single agent. Arch Dermatol 2006;142(2):166–72.

[93] Chmiel KD, Suan D, Liddle C, Nankivell B, Ibrahim R, Bautista C, et al. Resolution of severe ipilimumab-induced hepatitis after antithymocyte globulin therapy. J Clin Oncol 2011;29(9):e237–40.

[94] Gutenberg A, Landek-Salgado M, Tzou S, Lupi I, Geis A, Kimura H, et al. Autoimmune hypophysitis: expanding the differential diagnosis to CTLA-4 blockade. Expert Rev Endocrinology & Metabolism 2009;4(6):681–98.

[95] Dillard T, Yedinak CG, Alumkal J, Fleseriu M. Anti-CTLA-4 antibody therapy associated autoimmune hypophysitis: serious immune related adverse events across a spectrum of cancer subtypes. Pituitary 2010;13(1):29–38.

[96] Carpenter KJ, Murtagh RD, Lilienfeld H, Weber J, Murtagh FR. Ipilimumab-induced hypophysitis: MR imaging findings. AJNR Am J Neuroradiol 2009;30(9):1751–3.

[97] Kaehler KC, Egberts F, Lorigan P, Hauschild A. Anti-CTLA-4 therapy-related autoimmune hypophysitis in a melanoma patient. Melanoma Res 2009;19(5):333–4.

[98] Shaw SA, Camacho LH, McCutcheon IE, Waguespack SG. Transient hypophysitis after cytotoxic T lymphocyte-associated antigen 4 (CTLA4) blockade. J Clin Endocrinol Metab 2007;92(4):1201–2.

[99] Min L, Vaidya A, Becker C. Ipilimumab therapy for advanced melanoma is associated with secondary adrenal insufficiency: a case series. Endoc Pract 2011:1–13.

[100] Min L, Vaidya A, Becker C. Thyroid autoimmunity and ophthalmopathy related to melanoma biological therapy. Eur J Endocrinol 2011;164(2):303–7.

[101] Bashey A, Medina B, Corringham S, Pasek M, Carrier E, Vrooman L, et al. CTLA4 blockade with ipilimumab to treat relapse of malignancy after allogeneic hematopoietic cell transplantation. Blood 2009;113(7):1581–8.

[102] Fadel F, El Karoui K, Knebelmann B. Anti-CTLA4 antibody-induced lupus nephritis. N Engl J Med 2009;361(2):211–2.

[103] Beck KE, Blansfield JA, Tran KQ, Feldman AL, Hughes MS, Royal RE, et al. Enterocolitis in patients with cancer after antibody blockade of cytotoxic T-lymphocyte-associated antigen 4. J Clin Oncol 2006;24(15):2283–9.

[104] Hunter G, Voll C, Robinson CA. Autoimmune inflammatory myopathy after treatment with ipilimumab. Can J Neurol Sci 2009;36(4):518—20.

[105] Maur M, Tomasello C, Frassoldati A, Dieci MV, Barbieri E, Conte P. Posterior Reversible Encephalopathy Syndrome During Ipilimumab Therapy for Malignant Melanoma. J Clin Oncol 2011.

[106] Bompaire F, Mateus C, Taillia H, De Greslan T, Lahutte M, Sallansonnet-Froment M, et al. Severe meningo-radiculo-nevritis associated with ipilimumab. Invest New Drugs 2012.

[107] Bhatia S, Huber BR, Upton MP, Thompson JA. Inflammatory enteric neuropathy with severe constipation after ipilimumab treatment for melanoma: a case report. J Immunother 2009;32(2):203—5.

[108] Yang JC, Hughes M, Kammula U, Royal R, Sherry RM, Topalian SL, et al. Ipilimumab (anti-CTLA4 antibody) causes regression of metastatic renal cell cancer associated with enteritis and hypophysitis. J Immunother 2007;30(8):825—30.

[109] Gordon IO, Wade T, Chin K, Dickstein J, Gajewski TF. Immune-mediated red cell aplasia after anti-CTLA-4 immunotherapy for metastatic melanoma. Cancer Immunol Immunother 2009;58(8):1351—3.

[110] Ahmad S, Lewis M, Corrie P, Iddawela M. Ipilimumab-induced thrombocytopenia in a patient with metastatic melanoma. J Oncol Pharm Pract 2011.

[111] Akhtari M, Waller EK, Jaye DL, Lawson DH, Ibrahim R, Papadopoulos NE, et al. Neutropenia in a patient treated with ipilimumab (anti-CTLA-4 antibody). J Immunother 2009;32(3):322—4.

[112] Delyon J, Mateus C, Lambert T. Hemophilia A induced by ipilimumab. N Engl J Med 2011;365(18):1747—8.

[113] Phan GQ, Touloukian CE, Yang JC, Restifo NP, Sherry RM, Hwu P, et al. Immunization of patients with metastatic melanoma using both class I- and class II-restricted peptides from melanoma-associated antigens. J Immunother 2003;26(4):349—56.

[114] Blansfield JA, Beck KE, Tran K, Yang JC, Hughes MS, Kammula US, et al. Cytotoxic T-lymphocyte-associated antigen-4 blockage can induce autoimmune hypophysitis in patients with metastatic melanoma and renal cancer. J Immunother 2005;28(6):593—8.

[115] Ku GY, Yuan J, Page DB, Schroeder SE, Panageas KS, Carvajal RD, et al. Single-institution experience with ipilimumab in advanced melanoma patients in the compassionate use setting: lymphocyte count after 2 doses correlates with survival. Cancer 2010;116(7):1767—75.

[116] Dea Berman. Association of peripheral blood absolute lymphocyte count (ALC) and clinical activity in patients (pts) with advanced melanoma treated with ipilimumab. J Clin Oncol 2009;27(Abstract):3020.

[117] Yang AS, et al. CTLA-4 blockade with ipilimumab increases peripheral CD8+ T cells: Correlation with clinical outcomes. J Clin Oncol 2010;28(Abstract):2555.

[118] Hutloff A, Dittrich AM, Beier KC, Eljaschewitsch B, Kraft R, Anagnostopoulos I, et al. ICOS is an inducible T-cell co-stimulator structurally and functionally related to CD28. Nature 1999;397(6716):263—6.

[119] Burmeister Y, Lischke T, Dahler AC, Mages HW, Lam KP, Coyle AJ, et al. ICOS controls the pool size of effector-memory and regulatory T cells. J Immunol 2008;180(2):774—82.

[120] Liakou CI, Kamat A, Tang DN, Chen H, Sun J, Troncoso P, et al. CTLA-4 blockade increases IFNgamma-producing CD4+ICOShi cells to shift the ratio of effector to regulatory T cells in cancer patients. Proce Nat Acad Sci U S A 2008;105(39):14987—92.

[121] Chen H, Liakou CI, Kamat A, Pettaway C, Ward JF, Tang DN, et al. Anti-CTLA-4 therapy results in higher CD4+ICOShi T cell frequency and IFN-gamma levels in both nonmalignant and malignant prostate tissues. Proce Nat Acad Sci U S A 2009;106(8):2729—34.

[122] Carthon BC, Wolchok JD, Yuan J, Kamat A, Ng Tang DS, Sun J, et al. Preoperative CTLA-4 blockade: tolerability and immune monitoring in the setting of a presurgical clinical trial. Clin Cancer Res 2010;16(10):2861—71.

[123] Hirota K, Martin B, Veldhoen M. Development, regulation and functional capacities of Th17 cells. Semin Immunopathol 2010;32(1):3—16.

[124] Canderan G, Dellabona P. T helper 17 T cells do good for cancer immunotherapy. Immunotherapy 2010;2(1):21—4.

[125] Saskia JAM. Abstract B20: Immune vs. clinical response monitoring in patients with metastatic hormone-refractory prostate cancer receiving combined prostate GVAX and anti-CTLA4 immunotherapy. Clin Cancer Res 2010;16(7). Suppl. 1.

[126] Weber JS. Phase II trial of extended dose anti-CTLA-4 antibody ipilimumab (formerly MDX-010) with a multipeptide vaccine for resected stages IIIC and IV melanoma. J Clin Oncol 2009:27.

[127] Jungbluth AA, Chen YT, Stockert E, Busam KJ, Kolb D, Iversen K, et al. Immunohistochemical analysis of NY-ESO-1 antigen expression in normal and malignant human tissues. Int J Cancer 2001;92(6):856—60.

[128] Yuan J, Adamow M, Ginsberg BA, Rasalan TS, Ritter E, Gallardo HF, et al. Integrated NY-ESO-1 antibody and CD8+ T-cell responses correlate with clinical benefit in advanced melanoma patients treated with ipilimumab. Proc Natl Acad Sci U S A 2011.

[129] Hamid O, Schmidt H, Nissan A, Ridolfi L, Aamdal S, Hansson J, et al. A prospective phase II trial exploring the association between tumor microenvironment biomarkers and clinical activity of ipilimumab in advanced melanoma. J Transl Med 2011;9(1):204.

[130] Ji RR, Chasalow SD, Wang L, Hamid O, Schmidt H, Cogswell J, et al. An immune-active tumor microenvironment favors clinical response to ipilimumab. Cancer Immunol Immunother 2011.

[131] Del Vecchio M, Mortarini R, Tragni G, Di Guardo L, Bersani I, Di Tolla G, et al. T-cell activation and maturation at tumor site associated with objective response to ipilimumab in metastatic melanoma. J Clin Oncol 2011;29(32):e783—8.

[132] Hodi FS, Butler M, Oble DA, Seiden MV, Haluska FG, Kruse A, et al. Immunologic and clinical effects of antibody blockade of cytotoxic T lymphocyte-associated antigen 4 in previously vaccinated cancer patients. Proc Natl Acad Sci U S A 2008;105(8):3005—10.

[133] Klein O, Ebert LM, Nicholaou T, Browning J, Russell SE, Zuber M, et al. Melan-A-specific cytotoxic T cells are associated with tumor regression and autoimmunity following treatment with anti-CTLA-4. Clin Cancer Res 2009;15(7):2507—13.

[134] Small EJ, Tchekmedyian NS, Rini BI, Fong L, Lowy I, Allison JP. A pilot trial of CTLA-4 blockade with human anti-CTLA-4 in patients with hormone-refractory prostate cancer. Clin Cancer Res 2007;13(6): 1810—5.

[135] Small E, Higano C, Tchekmedyian N, Sartor O, Stein B, Young R, et al. Randomized phase II study comparing 4 monthly doses of ipilimumab (MDX-010) as a single agent or in combination with a single dose of docetaxel in patients with hormone-refractory prostate cancer. Journal of Clinical Oncology. ASCO Annual Meeting Proceedings Part I 2006;vol. 24:4609. No 18S (June 20 Supplement)2006.

[136] Fong L, Kwek SS, O'Brien S, Kavanagh B, McNeel DG, Weinberg V, et al. Potentiating endogenous antitumor immunity to prostate cancer through combination immunotherapy with CTLA4 blockade and GM-CSF. Cancer Res 2009;69(2):609—15.

[137] Slovin SF, Beer TM, Higano CS, Tejwani S, Hamid O, Picus J, et al. Initial phase II experience of ipilimumab (IPI) alone and in combination with radiotherapy (XRT) in patients with metastatic castration-resistant prostate cancer (mCRPC). J Clin Oncol 2009;27: 15s, (Suppl; abstr 5138).

[138] Mohebtash M, Madan RA, Arlen PM, Rauckhorst M, Tsang KY, Cereda V, et al. Phase I trial of targeted therapy with PSA-TRICOM vaccine (V) and ipilimumab (ipi) in patients (pts) with metastatic castration-resistant prostate cancer (mCRPC). J Clin Oncol 2009;27: 15s, (Suppl; abstr 5144).

[139] van den Eertwegh AJ, Versluis J, van den Berg HP, Santegoets SJ, van Moorselaar RJ, van der Sluis TM, et al. Combined immunotherapy with granulocyte-macrophage colony-stimulating factor-transduced allogeneic prostate cancer cells and ipilimumab in patients with metastatic castration-resistant prostate cancer: a phase 1 dose-escalation trial. Lancet Oncol 2012.

[140] Madan RA, Mohebtash M, Arlen PM, Vergati M, Rauckhorst M, Steinberg SM, et al. Ipilimumab and a poxviral vaccine targeting prostate-specific antigen in metastatic castration-resistant prostate cancer: a phase 1 dose-escalation trial. Lancet Oncol 2012.

[141] Lynch TJ, Bondarenko IN, Luft A, Serwatowski P, Barlesi F, Chacko RT, et al. Phase II trial of ipilimumab (IPI) and paclitaxel/carboplatin (P/C) in first-line stage IIIb/IV non-small cell lung cancer (NSCLC). J Clin Oncol 2010;28: 15s (Suppl; abstr 7531).

[142] Ansell SM, Hurvitz SA, Koenig PA, LaPlant BR, Kabat BF, Fernando D, et al. Phase I study of ipilimumab, an anti-CTLA-4 monoclonal antibody, in patients with relapsed and refractory B-cell non-Hodgkin lymphoma. Clin Cancer Res 2009;15(20):6446—53.

[143] Royal RE, Levy C, Turner K, Mathur A, Hughes M, Kammula US, et al. Phase 2 trial of single agent Ipilimumab (anti-CTLA-4) for locally advanced or metastatic pancreatic adenocarcinoma. J Immunother 2010;33(8):828—33.

[144] Sanderson K, Scotland R, Lee P, Liu D, Groshen S, Snively J, et al. Autoimmunity in a phase I trial of a fully human anti-cytotoxic T-lymphocyte antigen-4 monoclonal antibody with multiple melanoma peptides and Montanide ISA 51 for patients with resected stages III and IV melanoma. J Clin Oncol 2005;23(4):741—50.

[145] Balachandran VP, Cavnar MJ, Zeng S, Bamboat ZM, Ocuin LM, Obaid H, et al. Imatinib potentiates anti-tumor T cell responses in gastrointestinal stromal tumor through the inhibition of Ido. Nat Med 2011;17(9):1094—100.

[146] Postow M, Callahan M, Barker C, Yamada Y, J Y, S K, et al. Immunologic Correlates of an Abscopal Effect in a Patient with Melanoma. N Engl J Med 2012;366(10):925—31.

CHAPTER 20

Recombinant TRICOM-based Therapeutic Cancer Vaccines: Lessons Learned

Jeffrey Schlom, James W. Hodge, Claudia Palena, John W. Greiner, Kwong-Yok Tsang, Benedetto Farsaci, Ravi A. Madan, James L. Gulley
Laboratory of Tumor Immunology and Biology, Center for Cancer Research, National Cancer Institute, National Institutes of Health, Bethesda, MD USA

I. THE CHOICE OF RECOMBINANT POXVIRAL VECTORS

309

The goal of cancer vaccines is to develop strategies that enhance the immunogenicity of weakly immunogenic tumor-associated antigens (TAAs). With time, when long-term safety profiles of these vaccines are established, these same vaccines could potentially be used for prevention of cancers in high-risk populations and eventually for the general population. Vaccinia viruses are among the most immunogenic viruses known; vaccinia was the agent used in the worldwide eradication of smallpox and has been administered to over 1 billion humans. Vaccinia and other members of the poxvirus family are attractive vaccine vectors for numerous reasons (Table 20.1).

II. DEVELOPMENT OF PRECLINICAL MODELS

One of the most widely expressed TAAs is carcinoembryonic antigen (CEA) [1]. One of the issues addressed early on was to optimize induction of CEA-specific CD4+ and CD8+ T-cell responses in a host tolerant to CEA and in which CEA is a self-antigen. Since mice do not express human CEA, CEA transgenic (Tg) mice were employed [2]. These mice express CEA, as do humans, in fetal tissue and in some adult gut tissues. They also express CEA in sera at levels similar to patients with CEA positive tumors. The challenge was to define the best delivery system to break tolerance to CEA in these mice, and to go on to kill tumors engineered to express human CEA. A recombinant vaccinia expressing the CEA transgene (designated rV-CEA) was constructed and demonstrated superiority to other forms of CEA-targeted therapy [3,4]. Subsequent studies [4] also demonstrated the superiority of rV-CEA vs. CEA protein in inducing antitumor responses. This study and numerous others have dispelled the belief of "antigenic competition" in using poxvirus vectors—i.e., that the poxviral epitopes would interfere with the TAA transgene epitopes for T-cell activation [5].

Cancer Immunotherapy. http://dx.doi.org/10.1016/B978-0-12-394296-8.00020-8

TABLE 20.1 Properties of Recombinant Poxviral Vaccine Vectors

- Vectors
Vaccinia (rV-)
  - elicits a strong immune response
  - host induced immunity limits its continuous use
  - MVA (replication defective)
Avipox (fowlpox rF-, ALVAC)
  - derived from avian species
  - safe; does not replicate
  - can be used repeatedly with little if any host neutralizing immunity
- Can insert multiple transgenes
- Do not integrate into host DNA
- Efficiently infect antigen-presenting cells including dendritic cells

A. Diversified prime and boost regimens

The intense immunogenicity of the replication-competent vaccinia virus also serves to limit the number of inoculations. Preclinical and clinical studies have shown that in a vaccinia-immune host, i.e., a patient who had received a prior smallpox vaccine, recombinant vaccinia can be given only once or twice, to enhance immunogenicity to TAA transgenes [6,7]. Subsequently, host immunity to vaccinia is more potent than the host's ability to mount immunity to the transgene. Recombinant avian poxviruses (avipox) such as fowlpox (rF-) or canarypox (ALVAC) have been used to potentiate immunity to transgenes following rV-priming. The use of a diversified immunization schema in CEA Tg mice using rV-CEA as a prime followed by multiple boosts with avipox CEA was shown to be superior to the use of either vector alone in eliciting CEA-specific T-cell responses [6,8].

III. T-CELL CO-STIMULATION: DEVELOPMENT OF TRICOM VECTORS

The generation of a robust host response to a weak "self-antigen" such as a TAA requires at least two signals (discussed in Chapters 2, 4). B7.1 (CD80) is one of the most studied co-stimulatory molecules in its interaction with its CD28 ligand on T cells. An rV-B7.1 vector was constructed and shown to faithfully express B7.1 transgenes. Studies then demonstrated that the admixing of rV-CEA with rV-B7.1 resulted in enhanced CEA-specific T-cell responses and antitumor immunity compared to either vector alone [9,10]. Additional studies were conducted with recombinant vaccinia viruses containing other T-cell co-stimulatory molecules including LFA-3, CD70, ICAM-1, 4-1BBL, and OX-40L [11–14]. Each was shown to enhance antigen-specific T-cell responses, but the combined use of three specific co-stimulatory molecules (B7.1, ICAM-1, and LFA-3) acted synergistically to further enhance antigen-specific T-cell responses (Figure 20.1). Each molecule binds to a different ligand on T cells and is known to signal through different pathways. This TRIad of CO-stimulatory Molecules has been designated TRICOM (Table 20.2). Attempts to add a fourth co-stimulatory molecule resulted in either a minimal enhancement or reduced immunogenicity to the TAA transgene.

Evaluation of different vaccine strategies [6,15] in the stringent CEA Tg animal model demonstrated that (a) a diversified vaccination protocol consisting of primary vaccination with rV-CEA-TRICOM followed by boosting with rF-CEA-TRICOM is more efficacious than homogeneous vaccination with either vector and more efficacious than the use of these vectors with one or no co-stimulatory molecules (Figure 20.2); (b) continued boosting with vaccine is required to maintain CEA-specific T-cell responses, and boosting with rF-CEA-TRICOM is superior to boosting with rF-CEA; and (c) the use of cytokines, such as local granulocyte

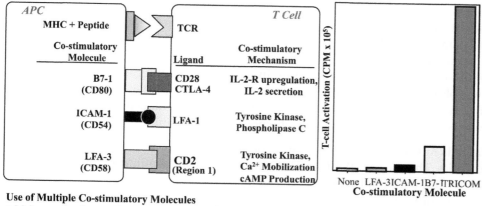

Use of Multiple Co-stimulatory Molecules
- Major co-stimulatory effect must be on the T cell
- No overlap of T-cell ligands
- No redundancy of co-stimulatory mechanisms

FIGURE 20.1
The three co-stimulatory molecules in TRICOM (B7.1, ICAM-1 and LFA-3) act synergistically in enhancing antigen-specific T-cell responses. Each molecule has a distinct ligand on T cells.

TABLE 20.2	TRICOM: TRIad of CO-stimulatory Molecules
Co-stimulatory Molecule	**Ligand on T cell**
B7.1 (CD80)	CD28/CTLA-4
ICAM-1 (CD54)	LFA-1
LFA-3 (CD58)	CD2

TRICOM = B7-1/ICAM-1/LFA-3
CEA/TRICOM = CEA/B7-1/ICAM-1/LFA-3
CEA/MUC-1/TRICOM = CEA/MUC-1/B7-1/ICAM-1/LFA-3 (PANVAC)
PSA/TRICOM = PSA/B7-1/ICAM-1

All vaccines contain: rV- as a prime vaccine
avipox (fowlpox, rF-) as multiple booster vaccines

CEA, MUC-1, and PSA transgenes all contain enhancer agonist

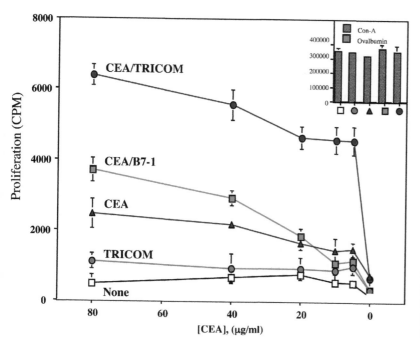

FIGURE 20.2
CEA-specific lymphoproliferation of T cells from CEA-Tg mice vaccinated with TRICOM vectors (without the CEA transgene); rV-, rF-CEA; rV-, rF-CEA-B7.1; or rV-, rF-CEA-TRICOM vectors. *Adapted from ref. [6].*

311

macrophage colony-stimulating factor (GM-CSF), in combination with vaccine enhanced antitumor activity. These strategies were combined to optimally treat CEA-expressing carcinoma liver metastases in CEA Tg mice [6,15]. Several preclinical studies have also supported the concept of intratumoral vaccination employing vectors expressing transgenes for both a TAA and TRICOM [16–20]. Despite CEA expression in some normal adult gastrointestinal tissues, no toxicity was observed in CEA-TRICOM–vaccinated mice. These studies and others [6,21,22] demonstrated that a balance can indeed be achieved between the induction of an antitumor immune response to a self-antigen, and the absence of autoimmunity.

Modified Vaccinia Ankara (MVA) is a replication defective form of vaccinia virus with reduced potential toxicities. The use of rMVA-CEA-TRICOM in a diversified prime and boost vaccine regimen with rF-CEA-TRICOM boosts induced similar levels of both CD4+ and CD8+ T-cell responses specific for CEA and antitumor activity to that seen with rV-CEA-TRICOM prime and rF-CEA-TRICOM boost [23,24].

High avidity cytotoxic T lymphocytes (CTLs) are most effective at clearing viruses and cancer cells. The TRICOM vaccine enhances the magnitude of the avidity of T cells generated and the combination strategy enhances the antitumor effects [16,25].

A. TRICOM infection of dendritic cells and other antigen-presenting cells

Dendritic cells (DCs) express several co-stimulatory molecules and are believed to be the most potent APCs (Chapter 5). One study [26] was designed to determine if infecting DCs with TRICOM vectors enhances their capacity to stimulate T-cell responses. Peptide-pulsed DCs infected with rF-TRICOM or rV-TRICOM induced CTL activity *in vivo* to a markedly greater extent than peptide-pulsed DCs ($P = 0.001$ in both).

While DCs are arguably the most potent APCs, limitations exist in their use as vaccines due to issues involving lot variability and production cost. Studies [27] have demonstrated that a generic APC population, murine splenocytes, can be made more efficient as APCs by infection with either rF-TRICOM(mu) or rV-TRICOM vectors(mu); this led to significant improvement in APC capabilities including: the amount of signal 1 needed to activate naive T cells, and a reduction in the APC numbers required to activate T cells.

Human DCs will vary among different donors and in terms of expression of different phenotypic markers, including co-stimulatory molecules. However, rF-TRICOM can efficiently infect human DCs of different states of maturity and hyperexpress each of the three co-stimulatory molecules [28]. rF-TRICOM–infected DCs were shown to be more effective than peptide-pulsed DCs in activating T cells to 9-mer peptides of CEA and prostate-specific antigen (PSA).

Human B cells can also be efficiently infected by an rF-TRICOM to markedly increase surface expression of B7.1, ICAM-1 and LFA-3. Peptide-pulsed rF-TRICOM–infected B cells were highly efficient in activating antigen-specific human T cells and shown to be superior to the use of CD40L in enhancing APC potency [29]. *Ex vivo*–generated antigen-specific T cells activated in this manner might be applied to novel vaccine protocols.

B. TRICOM infection of human tumor cells as a vaccine platform

Chronic lymphocytic leukemia (CLL) is a disease of CD5+ B lymphocytes that are inefficient APCs. Their poor ability to present antigens to T cells, largely due to an inadequate co-stimulatory capacity, is manifested as a failure to stimulate proliferation of both allogeneic and autologous T cells. Proliferation of allogeneic and autologous T cells was observed when rMVA-TRICOM–infected CLL cells were used as stimulators in proliferation assays [30,31]. CTLs generated *in vitro* by stimulation of autologous T cells with rMVA-TRICOM–infected CLL cells showed cytotoxicity against unmodified/uninfected CLL cells. These findings suggested that the use of CLL cells infected *ex vivo* with rMVA-TRICOM or direct injection of rMVA-TRICOM in patients with CLL has potential for the immunotherapy of CLL. A subsequent study [32] comparing rMVAs encoding CD40L or TRICOM for their ability to enhance the immunogenicity of CLL cells showed differential responses among patients to each vector in terms of induction of autologous T-cell responses. This study supported the rationale for the use of CLL cells modified *ex vivo* with prespecified recombinant MVA vectors as a whole tumor-cell vaccine for immunotherapy in CLL patients.

C. The importance of antigen cascade in vaccine-mediated therapeutic responses

Studies were undertaken [16,18] to determine the range of specific immune responses associated with vaccination-mediated tumor regression. CEA Tg mice bearing CEA$^+$ tumors were vaccinated with the CEA-TRICOM s.c./i.t. regimen, and antitumor (Figure 20.3, top panel) and T-cell immune responses were assessed. These studies showed that CEA was needed to be present in both the vaccine and the tumor for therapeutic effects. T cell responses could be detected not only to CEA encoded in the vaccine but also to other antigens expressed on the tumor itself: wild-type p53 and an endogenous retroviral epitope of gp70 (Figure 20.3, middle panel). Moreover, the magnitude of CD8+ T-cell immune responses to gp70 was far greater than that induced to CEA or p53. Finally, the predominant T-cell population infiltrating the regressing CEA$^+$ tumor after therapy was specific for gp70 (Figure 20.3, middle panel). Challenge of cured mice with tumors expressing CEA, gp70, both, or none showed that the predominant antitumor effect was due to gp70, i.e., the cascade antigen (Figure 20.3, lower panel). These studies showed that the breadth and magnitude of antitumor immune cascades to multiple antigens can be critical in the therapy of established tumors.

IV. CLINICAL TRIALS

A. Pan carcinoma (nonprostate) clinical trials

Several clinical studies were first carried out using the following vaccines: rV-CEA, avipox-CEA, avipox-CEA-B7.1. These studies showed both safety, the advantage of the vaccinia prime/ avipox booster regimen, and preliminary evidence of clinical benefit in carcinoma patients [33–39]. In clinical trials with avipox-CEA-B7.1 [34,38,39], several patients experienced clinically stable disease that correlated with increasing CEA-specific precursor T cells. All of the patients had evidence of leukocytic infiltration and CEA expression in vaccine biopsy sites. The number of prior chemotherapy regimens was negatively correlated with the generation of a T-cell response, whereas a positive correlation was observed between the number of months from the last chemotherapy regimen and the T-cell response. Avipox-CEA-B7.1 was thus shown to be safe in patients with advanced recurrent adenocarcinomas that express CEA, and is associated with disease stabilization for up to 13 months.

B. TRICOM-based vaccines: clinical studies (nonprostate)

Three of the most widely studied human TAAs are CEA, mucin-1 (MUC-1), and PSA. CEA is overexpressed in a wide range of human carcinomas, including gastrointestinal, breast, lung, pancreatic, medullary thyroid, ovarian, and prostate. MUC-1 is a tumor-associated mucin, which is overexpressed and hypoglycosylated in all human carcinomas as well as in acute myeloid leukemia (AML) and multiple myeloma. The elegant studies of Kufe and colleagues [40,41] as well as others have demonstrated that the C-terminus of MUC-1 functions as an oncogene.

We conducted the first TRICOM trial in humans [42] with rV-, rF-CEA-TRICOM vaccines (also including an enhancer agonist epitope within the CEA gene) (Figure 20.4). Twenty-three patients (40%) had stable disease for at least 4 months, with 14 (24%) of these patients having prolonged stable disease (>6 months). Eleven patients had decreasing or stable serum CEA,

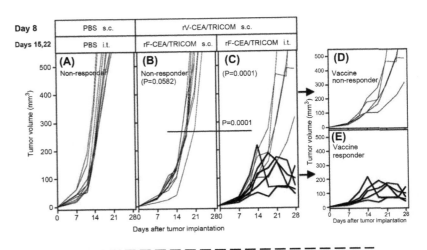

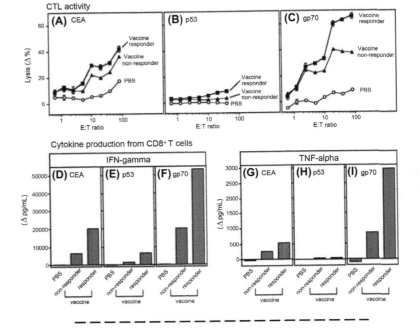

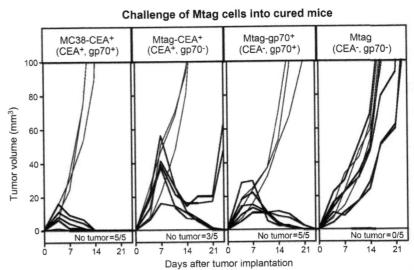

314

FIGURE 20.3

CEA-TRICOM vaccination induces antitumor activity and antigen cascade. **Top panel:** CEA-Tg mice were transplanted s.c. with MC38-CEA$^+$ tumors on day 0 ($n = 10$). A. control mice were vaccinated with PBS vehicle s.c. on day 8 and intratumorally (i.t.) on days 15 and 22. B. mice were vaccinated s.c. with rV-CEA=TRICOM on day 8 and then boosted s.c. with rF-CEA-TRICOM on days 15 and 22. C. mice were vaccinated s.c. with rV-CEA-TRICOM on day 8 and then boosted i.t. with rF-CEA-TRICOM on days 15 and 22. P values on day 28 compared with the PBS control group. Mice in C were separated into two groups (D and E) based on the tumor volume at day 28 and were used for subsequent immunologic analyses after tumor transplantation. **Middle panel:** Induction of CD8$^+$ T-cell responses to CEA, p53, and gp70 after the CEA-TRICOM s.c. prime/intratumoral (i.t.) boost vaccine regimen. Splenic lymphocytes from CEA-Tg mice were used 29 days after tumor transplantation. A. CEA-specific CTL activity. B. p53-specific CTL activity. C. gp70-specific CTL activity. Control mice treated with PBS (○), nonresponders to CEA/TRICOM s.c./i.t. vaccine therapy (▲), and responders to CEA/TRICOM s.c./i.t. vaccine therapy (■). D–F. antigen-specific IFN-γ production from CD8$^+$ T cells. G–I. antigen-specific tumor necrosis factor-α production from CD8$^+$ T cells. **Bottom panel:** CEA-Tg mice were vaccinated s.c. with rV-CEA-TRICOM on day 8 and then boosted s.c. with rF-CEA=TRICOM on days 15, 22, and 29. Cured mice after the therapy were challenged with tumor cells (3 × 10^5) 88 days after tumor implantation ($n = 5$, bold lines). Cured mice were challenged with tumor cells that were either CEA$^+$gp70$^+$, CEA$^+$gp70$^-$, CEA$^-$gp70$^+$, or CEA$^-$gp70$^-$. The results demonstrate that some of the antitumor effects can be attributed to CEA in the original vaccination, but the most potent antitumor effects are those directed against the tumor-associated cascade antigen gp70 not in the vaccine. As a control, age/sex-matched CEA-Tg mice were implanted with same tumors (thin lines). *Adapted from ref. [18].*

TRICOM Vaccines

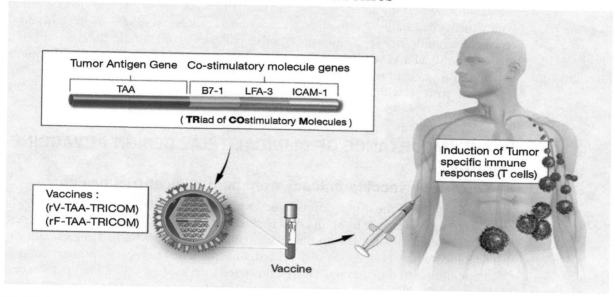

FIGURE 20.4

Representation of the "off-the-shelf" nature of TRICOM vaccines containing tumor-associated antigen (TAA) and co-stimulatory molecule transgenes. Prime and booster vaccinations are given subcutaneously.

and one patient had a pathologic complete response. Enhanced CEA-specific T-cell responses were observed in the majority of patients tested.

We then conducted a pilot study [43] of 25 patients treated with the poxviral vaccine regimen consisting of the genes for CEA and MUC-1, along with TRICOM, engineered into vaccinia (PANVAC-V) as a prime vaccination and into fowlpox (PANVAC-F) as a booster vaccination. The vaccine regimen was well tolerated. Immune responses to MUC-1 and/or CEA were seen following vaccination in nine of 16 patients tested. A breast cancer patient had a confirmed decrease of >20% in the size of large liver metastases, and a patient with clear cell ovarian cancer and symptomatic ascites had a durable (18-month) clinical response radiographically and biochemically (Figure 20.5).

Another study [44] was conducted to obtain preliminary evidence of clinical response in metastatic breast and ovarian cancer patients with PANVAC. Twenty-six patients were enrolled and given monthly vaccinations. These patients were heavily pretreated, with 21 of 26 patients having had three or more prior chemotherapy regimens. Side effects were largely limited to

315

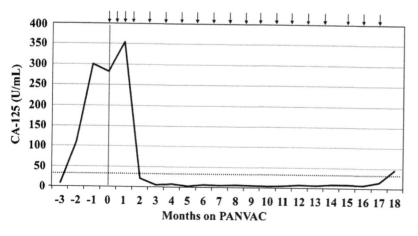

FIGURE 20.5

Serum CA-125 levels from a 42-year-old patient with platinum-refractory clear cell ovarian cancer who received PANVAC-V on day 1, followed by multiple boosts with PANVAC-F (vaccinations designated by arrows). The CA-125 level decreased from a peak of 351 to <10 units/mL until 18 months on study. *Adapted from ref. [43].*

mild injection-site reactions. For the 12 breast cancer patients enrolled, median time to progression was 2.5 months (1–37+) and median overall survival (OS) was 13.7 months. Four patients had stable disease. One patient had a complete response by RECIST and remained on study for over 37 months. Another patient with metastatic disease confined to the mediastinum had a 17% reduction in mediastinal mass and was on study for 10 months. Patients with stable or responding disease had fewer prior therapies and lower tumor marker levels than patients with no evidence of response. Further studies to confirm these results are warranted.

V. THE IMPORTANCE OF CLINICAL TRIAL DESIGN IN VACCINE THERAPY

A. Separating vaccine efficacy from poor clinical trial design

A classic example of the distinction between a vaccine's potential efficacy and a poor clinical trial design was evidenced by an ill-conceived corporate Phase III trial with PANVAC. Vaccine was administered to patients with metastatic pancreatic cancer who had already failed prior gemcitabine therapy [45]. As many predicted, this trial failed to meet its primary endpoint of OS. Poor clinical trial design was clearly illustrated by a median OS of less than 3 months in this patient population. Numerous randomized trials of various FDA-approved and experimental drug combinations have failed to extend survival in this patient population of second-line pancreatic cancer. As evidenced by the PANVAC trials completed and ongoing showing evidence of clinical benefit, the failure of a Phase III vaccine trial in second-line therapy of pancreatic cancer should foremost be considered a failure in clinical trial design employing an inappropriate patient population for vaccine monotherapy.

B. The importance of tumor volume

A clinical trial employing the CEA-TRICOM vaccine platform in colorectal cancer patients with large volume liver metastases showed no evidence of patient benefit [42]. These findings are in contrast to recent results from a trial to evaluate the CEA-MUC1-TRICOM (PANVAC) vaccine in colorectal cancer patients following metastasectomy (surgical removal) of liver or lung metastases. In this multicenter trial [46,47], 74 patients with no evidence of disease after resection and completion of their physician-determined perioperative chemotherapy were vaccinated with PANVAC (i.e., with vaccine alone or with vaccine-modified DCs). Data from a prospectively registered, comparable contemporary control group of colorectal cancer patients who had undergone metastasectomy ($n = 161$) were also available [46,47]. The 2-year relapse-free survival was similar in all groups: 50% for the DC-PANVAC group, 56% for the PANVAC group, and 55% for the contemporary control group. However, the 2-year OS was 95% for the vaccinated group and 75% for the contemporary control group; after approximately 40 months of follow-up, 67 of 74 (90%) of the vaccinated patients survived vs. approximately 47% OS in the contemporary control group; the data for 3- to 5-year survival of colorectal cancer patients after metastasectomy in five other trials ranges from 28% to 58% [48–53]. A randomized trial is necessary to confirm these results. It is of interest, however, that this was yet another example of a vaccine trial that showed little or no evidence of an improvement in relapse-free survival, yet had an apparent benefit in OS.

VI. PROSTATE CANCER CLINICAL TRIALS

While the vast majority of prior and ongoing vaccine trials have been conducted in patients with metastatic melanoma, several characteristics render prostate cancer a prototype disease for the evaluation of therapeutic cancer vaccines: [54] (a) time is often required to generate a sufficient immune response capable of curtailing disease growth. Prostate cancer is generally an indolent disease that may not lead to metastatic disease or death for over a decade or more; (b) prostate cancer cells express a variety of well-characterized TAAs; (c) the serum marker PSA can be used to identify patients with minimal tumor burden and those responding to therapy; and (d) a well-defined nomogram, the Halabi nomogram [55], can be used at presentation of metastatic disease to predict probable response to standard-of-care chemotherapy and/or hormone therapy.

Several clinical studies were first conducted using rV-PSA alone, and then with rV-PSA as a prime and rF-PSA as booster vaccinations [56–58]. A Phase II clinical trial was conducted [7] to evaluate the feasibility, tolerability and efficacy of the prime/boost vaccine strategy in patients with biochemical progression after local therapy for prostate cancer. The induction of PSA-specific immunity was also evaluated. The multicenter clinical trial [7] was conducted by the Eastern Cooperative Oncology Group and 64 patients were randomly assigned to receive (a) four vaccinations with rF-PSA (FFFF), (b) three rF-PSA vaccines followed by one rV-PSA vaccine (FFFV), or (c) one rV-PSA vaccine followed by three rF-PSA vaccines (VFFF). The median time to PSA and/or clinical progression was 9.2 months in the FFFF cohort, and 9.0 months in the FFFV cohort, and had not been reached in the VFFF cohort. An update [59,60] on this trial with a median follow-up of 50 months, moreover, revealed a median time to PSA progression of 9.2 and 9.1 months for the FFFF and FFFV cohorts, respectively, and 18.2 months for the VFFF cohort.

A. PSA-TRICOM (PROSTVAC) studies

A Phase I study was first conducted to evaluate the clinical safety of rV-, rF-PSA-TRICOM (PROSTVAC) in patients with prostate cancer [61]. A Phase II trial of rV, rF-PSA-TRICOM (PROSTVAC) in patients with metastatic castration-resistant prostate cancer (mCRPC) was then conducted to investigate the influence of GM-CSF with vaccine, and the influence of immunologic and prognostic factors on median OS [62]. Thirty-two patients were vaccinated once with rV-PSA-TRICOM and received boosters with rF-PSA-TRICOM. Twelve of the patients showed declines in serum PSA post-vaccination and two of 12 showed decreases in index lesions. Median OS was 26.6 months (predicted median OS by the Halabi nomogram was 17.4 months). Patients with greater PSA-specific T-cell responses showed a trend ($P = 0.055$) toward enhanced survival (Figure 20.6). There was no difference in T-cell responses or survival in cohorts of patients receiving GM-CSF versus no GM-CSF. In a contemporary Phase II trial conducted at the same institution (NCI), the Halabi nomogram accurately predicted survival in a similar patient population receiving the standard-of-care drug docetaxel (Table 20.3). In the vaccine trial, patients with a Halabi predicted survival (HPS) [55] of <18 months (median predicted 12.3 months) had an actual median OS of 14.6 months, while those with an HPS of ≥18 months (median predicted survival 20.9 months) will meet or exceed 37.3 months, with 12 of 15 patients living longer than predicted ($P = 0.035$) (Table 20.3, Figure 20.7). Regulatory T-cell (Treg) suppressive function was shown to decrease following vaccine in patients surviving longer than predicted, and increase in patients surviving less than predicted. Trends were also observed in analyzing effector:Treg (CD4+CD25+CD127-FoxP3+CTLA4+) ratio post- versus pre-vaccination with OS versus HPS. This hypothesis-generating study provided evidence that patients with more indolent mCRPC (HPS ≥18 months) may best benefit from vaccine therapy.

rV, rF-PSA-TRICOM (PROSTVAC-VF) was further evaluated for prolongation of progression-free survival (PFS) and OS in a 43-center randomized, controlled, and blinded Phase II study [63]. In total, 125 patients with minimally symptomatic mCRPC were randomly assigned. Patients were allocated (2:1) to PROSTVAC-VF plus GM-CSF or to control empty vectors plus saline injections. Eighty-two patients received PROSTVAC-VF and 40 received control vectors. Patient characteristics were similar in both groups. The primary end point was PFS, which was similar in the two groups ($P = 0.6$). However, at 3 years post-study, PROSTVAC-VF patients had a better OS with 25 (30%) of 82 alive versus 7 (17%) of 40 controls, longer median survival by 8.5 months (25.1 vs. 16.6 months for controls), an estimated hazard

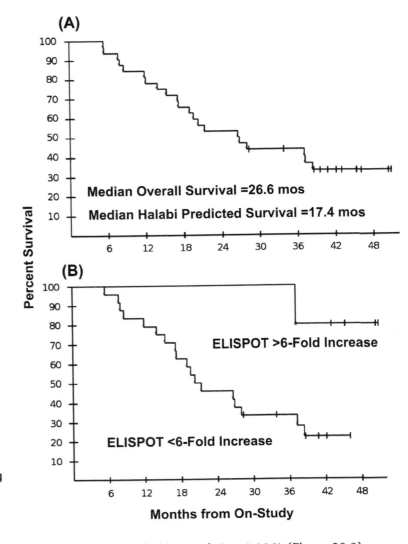

FIGURE 20.6

A. The Kaplan-Meier curve for the patients ($n = 32$) with metastatic prostate cancer vaccinated with rV-, rF-PSA-TRICOM (PROSTVAC) demonstrates (panel A) a median overall survival (OS) of 26.6 months. B. There was a strong trend in the ability to mount a 6-fold increase in PSA–T cells post-vaccine and an increase in OS. *Adapted from ref. [62].*

318

ratio of 0.56 (95% CI, 0.37 to 0.85), and stratified log-rank $P = 0.0061$ (Figure 20.8). PROSTVAC-VF immunotherapy was thus well tolerated and associated with a 44% reduction in the death rate and an 8.5-month improvement in median OS in men with mCRPC. These provocative data provided evidence of clinically meaningful benefit but need to be confirmed in a 1,200-patient ongoing Phase III study.

It has been hypothesized that vaccine therapy will have significant benefit in patients with minimal disease recurrence. In order to begin to test this idea, we treated hormone naive patients ($n = 50$) with micro-metastatic disease with PROSTVAC [64]. Among 29 patients with follow-up >6 months, the PSA progression-free rate at 6 months (the primary endpoint) was 66%. Pre-treatment PSA slope was 0.17 log PSA/month (median PSA doubling time (PSADT) 4.4 months), in contrast to the on-treatment slope of 0.12 log PSA/month (median PSADT 7.7 months), $p = 0.002$. PSA-TRICOM can thus be administered safely in the multi-institutional cooperative group setting to patients with minimal disease volume [64].

VII. TRICOM VACCINES ALSO CONTAIN TUMOR ANTIGEN AGONIST EPITOPES

We have modified specific epitopes of PSA, CEA, and MUC-1 to enhance their ability to generate human CD8+ T-cell responses. The resultant T cells, however, must maintain their ability to recognize the native configuration of the peptide-MHC interaction on the tumor cell

TABLE 20.3 Predicted Survival of Patients With Metastatic Prostate Cancer by Halabi Nomogram vs. Actual Overall Survival

	All patients	Patients with HPS <18 months	Patients with HPS ≥18 months
Vaccine: PROSTVAC (n = 32)			
Median survival predicted by Halabi model (months)	17.4	12.3	20.9
Actual median overall survival (months)	26.6	14.6	≥ 37.3 not reached*
Patients surviving longer than predicted by Halabi nomogram	22 of 32 (69%)	10 of 17 (59%)	12 of 15 (80%)
p value**			p = 0.035
Difference*** (months)	9.2	2.3	≥16.4
Docetaxel[a] therapy (n = 22)			
Median survival predicted by Halabi model (months)	16.5	13.0	21.0
Actual median overall survival (months)	15.5	15.4	16.9
Patients surviving longer than predicted by Halabi nomogram	11 of 22 (50%)	8 of 13 (62%)	3 of 9 (33%)
Difference*** (months)	(−1.0)	2.4	(−4.1)

HPS, Halabi predicted survival.

Adapted from ref. [62].

*Median overall survival based on failures to date will meet or exceed 37.3 months.

**The two-tailed p-value is based on an exact binomial test, with p = 0.5 as the fraction living longer than expected if this were a random occurrence.

***The difference in months denotes the amount by which the actual median overall survival (actuarial) exceeds the arithmetic median survival predicted by Halabi nomogram.

[a]Docetaxel administered weekly for 3 of 4 weeks.

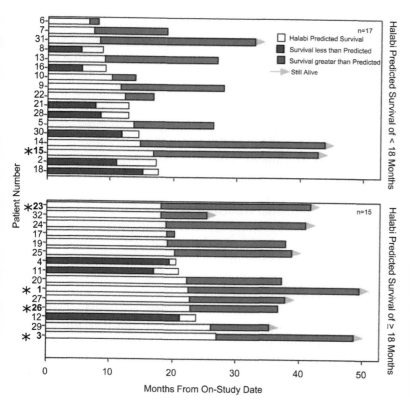

FIGURE 20.7

Results of a Phase II study of patients with metastatic prostate cancer receiving PROSTVAC vaccination. The graph depicts actual overall survival (OS), predicted OS (open bar) and whether or not an individual survived greater than (darkened area to the right) or less than (darkened area to the left) the Halabi predicted survival. In addition, arrows demonstrate patients who were alive at time of analysis. Asterisks depict >6-fold PSA—T-cell responses. Adapted from ref. [62].

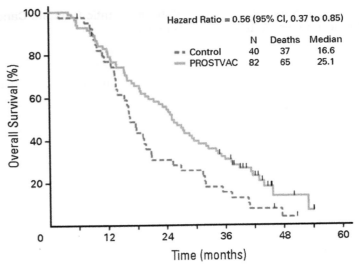

FIGURE 20.8

Overall survival (OS) of a 43-center placebo-controlled randomized Phase II study of PROSTVAC vaccination. Kaplan-Meier estimator for PROSTVAC (rV-, rF-PSA-TRICOM) arm is shown as a solid line and estimator for the control arm is a dashed line. The small vertical tic marks show the censoring times. The estimated median OS is 25.1 months for the PROSTVAC arm and 16.6 months for the control arm ($P = 0.006$). *Adapted from ref. [63].*

target. The clinical studies described above using rV-, rF-PSA-TRICOM vectors contain a PSA enhancer agonist epitope, and those using rV, rF-CEA-MUC 1-TRICOM contain enhancer epitopes for both CEA and MUC-1.

VIII. TRICOM VACCINATION AFFECTS TUMOR GROWTH RATES

In patients who are treated with traditional cytotoxic agents, it is widely believed that improved time to progression is a prerequisite for improved OS. A recent study [65] evaluated tumor regression and growth rates in four chemotherapy trials and one vaccine trial in patients with mCRPC. Figure 20.9 illustrates the growth rate constants defined in that study. Cytotoxic agents affect the tumor only during the period of administration; soon after the drug is discontinued, because of drug resistance or toxicity, antitumor activity ceases and the growth of the tumor increases (Figure 20.9A, line b). With vaccine therapy, the mechanism of action and kinetics of clinical response appear to be very different [65]. Therapeutic vaccines do not directly target the tumor; rather, they target the immune system. Immune responses often take time to develop and can potentially be enhanced by continued booster vaccinations; any resulting tumor cell lysis can lead to cross-priming of additional TAAs, thus broadening the immune repertoire (a phenomenon known as antigen cascade or epitope spreading). This broader, and perhaps more relevant, immune response may also take some time to develop. Although a vaccine may not induce any substantial reduction in tumor burden, vaccines as monotherapy have the potential to apply antitumor activity over a long period, resulting in a slower tumor growth rate (Figure 20.9A, line c). This deceleration in growth rate may continue for months or years and, more importantly, through subsequent therapies. This process can thus lead to clinically significant improved OS, often with little or no difference in time to progression and a low rate of, or lack of, objective response (Figure 20.9A, line c). Thus, treating patients with a vaccine when they have a lower tumor burden, as compared with a greater tumor burden, may result in far better outcomes (Figure 20.9B, line d vs. line e). It is hypothesized that the combined use of vaccine and cytotoxic therapy (Figure 20.9C) may result in both tumor regression (via the cytotoxic therapy) and reduced tumor growth rate (via vaccine therapy) [65–68]. These concepts will be discussed below. Thus, early clinical trials with vaccine may have been terminated prematurely with the observance of tumor progression

(A)

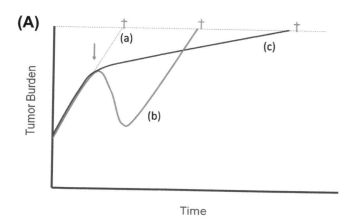

(B)

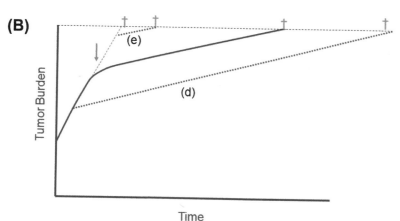

FIGURE 20.9

Tumor growth rates following chemotherapy vs. vaccine therapy. Adapted from data in refs. [65,66,91,92]. A. Growth rate of tumor if no therapy is initiated (line a). An examination of five clinical trials (four with chemotherapy and one with PSA-TRICOM (PROSTVAC) vaccine) in patients with metastatic prostate cancer demonstrated that with the use of chemotherapy there was an initial tumor reduction, but that the growth rate of tumors at relapse (line b) was similar to the initial tumor growth rate prior to therapy; this is contrasted with the reduction in tumor growth rate following vaccine therapy (line c). Thus for patients with little or any tumor reduction (and thus virtually no increase in time to progression), an increase in survival was observed. (†) denotes time to death. B. This phenomenon could potentially be enhanced if vaccine therapy is initiated earlier in disease progression or in patients with low tumor burden metastatic disease (line d), but would have minimal effect in patients with large tumor burden (line e). C. Additional therapies received with vaccine may take advantage of both modalities.

321

(C)

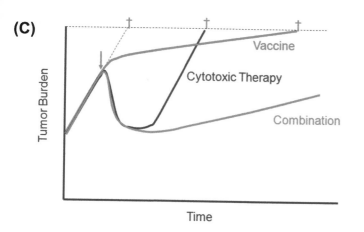

before sufficient vaccine boosts could be administered. This phenomenon has actually led to modifications in how vaccine clinical trials are now designed and to new "immune response criteria" for immunotherapy [69].

IX. INTRATUMORAL VACCINATION: CLINICAL STUDIES

Studies were carried out to evaluate the intratumoral (i.t.) effects of rV-TRICOM [70,71]. In a dose escalation Phase I clinical trial in patients ($n = 13$) with metastatic melanoma, there was a 30.7% objective clinical response, with one patient achieving a complete response for more than 22 months. Patients who failed to respond to vaccination but received high-dose IL-2 had a trend toward improved survival. Collectively, these results confirmed the safety profile and feasibility of direct injection of rV-TRICOM in patients with established tumors.

A study was also conducted to define the level of safety of intraprostatic (i.p.) TRICOM-based vaccine administration [72]. Secondary goals were immunologic and tumor response. Twenty-one patients with locally recurrent prostate cancer after radiation were enrolled into five cohorts and received initial vaccination with s.c. rV-PSA-TRICOM and booster i.p. rF-PSA-TRICOM. Cohorts 3–5 also received i.p. rF-GM-CSF. Cohort 5 received concurrent s.c. and i.p. boosters. Patients had pre- and post-treatment prostate biopsies. Tumor infiltrate was evaluated when adequate tissue was available. Only one grade 3 toxicity occurred, a transient fever. Eighteen of 21 patients had stable or improved PSA on study. Sixteen of 21 patients had stable or improved PSA doubling time. A paired t-test of 13 biopsies pre- and post-vaccination showed increases in tumor immunologic infiltrates of CD3+, CD4+, and CD8+ T cells. Intraprostatic administration of PSA-TRICOM was thus shown to be safe and feasible, and to generate a substantial immune response with improved PSA kinetics, and with intense post-vaccination immune infiltrates in the majority of patients.

X. COMBINATION THERAPIES—PRECLINICAL STUDIES

A. Vaccine in combination with inhibitors of immune suppression

We have demonstrated [73] a biological synergy between TRICOM vaccination and CTLA-4 blockade. The synergy was very much dependent on the temporal relationship of scheduling of the two agents.

B. Vaccine/vaccine combinations

Using recombinant TRICOM and yeast (*Saccharomyces cerevisiae*) vaccines, studies evaluated T-cell populations induced by these two diverse platforms in terms of serum cytokine response, T-cell gene expression, T-cell receptor phenotype, and antigen-specific cytokine expression [74]. T-cell avidity and T-cell antigen-specific tumor cell lysis demonstrated that vaccination with rV,rF-CEA-TRICOM or heat-killed yeast-CEA elicits T-cell populations with both shared and unique phenotypic and functional characteristics. Furthermore, both the antigen and the vector played a role in the induction of distinct T-cell populations. These studies [74] thus provide the rationale for future clinical studies investigating concurrent administration of different vaccine platforms targeting a single antigen.

C. Vaccine and radiation synergy

A biological synergy has been demonstrated between local radiation of tumor and vaccine therapy [75,76]. CEA Tg mice with developing MC38 murine carcinoma cells transfected with CEA were treated with rV-, rF-CEA-TRICOM. One dose of 8-Gy radiation to tumor induced upregulation of the death receptor Fas (CD95) *in situ* for up to 11 days. When vaccine therapy and local radiation of tumor were used in combination, dramatic and significant cures were achieved [75,76]. This was shown to be mediated by the engagement of the Fas/Fas ligand pathway.

Radiolabeled MAbs have demonstrated measurable antitumor effects in hematologic malignancies. This outcome has been more difficult to achieve for solid tumors due, for the most part, to difficulties in delivering sufficient quantities of MAb to the tumor mass. A single dose of Y-90-labeled anti-CEA MAb, in combination with CEA-TRICOM vaccine therapy, however, resulted in a statistically significant increase in survival in tumor-bearing mice over vaccine or MAb alone [77].

A study [78] was then designed to determine whether radiation would also sensitize human tumor cells to T-cell-mediated killing. Twenty-three human carcinoma cell lines (12 colon, 7 lung, and 4 prostate) were examined for their response to nonlytic doses of radiation. Seventy-two hours post-irradiation, changes in surface expression of Fas, as well as expression of other

Treatment of LnCaP prostate cancer cells with palliative doses of ^{153}Sm results in the upregulation of MHC class I and Fas

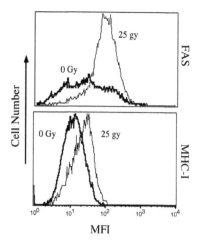

MFI

Treatment of LnCaP prostate cancer cells with palliative doses of ^{153}Sm results in the upregulation of TAAs

Tumor antigen genes

	0 Gy	25 Gy
PSA	1	2.79
PSMA	1	4.14
PAP	1	29.0
CEA	1	10.3
MUC-1	1	3.67

Treatment of LnCaP prostate cancer cells with palliative doses of ^{153}Sm results in increased sensitivity to multiple CTLs

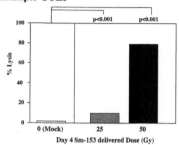

Day 4 Sm-153 delivered Dose (Gy)

FIGURE 20.10

Treatment of LnCaP prostate cells with palliative levels of samarium-153-ethylenediaminetetramethylene-phosphonate ((153)Sm-EDTMP; Quadramet) modulates phenotype, upregulates tumor-associated antigen, and increases sensitivity to antigen-specific CTL killing. *Adapted from ref. [79].*

surface molecules involved in T-cell-mediated immune attack such as ICAM-1, MUC-1, CEA, and MHC class I, were examined. Twenty-one of the 23 (91%) cell lines upregulated one or more of these surface molecules post-irradiation. Furthermore, five of five irradiated CEA+/A2+ colon tumor cells lines demonstrated significantly enhanced killing by CEA-specific HLA-A2—restricted CD8+ CTLs compared with nonirradiated counterparts. Overall, the results of this study suggested that nonlethal doses of radiation can be used to make human tumors more amenable to T-cell attack. Another study [79] explored the possibility that exposure to palliative doses of a radiopharmaceutical agent could also alter the phenotype of tumor cells to render them more susceptible to T-cell-mediated killing. LNCaP tumor cells exposed to (153)Sm-EDTMP, which is used in cancer patients to treat pain due to bone metastasis, also upregulated the surface molecules Fas, CEA, MUC-1, MHC class I, and ICAM-1, and rendered LNCaP cells more susceptible to killing by CTLs specific for PSA, CEA, and MUC-1 (Figure 20.10).

D. Vaccines in combination with chemotherapy

Taxanes comprise some of the most widely used cancer chemotherapeutic agents. This drug family is commonly used to treat breast, prostate, and lung cancers, among others. One study [80] showed that (a) docetaxel modulates CD4+, CD8+, CD19+, natural killer cell, and Treg populations in non-tumor-bearing mice; (b) docetaxel enhances CD8+ but not CD4+ response to CD3 cross-linking; and (c) docetaxel combined with CEA-TRICOM vaccination is superior to either agent alone at reducing tumor burden.

E. Vaccine in combination with small molecule targeted therapies

Small molecule BCL-2 inhibitors are being examined as monotherapy in Phase I/II clinical trials for several types of tumors. Activated mature CD8+ T lymphocytes were shown [81] to be more resistant to GX15-070 as compared to early-activated cells. *In vivo*, GX15-070 was given after vaccination so as to not negatively impact the induction of vaccine-mediated immunity; this resulted in increased intratumoral activated CD8+:Treg ratio and significant reduction of pulmonary tumor nodules (Figure 20.11).

323

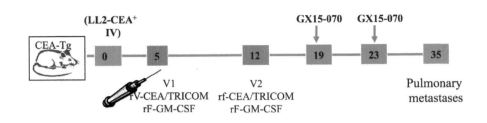

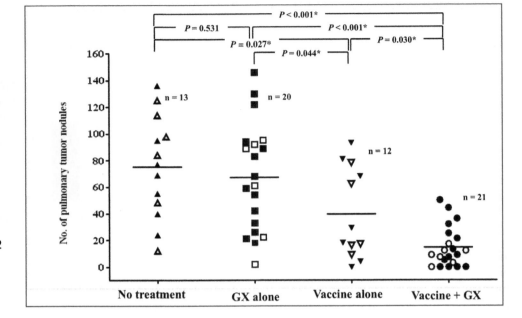

FIGURE 20.11
Antitumor effects of CEA-TRICOM vaccine in combination with a BCL-2 inhibitor via exploiting the differential effect of the pan BCL-2 inhibitor on Tregs vs. effector cells. *Adapted from ref. [81].*

A study [82] has investigated the immunomodulatory effects of sunitinib to rationally design a combinational platform with TRICOM vaccination. The effect of differently timed combinations of sunitinib and CEA-TRICOM in CEA Tg mice was evaluated. *In vivo*, one cycle of sunitinib caused bimodal immune effects: (a) decreased regulatory cells during the 4 weeks of treatment and (b) an immune-suppression rebound during the 2 weeks of treatment interruption. Continuous sunitinib followed by vaccine increased intratumoral infiltration of antigen-specific T lymphocytes, decreased immunosuppressant Tregs and myeloid-derived suppressor cells, reduced tumor volumes and increased survival (Figure 20.12). The immunomodulatory activity of continuous sunitinib can thus create a more immune-permissive environment for combination therapy with vaccine.

XI. COMBINATION THERAPIES—CLINICAL STUDIES

Several hypothesis-generating clinical trials were first conducted with rV-PSA admixed with rV-B7.1 followed by rF-PSA boosts as the vaccine regimen in combination with hormonal therapy, radiation, and chemotherapy [83–86].

A. Vaccine plus hormonal therapy

Forty-two nonmetastatic prostate cancer patients were randomized to receive vaccine (rV-PSA + rV-B7.1 followed by rF-PSA boosts) vs. second-line antiandrogen therapy with nilutamide [84]. Of the patients in the nilutamide arm, eight had vaccine added at the time of PSA progression. Median time to treatment failure with combined therapy was 5.2 months, with a median duration from study entry of 15.9 months. Of the patients in the vaccine arm, 12 had nilutamide added at the time of PSA progression. Median time to treatment failure with combined therapy was 13.9 months and a median of 25.9 months from initiation of therapy.

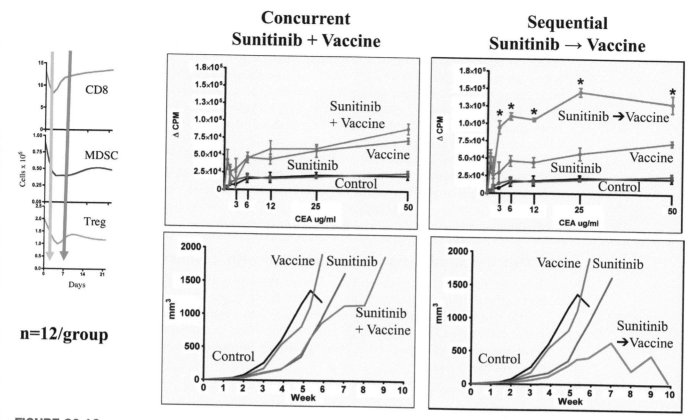

FIGURE 20.12

The importance of dose scheduling in the use of the small molecule inhibitor sunitinib in combination with CEA-TRICOM vaccine. Enhanced antigen-specific T-cell responses and antitumor activity were observed when sunitinib was given prior to vaccine as compared to giving both agents concurrently. This was due to the modulation of Tregs by sunitinib, rendering more efficacious vaccine activity. *Adapted from ref. [82].*

325

A subsequent survival analysis at 6.5 years from the initiation of therapy on this trial with a median potential follow-up of 4.4 years was reported [86]. Median survival exhibited a trend toward improvement for patients initially randomized to the vaccine arm (median, 5.1 versus 3.4 years). These data suggested that patients with more indolent disease may derive greater clinical benefit from vaccine alone or vaccine before second-line hormone therapy compared with hormone therapy alone or hormone therapy followed by vaccine. A study is currently enrolling patients with nonmetastatic CRPC on testosterone suppression therapy who have a rising PSA. The first 26 patients enrolled were evaluated. Median time to progression was 223 days for flutamide + PSA-TRICOM vs. 85 days for flutamide alone [87].

B. Vaccine plus chemotherapy

Twenty-eight patients with metastatic androgen-independent prostate cancer were randomized to receive either vaccine (rV-PSA + rV-B7.1 prime followed by rF-PSA boosters) and weekly docetaxel, or vaccine alone [83]. The median increase in these T-cell precursors to PSA was 3.33-fold in both arms following 3 months of therapy. In addition, immune responses to other prostate cancer-associated tumor antigens were also detected post-vaccination. This was the first clinical trial to show that docetaxel can be administered safely with vaccine without inhibiting vaccine-mediated T-cell responses. Based on these findings, a randomized multicenter study was initiated evaluating docetaxel vs. docetaxel plus PANVAC vaccine (rV-, rF-CEA-MUC1-TRICOM) in patients (*n* = 48) with metastatic breast carcinoma. Preliminary findings [88] to date indicate a substantial increase in time to progression in the combination arm vs. the docetaxel alone arm.

C. Vaccine plus radiation therapy

Many patients with clinically localized prostate cancer develop biochemical failure despite excellent local therapy, perhaps due to occult metastatic disease. Thirty patients were randomized into vaccine (rV-PSA + rV-B7.1 prime followed by rF-PSA boosters) plus radiotherapy or radiotherapy-only arms [85]. Thirteen of 17 patients in the combination arm had increases in PSA-specific T cells of at least 3-fold versus no detectable increases in the radiotherapy-only arm ($P < 0.0005$). There was also evidence of *de novo* generation of T cells to well-described prostate-associated antigens not found in the vaccine, providing indirect evidence of immune-mediated tumor killing [85]. Another study [89] in men with localized prostate cancer investigated whether the vaccination with rV-PSA/rV-B7.1 prime and rF-PSA boosters induced immune responses to additional TAAs. Western blotting revealed treatment-associated autoantibody responses in 15 of 33 (45.5%) patients treated with vaccine + radiotherapy versus 1 of 8 (12.5%) treated with radiation alone.

D. TRICOM vaccination in combination with ipilimumab

A recently completed study in mCRPC demonstrated that when ipilimumab (anti-CTLA4 MAb) was combined with PSA-TRICOM at escalating doses, the median survival was 34 months, which compares favorably to previous vaccine trials in mCRPC that resulted in median survivals of approximately 26 months [90]. These and other data support the rationale for randomized studies employing immune checkpoint inhibitors in combination with TRICOM-based vaccines.

XII. LESSONS LEARNED AND MOVING FORWARD

Numerous lessons have been learned in the preclinical and clinical studies employing the TRICOM viral vector platform. These include: (a) the diversified vaccination schema of rV-prime followed by multiple rF-boosters is superior to the exclusive use of either vector alone; (b) the inclusion of the triad of co-stimulatory molecules into vectors along with the TAA(s) not only enhances antigen-specific T-cell numbers but also T-cell avidity; (c) an extremely good safety profile has been achieved in numerous preclinical and clinical studies with no evidence of autoimmunity; (d) dendritic cells, B cells and tumor cells can all be made more immunogenic with the infection of TRICOM vectors; (e) one can break tolerance and induce antigen-specific T-cell responses in carcinoma patients by the inclusion of the TAAs PSA, CEA or MUC-1 into TRICOM vaccine; (f) when employed as a monotherapy, patients most likely to benefit are those with more indolent disease and/or lower metastatic tumor burden; (g) TRICOM vaccination can alter the growth rate of tumor resulting in prolonged survival; thus as a monotherapy, survival is the most appropriate clinical endpoint; (h) preclinical studies have defined the importance of scheduling of vaccines when used in combination with other forms of therapy including small molecule targeted therapeutics; (i) TRICOM-based vaccines can be used safely and with evidence of clinical benefit in clinical trials in combination with certain chemotherapeutic agents, radiation, hormonal therapies, and checkpoint inhibitors; and (j) multicenter randomized Phase II and now Phase III trials can be carried out efficiently with the "off-the-shelf" TRICOM vaccine platform. The studies outlined here and in recent reviews [54,66–68,91,92] highlight how TRICOM-based vaccines can potentially be employed as monotherapy and with numerous standard-of-care therapies in the management of different stages of numerous cancer types.

References

[1] Schlom J, Tsang KY, Hodge JW, Greiner JW. Carcinoembryonic antigen as a vaccine target. In: Rees RC, Robins A, editors. Cancer Immunology: Immunology in Medicine Series. Norwell, MA: Kluwer Academic Publishers; 2001. p. 73–100.

[2] Clarke P, Mann J, Simpson JF, Rickard-Dickson K, Primus FJ. Mice transgenic for human carcinoembryonic antigen as a model for immunotherapy. Cancer Res 1998;58(7):1469–77.

[3] Irvine K, Kantor J, Schlom J. Comparison of a CEA-recombinant vaccinia virus, purified CEA, and an anti-idiotypic antibody bearing the image of a CEA epitope in the treatment and prevention of CEA-expressing tumors. Vaccine Res 1993;2:79–94.

[4] Kass E, Schlom J, Thompson J, Guadagni F, Graziano P, Greiner JW. Induction of protective host immunity to carcinoembryonic antigen (CEA), a self-antigen in CEA transgenic mice, by immunizing with a recombinant vaccinia-CEA virus. Cancer Res 1999;59(3):676–83.

[5] Larocca C, Schlom J. Viral vector-based therapeutic cancer vaccines. Cancer J 2011;17(5):359–71.

[6] Aarts WM, Schlom J, Hodge JW. Vector-based vaccine/cytokine combination therapy to enhance induction of immune responses to a self-antigen and antitumor activity. Cancer Res 2002;62(20):5770–7.

[7] Kaufman HL, Wang W, Manola J, DiPaola RS, Ko YJ, Sweeney C, et al. Phase II randomized study of vaccine treatment of advanced prostate cancer (E7897): a trial of the Eastern Cooperative Oncology Group. J Clin Oncol 2004;22(11):2122–32.

[8] Hodge JW, McLaughlin JP, Kantor JA, Schlom J. Diversified prime and boost protocols using recombinant vaccinia virus and recombinant non-replicating avian pox virus to enhance T-cell immunity and antitumor responses. Vaccine 1997;15(6-7):759–68.

[9] Hodge JW, McLaughlin JP, Abrams SI, Shupert WL, Schlom J, Kantor JA. Admixture of a recombinant vaccinia virus containing the gene for the costimulatory molecule B7 and a recombinant vaccinia virus containing a tumor-associated antigen gene results in enhanced specific T-cell responses and antitumor immunity. Cancer Res 1995;55(16):3598–603.

[10] Kalus RM, Kantor JA, Gritz L, Gomez Yafal A, Mazzara GP, Schlom J, et al. The use of combination vaccinia vaccines and dual-gene vaccinia vaccines to enhance antigen-specific T-cell immunity via T-cell costimulation. Vaccine 1999;17(7-8):893–903.

[11] Kudo-Saito C, Hodge JW, Kwak H, Kim-Schulze S, Schlom J, Kaufman HL. 4-1BB ligand enhances tumor-specific immunity of poxvirus vaccines. Vaccine 2006;24(23):4975–86.

[12] Lorenz MG, Kantor JA, Schlom J, Hodge JW. Anti-tumor immunity elicited by a recombinant vaccinia virus expressing CD70 (CD27L). Hum Gene Ther 1999;10(7):1095–103.

[13] Lorenz MG, Kantor JA, Schlom J, Hodge JW. Induction of anti-tumor immunity elicited by tumor cells expressing a murine LFA-3 analog via a recombinant vaccinia virus. Hum Gene Ther 1999;10(4):623–31.

[14] Uzendoski K, Kantor JA, Abrams SI, Schlom J, Hodge JW. Construction and characterization of a recombinant vaccinia virus expressing murine intercellular adhesion molecule-1: induction and potentiation of antitumor responses. Hum Gene Ther 1997;8(7):851–60.

[15] Grosenbach DW, Barrientos JC, Schlom J, Hodge JW. Synergy of vaccine strategies to amplify antigen-specific immune responses and antitumor effects. Cancer Res 2001;61(11):4497–505.

[16] Kudo-Saito C, Garnett CT, Wansley EK, Schlom J, Hodge JW. Intratumoral delivery of vector mediated IL-2 in combination with vaccine results in enhanced T cell avidity and anti-tumor activity. Cancer Immunol Immunother 2007;56(12):1897–910.

[17] Kudo-Saito C, Schlom J, Hodge JW. Intratumoral vaccination and diversified subcutaneous/intratumoral vaccination with recombinant poxviruses encoding a tumor antigen and multiple costimulatory molecules. Clin Cancer Res 2004;10(3):1090–9.

[18] Kudo-Saito C, Schlom J, Hodge JW. Induction of an antigen cascade by diversified subcutaneous/intratumoral vaccination is associated with antitumor responses. Clin Cancer Res 2005;11(6):2416–26.

[19] Kudo-Saito C, Wansley EK, Gruys ME, Wiltrout R, Schlom J, Hodge JW. Combination therapy of an orthotopic renal cell carcinoma model using intratumoral vector-mediated costimulation and systemic interleukin-2. Clin Cancer Res 2007;13(6):1936–46.

[20] Slavin-Chiorini DC, Catalfamo M, Kudo-Saito C, Hodge JW, Schlom J, Sabzevari H. Amplification of the lytic potential of effector/memory CD8+ cells by vector-based enhancement of ICAM-1 (CD54) in target cells: implications for intratumoral vaccine therapy. Cancer Gene Ther 2004;11(10):665–80.

[21] Greiner JW, Zeytin H, Anver MR, Schlom J. Vaccine-based therapy directed against carcinoembryonic antigen demonstrates antitumor activity on spontaneous intestinal tumors in the absence of autoimmunity. Cancer Res 2002;62(23):6944–51.

[22] Zeytin HE, Patel AC, Rogers CJ, Canter D, Hursting SD, Schlom J, et al. Combination of a poxvirus-based vaccine with a cyclooxygenase-2 inhibitor (celecoxib) elicits antitumor immunity and long-term survival in CEA.Tg/MIN mice. Cancer Res 2004;64(10):3668–78.

[23] Hodge JW, Higgins J, Schlom J. Harnessing the unique local immunostimulatory properties of modified vaccinia Ankara (MVA) virus to generate superior tumor-specific immune responses and antitumor activity in a diversified prime and boost vaccine regimen. Vaccine 2009;27(33):4475–82.

[24] Hodge JW, Poole DJ, Aarts WM, Gomez Yafal A, Gritz L, Schlom J. Modified vaccinia virus ankara recombinants are as potent as vaccinia recombinants in diversified prime and boost vaccine regimens to elicit therapeutic antitumor responses. Cancer Res 2003;63(22):7942–9.

[25] Hodge JW, Chakraborty M, Kudo-Saito C, Garnett CT, Schlom J. Multiple costimulatory modalities enhance CTL avidity. J Immunol 2005;174(10):5994–6004.

[26] Hodge JW, Rad AN, Grosenbach DW, Sabzevari H, Yafal AG, Gritz L, et al. Enhanced activation of T cells by dendritic cells engineered to hyperexpress a triad of costimulatory molecules. J Natl Cancer Inst 2000;92(15):1228–39.

[27] Hodge JW, Grosenbach DW, Rad AN, Giuliano M, Sabzevari H, Schlom J. Enhancing the potency of peptide-pulsed antigen presenting cells by vector-driven hyperexpression of a triad of costimulatory molecules. Vaccine 2001;19(25-26):3552–67.

[28] Zhu M, Terasawa H, Gulley J, Panicali D, Arlen P, Schlom J, et al. Enhanced activation of human T cells via avipox vector-mediated hyperexpression of a triad of costimulatory molecules in human dendritic cells. Cancer Res 2001;61(9):3725–34.

[29] Palena C, Zhu M, Schlom J, Tsang KY. Human B cells that hyperexpress a triad of costimulatory molecules via avipox-vector infection: an alternative source of efficient antigen-presenting cells. Blood 2004;104(1):192–9.

[30] Litzinger MT, Foon KA, Sabzevari H, Tsang KY, Schlom J, Palena C. Chronic lymphocytic leukemia (CLL) cells genetically modified to express B7-1, ICAM-1, and LFA-3 confer APC capacity to T cells from CLL patients. Cancer Immunol Immunother 2009;58(6):955–65.

[31] Palena C, Foon KA, Panicali D, Yafal AG, Chinsangaram J, Hodge JW, et al. Potential approach to immunotherapy of chronic lymphocytic leukemia (CLL): enhanced immunogenicity of CLL cells via infection with vectors encoding for multiple costimulatory molecules. Blood 2005;106(10):3515–23.

[32] Litzinger MT, Foon KA, Tsang KY, Schlom J, Palena C. Comparative analysis of MVA-CD40L and MVA-TRICOM vectors for enhancing the immunogenicity of chronic lymphocytic leukemia (CLL) cells. Leuk Res 2010;34(10):1351–7.

[33] Arlen P, Tsang KY, Marshall JL, Chen A, Steinberg SM, Poole D, et al. The use of a rapid ELISPOT assay to analyze peptide-specific immune responses in carcinoma patients to peptide vs. recombinant poxvirus vaccines. Cancer Immunol Immunother 2000;49(10):517–29.

[34] Horig H, Lee DS, Conkright W, Divito J, Hasson H, LaMare M, et al. Phase I clinical trial of a recombinant canarypoxvirus (ALVAC) vaccine expressing human carcinoembryonic antigen and the B7.1 co-stimulatory molecule. Cancer Immunol Immunother 2000;49(9):504–14.

[35] Marshall JL, Hawkins MJ, Tsang KY, Richmond E, Pedicano JE, Zhu MZ, et al. Phase I study in cancer patients of a replication-defective avipox recombinant vaccine that expresses human carcinoembryonic antigen. J Clin Oncol 1999;17(1):332–7.

[36] Marshall JL, Hoyer RJ, Toomey MA, Faraguna K, Chang P, Richmond E, et al. Phase I study in advanced cancer patients of a diversified prime-and-boost vaccination protocol using recombinant vaccinia virus and recombinant nonreplicating avipox virus to elicit anti-carcinoembryonic antigen immune responses. J Clin Oncol 2000;18(23):3964–73.

[37] Tsang KY, Zaremba S, Nieroda CA, Zhu MZ, Hamilton JM, Schlom J. Generation of human cytotoxic T cells specific for human carcinoembryonic antigen epitopes from patients immunized with recombinant vaccinia-CEA vaccine. J Natl Cancer Inst 1995;87(13):982–90.

[38] von Mehren M, Arlen P, Gulley J, Rogatko A, Cooper HS, Meropol NJ, et al. The influence of granulocyte macrophage colony-stimulating factor and prior chemotherapy on the immunological response to a vaccine (ALVAC-CEA B7.1) in patients with metastatic carcinoma. Clin Cancer Res 2001;7(5):1181–91.

[39] von Mehren M, Arlen P, Tsang KY, Rogatko A, Meropol N, Cooper HS, et al. Pilot study of a dual gene recombinant avipox vaccine containing both carcinoembryonic antigen (CEA) and B7.1 transgenes in patients with recurrent CEA-expressing adenocarcinomas. Clin Cancer Res 2000;6(6):2219–28.

[40] Kufe DW. Mucins in cancer: function, prognosis and therapy. Nat Rev Cancer 2009;9(12):874–85.

[41] Raina D, Kosugi M, Ahmad R, Panchamoorthy G, Rajabi H, Alam M, et al. Dependence on the MUC1-C oncoprotein in non-small cell lung cancer cells. Mol Cancer Ther 2011;10(5):806–16.

[42] Marshall JL, Gulley JL, Arlen PM, Beetham PK, Tsang KY, Slack R, et al. Phase I study of sequential vaccinations with fowlpox-CEA(6D)-TRICOM alone and sequentially with vaccinia-CEA(6D)-TRICOM, with and without granulocyte-macrophage colony-stimulating factor, in patients with carcinoembryonic antigen-expressing carcinomas. J Clin Oncol 2005;23(4):720–31.

[43] Gulley JL, Arlen PM, Tsang KY, Yokokawa J, Palena C, Poole DJ, et al. Pilot study of vaccination with recombinant CEA-MUC-1-TRICOM poxviral-based vaccines in patients with metastatic carcinoma. Clin Cancer Res 2008;14(10):3060–9.

[44] Mohebtash M, Tsang KY, Madan RA, Huen NY, Poole DJ, Jochems C, et al. A pilot study of MUC-1/CEA/TRICOM poxviral-based vaccine in patients with metastatic breast and ovarian cancer. Clin Cancer Res 2011;17(22):7164–73.

[45] Madan RA, Arlen PM, Gulley JL. PANVAC-VF: poxviral-based vaccine therapy targeting CEA and MUC1 in carcinoma. Expert Opin Biol Ther 2007;7(4):543–54.

[46] Lyerly HK, Hobeika A, Niedzwiecki D, Osada T, Marshall J, Garrett CR, et al. A dendritic cell-based vaccine effects on T-cell responses compared with a viral vector vaccine when administered to patients following resection of colorectal metastases in a randomized Phase II study. American Society of Clinical Oncology 2011 Annual Meeting. J Clin Oncol 2011;29 (Suppl.) (abstr 2533).

[47] Morse M, Niedzwiecki D, Marshall J, Garrett CR, Chang DZ, Aklilu M, et al. Survival rates among patients vaccinated following resection of colorectal cancer metastases in a Phase II randomized study compared with contemporary controls. American Society of Clinical Oncology 2011 Annual Meeting. J Clin Oncol 2011;29 (Suppl.) (abstr 3557).

[48] Andres A, Majno PE, Morel P, Rubbia-Brandt L, Giostra E, Gervaz P, et al. Improved long-term outcome of surgery for advanced colorectal liver metastases: reasons and implications for management on the basis of a severity score. Ann Surg Oncol 2008;15(1):134–43.

[49] Arru M, Aldrighetti L, Castoldi R, Di Palo S, Orsenigo E, Stella M, et al. Analysis of prognostic factors influencing long-term survival after hepatic resection for metastatic colorectal cancer. World J Surg 2008;32(1):93–103.

[50] Choti MA, Sitzmann JV, Tiburi MF, Sumetchotimetha W, Rangsin R, Schulick RD, et al. Trends in long-term survival following liver resection for hepatic colorectal metastases. Ann Surg 2002;235(6):759–66.

[51] House MG, Ito H, Gonen M, Fong Y, Allen PJ, DeMatteo RP, et al. Survival after hepatic resection for metastatic colorectal cancer: trends in outcomes for 1,600 patients during two decades at a single institution. J Am Coll Surg 2010;210(5):744–52.

[52] Pawlik TM, Scoggins CR, Zorzi D, Abdalla EK, Andres A, Eng C, et al. Effect of surgical margin status on survival and site of recurrence after hepatic resection for colorectal metastases. Ann Surg 2005;241(5):715–22, discussion 22–24.

[53] Sasaki A, Iwashita Y, Shibata K, Matsumoto T, Ohta M, Kitano S. Analysis of preoperative prognostic factors for long-term survival after hepatic resection of liver metastasis of colorectal carcinoma. J Gastrointest Surg 2005;9(3):374–80.

[54] Madan RA, Mohebtash M, Schlom J, Gulley JL. Therapeutic vaccines in metastatic castration-resistant prostate cancer: principles in clinical trial design. Expert Opin Biol Ther 2010;10(1):19–28.

[55] Halabi S, Small EJ, Kantoff PW, Kattan MW, Kaplan EB, Dawson NA, et al. Prognostic model for predicting survival in men with hormone-refractory metastatic prostate cancer. J Clin Oncol 2003;21(7):1232–7.

[56] Eder JP, Kantoff PW, Roper K, Xu GX, Bubley GJ, Boyden J, et al. A phase I trial of a recombinant vaccinia virus expressing prostate-specific antigen in advanced prostate cancer. Clin Cancer Res 2000;6(5):1632–8.

[57] Gulley J, Chen AP, Dahut W, Arlen PM, Bastian A, Steinberg SM, et al. Phase I study of a vaccine using recombinant vaccinia virus expressing PSA (rV-PSA) in patients with metastatic androgen-independent prostate cancer. Prostate 2002;53(2):109–17.

[58] Sanda MG, Smith DC, Charles LG, Hwang C, Pienta KJ, Schlom J, et al. Recombinant vaccinia-PSA (PROSTVAC) can induce a prostate-specific immune response in androgen-modulated human prostate cancer. Urology 1999;53(2):260–6.

[59] Kaufman HL, Wang W, Manola J, DiPaola RS, Ko YJ, Sweeny CJ, et al. Phase II prime/boost vaccination using poxviruses expressing PSA in hormone dependent prostate cancer: follow-up clinical results from ECOG 7897. American Society of Clinical Oncology 2005 Annual Meeting. J Clin Oncol 2005;23(Suppl.) (abstr 4501).

[60] Schlom J, Gulley JL, Arlen PM. Paradigm shifts in cancer vaccine therapy. Exp Biol Med (Maywood) 2008;233(5):522–34.

[61] Arlen PM, Skarupa L, Pazdur M, Seetharam M, Tsang KY, Grosenbach DW, et al. Clinical safety of a viral vector based prostate cancer vaccine strategy. J Urol 2007;178(4 Pt 1):1515–20.

[62] Gulley JL, Arlen PM, Madan RA, Tsang KY, Pazdur MP, Skarupa L, et al. Immunologic and prognostic factors associated with overall survival employing a poxviral-based PSA vaccine in metastatic castrate-resistant prostate cancer. Cancer Immunol Immunother 2010;59(5):663–74.

[63] Kantoff PW, Schuetz TJ, Blumenstein BA, Glode LM, Bilhartz DL, Wyand M, et al. Overall survival analysis of a phase II randomized controlled trial of a Poxviral-based PSA-targeted immunotherapy in metastatic castration-resistant prostate cancer. J Clin Oncol 2010;28(7):1099–105.

[64] DiPaola RS, Chen Y, Bubley GJ, Hahn NM, Stein M, Schlom J, et al. A phase II study of PROSTVAC-V (vaccinia)/TRICOM and PROSTVAC-F (fowlpox)/TRICOM with GM-CSF in patients with PSA progression after local therapy for prostate cancer: results of ECOG 9802. American Society of Clinical Oncology 2009. Genitourinary Cancers Symposium (abstr 108).

[65] Stein WD, Gulley JL, Schlom J, Madan RA, Dahut W, Figg WD, et al. Tumor regression and growth rates determined in five intramural NCI prostate cancer trials: the growth rate constant as an indicator of therapeutic efficacy. Clin Cancer Res 2011;17(4):907–17.

[66] Gulley JL, Madan RA, Schlom J. The impact of tumour volume on potential efficacy of therapeutic vaccines [review]. Curr Oncol 2011;18(3):e150–e7.

[67] Madan RA, Gulley JL, Fojo T, Dahut WL. Therapeutic cancer vaccines in prostate cancer: the paradox of improved survival without changes in time to progression. Oncologist 2010;15(9):969–75.

[68] Gulley JL, Arlen PM, Hodge JW, Schlom J. Vaccines and immunostimulants. In: Hong WH, editor. Holland-Frei Cancer Medicine 8. Shelton, CT: People's Medical Publishing House-USA; 2010. p. 725–36.

[69] Hoos A, Eggermont AM, Janetzki S, Hodi FS, Ibrahim R, Anderson A, et al. Improved endpoints for cancer immunotherapy trials. J Natl Cancer Inst 2010;102(18):1388–97.

[70] Kaufman HL, Cohen S, Cheung K, DeRaffele G, Mitcham J, Moroziewicz D, et al. Local delivery of vaccinia virus expressing multiple costimulatory molecules for the treatment of established tumors. Hum Gene Ther 2006;17(2):239–44.

[71] Kaufman HL, Deraffele G, Mitcham J, Moroziewicz D, Cohen SM, Hurst-Wicker KS, et al. Targeting the local tumor microenvironment with vaccinia virus expressing B7.1 for the treatment of melanoma. J Clin Invest 2005;115(7):1903–12.

[72] Heery CR, Pinto PA, Schlom J, Tsang KY, Madan RA, Poole D, et al. Intraprostatic PSA-TRICOM vaccine administration in patients with locally recurrent prostate cancer. American Society of Clinical Oncology 2011 Annual Meeting. J Clin Oncol 2011;29 (Suppl.) (abstr 2530).

[73] Chakraborty M, Schlom J, Hodge JW. The combined activation of positive costimulatory signals with modulation of a negative costimulatory signal for the enhancement of vaccine-mediated T-cell responses. Cancer Immunol Immunother 2007;56(9):1471–84.

[74] Boehm AL, Higgins J, Franzusoff A, Schlom J, Hodge JW. Concurrent vaccination with two distinct vaccine platforms targeting the same antigen generates phenotypically and functionally distinct T-cell populations. Cancer Immunol Immunother 2010;59(3):397–408.

[75] Chakraborty M, Abrams SI, Coleman CN, Camphausen K, Schlom J, Hodge JW. External beam radiation of tumors alters phenotype of tumor cells to render them susceptible to vaccine-mediated T-cell killing. Cancer Res 2004;64(12):4328–37.

[76] Kudo-Saito C, Schlom J, Camphausen K, Coleman CN, Hodge JW. The requirement of multimodal therapy (vaccine, local tumor radiation, and reduction of suppressor cells) to eliminate established tumors. Clin Cancer Res 2005;11(12):4533–44.

[77] Chakraborty M, Gelbard A, Carrasquillo JA, Yu S, Mamede M, Paik CH, et al. Use of radiolabeled monoclonal antibody to enhance vaccine-mediated antitumor effects. Cancer Immunol Immunother 2008;57(8):1173–83.

[78] Garnett CT, Palena C, Chakraborty M, Tsang KY, Schlom J, Hodge JW. Sublethal irradiation of human tumor cells modulates phenotype resulting in enhanced killing by cytotoxic T lymphocytes. Cancer Res 2004;64(21):7985–94.

[79] Chakraborty M, Wansley EK, Carrasquillo JA, Yu S, Paik CH, Camphausen K, et al. The use of chelated radionuclide (samarium-153-ethylenediaminetetramethylenephosphonate) to modulate phenotype of tumor cells and enhance T cell-mediated killing. Clin Cancer Res. 2008;14(13):4241–9.

[80] Garnett CT, Schlom J, Hodge JW. Combination of docetaxel and recombinant vaccine enhances T-cell responses and antitumor activity: effects of docetaxel on immune enhancement. Clin Cancer Res. 2008;14(11):3536–44.

[81] Farsaci B, Sabzevari H, Higgins JP, Di Bari MG, Takai S, Schlom J, et al. Effect of a small molecule BCL-2 inhibitor on immune function and use with a recombinant vaccine. Int J Cancer 2010;127(7):1603–13.

[82] Farsaci B, Higgins JP, Hodge JW. Consequence of dose scheduling of sunitinib on host immune response elements and vaccine combination therapy. Int J Cancer 2012;130(8):1948–59.

[83] Arlen PM, Gulley JL, Parker C, Skarupa L, Pazdur M, Panicali D, et al. A randomized phase II study of concurrent docetaxel plus vaccine versus vaccine alone in metastatic androgen-independent prostate cancer. Clin Cancer Res. 2006;12(4):1260–9.

[84] Arlen PM, Gulley JL, Todd N, Lieberman R, Steinberg SM, Morin S, et al. Antiandrogen, vaccine and combination therapy in patients with nonmetastatic hormone refractory prostate cancer. J Urol 2005;174(2):539–46.

[85] Gulley JL, Arlen PM, Bastian A, Morin S, Marte J, Beetham P, et al. Combining a recombinant cancer vaccine with standard definitive radiotherapy in patients with localized prostate cancer. Clin Cancer Res. 2005;11(9):3353–62.

[86] Madan RA, Gulley JL, Schlom J, Steinberg SM, Liewehr DJ, Dahut WL, et al. Analysis of overall survival in patients with nonmetastatic castration-resistant prostate cancer treated with vaccine, nilutamide, and combination therapy. Clin Cancer Res. 2008;14(14):4526–31.

[87] Bilusic M, Gulley J, Heery C, et al. A randomized phase II study of flutamide with or without PSA-TRICOM in nonmetastatic castration-resistant prostate cancer. American Society of Clinical Oncology 2011 Genitourinary Symposium. J Clin Oncol 2011;29 (Suppl. 7.) (abstr 163).

[88] Mohebtash M, Madan RA, Gulley JL, Jones J, Pazdur M, Rauckhorst M, et al. PANVAC vaccine alone or with docetaxel for patients with metastatic breast cancer. American Society of Clinical Oncology 2008 Annual Meeting. J Clin Oncol 2008;26(Suppl.) (abstr 3035).

[89] Nesslinger NJ, Ng A, Tsang KY, Ferrara T, Schlom J, Gulley JL, et al. A viral vaccine encoding prostate-specific antigen induces antigen spreading to a common set of self-proteins in prostate cancer patients. Clin Cancer Res 2010;16(15):4046—56.

[90] Madan RA, Mohebtash M, Arlen PM, Vergati M, Rauckhorst M, Steinberg SM, et al. Ipilimumab and a poxviral vaccine targeting prostate-specific antigen in metastatic castration-resistant prostate cancer: a phase 1 dose-escalation trial. Lancet Oncol 2012;13:501—8.

[91] Schlom J. Therapeutic cancer vaccines: current status and moving forward. J Natl Cancer Inst 2012;104(8): 599—613.

[92] Madan RA, Bilusic M, Heery C, Schlom J, Gulley JL. Clinical evaluation of TRICOM vector therapeutic cancer vaccines. Semin Oncol 2012;39(3):296—304.

CHAPTER 21

Adjuvant Strategies for Vaccines

The Use of Adjuvants within the Cancer Vaccine Setting

Claire Hearnden, Ed C. Lavelle
Adjuvant Research Group, School of Biochemistry and Immunology, Trinity Biomedical Sciences Institute, Trinity College Dublin, Dublin 2, Ireland

I. INTRODUCTION

The immune system and tumor cells have a complex interplay whereby leukocytes and tumor cells are in a constant battle. The tumor microenvironment is dynamic and the immune system can determine whether premalignant lesions develop into aggressive cancers. It has been known since the 1940s that mice immunized with irradiated cancer cells show resistance to subsequent challenges with corresponding viable cancer cells [1]. This implies that cancers are immunogenic and that an optimal antitumor cell immune response can inhibit tumor growth.

Vaccination is a means by which the immune response can be "taught" how to respond to antigens. Indeed, vaccination has led to the eradication of smallpox and greatly reduced the incidence of many diseases including polio. In the context of cancer it has been suggested that people who are predisposed to tumor growth could be protected via therapeutic or prophylactic vaccine strategies [2]. The advantages of cancer vaccines over other therapies include increased specificity to tumor cells, reduced toxicity and more robust long-term effects [3].

II. WHY ADJUVANTS WORK

Vaccination aims to provide a stimulus that will generate an appropriate long-term protective immune response [4]. To generate such a response the host must be exposed to the antigen in a controlled way that will facilitate immune recognition, activation and memory generation. This process is dependent on antigen-presenting cells (APCs), particularly dendritic cells (DCs), which capture tumor antigens, process them and display the resulting peptide epitopes in an immunogenic context to stimulate T cells [5].

Most antigens do not induce a protective T-cell response when administered by themselves as a vaccine. Adjuvants are substances that can be incorporated into vaccines to enhance the magnitude, breadth and quality of the immune response to antigens. Adjuvants were first described by Ramon as "substances used in combination with a specific antigen that produce more immunity than the antigen alone" [6]. Despite extensive research, in most cases the precise mechanism of adjuvanticity remains unknown and it is because of this that Charles Janeway once referred to adjuvants as "the dirty little secret of immunologists."

Cancer Immunotherapy. http://dx.doi.org/10.1016/B978-0-12-394296-8.00021-X

Adjuvants comprise a diverse group of compounds whose proposed roles range from carriers/antigen depots to immunostimulatory/immunomodulatory molecules [7]. There are many advantages of using adjuvants in vaccine formulations including their ability to promote cell-mediated immunity, to serve as an antigen depot and reduce the amount of antigen necessary in vaccines for protection ("dose sparing") and also to reduce the number of vaccinations required to induce an effective immune response [8]. Ultimately, adjuvants are required to activate DCs and promote effective uptake, processing and presentation of antigen to T cells in secondary lymphoid organs, thereby stimulating powerful antigen-specific immune responses [9].

Pathogens are recognized by DCs through the range of pattern recognition receptors (PRR) that can be found on the cell surface as well as in the cytosol, and have evolved to recognize particular patterns on pathogens that are conserved across several species termed PAMPs (Pathogen Associated Molecular Patterns) [10]. These PAMPs can be purified or synthesized and used as adjuvants. Different PRR recognize specific types of PAMPs and are broadly grouped by structure. Prominent PRR include mannose-binding lectin, pulmonary surfactant protein, C-reactive protein, Toll-like receptors (TLRs), C-type lectin receptors (CLRs), Nod-like receptors (NLRs), Rig-I like receptors (RLRs) and MX proteins.

Charles Janeway demonstrated that the adaptive immune responses generated against infectious microorganisms are dependent on the initial innate immune responses upon exposure to the pathogen [11]. Upon recognition of PAMPs, DCs become activated, a process termed maturation, and begin to upregulate co-stimulatory molecules, process antigens and present these antigens to T cells, thus initiating adaptive immunity [11]. Thus, DCs bridge the divide between innate and adaptive immunity. This led to the rational design of adjuvants that can target specific receptors and generate adaptive immune responses, as well as adjuvants that are not immunostimulatory themselves, but are capable of modulating the immune system in a particular way.

III. TUMOR-ASSOCIATED ANTIGENS AND THE NEED FOR ADJUVANTS IN CANCER VACCINES

The rationale for therapeutic vaccines in cancer began in the 1950s when it was demonstrated that transformed tumor cells express antigens called tumor-associated antigens (TAAs) that are not found on normal cells [12–14]. Since these endogenous TAAs are not expressed by normal cells, they have potential as antigens that could be presented to DCs. For example, malignant melanomas, which are one of the most aggressive malignancies in humans, express many TAAs that can be recognized by T cells. These TAAs include gp100, Melan-A/Mart-1, tyrosinase, MAGE-A1, and NY-ESO [15]. However, tumors are capable of modulating the immune response to facilitate their own growth, most notably through their ability to downregulate the expression of TAAs, secrete inhibitory molecules and reduce the expression of co-stimulatory molecules, thus making tumor cells poorly immunogenic [12,16].

An important aspect of cancer immunotherapy is developing appropriate adjuvants for cancer vaccines to enable the immune system to mount an effective TAA-specific response. The nature of the adjuvant used can determine the type of immune response generated against the antigen. When a DC is activated, or matures, as well as upregulating co-stimulatory molecules it upregulates receptors that allow it to migrate to the lymph nodes and here the DC displays antigen complexes on its cell surface. The nature of the antigen and adjuvant can influence whether peptides are displayed on major histocompatibility complex (MHC) class I (MHCcI) or MHC class II (MHCcII) and the type of T-cell response that will be generated. MHCcI usually display peptides derived from proteins synthesized in the cytosol, such as those from viruses or endogenous TAAs. MHCcII bind peptides derived from intracellular vesicles, for example those containing pathogens internalized by phagocytosis. MHCcI complexes are recognized by T cells expressing CD8 molecules on their surface (CD8$^+$ cytotoxic T lymphocyte

(CTL)) and MHCcII complexes are recognized by T cells expressing CD4 molecules on their surface (CD4$^+$ T-helper cells). A process referred to as *cross-presentation* enables DCs to promote a CTL response against exogenous antigens by delivering them to MHCcI molecules, a process which is critical for immunity against tumor cells and virus-infected cells [17,18,19]. CD4 T-helper (Th) cells are categorized into various subsets including Th1, Th2 and Th17 cells. The cytokines that DCs secrete following maturation and subsequent T-cell activation polarize the different T-cell subsets; for example, IFN-γ is a Th1 polarizing cytokine and IL-4 a Th2 polarizing cytokine [20].

Regulatory T (Treg) cells represent approximately 5–10% of peripheral Th cells and are characterized by their ability to suppress components of the immune system including T-cell responses [12]. There are two types of Treg cells, those that are produced in the thymus and are functionally mature, and those that can be recruited from the periphery and induced to become Treg cells. Treg cells selectively recruited to the tumor site will be activated by mature DCs and since inducible Treg cells are highly specific for antigens, they have the ability to exert T-cell suppression in an antigen-dependent manner [21,22].

Efficient delivery of TAA to DCs requires an adjuvant so that the DC can mature and elicit effective antitumor immunity [23]. DCs' need to be activated by adjuvants as targeted antigen does not generate an effective antitumor immune response [24–26]. Antitumor activity is strongly dependent on CTL, which have been shown previously to secrete IFN-γ and also to possess cytolytic ability [25,27–29]. CD4$^+$ T cells with a Th1 phenotype also have a role in preventing tumor growth although the need for Th1 cells may be TAA specific [23]. Therefore, induction of a CTL response coupled with pro-inflammatory stimuli such as IFN-γ, IL-12p70 and TNF-α which can polarize a Th1 type response is critical for the development of an effective antitumor therapeutic vaccine (Figure 21.1) [8,30,31].

Although a cellular immune response is crucial for antitumor immunity, studies have also shown that humoral responses can provide protection. Vaccination of HER-2/neu mice, a mouse model of metastatic breast cancer using the oncogenic TAA HER-2, with IL-12 and allogeneic mammary carcinoma cells expressing p185(neu) prevented tumor onset independently of CTL by anti-p185(neu) antibodies [32]. Similarly, Park et al. found that in transgenic BALB-neuT HER-2 mice, a transgenic BALB/c mouse model for the *neu* oncogene, development of spontaneous HER-2 positive carcinomas was independent of CD8$^+$ T cells. Importantly CD4$^+$ T cells were required only early in the immediate post-vaccination period to induce anti-HER-2 Abs, which were both necessary and sufficient for protection [33].

A caveat with developing cancer vaccines is that TAAs are self antigens that are over-expressed. This means that there may be preexisting tolerance for these antigens within the immune

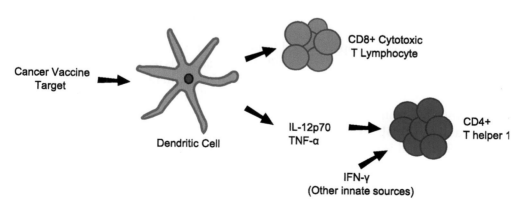

FIGURE 21.1
Cancer vaccines, as with most vaccines, target dendritic cells. The immunological correlate of protective immunity in cancer is a CD8+ cytotoxic T-lymphocyte response and a cytokine response made up of IFN-γ, IL-12p70 and TNF-α which promote a Th1 T-cell response.

system. In order to overcome the tolerance, both humoral and cellular immunity may be required. Reilly et al., using mice tolerant to the oncogene neu, found that neu-specific IgG alone was insufficient for protection against challenge and a combined cellular and humoral response was required for effective antitumor immunity [34].

IV. IMMUNOSTIMULATORY ADJUVANTS

It is critical that the adjuvants administered in vaccines are safe, well tolerated, biodegradable and can promote long-lasting protective immunity [35]. For this reason adjuvants must be very well characterized, both physically and chemically. Adjuvants can be roughly divided into immunostimulatory adjuvants, those that are capable of interacting directly with specific receptors on APCs, and particulate vaccine adjuvants, that are capable of delivering antigen to APCs, particularly DCs [36].

A. Pathogen derived immunostimulatory adjuvants

A primary aim of cancer vaccines is to induce DC maturation so that tumor antigens can be presented to T cells and break TAA tolerance [2,37]. DC activated via PRR have an enhanced capacity to present peptides to T cells and generate antigen-specific responses [38]. For example, CG-enriched oligodeoxynucleotides (CpG) engage TLR9 and induce DC maturation, a process characterized by increased surface expression of CD80, CD86 and MHCcII and also secretion of a range of pro-inflammatory cytokines [39,40]. Unmethylated CpG motifs are abundant in mycobacterial DNA and induce a Th1 immune response. Synthetic oligodeoxynucleotides containing CpG motifs have been used with a CTL peptide epitope from the RNEU (rat HER-2/ *neu* gene product) sequence (p66) as a vaccine therapy in a mouse model for spontaneous breast tumors [41]. Vaccination with peptide in combination with CpG was effective in promoting CTL responses and subsequent antitumor activity. However, this was dependent on combined Treg-cell suppression and multiple booster vaccinations [41].

CpG motifs have also been used in other vaccine strategies, including exposure of tumor B cells to CpG *ex vivo* and injection into the host as a whole cell tumor vaccine. Intratumoral vaccination with CpG in combination with cytotoxic chemotherapy has also been used [42]. Interestingly, direct intratumoral immunization induced a CTL response whereas vaccination with CpG-loaded tumor B cells resulted in an antitumor response mediated by CD4$^+$ T cells [42].

Some studies have shown that encapsulation of CpG motifs in liposomes enhances the immunostimulatory activity of the ligand by targeting it directly to DCs for uptake and processing [43]. In models of thymoma and melanoma this approach generated adaptive immune responses against co-administered TAAs after subcutaneous immunization with liposomes containing CpG motifs [43].

3-O-desacyl-4′-monophosphoryl lipid A (MPL) is derived from the detoxified LPS of the Gram-negative bacterium *Salmonella Minnesota* and is recognized by TLR4. Importantly, MPL® is significantly less toxic then LPS so is safe for use in humans, but it also retains its adjuvant properties [44–46]. MPL® promotes cell-mediated immunity with a predominantly Th1 profile in addition to CTL responses and is currently the only TLR ligand in licensed human vaccines [8,46]. MPL® is used in combination with aluminum salt as Adjuvant System 04 (ASO4) and is included in two licensed vaccines, the human papillomavirus (HPV) vaccine Cervarix® and the Hepatitis B virus (HBV) vaccine Fendrix.®

Due to the success of MPL a new generation of TLR4 agonists is being developed, including aminoalkyl glucosamimide phosphates (AGPs) and a synthetic LPS mimetic RC-529.

The double-stranded RNA mimic and TLR3 ligand polyinosinic polycytidylic acid (poly(I:C)) has also been investigated as a potential cancer adjuvant [47]. As a synergistic strategy for DC maturation, poly(I:C) has been combined with an agonistic anti-CD40 antibody which mimics CD40L functions [48–50]. Using these adjuvants with OVA as an antigen in prophylactic vaccination experiments induced both CD8$^+$ and CD4$^+$ responses, and in a challenge model 94% of animals immunized with poly(I:C) and anti-CD40 in combination with OVA were protected against tumor growth in an E.G7-OVA thymoma model [51].

The same group working on the B16-OVA melanoma model also found that the combination of poly(I:C) and anti-CD40 was ineffective. However, a combination approach relying on synergy between poly(I:C), anti-CD40 and the TLR7 ligand, Imiquimoid, with OVA coupled to the extra domain A of the TLR4 ligand, fibronectin (EDA), led to a complete block of tumor growth and protection against rechallenge with B16-OVA cells [37]. Interestingly, mice were also protected against challenge with B16.F10 tumor cells, which do not express OVA and 80% of mice remained tumor free for up to 80 days later, indicating that the adjuvant combination vaccine not only induces responses against the administered antigen, but also against other antigens expressed by tumor cells [37].

While TLRs are not the only PRR which are current cancer vaccine adjuvant targets, they are the best defined. CLRs are involved in the recognition of carbohydrate entities. For example, the CLR Mincle is a ligand for the mycobacterial cord factor/trehalose dimycolate which promotes Th1/Th17 responses [52,53]. Other PRR such as RLRs and intracellular DNA-sensing receptors are less well characterized and may have important roles in adjuvanticity that are being resolved.

Strategies to activate both cell surface and intracellular PRR simultaneously have also shown promise. Flagellin is the main component of the bacterial flagellum and is recognized by the immune system through TLR5 on the cell surface as well as cytosolic Nod-like receptors (NLRs). Expression of flagellin within tumor cells was shown to clear these cells through TLR5-mediated activation of macrophages in addition to TLR5 and NLRC4 (NOD-, LRR- and CARD-containing 4)/NAIP5 (neuronal apoptosis inhibitory protein 5) mediated priming of antitumor CD4$^+$ and CD8$^+$ T cells [54]. Although using flagellin as an adjuvant is still at an early stage, it is clear that this TLR agonist has potential as an effective antitumor vaccination strategy.

B. QS21

Saponins come from the bark, stem, roots and flowers of many plant species and are made up of sterol glycosides and triterpenoid glycosides and were named due to their detergent nature [55]. Saponin fractions from the South American tree *Quillaja saponaria* have been isolated and shown to have potent adjuvant properties [56]. Kensil et al. purified numerous fractions and found fraction 21 (QS21), a mixture of soluble triterpene glycosides, to have exceptional adjuvant properties for a range of antigens [55,57].

QS21 has been used as an adjuvant with various cell surface gangliosides whose expression is upregulated in the process of malignant transformation of cancers [58]. Immunization with gangliosides alone (including the monosialoganglioside GM2 and the disialo gangliosides GD2 and GD3) failed to induce production of antigen-specific antibodies [59]. Induction of IgG antibodies against carbohydrate antigens such as gangliosides requires a CD4$^+$ Th cell response so that isotype class switching of immunoglobulins occurs. The optimal approach for induction of antibodies against gangliosides requires covalent attachment of the tumor antigen to an immunogenic carrier molecule such as keyhole limpet hemocyanin (KLH), in addition to the use of a potent adjuvant. Helling et al. showed that the conjugate GM2-KLH in combination with QS-21 elicited significant CD4$^+$ Th-cell responses, higher antibody titers, a longer-lasting GM2-specific IgM antibody response, and also an IgG response (isotype IgG1 and IgG3) [58]. Kim et al. screened 19 different adjuvants including CpG ODN, Ginseng saponin and MPL, in combination with either the MUC1 peptide or GD3 ganglioside tumor antigens and found that QS-21 was the most effective adjuvant [60]. Interestingly, the authors did not detect strong T-cell responses to the TAA themselves but potent KLH-specific T-cell responses appeared to lead to higher levels of antibody against the conjugated antigens [61]. Further studies determined that, although QS-21 is effective as an adjuvant when used alone, it is more effective when used in combination with other adjuvants such as CpG, MPL, Titermax and MoGM-CSF, highlighting the potential of adjuvant combinations in cancer vaccines [61].

C. Heat shock proteins

Heat Shock Proteins (HSP) are chaperones that bind a wide repertoire of peptides, including antigenic peptides. They are endogenous molecules that can be captured by DCs when released from a cell, and can present HSP-associated peptides on MHCcI by cross presentation [62–64]. Although the proteins are involved in numerous physiological processes and can bind various peptides, this approach typically promotes CTL and antibody responses, the specificity of which is dependent on the peptide being chaperoned [64,65]. If HSP are stripped of their associated peptides their ability to induce protection is lost [64,66]. Interestingly, HSPs were the first adjuvants of mammalian origin described [67].

Cancer-derived HSP-peptide complexes have been used to elicit regression and even cure of preexisting cancers in mice [1,68]. Since HSPs chaperone the antigenic repertoire of the cells from which they are purified, cancer-derived HSP preparations permit access to the antigenic fingerprint of a cancer cell and are capable of eliciting potent T-cell responses against the cells from which they are purified [68,69].

Prophylactic immunization experiments in mice with the HSPs GP96 and HSP70 showed specificity in treating established tumors [69]. Human HSP70-mediated T-cell activation was shown to occur *in vitro* via recognition by MHC molecules of the matched DCs pulsed with the melanoma-derived HSP70 and was strictly dependent on the presence of peptides chaperoned by HSP [65]. Clinical studies have generated mixed results.

Autologous, patient-derived gp96-peptide complexes elicited tumor-specific T-cell responses in HSP-vaccinated cancer patients [70]. However, a Phase III trial comparing autologous, tumor-derived gp96 peptide complexes (vitespen) with the current best treatment for stage IV melanoma found that only a subset of patients with early stage disease that received a large number of vitespen injections survived longer [71]. A separate Phase III trial focusing on renal cell carcinoma found that delivery of the gp96 peptide complex as an adjuvant to patients with high risk of recurrence was ineffective with regard to recurrence-free survival compared to patients who received no treatment [72].

Current strategies in adjuvant development of HSP involve extracting HSP-protein complexes from both patient-derived and established cancer cells and exposing them *ex vivo* to healthy donor DCs for 5 days. The enriched antigenic peptides, bound to HSP, from the DC-tumor cell mix are then extracted using an anti-HSP antibody and used to stimulate T cells [73]. DCs can be mixed with different types of cancer cells *ex vivo*. The DC loaded with HSP-bound peptides are capable of inducing polyclonal CTLs that kill tumor cells from which the HSP was extracted, as well as tumor cells with shared antigen and restriction elements [73].

V. PARTICULATE VACCINE ADJUVANTS

Particulate adjuvants do not generally contain specific agonists for PRR yet are still capable of promoting innate and subsequently adaptive immunity. How they accomplish this is not fully understood but proposed mechanisms include depot formation, release of danger signals, controlled antigen release, and/or inflammasome activation [74].

A. EMULSIONS

The first use of emulsions as adjuvants can be traced back to 1916 when LeMoignic Pinoy used a water and Vaseline emulsion containing inactivated *Salmonella typhimurium*. Since then emulsion adjuvants have diversified slightly but still remain the same in essence. Emulsions make antigens particulate in nature through aggregate formation [75].

One of the most widely used adjuvants was developed by Freund in the 1930s. This adjuvant is a paraffin-oil based emulsion that can contain heat-killed *Mycobacteria*. Freund's adjuvant is an example of a water-in-oil (W/O) emulsion. W/O emulsions consist of water droplets containing antigen that are surrounded by a continuous oil phase and have been found to be very efficient in enhancing immune responses. However, Freund's adjuvants are too toxic for use in humans.

Alternative W/O emulsions with better safety profiles such as ISA 51 and ISA 720 have been developed using specific surfactants and refined oils. ISA 51 is a mineral-oil based emulsion while ISA 720 contains the animal or vegetable oil squalene [76,77]. Although both ISA 51 and ISA 720 can lead to the development of mild to moderate local reactions, where the benefit outweighs the risk these adjuvants have been used in both therapeutic and prophylactic vaccines [77].

The ability of Montanide ISA 51 to promote T-cell responses appears to be dependent on the surfactant composition. For example, a clinical trial for melanoma involved an ISA 51 formulation that included a surfactant containing the fatty acid, oleic acid, which comes from beef tallow. Due to the possible risk of prions in beef tallow, the use of beef oleic acid was discontinued in 2006 and was substituted with oleic acid of olive origin. However, when patients were immunized with the same peptide emulsified in the new vegetable oleic acid-based Montanide ISA 51 (ISA 51 VG) there appeared to be less adjuvanticity as measured by a reduction in peptide-specific T cells and local skin inflammation at the injection site [78]. O'Neill et al. have shown that ISA 51 VG is well tolerated in humans. Indeed, when immunized with six HLA-A2 antigens and KLH, KLH-specific CD4$^+$ T cells were generated which secreted the Th1 cytokines IFN-γ, TNF-α and IL-2. Hence the potential of this adjuvant in cancer vaccines should not be underestimated [79].

Oil-in-water (O/W) emulsions were developed as an alternative to W/O emulsion adjuvants, and are composed of antigen in a water phase with oil droplets. O/W emulsions have a far superior safety profile due to the reduced oil content. MF59^{TM} is an O/W emulsion which is composed of squalene with Tween 80 and Span 85 as surfactants. It appears to work by acting as an antigen depot, which in turn causes an influx of granulocytes to the site of injection, as well as an increase in endocytosis and increased expression of markers indicative of DC maturation (MHCcII, CD86, CD83, CCR7) [35,80]. MF59^{TM} has been used extensively as an adjuvant in vaccines against infectious diseases such as herpes simplex virus (HSV), HBV, and human immunodeficiency virus (HIV). However, its ability to induce a protective response in cancer has yet to be tested [8].

B. ISCOMs

Immunostimulating complexes or ISCOMs are spherical cage-like particles, approximately 40nm in diameter, and were first described in 1984 by Morein et al. [81]. They are capable of promoting long-lasting functional antibody responses as well as powerful T-cell responses, including enhanced cytokine secretion and CTL activation which, as mentioned earlier, is critical in controlling cancer [82,83]. Studies have shown that ISCOMs can be efficiently phagocytosed and activate DCs, leading to the development of an immune response [84−86].

ISCOMs can be composed of several different materials and tend to be subdivided into two main types, classical ISCOMs and the ISCOMATRIX.® Classical ISCOMs are made up of saponins from *Quillaia saponaria*, cholesterol, phospholipid and amphipathic protein, and were originally designed to incorporate viral components, thus making them extremely immunogenic [81]. The difference between ISCOMATRIX® and classical ISCOMs is that the protein component and antigen which are incorporated into ISCOMs can be mixed together with ISCOMATRIX.®

Since pancreatic carcinoma cells can be recognized by T cells, a method to overcome immunotolerance in patients with pancreatic cancer would be of huge benefit [87]. TAA require cross presentation on MHCcI by DC to activate CTL, a task which is effectively performed by ISCOMs. Studies using ISCOMs as adjuvants for pancreatic cancer vaccines have had varying degrees of success. Injection of NY-ESO-1 (a highly immunogenic antigen expressed in several malignancies) with ISCOMATRIX® in patients with resected malignant melanoma generated a broad cellular immune response with an excellent safety profile in an initial study [88]. However, in a follow-up study of patients with advanced malignant melanoma injected with NY-ESO-1 and ISCOMATRIX,® antibodies were present but a T-cell response capable of overcoming the tumor-induced immune suppression in patients was lacking [89]. In a mouse orthotopic model of pancreatic carcinoma, a similar antigen-specific immunosuppression rendered the ISCOM vaccine ineffective as a therapeutic strategy. However, when the TLR agonist CpG was added to the ISCOM vaccine, superior CTL priming was generated and tumor-induced immunosuppression was broken [90].

C. Mineral salts

Adjuvants containing aluminum have been used in numerous different types of vaccines for decades, yet their exact mechanism of action still remains elusive. Aluminum potassium phosphate (Alum-phos) and aluminum hydroxide (commonly called "alum") are the most common mineral salts currently being used and are licensed for use in several vaccines including Diptheria-Pertussis-Tetanus, *Haemophilus influenza* B and human papillomavirus (HPV) [91]. It has been proposed that alum principally works as an antigen "depot," thus allowing prolonged exposure of the antigen to the immune system [92−96]. However, since alum is a potent inducer of humoral immunity but is less effective in promoting cell-mediated immunity, its use in cancer vaccines is limited.

D. Biodegradable microparticles

340

Controlled release vaccine delivery can be effectively achieved by the use of biodegradable microparticles such as poly (lactide-co-glycolide) (PLGA) particles. PLGA is a Food and Drugs Administration (FDA) approved polymer that is degraded into lactic acid and glycolic acid, which are normal metabolites and well tolerated in the human body [17]. PLG microparticles are prime candidates for development of vaccine adjuvants as they are biodegradable *in vivo* and their half-life can range from days to years depending on their composition. Antigens, as well as other adjuvants, can be encapsulated within PLG particles and released into the processing pathways for presentation on MHC class I and II. These systems have been shown to effectively increase antibody titers compared to antigen/adjuvant alone [97−99].

The advantages of using PLGA particles include their ability to target DCs while protecting antigen from degradation and from entering the systemic circulation, their ability to efficiently facilitate antigen cross presentation and to facilitate co-delivery of various immunomodulators to DCs [17].

In the mouse B16 tumor model, tyrosine related protein-2 (TRP2) is over-expressed. Hamdy et al. encapsulated this antigen, along with 7-acyl lipid A (a synthetic derivative of lipid A from MPL which has comparable immunostimulatory effects to MPL) within PLGA microparticles and observed a TRP2-specific CTL response that correlated with a therapeutic antitumor response [100]. They also found that the immunosuppressive milieu of the tumor microenvironment was overcome, an event characterized by an increase in characteristic Th1 cytokines such as IFN-γ, IL-6, IL-12 and TNF-α and a decrease in the tumor-promoting factor vascular endothelial growth factor (VEGF) [100].

Schlosser et al. found that co-encapsulation of poly I:C and CpG oligonucleotides within the same PLGA microparticle was more effective for generating cross priming and a CTL response than encapsulation of either adjuvant alone [101]. Heit et al. also used the co-encapsulation method for CpG ODNs and their antigen, OVA, in PLGA particles and found that the expansion of antigen-specific $CD4^+$ and $CD8^+$ T cells generated a protective and therapeutic effect towards mouse melanoma tumor cells [102].

E. Other particulate vaccine adjuvants

Based on the ability of viruses to efficiently penetrate cells, virus-like particles (VLP) and virosomes have been developed as adjuvant vectors to present and deliver antigens to immune cells. These particles range from 20—100nm in size (the average cell being 10μm), consist of self-assembling viral envelope proteins and lack the ability to replicate and infect cells as they do not contain any viral nucleic acids [103]. Importantly, they are capable of stimulating both cell-mediated and humoral immunity through their highly repetitive surfaces composed of viral proteins [104—106]. VLP can be manipulated in such a way that other PAMPs can be incorporated within them, making them capable of targeting specific PRR and hence dictating the type of immune response induced [107].

The role for infectious agents, particularly viruses, as causative agents of cancer is substantial [108,109]. The bacterium *Heliobacter pylori* colonizes the gastric epithelium and is a strong risk factor for noncardia gastric adenocarcinoma. Worldwide, 5.5% of cancers are attributed to *H. pylori* [109]. Viruses such as Hepatitis B and C and Epstein-Barr virus can cause liver cancer and Burkitt's lymphoma, respectively. In fact, Hepatitis B is responsible for half of all liver cancers and Hepatitis C causes 30% of liver cancers. Vaccines against such infectious agents implicated in the development of cancer are currently being developed, the most successful of which is the HPV cervical cancer vaccine. Developing vaccines and adjuvants for these types of cancers can involve different approaches as a prophylactic rather than a therapeutic approach is feasible and neutralizing antibodies are a key requirement. This type of cancer vaccine will target the pathogen that causes the cancer, rather than the cancer itself.

The human papillomaviruses (HPVs) are a group of viruses which can cause benign and malignant lesions of the skin and the mucosa. There are 12 types of HPV that are known to cause cervical cancer, and infection with at least one of these HPV types is required for cervical cancer to develop [110]. HPV-16 and HPV-18 are most virulent and account for approximately 70% of cervical neoplasms [111]. Gardasil® and Cervarix® are prophylactic vaccines against HPV that are currently licensed. Gardasil® is a VLP-based vaccine composed of LI (a major capsid protein) from several HPV serotypes (6,11,16,18) and uses aluminum hydroxy-phosphate sulphate as its adjuvant (Table 21.1) [112]. Antibody responses are critical for immunity against these viruses and alum adjuvants are extremely effective at generating humoral immunity. Gardasil® vaccine has been shown to reduce HPV infection by 90% [112]. Cervarix® is a bivalent vaccine against HPV serotypes 16 and 18 and uses a GSK adjuvant system called AS04 which is composed of alum and MPL (Table 21.1). Further studies have shown that the vaccines are immunogenic 4 years after vaccination and that it confers cross-protection for other HPV types including HPV 45 and HPV 31 [110].

Other particulate vaccine adjuvants include liposomes, which are particulate structures composed of either natural or synthetic phospholipids. They were developed by Alec Bangham who extracted lipids from egg yolk and described the formation of a double-layered bubble the size of a cell when these lipids were added to an aqueous solution. Incorporating antigen into liposomes leads to increased antibody titers, and this is why so much work has gone into designing liposomes that are stable in the bloodstream and can target specific cells of the immune system to generate a particular immune response [113—115].

Stimuvax® is a liposome-based vaccine containing MPL which was developed for the treatment of non-small cell lung cancer, but has also been tested on breast cancers and multiple myelomas. MUC1 is a membrane protein of mucin-secreting epithelial cells and

TABLE 21.1 Currently Licensed Cancer Vaccines and their Adjuvant Components

Vaccine	Application	Adjuvant
Cervarix®	Prophylactic vaccine against cervical cancer caused by HPV virus strains 16 and 18	AS04 (GSK adjuvant system composed of Alum and MPL).
Gardasil®	Prophylactic recombinant vaccine composed of virus-like particles derived from the L1 capsid proteins of HPV virus strains 6, 11, 16 and 18.	Aluminum Hydroxyphosphate Sulfate.
Sipuleucel-T	Treatment vaccine for men with metastatic prostate cancer.	Leukapheresis involving stimulation with prostatic acid phosphatase (PAP) antigen and GM-CSF.

is over-expressed in 60% of lung cancers [116]. Stimuvax® targets this TAA using a lyophilized preparation of the 25-amino-acid BLP25 lipopeptide, MPL and three lipids (cholesterol, dimyristoyl phosphatidylglycerol and dipalmitoyl phosphatidylcholine) [117]. After a patient participating in a Phase II exploratory clinical trial with the therapeutic cancer vaccine developed encephalitis, clinical trials were halted. However, the study has been reintroduced and is currently recruiting for a Phase III trial with predicted completion in 2018 [117].

F. Combination vaccine adjuvants

The advances in biotechnology, molecular biology and immunology have enabled the rational development of well-defined, PAMP-based adjuvants. This, along with developments in synthetic chemistry and particulates which are capable of activating the immune system, has enabled the advancement of combination vaccine adjuvants.

Combining different adjuvants allows for a tailored immune response to be optimized. Advantages of these types of adjuvant strategies can include the ability to promote the development of heterologous antibodies that have increased cross reactivity among strains of pathogens, more effective T-cell responses and more potent functional antibodies. Although the process of combining adjuvants with other immunostimulatory components is not new, it is only recently that these types of adjuvants have been licensed [35].

GlaxoSmithKline (GSK) has been the front-runner in combination adjuvant development. Their adjuvant system (AS) portfolio is composed of various mixtures of classical adjuvants combined with other immunomodulators (Table 21.2) [118]. AS04 is a combination of MPL and alum and is used in the Fendrix® and Cervarix® vaccines that are currently on the market. Indeed there are several other AS combinations that are in clinical trials for infectious diseases such as malaria as well as some cancers.

As mentioned in Section D, biodegradable microparticles can enhance the immune response to associated antigens and adjuvants. It has been shown that PLG-encapsulated CpG promotes higher antibody titers and enhanced T-cell responses compared with soluble CpG [97,98].

VI. DC PRIMING *IN VIVO* VERSUS *EX VIVO*

Activation or priming of DCs is a key objective of the adjuvants mentioned above as these cells have a unique ability for antigen acquisition and display, leading to the generation of antigen-specific immune responses [17]. However, it should be recognized that in addition to *in vivo* methods of doing this, including injecting irradiated cytokine secreting whole tumor cells

TABLE 21.2 Combination Adjuvants that are Licensed or are Currently in Clinical Trials

Name	Company	Class	Indications	Stage
AS01	GSK	MPL + liposomes + QS21	Malaria	Phase III [118]
AS02	GSK	MPL + O/W emulsion + QS21	Malaria	Phase III [118]
AS03	GSK	α-tocopherol + O/W emulsion	Pandemic Influenza	Licensed (EU) [118]
AS04	GSK	MPL + Aluminum hydroxide	HBV (Fendrix), HPV (Cervarix)	Licensed (EU) [118]
AS15	GSK	ASO1 + CpG	Metastatic breast cancer	Phase I [118]
L-BLP25	Merck	Liposomes + MPL	Non-small cell lung cancer	Phase III [117]
IC31	Intercell	Anti-microbial peptide KLK & oligodeoxynocleotide ODN1a	Tuberculosis	Phase I*

*(http://www.intercell.com/main/forvaccperts/product-pipeline/)

which DCs can then phagocytose, and vaccinating with certain adjuvant combinations, there are also strategies being employed to prime DCs *ex vivo* [5]. One method involves isolating DCs from patients' blood, loading them with tumor antigens in culture medium, treating the cells with various stimuli to induce maturation and injecting them back into the patient [17,119]

Tumor cells already killed by chemotherapy or targeted therapies also have the potential to facilitate DC priming *in situ* [5]. Using patient-derived TAA and synthetic peptides derived from TAA, a DC focused immunotherapy can be achieved that induces antitumor effector cells [2,41]. As with *in vivo* targeting of DCs, adjuvants can be used in an *ex vivo* setting to optimize the type of DC-induced immune response generated against cancer. Advantages of *ex vivo* DC activation compared to *in vivo* activation is that the activation status can be determined before intratumoral injection [120].

Shibata and colleagues used an *ex vivo* method in mice to mature DCs by infecting them with recombinant Sendai virus (SeV) [120]. When these mature DCs were injected intratumorally to a B16F1 melanoma, the tumors were eliminated and the mice survived. The effect was enhanced by expressing IFN-β in DCs (SeV-murine IFN-β) and this approach could render the established low malignancy tumors dormant [120].

A recent study compared *in vivo* DC-targeting with priming *ex vivo* antigen-loaded DCs [28]. A vaccine composed of anti-DEC-205-OVA in the presence of CD40 monoclonal antibodies prevented B16 OVA tumor growth in a mouse model whereas *ex vivo* OVA-loaded mature DCs did not protect against tumor growth [28].

PROVENGE® (Sipuleucel-T) is an FDA-approved DC vaccine against metastatic, castration-resistant prostate cancer, designed to stimulate T cells specific for prostatic acid phosphatase (PAP) which is over-expressed in prostate carcinoma cells. This therapy involves the culture of a patient's own DCs with a fusion protein of PAP fused to granulocyte–macrophage colony-stimulating factor (GMCSF), a cytokine which can activate immune cells [121]. The DCs are then infused back into the patient and the hypothesis is that the primed DCs are capable of activating T cells that recognize the PAP antigen [122]. Patients showed increased survival with this therapy; however, the median improved survival was only 4 months and no effect on time to disease progression was observed [123]. The vaccine has come under some criticism due to the fact that there is a lack of direct antitumor responses to the treatment, the increased survival found was strongly related to the age of the patient and that the placebo was not directly

343

comparable to the treatment group. It is important that the exact mechanisms of action of the vaccine are determined [124].

Although these recent developments are encouraging, *ex vivo* targeting has encountered several issues. *Ex vivo* targeted DCs that have been re-infused do not migrate to the lymph nodes very efficiently, with only 3–5% able to present antigen to T cells [125]. Other limitations are that only certain subsets of DCs can be isolated and cultured *in vitro*. Furthermore, DCs that are used in this treatment must come from each individual patient and must be put back into the same patient, thus making the strategy time consuming and costly [17]. For these reasons, *in vivo* targeting of DCs through the development of cancer vaccines and adjuvants seems a more robust option [123].

VII. CONCLUSIONS

The importance of choosing the right adjuvant in vaccines cannot be overestimated. An adjuvant can determine the immunophenotype and consequently the efficacy of the vaccine [74]. In terms of adjuvant development, the acceptable tolerability profile for a therapeutic cancer vaccine may be different from a prophylactic vaccine to be used in infants. Currently this is not a consideration in safety procedures by both the FDA and the EMA, which will severely limit the development of adjuvants that have potential within a therapeutic vaccine setting [35]. In certain circumstances a degree of adjuvant-mediated toxicity may be acceptable if the overall result is effective antitumor immunity [123].

Tumors are known to interfere with DC function and hence designing a vaccine is not straightforward [126]. Correct adjuvant design involves selecting an appropriate stimulus to bring about DC maturation that generates strong helper and cytotoxic T-cell immunity [126]. In cancer vaccines, adjuvants that elicit CTL accompanied by a Th1 response will be the most effective and hence should be prioritized in current clinical research settings.

References

[1] Srivastava PK, Menoret A, Basu S, Binder RJ, McQuade KL. Heat Shock Proteins Come of Age: Primitive Functions Acquire New Roles in an Adaptive World. Immunity 1998;8:657–65.

[2] Palucka K, Ueno H, Banchereau J. Recent developments in cancer vaccines. J Immunol 2011;186:1325–31.

[3] Schuster M, Nechansky A, Kircheis R. Cancer immunotherapy. Biotechnol J 2006;1:138–47.

[4] Pulendran B, Ahmed R. Translating innate immunity into immunological memory: implications for vaccine development. Cell 2006;124:849–63.

[5] Vanneman M, Dranoff G. Combining immunotherapy and targeted therapies in cancer treatment. Nat Rev Cancer 2012;12:237–51.

[6] Ramon G. Sur la toxine et sur l'anatoxine diphtheriques. Annales de l'Institut Pasteur 1924;38:1–10.

[7] Guy B. The perfect mix: recent progress in adjuvant research. Nat Rev Microbiol 2007;5:505–17.

[8] Dubensky TW, Reed SG. Adjuvants for cancer vaccines. Semin Immunol 2010;22:155–61.

[9] Cluff CW. Monophosphoryl lipid A (MPL) as an adjuvant for anti-cancer vaccines: clinical results. Adv Exp Med Biol 2009;667:111–23.

[10] Takeuchi O, Akira S. Pattern recognition receptors and inflammation. Cell 2010;140:805–20.

[11] Janeway CA, Medzhitov R. Innate immune recognition. Annu Rev Immunol 2002;20:197–216.

[12] Pandolfi F, Cianci R, Pagliari D, et al. The Immune Response to Tumors as a Tool toward Immunotherapy. Clin Develop Immunol 2011;2011:894704.

[13] Foley EJ. Antigenic properties of methylcholanthrene-induced tumors in mice of the strain of origin. Cancer Resear 1953;13:835–7.

[14] Prehn RT, Main JM. Immunity to methylcholanthrene-induced sarcomas. J Natl Cancer Institute 1957;18:769–78.

[15] Dunn IS, Haggerty TJ, Kono M, et al. Enhancement of human melanoma antigen expression by IFN-beta. J Immunol 2007;179:2134–42.

[16] Smith MEF. Loss of HLA-A, B, C Allele Products and Lymphocyte Function-Associated Antigen 3 in Colorectal Neoplasia. Pro Natl Acad Sci 1989;86:5557—61.

[17] Hamdy S, Haddadi A, Hung RW, Lavasanifar A. Targeting dendritic cells with nano-particulate PLGA cancer vaccine formulations. Adv Drug Deliv Rev 2011;63:943—55.

[18] Norbury CC, Malide D, Gibbs JS, Bennink JR, Yewdell JW. Visualizing priming of virus-specific CD8+ T cells by infected dendritic cells in vivo. Nat Immunol 2002;3:265—71.

[19] Norbury CC, Basta S, Donohue KB, et al. CD8+ T cell cross-priming via transfer of proteasome substrates. Science (New York, NY) 2004;304:1318—21.

[20] Kaech SM, Wherry EJ, Ahmed R. Effector and memory T-cell differentiation: implications for vaccine development. Nat Rev Immunol 2002;2:251—62.

[21] Nishikawa H, Sakaguchi S. Regulatory T cells in tumor immunity. Int J Cancer 2010;127:759—67.

[22] Bonertz A, Weitz J, Pietsch D-HK, et al. Antigen-specific Tregs control T cell responses against a limited repertoire of tumor antigens in patients with colorectal carcinoma. J Clin Invest 2009;119:3311—21.

[23] Caminschi I, Maraskovsky E, Heath R. Targeting dendritic cells in vivo for cancer therapy. Frontiers in Immunology 2012;3:1—13.

[24] Van Broekhoven CL, Parish CR, Demangel C, Britton WJ, Altin JG. Targeting dendritic cells with antigen-containing liposomes: a highly effective procedure for induction of antitumor immunity and for tumor immunotherapy. Cancer Res 2004;64:4357—65.

[25] Mahnke K, Qian Y, Fondel S, Brueck J, Becker C, Enk AH. Targeting of antigens to activated dendritic cells in vivo cures metastatic melanoma in mice. Cancer Res 2005;65:7007—12.

[26] Dickgreber N, Stoitzner P, Bai Y, et al. Targeting antigen to MHC class II molecules promotes efficient cross-presentation and enhances immunotherapy. J Immunol (Baltimore, Md : 1950) 2009;182:1260—9.

[27] Wei H, Wang S, Zhang D, et al. Targeted delivery of tumor antigens to activated dendritic cells via CD11c molecules induces potent antitumor immunity in mice. Clin Cancer Res 2009;15:4612—21.

[28] Bonifaz LC, Bonnyay DP, Charalambous A, et al. In vivo targeting of antigens to maturing dendritic cells via the DEC-205 receptor improves T cell vaccination. J Exp Med 2004;199:815—24.

[29] Hishii M, Kurnick JT, Ramirez-Montagut T, Pandolfi F. Studies of the mechanism of cytolysis by tumour-infiltrating lymphocytes. Clin Exp Immunol 1999;116:388—94.

[30] Pulendran B. Modulating vaccine responses with dendritic cells and Toll-like receptors. Immunol Rev 2004;199:227—50.

[31] Kennedy R, Celis E. Multiple roles for CD4+ T cells in anti-tumor immune responses. Immunol Rev 2008;222:129—44.

[32] Nanni P, Landuzzi L, Nicoletti G, et al. Immunoprevention of mammary carcinoma in HER-2/neu transgenic mice is IFN-gamma and B cell dependent. J Immunol (Baltimore, Md : 1950) 2004;173:2288—96.

[33] Park JM, Terabe M, Sakai Y, et al. Early role of CD4+ Th1 cells and antibodies in HER-2 adenovirus vaccine protection against autochthonous mammary carcinomas. J Immunol 2005;174:4228—36.

[34] Reilly RT, Machiels JP, Emens LA, et al. The collaboration of both humoral and cellular HER-2/neu-targeted immune responses is required for the complete eradication of HER-2/neu-expressing tumors. Cancer Res 2001;61:880—3.

[35] O'Hagan DT, De Gregorio E. The path to a successful vaccine adjuvant—'the long and winding road'. Drug discovery today 2009;14:541—51.

[36] O'Hagan DT, Singh M. Microparticles as vaccine adjuvants and delivery systems. Expert Rev vaccines 2003;2:269—83.

[37] Aranda F, Llopiz D, Díaz-Valdés N, et al. Adjuvant combination and antigen targeting as a strategy to induce polyfunctional and high-avidity T-cell responses against poorly immunogenic tumors. Cancer Res 2011;71: 3214—24.

[38] Kaisho T, Akira S. Toll-like receptors as adjuvant receptors. Biochim Biophys Acta 2002;1589:1—13.

[39] Haining WN, Davies J, Kanzler H, et al. CpG oligodeoxynucleotides alter lymphocyte and dendritic cell trafficking in humans. Clin Cancer Res 2008;14:5626—34.

[40] Jahrsdorfer B, Hartmann G, Racila E, et al. CpG DNA increases primary malignant B cell expression of costimulatory molecules and target antigens. J Leukoc Biol 2001;69:81—8.

[41] Nava-Parada P, Forni G, Knutson KL, Pease LR, Celis E. Peptide vaccine given with a Toll-like receptor agonist is effective for the treatment and prevention of spontaneous breast tumors. Cancer Res 2007;67:1326—34.

[42] Goldstein MJ, Varghese B, Brody JD, et al. A CpG-loaded tumor cell vaccine induces antitumor CD4+ T cells that are effective in adoptive therapy for large and established tumors. Blood 2011;117:118—27.

[43] de Jong S, Chikh G, Sekirov L, et al. Encapsulation in liposomal nanoparticles enhances the immunostimulatory, adjuvant and anti-tumor activity of subcutaneously administered CpG ODN. Cancer Immunol Immunother 2007;56:1251—64.

[44] Ulrich J, Myers K. Monophosphoryl lipid A as an adjuvant. Past experiences and new directions. In: Vaccine Design: the subunit and adjuvant approach; 1995. p. 495−524.

[45] Persing D, Coler R, Lacy M, et al. Taking toll: lipid A mimetics as adjuvants and immunomodulators. Trends Microbiol 2002;10:S32−7.

[46] Didierlaurent AM, Morel S, Lockman L, et al. AS04, an aluminum salt- and TLR4 agonist-based adjuvant system, induces a transient localized innate immune response leading to enhanced adaptive immunity. J Immunol 2009;183:6186−97.

[47] Alexopoulou L, Holt AC, Medzhitov R, Flavell RA. Recognition of double-stranded RNA and activation of NF-kappaB by Toll-like receptor 3. Nature 2001;413:732−8.

[48] Warger T, Osterloh P, Rechtsteiner G, et al. Synergistic activation of dendritic cells by combined Toll-like receptor ligation induces superior CTL responses in vivo. Blood 2006;108:544−50.

[49] Whitmore MM, DeVeer MJ, Edling A, et al. Synergistic activation of innate immunity by double-stranded RNA and CpG DNA promotes enhanced antitumor activity. Cancer Res 2004;64:5850−60.

[50] Ahonen CL, Doxsee CL, McGurran SM, et al. Combined TLR and CD40 triggering induces potent CD8+ T cell expansion with variable dependence on type I IFN. J Exp Med 2004;199:775−84.

[51] Llopiz D, Dotor J, Zabaleta A, et al. Combined immunization with adjuvant molecules poly(I: C) and anti-CD40 plus a tumor antigen has potent prophylactic and therapeutic antitumor effects. Cancer Immunol Immunother 2008;57:19−29.

[52] Schoenen H, Bodendorfer B, Hitchens K, et al. Cutting edge: Mincle is essential for recognition and adjuvanticity of the mycobacterial cord factor and its synthetic analog trehalose-dibehenate. J Immunol (Baltimore, Md : 1950) 2010;184:2756−60.

[53] Ishikawa E, Ishikawa T, Morita YS, et al. Direct recognition of the mycobacterial glycolipid, trehalose dimycolate, by C-type lectin Mincle. J Exp Med 2009;206:2879−88.

[54] Garaude J, Kent A, van Rooijen N, Blander JM. Simultaneous targeting of toll- and nod-like receptors induces effective tumor-specific immune responses. Sci Transl Med 2012;4:120. ra16.

[55] Kensil C, Patel U, Lennick M, Marciani D. Separation and characterization of saponins with adjuvant activity from Quillaja saponaria Molina cortex. J Immunol 1991;146:431−7.

[56] Sun H-X, Xie Y, Ye Y- P. Advances in saponin-based adjuvants. Vaccine 2009;27:1787−96.

[57] Ragupathi G, Gardner JR, Livingston PO, Gin DY. Natural and synthetic saponin adjuvant QS-21 for vaccines against cancer. Exp Rev Vaccin 2011;10:463−70.

[58] Helling F, Zhang S, Shang A, et al. GM2-KLH conjugate vaccine: increased immunogenicity in melanoma patients after administration with immunological adjuvant QS-21. Cancer Res 1995;55:2783−8.

[59] Livingston PO, Natoli E, Calves M, Stockert E, Oettgen HF, Old LJ. Vaccines containing purified GM2 ganglioside elicit GM2 antibodies in melanoma patients. Proc Natl Acad Sci 1987;84:2911−5.

[60] Kim SK, Ragupathi G, Musselli C, Choi S-J, Park YS, Livingston PO. Comparison of the effect of different immunological adjuvants on the antibody and T-cell response to immunization with MUC1-KLH and GD3-KLH conjugate cancer vaccines. Vaccine 1999;18:597−603.

[61] Kim SK, Ragupathi G, Cappello S, Kagan E, Livingston PO. Effect of immunological adjuvant combinations on the antibody and T-cell response to vaccination with MUC1−KLH and GD3−KLH conjugates. Vaccine 2000;19:530−7.

[62] Nencioni A, Grüenbach F, Patrone F, Brossart P. Anticancer vaccination strategies. Annals of oncology : official journal of the European Society for Medical Oncology / ESMO 2004;15(Suppl. 4). iv153−60.

[63] Arnold D, Faath S, Rammensee H, Schild H. Cross-priming of minor histocompatibility antigen-specific cytotoxic T cells upon immunization with the heat shock protein gp96. J Exp Med 1995;182:885−9.

[64] Suto R, Srivastava P. A mechanism for the specific immunogenicity of heat shock protein-chaperoned peptides. Science 1995;269:1585−8.

[65] Castelli C, Ciupitu A, Rini F, et al. Human heat shock protein 70 peptide complexes specifically activate antimelanoma T cells. Cancer Res 2001;61:222−7.

[66] Udono H. Cellular Requirements for Tumor-Specific Immunity Elicited by Heat Shock Proteins: Tumor Rejection Antigen gp96 Primes CD8+ T Cells in vivo. Proc Natl Acad Sci 1994;91:3077−81.

[67] Blachere N, Li Z, Chandawarkar R, et al. Heat shock protein-peptide complexes, reconstituted in vitro, elicit peptide-specific cytotoxic T lymphocyte response and tumor immunity. J Exp Med 1997;186:1315−22.

[68] Srivastava PK. Immunotherapy for human cancer using heat shock protein-peptide complexes. Curr Oncol Rep 2005;7:104−8.

[69] Tamura Y, Peng P, Liu K, Daou M, Srivastava PK. Immunotherapy of tumors with autologous tumor-derived heat shock protein preparations. Science 1999;278:117−20.

[70] Rivoltini L, Castelli C, Carrabba M, et al. Human tumor-derived heat shock protein 96 mediates in vitro activation and in vivo expansion of melanoma- and colon carcinoma-specific T cells. J Immunol 2003;171: 3467–74.

[71] Testori A, Richards J, Whitman E, et al. Phase III comparison of vitespen, an autologous tumor-derived heat shock protein gp96 peptide complex vaccine, with physician's choice of treatment for stage IV melanoma: the C-100-21 Study Group. J Clin Oncol 2008;26:955–62.

[72] Wood C, Srivastava P, Bukowski R, et al. An adjuvant autologous therapeutic vaccine (HSPPC-96; vitespen) versus observation alone for patients at high risk of recurrence after nephrectomy for renal cell carcinoma: a multicentre, open-label, randomised phase III trial. Lancet 2008;372:145–54.

[73] Gong J, Zhang Y, Durfee J, et al. A Heat Shock Protein 70-Based Vaccine with Enhanced Immunogenicity for Clinical Use. J Immunol 2009;184:488–96.

[74] Schijns VEJC, Lavelle EC. Trends in vaccine adjuvants. Exp Rev Vaccin 2011;10:539–50.

[75] Morse MA, Clay TM, Lyerly HK. Handbook of cancer vaccines, Volume 1., 204AD.

[76] Aucouturier J, Dupuis L, Ganne V. Adjuvants designed for veterinary and human vaccines. Vaccine 2001;19:2666–72.

[77] Aucouturier J, Ascarateil S, Dupuis L. The use of oil adjuvants in therapeutic vaccines. Vaccine 2006;24:S44–5.

[78] Rosenberg SA, Yang JC, Kammula US, et al. Different adjuvanticity of incomplete freund's adjuvant derived from beef or vegetable components in melanoma patients immunized with a peptide vaccine. J Immunother; 33: 626–9

[79] O'Neill D, Adams S, Goldberg J, et al. Comparison of the immunogenicity of Montanide ISA 51 adjuvant and cytokine-matured dendritic cells in a randomized controlled clinical trial of melanoma vaccines. J Clin Oncol 2009;27:15s.

[80] Seubert A, Monaci E, Pizza M, O'Hagan DT, Wack A. The adjuvants aluminum hydroxide and MF59 induce monocyte and granulocyte chemoattractants and enhance monocyte differentiation toward dendritic cells. J Immunol 2008;180:5402–12.

[81] Morein B, Sundquist B, Höglund S, Dalsgaard K, Osterhaus A. Iscom, a novel structure for antigenic presentation of membrane proteins from enveloped viruses. Nature 1984;308:457–60.

[82] Barr IG, Mitchell GF. ISCOMs (immunostimulating complexes): the first decade. Immunol Cell Biol 1996;74:8–25.

[83] Claassen I, Osterhaus A. The iscom structure as an immune-enhancing moiety: experience with viral systems. Resear Immunol 1992;143:531–41.

[84] Villacres-Eriksson M, Bergström-Mollaoglu M, Kåberg H, Lövgren K, Morein B. The induction of cell-associated and secreted IL-1 by iscoms, matrix or micelles in murine splenic cells. Clin Exp Immunol 1993;93:120–5.

[85] Behboudi S, Morein B, Villacres-Eriksson M. In vivo and in vitro induction of IL-6 by Quillaja saponaria molina triterpenoid formulations. Cytokine 1997;9:682–7.

[86] Behboudi S, Morein B, Villacres-Eriksson M. In vitro activation of antigen-presenting cells (APC) by defined composition of Quillaja saponaria Molina triterpenoids. Clin Exp Immunol 1996;105:26–30.

[87] Schmitz-Winnenthal FH, Volk C, Z'graggen K, et al. High frequencies of functional tumor-reactive T cells in bone marrow and blood of pancreatic cancer patients. Cancer Res 2005;65:10079–87.

[88] Davis ID, Chen W, Jackson H, et al. Recombinant NY-ESO-1 protein with ISCOMATRIX adjuvant induces broad integrated antibody and CD4+ and CD8+ T cell responses in humans. Proc Natl Acad Sci USA 2004;101:10697–702.

[89] Nicholaou T, Ebert LM, Davis ID, et al. Regulatory T-cell-mediated attenuation of T-cell responses to the NY-ESO-1 ISCOMATRIX vaccine in patients with advanced malignant melanoma. Clin Cancer Res 2009;15:2166–73.

[90] Jacobs C, Duewell P, Heckelsmiller K, et al. An ISCOM vaccine combined with a TLR9 agonist breaks immune evasion mediated by regulatory T cells in an orthotopic model of pancreatic carcinoma. Int J Cancer 2011;128:897–907.

[91] Clements CJ, Griffiths E. The global impact of vaccines containing aluminium adjuvants. Vaccine 2002;20:S24–33.

[92] Jordan MB, Mills DM, Kappler J, Marrack P, Cambier JC. Promotion of B cell immune responses via an alum-induced myeloid cell population. Science 2004;304:1808–10.

[93] McKee AS, MacLeod M, White J, Crawford F, Kappler JW, Marrack P. Gr1+IL-4-producing innate cells are induced in response to Th2 stimuli and suppress Th1-dependent antibody responses. Int Immunol 2008;20:659–69.

[94] Wang H-B, Weller PF. Pivotal advance: eosinophils mediate early alum adjuvant-elicited B cell priming and IgM production. J Leukoc Biol 2008;83:817–21.

[95] Glenny A, Pope C. The antigenic effect of intravenous injection of diphtheria toxin. J Pathol Bacteriol 1925;28:273—8.

[96] Glenny A, Buttle G, Stevens M. Rate of disappearance of diptheria toxoid injected into rabbits and guinea pigs: toxoid precipitated with alum. J Pathol Bacteriol 1931;34:267—75.

[97] Malyala P, Chesko J, Ugozzoli M, et al. The potency of the adjuvant, CpG oligos, is enhanced by encapsulation in PLG microparticles. J Pharma Sci 2008;97:1155—64.

[98] Kazzaz J, Singh M, Ugozzoli M, Chesko J, Soenawan E, O'Hagan DT. Encapsulation of the immune potentiators MPL and RC529 in PLG microparticles enhances their potency. J Control Release 2006;110: 566—73.

[99] Waeckerle-Men Y, Allmen EU-von Gander B, et al. Encapsulation of proteins and peptides into biodegradable poly(D, L-lactide-co-glycolide) microspheres prolongs and enhances antigen presentation by human dendritic cells. Vaccine 2006;24:1847—57.

[100] Hamdy S, Molavi O, Ma Z, et al. Co-delivery of cancer-associated antigen and Toll-like receptor 4 ligand in PLGA nanoparticles induces potent CD8+ T cell-mediated anti-tumor immunity. Vaccine 2008;26: 5046—57.

[101] Schlosser E, Mueller M, Fischer S, et al. TLR ligands and antigen need to be coencapsulated into the same biodegradable microsphere for the generation of potent cytotoxic T lymphocyte responses. Vaccine 2008;26:1626—37.

[102] Heit A, Schmitz F, Haas T, Busch DH, Wagner H. Antigen co-encapsulated with adjuvants efficiently drive protective T cell immunity. Eur J Immunol 2007;37:2063—74.

[103] Scheerlinck J-PY, Greenwood DLV. Virus-sized vaccine delivery systems. Drug Discovery Today 2008;13:882—7.

[104] Glück R, Moser C, Metcalfe IC. Influenza virosomes as an efficient system for adjuvanted vaccine delivery. Expert Opin Biol Ther 2004;4:1139—45.

[105] Grgacic EVL, Anderson DA. Virus-like particles: passport to immune recognition. Methods 2006;40:60—5.

[106] Huckriede A, Bungener L, Stegmann T, et al. The virosome concept for influenza vaccines. Vaccine 2005;23(Suppl. 1):S26—38.

[107] Bachmann MF, Jennings GT. Vaccine delivery: a matter of size, geometry, kinetics and molecular patterns. Nat Rev Immunol 2010;10:787—96.

[108] de Martel C, Franceschi S. Infections and cancer: established associations and new hypotheses. Crit Rev Oncol/Hematol 2009;70:183—94.

[109] Parkin DM. The global health burden of infection-associated cancers in the year 2002. Int J Cancer 2006;118:3030—44.

[110] Harper DM, Franco EL, Wheeler CM, et al. Sustained efficacy up to 4.5 years of a bivalent L1 virus-like particle vaccine against human papillomavirus types 16 and 18: follow-up from a randomised control trial. Lancet 2006;367:1247—55.

[111] Smith JS, Lindsay L, Hoots B, et al. Human papillomavirus type distribution in invasive cervical cancer and high-grade cervical lesions: a meta-analysis update. Int J Cancer 2007;121:621—32.

[112] Villa LL, Costa RLR, Petta CA, et al. Prophylactic quadrivalent human papillomavirus (types 6, 11, 16, and 18) L1 virus-like particle vaccine in young women: a randomised double-blind placebo-controlled multicentre phase II efficacy trial. Lancet Oncol 2005;6:271—8.

[113] Maruyama K, Okuizumi S, Ishida O, Yamauchi H, Kikuchi H, Iwatsuru M. Phosphatidyl polyglycerols prolong liposome circulation in vivo. Inter J Pharma 1994;111:103—7.

[114] Foged C, Arigita C, Sundblad A, Jiskoot W, Storm G, Frokjaer S. Interaction of dendritic cells with antigen-containing liposomes: effect of bilayer composition. Vaccine 2004;22:1903—13.

[115] Allison A, Gregoriadis G. Liposomes as immunological adjuvants. Nature 1974;252. 252—252.

[116] Morgensztern D, Goodgame B, Govindan R. Vaccines and Immunotherapy for non-small cell lung cancer. J Thorac Oncol 2010;5:S463—5.

[117] Wu Y-L, Park K, Soo RA, et al. INSPIRE: A phase III study of the BLP25 liposome vaccine (L-BLP25) in Asian patients with unresectable stage III non-small cell lung cancer. BioMed Central Cancer 2011;11:430.

[118] Garçon N, Chomez P, Van Mechelen M. GlaxoSmithKline Adjuvant Systems in vaccines: concepts, achievements and perspectives. Exp Rev Vaccin 2007;6:723—39.

[119] Tacken PJ, de Vries IJM, Torensma R, Figdor CG. Dendritic-cell immunotherapy: from ex vivo loading to in vivo targeting. Nat Rev Immunol 2007;7:790—802.

[120] Shibata S, Okano S, Yonemitsu Y, et al. Induction of Efficient Antitumor Immunity Using Dendritic Cells Activated by Recombinant Sendai Virus and Its Modulation by Exogenous IFN-beta Gene. J Immunol 2006;177:3564—76.

[121] Kantoff P, Higano C, Shore N, et al. Sipuleucel-T Immunotherapy for castration-resistant prostate cancer. New Engl J Med 2010;363:411—22.

[122] Sonpavde G, Di Lorenzo G, Higano CS, Kantoff PW, Madan R, Shore ND. The role of sipuleucel-T in therapy for castration-resistant prostate cancer: a critical analysis of the literature. Eur Urol 2012;61:639—47.

[123] Madorsky-Rowdo FP, Lacreu ML, Mordoh J. Melanoma vaccines and modulation of the immune system in the clinical setting: building from new realities. Frontiers in immunology 2012;3:103.

[124] Huber ML, Haynes L, Parker C, Iversen P. Interdisciplinary critique of sipuleucel-T as immunotherapy in castration-resistant prostate cancer. J Nat Cancer Inst 2012;104:273—9.

[125] De Vries IJM, Lesterhuis WJ, Scharenborg NM, et al. Maturation of dendritic cells is a prerequisite for inducing immune responses in advanced melanoma patients. Clin Cancer Res 2003;9:5091—100.

[126] Steinman RM. Decisions About Dendritic Cells: Past, Present, and Future, http://www.annualreviews.org/doi/abs/10.1146/annurev-immunol-100311-102839, 2011. (accessed 26 Jan2012).

Improving Immunotherapeutic Responses

Epigenetic Approaches: Emerging Role of Histone Deacetylase Inhibitors in Cancer Immunotherapy

Eva Sahakian, Karrune Woan, Alejandro Villagra, Eduardo M. Sotomayor
Department of Immunology and Malignant Hematology, H. Lee Moffitt Cancer Center & Research Institute, Tampa, FL USA

I. INTRODUCTION

During the past several years, studies in experimental models as well as in humans have provided sufficient evidence supporting the conclusion that tumor-induced T-cell tolerance represents a significant barrier to harness effective antitumor immunity [1—4]. Important lessons learned from these studies point to manipulation of the inflammatory status of immune cells and tumor cells as an enticing strategy to overcome tolerogenic mechanisms in cancer [5—8]. Such knowledge has already been translated into immunotherapeutic approaches, that after many years of unsuccessful attempts, have finally achieved the long elusive goal of cancer immunotherapy, i.e., generation of clinically significant antitumor immune responses that are improving the outcome of patients [9—11].

Despite these success stories, a large majority of cancer patients will still succumb to their disease, highlighting the need for continued understanding of the mechanisms regulating antitumor immune responses, not only at the genetic, but also, as presented in this chapter, at the epigenetic level. Indeed, a significant effort is being devoted to unveil the mechanisms regulating pro-inflammatory and anti-inflammatory genes in their natural setting, the chromatin substrate [12]. Among these, chromatin modification by acetylation/deacetylation has gained particular attention given its important role in regulation of gene transcription, including genes involved in the inflammatory response [13]. In general, while histone acetylation mediated by histone acetyl transferases (HATs) results in transcriptionally active chromatin, histone deacetylation mediated by histone deacetylases (HDACs) leads to an inactive chromatin and gene repression [14]. In this review, we summarize the emerging role of specific HDACs in regulation of inflammatory responses and how such knowledge is helping not only to better explain the divergent inflammatory effects of the current generation of histone deacetylase inhibitors (HDI), but also in providing the proper framework for the development of more selective inhibitors that either alone or in combination with other immunotherapeutic agents might overcome tolerance to tumor antigens and elicit more effective and durable antitumor immunity.

Cancer Immunotherapy. http://dx.doi.org/10.1016/B978-0-12-394296-8.00022-1

II. TUMOR-INDUCED TOLERANCE IS A SIGNIFICANT BARRIER FOR CANCER IMMUNOTHERAPY

It is now well recognized that antigen encounter in the periphery by cells of the immune system does not necessarily lead to immune activation and can result instead immunological unresponsiveness [15]. Bone marrow-derived (BM-derived) antigen presenting in cells (APCs) lie at the junction of this critical choice of the immune system. These cells have been shown to capture and present peptide antigens derived from dying cells to antigen-specific T cells, interactions that can lead to initiation of either T-cell priming [16] or T-cell tolerance [17,18]. These opposing T-cell outcomes are greatly influenced by the environmental surroundings in which the APC originally encountered the antigen. For instance, if an antigen is encountered in an inflammatory environment, this will cause APC maturation to a functional status that ultimately will lead to effective activation of T cells (Figure 22.1A). In contrast, in the absence of inflammatory factors, or in the presence of anti-inflammatory molecules, BM-derived APCs will express lower levels of MHC, co-stimulatory molecules, and other adhesion molecules essential for effective T-cell priming, inducing instead T-cell unresponsiveness, a default outcome that characterizes how the immune system normally responds to self-antigens expressed in the periphery [19] (Figure 22.1B).

The latter scenario—absence or minimal inflammatory environment—also exemplifies how BM-derived APCs likely encounter tumor antigens *in vivo*, an event that harmfully (for the host) will be conducive to T-cell tolerance toward tumor antigens rather than T-cell activation. Adding complexity to this sobering scenario, as tumor develops, its microenvironment not only fails in providing inflammatory signals needed for effective APC maturation/activation, but produces immunosuppressive factors (IL-10, TGF-β, and VEGF among others) or attracts cells with

354

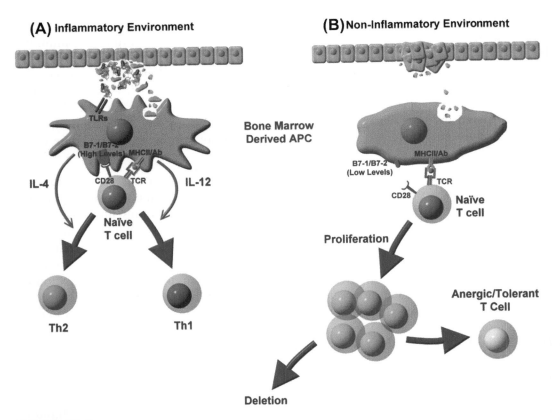

FIGURE 22.1
APCs dictate T-cell activation vs. tolerance. Antigen-presenting cells are key regulators of adaptive, cellular immunity. Depending on the context under which APCs encounter antigen, inflammatory (A) or non-inflammatory (B) milieu, they can either drive immunity (A) or tolerance (B), respectively.

immunoregulatory properties (Tregs, myeloid derived suppressor cells) that negatively influence APC function even further [1]. Consequently, APCs from the non-inflammatory or even "hostile" tumor microenvironment are comparatively inefficient at priming protective responses, inducing T-cell anergy towards tumor antigens [20].

Conversion of this T-cell encounter with tumor antigen/APC from a tolerizing event into a priming event has emerged as a desirable goal. A proof of principle supporting this approach was provided by the findings that manipulation of the inflammatory/activation status of the APC via CD40 ligation [21], or through inhibition of pathways that negatively impact inflammation, such as STAT3 [5], could convert T-cell tolerance into T-cell priming in the tumor-bearing host. These results also underlined the intrinsic plasticity of the APC to become activating or tolerogenic, a property influenced by the presence—or not—of inflammatory signals at the site of antigen encounter.

Continued identification of genetic and epigenetic mechanism(s) regulating pro- and anti-inflammatory pathways in the APC would offer further insights into how these cells influence T-cell function and might reveal novel targets to overcome the obstacle that tolerance has imposed to cancer immunotherapy. For example, it is now well-known that accessibility to DNA by molecules involved in transcriptional regulation, including cis-acting transcription factors (e.g., STAT3), is dependent on chromatin structure, composition and flexibility [22]. These processes are highly regulated by specific proteins, collectively named as "readers," which interact with specific chromatin modifications through bromo- and chromo-domains, as an example [23]. The "chromatin landscape" for these "readers" is influenced by other groups of proteins known as "writers" or "erasers" of histone marks [24]. In particular, chromatin modifications by acetylation/deacetylation of histone tails have been demonstrated to play an important role in the regulation of genes involved in the inflammatory response [13]. It is plausible, therefore, that dynamic and reversible changes at the chromatin level and as a result, dynamic changes in expression of inflammatory and/or anti-inflammatory genes, might contribute to the intrinsic plasticity of the APC to determine T-cell activation versus T-cell tolerance.

III. EPIGENETICS AND CANCER

Conventionally, cancer has been seen as a genetic disease. However, it is now realized that other factors such as epigenetic changes can also influence the initiation, progression and aggressiveness of cancer cells. Epigenetics refers to functionally significant changes in gene expression that do not include a change in the nucleotide sequence [25]. The heritability of specific expression profiles is mediated by modifications at the DNA and protein levels. Among them, methylation of cytosine bases in DNA, microRNA (miRNA), post-translational modifications of histone proteins and changes in the positioning of nucleosomes along the DNA are considered the most important [26]. These modifications, collectively named as the *epigenome*, provide singular variations among different cell types without interfering with the coding DNA sequence.

Almost all epigenetic heritable signatures began early during cellular differentiation and reach a steady state according to the stage of development [26]. Therefore, changes in this epigenetic pattern, as seen in cancer, will promote loss or gaining of cellular functions, not naturally assigned to a specific cell type. The most described epigenetic-based deregulations are those leading to abnormal proliferation and apoptosis of cancer cells. However, there is growing evidence suggesting that cells with oncogenic potential can evade host defenses earlier during cancer development, escaping immune recognition and transforming into malignant cells [27,28]. For many years, the study of tumor escape mechanisms has mainly focused on genetic mutations of immune and apoptotic-related genes. However, data gathered over the past few years indicates that epigenetic silencing may be as frequent as mutations in the process of gene inactivation [26]. Epigenetic aberrations, unlike genetic mutations, are potentially reversible and can be restored to their normal state by epigenetic therapy. These observations highlight the potential of epigenetic modifiers as promising approaches for cancer immunotherapy.

One epigenetic target that has shown promise in cancer immunotherapy is HDACs, which is the topic of this review. In eukaryotic cells, DNA is wrapped around small positively charged proteins known as histones to form the basic chromatin building block, the nucleosome [29]. The conformation of nucleosomes is highly dynamic, mainly due to variations in the interaction between histones and DNA. Important to mention are the dynamic and reversible chemical modifications generated by a heterogeneous group of proteins known as histone "writers" or "erasers" [24,30]. These antagonistic sets of enzymes attach or remove a chemical group upon histones in a site-specific manner. Among them, enzymes involved in methylation, acetylation, ubiquitination, phosphorylation, proline-isomerization, ADPribosylation, or those that modify histones by other means such as citrullination or proteolytic cleavage are important [31]. One of the most studied histone modifications is the acetylation of lysine at the N-terminal tails of histones. In an unmodified state, the highly positive N-terminal end of histones provides for a more compacted structure through interactions with the negatively charged DNA backbone. This generates an obstacle for the binding of transcription factors and the recruitment of other proteins that need to read the nucleosomes to exert their transcriptional functions. In this context, acetylation of histones neutralizes these positive charges, promoting a relaxed nucleosome conformation and allowing the binding of various proteins, including transcription factors. These acetyl modifications are introduced by histone acetyltransferases (HATs) ("writers"), a heterogeneous group of proteins often found in multiprotein co-activation complexes that can be selectively recruited to particular DNA sequences [32]. Conversely, acetyl modifications can be removed by HDACs ("erasers"). The 18 HDACs identified in humans are subdivided into two families: the classical HDAC family of zinc-dependent metalloproteins, composed of classes I, II and IV; and the NAD^+-dependent Class III sirtuin family of HDACs, which are not within the scope of this review. Class I HDACs (HDAC1, 2, 3 and 8) are most closely related to the yeast deacetylase RPD3. Class II HDACs encompass HDAC 4, 5, 6, 7, 9, and 10, sharing homology with the yeast deacetylase HDA1. Finally, the newest HDAC identified, HDAC11, is the sole member of Class IV, and does not share homology with either RPD3 or HDA1 [33]. Shown in Table 20.1 is a summary of our current knowledge of the zinc-dependent HDACs.

Despite their name, it is now well known that some HDACs can also target a variety of non-histone proteins [34], and proteins considered as HDACs (e.g., HDAC6) display minimal or no histone deacetylase activity at all. Thus, the denomination "HDAC" is merely historic and does not reflect accurately the physiological and broader role of these proteins in cell biology. For instance, HDACs deacetylate nonhistone proteins involved in several cellular processes, including proteins linked to structural, metabolic signaling as well as immune responses. Of note, a large number of transcription factors are regulated by HDACs, positioning this family of proteins as indirect regulators of gene expression. Functionally, deacetylation by HDACs has different outcomes in their protein targets. For example, deacetylation can diminish the ability of transcription factors to bind DNA (i.e., p53 [35], STAT3 [36], GATA1 [37], and E2F1 [38]), or conversely, increase its DNA binding (i.e., YY1 [39], HMG [40] and p65 [41]). Additionally, the acetylation status of some proteins controls their interaction with other proteins, as observed with the acetylation of STAT3 [36] and the estrogen receptor-α [42]. HDACs have been also shown to regulate the transcriptional activity and protein stability of p53 [35], androgen receptor [43], and E2F [44]. Finally, HDACs can also regulate the function of proteins involved in cell structure and intracellular trafficking. In this group, it is important to mention the role of HDAC6 in the regulation of the molecular chaperone Hsp90 [45] and the cytoskeletal protein α-tubulin [46].

As can be gathered from above, significant advances have been made in the understanding of the biology of HDACs in nonimmune cells. In recent years, however, it has become clear that

HDACs also play important regulatory roles in cells of the immune system. As such, the role of specific HDACs goes beyond their initially described effects on histones and encompass now more complex regulatory functions that are dependent upon HDAC tissue expression profile, cellular compartment distribution, stage of cellular differentiation and pathophysiological conditions [34,47–49].

IV. ROLE OF SPECIFIC HDACS IN IMMUNITY: MOLECULAR SIGNALING AND PATHWAYS

The dynamic production of pro- and anti-inflammatory mediators by the APC during the interface with T cells has been shown to influence the initiation, magnitude and the duration of an immune response [50]. IL-12 and IL-10, cytokines with divergent inflammatory properties, are central in the regulation of these dynamic changes and in maintaining a delicate balance to prevent autoimmune attack while allowing an efficient immune response against foreign antigens. For instance, IL-12 is essential for resistance against infections, but elevated levels could result in autoimmunity [51]. Conversely, IL-10 plays a key role in tolerance induction by keeping immune responses at check and preventing self-tissue damage [52–54]. Recently, it has been shown that cytokine production by the APC is regulated by changes in the acetylation status of gene promoters [55,56]. Given this emerging knowledge, our group as well as others have focused attention into understanding how dynamic changes at the chromatin level induced by HDACs and, as a result, dynamic regulation of inflammatory or anti-inflammatory genes might influence immune responses and, in particular, the critical decision of the APC to determine T-cell activation versus T-cell tolerance to tumor antigens. Below we summarize the current knowledge of the role of specific HDACs in regulation of immune responses.

A. Class I HDACs

357

Among the members of class I HDACs, HDAC1 has been identified as a key regulator of cyclin-dependent-kinase (CDK) inhibitors p21 and p27 [57] which are instrumental for proper cell cycle progression and as such appealing targets for cancer therapy [58,59]. HDAC1 knockout (KO) mice were generated but were embryonic lethal at very early stages of development [58]. Immunological targets of HDAC1 consist of IL-1 [60], IL-2 [61], IL-12 [62], IL-5 [63], IFN-β [64], IFN-γ [65], IL-4 [66], signal transducer and activator of transcription 5 (STAT5) [67], STAT3 [36], MHC class I-related chain A, B (MIC-A/B) [68], and major histocompatibility complex class I (MHC I) [69]. Immune diseases such as rheumatoid arthritis (RA) [70], systemic lupus erythematosis (SLE) [71], juvenile idiopathic arthritis (JIA) [72], and multiple sclerosis (MS) [73] are associated with HDAC1. HDAC2 is mainly involved in modulating the growth response of cartilage and cardiac muscle, and mice deficient for HDAC2 survived until perinatal period [74]. Immunological targets of HDAC2 consist of IFN-γ [65], IL-4 [66], STAT3 [36], granulocyte macrophage colony-stimulating factor (GM-CSF) [75], and MHC class II trans-activator (CIITA) [76]. HDAC2 has been associated with chronic obstructive pulmonary disease (COPD) [77], muscular dystrophy (MD) [78] and RA [79]. HDAC3, another member of this class, is involved in cell cycle progression and cell cycle-dependent DNA damage control. Inactivation of this enzyme is embryonic lethal and causes delay and inefficiency in cell cycle progression [80]. Immunological targets of HDAC3 consist of IL-4 [66], STAT3 [36], STAT1 [81], IFN-β [64], pro-IL-6 [82], GATA-binding protein 1 (GATA1) [83], GATA2 [84], and GATA3 [85]. HDAC3 has been associated with systemic sclerosis (SS) [86] and SLE [71]. HDAC3 KO mice are embryonic lethal owing to defects in gastrulation [87]. HDAC1, 2 and 3 have been directly involved in the regulation of STAT3 activity through the acetylation of Lys 685 [36], and recently, Icardi et al., demonstrated that HDAC1 and HDAC2 differentially modulate STAT activity in response to type I interferons (JAK/STAT pathway dependent) influencing the transcription of STAT3-dependent genes [88]. Given the aberrant activation of STAT3 in multiple human cancers and its role as a negative regulator of antitumor immune responses [89,90], HDACs controlling STAT3 activity are appealing targets for tumor immunotherapy. The last member of class I HDACs, HDAC8 was early identified as a regulator of the expression of the MHC class I promoter [91]. HDAC8 has also been identified to repress the expression of IFN-β gene [64]. HDAC8 KO mice are perinatal lethal due to skull instability [92].

B. Class IIA HDACs

Members of class IIA HDAC family are known for their involvement in repression of cell growth in cardiomiocytes (HDAC5 and 9) [93] and chondrocytes (HDAC4) [94]. HDAC4 KO mice die within the first week of life due to ectopic ossification of endochondral cartilage [94]. Previous studies by Watamoto et al. have demonstrated that HDAC4 directly interacts with GATA1 [83]. HDAC5 KO mice developed cardiac hypertrophy [93]; however, the phenotype does not cause any immunological aberrations. Immunological targets of HDAC5 consist of GATA1 regulating erythropoiesis [83] and IL-8 to which HDAC5 is recruited to the promoter. However, little is known about its regulatory effect [95]. HDAC7, also a member of this class of HDACs, has been identified to be important in maintaining vascular integrity via repression of matrix metalloproteinase 10 (MMP10) [96]. Interestingly, Li et al., reported that transcriptional repression by the FOXP3 transcription factor, a key molecule in regulatory T cells (Tregs), involves a histone acetyltransferase-deacetylase complex containing the "writer" histone acetyltranferase (HAT) TIP60 (Tat-interactive protein, 60 kDa) and the "erasers" HDAC7 and HDAC9 [97]. Additionally, regulation of IL-2 production in T cells requires a minimum level of FOXP3 ensemble including native TIP60 and HDAC7. Of note, FOXP3 association with HDAC9 is antagonized by T-cell stimulation (CD28) and can be restored by the HDAC inhibitor TSA [97]. The important role of HDAC7 in the regulation of FOXP3 and Treg function has been recently highlighted by Bettini et al., who showed that reduced interaction between FOXP3, TIP60, HDAC7 and the Ikaros family zinc finger 4, Eos, resulted in reduced FOXP3 acetylation and decreased FOXP3-mediated gene repression, particularly at the level of the IL-2 promoter. Such a loss of FOXP3-driven epigenetic modification resulted in less suppressive Tregs and increased predisposition to autoimmunity [98]. In addition to its role in Treg function, HDAC7 is highly expressed in cytotoxic T lymphocytes (CTLs). Of note, continued phosphorylation of HDAC7 was associated with export of this transcriptional repressor from the nucleus and increased expression of genes encoding key cytokines, cytokine receptors and adhesion molecules that are critical in CTL function. Conversely, dephosphorylation of HDAC7 resulted in its accumulation in the nucleus, gene suppression and impaired CTL function [99].

Unlike, HDAC7 KO mice that are embryonic lethal [96], HDAC9 KO mice are viable but develop cardiac hypertrophy [100]. It has also been suggested that changes in the expression of HDAC9 in Tregs alter suppression in SLE disease [71]. Studies have demonstrated that HDAC9 seems predominantly important in regulating FOXP3-dependent suppression [101]. Notably, FOXP3 acetylation enhances the binding of FOXP3 to IL-2 promoter and suppression of endogenous production of IL-2 [102].

C. Class IIB HDACs

HDAC6 is the largest HDAC protein identified (1215aa) and the only HDAC having two different, independently active deacetylase domains [103]. Initial characterization of this HDAC assigned its localization and function to the cytoplasmic compartment [46,104]. However, recent reports showed that HDAC6 is also present in the nucleus [105,106]. The "HDAC activity" of HDAC6 is questioned given scarce in vitro reports demonstrating its "histone" deacetylase activity [107] and the lack of strong evidence pointing to histones as enzymatic substrates for HDAC6.

In spite of its weak histone deacetylase activity, HDAC6 has been found to regulate the acetylation of several proteins including α-tubulin, Hsp90, and cortactin [108]. HDAC6 is therefore recognized as a key regulator of cytoskeletal dynamics, cell migration and cell–cell interactions [109]. Importantly, emerging evidence also implicates this HDAC in the regulation of immune responses, in particular at the level of the APC/T-cell immune synapse [110], Treg modulation [111] and as recently found by our group, a key regulator of the production of the immunosuppressive cytokine IL-10 (Cheng et al. Submitted). The latter finding is of interest, given that HDAC6 has been shown to interact with HDAC11 *in vitro*, an HDAC recently found to be a transcriptional repressor of IL-10 gene expression in APCs [112]. Thus, HDAC6 might be a novel target to therapeutically inhibit the production of IL-10 and tip the balance towards the generation of inflammatory APCs able of inducing T-cell activation rather than T-cell tolerance. The availability of isotype-selective HDAC6 inhibitors already being evaluated in human malignancies [113] points to HDAC6 as an attractive target for cancer immunotherapy. HDAC6 KO mice are viable, but they exhibit hyperacetylated tubulin [114].

HDAC10 is the other member of the class IIB HDAC family [115]. The expression level of this HDAC was found to be decreased in patients with aggressive lung cancer [116], suggesting that HDAC10 might be important in maintaining normal cell growth/function. HDAC10 is able to associate with several other HDACs. Therefore it might function as a recruiter rather than as a deacetylase [33]. Fundamental understanding of its function in nonimmune as well as immune cells remains to be elucidated.

D. Class IV HDAC

HDAC11, a 39 kDa protein encoded by chromosome 3, is the latest identified member of the histone deacetylase family [117]. This HDAC is localized mainly in the nucleus and its expression seems to be tissue specific with higher expression in brain, heart, skeletal muscle and kidney [117]. Although the enzymatic activity and tissue distribution of HDAC11 has been studied [117,118], little was known about the functional role of this HDAC until our discovery that HDAC11 is an important transcriptional repressor of IL-10 gene expression [112].

We demonstrated that HDAC11, by interacting at the chromatin level with the IL-10 promoter downregulates IL-10 transcription in murine and human APCs. Such an effect not only determined the inflammatory status of these cells but also influenced priming versus tolerance of antigen-specific CD4$^+$ T cells [112]. For instance, in APCs overexpressing HDAC11 we found a significant decrease of H3 and H4 acetylation, at the level of the IL-10 gene promoter which was associated with diminished recruitment of the transcriptional activators STAT3 and Sp1, perhaps as a reflection of their decreased accessibility to a less acetylated and, therefore, more compacted chromatin. The enzymatic activity of HDAC11 was needed in the above process, since over-expression of an HDAC11 mutant with a deleted deacetylase domain failed to inhibit IL-10 gene expression. Conversely, in APCs in which HDAC11 was knocked-down by shRNA, we observed an opposite outcome, i.e., enhanced IL-10 gene transcriptional activity. In cells lacking HDAC11, we found an increase in H3 and H4 acetylation that was accompanied by an enhanced recruitment of the transcriptional activators Sp1 and STAT3 to the IL-10 promoter. The significance of these findings lies at several levels: *first*, it provided a physiological role for HDAC11; *second*, HDAC11 by inducing dynamic changes at the chromatin level regulates the expression of IL-10 (and perhaps other genes involved in the inflammatory response), an effect that might explain—at least in part—the plasticity of the APC to determine T-cell activation versus T-cell tolerance; *third*, HDAC11 represents a novel molecular target to potentially influence immune activation versus immune tolerance, a critical decision with significant implications for cancer immunotherapy.

Finally, recent studies have shown that HDAC11 regulates the expression of OX40L in Hodgkin's lymphoma (HL) cell lines. Indeed, by knocking down HDAC11 with small

TABLE 22.1 Classes of HDACs

Class		Size (AA)	Deacetylase Domain (PF00850)	Protein Structure	Localization	Chromosome Location	Complex	Knock-out Phenotype	Aberrations in Immune Diseases	Immunological targets
HDAC1	I	482	5-384	N/A	Nuc.	1p34	Sin3, Nurd, CoREST	Embrionic lethal (e10.5). Proliferation defects and general growth retardation.	RA SLE JIA MS	IL-1, IL-2, IL-12, II-5, INF-b, INF-g, IL-4, STAT5, STAT3
HDAC2	I	488	23-319	3MAX (2.05A) Bressi et al, 2010	Nuc.	6q21	Sin3, Nurd, CoREST	Perinatal lethal. Cardiac malformations.	RA COPD MD	GM-CSF, IFN-γ, IL-4, STAT3
HDAC3	I	428	19-314	N/A	Nuc.	5q31	N-CoR	Embrionic lethal (e9.5). Gastrulation defects	SLE SS	IL-4, pro-IL-16, STAT3, STAT1, GATA1, GATA2, GATA3, NFκβ
HDAC8	I	377	28-322	2V5W (2.00A) Vannini et al, 2007	Nuc.	Xq13	-	Perinatal lethal. Skull instability.	N/A	INF-β
HDAC4	IIa	1084	671-992	2VQM (1.80A) Bottomley et al, 2008	Nuc./Cyt.	2q37.3	N-CoR, MEF2	Perinatal lethal. Ectopic ossification of endochondral cartilage.	MS	GATA1
HDAC5	IIa	1122	700-1022	N/A	Nuc./Cyt.	17q21	N-CoR, MEF2	Non lethal. Cardiac hypertrophy.	N/A	IL-8, GATA1
HDAC7	IIa	952	538-859	3COZ (2.10A) Schuetz et al, 2008	Nuc./Cyt.	12q13.1	N-CoR, Sin3 MEF2	Embrionic lethal. Endothelial cells missfunction.	SLE	IL-2, FOXP3
HDAC9	IIa	1011	651-972	N/A	Nuc./Cyt.	7p21.1	N-CoR, MEF2	Non lethal. Cardiac hypertrophy.	SLE	IL-2, FOXP3
HDAC6	IIb	1215	104-402 495-798	N/A	Nuc./Cyt.	Xp11.23	HDAC11	Non lethal.	MS	IFN-β
HDAC10	IIb	669	25-321	N/A	Nuc./Cyt.	22q13.31	N-CoR	Non lethal.	N/A	-
HDAC11	IV	347	30-318	N/A	Nuc./Cyt.	3p25.1	HDAC6	Non lethal. Unpublished phenotype	N/A	IL-10

RA: Rheumatoid Arthritis, SLE: Systemic Lups Erythematosus, JIA: Juvenile Idioathic Arthritis, MS: Multiple Sclerosis, COPD: Chronic Obstructive Pulmonary Disease, SS: Systemic Syndrome, N/A: Not Available, Nuc.: Nuclear, Cyt.: Cytoplasmic.

Bressi JC, Jennings AJ, Skene R, Wu Y, Melkus R, De Jong R, et al. Exploration of the HDAC2 foot pocket: Synthesis and SAR of substituted N-(2-aminophenyl)benzamides. Bioorg Med Chem Lett. 2010; 20(10): 4.

Vannini A, Volpari C, Gallinari P, Jones P, Mattu M, Carfi A, et al. Substrate binding to histone deacetylases as shown by the crystal structure of the HDAC8-substrate complex. EMBO Rep. 2007; 8(9): 879-84.

Bottomley MJ. Structures of protein domains that create or recognize histone modifications. EMBO Rep. 2004; 5: 464.

Schuetz A, Min J, Allali-Hassani A, Schapira M, Shuen M, Loppnau P, et al. Human HDAC7 harbors a class IIa histone deacetylase-specific zinc binding motif and cryptic deacetylase activity. J Biol Chem. 2008; 283(17): 11355-63.

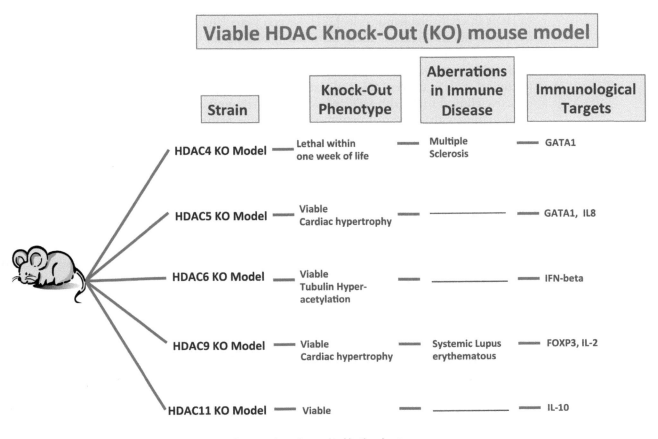

FIGURE 22.2
Characteristics of viable HDAC KO mouse models. Specific phenotypes, immunologic targets, and implicated immunopathologies are depicted.

interfering RNAs (siRNAs), Younes and colleagues found a significant upregulation of OX40L in HL cells. Given that engagement of OX40L with the OX40 receptor is essential for the generation of antigen-specific memory T cells and that OX40L can inhibit the generation of IL-10-producing Tregs, specific inhibition of HDAC11 has emerged as an appealing strategy to augment T-cell immunity in patients with HL [119].

Shown in Table 22.1 and Figure 22.2 are the known immunological targets of HDACs as well as the phenotype of mice with genetic disruption of specific HDACs.

V. HDIs

A. HDI in cancer treatment

HDIs are a heterogeneous group of chemical compounds with the capacity to inhibit the enzymatic activity of HDACs. The chemical structure of these compounds falls into six different groups: short-chain fatty acids (e.g., valproic acid), hydroxamates (e.g., TSA, SAHA), benzamides (e.g., MS-275), cyclic tetrapeptides (e.g., depsipeptide), electrophilic ketones (e.g., trifluoromethylketone), and miscellaneous compounds (e.g., MGCD0103). The inhibitory activity of the majority of HDIs is due to their interaction with the active zinc site at the catalytic pocket of HDACs, as demonstrated by crystallographic studies of HDAC/HDI interactions (Table 22.1). These compounds were first used clinically for the treatment of neurologic conditions such as epilepsy long before their mechanisms of action were understood [120]. Nearly four decades ago, Leder and colleagues observed an antiproliferative effect of HDIs in erythroleukemic cells [121]. Several years later, Yoshida et al. found that in a number of cell lines, including mammary gland tumor cells, TSA treatment resulted in inhibition of HDACs as evidenced by increased histone acetylation [122]. Following these earlier observations, a number of HDI have been designed, and several of them have advanced to clinical trials in cancer [48]. The National Cancer Institute (NCI) maintains a complete list of active clinical trials with HDI (www.clinicaltrials.gov) either as a single agent or in combination with other treatment modalities. Some of the HDIs evaluated in clinical trials are Belinostat (PXD101), Givinostat (ITF2357), Panobinostat (LBH589), Vorinostat (SAHA, MK0683), Valproic acid, Romidepsin (FK2288, FR901228), CHR 2845, JNJ-26481585 and the HDAC6 selective inhibitor ACY1215 [48,113]. Of note, the U.S Food and Drug Administration (FDA) approved Vorinostat (Zolinza) [123] and Romidepsin (Istodax) [124] for the treatment of patients with refractory cutaneous T-cell lymphoma (CTCL). Furthermore, resminostat, a sulfonylpyrrole hydroxamate, has been recently granted orphan drug status for the treatment of patients with multiple myeloma [125].

Extensive preclinical work and data obtained from correlative studies in cancer patients treated with HDIs have provided important insights into their antitumor effects. For instance, it is now well established that all HDIs inhibit proliferation of malignant cells *in vitro* by inducing cell cycle arrest and apoptosis [126]. Furthermore, some HDIs also demonstrated significant antitumor activity in preclinical animal models as well as in recently completed clinical trials, in particular for patients with T-cell malignancies. An additional advantage of HDIs as anti-cancer agents is their selectivity upon transformed cells, with normal cells being more resistant to the inhibitory effects of these drugs [127].

B. HDI in the treatment of autoimmune disorders

Currently, about 5% of the western world population are being affected by approximately 80 different autoimmune disorders [128]. Immunosuppressive drugs such as steroids and cyclosporine are commonly used agents for the treatment of autoimmune diseases. Of note, Phase I and Phase II clinical trials in patients treated with HDIs (e.g., valproic acid, SAHA, MS-275, and ITF2357) showed an increased incidence of infections in the absence of neutropenia [129,130], suggesting that perhaps these compounds display immunosuppressive properties. Given these findings, HDIs were evaluated in preclinical studies of systemic lupus erythematous (SLE) [71], rheumatoid arthritis (RA), juvenile idiopathic arthritis (JIA) [131–133], systemic sclerosis [134], multiple sclerosis (MS) [135], ulcerative colitis (UC) [136] and psoriasis [137]. All these studies have highlighted the anti-inflammatory properties of HDIs leading to lessening of the autoimmune damage that characterizes these disorders. In SLE, for instance, epigenetic modifications affect a substantial number of genes [138] involved in pathways controlling immune cell development and function, such as lymphocyte differentiation (PDCD1, IKZF1, IKZF3), apoptotic cell death (PARP, CRP, ATG5), cytokine signaling (STAT4, IRF5, TNFSF4), and complement activation (C1q, C2, C24a, C4b) [139,140]. Of note, the pan-HDI, TSA was shown to reverse the skewed expression of CD40 ligand, IL-10 and IFN-γ in lupus T cells [141]. TSA treatment also led to lessening of disease activity in a rat model of RA due to inhibition of the inflammatory cytokines IL-1, IL-6, and TNF-α as well as upregulation of CDK inhibitors (p16^{INK4a} and p21$^{WAF1/Cip1}$) in diseased joints [142]. Abrogation of HDAC enzymatic activity can also alter the immunopathology of RA and other immune-mediated inflammatory diseases through both epigenetic dependent or independent processes [143,144].

C. Antitumor immune effects triggered by HDI: Implications for cancer immunotherapy

Given the anti-inflammatory properties of HDIs it was quite unlikely that they would find a place in the cancer immunotherapy armamentarium. Surprisingly, several studies have demonstrated that HDIs can augment the immunogenicity of tumor cells and enhance the antitumor properties of immune cells. First, studies by Tomasi's group showed that treatment of melanoma cells with HDIs augments their antigen-presenting capabilities leading to activation of IFN-γ secreting T cells via the Class I pathway [145,146]. HDIs can also enhance the expression of specific receptors in tumor cells such as stress-related ligands, MIC-A and MIC-B, which ligate to NKG2D on CD8$^+$ cytotoxic T lymphocytes (CTLs) and natural killer (NK) cells and promotes immune recognition of tumor cells [147]. Second, recent studies have shown that HDIs induce upregulation of OX40L in Hodgkin's lymphoma (HL) cells. Given that engagement of OX40L expressed by malignant cells with the OX40 receptor is essential for generation of antigen-specific memory T cells and for inhibition of IL-10-producing Tregs, this effect of HDI upon OX40L expression might also promote strong T-cell responses against HL cells [119].

Regarding the effects of HDIs upon immune cells, Vo *et al.* recently demonstrated that *in vivo* treatment of tumor-bearing mice with the pan-HDI LAQ824, enhanced the antitumor activity of adoptively transferred antigen-specific T cells [148]. Similarly, our group has shown that LAQ824, by inhibiting IL-10 and increasing the expression of B7.2 and the production of several pro-inflammatory factors, induced inflammatory APCs that effectively activated antigen-specific CD4$^+$ T cells and reinstated the responsiveness of tolerant T cells. These positive effects of LAQ824 were also exhibited by other members of the hydroxamic acid family like LBH589, TSA and SAHA, but not by the more selective HDI MS-275, which primarily targets Class I HDACs [149]. In addition, HDIs have also been demonstrated to induce a favorable antitumor immune response in Hodgkin's lymphoma by downregulating the expression and secretion of thymus and activation-regulated chemokine (TARC/CCL17) in Reed-Sternberg (RS) cells and dendritic cells *in vitro* and by favoring a pro-inflammatory Th1-type response [150].

Mechanistically, it has been shown that cytokine production is greatly regulated at the chromatin level by alterations in the acetylation status of the gene promoter. For example, changes in the chromatin structure of the IL-10 promoter in T cells differentiated into the T$_H$1 or T$_H$2 phenotype closely regulate IL-10 expression [151]. In macrophages, increased acetylation of the IL-10 promoter has been associated with enhanced transcriptional activity [55]. Conversely, we demonstrated that decreased acetylation of the IL-10 promoter was associated with decreased IL-10 transcriptional activity in murine and human APCs [112]. Given the above, we expected that treatment of APCs *in vitro* with the HDI LAQ824 would result in increased histone acetylation and increased IL-10 production. Although an increased global acetylation of histones H3 and H4 was observed in cells treated with LAQ824, an opposite outcome was observed at the level of the IL-10 gene promoter in LAQ824-treated cells. Unexpectedly, diminished H3 and H4 acetylation at the IL-10 promoter was seen at all evaluated time-points in treated macrophages. This decrease in histone acetylation, which occurred early, decreased recruitment of the transcriptional activators STAT3 and Sp1 to the IL-10 gene promoter. It is probable that a more compacted chromatin due to diminished histone acetylation in the IL-10 promoter region might block the access of these transcriptional activators to the promoter region, resulting in the decreased IL-10 gene transcriptional activity observed in LAQ824-treated APCs. Kinetic analysis of H3 and H4 acetylation provided some clues as to why this might be occurring. In macrophages pretreated with LAQ824 and then stimulated with LPS, we observed an initial acetylation of H3 and H4 that reaches its peak at one hour poststimulation. However, the extent of these changes was greatly lower than in macrophages treated with LPS only. Following this peak acetylation, we observed a rapid abrogation of such a response in cells treated with HDI, suggesting either an absence of stimuli to support H3 and H4 acetylation and/or the initiation of counter-regulatory mechanism(s) that lessened the degree of H3 and H4 acetylation observed in cells treated with LPS alone. Of particular interest was the finding of enhanced recruitment of the transcriptional repressors PU.1 and HDAC11 to the IL-10 gene promoter. It is plausible therefore that recruitment of these two repressors might represent a counter-regulatory mechanism triggered by HDI to diminish H3 and H4 acetylation and block the sequence of events that lead to IL-10 gene transcriptional activation. Supporting the above, we have found that over-expression of HDAC11 in the macrophage cell line RAW264.7 resulted in decreased H3 and H4 acetylation of the IL-10 gene promoter and inhibition of IL-10 gene transcriptional activity [112]. Interestingly, Bradbury *et al.* have found that treatment of myeloid leukemic blasts with TSA resulted in a 60- to 200-fold induction of HDAC11 mRNA expression [118]. Such an effect of HDIs upon HDAC11 expression might explain the increased recruitment of this specific HDAC to the IL-10 gene promoter in cells treated with LAQ824. Needless to say, the mechanism(s) of increased HDAC11 expression with in HDI-treated APCs, remains to be elucidated.

VI. CONTROVERSY: ARE HDIs PRO- OR ANTI-INFLAMMATORY DRUGS?

We are left to explain the divergent effects of HDIs as anti-inflammatory as well as pro-inflammatory drugs. One potential explanation may lie in the lack of selectivity of the majority of the HDIs currently in use. Most are pan-HDI that can target any of the three classes of zinc-dependent HDACs. In addition, they have differing potencies against specific substrates, with IC50s that are indeed different for each HDAC.

As described in this chapter, emerging data points to particular HDACs as being endowed with pro-inflammatory properties (i.e., HDAC11 negatively regulates the anti-inflammatory cytokine IL-10), while other HDACs are important in regulation of anti-inflammatory pathways (HDAC6 in Tregs and APCs). As such, depending on the potency and relative IC50s of the pan-HDI for their HDAC targets, one particular HDI might be more prone to exert anti-inflammatory effects while other HDIs might instead trigger a pro-inflammatory effect. For example, we have found that the pan-HDIs LBH589, LAQ824 and SAHA induce pro-inflammatory APCs *in vitro*. Although these HDIs belong to the same family of hydroxamic acid compounds, their pro-inflammatory effects and their ability to inhibit IL-10 differs significantly, with LAQ824 and LBH589 being more potent IL-10 inhibitors than SAHA [149]. In contrast, others have found that SAHA attenuated inflammatory responses in DCs through IDO-dependent mechanisms and also decreased the severity of graft-versus-host disease (GvHD) in a murine allogeneic bone marrow transplantation model [152,153]. Several differences between these studies and ours may explain these seemingly conflicting results. First, in our *in vitro* system we used macrophages that were treated with HDI and LPS given at the same time. In their study, DCs primarily were pretreated with SAHA prior to stimulation with TLR agonist. Second, they found that SAHA treatment did not induce significant changes in the production of IL-10 by DCs. Supporting their observation, we have also found that among all the members of the hydroxamic family of HDIs, SAHA was the weakest inhibitor of IL-10 production in macrophages which might explain, at least in part, the divergent effects of these HDIs upon the inflammatory status of APCs.

Emerging evidence points to the timing of administration of the HDI in influencing cellular responses to inflammatory stimuli such as TLR agonists [149,154]. Kinetic studies in macrophages have revealed an initial induction of pro-inflammatory cytokines, followed by production of anti-inflammatory mediators such as IL-10 in response to LPS stimulation [149]. It is plausible that, in our experiments, the concomitant administration of HDI with LPS did not provide sufficient time for the drug to modulate pro-inflammatory genes. Instead, by negatively influencing the expression of anti-inflammatory genes (like IL-10) late during the inflammatory response, HDI treatment might perpetuate a pro-inflammatory reaction in the absence of counter-regulatory anti-inflammatory mechanisms. Conversely, pretreatment with HDIs, as in the studies by Reddy and colleagues

[152,153] might preferentially dampen the initial pro-inflammatory response more so than the late anti-inflammatory response, leading to the observed anti-inflammatory status of APCs.

Another possible explanation for the pleiotropic effects of HDIs upon inflammatory responses might be related to the emerging context-dependent and cell-intrinsic roles of specific HDACs. For transcriptional regulation, this could be due to the fact that HDACs do not possess any intrinsic DNA binding capacity. Therefore, HDACs rely on particular *cis*-acting elements which comprise the co-repressor complex. It is plausible that pan-HDI might exert different effects upon complexes involved in the transcriptional regulation of inflammatory and/or anti-inflammatory genes resulting in divergent outcomes. For regulation of nonhistone targets such as those influenced by HDAC6, the opposite effects of HDIs may be related to their differential effects upon different immune cell populations and/or substrate targets. For instance, HDAC6 inhibition has been shown to enhance immune synapse formation between CD8+ T cells and APCs, thereby improving T-cell immunity. Conversely, HDAC6 inhibition also augments the immunosuppressive function of Tregs, leading to immune tolerance rather than T-cell activation. Therefore, depending on the predominant effect of pan-HDIs or even isotype-selective HDAC6 inhibitors upon one cell type versus the other, the outcome of a T-cell mediated immune response *in vivo* might be quite opposing. Furthermore, the differential cellular expression of HDAC6 target protein such as FOXP3 and/or tubulin might play a role in the divergent outcomes that have been observed. For instance, FOXP3 might not be relevant for CTL-APC interactions and as such the predominant effect of HDIs will be at the level of enhancing the immunological synapse leading to T-cell immunity. In sharp contrast, if HDIs mainly affect the acetylation status of FOXP3, a critical molecule for Treg function, the overall effect might be enhanced immune suppression.

An interesting concept that is emerging in the field is that the differential effects of specific HDACs in immune cells might be amplified across different immune compartments and environmental contexts. The observation that particular HDACs might have opposing effects upon T-cell subsets or among different immune cell populations provide an explanation for the lack of overt immune pathologies in mice with genetic disruption of specific HDACs. For instance, we have recently found that while T cells from HDAC11 KO mice are hyperreactive and prone to trigger autoimmunity and antitumor effects when adoptively transferred into wild type recipients, myeloid cells from these same HDAC11 KO mice are more immunosuppressive. As a result of this counterbalance, HDAC11 KO mice are viable and develop neither overt autoimmunity nor an immunosuppressive phenotype (unpublished data). From an evolutionarily point of view, these opposing effects of specific HDACs might provide a fine balance that prevents either exuberant autoimmunity or immune suppression. It is plausible, therefore, that HDAC inhibition may serve primarily to modulate extreme immune responses. That is, in the setting of autoimmunity, HDIs may temper the aberrant function of some immune cells, while in cancer HDIs might disrupt excessively redundant immunosuppressive networks.

Taken together, we are in the infancy of our understanding of the role of specific HDACs in regulation of immune responses and how pan-HDI might influence these HDAC-mediated regulatory pathways. Much work is still needed to tease out the mechanisms by which HDIs influence inflammatory responses in cancer, autoimmunity, and transplantation. However, a significant obstacle to be faced relates to the pleiotropic effects and pan-HDAC inhibitory activity of the current generation of HDIs. Their lack of selectivity for individual enzymes results in a myriad of cellular effects that would make dissection of the relevant mechanism(s)/target(s) in immune cells a barrier difficult to overcome. To complicate things even further specific HDACs also influence the function of nonhistone proteins and display regulatory functions that are dependent on their tissue expression, cellular compartment distribution and/or stage of cellular differentiation (Figure 22.3). The alternative strategy of

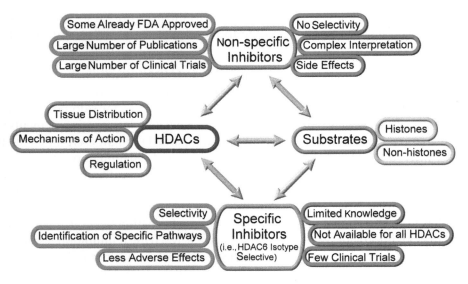

FIGURE 22.3
Effect of HDIs on HDACs and their substrates. Unique characteristics of HDACs (purple) mediate substrate-specific effects (blue). There are a multitude of both nonspecific (top) and specific inhibitors (bottom), each category having distinct advantages (green) and disadvantages and limitations (red).

better understanding the role of specific HDACs in immune regulation as a first step to unveil molecular mechanisms is already leading to the rational design of more specific HDIs (Figure 22.3 bottom). Although a particular HDAC may have opposing effects depending on the cell and context, an increased knowledge of the substrate-specificity of each HDAC will nevertheless enable the rational design of more selective and perhaps less toxic epigenetic-based approaches to effectively harness antitumor immune responses. Needless to say, future studies will determine which will be the optimal HDAC to target, in which cell, and under what conditions (e.g., dosing, regimen, and sequence of combination approaches) in cancer patients.

VII. CONCLUSIONS

Within the last decade, HDIs have been recognized to have regulatory effects on the immunobiology of cells in autoimmune and inflammatory diseases as well as in cancer [155]. The often times paradoxical effects of HDIs exerting both pro- and anti-inflammatory effects may stem from the fact that a majority of HDIs currently in use are pan-HDIs that inhibit all three classes of zinc-dependent HDACs. Undoubtedly, mechanistic insights into these contradictory effects in cancer, autoimmunity, and other pathologies will lead to the development of more targeted therapeutics to regulate specific targets and pathways. It is important to recognize that the use of HDIs in the treatment of cancer is affecting not only the proliferation and survival of cancer cells, but also many other pathways, including those related to immunological networks.

References

[1] Rabinovich GA, Gabrilovich D, Sotomayor EM. Immunosuppressive Strategies that are Mediated by Tumor Cells. Annu Rev Immunol 2007;25(1):267—96.

[2] Munn DH, Sharma MD, Lee JR, Jhaver KG, Johnson TS, Keskin DB, et al. Potential regulatory function of human dendritic cells expressing indoleamine 2,3-dioxygenase. Science 2002;297(5588):1867—70.

[3] Staveley-O'Carroll K, Sotomayor E, Montgomery J, Borrello I, Hwang L, Fein S, et al. Induction of antigen-specific T cell anergy: An early event in the course of tumor progression. Proc Natl Acad Sci U S A 1998;95(3):1178—83.

[4] Bogen B, Munthe L, Sollien A, Hofgaard P, Omholt H, Dagnaes F, et al. Naive CD4+ T cells confer idiotype-specific tumor resistance in the absence of antibodies. Eur J Immunol 1995;25(11):3079−86.

[5] Cheng F, Wang HW, Cuenca A, Huang M, Ghansah T, Brayer J, et al. A critical role for Stat3 signaling in immune tolerance. Immunity 2003;19(3):425−36.

[6] Evel-Kabler K, Song XT, Aldrich M, Huang XF, Chen SY. SOCS1 restricts dendritic cells' ability to break self tolerance and induce antitumor immunity by regulating IL-12 production and signaling. J Clin Invest 2006;116(1):90−100.

[7] Horna P, Sotomayor EM. Cellular and molecular mechanisms of tumor-induced T-cell tolerance. Curr Cancer Drug Targets 2007;7(1):41−53.

[8] Song XT, Evel-Kabler K, Shen L, Rollins L, Huang XF, Chen SY. A20 is an antigen presentation attenuator, and its inhibition overcomes regulatory T cell-mediated suppression. Nat Med 2008;14(3):258−65.

[9] Brahmer JR, Tykodi SS, Chow LQM, Hwu W-J, Topalian SL, Hwu P, et al. Safety and Activity of Anti−PD-L1 Antibody in Patients with Advanced Cancer. N Engl J Med 2012;366(26):2455−65.

[10] Topalian SL, Hodi FS, Brahmer JR, Gettinger SN, Smith DC, McDermott DF, et al. Safety, Activity, and Immune Correlates of Anti−PD-1 Antibody in Cancer. N Engl J Med 2012;366(26):2443−54.

[11] Pardoll DM. The blockade of immune checkpoints in cancer immunotherapy. Nat Rev Cancer 2012;12(4):252−64.

[12] Georgopoulos K. From immunity to tolerance through HDAC. Nat Immunol 2009;10(1):13−4.

[13] Foster SL, Hargreaves DC, Medzhitov R. Gene-specific control of inflammation by TLR-induced chromatin modifications. Nature 2007;447(7147):972−8.

[14] Glozak MA, Seto E. Histone deacetylases and cancer. Oncogene 2007;26(37):5420−32.

[15] Pardoll D. Does the immune system see tumors as foreign or self? Annu Rev Immunol 2003;21:807−39.

[16] Huang AY, Golumbek P, Ahmadzadeh M, Jaffee E, Pardoll D, Levitsky H. Role of bone marrow-derived cells in presenting MHC class I-restricted tumor antigens. Science 1994;264(5161):961−5.

[17] Adler AJ, Marsh DW, Yochum GS, Guzzo JL, Nigam A, Nelson WG, et al. CD4(+) T cell tolerance to parenchymal self-antigens requires presentation by bone marrow-derived antigen-presenting cells [In Process Citation]. J Exp Med 1998;187(10):1555−64.

[18] Sotomayor EM, Borrello I, Rattis FM, Cuenca AG, Abrams J, Staveley-O'Carroll K, et al. Cross-presentation of tumor antigens by bone marrow-derived antigen-presenting cells is the dominant mechanism in the induction of T-cell tolerance during B-cell lymphoma progression. Blood 2001;98(4):1070−7.

[19] Steinman RM, Hawiger D, Nussenzweig MC. Tolerogenic dendritic cells. Annu Rev Immunol 2003;21:685−711.

[20] Cuenca A, Cheng F, Wang H, Brayer J, Horna P, Gu L, et al. Extra-Lymphatic Solid Tumor Growth Is Not Immunologically Ignored and Results in Early Induction of Antigen-Specific T-Cell Anergy: Dominant Role of Cross-Tolerance to Tumor Antigens. Cancer Res 2003;63(24):9007−15.

[21] Sotomayor EM, Borrello I, Tubb E, Rattis FM, Bien H, Lu Z, et al. Conversion of tumor-specific CD4+ T-cell tolerance to T-cell priming through in vivo ligation of CD40. Nat Med 1999;5(7):780−7.

[22] Travers AA, Vaillant C, Arneodo A, Muskhelishvili G. DNA structure, nucleosome placement and chromatin remodelling: a perspective. Biochem Soc Trans 2012;40(2):335−40.

[23] Yun M, Wu J, Workman JL, Li B. Readers of histone modifications. Cell Res 2011;21(4):564−78.

[24] Arrowsmith CH, Bountra C, Fish PV, Lee K, Schapira M. Epigenetic protein families: a new frontier for drug discovery. Nat Rev Drug Discov 2012;11(5):384−400.

[25] Berger SL, Kouzarides T, Shiekhattar R, Shilatifard A. An operational definition of epigenetics. Genes Dev 2009;23(7):781−3.

[26] Sharma S, Kelly TK, Jones PA. Epigenetics in cancer. Carcinogenesis 2010;31(1):27−36.

[27] Miremadi A, Oestergaard MZ, Pharoah PDP, Caldas C. Cancer genetics of epigenetic genes. Hum Mol Genet 2007;16(R1):R28−49.

[28] Schreiber RD, Old LJ, Smyth MJ. Cancer Immunoediting: Integrating Immunity's Roles in Cancer Suppression and Promotion. Science 2011;331(6024):1565−70.

[29] Luger K, Mader AW, Richmond RK, Sargent DF, Richmond TJ. Crystal structure of the nucleosome core particle at 2.8[thinsp]A resolution. Nature 1997;389(6648):251−60.

[30] Suganuma T, Workman J. Signals and Combinatorial Functions of Histone Modifications. Annu Rev Biochem 2011;80:27.

[31] Bannister AJ, Kouzarides T. Regulation of chromatin by histone modifications. Cell Res 2011;21(3):381−95.

[32] Lee KK, Workman JL. Histone acetyltransferase complexes: one size doesn't fit all. Nat Rev Mol Cell Biol 2007;8(4):284−95.

[33] de Ruijter AJM, van Gennip AH, Caron HN, Kemp S, van Kuilenburg ABP. Histone deacetylases (HDACs): characterization of the classical HDAC family. Biochem J 2003;370(3):737−49.

367

[34] Glozak MA, Sengupta N, Zhang X, Seto E. Acetylation and deacetylation of non-histone proteins. Gene 2005;363:15−23.

[35] Gu W, Roeder RG. Activation of p53 sequence-specific DNA binding by acetylation of the p53 C-terminal domain. Cell 1997;90(4):595−606.

[36] Z-l Yuan. Guan Y-j, Chatterjee D, Chin YE. Stat3 Dimerization Regulated by Reversible Acetylation of a Single Lysine Residue. Science 2005;307(5707):269−73.

[37] Boyes J, Byfield P, Nakatani Y, Ogryzko V. Regulation of activity of the transcription factor GATA-1 by acetylation. Nature 1998;396(6711):594−8.

[38] Marzio G, Wagener C, Gutierrez MI, Cartwright P, Helin K, Giacca M. E2F Family Members Are Differentially Regulated by Reversible Acetylation. J Biol Chem 2000;275(15):10887−92.

[39] Yao Y-L, Yang W-M, Seto E. Regulation of Transcription Factor YY1 by Acetylation and Deacetylation. Mol Cell Biol 2001;21(17):5979−91.

[40] Munshi N, Merika M, Yie J, Senger K, Chen G, Thanos D. Acetylation of HMG I(Y) by CBP Turns off IFNβ Expression by Disrupting the Enhanceosome. Mol Cell 1998;2(4):457−67.

[41] Kiernan R, Brès V, Ng RWM, Coudart M-P, El Messaoudi S, Sardet C, et al. Post-activation Turn-off of NF-κB-dependent Transcription Is Regulated by Acetylation of p65. J Biol Chem 2003;278(4):2758−66.

[42] Kawai H, Li H, Avraham S, Jiang S, Avraham HK. Overexpression of histone deacetylase HDAC1 modulates breast cancer progression by negative regulation of estrogen receptor α. Int J Cancer 2003;107(3):353−8.

[43] Gaughan L, Logan IR, Neal DE, Robson CN. Regulation of androgen receptor and histone deacetylase 1 by Mdm2-mediated ubiquitylation. Nucleic Acids Res 2005;33(1):13−26.

[44] Martinez-Balbas MA, Bauer U-M, Nielsen SJ, Brehm A, Kouzarides T. Regulation of E2F1 activity by acetylation. Embo J 2000;19(4):662−71.

[45] Kovacs JJ, Murphy PJM, Gaillard S, Zhao X, Wu J-T, Nicchitta CV, et al. HDAC6 Regulates Hsp90 Acetylation and Chaperone-Dependent Activation of Glucocorticoid Receptor. Mol Cell 2005;18(5):601−7.

[46] Hubbert C, Guardiola A, Shao R, Kawaguchi Y, Ito A, Nixon A, et al. HDAC6 is a microtubule-associated deacetylase. Nature 2002;417(6887):455−8.

[47] Woan KV, Sahakian E, Sotomayor EM, Seto E, Villagra A. Modulation of antigen-presenting cells by HDAC inhibitors: implications in autoimmunity and cancer. Immunol Cell Biol 2012;90(1):55−65.

[48] Villagra A, Sotomayor EM, Seto E. Histone deacetylases and the immunological network: implications in cancer and inflammation. Oncogene 2010;29(2):157−73.

[49] Minucci S, Pelicci PG. Histone deacetylase inhibitors and the promise of epigenetic (and more) treatments for cancer. Nat Rev Cancer 2006;6:38−51.

[50] Napolitani G, Rinaldi A, Bertoni F, Sallusto F, Lanzavecchia A. Selected Toll-like receptor agonist combinations synergistically trigger a T helper type 1-polarizing program in dendritic cells. Nat Immunol 2005;6:769.

[51] Trinchieri G. Interleukin-12 and the regulation of innate resistance and adaptive immunity. Nat Rev Immunol 2003;3(2):133−46.

[52] Li MO, Flavell RA. Contextual regulation of inflammation: a duet by transforming growth factor-beta and interleukin-10. Immunity 2008;28(4):468−76.

[53] Rubtsov YP, Rasmussen JP, Chi EY, Fontenot J, Castelli L, Ye X, et al. Regulatory T cell-derived interleukin-10 limits inflammation at environmental interfaces. Immunity 2008;28(4):546−58.

[54] Moore KW, de Waal Malefyt R, Coffman RL, O'Garra A. Interleukin-10 and the interleukin-10 receptor. Annu Rev Immunol 2001;19(1):683−765.

[55] Zhang X, Edwards JP, Mosser Dynamic DM, Transient. Remodeling of the Macrophage IL-10 Promoter during Transcription. J Immunol 2006;177(2):1282−8.

[56] Yao Y, Li W, Kaplan MH, Chang CH. Interleukin (IL)-4 inhibits IL-10 to promote IL-12 production by dendritic cells. J Exp Med 2005;201(12):1899−903.

[57] Lagger S, Meunier D, Mikula M, Brunmeir R, Schlederer M, Artaker M. Crucial function of histone deacetylase 1 for differentiation of teratomas in mice and humans. Embo J 2010;29:3992−4007.

[58] Lagger G, O'Carroll D, Rembold M, Khier H, Tischler J, Weitzer G. Essential function of histone deacetylase 1 in proliferation control and CDK inhibitor repression. Embo J 2002;21:2672−81.

[59] Khan O, La Thangue NB. HDAC inhibitors in cancer biology: emerging mechanisms and clinical applications. Immunol Cell Biol 2012;90(1):85−94.

[60] Enya K, Hayashi H, Takii T, Ohoka N, Kanata S, Okamoto T, et al. The interaction with Sp1 and reduction in the activity of histone deacetylase 1 are critical for the constitutive gene expression of IL-1 alpha in human melanoma cells. J Leukoc Biol 2008;83(1):190−9.

[61] Wang J, Lee S, Teh CE-Y, Bunting K, Ma L, Shannon MF. The transcription repressor, ZEB1, cooperates with CtBP2 and HDAC1 to suppress IL-2 gene activation in T cells. Int Immunol 2009;21(3):227−35.

[62] Lu J, Sun H, Wang X, Liu C, Xu X, Li F, et al. Interleukin-12 p40 promoter activity is regulated by the reversible acetylation mediated by HDAC1 and p300. Cytokine 2005;31(1):46—51.

[63] Jee YK, Gilmour J, Kelly A, Bowen H, Richards D, Soh C, et al. Repression of interleukin-5 transcription by the glucocorticoid receptor targets GATA3 signaling and involves histone deacetylase recruitment. J Biol Chem 2005;280(24):23243—50.

[64] Nusinzon I, Horvath Positive CM, Negative. Regulation of the Innate Antiviral Response and Beta Interferon Gene Expression by Deacetylation. Mol Cell Biol 2006;26(8):3106—13.

[65] Chang S, Collins PL, Aune TM. T-Bet Dependent Removal of Sin3A-Histone Deacetylase Complexes at the Ifng Locus Drives Th1 Differentiation. J Immunol 2008;181(12):8372—81.

[66] Valapour M, Jia G, John TS, Judith K, Antonella C, Vincenzo C, et al. Histone deacetylation inhibits IL4 gene expression in T cells. J Allergy Clin Immunol 2002;109(2):238—45.

[67] Xu M, Nie L, Kim SH, Sun XH. STAT5-induced Id-1 transcription involves recruitment of HDAC1 and deacetylation of C/EBPbeta. Embo J 2003;22(4):893—904.

[68] Kato N, Tanaka J, Sugita J, Toubai T, Miura Y, Ibata M, et al. Regulation of the expression of MHC class I-related chain A, B (MICA, MICB) via chromatin remodeling and its impact on the susceptibility of leukemic cells to the cytotoxicity of NKG2D-expressing cells. Leukemia 2007;21(10):2103—8.

[69] Khan AN, Gregorie CJ, Tomasi TB. Histone deacetylase inhibitors induce TAP, LMP, Tapasin genes and MHC class I antigen presentation by melanoma cells. Cancer Immunol Immunother 2008;57(5):647—54.

[70] Kawabata T, Nishida K, Takasugi K, Ogawa H, Sada K, Kadota Y, et al. Increased activity and expression of histone deacetylase 1 in relation to tumor necrosis factor-alpha in synovial tissue of rheumatoid arthritis. Arthritis Res Ther 2010;12(4):R133.

[71] Reilly CM, Regna N, Mishra N. HDAC inhibition in lupus models. Mol Med 2011;17(5-6):417—25.

[72] Leoni F, Fossati G, Lewis EC, Lee JK, Porro G, Pagani P. The histone deacetylase inhibitor ITF2357 reduces production of pro-inflammatory cytokines in vitro and systemic inflammation in vivo. Mol Med 2005;11:1—15.

[73] Faraco G, Cavone L, Chiarugi A. The therapeutic potential of HDAC inhibitors in the treatment of multiple sclerosis. Mol Med 2011;17(5-6):442—7.

[74] Montgomery RL, Davis CA, Potthoff MJ, Haberland M, Fielitz J, Qi X, et al. Histone deacetylases 1 and 2 redundantly regulate cardiac morphogenesis, growth, and contractility. Genes Dev 2007;21(14):1790—802.

[75] Ito K, Barnes PJ, Adcock IM. Glucocorticoid Receptor Recruitment of Histone Deacetylase 2 Inhibits Interleukin-1beta -Induced Histone H4 Acetylation on Lysines 8 and 12. Mol Cell Biol 2000;20(18): 6891—903.

[76] Kong X, Fang M, Li P, Fang F, Xu Y. HDAC2 deacetylates class II transactivator and suppresses its activity in macrophages and smooth muscle cells. J Mol Cell Cardiol 2009;46(3):292—9.

[77] Marwick JA, Ito K, Adcock IM, Kirkham PA. Oxidative stress and steroid resistance in asthma and COPD: pharmacological manipulation of HDAC-2 as a therapeutic strategy. Expert Opin Ther Targets 2007;11(6):745—55.

[78] Minetti GC, Colussi C, Adami R, Serra C, Mozzetta C, Parente V, et al. Functional and morphological recovery of dystrophic muscles in mice treated with deacetylase inhibitors. Nat Med 2006;12(10):1147—50.

[79] Huber LC, Brock M, Hemmatazad H, Giger OT, Moritz F, Trenkmann M, et al. Histone deacetylase/acetylase activity in total synovial tissue derived from rheumatoid arthritis and osteoarthritis patients. Arthritis Rheum 2007;56(4):1087—93.

[80] Montgomery RL, Potthoff MJ, Haberland M, Qi X, Matsuzaki S, Humphries KM, et al. Maintenance of cardiac energy metabolism by histone deacetylase 3 in mice. J Clin Invest 2008;118(11):3588—97.

[81] KrÃmer OH, Knauer SK, Greiner G, Jandt E, Reichardt S, GÃhrs K-H, et al. A phosphorylation-acetylation switch regulates STAT1 signaling. Genes Dev 2009;23(2):223—35.

[82] Zhang Y, Tuzova M, Xiao Z-XJ, Cruikshank WW, Center DM. Pro-IL-16 Recruits Histone Deacetylase 3 to the Skp2 Core Promoter through Interaction with Transcription Factor GABP. J Immunol 2008;180(1): 402—8.

[83] Watamoto K, Towatari M, Ozawa Y, Miyata Y, Okamoto M, Abe A, et al. Altered interaction of HDAC5 with GATA-1 during MEL cell differentiation. Oncogene 2003;22(57):9176—84.

[84] Ozawa Y, Towatari M, Tsuzuki S, Hayakawa F, Maeda T, Miyata Y, et al. Histone deacetylase 3 associates with and represses the transcription factor GATA-2. Blood 2001;98(7):2116—23.

[85] Chen GY, Osada H, Santamaria-Babi LF, Kannagi R. Interaction of GATA-3/T-bet transcription factors regulates expression of sialyl Lewis X homing receptors on Th1/Th2 lymphocytes. Proc Natl Acad Sci U S A 2006;103(45):16894—9.

[86] Kuwatsuka Y, Ogawa F, Iwata Y, Komura K, Muroi E, Hara T, et al. Decreased levels of autoantibody against histone deacetylase 3 in patients with systemic sclerosis. Autoimmunity 2009;42(2):120—5.

369

[87] Bhaskara S, Chyla BJ, Amann JM, Knutson SK, Cortez D, Sun Z-W, et al. Deletion of Histone Deacetylase 3 Reveals Critical Roles in S Phase Progression and DNA Damage Control. Mol Cell 2008;30(1):61—72.

[88] Icardi L, Lievens S, Mori R, Piessevaux J, De Cauwer L, De Bosscher K, et al. Opposed regulation of type I IFN-induced STAT3 and ISGF3 transcriptional activities by histone deacetylases (HDACS) 1 and 2. FASEB J 2012;26(1):240—9.

[89] Kortylewski M, Kujawski M, Wang T, Wei S, Zhang S, Pilon-Thomas S, et al. Inhibiting Stat3 signaling in the hematopoietic system elicits multicomponent antitumor immunity. Nat Med 2005;11(12):1314—21.

[90] Wang T, Niu G, Kortylewski M, Burdelya L, Shain K, Zhang S, et al. Regulation of the innate and adaptive immune responses by Stat-3 signaling in tumor cells. Nat Med 2004;10(1):48—54.

[91] Li H, Ou X, Xiong J, Wang T. HPV16E7 mediates HADC chromatin repression and downregulation of MHC class I genes in HPV16 tumorigenic cells through interaction with an MHC class I promoter. Biochem Biophys Res Commun 2006;349(4):1315—21.

[92] Haberland M, Mokalled MH, Montgomery RL, Olson EN. Epigenetic control of skull morphogenesis by histone deacetylase 8. Genes Dev 2009;23(14):1625—30.

[93] Chang S, McKinsey TA, Zhang CL, Richardson JA, Hill JA, Olson EN. Histone Deacetylases 5 and 9 Govern Responsiveness of the Heart to a Subset of Stress Signals and Play Redundant Roles in Heart Development. Mol Cell Biol 2004;24(19):8467—76.

[94] Vega RB, Matsuda K, Oh J, Barbosa AC, Yang X, Meadows E, et al. Histone Deacetylase 4 Controls Chondrocyte Hypertrophy during Skeletogenesis. Cell 2004;119(4):555—66.

[95] Schmeck B, Lorenz J, N'Guessan PD, Opitz B, van Laak V, Zahlten J, et al. Histone Acetylation and Flagellin Are Essential for Legionella pneumophila-Induced Cytokine Expression. J Immunol 2008;181(2):940—7.

[96] Chang S, Young BD, Li S, Qi X, Richardson JA, Olson EN. Histone Deacetylase 7 Maintains Vascular Integrity by Repressing Matrix Metalloproteinase 10. Cell 2006;126(2):321—34.

[97] Li B, Samanta A, Song X, Iacono KT, Bembas K, Tao R, et al. FOXP3 interactions with histone acetyltransferase and class II histone deacetylases are required for repression. Proc Natl Acad Sci U S A 2007;104(11):6.

[98] Bettini ML, Pan F, Bettini M, Finkelstein D, Rehg JE, Floess S, et al. Loss of epigenetic modification driven by the Foxp3 transcription factor leads to regulatory T cell insufficiency. Immunity 2012;36(5):717—30.

[99] Navarro MN, Goebel J, Feijoo-Carnero C, Morrice N, Cantrell DA. Phosphoproteomic analysis reveals an intrinsic pathway for the regulation of histone deacetylase 7 that controls the function of cytotoxic T lymphocytes. Nat Immunol 2011;12(4):352—61.

[100] Zhang CL, McKinsey TA, Chang S, Antos CL, Hill JA, Olson EN. Class II Histone Deacetylases Act as Signal-Responsive Repressors of Cardiac Hypertrophy. Cell 2002;110(4):479—88.

[101] Tao R, de Zoeten EF, Ozkaynak E, Chen C, Wang L, Porrett PM, et al. Deacetylase inhibition promotes the generation and function of regulatory T cells. Nat Med 2007;13(11):1299—307.

[102] de Zoeten EF, Wang L, Sai H, Dillmann WH, Hancock WW. Inhibition of HDAC9 increases T regulatory cell function and prevents colitis in mice. Gastroenterology 2010;138(2):583—94.

[103] Grozinger CM, Hassig CA, Schreiber SL. Three proteins define a class of human histone deacetylases related to yeast Hda1p. Proc Natl Acad Sci U S A 1999;96(9):6.

[104] Verdel A, Curtet S, Brocard MP, Rousseaux S, Lemercier C, Yoshida M, et al. Active maintenance of mHDA2/mHDAC6 histone-deacetylase in the cytoplasm. Curr Biol 2000;10(12):747—9.

[105] Palijan A, Fernandes I, Bastien Y, Tang L, Verway M, Kourelis M, et al. Function of Histone Deacetylase 6 as a Cofactor of Nuclear Receptor Coregulator LCoR. J Biol Chem 2009;284(44):30264—74.

[106] Toropainen S, Väisänen S, Heikkinen S, Carlberg C. The Down-regulation of the Human MYC Gene by the Nuclear Hormone 1[alpha],25-dihydroxyvitamin D3 is Associated with Cycling of Corepressors and Histone Deacetylases. J Mol Biol 2010;400(3):284—94.

[107] Todd PK, Oh SY, Krans A, Pandey UB, Di Prospero NA, Min K-T, et al. Histone Deacetylases Suppress CGG Repeatâ Induced Neurodegeneration Via Transcriptional Silencing in Models of Fragile X Tremor Ataxia Syndrome. PLoS Genet 2010;6(12):e1001240.

[108] Valenzuela-Fernández A, Cabrero JR, Serrador JM, Sánchez-Madrid F. HDAC6: a key regulator of cytoskeleton, cell migration and cell-cell interactions. Trends Cell Biol 2008;18(6):291—7.

[109] Aldana-Masangkay GI, Sakamoto KM. The role of HDAC6 in cancer. J Biomed Biotechnol 2010;2011:875824.

[110] Serrador JM, Cabrero JR, Sancho D, Mittelbrunn M, Urzainqui A, Sanchez-Madrid F. HDAC6 deacetylase activity links the tubulin cytoskeleton with immune synapse organization. Immunity 2004;20(4):417—28.

[111] de Zoeten EF, Wang L, Butler K, Beier UH, Akimova T, Sai H, et al. Histone deacetylase 6 and heat shock protein 90 control the functions of Foxp3(+) T-regulatory cells. Mol Cell Biol 2011;31(10):2066—78.

[112] Villagra A, Cheng F, Wang HW, Suarez I, Glozak M, Maurin M, et al. The histone deacetylase HDAC11 regulates the expression of interleukin 10 and immune tolerance. Nat Immunol 2009;10(1):92—100.

[113] Santo L, Hideshima T, Kung AL, Tseng JC, Tamang D, Yang M, et al. Preclinical activity, pharmacodynamic, and pharmacokinetic properties of a selective HDAC6 inhibitor, ACY-1215, in combination with bortezomib in multiple myeloma. Blood 2012;119(11):2579—89.

[114] Zhang Y, Kwon S, Yamaguchi T, Cubizolles F, Rousseaux S, Kneissel M, et al. Mice lacking histone deacetylase 6 have hyperacetylated tubulin but are viable and develop normally. Mol Cell Biol 2008;28(5): 1688—701.

[115] Kao H-Y, Lee C-H, Komarov A, Han CC, Evans RM. Isolation and Characterization of Mammalian HDAC10, a Novel Histone Deacetylase. J Biol Chem 2002;277(1):187—93.

[116] Osada H, Tatematsu Y, Saito H, Yatabe Y, Mitsudomi T, Takahashi T. Reduced expression of class II histone deacetylase genes is associated with poor prognosis in lung cancer patients. Int J Cancer 2004;112: 26—32.

[117] Gao L, Cueto MA, Asselbergs F, Atadja Cloning P, Characterization Functional. of HDAC11, a Novel Member of the Human Histone Deacetylase Family. J Biol Chem 2002;277(28):25748—55.

[118] Bradbury CA, Khanim FL, Hayden R, Bunce CM, White DA, Drayson MT, et al. Histone deacetylases in acute myeloid leukaemia show a distinctive pattern of expression that changes selectively in response to deacetylase inhibitors. Leukemia 2005;19(10):1751—9.

[119] Buglio D, Khaskhely NM, Voo KS, Martinez-Valdez H, Liu Y-J, Younes A. HDAC11 plays an essential role in regulating OX40 ligand expression in Hodgkin lymphoma. Blood 2011;117(10):8.

[120] Shoji M, Ninomiya I, Makino I, Kinoshita J, Nakamura K, Oyama K, et al. Valproic acid, a histone deacetylase inhibitor, enhances radiosensitivity in esophageal squamous cell carcinoma. Int J Oncol 2012;40(6): 2140—6.

[121] Leder A, S O, P L. Differentiation of erythroleukemic cells in the presence of inhibitors of DNA synthesis. Science 1975;190:893—4.

[122] Yoshida M, Kijima M, Akita M, Beppu T. Potent and specific inhibition of mammalian histone deacetylase both in vivo and in vitro by trichostatin A. J Biol Chem 1990;265(28):17174—9.

[123] Marks PA, Breslow R. Dimethyl sulfoxide to vorinostat: development of this histone deacetylase inhibitor as an anticancer drug. Nat Biotech 2007;25(1):84—90.

[124] Piekarz RL, Frye R, Turner M, Wright JJ, Allen SL, Kirschbaum MH, et al. Phase II multi-institutional trial of the histone deacetylase inhibitor romidepsin as monotherapy for patients with cutaneous T-cell lymphoma. J Clin Oncol 2009;27(32):5410—7.

[125] Mandl-Weber S, Meinel FG, Jankowsky R, Oduncu F, Schmidmaier R, Baumann P. The novel inhibitor of histone deacetylase resminostat (RAS2410) inhibits proliferation and induces apoptosis in multiple myeloma (MM) cells. Br J Haematol 2010;149(4):518—28.

[126] Marks PA, Richon VM, Rifkind RA. Histone Deacetylase Inhibitors: Inducers of Differentiation or Apoptosis of Transformed Cells. J Natl Cancer Inst 2000;92(15):1210—6.

[127] Dokmanovic M, Clarke C, Histone Deacetylase Inhibitors Marks PA, Overview, PerspectivesMol. Cancer Res 2007;5:981.

[128] Shapira Y, Agmon-Levin N, Shoenfeld Y. Defining and analyzing geoepidemiology and human autoimmunity. J Autoimmun 2010;34(3):J168—77.

[129] Kelly WK, O'Connor OA, Krug LM, Chiao JH, Heaney M, Curley T, et al. Phase I Study of an Oral Histone Deacetylase Inhibitor, Suberoylanilide Hydroxamic Acid, in Patients With Advanced Cancer. J Clin Oncol 2005;23(17):3923—31.

[130] Galli M, Salmoiraghi S, Golay J, Gozzini A, Crippa C, Pescosta N, et al. A phase II multiple dose clinical trial of histone deacetylase inhibitor ITF2357 in patients with relapsed or progressive multiple myeloma. Ann Hematol 2010;89(2):185—90.

[131] Grabiec AM, Reedquist KA. Histone deacetylases in RA: epigenetics and epiphenomena. Arthritis Res Ther 2010;12(5):142.

[132] Leoni F, Fossati G, Lewis EC, Lee JK, Porro G, Pagani P, et al. The histone deacetylase inhibitor ITF2357 reduces production of pro-inflammatory cytokines in vitro and systemic inflammation in vivo. Mol Med 2005;11(1-12):1—15.

[133] Vojinovic J, Damjanov N. HDAC inhibition in rheumatoid arthritis and juvenile idiopathic arthritis. Mol Med 2011;17(5-6):397—403.

[134] Qi Q, Guo Q, Tan G, Mao Y, Tang H, Zhou C, et al. Predictors of the scleroderma phenotype in fibroblasts from systemic sclerosis patients. J Eur Acad Dermatol Venereol 2009;23(2):160—8.

[135] Mastronardi FG, Noor A, Wood DD, Paton T, Moscarello MA. Peptidyl argininedeiminase 2 CpG island in multiple sclerosis white matter is hypomethylated. J Neurosci Res 2007;85(9):2006—16.

[136] Glauben R, Siegmund B. Inhibition of histone deacetylases in inflammatory bowel diseases. Mol Med 2011;17(5-6):426—33.

371

[137] Zhang K, Zhang R, Li X, Yin G, Niu X. Promoter methylation status of p15 and p21 genes in HPP-CFCs of bone marrow of patients with psoriasis. Eur J Dermatol 2009;19(2):141–6.

[138] D'Cruz DP, Khamashta MA, Hughes GR. Systemic lupus erythematosus. Lancet 2007;369(9561):587–96.

[139] Rahman A, Isenberg DA. Systemic lupus erythematosus. N Engl J Med 2008;358(9):929–39.

[140] Moser KL, Kelly JA, Lessard CJ, Harley JB. Recent insights into the genetic basis of systemic lupus erythematosus. Genes Immun 2009;10(5):373–9.

[141] Mishra N, Brown DR, Olorenshaw IM, Kammer GM. Trichostatin A reverses skewed expression of CD154, interleukin-10, and interferon-gamma gene and protein expression in lupus T cells. Proc Natl Acad Sci U S A 2001;98(5):2628–33.

[142] Chung YL, Lee MY, Wang AJ, Yao LF. A therapeutic strategy uses histone deacetylase inhibitors to modulate the expression of genes involved in the pathogenesis of rheumatoid arthritis. Mol Ther 2003;8(5):707–17.

[143] Grabiec AM, Krausz S, de Jager W, Burakowski T, Groot D, Sanders ME, et al. Histone deacetylase inhibitors suppress inflammatory activation of rheumatoid arthritis patient synovial macrophages and tissue. J Immunol 2010;184(5):2718–28.

[144] Maciejewska Rodrigues H, Jungel A, Gay RE, Gay S. Innate immunity, epigenetics and autoimmunity in rheumatoid arthritis. Mol Immunol 2009;47(1):12–8.

[145] Tomasi TB, Magner WJ, Khan AN. Epigenetic regulation of immune escape genes in cancer. Cancer Immunol Immunother 2006;55(10):1159–84.

[146] Khan A, Tomasi T. Histone deacetylase regulation of immune gene expression in tumor cells. Immunol Res 2008;40(2):164–78.

[147] Setiadi AF, Omilusik K, David MD, Seipp RP, Hartikainen J, Gopaul R, et al. Epigenetic enhancement of antigen processing and presentation promotes immune recognition of tumors. Cancer Res 2008;68(23):9601–7.

[148] Vo DD, Prins RM, Begley JL, Donahue TR, Morris LF, Bruhn KW, et al. Enhanced Antitumor Activity Induced by Adoptive T-Cell Transfer and Adjunctive Use of the Histone Deacetylase Inhibitor LAQ824. Cancer Res 2009;69(22):8693–9.

[149] Wang H, Cheng F, Woan K, Sahakian E, Merino O, Rock-Klotz J, et al. Histone Deacetylase Inhibitor LAQ824 Augments Inflammatory Responses in Macrophages through Transcriptional Regulation of IL-10. J Immunol 2011;186(7):11.

[150] Buglio D, Georgakis GV, Hanabuchi S, Arima K, Khaskhely NM, Liu Y-J, et al. Vorinostat inhibits STAT6-mediated TH2 cytokine and TARC production and induces cell death in Hodgkin lymphoma cell lines. Blood 2008;112(4):1424–33.

[151] Im SH, Hueber A, Monticelli S, Kang KH, Rao A. Chromatin-level regulation of the IL10 gene in T cells. J Biol Chem 2004;279(45):46818–25.

[152] Reddy P, Sun Y, Toubai T, Duran-Struuck R, Clouthier SG, Weisiger E, et al. Histone deacetylase inhibition modulates indoleamine 2,3-dioxygenase-dependent DC functions and regulates experimental graft-versus-host disease in mice. J Clin Invest 2008;118(7):2562–73.

[153] Reddy P, Maeda Y, Hotary K, Liu C, Reznikov LL, Dinarello CA, et al. Histone deacetylase inhibitor suberoylanilide hydroxamic acid reduces acute graft-versus-host disease and preserves graft-versus-leukemia effect. Proc Natl Acad Sci U S A 2004;101(11):3921–6.

[154] Bode KA, Schroder K, Hume DA, Ravasi T, Heeg K, Sweet MJ, et al. Histone deacetylase inhibitors decrease Toll-like receptor-mediated activation of proinflammatory gene expression by impairing transcription factor recruitment. Immunology 2007;122(4):596–606.

[155] Szyf M. Epigenetic therapeutics in autoimmune disease. Clin Rev Allergy Immunol 2010;39(1):62–77.

CHAPTER 23

Molecular Profiling of Immunotherapeutic Resistance

Davide Bedognetti[1,2], Ena Wang[1], Marimo Sato-Matsushita[1,4], Francesco M Marincola[1,5], Maria Libera Ascierto[1,2,3]

[1]Infectious Disease and Immunogenetics Section (IDIS), Department of Transfusion Medicine (DTM), FOCIS Center of Excellence, Clinical Center (CC) and Trans-National Institutes of Health (NIH) Center for Human Immunology (CHI), NIH, Bethesda, MD USA
[2]Department of Internal Medicine (DiMI), University of Genoa, Genoa, Italy
[3]Center of Excellence for Biomedical Research (CEBR), University of Genoa, Genoa, Italy
[4]Institute of Medical Science, The University of Tokyo, Tokyo, Japan
[5]Sidra Medical and Research Centre, Doha, Qatar

I. INTRODUCTION—THE BEDSIDE TO BENCH AND BACK (BB&B) APPROACH TO TUMOR IMMUNOLOGY: *IN VIVO VERITAS*

In medicine, we call *Bedside to Bench and Back* a translational approach to medical problems based on the direct study of humans [1–6]. From a philosophical point of view, the *Bedside to Bench and Back* integrates a sequential observationalist-inductivist account of science (from *Bedside to Bench*) with deductive methods and critical rationalism (*and Back*). Although it could sound semantically complicated, it represents, from our point of view, the most natural, simple, and effective approach to the complexity of human diseases.

The observationalist-inductivist reasoning is a process of using observations to develop general principles about a specific subject [7]. A group of similar specimens, events, or subjects are first observed and studied; findings from the observations are then used to make broad statements about the subjects (patients) that were examined (from *Bedside*). These statements may then become laws of nature or theories. In the *Bedside to Bench and Back* approach, descriptive discovery-generating investigations are aimed at defining a theory able to explain the target observation (clinical question, generated at the patient bed). These theories are then renamed as "hypotheses" and are pretested through a deductive approach which moves from "theory" (hypothesis) to observations or findings through the design of hypothesis-driven investigations that could be pretested *ex vivo*, *in vitro* or *in vivo* in animals models (to *Bench*) but need to be conclusively validated (tested) in humans (and *Back* (to the bedside)). The last step fits some concepts raised by critical rationalism [8]. With critical rationalism, the philosopher Karl Popper argued that scientific theories were often generated by the creative imagination linked to the specific cultural setting, and they are irreducibly conjectural or hypothetical. Logically, no number of positive outcomes at the level of experimental testing can confirm a scientific theory, but a single counterexample is (conceptually) logically decisive. According to critical rationalism a theory should be considered scientific if, and only if, it is (conceptually) falsifiable (Wikipedia: http://en.

Cancer Immunotherapy. http://dx.doi.org/10.1016/B978-0-12-394296-8.00023-3

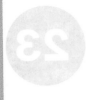
wikipedia.org/wiki/Critical_rationalism). Some implications of this interesting point of view are that a theory is better than another one if it is less likely to be true (i.e., if it contains a higher amount of information that determines a greater chance to be falsified). Paradoxically, even a highly unlikely theory that clashes with current observations (for example, "all the sheep are black") must be preferred to one that fits observations perfectly, but is highly probable (such as "all sheep have a color"). We recognize that scientific theories of human biology are unlikely to turn out to be true, due to the lack of adequate algorithms able to decodify stochastic systems with a number of hidden variables and to handle biases due to multidimensionality of the data produced by modern high-throughput technologies. However, those theories should be at least scientific or, in other words, falsifiable in nature.

For this reason, planning of the final step *and Back* (to Bedside) is necessary since hypotheses (theories) generated from humans can be conclusively validated (but more important falsified) only in humans and not in animals. This process should determine the continued selection of more informative theories.

In translational medicine, this last logical step could be represented by the design of clinical-translational studies assessing the therapeutic approach developed *in vitro* and pretested in animal models, but based on conclusion generated by relevant, and informative, observations in humans.

Although it could appear obvious that the conclusive solution of clinical questions should be sought by studying humans, this does not seem the case, especially for certain branches of medicine, including oncology and, in particular, tumor immunology.

A prodromic *Bedside to Bench and Back* approach led William Coley in the 1890s to define a hypothesis that represents the basis of modern immunotherapy. Starting from direct observation that spontaneous tumor regression often followed infective episodes, Coley injected bacterial products (also known as Coley's toxin or Coley's vaccine) directly into tumor, achieving dramatic response in some cases [9,10]. A hundred years later, modern medicine has conclusively demonstrated that the passive or active elicitation of the immune system can be pursued as effective cancer therapy [11–14].

However, in the last 20 years, a flurry of clinical trials and basic research not accompanied by an adequate number of observational bias-free studies has led to a disharmonic growth of scientific knowledge [3,15]. As a consequence, a myriad of non-evidence-based hypotheses have interacted, in a competitive manner, with the few evidence-based hypotheses generated from the combination of observational and mechanistic investigations in humans leading to the accumulation of clinical breakdown and "mysterious" successes [11,15,16]. It is curious, for example, that the only vaccine approved so far by the FDA for the treatment of metastatic cancer patients prolonged the overall survival without any impact on either progression-free survival nor on tumor regression [17]. As for oncoimmunology, there is a tremendous lack of studies assessing the phenomenon of immune-mediated tumor rejection where it occurs (i.e., in the tumor).

In addition to the intrinsic practical difficulties related to the accessibility of tumor sites in humans and the collection and storage of human samples, the idea that the reasons "why" tumor rejection occur could be found by bypassing the characterization of "how" this phenomenon occurs has certainly contributed to the delay in the identification of the appropriate target mechanisms. This has contributed to the delay in the development of more effective cancer treatments.

Considering the advanced development of biomedical technologies, the first step of a strategy aimed at decrypting the dynamism of tumor–host interplay should consist (conceptually) in the design of translational studies covering genomic, epigenomic, transcriptomic and proteomic analyses at different time-points in relation to treatment by collecting different biological samples including, at least, tumor and blood samples. Although findings from such an approach are not available yet, the use of whole genome gene expression profiling (microarray), which allows us to catch in real-time the physiology of disease by simultaneously ascertaining the expression of thousands of human genes, has led to intriguing hypotheses of "how" tumor rejection occurs. Here, we will describe results of such studies focusing on our work and referring to the information derived from investigations from other groups who assessed tumor—host interactions through similar approaches.

II. STRATEGIES TO IDENTIFY MOLECULAR PATHWAYS ASSOCIATED WITH IMMUNORESPONSIVENESS AND IMMUNORESISTANCE FOLLOWING IMMUNOTHERAPY

In the 1980s, almost 100 years after Coley's observation, data from clinical trials employing pro-inflammatory cytokines (interleukin-(IL)-2 and interferon-(IF)-α) for the treatment of metastatic cancer patients conclusively demonstrated that the elicitation of immune response can trigger, in some cases, an efficient antitumor response [18–22]. A decade after, the description of tumor antigens recognized by autologous T cells (tumor antigens: TAs), followed by the molecular characterization of human cancer-specific epitopes, provided evidence that CD8+ T cells can recognize and eventually kill cancer cells [23,24]. The subsequent natural step was the development of anticancer vaccines [13,25–28]. The induction *in vivo* of a clonal expansion of CD8+ T cells that could selectively recognize cancer cells offered an incredible opportunity to study the dynamics of antitumor response. Together with the evidence that cancer vaccine could trigger tumor rejection, the discrepancy between clinical and immunologic end-point response represents one of the most important lessons learned from vaccination studies. In fact, results of clinical trials testing TA-based vaccines showed that this strategy is extremely effective in inducing cancer cell-specific cellular responses, which are, however, only rarely followed by a clinically detectable tumor rejection [16].

The observation that the generation of TA-specific immune responses may represent a necessary but not sufficient condition for the induction of cancer rejection has led to the development of novel approaches capable of investigating events downstream of the TA-specific T-cell generation and of catching tumor—host dynamism in its globality by studying the tumor microenvironment. The first step of our strategy was to apply high-throughput discovery-driven approaches by profiling *ex vivo* at different time points tumor biopsies from patients treated with immunotherapy. A discovery-driven *Bedside to Bench* approach was needed, since too many "hypotheses" largely based on animal models were available and, as a matter of fact, no single solid (falsifiable) hypotheses based on results from experimental human investigations that could have been prospectively tested in humans existed.

Using this approach we tried to assess the following questions:

1) Which molecular pathways are activated in tumor (intended as host/tumor interaction) following immunotherapy?
2) Which molecular pathways are activated in tumors undergoing regression as compared to treatment-resistant tumors following immunotherapy?
3) Which molecular pathways can identify tumor lesions more likely to respond to immunotherapy?

The first two questions try to identify mechanistic signatures that provide proof of mechanism of action of a given agent/agent combination or the occurrence of a certain phenomenon (e.g., tumor regression or tumor progression). The third one seeks to define predictive signatures, which are signatures that classify lesions (patients) that are more likely to be sensitive or resistant to a specific treatment.

Predictive signatures could be assessed by the analysis of tumor biopsies at a single time point (i.e., before treatment) and major limiting factors for these analyses are an adequate preservation of samples for a gene expression profile and, as for its validation, the need for large and homogeneous sample sizes and a standardized procedure. However, a meaningful determination of mechanistic signatures also requires the collection of tumor samples at different time points, which is possible only if the target lesion is not removed. Toward this purpose we developed and validated a refined technology for linear amplification of mRNA species, which allows the evaluation of transcriptional profiling using microarray technology by the utilization of minimal starting material, such as that obtained by fine-needle aspirated (FNAs) [29]. We therefore conducted a series of investigations where gene expression profiling was assessed in tumor lesions biopsied at consecutive time points (i.e., pre- and posttreatment, at a time when immune rejection is likely to occur). Applying this strategy, we studied melanoma patients treated with an interleukin-(IL)-2 based approach and basal cell carcinoma treated with imiquimod (a Toll-like receptor agonist) [30—35].

III. THE EMERGING OF A MORE FALSIFIABLE, INFORMATIVE AND PREFERRED THEORY: THE IMMUNOLOGIC CONSTANT OF REJECTION (ICR)

Although several speculations could be made to explain why cancer cells escape the host immune system, we observed that the activation of common and nonredundant inflammatory pathways are necessary for the occurrence of immune-mediated tumor rejection, while resistance to treatment is associated with the lack of their coordinate activation [30—35]. Lesions undergoing regression upon therapy display a powerful acute inflammatory process sustained by the activation of specific pro-inflammatory pathways [31,32,34—36]. This is in line with the observation that during IL-2 therapy these lesions become tender and swell before regression and, similarly, basal cell carcinomas become extremely inflamed during treatment with imiquimod (a Toll-like-treceptor-(TLR)-7 agonist), while the surrounding skin remains unaffected. Interestingly, by studying transcriptomic changes in peripheral mononuclear cell (PBMC), one of the main mechanisms of action of IL-2 *in vivo* seems to be the induction of an inflammatory status through the direct and indirect induction of the same pathways whose activation mediate the switch from chronic to acute inflammation-sustaining immune-mediated tumor rejection [30,32,33]. Similar pathways responsible for the activation of this acute (and specific) inflammatory process observed in post-treatment rejecting lesions are found partially pre-activated in lesions more likely to respond to treatment, suggesting that tumors intrinsically unable to display a polarized inflammatory status are also quite refractory to switch on those pathways following treatment [34,35]. Others [37] observed similar patterns by studying biopsies of tissues suffering chronic graft versus host disease and similar patterns were observed in the liver during clearance of HCV infection [38—42]. Several authors described the presence of these pathways in organs from transplant patients undergoing allograft rejections, recently summarized in a meta-analysis conducted by our group [43], and similar signatures were observed in the destructive phases of acute cardiovascular events, [44,45] chronic obstructive pulmonary disease, [46] and placental villitis [47].

Epidemiological and observational studies in humans have repetitively shown that chronic inflammation promotes tumorigenesis [48]. However, the presence of immune cells in tumor lesions has often been seen in a simplistic way as the proof of the protumorigenic effect of tumor inflammation [49—51]. When a temporal dimension is added to the static observation and established inflammatory tumors are removed and patients are prospectively followed, intriguing hypotheses on the role of tumor inflammation in counteracting tumor spreading and progression emerge [51,52].

Large retrospective studies involving more than 1000 patients for each cancer site have conclusively shown that the presence of a T-cell infiltrate is a favorable prognostic factor for melanoma [53], breast [54] ovarian [55] and colorectal cancer patients [49,56,57]. Since these studies were designed to detect prognostic biomarkers (i.e., biomarkers predictive of clinical benefit independently to the treatment administered), but a considerable number of patients were treated with adjuvant chemotherapy (breast and cancer patients), hormonotherapy (breast cancer patients), or immunotherapy (melanoma patients), it is not clear whether this inflammatory status could have also optimized the efficacy of the treatment administered or rather if it could have limited the tumor spreading or both. Notably, however, T-cell infiltrate has been found to predict the efficacy of neoadjuvant therapy in breast cancer patients, suggesting that antitumor immune response is an important chemotherapeutic adjuvant [58].

Only in the last 5–7 years, however, have scientific advances explained and dissected these broad observations more in-depth by giving molecular precision to this phenomenon [49,56,57,59–66]. These studies, in combination with those that have defined mechanistic and predictive molecular biomarkers in cancer immunotherapy and with those that have assessed other conditions of immune-mediated rejection, led to the definition of a more informative (i.e., more falsifiable, and therefore preferred) theory on the phenomenon of the immunomediated tissue destruction process: the immunologic constant of rejection (ICR).

High-throughput gene expression profile studies revealed that mechanistic and predictive molecular pathways observed in the immunotherapeutic setting almost perfectly overlap with those that are described to be associated with the development of allograft rejection [65], and with the decreased risk of relapse and/or survival after primary tumor excision in colorecal cancer [56,57,61,64], and, more recently, also in melanoma [67] and breast cancer [65,66].

These inflammatory pathways illustrate a process characterized by the coordinated modular activation of interferon-stimulated genes (ISGs) toward a T-helper 1 polarization, the recruitment of cytotoxic cells through the massive production of specific chemokine ligands (CXCR3 and CCR5 ligands), and the activation of immune effector function (IEF) genes (granzyme, granulysis and perforin; genes expressed by NK cells and CD8+ and T helper-1 CD4+ cells upon activation). We defined these modules, which we called the ICR pathways (Figure 23.1), as follows:

1. IFN-γ module → STAT-1/IRF-1/IFN-γ-stimulated genes pathway
2. Specific T helper-1/NK chemokine module → CXCR3/CXCR3 ligand (CXCL9, -10, and -11) and CCR5/CCR5 ligand (CCL3, -4, and -5) pathway
3. Immuno-effector function module → Granzyme/Perforin/Granulisin/TIA-1 pathway

Strikingly, all the immunotherapeutic approaches assessed so far seem to act through the common induction of the ICR modules, and the degree of activation correlates with their antitumor activity. The lack of their pre-activation configures a non-inflammatory cancer phenotype that is not only more resistant to immunotherapeutic treatments but that is also characterized by a poor prognosis (Figure 23.1).

In this chapter we will provide evidence in favor of this hypothesis by referring to investigations performed in humans. These observations indicate the centrality of these pathways in the achievement of an efficient and disruptive tissue destruction reaction and encourages the development of an approach targeting (directly or indirectly) these mechanisms as a strategy to overcome immunotherapeutic resistances.

IV. UNDERSTANDING THE MECHANISM OF ACTIONS OF IMMUNOTHERAPEUTIC AGENTS THROUGH GENE EXPRESSION PROFILING

A. Imiquimod

Imiquimod belongs to a family of synthetic small nucleotide-like molecules with potent pro-inflammatory activity mediated through TLR-7 signaling. TLR-7 plays a fundamental role in pathogen recognition and in the activation of innate immunity. This drug targets

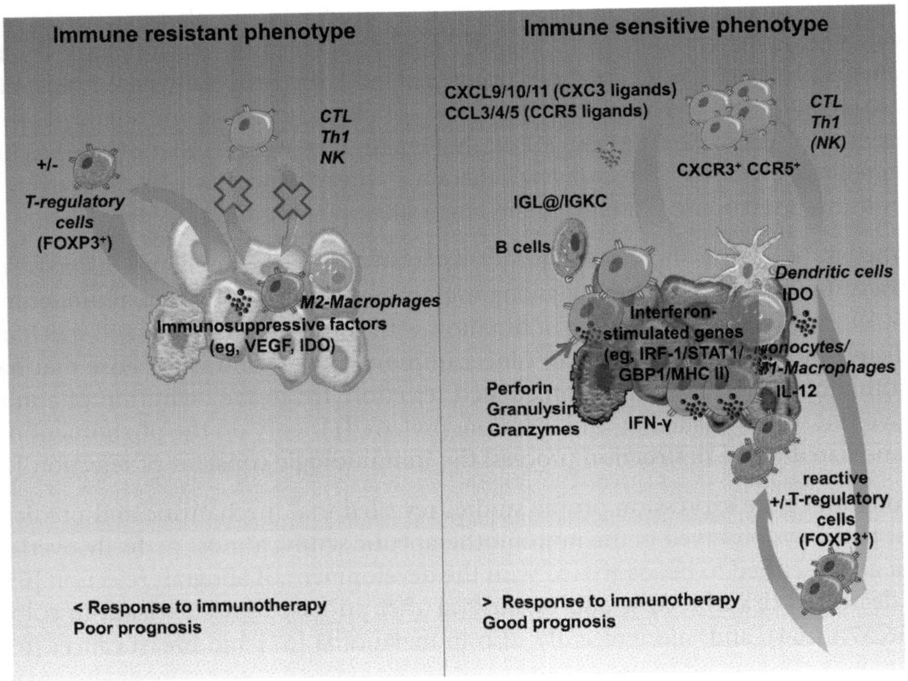

FIGURE 23.1

Immune resistant and immune sensitive cancer phenotypes. The first phenotype is characterized by an immune-resistant phenotype. This quiescent phenotype, which does not express the activation of interferon-stimulated genes and where immune infiltrates are scant and/or display a suppressive phenotype (T-regulatory cells, M2 macrophages) without the activation of immune-effector functions, features a poor outcome and scarce response to immunotherapy. The second is characterized by a polarized T helper-1 inflammatory status driven by interferon-γ stimulated (e.g., IRF-1, STAT1, GBP1, MHC II) genes with production of specific chemoattractants (CXCR3 and CCR5 ligands) and partial activation of the immune-effector function genes (perforin, granzymes, TIA-1, granulysin). This latter phenotype can also be characterized by the activation of B-cell lymphocytes and by counter-activation of suppressive mechanisms (e.g., FOXP3, IDO) and is distinguished by a more favorable prognosis and a better response to immunotherapy.

predominantly TLR-7 (and 8) expressing plasmacytoid dendritic cells with consequent recruitment of other dendiritic cells, macrophages and (eventually) the induction of a T/NK mediated response. It is currently only approved for the local treatment of basal cell carcinoma, since its toxicity prevents systemic administration. The high response rate associated with imiquimod, combined with the easily accessibility of BCC lesions, makes this topical administration an outstanding model for the study of the mechanism of immune-mediated tumor rejection [31]. This model emphasizes the quantitative aspects of immunotherapy suggesting that the high concentrations of immune stimulator that could be achieved with a topical treatment could shift the balance between host and cancer cell interactions in favor of the host by local manipulations of the microenvironment that cannot be easily and specifically achieved through systemic administration due to its toxic effect.

Even though the direct and immediate consequence of the TLR-7 (and 8) stimulation by imiquimod is the mediation of the type I IFN (i.e., IFN-α/β) cascade [68], it is not clear whether this pathway is solely responsible for all the downstream effects ultimately resulting in tumor rejection. Thus, we conducted a prospective, randomized, placebo-controlled double-blinded trial comparing the gene expression profile of paired punch biopsies pre- and posttreatment (approximately 1 day after the last dose administered) [31]. The result of this study, which enrolled 36 patients, demonstrated that the eradication of BCC is a complex multifactorial phenomenon. Of 637 genes specifically induced by imiquimod, only a minority (98 genes) were canonical type I IFN-induced ISGs while the rest portrayed additional immunological functions predominantly involving innate and adaptive immune effector mechanisms. However, IFN-γ transcription was more prevalent than IFN-α transcription. The abundance of IFN-γ suggests that pDCs trigger other immune functions through the production of IFN-α, which in turn activates T and NK cells, selective producers of IFN-γ. Other relevant IFN-γ stimulated genes were class I and class II HLAs, C1QA (complement component 1a) and STAT-1. CXCR3 and CXCR3 ligands (CXCL9 and -10) and CCR5 ligands (CCL3 and -4), were also overinduced. These chemokines represent the major chemotactic factor for T helper-1 cells, activated CD8+ and NK cells, which express both CXCR3 and CCR5. Moreover, the upregulation of cytokine and corresponding receptors within the common γ chain receptor (IL-15 and IL-15 receptor α chain, the IL-2/IL-15 receptor β chain and the common γ chain itself) suggests early activation of NK and CD8+ T cells within the tumor microenvironment, also corroborated by the evidence of the activation NK and CD8+ T cells' cytotoxic mechanisms (granzymes, perforin, granulysin, NK4 and caspases). Immunohistochemistry confirmed the presence of CD8+ T and NK cells within treated lesions, supporting the aforementioned interpretation of gene-expression data.

B. Interleukin-2 (IL-2)

IL-2 has been used in oncology for more than 20 years and it is the only cytokine approved by the FDA for the treatment of metastatic patients. However, its mechanism of action is still not completely understood. We characterized the molecular changes associated with the administration of this cytokine in a series of proteomic and genomic studies assessing gene profile in tumor metastases, PBMC, as well as the modification of peripheral soluble factors in metastatic melanoma patients receiving intravenous IL-2 (720,000 IU/kg, every 8 hours) [30,32,33].

Although our proteomic analyses showed that cytokine patterns varied quantitatively among patients (and could be explained by the different repertoire of immune polymorphism(s) affecting individual responses to immune stimulation), some general concepts emerged. Time course experiments in PBMC *in vitro* and *ex vivo* concordantly suggested that the 3-hour time point provides the most comprehensive overview of the transcriptional changes following IL-2 administration. Moreover, most of the systemic signs of IL-2 are apparent after about 3 hours of its administration, suggesting that the peak of soluble factors is reached at that time point. These considerations led us to choose the 3-hour time point for both the transcriptomic and proteomic analyses. Longitudinal analyses were performed on samples collected after the first and the fourth administration, where the fourth dose was selected as a later time point since it was likely to be reached by most patients before discontinuation due to the toxic effects. As for the soluble factors, we observed that administration of IL-2 induces a cytokine storm after just the first administration, where most of the cytokines investigated (e.g., IFN-γ, IL-10, and TNF-α) increased significantly compared with the baseline value. CXCR3 ligands (i.e., CXCL9, 10 and 11) and CCR5 ligands (i.e., CCL3 and CCL4) were found among the chemokines that significantly increased during the first dose. Although most of the soluble factors increased over time, only six decreased from the first to the fourth dose, including CCR5 ligands (i.e., CCL4, and CCL5). This is intriguing and could help to explain some paradoxical phenomena that were observed by studying the trafficking of tumor infiltrating lymphocytes adoptively transferred in conjunction with the administration of IL-2 (see below) [69]. Similarly, the gene-expression profile of PBMC obtained 3 hours after IL-2 administration showed an upregulation of several IFN-γ inducible genes (e.g., GBP1 and GBP2), including CXCR3 and CCR5 ligands (CXCL10 and CCL4, respectively). These genes were consistently upregulated both in PBMC from patients receiving IL-2 and in PBMC stimulated with the IL-2 *in vitro* at the same time point (i.e., 3 hours after IL-2 administration).

The administration of IL-2 is followed by a dramatic change in leukocyte proportion, characterized by a rapid clearance of lymphocytes and monocytes (but not of neutrophils) within one hour after its administration [33]. Although the density gradient separation almost completely compensated for this shift by eliminating polymorphonuclear cells and leaving a mononuclear population cell comparable with that before treatment, the consistent upregulation of several IFN-γ stimulated genes *in vivo* suggests that they reflect a real activatory status induced by IL-2 administration rather than a shift in cell proportion.

Even though it was suggested that the rapid clearance of lymphocytes following IL-2 administration is due to an increase of the endothelial permeability inducing cell migration into extravascular spaces including tumor sites [70], the study of the microenvironment performed by profiling FNAs of melanoma metastases before therapy and 3 hours after the first and fourth dose of treatment, did not confirm that lymphocytes migrate (at these early time points) into tumor sites [32]. The results of this study surprisingly suggested that, contrary to what was previously believed, IL-2 has little effect on proliferation or migration of T cells at tumor site. The evaluation within tumor metastases of the genes that were consistently modulated on PBMC following IL-2 administration revealed that only a subset of genes was also consistently upregulated in tumor metastases. These genes codify for IFN-γ stimulated genes (i.e., GBP1) and pro-inflammatory chemokines (i.e., CCL2, CCL7 (CCR2 ligands), CCL3, CCL4 (CCR5 ligands), CXCL9, CXCL10 (CXCR3 ligands)), which regulate chemotaxis of monocytes, NK cells and activated T CD8+ and T helper-1 cells. These arrays of cytokines are characteristic of M1 polarized macrophages, which exert a powerful inflammatory function. Other genes specifically activated in tumor metastases included cytokine receptors (e.g., IL-2R beta and IFN-γ receptor alpha chain), adhesion molecules associated with mononuclear cell migration (e.g., CD62 and V-CAM1), activation of immune effector functions associated with the cytotoxic mechanisms in monocytes (calgranulin, grancalcin), NK and activated T cells (NK4; natural killer receptor 4, NKG5; granulysin), and several other genes associated with IFN-γ activity, such as HLA class II molecules and interferon-regulatory-factor-(IRF)-1. These may in turn contribute to epitope spreading through killing of cancer cells, with consequent uptake of shed antigens and presentation to adaptive immune cells. However, this upregulation was not accompanied by a parallel activation of genes constitutively expressed by immune cells (i.e., CD3, CD4, CD8, CD10, TCR associated genes, CD20, CD11, CD14, CD16 FC-gamma, and CD83), providing evidence against a migration of immune cells at tumor sites at earlier time points. These data derived from the study of 16 melanoma metastases from 6 patients treated at the NCI. Even though the genes included in the array at that time were limited (about 6,000 genes), these observations were recently confirmed in an independent cohort of patients treated with IL-2 using a more comprehensive platform [34]. This second (prospective) investigation identified about 350 genes differentially expressed between pre- and post-treatment lesions. The pathway analysis confirmed activation of molecular pathways associated with macrophage activation including CCR5 signaling pathway (top immunological pathway) as well as pathways associated with IL-17, probably missed in our previous analyses due to the limited number of genes included in earlier platforms. Altogether these findings suggest that the main role of IL-2 is the activation of innate mechanisms driven by monocytes and eventually sustained by NK, and the tumor infiltrating lymphocytes, which in concert can initiate an inflammatory chemotactic cascade, orchestrated by the activation of the IFN-γ pathway and inducing release of related specific chemotactic ligands, with consequent polarized (T helper 1) recruitment of other immune cells later on.

Recently, in collaboration with Kaufman's group, we identified high levels of serum vascular endothelial growth factor (VEGF) and fibronectin as predictor factors of IL-2 therapy in metastatic melanoma/renal cell carcinoma patients [71]. This data, originated through a high-throughput proteomic approach, fit with several observations which suggest that, beyond the angiogenic activity, VEGF can act as an immune suppressant by blocking maturation of dendritic cells [72] or by inhibiting effective priming of T-cell response [73].

C. Adoptive therapy

Adoptive therapy is a promising treatment for patients with metastatic melanoma, with a rate of durable complete remission (CR) up to 20% according to phase II trials [12]. In this procedure, TILs are expanded and activated *ex vivo*, and then re-infused into the patients in combination with high-dose interleukin-(IL)-2. The kinetic of infused TILs can be investigated by labeling TILs just before the re-infusion, concomitant with the IL-2 administration. Studies where TILs were labeled with Indium 111 showed that localization at tumor site is a necessary, although not sufficient, condition for the induction of tumor regression [74]. However, TILs migration at the tumor site does not follow a linear kinetic [75]. After two hours of their infusion, which was immediately followed by the administration of IL-2, TILs massively localized in lung, spleen and liver but not at tumor sites. TIL migration into tumor sites was detectable 24 or 48 hours after the infusion, in concomitance with a partial clearance of the TILs from the lung. The migration of TILs further increases over time during the following week of follow-up, and, in some patients, new foci of tumors were evident only well beyond the 48 hours, suggesting a delayed migration or a recirculation [75]. Although TILs were documented by gamma camera, histopathological examination did not detect a predominance of lymphoid infiltrate in any patients' biopsies, confirming that the TIL migration is moderate also at these intermediate-early time points [75].

Because we showed that the transcriptional changes in cytokine/chemokine genes of PBMCs induced by IL-2 are followed by the secretion of the corresponding soluble factor, it is connectible that these cells represent an important source (either by degranulation or *de novo* synthesis) of the cytokines and chemokines detected in the serum following IL-2 administration. However, because there is neither evidence of migration of PBMC at the tumor site at early time points after IL-2 administration, nor evidence of the induction of apoptosis, it is clear that their disappearance is due to the compartmentalization of lymphocytes/monocytes in peripheral organs. These data need to be integrated with the observation that the selective depletion of lymphocytes and monocytes following IL-2 administration could not merely be explained by the increase of endothelium permeability with consequent extravasation into extravascular sites, which would determine also the clearance of polymorphic nuclear cells. It is possible, instead, that this compartmentalization is mediated by the release of specific chemokines (primarily CXCR3 and CCR5 ligands) from peripheral organs (e.g., spleen, lung and liver) by the resident immune cells as well as by the stromal cells following IL-2 administration.

Intriguingly, by analyzing a large cohort of 142 patients treated with IL-2, we recently noted that the downregulation of CXCR3 and CCR5 receptors in TILs due to the downregulation of and/or to the presence of common polymorphism (CCR5 Δ32, which codifies for a nonfunctionant receptor), correlates with the frequency and the degree of response [69]. It is tempting to hypothesize that a reduced, but not absent, expression of these receptors prevents their earlier sequestration by extratumor sites. Noteworthy, while modification of tumor environment increases progressively over time, CCR5 ligands in serum decreased over the 24 hours and this time point also coincides with the clearance of TIL in the lung. It is possible that at this time point the peripheral organ vs. tumor chemo-attractive coefficient becomes unbalanced in favor of tumor (which in any case contributes in minimal part to the overall concentration of these ligands in peripheral blood), with consequent tumor trafficking of those TILs that, in view of their relatively low expression of CXC3 and CCR5 ligands, were spared by early peripheral sequestration and can migrate into the tumor later on, when the cytokine storm has subsided and the tumor remains the main tissue maintaining expression of chemokines.

V. UNDERSTANDING THE IMMUNE-MEDIATED TUMOR REJECTION THROUGH GENE EXPRESSION PROFILING

Although the studies described above [30–33] assessing intratumoral gene-expression profile gave an overview of the molecular changes following immunotherapy, they were not designed to detect differences between responder and not-responder lesions. Notably, however, a particular subset of genes whose expression appeared to be associated with clinical response to IL-2 was already noted one decade ago. This lesion was characterized by an extreme post-treatment activation (as compared with the other lesions) of ISGs preferentially induced by IFN-γ/interferon-regulatory factor-1 (IRF-1)/signal transducers and activator of transcription (STAT-1) pathway, including the expression of human HLA class I and II and genes associated with effector function: nucleolysin cytotoxic granule (TIAR), NK4 and granulysin [32]. Although this observation was based on the analysis of a single paradigmatic responding lesion, its relevance was confirmed by a second set of investigations conducted by our group [34–36] and (most recently) by others [76] that assessed this relevant issue in detail. Altogether, this second set of investigations corroborates on one hand that the downstream effect of various immunotherapies is the induction of a polarized inflammation through the activation of defined and poorly redundant pathways and on the other they clarify that a powerful and coordinated activation of all these pathways is a necessary requirement for the induction of tumor rejection, being the degree of this switch correlated with clinical response. By profiling 37 pre- and post-treatment FNAs (at least after one course of treatment) from patients treated with IL-2 high dose and various vaccination schedules (e.g., MART-1/GP-100 vaccines), we showed that tumor clearance (achievement of complete remission) is associated with the induction of a turbulent inflammatory reaction, while minimal changes were observed among the nonresponding lesions [35]. The number of genes differentially expressed pre- and post-treatment by the nine lesions undergoing complete remission later on was significantly elevated and most of them were immune-related, while the number of genes differentially expressed after treatment in the 14 paired nonresponding lesions was close to that expected by chance and not statistically significant. The most upregulated gene in the complete responding lesions was the interferon-regulatory-factor 1 (IRF-1) a key transcription factor activated during the I IFN-γ cascade and responsible for the transcription of CXCL9, -10, 11 (CXCR3 ligands) and CCL5 (CCR5 ligand). This was a retrospective-prospective study employing arrays that contained a limited number of genes (around 6,000) and the samples were collected within clinical trials at the NCI and retrospectively analyzed when material was available.

In a second clinical-translational prospective trial, we assessed, through a whole-genome gene expression analysis, 30 pre/post FNAs samples from 13 melanoma patients homogenously treated with high dose IL-2 at the University of Virginia [34]. The prospective design of the study allows the collection of the sample within homogenous time points (i.e., 3 hours after the first and the fourth dose of IL-2 administration). Class comparison in this case was made between patients with clinical response (complete remission, partial remission or stable disease) and those that progressed.

This study confirmed that the activation of the ICR pathways (activation of IFN-γ-stimulated genes, induction of specific chemokine-ligand genes, and activation of the immune-effector functions) is the key mechanism of action of the IL-2 and that a powerful induction of IFN-γ cascade is indispensable for the achievement of clinical result.

Another confirmation of the relevance of the induction of ICR came recently from our whole-genome gene expression analyses of two rare and paradigmatic cases of mixed response patients [36]. The intra-patients correction allows exclusion from the tumor/host algorithm modulatory variables related to the host's genetic background. The comparisons between 10 regressing and 5 progressing melanoma metastases obtained from two patients treated with either autologous vaccination (M-VAX) or IFN-α revealed 167 genes differentially expressed between the two groups, most of which associated with antigen presentation and acute immune response [36]. A massive and coordinated overexpression of all the ICR pathways in the regressing metastases as compared with the progressing ones was evident. In details, IFN-γ stimulated genes (e.g., STAT-1, IRF-1, and -5, HLA class I and II, GBP-1, TAP-1), CCR5 ligand genes (i.e., CCL3, and 4) and immune-effector genes associated with T and NK functions (FCGR3A (CD16a), LCP1, CD3, CD2, CD48, LY9) were among the most upregulated genes in the regressing lesions. In addition, quantitative expression analysis of HLA-A, B and C genes confirmed a higher HLA expression in the regressing versus the progressing lesions. The prevalence of T cells infiltrated in the regressing metastases was confirmed by immune-histochemistry analyses. Since lesions were excised weeks or months after treatment administration, these data confirmed that, in the contest of immune-mediated tissue destruction following immunotherapy administration, the migration of immune cells at the tumor site is only a late, yet necessary, event. However, there were no significant differences between regressing metastases collected after IFN-α versus those after vaccination, providing direct evidence that tissue destruction triggered by different stimula converges into a unique mechanism. The final results of an independent investigation assessing molecular changes in tumor metastases from melanoma patients treated with ipilimumab corroborate the existence of this convergent phenomenon. Ji et al. [76] applied whole-genome gene expression profile to the study of melanoma metastases from 45 patients treated with ipilimumab (a mAb specific to CTLA-4, an inhibitory receptor expressed by T cells, recently approved for the treatment of metastatic disease). Biopsies (although not paired as for our study) were collected before and 1 or 3 days after the second administration of ipilimumab, which was administered 3 weeks after the first dose. Class comparison between pre- vs. post-treatment metastases detected 376 genes differentially expressed between the two groups. The increase of the mean expression of these genes was larger in patients who experienced clinical benefit (i.e., complete response, partial response or prolonged stable disease) compared with those from patients that did not benefit from the treatment. Again, the top functional biological process under-lined by these genes was the inflammatory response. Interestingly, also B-cell signatures were detected, which have been recently associated with other immune-mediated tissue destruction processes (e.g., allograft rejection) [43,77]. At the single-gene level, among the 25 genes with the higher post vs pre-treatment fold increase in patients who experienced clinical benefit, most were immune-related and included the ICR pathways (e.g., CXCL11, GZMA, GZMB, GZMK, PRF1, GNLY, TLR8). There was also an increase of T-cell markers (i.e., CD3E and CD8) suggesting a T-cell migration at this relatively late time point. In concordance with our early observations, the post- vs. pre-treatment gene expression change was larger in the responder patients [76], confirming that the induction of a turbulent and polarized inflammatory reaction is necessary for the induction of tumor regression.

VI. PREDICTING IMMUNE RESPONSIVENESS TO IMMUNOTHERAPEUTICS THROUGH GENE EXPRESSION PROFILING

By collecting clinical information regarding lesions from which FNA samples had been serially obtained, we observed that lesions were separated according to their clinical response to immunization (peptide vaccination combined with high-dose IL-2 administration in the first study and IL-2 alone in the following prospective investigation) and transcriptional profile identified gene predictors of immune responsiveness [34,35]. In particular, the identification of the overexpression of several pro-inflammatory genes as a predictor of immune responsiveness suggested that tumors more likely to respond to immunotherapy are chronically inflamed before treatment.

These genes were represented by interferon-related genes (e.g., interferon-regulatory-factor-(IRF)-2, IF127) and genes associated with immune-effector functions (e.g., TIA-1, a cytolitic granule component responsible for killing of CTL targets) [35]. When a comprehensive whole-genome gene expression profiling was performed, the top functional pathways associated with clinical response (among all the archived canonical pathways) individuated by Ingenuity Pathway Analysis Software in pre-treatment lesions were associated with immune-mediated tissue destruction (i.e., systemic lupus erythematosus signaling, role of NFAT in immune response, G-beta gamma signaling, allograft rejection signaling, autoimmune thyroiditis signaling, phospholipase C signaling, and type I diabetes signaling), centered on IFN-γ signaling [34,35]. Also B-cell signatures (i.e., IgG mRNA expression) were associated with immune responsiveness. Interestingly, B-cell signatures have been recently associated with good prognosis in breast [66], colon and non-small lung cancer patients [78] and are also associated with immune-mediated tissue destruction, as mentioned above [43].

Similarly, by profiling pre-treatment biopsies of metastatic melanoma patients treated with peptide vaccination and IL-12, Gajewski et al. showed that the overexpression of CXCR3 and CCR5 ligands (i.e., CXCL9, -10 and CCL4, 5, respectively) correlated with clinical benefit (response or clinical stabilization) and was associated with the presence of CD8$^+$ cells expressing CCR5 and CXCR3 [79−81].

The same group also found that a similar inflammatory profile including specific chemokines, T-cell markers and interferon-related genes was associated with clinical benefit in metastatic melanoma patients treated with a dendritic cell-based vaccine [82]. The EORTC MAGE-A3 vaccine trial independently confirmed the high expression of CCL5 and CXCL9, 10 in this setting of patients [52,81,83,84]. Most of the genes included in this signature (GS) were immune-related (e.g., ICOS, IFN-γ, CD20). The signature was also associated with clinical benefit when tested within a MAGE-A3 trial in non-small-cell lung cancer [85], corroborating the hypothesis that cancers segregate into different immune categories independent from their tissue derivation [65].

Additionally, Sullivan et al. found that a signature characterized by immune-related genes is predictive of favorable outcome in melanoma patients treated with high-dose IL-2 [86,87].

The recent results of the study of Ji et al. evaluating gene expression profiling in melanoma patients treated with ipilimumab confirmed the relevance of the ICR as predictive biomarkers of responsiveness independently from the type of immunotherapy used.

Among the top 22 genes upregulated in responding patients comparing with the nonresponding ones were CD8A, MHC class II (IFN-γ/T helper-1 genes), CCL4, and -5 (CCR5 ligands), CCL9, 10, and 11 (CXCR3 ligands), NKG7, GZMB and PRF1 (immune-effector genes).

All the top 10 canonical pathways (i.e., those identified by Ingenuity Pathway Analysis Software) identified were immune-related, and centered on IFN-γ signaling. Even more, seven of them (i.e., antigen-presentation pathway, allograft rejection signaling, Type I diabetes signaling, autoimmune thyroid disease signaling, graft versus host disease signaling, systemic lupus erythematosus signaling, and primary immunodeficiency signaling) were included in the 10 canonical pathways identified through the same software in our study comparing post-IL-2 responder vs. nonresponder lesions, which in turn overlapped with those identifying pre-treatment responder lesions [34]. This analogy is impressive and encouraging considering all the possible combinations that could have been generated by the analysis of the entire human transcriptome. B-cell related genes (e.g., IGL@) were also found upregulated in responding lesions, corroborating again our previous observation [34]. Interestingly, IDO1 (indolamine 2,3-deoxygenase, inhibiting T-cell response) was also overexpressed in pre-treatment responding lesions.

Gajewski et al. observed that tumors with inflammatory phenotype overexpress genes associated with immunosuppressive mechanisms, including IDO, B7-H1/PD-L1 (providing a co-inhibitory signal to T cells) and FOXP3 (T-regulatory cell markers), suggesting an ongoing immune response in the tumor microenvironment concomitant with tumor escape mechanisms [81,88]. However, Hamid et al., showed that the pre-treatment FOXP3 expression and IDO (evaluated by immunohistochemistry) by tumor infiltrating immune cells is positively associated with clinical outcome in melanoma patients treated with ipilimumab [89].

In order to interpret these findings, it should be taken into account that IDO1 is an IFN-γ inducible gene [90], and this overexpression could be due to the excess of IFN-γ consequent to the T helper-1 infiltration. In addition, IDO exerts pleiotropic functions and should not be considered as a merely immunosuppressive enzyme [90]. IDO in fact can mediate pro-inflammatory mechanisms, in particular those driven by autoreactive B cells, as shown by several mechanistic studies performed by Prendergast and colleagues [90−92].

As for FOXP3, several independent studies recently observed a paradoxical association between the infiltration of colon cancer by T cells expressing the T-regulatory cell marker FOXP3 and favorable prognosis after primary tumor excision or after chemo- or chemo-immunotherapy in advanced stages [64,93−95], in contrast with that observed in other type of cancers, as recently reviewed by Ladoire et al [96]. However, more than the total number of bona fide T-regulatory cells (FOXP3+), it seems that the analysis of the ratio between these immune-suppressive and the immune-effector T cells can provide more useful information about tumor immune responsiveness. Yoon et al. [97], for example, showed that, in colon cancer, T-regulatory cells represent a favorable prognostic marker only in absence of a dense CD8+ T-cell infiltrate.

Although the presence of T-regulatory cells could be interpreted as a counter-regulatory response after a powerful immune reaction, the evidence that CD4+ T cells can transiently express FOXP3 without acquisition of suppressive functions [98,99] and that CD8+ FOXP3+ T cells with effector function were detected in the context of an effective antitumor response [100] suggest caution in the interpretation of the aforementioned results in absence of functional cell-specific analyses. Even more, tumor cells can express both FOXP3 and IDO, adding complexity to the interpretation of these correlative studies. Brody et al., for example, showed an upregulation of IDO by melanoma cells accompanied by the presence of FOXP3+ T-regulatory cells and associated with poor survival by analyzing lesions from 25 metastatic melanoma patients, suggesting IDO upregulation as a possible immune escaping mechanism [101,102]. Since the authors neither report the response rate nor the characteristics of the treatment administrated, it is not clear if the association with poor survival was due to a more aggressive phenotype (prognostic biomarker) rather than to a lack of treatment responsiveness (predictive biomarkers).

VII. LINKAGE BETWEEN AUTOIMMUNITY AND TUMOR REJECTION

Intriguingly, clinical manifestations of autoimmunity (e.g., vitiligo, thyroiditis, enterocolitis) following treatment administration are highly correlated with favorable outcome in metastatic melanoma patients treated with the anti-CTLA-4 mAb ipilimumab [103,104], high-dose IL-2 [19] and vaccination [105]. In high-risk melanoma patients treated with high-dose IFN-α, post-treatment clinical and/or molecular manifestation of autoimmunity were found to be associated with diminished risk of deaths or relapse in the Hellenic IFN trial [106]. However, the development of autoimmunity as a predictive biomarker of response to IFN-α is now debated. In fact, the integrated analysis of the EORTC and the Nordic IFN trials showed a lack of significant correlation between the appearance of auto-antibodies and clinical outcomes when a guarantee-time bias correction was applied [107,108]. Another link between autoimmunity and response to immunotherapy is represented by the fact that studies analyzing the correlation between peripheral immune response and clinical response after vaccination in melanoma patients showed that nonresponders did not generate reactivity to epitopes other than those used for vaccination, while patients that developed a clinical response displayed with high frequency reactivity to antigens that were not included in the vaccination [109−112]. This phenomenon, called determinant spreading, is characteristic of autoimmune diseases and is the basis of continuing pathologic tissue destruction.

In this context, the presence of determinant spreading could be interpreted as the result of an effective tissue destruction with consequent cross-priming mediated by local antigen-presenting cells, thereby representing a mechanistic (and predictive) biomarker of response to immunotherapy [112,113].

We recently observed that IRF-5 polymorphisms associated with the development of lupus erythematous influence the strength of the antitumor response to adoptive therapy, underlining the genetic linkage between the predispositions to develop different immune-mediated tissue destruction processes [114]. Even more, the observation that IRF-5 polymorphism-specific signatures detected in melanoma cell lines can be used to predict responsiveness to adoptive therapy of the parental metastases suggests that a host's genetics can directly modulate the intrinsic cancer biology besides modulating the reaction of the host's immune cells to immunotherapy [114].

VIII. UNDERSTANDING THE ORIGIN OF THE IMMUNE-SIGNATURE AND FUTURE DIRECTIONS

Although molecular profiling studies have clearly defined two cancer "personalities" independent of their "social" origins (i.e., the tissue from which they derive), it is not clear which factors determine these traits and, if any, which one plays a pivotal role. It is presently unclear which one among the genetics of the host, the genetics of cancer cells, and host environment plays a dominant/driving role. These variables are closely related considering that, for example, the genetics of cancer cells bears also on the genetics of the individual and that host environment (e.g., exposure to viral infections) can modify cancer genetics as well as the phonotypical traits of the host.

The transcriptional profile of the whole tumor tissue cannot clarify the sources of cells expressing the immune genes. Even if it is assumed that the activation of the immune-effector genes detected in these studied mostly reflect the activation/presence of immune cells, we observed that pancreatic and melanoma cell lines could be segregated in different categories according to the intrinsic activation of interferon-stimulated-genes including interferon-regulatory-factors [115,116].

The correlation between the signature detected *in vivo* and *in vitro* is, however, not linear. When we correlated the expression of CXCR3 and CCR5 ligands between 15 melanoma tumor cell lines and the parental tumor tissue we did not find any significant correlation between the *in vivo* and *in vitro* data [117]. In addition, among the melanoma cell lines, there was no correlation between gene copy number and the corresponding gene expression [117]. However, when we applied the gene signatures obtained by the class comparisons of melanoma cell lines according to pSTAT1 and pSTAT3 (key molecules involved in the IFN signaling) levels to the parental metastases, we observed that the same signatures approximated the results observed in cell lines [118]. Altogether these findings suggest that the origin of the immune signature in some tumors is a complex, nonlinear, multifactorial and dynamic *in vivo* phenomenon but also support the notion that it is at least in part determined by the intrinsic biology of cancer cells.

We recently identified a list of 968 genes (genomic delegates) that display correlation between copy number and gene expression in melanoma tumor cell lines and were also correlated with the gene expression of the parental tumor metastases [116]. When we used these genes to reclassify tumor metastases, we observed that they segregate in two main categories, of which one is characterized by a T helper-1/1IFN-γ phenotype. Again, this observation suggests the existence of a stable trait of melanoma genetics that can in turn modulate immune reaction *in vivo* with consequent lack of linearity between *in vivo* and *ex vivo* transcripts of the immune-related genes. Interestingly, Curtis et al. showed that a particular breast cancer *in vivo* phenotype characterized by a flat copy number landscape is associated with an enrichment of ICR genes and, in turn, with a favorable prognosis [119]. Although this finding could be explained in part by the fact that a lack of copy number aberrations could represent the effect of a dilution of cancer aberrations consequent to an enrichment of immune-cell germinal DNA, this observation is intriguing and could support the driving role of cancer-cell genetics in determining the *in vivo* immune phenotype.

From a technical point of view, laser microdissection could be useful to deconvolute the cell-specific origin of the gene signatures observed. However, it presents several technical challenges since microdissection is extremely difficult when immune cells have a pattern of diffuse infiltration, and the total RNA obtained is extremely limited and does not allow in general the performance of a comprehensive gene-expression analysis. This technique could be rather useful to test a panel of selected genes using multi-PCR platforms, which requires an extremely limited number of cells.

We believe that next-generation studies based on Whole Genome Analysis through DNA/RNA sequencing characterizing somatic and germinal mutations/polymorphisms, integrated with gene-expression profiling, microRNA and proteomic analysis, will shed some light on this matter. Data from this approach and focusing on this central question are unavailable yet. We are currently investigating through a genome-wide association study the relevance of host polymorphisms and cancer cell genetics in determining the likelihood of response to immunotherapy in melanoma patients and in driving the immune-friendly personality of cancer.

IX. CONCLUSION

In summary, the development of high-throughput technology and its use in pioneer studies within humans has unveiled novel and paradoxical relations between cancer and immune systems, allowing the determination of promising biomarkers of immunoresponsiveness. It is becoming clear that tumors can be segregated into at least two categories. One of them bears an inflammatory signature characterized by the activation of the following modules: 1) IFN-γ/ T helper-1 module (STAT-1/IRF-1/IFN-γ-stimulated genes pathway); 2) The specific cytotoxic recruitment module (CXCR3/CXCR3 ligand and CCR5/CCR5 ligand pathway) and the immuno-effector function module (Granzyme/Perforin/Granulisin/TIA-1 pathway). This phenotype, which can also be characterized by the counter-activation of suppressive mechanisms, is distinguished by a more favorable history and a better response to immunotherapy (Table 23.2). Future research should better define whether it depends on the genetic makeup of individuals bearing the disease or whether it is due to somatic mutations within cancer cells. It is also unknown whether a counterpart of these intratumoral perturbations could be found within peripheral immune cells. We believe that future clinical-translational studies involving novel available technologies (e.g., deep sequencing) comparing tumor tissue characteristics with the peripheral circulation, along

387

TABLE 23.1 Post-treatment molecular pathways activated by immunotherapeutic agents and associated with treatment response individuated by gene-expression profiling

	Immunologic Constant of Rejection Pathways			Ref
	STAT-1 IRF-1/IFN-γ-SG pathway	CXCR3/CXCL9, -10, -11 CCR5/CCL3, -4,- 5 pathway	Granzyme Perforin Granulisin/TIA-1 pathway	
IL-2/IFN-α based treatment/vaccination (Melanoma)	+	+	+	[34—36]
Ipilimumab (Melanoma)	+	+	+	[76]
Imiquimod (Basal Cell Carcinoma)	+	+	+	[31]

TABLE 23.2 Pre-treatment molecular pathways predictive of immunoresponsiveness individuated by gene expression profiling

	Immunologic Constant of Rejection Pathways			Emerging Bio-markers			Ref
	T helper-1 polarization			T-regulatory cell/Immunosuppressive mechanisms		B cells	
	STAT-1 IRF-1/IFN-γ-SG pathway	CXCR3/CXCL9, -10, -11 CCR5/CCL3, -4, -5 pathway	Granzyme Perforin Granulisin/TIA-1 pathway	IDO	FOXP3	IGL@/IGKC	
IL-2 based treatment/vaccination (Melanoma)	+	+	+			+	[34,35,117]
Ipilimumab (Melanoma)	+	+	+	+	+	+	[89,76]
IL-12 and vaccination (Melanoma)	+	+		+	+		[79–81]
MAGE-3 vaccine (Lung Cancer and Melanoma)	+	+					[81,83,85]

IFN-γ-SG : IFN-γ stimulated genes

with clinical data, will be key to better characterized cancers. In parallel, in view of the substantial lack of standardized procedures that combine the variable assay protocols across laboratories, the procedures for the definition of a reliable immune-score useful for patient stratification need to be harmonized, as discussed elsewhere [52,120−124].

We believe that strategies aimed at targeting the tumor microenvironment through the enhancement of the described pathways [125], combined with the approaching next-generation cellular therapies capable of generating T cells with higher affinity to cancer antigens [126,127], or with a higher self-renewal and antitumor potential [128,129], could have a dramatic impact on this field in the near future.

ACKNOWLEDGMENTS

Researches performed in the Infectious Disease and Immunogenetics Section (Marincola's Lab) are supported by the NIH Intramural Research Program. Dr Bedognetti's researches were also supported by the Conquer Cancer Foundation of the American Society of Clinical Oncology (2011 Young Investigator Award). Dr. Bedognetti thanks Dr. Pietro Blandini (U.C. Sampdoria, Genoa, Italy) and Dr. Italia Grenga for insightful suggestions. Dr. Bedognetti dedicates this manuscript to Irina.

References

[1] Lindahl S, Marincola FM. Translational medicine, Encyclopedia Britannica; 2012. in press.

[2] Marincola FM. In support of descriptive studies; relevance to translational research. J Transl Med 2007;5:21.

[3] Marincola FM. The trouble with translational medicine. J Intern Med 2011;270(2):123−7.

[4] Marincola FM. Translational Medicine: A two-way road. J Transl Med 2003;1(1):1.

[5] Nussenblatt RB, Marincola FM, Schechter AN. Translational medicine−doing it backwards. J Transl Med 2010;8:12.

[6] BB&B -Bedside to Bench & Back Lecture Series. [cited; Available from, http://www.nhlbi.nih.gov/resources/chi/meetings/bedside.htm.

[7] Achinstein P. General Introduction. Science Rules: A Historical Introduction to Scientific Methods. Johns Hopkins University Press; 2004. p. 1−5.

[8] Popper K. The Logic of Scientific Discovery. New York, NY: Routledge Classics; 2002.

[9] Coley WB. II. Contribution to the Knowledge of Sarcoma. Ann Surg 1891;14(3):199−220.

[10] Coley WB. II. Injury as a Causative Factor in Cancer (Continued). Ann Surg 1911;53(5):615−50.

[11] Bedognetti D, Wang E, Sertoli MR, Marincola FM. Gene-expression profiling in vaccine therapy and immunotherapy for cancer. Expert Rev Vaccines 2010;9(6):555−65.

[12] Rosenberg SA, Yang JC, Sherry RM, Kammula US, Hughes MS, Phan GQ, et al. Durable complete responses in heavily pretreated patients with metastatic melanoma using T-cell transfer immunotherapy. Clin Cancer Res 2011;17(13):4550−7.

[13] Schwartzentruber DJ, Lawson DH, Richards JM, Conry RM, Miller DM, Treisman J, et al. gp100 peptide vaccine and interleukin-2 in patients with advanced melanoma. N Engl J Med 2011;364(22):2119−27.

[14] Hodi FS, O'Day SJ, DFMcDermott, Sosman JA, Haanen JB, et al. Improved survival with ipilimumab in patients with metastatic melanoma. N Engl J Med 2010;363(8):711−23.

[15] Bedognetti D, Wang E, Sertoli MR, F.M. M. Melanoma and biomarkers of immunoresponsiveness. In: "Emerging therapeutics for melanoma. FM Marincola PAaJKE, Future Science Group, 2011. Melanoma and biomarkers of immunoresponsiveness. In: Emerging therapeutics for melanoma. Future Science Group; 2012.

[16] Bedognetti D, Balwit JM, Wang E, Disis ML, Britten CM, Delogu LG, et al. SITC/iSBTc Cancer Immunotherapy Biomarkers Resource Document: Online resources and useful tools - a compass in the land of biomarker discovery. J Transl Med 2011;9.

[17] Kantoff PW, Higano CS, Shore ND, Berger ER, Small EJ, Penson DF, et al. Sipuleucel-T immunotherapy for castration-resistant prostate cancer. N Engl J Med 2010;363(5):411−22.

[18] Atkins MB, Lotze MT, Dutcher JP, Fisher RI, Weiss G, Margolin K, et al. High-dose recombinant interleukin 2 therapy for patients with metastatic melanoma: analysis of 270 patients treated between 1985 and 1993. J Clin Oncol 1999;17(7):2105−16.

[19] Atkins MB, Mier JW, Parkinson DR, Gould JA, Berkman EM, Kaplan MM. Hypothyroidism after treatment with interleukin-2 and lymphokine-activated killer cells. N Engl J Med 1988;318(24):1557−63.

[20] Mazumder A, Rosenberg SA. Successful immunotherapy of natural killer-resistant established pulmonary melanoma metastases by the intravenous adoptive transfer of syngeneic lymphocytes activated in vitro by interleukin 2. J Exp Med 1984;159(2):495—507.

[21] Kirkwood JM, Tarhini AA, Panelli MC, Moschos SJ, Zarour HM, Butterfield LH, et al. Next generation of immunotherapy for melanoma. J Clin Oncol 2008;26(20):3445—55.

[22] Kirkwood JM, Ernstoff MS, Davis CA, Reiss M, Ferraresi R, Rudnick SA. Comparison of intramuscular and intravenous recombinant alpha-2 interferon in melanoma and other cancers. Ann Intern Med 1985;103(1): 32—6.

[23] van der Bruggen P, Traversari C, Chomez P, Lurquin C, De Plaen E, Van den Eynde B, et al. A gene encoding an antigen recognized by cytolytic T lymphocytes on a human melanoma. Science 1991; 254(5038):1643—7.

[24] Traversari C, van der Bruggen P, Luescher IF, Lurquin C, Chomez P, Van Pel A, et al. A nonapeptide encoded by human gene MAGE-1 is recognized on HLA-A1 by cytolytic T lymphocytes directed against tumor antigen MZ2-E. J Exp Med 1992;176(5):1453—7.

[25] Belli F, Testori A, Rivoltini L, Maio M, Andreola G, Sertoli MR, et al. Vaccination of metastatic melanoma patients with autologous tumor-derived heat shock protein gp96-peptide complexes: clinical and immuno-logic findings. J Clin Oncol 2002;20(20):4169—80.

[26] Marincola FM, Ferrone S. Immunotherapy of melanoma: the good news, the bad ones and what to do next. Semin Cancer Biol 2003;13(6):387—9.

[27] Marincola FM, Jaffee EM, Hicklin DJ, Ferrone S. Escape of human solid tumors from T-cell recognition: molecular mechanisms and functional significance. Adv Immunol 2000;74:181—273.

[28] Marincola FM, Wang E, Herlyn M, Seliger B, Ferrone S. Tumors as elusive targets of T-cell-based active immunotherapy. Trends Immunol 2003;24(6):335—42.

[29] Wang E, Miller LD, Ohnmacht GA, Liu ET, Marincola FM. High-fidelity mRNA amplification for gene profiling. Nat Biotechnol 2000;18(4):457—9.

[30] Panelli MC, Martin B, Nagorsen D, Wang E, Smith K, Monsurro V, et al. A genomic- and proteomic-based hypothesis on the eclectic effects of systemic interleukin-2 administration in the context of melanoma-specific immunization. Cells Tissues Organs 2004;177(3):124—31.

[31] Panelli MC, Stashower ME, Slade HB, Smith K, Norwood C, Abati A, et al. Sequential gene profiling of basal cell carcinomas treated with imiquimod in a placebo-controlled study defines the requirements for tissue rejection. Genome Biol 2007;8(1):R8.

[32] Panelli MC, Wang E, Phan G, Puhlmann M, Miller L, Ohnmacht GA, et al. Gene-expression profiling of the response of peripheral blood mononuclear cells and melanoma metastases to systemic IL-2 administration. Genome Biol 2002;3(7). RESEARCH0035.

[33] Panelli MC, White R, Foster M, Martin B, Wang E, Smith K, et al. Forecasting the cytokine storm following systemic interleukin (IL)-2 administration. J Transl Med 2004;2(1):17.

[34] Weiss GR, Grosh WW, Chianese-Bullock KA, Zhao Y, Liu H, Slingluff Jr CL, et al. Molecular insights on the peripheral and intratumoral effects of systemic high-dose rIL-2 (aldesleukin) administration for the treatment of metastatic melanoma. Clin Cancer Res 2011;17(23):7440—50.

[35] Wang E, Miller LD, Ohnmacht GA, Mocellin S, Perez-Diez A, Petersen D, et al. Prospective molecular profiling of melanoma metastases suggests classifiers of immune responsiveness. Cancer Res 2002;62(13): 3581—6.

[36] Carretero R, Wang E, Rodriguez AI, Reinboth J, Ascierto ML, Engle AM, et al. Regression of melanoma metastases after immunotherapy is associated with activation of antigen presentation and interferon-mediated rejection genes. Int J Cancer 2011.

[37] Imanguli MM, Swaim WD, League SC, Gress RE, Pavletic SZ, Hakim FT. Increased T-bet+ cytotoxic effectors and type I interferon-mediated processes in chronic graft-versus-host disease of the oral mucosa. Blood 2009;113(15):3620—30.

[38] Bigger CB, Brasky KM, Lanford RE. DNA microarray analysis of chimpanzee liver during acute resolving hepatitis C virus infection. J Virol 2001;75(15):7059—66.

[39] He XS, Ji X, Hale MB, Cheung R, Ahmed A, Guo Y, et al. Global transcriptional response to interferon is a determinant of HCV treatment outcome and is modified by race. Hepatology 2006;44(2):352—9.

[40] Feld JJ, Nanda S, Huang Y, Chen W, Cam M, Pusek SN, et al. Hepatic gene expression during treatment with peginterferon and ribavirin: Identifying molecular pathways for treatment response. Hepatology46 2007;(5)::1548—63.

[41] Nanda S, Havert MB, Calderon GM, Thomson M, Jacobson C, Kastner D, et al. Hepatic transcriptome analysis of hepatitis C virus infection in chimpanzees defines unique gene expression patterns associated with viral clearance. PloS one 2008;3(10):e3442.

[42] Asselah T, Bieche I, Narguet S, Sabbagh A, Laurendeau I, Ripault MP, et al. Liver gene expression signature to predict response to pegylated interferon plus ribavirin combination therapy in patients with chronic hepatitis C. Gut 2008;57(4):516—24.

[43] Spivey TL, Uccellini L, Ascierto ML, Zoppoli G, De Giorgi V, Delogu LG, et al. Gene expression profiling in acute allograft rejection: challenging the immunologic constant of rejection hypothesis. J Transl Med 2011;9:174.

[44] Zhao DX, Hu Y, Miller GG, Luster AD, Mitchell RN, Libby P. Differential expression of the IFN-gamma-inducible CXCR3-binding chemokines, IFN-inducible protein 10, monokine induced by IFN, and IFN-inducible T cell alpha chemoattractant in human cardiac allografts: association with cardiac allograft vasculopathy and acute rejection. J Immunol 2002;169(3):1556—60.

[45] Okamoto Y, Folco EJ, Minami M, Wara AK, Feinberg MW, Sukhova GK, et al. Adiponectin inhibits the production of CXC receptor 3 chemokine ligands in macrophages and reduces T-lymphocyte recruitment in atherogenesis. Circ Res 2008;102(2):218—25.

[46] Costa C, Rufino R, Traves SL, Lapa ESJR, Barnes PJ, Donnelly LE. CXCR3 and CCR5 chemokines in induced sputum from patients with COPD. Chest 2008;133(1):26—33.

[47] Kim MJ, Romero R, Kim CJ, Tarca AL, Chhauy S, LaJeunesse C, et al. Villitis of unknown etiology is associated with a distinct pattern of chemokine up-regulation in the feto-maternal and placental compartments: implications for conjoint maternal allograft rejection and maternal anti-fetal graft-versus-host disease. J Immunol 2009;182(6):3919—27.

[48] Trinchieri G. Cancer and inflammation: an old intuition with rapidly evolving new concepts. Annu Rev Immunol 2012;30:677—706.

[49] Fridman WH, Galon J, Pages F, Sautes-Fridman C, Kroemer G. Prognostic and predictive impact of intra- and peritumoral immune infiltrates. Cancer Res 2011;71(17):5601—5.

[50] Wang E, Worschech A, Marincola FM. The immunologic constant of rejection. Trends Immunol 2008;29(6):256—62.

[51] Ascierto ML, De Giorgi V, Liu QZ, Bedognetti D, Spivey TL, Murtas D, et al. An immunologic portrait of cancer. J Transl Med 2011;9.

[52] Ascierto PA, De Maio E, Bertuzzi S, Palmieri G, Halaban R, Hendrix M, et al. Future perspectives in melanoma research. Meeting report from the "Melanoma Research: a bridge Naples-USA. Naples, December 6th-7th 2010". J Transl Med 2011;9:32.

[53] Azimi F, Scolyer RA, Rumcheva P, Moncrieff M, Murali R, McCarthy SW, et al. Tumor-infiltrating lymphocyte grade is an independent predictor of sentinel lymph node status and survival in patients with cutaneous melanoma. J Clin Oncol 2012;30(21):2678—83.

[54] Mahmoud SM, Paish EC, Powe DG, Macmillan RD, Grainge MJ, Lee AH, et al. Tumor-infiltrating CD8+ lymphocytes predict clinical outcome in breast cancer. J Clin Oncol 2011;29(15):1949—55.

[55] Hwang WT, Adams SF, Tahirovic E, Hagemann IS, Coukos G. Prognostic significance of tumor-infiltrating T cells in ovarian cancer: a meta-analysis. Gynecol Oncol 2012;124(2):192—8.

[56] Galon J, Costes A, Sanchez-Cabo F, Kirilovsky A, Mlecnik B, Lagorce-Pages C, et al. Type, density, and location of immune cells within human colorectal tumors predict clinical outcome. Science 2006;313(5795):1960—4.

[57] Pages F, Berger A, Camus M, Sanchez-Cabo F, Costes A, Molidor R, et al. Effector memory T cells, early metastasis, and survival in colorectal cancer. N Engl J Med 2005;353(25):2654—66.

[58] Denkert C, Loibl S, Noske A, Roller M, Komor M, et al. Tumor-associated lymphocytes as an independent predictor of response to neoadjuvant chemotherapy in breast cancer. J Clin Oncol 2010;28(1):105—13.

[59] Camus M, Tosolini M, Mlecnik B, Pages F, Kirilovsky A, Berger A, et al. Coordination of intratumoral immune reaction and human colorectal cancer recurrence. Cancer Res 2009;69(6):2685—93.

[60] Galon J, Fridman WH, Pages F. The adaptive immunologic microenvironment in colorectal cancer: a novel perspective. Cancer Res 2007;67(5):1883—6.

[61] Mlecnik B, Tosolini M, Charoentong P, Kirilovsky A, Bindea G, Berger A, et al. Biomolecular network reconstruction identifies T-cell homing factors associated with survival in colorectal cancer. Gastroenterology 2010;138(4):1429—40.

[62] Mlecnik B, Tosolini M, Kirilovsky A, Berger A, Bindea G, Meatchi T, et al. Histopathologic-based prognostic factors of colorectal cancers are associated with the state of the local immune reaction. J Clin Oncol 2011;29(6):610—8.

[63] Pages F, Kirilovsky A, Mlecnik B, Asslaber M, Tosolini M, Bindea G, et al. In situ cytotoxic and memory T cells predict outcome in patients with early-stage colorectal cancer. J Clin Oncol 2009;27(35):5944—51.

[64] Tosolini M, Kirilovsky A, Mlecnik B, Fredriksen T, Mauger S, Bindea G, et al. Clinical impact of different classes of infiltrating T cytotoxic and helper cells (Th1, th2, treg, th17) in patients with colorectal cancer. Cancer Res 2011;71(4):1263—71.

[65] Ascierto ML, De Giorgi V, Liu Q, Bedognetti D, Spivey TL, Murtas D, et al. An immunologic portrait of cancer. J Transl Medicine 2011. in press.

[66] Ascierto ML, Kmieciak M, Idowu MO, Manjili R, Zhao Y, Grimes M, et al. A signature of immune function genes associated with recurrence-free survival in breast cancer patients. Breast Cancer Res Treat 2012;131(3):871–80.

[67] McGray AJ, DBernard, Hallett R, Kelly R, Jha M, Gregory C, et al. Combined vaccination and immunostimulatory antibodies provides durable cure of murine melanoma and induces transcriptional changes associated with positive outcome in human melanoma patients. Oncoimmunology 2012;1(4):419–31.

[68] Urosevic M, Maier T, Benninghoff B, Slade H, Burg G, Dummer R. Mechanisms underlying imiquimod-induced regression of basal cell carcinoma in vivo. Arch Dermatol 2003;139(10):1325–32.

[69] Bedognetti D, Uccellini L, Wang E, Dudley ME, Pos Z, Ascierto ML, et al. Evaluation of CXCR3 and CCR5 Polymorphisms and Gene-Expression as Predictive Biomarkers of Clinical Response to Adoptive Therapy in Melanoma Patients. J Immunother 2010;33(8):860.

[70] Cotran RS, Pober JS, Gimbrone Jr MA, Springer TA, Wiebke EA, Gaspari AA, et al. Endothelial activation during interleukin 2 immunotherapy. A possible mechanism for the vascular leak syndrome. J Immunol 1988;140(6):1883–8.

[71] Sabatino M, Kim-Schulze S, Panelli MC, Stroncek D, Wang E, Taback B, et al. Serum vascular endothelial growth factor and fibronectin predict clinical response to high-dose interleukin-2 therapy. J Clin Oncol 2009;27(16):2645–52.

[72] Gabrilovich DI, Chen HL, Girgis KR, Cunningham HT, Meny GM, Nadaf S, et al. Production of vascular endothelial growth factor by human tumors inhibits the functional maturation of dendritic cells. Nat Med 1996;2(10):1096–103.

[73] Ohm JE, Gabrilovich DI, Sempowski GD, Kisseleva E, Parman KS, Nadaf S, et al. VEGF inhibits T-cell development and may contribute to tumor-induced immune suppression. Blood 2003;101(12):4878–86.

[74] Pockaj BA, Sherry RM, Wei JP, Yannelli JR, Carter CS, Leitman SF, et al. Localization of 111indium-labeled tumor infiltrating lymphocytes to tumor in patients receiving adoptive immunotherapy. Augmentation with cyclophosphamide and correlation with response. Cancer 1994;73(6):1731–7.

[75] Fisher B, Packard BS, Read EJ, Carrasquillo JA, Carter CS, Topalian SL, et al. Tumor localization of adoptively transferred indium-111 labeled tumor infiltrating lymphocytes in patients with metastatic melanoma. J Clin Oncol 1989;7(2):250–61.

[76] Ji RR, Chasalow SD, Wang L, Hamid O, Schmidt H, Cogswell J, et al. An immune-active tumor microenvironment favors clinical response to ipilimumab. Cancer Immunol Immunother CII 2012;61(7):1019–31.

[76] Ji RR, Chasalow SD, Wang L, Hamid O, Schmidt H, Cogswell J, et al. An immune-active tumor microenvironment favors clinical response to ipilimumab. Cancer Immunol Immunother (CII) 2012;61(7):1019–31.

[77] Sarwal M, Chua MS, Kambham N, Hsieh SC, Satterwhite T, Masek M, et al. Molecular heterogeneity in acute renal allograft rejection identified by DNA microarray profiling. N Engl J Med 2003;349(2):125–38.

[78] Schmidt M, Hellwig B, Hammad S, Othman A, Lohr M, Chen Z, et al. A comprehensive analysis of human gene expression profiles identifies stromal immunoglobulin kappa C as a compatible prognostic marker in human solid tumors. Clin Cancer Res 2012;18(9):2695–703.

[79] Gajewski T, Meng Y, Harlin H. Chemokines expressed in melanoma metastases associated with T cell infiltration. J Clin Oncol 2007:25.

[80] Harlin H, Meng Y, Peterson AC, Zha Y, Tretiakova M, Slingluff C, et al. Chemokine expression in melanoma metastases associated with CD8+ T-cell recruitment. Cancer Res 2009;69(7):3077–85.

[81] Gajewski TF, Fuertes M, Spaapen R, Zheng Y, Kline J. Molecular profiling to identify relevant immune resistance mechanisms in the tumor microenvironment. Curr Opin Immunol 2011;23(2):286–92.

[82] Gajewski TF, Zha Y, Thurner B, Schuler G. Association of gene expression profile in metastatic melanoma and survival to a dendritic cell-based vaccine. J Clin Oncol 2009;29(15).

[83] Louahed O, Gruselle O, Gaulis S, Coche T, Eggermont AM, Kruit W, et al. Expression of defined genes identified by pretreatment tumor profiling: Association with clinical responses to the GSK MAGE- A3 immunotherapeutic in metastatic melanoma patients (EORTC 16032-18031). J Clin Oncol 2008:26.

[84] Tahara H, Sato M, Thurin M, Wang E, Butterfield LH, Disis ML, et al. Emerging concepts in biomarker discovery; the US-Japan Workshop on Immunological Molecular Markers in Oncology. J Transl Med 2009;7:45.

[85] Vansteenkiste JF, Zielinski M, Dahabreh IJ, Linder A, Lehmann F, Gruselle O, et al. Association of gene expression signature and clinical efficacy of MAGE-A3 antigen-specific cancer immunotherapeutic (ASCI) as adjuvant therapy in resected stage IB/II non-small cell lung cancer (NSCLC). J Clin Oncol 2008:26.

[86] Sullivan RJ, Hoshida Y, Brunet J, Tahan S, Aldridge J, Kwabi C, et al. A single center experience with high-dose (HD) IL-2 treatment for patients with advanced melanoma and pilot investigation of a novel gene expression signature as a predictor of response. J Clin Oncol 2009:27.

[87] Sznol M. Molecular markers of response to treatment for melanoma. Cancer J 2011;17(2):127—33.

[88] Gajewski TF, Louahed J, Brichard VG. Gene signature in melanoma associated with clinical activity: a potential clue to unlock cancer immunotherapy. Cancer J 2010;16(4):399—403.

[89] Hamid O, Schmidt H, Nissan A, Ridolfi L, Aamdal S, Hansson J, et al. A prospective phase II trial exploring the association between tumor microenvironment biomarkers and clinical activity of ipilimumab in advanced melanoma. J Transl Med 2011;9:204.

[90] Muller AJ, Mandik-Nayak L, Prendergast GC. Beyond immunosuppression: reconsidering indoleamine 2,3-dioxygenase as a pathogenic element of chronic inflammation. Immunotherapy 2010;2(3):293—7.

[91] Prendergast GC, Chang MY, Mandik-Nayak L, Metz R, Muller AJ. Indoleamine 2,3-dioxygenase as a modifier of pathogenic inflammation in cancer and other inflammation-associated diseases. Curr Med Chem 2011;18(15):2257—62.

[92] Scott GN, DuHadaway J, Pigott E, Ridge N, Prendergast GC, Muller AJ, et al. The immunoregulatory enzyme IDO paradoxically drives B cell-mediated autoimmunity. J Immunol 2009;182(12):7509—17.

[93] Correale P, Rotundo MS, Del Vecchio MT, Remondo C, Migali C, Ginanneschi C, et al. Regulatory (FoxP3+) T-cell tumor infiltration is a favorable prognostic factor in advanced colon cancer patients undergoing chemo or chemoimmunotherapy. J Immunother ;33(4)2010:435—41.

[94] Frey DM, Droeser RA, Viehl CT, Zlobec I, Lugli A, Zingg U, et al. High frequency of tumor-infiltrating FOXP3(+) regulatory T cells predicts improved survival in mismatch repair-proficient colorectal cancer patients. Int J Cancer 2010;126(11):2635—43.

[95] Salama P, Phillips M, Grieu F, Morris M, Zeps N, Joseph D, et al. Tumor-infiltrating FOXP3+ T regulatory cells show strong prognostic significance in colorectal cancer. J Clin Oncol 2009;27(2):186—92.

[96] Ladoire S, Martin F, Ghiringhelli F. Prognostic role of FOXP3+ regulatory T cells infiltrating human carcinomas: the paradox of colorectal cancer. Cancer Immunol Immunother CII. 2011;60(7):909—18.

[97] Yoon HH, Orrock JM, Foster NR, Sargent DJ, Smyrk TC, Sinicrope FA. Prognostic Impact of FoxP3+ Regulatory T Cells in Relation to CD8+ T Lymphocyte Density in Human Colon Carcinomas. PloS one 2012;7(8):e42274.

[98] Roncador G, Brown PJ, Maestre L, Hue S, Martinez-Torrecuadrada JL, Ling KL, et al. Analysis of FOXP3 protein expression in human CD4+CD25+ regulatory T cells at the single-cell level. Eur J Immunol 2005;35(6):1681—91.

[99] Walker MR, Kasprowicz DJ, Gersuk VH, Benard A, Van Landeghen M, Buckner JH, et al. Induction of FoxP3 and acquisition of T regulatory activity by stimulated human CD4+CD25- T cells. J Clin Invest 2003;112(9):1437—43.

[100] Le DT, Ladle BH, Lee T, Weiss V, Yao X, Leubner A, et al. CD8(+) Foxp3(+) tumor infiltrating lymphocytes accumulate in the context of an effective anti-tumor response. Int J Cancer 2011;129(3):636—47.

[101] Brody JR, Costantino CL, Berger AC, Sato T, Lisanti MP, Yeo CJ, et al. Expression of indoleamine 2,3-dioxygenase in metastatic malignant melanoma recruits regulatory T cells to avoid immune detection and affects survival. Cell Cycle 2009;8(12):1930—4.

[102] Prendergast GC, Metz R, Muller AJ. IDO recruits Tregs in melanoma. Cell Cycle 2009;8(12):1818—9.

[103] Beck KE, Blansfield JA, Tran KQ, Feldman AL, Hughes MS, Royal RE, et al. Enterocolitis in patients with cancer after antibody blockade of cytotoxic T-lymphocyte-associated antigen 4. J Clin Oncol 2006;24(15):2283—9.

[104] Phan GQ, Yang JC, Sherry RM, Hwu P, Topalian SL, Schwartzentruber DJ, et al. Cancer regression and autoimmunity induced by cytotoxic T lymphocyte-associated antigen 4 blockade in patients with metastatic melanoma. Proc Natl Acad Sci U S A 2003;100(14):8372—7.

[105] Phan GQ, Attia P, Steinberg SM, White DE, Rosenberg SA. Factors associated with response to high-dose interleukin-2 in patients with metastatic melanoma. J Clin Oncol 2001;19(15):3477—82.

[106] Gogas H, Ioannovich J, Dafni U, Stavropoulou-Giokas C, Frangia K, Tsoutsos D, et al. Prognostic significance of autoimmunity during treatment of melanoma with interferon. N Engl J Med 2006;354(7):709—18.

[107] Bouwhuis MG, Suciu S, Collette S, Aamdal S, Kruit WH, Bastholt L, et al. Autoimmune antibodies and recurrence-free interval in melanoma patients treated with adjuvant interferon. J Natl Cancer Inst 2009;101(12):869—77.

[108] Bouwhuis MG, Suciu S, Testori A, Kruit WH, Sales F, Patel P, et al. Phase III trial comparing adjuvant treatment with pegylated interferon Alfa-2b versus observation: prognostic significance of auto-antibodies—EORTC 18991. J Clin Oncol 2010;28(14):2460—6.

[109] Butterfield LH, Comin-Anduix B, Vujanovic L, Lee Y, Dissette VB, Yang JQ, et al. Adenovirus MART-1-engineered autologous dendritic cell vaccine for metastatic melanoma. J Immunother 2008;31(3):294–309.

[110] Butterfield LH, Ribas A, Dissette VB, Amarnani SN, Vu HT, Oseguera D, et al. Determinant spreading associated with clinical response in dendritic cell-based immunotherapy for malignant melanoma. Clin Cancer Res 2003;9(3):998–1008.

[111] Ribas A, Glaspy JA, Lee Y, Dissette VB, Seja E, Vu HT, et al. Role of dendritic cell phenotype, determinant spreading, and negative costimulatory blockade in dendritic cell-based melanoma immunotherapy. J Immunother 2004;27(5):354–67.

[112] Ribas A, Timmerman JM, Butterfield LH, Economou JS. Determinant spreading and tumor responses after peptide-based cancer immunotherapy. Trends Immunol 2003;24(2):58–61.

[113] Disis ML. Immunologic biomarkers as correlates of clinical response to cancer immunotherapy. Cancer Immunol Immunother CII. 2011;60(3):433–42.

[114] Uccellini L, De Giorgi V, Zhao Y, Tumaini B, Erdenebileg N, Dudley ME, et al. IRF5 gene polymorphisms in melanoma. J Transl Med 2012;10(1):170.

[115] Monsurro V, Beghelli S, Wang R, Barbi S, Coin S, Di Pasquale G, et al. Anti-viral state segregates two molecular phenotypes of pancreatic adenocarcinoma: potential relevance for adenoviral gene therapy. J Transl Med 2010;8:10.

[116] Spivey TL, De Giorgi V, Zhao YD, Bedognetti D, Pos Z, Liu QZ, et al. The stable traits of melanoma genetics: an alternate approach to target discovery. Bmc Genomics 2012:13.

[117] Bedognetti D, Tomei S, Spivey S, De Giorgi V, Ascierto ML, Wang E, et al. Evaluation of chemokine-ligand pathways in pretreatment tumor biopsies as predictive biomarker of response to adoptive therapy in metastatic melanoma patients. Journal of clinical oncology: official journal of the American Society of Clinical Oncology 2012 (Suppl; abstr 8756).

[118] De Giorgi V, Liu Q, Pos Z, Wunderlich J, Spivey TL, Uccellini L, et al. Genotypic, Phenotypic and Functional Analysis of Melanoma. J Immunother 2011;34:696 (abstract).

[119] Curtis C, Shah SP, Chin SF, Turashvili G, Rueda OM, Dunning MJ, et al. The genomic and transcriptomic architecture of 2,000 breast tumours reveals novel subgroups. Nature 2012;486(7403):346–52.

[120] Emens LA, Silverstein SC, Khleif S, Marincola FM, Galon J. Toward integrative cancer immunotherapy: targeting the tumor microenvironment. J Transl Med 2012;10:70.

[121] Fox BA, Schendel DJ, Butterfield LH, Aamdal S, Allison JP, Ascierto PA, et al. Defining the critical hurdles in cancer immunotherapy. J Transl Med 2011;9(1):214.

[122] Galon J, Pages F, Marincola FM, Thurin M, Trinchieri G, Fox BA, et al. The immune score as a new possible approach for the classification of cancer. J Transl Med 2012;10:1.

[123] Fridman WH, Pages F, Sautes-Fridman C, Galon J. The immune contexture in human tumours: impact on clinical outcome. Nat Rev Cancer 2012;12(4):298–306.

[124] Ogino S, Galon J, Fuchs CS, Dranoff G. Cancer immunology—analysis of host and tumor factors for personalized medicine. Nat Rev Clin Oncol 2011;8(12):711–9.

[125] Muthuswamy R, Berk E, Junecko BF, Zeh HJ, Zureikat AH, Normolle D, et al. NF-kappaB hyperactivation in tumor tissues allows tumor-selective reprogramming of the chemokine microenvironment to enhance the recruitment of cytolytic T effector cells. Cancer Res 2012;72(15):3735–43.

[126] Porter DL, Levine BL, Kalos M, Bagg A, June CH. Chimeric antigen receptor-modified T cells in chronic lymphoid leukemia. N Engl J Med 2011;365(8):725–33.

[127] Scholler J, Brady TL, Binder-Scholl G, Hwang WT, Plesa G, Hege KM, et al. Decade-long safety and function of retroviral-modified chimeric antigen receptor T cells. Sci Transl Med 2012;4(132):132ra53.

[128] Gattinoni L, Lugli E, Ji Y, Pos Z, Paulos CM, Quigley MF, et al. A human memory T cell subset with stem cell-like properties. Nat Med 2011;17(10):1290–7.

[129] Gattinoni L, Klebanoff CA, Restifo NP. Paths to stemness: building the ultimate antitumour T cell. Nat Rev Cancer 2012;12(10):671–684.

CHAPTER 24

Immune Stimulatory Features of Classical Chemotherapy

W. Joost Lesterhuis[1], Anna K. Nowak[1,2], Richard A. Lake[1]
[1]National Centre for Asbestos Related Diseases and Tumor Immunology Group, School of Medicine and Pharmacology, University of Western Australia, Sir Charles Gairdner Hospital, Nedlands, WA, Australia
[2]Department of Medical Oncology, Sir Charles Gairdner Hospital Nedlands, WA, Australia

I. INTRODUCTION

Historically, clinical dogma has held that classical cancer chemotherapy could not be used in combination with immunotherapeutic approaches because of its myelosuppressive effect. However, as early as the 1970s a few preclinical studies indicated that there was a potential benefit to the immune response from cytotoxic cancer drugs. One of the first demonstrations of an immunogenic momentum of cancer chemotherapy was the finding that mice treated with 6-mercaptopurine in combination with a *Salmonella Paratyphi* B antigen vaccine displayed a marked lymphocyte hyperplasia, with an enhanced rather than decreased immune activation against the vaccinated antigen [1,2]. Several other studies at that time described how cancer patients often displayed a so-called "immunological overshoot phenomenon" during chemotherapy: their peripheral blood lymphocytes were more activated after chemotherapy treatment, as measured by PHA stimulation and thymidine incorporation, with the magnitude of the overshoot correlating with a better clinical outcome [3,4]. In parallel studies in animals, it was found that intratumoral treatment with anthracyclines or actinomycin-D but not the antimetabolites methotrexate or 5-FU resulted in systemic antitumor immunity [5]. The same was later shown for the topoisomerase inhibitor etoposide [6]. Cyclophosphamide was found to deplete suppressive lymphocytes and reverse immunological tolerance [7]. Lastly, a particularly interesting study, in retrospect, investigated the combined use of cisplatin with the yeast glucan zymosan (now known to be a ligand of Toll-like receptor 2), where the authors reported that the combination treatment resulted in a 50% higher cure rate than cisplatin treatment alone [8].

Based on these and other findings, Kleinerman and Zwelling proposed that in addition to the two main and recognized features that determined the success or failure of cancer cytotoxic drugs—toxic effect on tumor cells and damage to normal cells—there was a third feature that had been overlooked: *beneficial* effects on normal body functions, both immune and nonimmune [9]. Now, with more advanced biological assays available, a wealth of studies has begun to unravel the molecular basis of these previously observed effects. In addition, immune-modulating effects of other classes of cancer chemotherapeutics have been described with a better understanding of the molecular mechanisms underlying their activity [10]. Nevertheless, it seems that there are still many more questions than

Cancer Immunotherapy. http://dx.doi.org/10.1016/B978-0-12-394296-8.00024-5

answers, and we are only beginning to translate the findings of fundamental studies into clinical trials.

II. THE IMMUNOPOTENTIATING EFFECT OF CANCER CHEMOTHERAPY

A. Chemotherapy effects on tumor cell immunogenicity

The intention when treating a patient with chemotherapy is cancer cell death. In the last decade, the immunological consequences of chemotherapy-induced cell death have been shown to be diverse. First, tumor cell death results in tumor antigen-release, which subsequently can be acquired and processed by antigen-presenting cells for crosspresentation to cytotoxic T cells. Indeed, in our own studies we found that treatment of malignant mesothelioma-bearing animals with the nucleoside analog gemcitabine resulted in increased antigen crosspresentation and priming of tumor-specific CD8 cells [11,12], although B-cell function was impaired [13].

Recently, a number of studies have provided compelling evidence that the way tumor cells die upon chemotherapy treatment is of crucial importance for the resulting immunological effect (Figure 24.1) [14–17]. The group of Kroemer and Zitvogel found that when mice were injected with tumor cells that had been pretreated *in vitro* with specific chemotherapeutics, including the platinum compound oxaliplatin and the anthracycline doxorubicin, they were effectively vaccinated against a rechallenge with live tumor cells. Depletion experiments showed that this immunity was dependent on the presence of dendritic cells and CD8 T cells. Interestingly, immunogenic cell vaccines were not created when other cytotoxic drugs were used, such as mitomycin-C [14,16]. In subsequent studies, it was found that a critical feature to induce an immune response was the translocation of calreticulin to the plasma membrane. This molecular flag was described as providing an *"eat me"* signal that could be recognized by passing dendritic cells [14,18]. In addition, chemotherapy-induced dying tumor cells could also release alarm signals, including HMGB-1 and ATP, that activated dendritic cells through Toll-like receptor 4 (TLR4) and NLRP3-mediated inflammasome stimulation, respectively. These signals in turn induced the production of pro-inflammatory cytokines and promoted local T-cell responses to tumor-associated antigens released by the dying tumor cells [15,17].

The clinical relevance of these findings was underlined by retrospective studies of selected breast cancer patients who had received adjuvant treatment with anthracyclines. Patients with loss-of-function alleles for the respective receptors for HMGB-1 and ATP displayed a worse clinical outcome when compared to patients with the normal alleles. Another study by the same group showed that patients with colorectal cancer who carried a loss-of-function TLR4

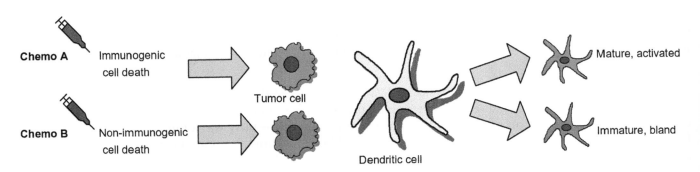

FIGURE 24.1

Immunogenic tumor cell death. It is now clear that the way chemotherapeutic drugs kill a tumor cell determines how that dying cell interacts with the immune system and whether the interaction will lead to an immune response. Immunogenic cell death induces DC maturation, allowing the DC to activate relevant T cells; in contrast, nonimmunogenic cell death is bland and does not activate the DC.

allele that resulted in a low-binding affinity for HMGB1 exhibited reduced progression-free and overall survival in response to oxaliplatin, as compared to patients carrying the normal TLR4 allele [19].

Importantly, not all chemotherapeutics induce all of the features of immunogenic cancer cell death. In fact, not all compounds within the same groups of cytotoxic drugs appear to have the same effects in this respect. For example, treatment with oxaliplatin results in calreticulin exposure, HMGB-1 and ATP release, but the other platinum compounds cisplatin and carboplatin do not appear to have this property. However, the lack of immunogenic cell death induction by cisplatin can be "repaired" by combining it with pharmacological ER stress inducers, which drive translocation of calreticulin from the ER to the plasma membrane [20]. Given the fact that cisplatin and carboplatin are much more widely used in the clinic than oxaliplatin, this approach holds promise for a wide array of different cancer types. However, these data were obtained *in vitro* and clinical studies demonstrating the actual value of this strategy in patients have yet to be published.

Another intriguing effect of some cytotoxic cancer drugs is their ability to sensitize tumor cells to T-cell-mediated cytotoxicity [21,22]. Cisplatin, doxorubicin and paclitaxel enhance the permeability of target cells to granzyme-B by upregulating mannose-6-phosphate receptors, thereby enhancing tumor cell killing by T cells [21]. Interestingly, the authors showed that not only tumor cells expressing the relevant antigen were destroyed by specific T cells, but also neighboring cancer cells that did not express the antigen, which in this case were lysed as "bystanders."

Other positive effects of chemotherapeutics on tumor cell immunogenicity include enhanced expression of tumor antigens by 5-FU, topoisomerase inhibitors and anthracylines and MHC I upregulation by gemcitabine (Table 24.1 and Figure 24.2) [23–25].

B. Chemotherapy effects on antigen-presenting cells

Recent work in murine models has demonstrated that several classes of cytotoxic drugs, such as taxanes, antifolates and anthracyclines, can have an activating effect on the antigen-presenting and T-cell-activating potential of dendritic cells [26]. Treatment with these drugs upregulates the antigen-processing machinery and co-stimulatory molecules on dendritic cells, as well as increases the expression of the pivotal T-cell-activating cytokine IL-12p70. However, it is important to point out that these data were obtained in mice treated with low, noncytotoxic doses of the drugs, and it has not yet been confirmed whether similar changes occur in human patients when treated with therapeutic doses of the compounds.

Using human dendritic cells and drug concentrations that relate to the peak values achieved in cancer patients, we have found that only platinum-based compounds can enhance the antigen-specific T-cell-stimulatory capacity of dendritic cells *in vitro*. This process occurs through a STAT6/PD-L2 dependent mechanism (see below) [27]. The differences in these findings may relate to the differences in drug concentrations, species or *in vitro* versus *in vivo* approaches that were used in these different studies.

Paclitaxel (but not the related taxane docetaxel) also appears to activate APC, possibly in the guise of an LPS mimetic that binds to the TLR4 accessory protein MD-2 in mice, but not humans [28,29]. This activation seems to occur through two pathways that are distinguished by their dependence or independence on TLR4 and MyD88 mechanisms [30]. However, in contrast to these potentially beneficial effects, there is evidence that paclitaxel-induced TLR4 signaling in TLR4-expressing human ovarian cancer cell-lines may enhance tumor survival and chemoresistance *in vitro* [31]. The net result for tumor control *in vivo* and the relevance of this pathway for the anticancer efficacy of paclitaxel has yet to be properly assessed.

TABLE 24.1 Immunological Effects of Different Classes of Cytotoxic Chemotherapy

Drug	Immunological Effect	Ref
Alkylating Agents		
DTIC/Temozolemide	Upregulation of T-cell-attracting chemokines by tumor cells, enhanced tumor antigen cross-priming, possibly immunogenic cell death, enhanced tumor sensitivity for T-cell-mediated lysis	[22,40,100,101]
Cyclophosphamide	Treg depletion, upregulation of tumor MHCI, Th17 skewing, deviation from Th2 response, promotion of homeostatic proliferation/activation, enhanced CTL-mediated killing *in vitro*	[43,44,46,60, 102–104]
Ifosfamide	*Impaired* CTL- (but not NK-) mediated cytotoxicity *in vitro* and *impaired* T-cell-stimulatory capacity of DCs	[105,106]
Melphalan	Skewing Th2 towards Th1 cytokine production by TILs, immunogenic cell death	[107,108]
Busulphan	Possibly preferential depletion of Treg	[109]
Clorambucil	*Impaired* NK- and CTL-mediated cytotoxicity *in vitro*	[104,108,110]
Carmustine	Possibly preferential depletion of Tregs*	[111,112]
Anti-Metabolites		
Metotrexate	DC activation, enhanced CTL-mediated killing *in vitro*	[26,104]
5-FU/Capecitabine	TAA upregulation, depletion of MDSCs, enhanced CTL-mediated killing *in vitro*, enhanced NK-mediated cytotoxicity *in vitro*, enhanced tumor sensitivity for T-cell-mediated lysis	[22,25,104,110,113]
Fludarabine	Treg depletion	[114]
Cytarabine	Enhanced CTL-mediated killing *in vitro*	[104]
Cladribine	*Impaired* NK-mediated cytotoxicity *in vitro*	[110]
6-Mercaptopurine	Enhanced CTL-mediated killing *in vitro*, enhanced NK-mediated cytotoxicity *in vitro*	[104,110]
Gemcitabine	Enhanced crosspresentation, Treg depletion, MDSC depletion, tumor MHC class I upregulation	[11,24,66,82]
Pemetrexed	no data	
Hydroxyurea	Enhanced CTL-mediated killing *in vitro*, enhanced NK-mediated cytotoxicity *in vitro*	[104,110]
Vinca Compounds		
Vincristine	DC activation, but *impaired* CTL-mediated killing *in vitro*	[26,104]
Vinblastine	DC activation, *Impaired* NK-mediated cytotoxicity *in vitro*	[26,110,115,116]
Vinorelbine	Enhanced CTL-mediated killing *in vitro*, but bystander-killing of immune cells by vinorelbine-treated tumor cells	[104,117]

Drug	Immune Stimulatory Features	References
Taxanes		
Paclitaxel	Reduced IL-10 and TGFβ-production by Treg, DC activation, enhanced tumor sensitivity for T-cell-mediated lysis, but *impaired* NK-cell-mediated cytotoxicity *in vitro*	[21,26,67,110]
Docetaxel	Increased IFN-γ production by CTLs, but *impaired* NK- and CTL-mediated cytotoxicity *in vitro*, depletion of MDSCs	[41,70,110]
Topoisomerase Inhibitors		
Etoposide	TAA upregulation, enhanced NK-mediated cytotoxicity *in vitro*	[23,110]
Irinotecan	Enhanced tumor sensitivity for T-cell-mediated lysis	[113]
Topotecan	TAA upregulation, enhanced CTL-mediated killing *in vitro*	[23,104,118]
Camptothecin	TAA upregulation	[23]
Cytotoxic Antibiotics		
Doxorubicin	Immunogenic cell death, TAA upregulation, DC activation, enhanced tumor sensitivity for T-cell-mediated lysis, enhanced NK-mediated cytotoxicity *in vitro*, but *impaired* CTL-mediated killing *in vitro*	[14,15,17,21,26,104,110]
Daunorubicin	TAA upregulation, enhanced CTL-mediated killing *in vitro*	[23,104]
Idarubicin	TAA upregulation, immunogenic cell death	[14,23]
Epirubicin	TAA upregulation, enhanced CTL-mediated killing *in vitro*, enhanced NK-mediated cytotoxicity *in vitro*	[23,104,110]
Mitomycin	DC activation with low doses, but skewing into *tolerogenic* DCs with high doses, and *impaired* CTL-mediated killing *in vitro*	[26,104,119]
Bleomycin	Possibly Treg depletion*, Enhanced NK-mediated cytotoxicity *in vitro*, but *impaired* CTL-mediated killing *in vitro*	[104,110,120]
Mitoxantrone	immunogenic cell death	[14]
Dactinomycine	no data	
Platinum-Based Compounds		
Cisplatin	Upregulation of T-cell-attracting chemokines by tumor cells, inactivation of STAT6 and subsequent downregulation of PD-L2, enhanced tumor sensitivity for T-cell-mediated lysis, enhanced CTL-mediated killing *in vitro*	[21,27,40,104,113]
Oxaliplatin	Immunogenic cell death through calreticulin-exposure, HMGB-1 and ATP secretion by dying cancer cells, inactivation of STAT6 and subsequent downregulation of PD-L2, but *impaired* CTL-mediated killing *in vitro*	[14,15,17,27,104]
Carboplatin	Inactivation of STAT6 and subsequent downregulation of PD-L2, enhanced CTL-mediated killing *in vitro*	[27,104]

*At the time Tregs could not be adequately characterized, due to a lack of markers such as Foxp3.

399

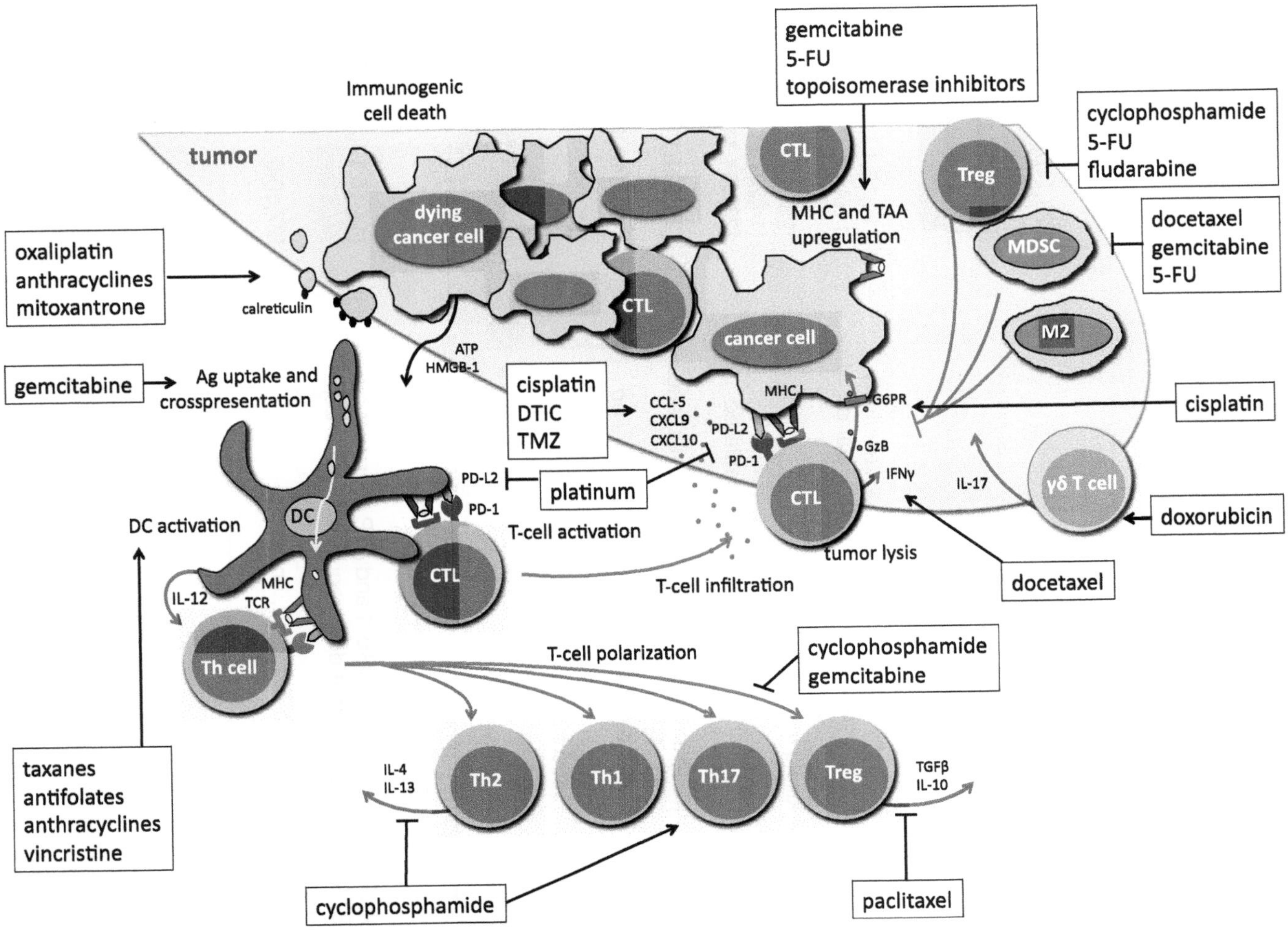

FIGURE 24.2
Effects of classic cytotoxic cancer chemotherapeutics on the tumor immune microenvironment. The immunological mechanisms of action of the drugs with the relevant references are discussed in detail in paragraph II and summarized in Table 24.1.

C. Chemotherapy effects on immune-effector cells

1. T CELLS

Ever since cytotoxic drugs first entered the clinic it has been assumed that they have a negative effect on the immune system. Patients treated with chemotherapy appeared highly susceptible to commensal bacterial infections that in general do not cause severe infections in healthy individuals. Not surprisingly, patients are particularly susceptible during the neutropenic phase of therapy, with high morbidity and even occasional mortality. Indeed, neutropenia is the dose-limiting toxicity of a number of cytotoxic agents or combinations. In addition, antibody responses during chemotherapy, such as after vaccination against viral diseases, are likely to be suboptimal [32]. In some cases, particularly in hematological malignancies, lymphocyte counts decrease dramatically and T-cell-mediated immunity is clearly impaired, resulting in severe fungal, yeast, viral and bacterial infections [33—35]. In the decades since the initial clinical development of chemotherapy, little attention has been paid to the effects of chemotherapy on T-cell function.

Recent evidence indicates that, although in some treatment schedules used for hematological malignancies T-cell responses indeed may be impaired, this does not seem to be the case for most cytotoxic drugs. In fact, for some drug combinations precisely the reverse situation may be true. In several studies in cancer patients, where vaccines were used in combination with cytotoxic drugs, *de novo* vaccine-induced tumor antigen-specific T- and B-cell responses were not impaired by the administration of the chemotherapy, and in fact in some cases these responses were even enhanced (listed in Table 24.2). Examples of drugs that have been found to positively affect vaccination outcome include doxorubicin, cyclophosphamide (though dependent on dosing), DTIC and platinum compounds (Table 24.2). In addition, there is convincing evidence that the period of lymphodepletion following nonmyeloablative chemotherapy allows for longer persistence of adoptively transferred T cells [36,37]. Whether this situation also holds true for outgrowth of *de novo*-induced endogenous tumor-specific T cells remains a question for future studies. Some animal studies show an enhanced preferential outgrowth of tumor antigen-specific T cells after chemotherapy-induced sub-myeloablative leucopenia that is followed by vaccination [38]. However, these findings could not be replicated in a human melanoma study that showed the frequency of tumor antigen-specific T cells remained low after vaccination, even though there was effective homeostatic proliferation of total lymphocyte populations and Epstein-Barr virus-specific T cells [39].

Additional information on the positive effects of chemotherapeutic agents on T-cell effector function has come from preclinical studies. Hong and colleagues investigated the effect of the alkylators dacarbazine and temozolomide and the platinum compound cisplatin on T-cell-attracting chemokines by melanoma cell lines *in vitro*, finding that CCL5 and the CXCR3 ligands CXCL9 and CXCL10 were all upregulated by chemotherapeutic treatment. Moreover, they found that these chemokines synergized in the treatment of a mouse model of melanoma, resulting in attraction of effector T cells into metastases and inhibition of tumor growth. Similarly, serial biopsies in melanoma patients who were treated with dacarbazine showed an increase of T-cell infiltration in chemotherapy-sensitive lesions, where the expression of these T-cell-attracting chemokines by melanoma was correlated with improved progression-free survival [40].

The taxane docetaxel has been reported to increase IFN-γ production by anti-CD3 stimulated CD8$^+$ T cells, but not CD4$^+$ T cells in a murine study. At the same time, the proliferative capacity of these T cells was unaltered by the drug. When colon cancer-bearing mice were treated with a carcinoembryonic antigen-based vaccine in combination with docetaxel, this combination treatment resulted in better tumor control than either treatment alone [41]. Enhanced amplification of vaccine-induced T cells also has been reported after administration of chemotherapy. For example, Rettig and colleagues found that gemcitabine increased the percentage of NY-ESO-1-specific T cells after vaccination in mice [42].

A much less studied immunological effect of chemotherapy involves the skewing of the T-cell repertoire in the tumor environment from a relatively ineffective Th2-helper response towards a more effective Th1 helper response. In fact, some very early animal studies showed that cyclophosphamide could induce such a switch [43,44]. Recently, we showed that platinum compounds can inactivate STAT6, the key regulator of Th2 responses, and indeed nonspecifically activated T cells of cancer patients produced more IFN-γ after treatment with platinum drugs, but whether this reflected a favorable skewing towards a Th1 phenotype remains to be proven [27,45]. Cyclophosphamide also appears to polarize T cells towards the pro-inflammatory Th17 phenotype, in both mouse models and cancer patients treated with a continuous low dose of the drug [46].

2. INNATE IMMUNE CELLS

Traditionally, T cells have been the main focus of attention in tumor immunology, but recent studies have emphasized the important role that other effector cells have in the tumor microenvironment, especially in the context of chemotherapy. Not only does this role concern immune cells with suppressive characteristics, such as myeloid-derived suppressive cells (MDSC) or M2 macrophages (discussed below), but also in effector cells that in principle can exert positive antitumor effects, such as B cells and neutrophils.

TABLE 24.2 Clinical Studies Investigating the Effect of Cytotoxic Cancer Drugs in Combination with Immunotherapeutic Approaches in Patients

Cytotoxic Drug	Vaccine / Immunotherapy	Cancer Type (n=)	Outcome	Trial Design	Ref
Chemotherapy/Vaccination Combination Trials					
Cyclophosphamide (300mg/m^2)	Class I/II TAA peptides	Melanoma (167)	Cyclophosphamide did not influence T-cell responses	Randomized phase I/II	[65]
Cyclophosphamide (200–350mg/m^2) Doxorubicine (15–35mg/m^2)	Irradiated Her2Neu$^+$ GM-CSF secreting allo-tumor cell-line	Breast cancer (28)	Doxorubicine highest dose and cyclophosphamide lowest dose enhanced DTH and humoral response	3x3 factorial dose-ranging study	[89]
Docetaxel	Vaccinia PSA/B7.1	Prostate cancer (28)	Docetaxel did not influence T-cell responses	Randomized phase II	[90]
5-FU + LV + irinotecan	ALVAC-CEA/B7.1	Colorectal cancer (118)	Chemotherapy did not affect CEA-specific T-cell responses after vaccination	Randomized phase I/II	[91]
DTIC	Class I TAA peptides + IFNα	Melanoma (36)	improved TAA-specific T-cell responses and broader T-cell repertoire in DTIC arm	Non-randomized phase I/II	[92,93]
Temozolemide	Telomerase peptide	Melanoma (25)	78% T-cell responsiveness (no direct comparative arm)	Single arm phase I/II	[94]
Gemcitabine	Class I Wilms tumor 1 peptide	Pancreatic or biliary tract cancer	Evidence for TAA-specific T-cell expansion in 59% of the patients	Single arm phase I	[95]
Cisplatin, vinblastin, cyclophosphamide (200mg/m^2)	EGF protein	NSCLC (20)	EGF-specific antibody responses were found in majority of patients	Single arm phase I/II	[96]
Temozolemide (500mg/m^2 per	EGFRvIII peptide	GBM (22)		Non-randomized phase II	[97]

5 days or 100mg/m² per 21 days)					
Oxaliplatin, capecitabine	DC+CEA	Colon cancer	DTH and humoral responses against peptide, but higher in dose-intensified group T-cell responses in DTH were not impaired. Increase in nonspecific T-cell activation after platinum drugs	Non-randomized phase I/II	[45]
Chemotherapy/Adoptive Transfer Combination Trials					
Cyclophosphamide 60mg/kg + Fludarabine ± TBI	TIL + IL-2	Melanoma (93)	High and durable response rates, long persistence of transferred T cells	3 single arm phase II studies	[36]
±Fludarabine	TAA-specific CTL clone	Melanoma (10)	Fludarabine pretreatment increased median *in vivo* persistence of CTL clone from 4.5 to 13 days	Single arm phase I/II study	[37]
Chemotherapy/Non-Specific Immunotherapy Combination Trials					
DTIC	Ipilimumab (3mg/kg)	Melanoma (72)	No immune-correlates. Response rate 14.3% DTIC+Ipi vs. 5.4% Ipi alone	Randomized phase II	[83]
DTIC	Ipilimumab (10mg/kg)	Melanoma (502)	3-year overall survival 20.8% DTIC + Ipi vs. 12.2% DTIC alone	Randomized phase III	[74]
Gemcitabine	Anti-CD40	Pancreatic cancer (21)	Several clinical responses. Unclear additive effect gemcitabine	Single arm Phase I	[98]
Carboplatin, paclitaxel	Ipilimumab (concurrent or sequential)	NSCLC (203)	Prolonged PFS for combination, sequential appeared better than concurrent	Randomized, double-blind, 3-arm phase II study	[99]

Nonstandard Abbreviations: TAA, Tumor-Associated Antigens; PSA, Prostate-Specific Antigen; DTH, Delayed-Type Hypersensitivity Reaction; NSCLC, Non-Small Cell Lung Cancer; EGF, Epidermal Growth Factor; EGFRvIII, Epidermal Growth Factor Receptor Variant III; GBM, Glioblastoma Multiforme; Ipi, Ipilimumab; TBI, Total Body Irradiation; TIL, Tumor-Infiltrating Lymphocytes

Many studies in the last 10–15 years that have investigated the role of neutrophils in cancer progression have found a tumor-promoting role for these cells. Specifically, granulocyte depletion has been reported to increase tumor infiltration of CD8+ T cells, inhibit tumor angiogenesis, and decrease tumor growth [47]. On the other hand, earlier studies have reported a beneficial effect of neutrophils in restricting tumor growth [48]. It appears that these conflicting data may be explained by the plasticity of neutrophils. Analogous to macrophages, neutrophils rely on the microenvironment for instructing signals, resulting in the generation of procarcinogenic N2 cells or anticarcinogenic N1 cells, with an important role for TGFβ in determining the balance between these cell types [49].

Since neutropenia is the most common toxicity associated with nearly all classical cytotoxic cancer drugs, it is tempting to speculate that the relative neutrophil "depletion" that occurs in these patients may for some part be responsible for the observed clinical effect. Intriguingly, in one large study carboplatin/paclitaxel-induced leucopenia was indeed associated with improved clinical outcome in patients with advanced ovarian cancer [50], and a meta-analysis found the same results for a wide array of cancer types [51]. Of course, this situation might also be explained by pharmacokinetic effects, such as differences in bioavailability of the drug and thus effective dose-intensity. At this point, while there are reasons to suspect immune inductive effects there are not yet data that can definitively substantiate the claim that depleting neutrophils by chemotherapy may contribute to its antitumor effects. For other innate immune cells, there is clear evidence from animal studies of a role in chemotherapy efficacy. The groups of Zitvogel and Smyth have found that the antitumor effects of antracyclines are compromised in γδ-T-cell knockout mice and that this effect was dependent on IL-17 production by these cells [52,53]. In these models, natural killer T cells (NKT cells) did not play a role in chemotherapy efficacy. Further studies in this burgeoning area are expected.

3. B CELLS

As for neutrophils, it also remains unclear whether B cells are friend or foe in the tumor microenvironment. In the last ten years or so, some evidence has accumulated showing that B cells deviate T-cell immune responses from a Th1 response towards a Th2 response that promotes tumor growth in several transgenic mouse models of *de novo* tumor development. These data have been reviewed in detail elsewhere [54]. However, the question of different roles for stimulatory and inhibitory B-cell subpopulations which may be highly relevant (e.g., regulatory B cells or Breg) has yet to receive significant attention in the context of cancer. Research from our group has demonstrated that, although CD4 and CD8 tumor-antigen specific T-cell responses were enhanced after gemcitabine treatment, B-cell function was clearly impaired [13], albeit by mechanisms yet to be understood.

D. Chemotherapy effects on suppressive networks

One of the lessons that can be learned from the plethora of vaccination studies performed over the last decade is that antigen-specific T-cell activation as a monotherapy is nearly always not enough to halt tumor progression. Although there are clear studies that have found a good correlation between response and the presence of vaccine-induced T cells, the majority of patients that have measurable antigen-specific T-cell responses do not show signs of tumor regression [10,55]. One of the key reasons for this failure almost certainly lies in the strong suppressive mechanisms erected by the tumor microenvironment, reflecting its mastery by tumor cells. These suppressive mechanisms of immune escape broadly consist of a) specific suppressive immune cells; b) suppressive molecules and metabolic properties of immune cells, tumor cells and stromal cells and c) soluble immune-modulating factors. Other chapters in this book as well as recent reviews cover these mechanisms in detail [56–58]. In the sections below, we focus on the effects of classic cancer chemotherapeutics on these immune suppressive pathways in the tumor microenvironment.

1. DEPLETION OF SUPPRESSIVE CELLS

As discussed in the introduction, one of the first discovered positive immunological effects of chemotherapy on the immune system was the discovery that cyclophosphamide could deplete Treg [7]. This immune stimulatory effect occurs in a dose-dependent manner with optimal Treg depletion, in the absence of impairing the T-cell effector pool at low doses [59–62]. Indeed, in several animal models as well as in patient studies, the strength of the induced immune response could be improved by combining immunotherapeutic approaches with cyclophosphamide [61,63,64]. One caveat to this otherwise uniform trend in response derives from the results a recently reported large randomized Phase II study in melanoma patients, where a multi-epitope peptide vaccination combined with low-dose cyclophosphamide did not show any beneficial effect on the vaccine-induced immune response, nor on clinical responses [65]. At the moment, several large clinical studies investigating low-dose cyclophosphamide with other immunotherapeutic approaches are ongoing, with both immunological and clinical endpoints. Thus, until the results of these studies are analyzed, the verdict on the value of cyclophosphamide in this setting still remains out.

Gemcitabine has also been reported to deplete Treg, albeit in a relatively modest manner and where the clinical relevance is unclear [66]. Interestingly, paclitaxel not only impairs the viability of Tregs, but also their production of the immunosuppressive cytokines TGFβ and IL-10 [67].

In addition to Tregs, myeloid-derived suppressor cells (MDSCs) also appear to be selectively depleted by some chemotherapeutics, including gemcitabine [68,69], 5-FU [69] and docetaxel [70]. The molecular mechanisms involved in these settings have not been described.

Less is known about the effect of cancer chemotherapeutics on tumor-promoting M2 macrophages. Studies from the Coussens group have demonstrated that paclitaxel enhances M2 macrophage infiltration of breast cancer by stimulating production of the monocyte-attracting cytokine CSF1 by mammary epithelial cells. Consistent with this observation, the efficacy of paclitaxel in a murine breast cancer model was improved significantly when the drug was combined with an antibody against CSF1 [71].

2. DOWNREGULATION OF SUPPRESSIVE MOLECULES

In recent years, an overwhelming amount of preclinical data has been generated on the different inhibitory molecules expressed by both immune cells and nonimmune cells, which presumably serve normally to prevent too much collateral damage in the context of effective, but also potentially destructive Th1 or Th17 immune responses [72]. So-called immune checkpoint molecules such as Cytotoxic T Lymphocyte Antigen (CTLA)-4 and Programmed Death receptor (PD)-1 have been successfully targeted in cancer patients using blocking antibodies. The anti-CTLA-4 antibody ipilimumab has demonstrated a survival benefit in metastatic melanoma on the basis of which it has been approved by the FDA for this indication [73,74]. The anti-PD-1 antibody MDX-1016 has shown some activity as monotherapy in Phase I studies and has now entered Phase II trials [75].

Little is known, however, about the effect of classic cytotoxic drugs on the expression and function of these inhibitory molecules. We recently found that platinum chemotherapeutics enhance the T-cell stimulatory potential of dendritic cells by downregulating PD-L2 in a STAT6-dependent manner [27]. The clinical relevance of these *in vitro* findings was substantiated by results of a retrospective study in patients with head and neck cancer who had been treated with cisplatinum-based chemoradiation: patients with STAT6-expressing tumors had a much better recurrence-free survival than patients with STAT6-negative tumors. Interestingly, the reverse was true for a matched cohort of patients that had been treated with radiotherapy alone. This observation suggests that STAT6 is part of an immune-deviating pathway that results in a poorer prognosis in patients with (head and neck) cancer, unless this pathway is abrogated by platinum chemotherapeutics. Importantly, although STAT6 appears to be constitutively phosphorylated in some tumors [76], this is probably not always the case, insofar as tumor cells can rely on IL-4, IL-13 or TSLP in the tumor microenvironment for STAT6 activation [57,77]. Thus, platinum-sensitivity may be at least partly determined by microenvironmental immune stimuli [78]. Given the implications for patient selection and combination therapies, further research should clarify whether this hypothesis is valid. In fact, not all is good with respect to platinum and the immune system, insofar as oxaliplatin was found to increase PD-L1 expression on plasmacytoid dendritic cells, thereby increasing an immune suppressive signal. Although TLR9-induced IFNα secretion was enhanced by oxaliplatin, the net result was decreased T-cell activation potential *in vitro* [79]. Future *in vivo* models and clinical studies in platinum-treated patients should clarify the net result of different mechanisms of action of platinum drugs on the immune system.

III. HOW CAN WE USE AND ENFORCE THE IMMUNOGENIC PROPERTIES OF CHEMOTHERAPEUTIC DRUGS?

Based on all the preclinical studies we can conclude that cancer chemotherapeutics can exert positive immunological effects. Two very important questions remain unanswered. First, how much of the observed clinical effect is truly determined by the immunological action of the drugs? And second, how can we exploit the immunological effects of chemotherapeutic treatments to increase their anticancer efficacy?

Addressing the first question, clinical studies suggest clearly that the immunological effects of chemotherapy are a significant part of their efficacy. As briefly mentioned above, a retrospective analysis of 338 colorectal cancer patients that had participated in a multi-institution, randomized clinical trial comparing up-front oxaliplatin-based combination chemotherapy versus sequential chemotherapy showed that patients harboring a loss-of-function allele for TLR4 displayed poorer progression-free and overall survival [19]. However, although the difference was significant, the effect was limited with an improvement in median progression-free survival from approximately 6 to 7–8 months. Investigating the effect of the same mutation, but in breast cancer patients who had been treated with doxorubicin in the adjuvant setting, the same group found a more pronounced negative effect of inadequate TLR4 or IL-1β signaling on overall survival [15,17]. However, since this concerns retrospective, observational, single-institution studies, these data need to be confirmed in prospective, controlled trials. This is also the case for our own study in head and neck cancer patients treated with cisplatin-based chemoradiation, in which STAT6 expression was correlated with an increased 3-year recurrence-free survival of 80% versus 48% for STAT6-negative tumors [27].

In addition, strong effects on survival in cancer patients have been found for the presence of different immune infiltrates in the tumor. However, in the majority of these clinical studies, treatments have not been confined to certain defined chemotherapy regimes, and markers found to correlate with survival must therefore be generally seen as prognostic, rather than predictive. While it goes beyond the scope of this chapter to review all those data, we refer the reader to an excellent recent review elsewhere [80].

Lastly, it is now clear that the efficacy of chemotherapeutics is impaired in animals that lack T-cell immunity, demonstrating a clear role for the adaptive immune response in anti-tumor efficacy of these drugs [81]. Such demonstrations make a strong case against concepts that took hold in the 1970s, based on findings of similar rates of spontaneous tumorigenesis in nude mice, that were unfortunately interpreted incorrectly at the time to mean that T-cell immunity exerts little effect on tumor outgrowth. Although at this moment the exact magnitude of the contribution of the immune system to the efficacy of cancer chemotherapy is not clear, it is now possible to conclude that there is certainly a significant effect.

With this conclusion, we come to the second question: how can we further exploit the immunogenic effects of classic cancer chemotherapy? Before being able to answer this question properly, we should preferably understand the most important immunological effects for the different drugs as listed in Table 24.2. For example, as discussed above, while treatment with gemcitabine can enhance tumor antigen crosspresentation by dendritic cells, it also triggers upregulation of tumor MHC class I expression and depletion of both regulatory T cells and myeloid-derived suppressor cells (Table 24.2) [11,24,66,82]. In order to design a clinical study that would optimally exploit the immunogenic momentum of gemcitabine, it would be useful to know which property is dominant. Additionally, it would be important to know which immunogenic pathways are saturated by chemotherapy and which ones could be further enhanced. For example, if antigen release and subsequent crosspresentation is the dominant immunogenic feature of gemcitabine that results in saturation with tumor antigen, it may not be logical to combine it with a vaccination approach.

One question is how much animal models will be able to teach us in this respect, since the amount of apoptosis induction that gemcitabine causes can differ considerably between mouse models and human cancer patients. Also, the type of T-cell response in the tumor microenvironment (e.g., Th1 vs. Th2) can differ between different mouse models, such that the immunological response to chemotherapeutic drugs may also differ. Nevertheless, while we do not yet fully grasp the dominant immunological features of different chemotherapeutics, given the expected additive effect of chemotherapy—immunotherapy combinations, and also the fact that several novel immunotherapeutic drugs are either already FDA approved or in a late stage of clinical development, it is likely that clinical research will outrun laboratory-based translational research in this arena. It therefore seems that, while ongoing investigations should decipher the most important immunological effects of different cytotoxic drugs, a more practical approach might also be followed, namely, to combine chemotherapy with immunological treatments that are (almost) available in the clinic, and that target the supposedly most prominent and important effector cell in the tumor—the T cell. Here the most obvious candidate is the recently FDA-approved monoclonal antibody against CTLA-4, ipilimumab, although other drugs such as anti-PD1 antibodies and IDO inhibitors are logical follow-up candidates to explore.

With regard to ipilimumab, a large Phase III trial in metastatic melanoma that combined anti-CTLA-4 with DTIC chemotherapy was reported recently. This study compared the combination therapy versus DTIC alone and it demonstrated a survival benefit for the combination therapy [74]. However, because there was no comparison to anti-CTLA-4 alone, the true added value of the DTIC chemotherapy could not be fully assessed. In a Phase II study that compared ipilimumab alone versus ipilimumab plus DTIC, but used lower (and less effective) dosages of anti-CTLA-4, there was a trend towards better disease control rate for the combination treatment, although this did not reach statistical significance [83]. Thus, based on published human studies, no definitive conclusion can be drawn on a possible synergistic effect of anti-CTLA-4 and chemotherapy. Additional Phase III studies to explore this question are currently accruing, such as in non-small cell lung cancer where investigations of paclitaxel/carboplatin with or without ipilimumab are being conducted (clinicaltrials.gov identifier NCT01285609, Table 24.1). The results of these studies are eagerly awaited.

We recently demonstrated in a murine mesothelioma model that treatment with gemcitabine chemotherapy in combination with anti-CTLA-4 blockade resulted in the induction of a potent antitumor immune response. Mice treated with the combination exhibited tumor regression and long-term protective immunity [84]. However, we found that the efficacy of the combination was dependent on the timing of administration of the two agents. Based on these results and the results from studies that combined anti-CTLA-4 with vaccines [85,86], we consider it very important to determine the optimal schedules in small pilot studies in animal models and cancer patients.

In addition, since treatment with anti-CTLA-4 sometimes gives rise to very severe autoimmune-related adverse events, with treatment-related deaths of $\sim 2\%$ [73], it is crucial to carefully monitor side effects when combining this drug with chemotherapeutic agents. This situation holds especially true for chemotherapy-induced side effects that may cause immune activation in themselves, such as for example mucositis of the gastrointestinal tract with irinotecan or kidney failure by cisplatin (the pathophysiology of which T cells play an important role [87]). A recent Phase I dose-escalating study investigating the combination of anti-CTLA-4 antibody tremelimumab in combination with the tyrosine kinase inhibitor sunitinib in 28 patients with metastatic renal cell cancer offers an illustrative example of the devastating toxicity that can potentially occur: 17 patients experienced grade 3–4 adverse events, 9 patients experienced a dose-limiting toxicity, of whom 4 patients had renal failure and 1 patient severe colitis, and there was 1 case of sudden death (although the latter may not have related to the study drugs) [88]. Although Phase I studies are designed in such a way that maximal safety for the patient is the primary consideration, it could be argued here that initial tests of the possible combinations in animal models first are warranted. Although animal models will not provide us with definite answers concerning whether severe toxicity will occur in humans, since the toxicity of both anti-CTLA-4 and the chemotherapeutics in general occur to a lesser extent in animal models, this shortcoming is not in our view a reason to skip such tests altogether, since they may at least offer some indication of the possible problems that may await clinicians and patients in exploring novel combinations, and they may also help guide the design of subsequent human studies.

In addition to anti-CTLA-4, there are several other candidate immunotherapeutic approaches that are in a late stage of development and that may potentially work in synergy with immuno-potentiating chemotherapy. These include (but are not limited to) agonistic antibodies against CD40 and OX40, blocking antibodies against the PD-1/PD-L pathway, vaccines, Toll-like receptor ligands and antibodies or small molecules that target TGFβ or IDO or other suppressive cytokines, growth factors and enzymes (Box 24.1). Future studies in both humans and animal models may show definitively whether or not the positive immunological effects of classic chemotherapeutics can be more fully exploited through combination with these immunotherapeutic treatment modalities, as an effective strategy to increase antitumor efficacy.

IV. CONCLUSIONS

It is now clear that classical chemotherapeutics exert positive immunological effects that may contribute to the clinical efficacy of these drugs in cancer. However, at this point we do not fully understand the magnitude of these effects: i.e., how many of the clinical effects seen in patients are caused by the immunological component of the mechanism of action of these drugs? Nor do we fully understand the mechanisms involved. To gain more insight into these matters, we need (preferably prospective) clinical trials that include an assessment of

BOX 24.2 KEY QUESTIONS FOR THE NEAR FUTURE

Which cytotoxic drugs have the most potent immunostimulating effect?

Which immunogenic properties are most dominant and should be targeted/exploited first?

Which chemo-immunotherapy combinations have a high chance for severe toxicity?

Can we predict which patients will respond best?

How do dosing and scheduling influence the immunological effects?

Do the tumors need to be chemo-sensitive?

immunological biomarkers, such as the discussed studies investigating the TLR4 or STAT6 pathways [19,27].

Regardless of the magnitude of the immunological effect of cancer cytotoxics, their immunological effects could likely be further exploited by combining these traditional drugs with various immunotherapeutic approaches (Box 24.2). Some of these immunotherapeutic approaches are already FDA approved or are in late-stage clinical development, allowing more rapid development of treatment combinations in clinical trials. Nevertheless, we suggest that before initiating classic Phase I human studies, both animal studies and in-depth small-scale clinical studies with immunological endpoints should be performed to investigate optimal scheduling and dosing of the separate components, and also to assess potential toxicities that could occur. In closing, we believe that the newly rediscovered immunopotentiating effects of classic chemotherapeutics may herald a new era in cancer treatment, by combining these drugs with immunotherapies to allow maximum synergy and maximum efficacy.

409

ACKNOWLEDGMENTS

The discussion of the literature in this book chapter is based on our own data and published literature accessible from PubMed using different combinations of the following key words: cancer, immune response, chemotherapy, cytotoxic, T cells, B cells, neutrophils, NK cells, NKT cells, dendritic cells, myeloid-derived suppressor cells, regulatory T cells, macrophages, depletion, tumor microenvironment, tumor antigens, vaccine, vaccination, adoptive transfer, CTLA-4, ipilimumab, PD-1, B7, toll-like receptor, lymphodepletion, immunogenic cell death, and all the chemotherapeutic names that have been listed in Table 24.1. We apologize to colleagues in the field for any papers that have been missed that would have been relevant to mention.

References

[1] Sterzl J. Inhibition of the inductive phase of antibody formation by 6-mercaptopurine examined by the transfer of isolated cells. Nature 1960;185:256−7.

[2] Reif AE. Immunity, cancer, and chemotherapy. Science 1966;154(3755):1475−8.

[3] Serrou B, Dubois JB. Immunological overshoot phenomenon following cancer chemotherapy: significance in prognosis evaluation of solid tumors. Biomedicine 1975;23(1):41−5.

[4] Harris J, Sengar D, Stewart T, Hyslop D. The effect of immunosuppressive chemotherapy on immune function in patients with malignant disease. Cancer 1976;37(Suppl. 2):1058−69.

[5] Bast Jr RC, Segerling M, Ohanian SH, Greene SL, Zbar B, Rapp HJ, et al. Regression of established tumors and induction of tumor immunity by intratumor chemotherapy. J Natl Cancer Inst 1976;56(4):829−32.

[6] Claessen AM, Bloemena E, Bril H, Meijer CJ, Scheper RJ. Locoregional administration of etoposide, but not of interleukin 2, facilitates active specific immunization in guinea pigs with advanced carcinoma. Cancer Res 1992;52(9):2440−6.

[7] Polak L, Turk JL. Reversal of immunological tolerance by cyclophosphamide through inhibition of suppressor cell activity. Nature 1974;249(458):654–6.

[8] Marx JL. Chemotherapy: renewed interest in platinum compounds. Science 1976;192(4241):774–5.

[9] Kleinerman E, Zwelling L. The Effect of cis-Diamminedichloroplatinum (II) on Immune Function in vitro and in vivo. Cancer Immunol Immunother 1982;12:191–6.

[10] Lesterhuis WJ, Haanen JB, Punt CJ. Cancer immunotherapy - revisited. Nat Rev Drug Discov 2011;10(8):591–600.

[11] Nowak AK, Lake RA, Marzo AL, Scott B, Heath WR, Collins EJ, et al. Induction of tumor cell apoptosis in vivo increases tumor antigen cross-presentation, cross-priming rather than cross-tolerizing host tumor-specific CD8 T cells. J Immunol 2003;170(10):4905–13.

[12] Nowak AK, Robinson BW, Lake RA. Synergy between chemotherapy and immunotherapy in the treatment of established murine solid tumors. Cancer Res 2003;63(15):4490–6.

[13] Nowak AK, Robinson BW, Lake RA. Gemcitabine exerts a selective effect on the humoral immune response: implications for combination chemo-immunotherapy. Cancer Res 2002;62(8):2353–8.

[14] Obeid M, Tesniere A, Ghiringhelli F, Fimia GM, Apetoh L, Perfettini JL, et al. Calreticulin exposure dictates the immunogenicity of cancer cell death. Nat Med 2007;13(1):54–61.

[15] Ghiringhelli F, Apetoh L, Tesniere A, Aymeric L, Ma Y, Ortiz C, et al. Activation of the NLRP3 inflammasome in dendritic cells induces IL-1beta-dependent adaptive immunity against tumors. Nat Med 2009;15(10):1170–8.

[16] Casares N, Pequignot MO, Tesniere A, Ghiringhelli F, Roux S, Chaput N, et al. Caspase-dependent immunogenicity of doxorubicin-induced tumor cell death. J Exp Med 2005;202(12):1691–701.

[17] Apetoh L, Ghiringhelli F, Tesniere A, Obeid M, Ortiz C, Criollo A, et al. Toll-like receptor 4-dependent contribution of the immune system to anticancer chemotherapy and radiotherapy. Nat Med 2007;13(9):1050–9.

[18] Clarke C, Smyth MJ. Calreticulin exposure increases cancer immunogenicity. Nat Biotechnol 2007;25(2):192–3.

[19] Tesniere A, Schlemmer F, Boige V, Kepp O, Martins I, Ghiringhelli F, et al. Immunogenic death of colon cancer cells treated with oxaliplatin. Oncogene 2009;29(4):482–91.

[20] Martins I, Kepp O, Schlemmer F, Adjemian S, Tailler M, Shen S, et al. Restoration of the immunogenicity of cisplatin-induced cancer cell death by endoplasmic reticulum stress. Oncogene 2011;30(10):1147–58.

[21] Ramakrishnan R, Assudani D, Nagaraj S, Hunter T, Cho HI, Antonia S, et al. Chemotherapy enhances tumor cell susceptibility to CTL-mediated killing during cancer immunotherapy in mice. J Clin Invest 2010;120(4):1111–24.

[22] Yang S, Haluska FG. Treatment of melanoma with 5-fluorouracil or dacarbazine in vitro sensitizes cells to antigen-specific CTL lysis through perforin/granzyme- and Fas-mediated pathways. J Immunol 2004;172(7):4599–608.

[23] Haggerty TJ, Dunn IS, Rose LB, Newton EE, Martin S, Riley JL, et al. Topoisomerase inhibitors modulate expression of melanocytic antigens and enhance T cell recognition of tumor cells. Cancer Immunol Immunother 2011;60(1):133–44.

[24] Liu WM, Fowler DW, Smith P, Dalgleish AG. Pre-treatment with chemotherapy can enhance the antigenicity and immunogenicity of tumours by promoting adaptive immune responses. Br J Cancer 2010;102(1):115–23.

[25] Correale P, Aquino A, Giuliani A, Pellegrini M, Micheli L, Cusi MG, et al. Treatment of colon and breast carcinoma cells with 5-fluorouracil enhances expression of carcinoembryonic antigen and susceptibility to HLA-A(*)02.01 restricted, CEA-peptide-specific cytotoxic T cells in vitro. Int J Cancer 2003;104(4):437–45.

[26] Shurin GV, Tourkova IL, Kaneno R, Shurin MR. Chemotherapeutic agents in noncytotoxic concentrations increase antigen presentation by dendritic cells via an IL-12-dependent mechanism. J Immunol 2009;183(1):137–44.

[27] Lesterhuis WJ, Punt CJ, Hato SV, Eleveld-Trancikova D, Jansen BJ, Nierkens S, et al. Platinum-based drugs disrupt STAT6-mediated suppression of immune responses against cancer in humans and mice. J Clin Invest 2011;121(8):3100–8.

[28] Ding AH, Porteu F, Sanchez E, Nathan CF. Shared actions of endotoxin and taxol on TNF receptors and TNF release. Science 1990;248(4953):370–2.

[29] Kawasaki K, Akashi S, Shimazu R, Yoshida T, Miyake K, Nishijima M. Mouse toll-like receptor 4.MD-2 complex mediates lipopolysaccharide-mimetic signal transduction by Taxol. J Biol Chem 2000;275(4):2251–4.

[30] Byrd-Leifer CA, Block EF, Takeda K, Akira S, Ding A. The role of MyD88 and TLR4 in the LPS-mimetic activity of Taxol. Eur J Immunol 2001;31(8):2448–57.

[31] Szajnik M, Szczepanski MJ, Czystowska M, Elishaev E, Mandapathil M, Nowak-Markwitz E, et al. TLR4 signaling induced by lipopolysaccharide or paclitaxel regulates tumor survival and chemoresistance in ovarian cancer. Oncogene 2009;28(49):4353–63.

[32] Ganz PA, Shanley JD, Cherry JD. Responses of patients with neoplastic diseases to influenza virus vaccine. Cancer 1978;42(5):2244–7.

[33] Bodey GP, Buckley M, Sathe YS, Freireich EJ. Quantitative relationships between circulating leukocytes and infection in patients with acute leukemia. Ann Intern Med 1966;64(2):328–40.

[34] Graham-Pole J, Willoughby ML, Aitken S, Ferguson A. Immune status of children with and without severe infection during remission of malignant disease. Br Med J 1975;2(5969):467–70.

[35] Mackall CL, Fleisher TA, Brown MR, Magrath IT, Shad AT, Horowitz ME, et al. Lymphocyte depletion during treatment with intensive chemotherapy for cancer. Blood 1994;84(7):2221–8.

[36] Rosenberg SA, Yang JC, Sherry RM, Kammula US, Hughes MS, Phan GQ, et al. Durable complete responses in heavily pretreated patients with metastatic melanoma using T-cell transfer immunotherapy. Clin Cancer Res 2011;17(13):4550–7.

[37] Wallen H, Thompson JA, Reilly JZ, Rodmyre RM, Cao J, Yee C. Fludarabine modulates immune response and extends in vivo survival of adoptively transferred CD8 T cells in patients with metastatic melanoma. PloS one 2009;4(3):e4749.

[38] Gameiro SR, Caballero JA, Higgins JP, Apelian D, Hodge JW. Exploitation of differential homeostatic proliferation of T-cell subsets following chemotherapy to enhance the efficacy of vaccine-mediated antitumor responses. Cancer Immunol Immunother 2011;60(9):1227–42.

[39] Laurent J, Speiser DE, Appay V, Touvrey C, Vicari M, Papaioannou A, et al. Impact of 3 different short-term chemotherapy regimens on lymphocyte-depletion and reconstitution in melanoma patients. J Immunother 2010;33(7):723–34.

[40] Hong M, Puaux AL, Huang C, Loumagne L, Tow C, Mackay C, et al. Chemotherapy induces intratumoral expression of chemokines in cutaneous melanoma, favoring T-cell infiltration and tumor control. Cancer Res 2011;71(22):6997–7009.

[41] Garnett CT, Schlom J, Hodge JW. Combination of docetaxel and recombinant vaccine enhances T-cell responses and antitumor activity: effects of docetaxel on immune enhancement. Clin Cancer Res 2008;14(11):3536–44.

[42] Rettig L, Seidenberg S, Parvanova I, Samaras P, Knuth A, Pascolo S. Gemcitabine depletes regulatory T-cells in human and mice and enhances triggering of vaccine-specific cytotoxic T-cells. Int J Cancer 2010.

[43] Matar P, Rozados VR, Gervasoni SI, Scharovsky GO. Th2/Th1 switch induced by a single low dose of cyclophosphamide in a rat metastatic lymphoma model. Cancer Immunol Immunother 2002;50(11):588–96.

[44] Inagawa H, Nishizawa T, Honda T, Nakamoto T, Takagi K, Soma G. Mechanisms by which chemotherapeutic agents augment the antitumor effects of tumor necrosis factor: involvement of the pattern shift of cytokines from Th2 to Th1 in tumor lesions. Anticancer Res 1998;18(5D):3957–64.

[45] Lesterhuis WJ, de Vries IJ, Aarntzen EA, de Boer A, Scharenborg NM, van de Rakt M, et al. A pilot study on the immunogenicity of dendritic cell vaccination during adjuvant oxaliplatin/capecitabine chemotherapy in colon cancer patients. Br J Cancer 2010;103(9):1415–21.

[46] Viaud S, Flament C, Zoubir M, Pautier P, LeCesne A, Ribrag V, et al. Cyclophosphamide induces differentiation of Th17 cells in cancer patients. Cancer Res 2011;71(3):661–5.

[47] Mantovani A, Cassatella MA, Costantini C, Jaillon S. Neutrophils in the activation and regulation of innate and adaptive immunity. Nat Rev Immunol 2011;11(8):519–31.

[48] Colombo MP, Ferrari G, Stoppacciaro A, Parenza M, Rodolfo M, Mavilio F, et al. Granulocyte colony-stimulating factor gene transfer suppresses tumorigenicity of a murine adenocarcinoma in vivo. J Exp Med 1991;173(4):889–97.

[49] Fridlender ZG, Sun J, Kim S, Kapoor V, Cheng G, Ling L, et al. Polarization of tumor-associated neutrophil phenotype by TGF-beta: "N1" versus "N2" TAN. Cancer Cell 2009;16(3):183–94.

[50] Lee CK, Gurney H, Brown C, Sorio R, Donadello N, Tulunay G, et al. Carboplatin-paclitaxel-induced leukopenia and neuropathy predict progression-free survival in recurrent ovarian cancer. Br J Cancer 2011;105(3):360–5.

[51] Shitara K, Matsuo K, Oze I, Mizota A, Kondo C, Nomura M, et al. Meta-analysis of neutropenia or leukopenia as a prognostic factor in patients with malignant disease undergoing chemotherapy. Cancer chemotherapy and pharmacology 2011;68(2):301–7.

[52] Mattarollo SR, Loi S, Duret H, Ma Y, Zitvogel L, Smyth MJ. Pivotal role of innate and adaptive immunity in anthracycline chemotherapy of established tumors. Cancer Res 2011;71(14):4809–20.

[53] Ma Y, Aymeric L, Locher C, Mattarollo SR, Delahaye NF, Pereira P, et al. Contribution of IL-17-producing gamma delta T cells to the efficacy of anticancer chemotherapy. J Exp Med 2011;208(3):491–503.

[54] Tan TT, Coussens LM. Humoral immunity, inflammation and cancer. Curr Opin Immunol 2007;19(2):209–16.

[55] Lesterhuis WJ, Aarntzen EH, De Vries IJ, Schuurhuis DH, Figdor CG, Adema GJ, et al. Dendritic cell vaccines in melanoma: from promise to proof? Crit Rev Oncol Hematol 2008;66(2):118–34.

[56] Gajewski TF. Failure at the effector phase: immune barriers at the level of the melanoma tumor microenvironment. Clin Cancer Res 2007;13(18 Pt 1):5256–61.

[57] Rozali EN, Hato SV, Robinson BW, Lake RA. W.J. L. Programmed Death-Ligand 2 in cancer-induced immune suppression. Clin Develop Immunol 2012. In press.

[58] Topalian SL, Drake CG, Pardoll DM. Targeting the PD-1/B7-H1(PD-L1) pathway to activate anti-tumor immunity. Curr Opin Immunol 2012.

[59] Diamantstein T, Willinger E, Reiman J. T-suppressor cells sensitive to cyclophosphamide and to its in vitro active derivative 4-hydroperoxycyclophosphamide control the mitogenic response of murine splenic B cells to dextran sulfate. A direct proof for different sensitivities of lymphocyte subsets to cyclophosphamide. J Exp Med 1979;150(6):1571–6.

[60] Lutsiak ME, Semnani RT, De Pascalis R, Kashmiri SV, Schlom J, Sabzevari H. Inhibition of CD4(+)25+ T regulatory cell function implicated in enhanced immune response by low-dose cyclophosphamide. Blood 2005;105(7):2862–8.

[61] Taieb J, Chaput N, Schartz N, Roux S, Novault S, Menard C, et al. Chemoimmunotherapy of tumors: cyclophosphamide synergizes with exosome based vaccines. J Immunol 2006;176(5):2722–9.

[62] van der Most RG, Currie AJ, Mahendran S, Prosser A, Darabi A, Robinson BW, et al. Tumor eradication after cyclophosphamide depends on concurrent depletion of regulatory T cells: a role for cycling TNFR2-expressing effector-suppressor T cells in limiting effective chemotherapy. Cancer Immunol Immunother 2009;58(8):1219–28.

[63] Liu JY, Wu Y, Zhang XS, Yang JL, Li HL, Mao YQ, et al. Single administration of low dose cyclophosphamide augments the antitumor effect of dendritic cell vaccine. Cancer Immunol Immunother 2007;56(10):1597–604.

[64] Malvicini M, Rizzo M, Alaniz L, Pinero F, Garcia M, Atorrasagasti C, et al. A novel synergistic combination of cyclophosphamide and gene transfer of interleukin-12 eradicates colorectal carcinoma in mice. Clin Cancer Res 2009;15(23):7256–65.

[65] Slingluff Jr CL, Petroni GR, Chianese-Bullock KA, Smolkin ME, Ross MI, Haas NB, et al. Randomized multicenter trial of the effects of melanoma-associated helper peptides and cyclophosphamide on the immunogenicity of a multipeptide melanoma vaccine. J Clin Oncol 2011;29(21):2924–32.

[66] Rettig L, Seidenberg S, Parvanova I, Samaras P, Knuth A, Pascolo S. Gemcitabine depletes regulatory T-cells in human and mice and enhances triggering of vaccine-specific cytotoxic T-cells. Int J Cancer 2011;129(4):832–8.

[67] Zhu Y, Liu N, Xiong SD, Zheng YJ, Chu YW. CD4+Foxp3+ regulatory T-cell impairment by paclitaxel is independent of toll-like receptor 4. Scandinavian journal of immunology 2011;73(4):301–8.

[68] Le HK, Graham L, Cha E, Morales JK, Manjili MH, Bear HD. Gemcitabine directly inhibits myeloid derived suppressor cells in BALB/c mice bearing 4T1 mammary carcinoma and augments expansion of T cells from tumor-bearing mice. Int Immunopharmacol 2009;9(7–8):900–9.

[69] Vincent J, Mignot G, Chalmin F, Ladoire S, Bruchard M, Chevriaux A, et al. 5-Fluorouracil selectively kills tumor-associated myeloid-derived suppressor cells resulting in enhanced T cell-dependent antitumor immunity. Cancer Res 2010;70(8):3052–61.

[70] Kodumudi KN, Woan K, Gilvary DL, Sahakian E, Wei S, Djeu JY. A novel chemoimmunomodulating property of docetaxel: suppression of myeloid-derived suppressor cells in tumor bearers. Clin Cancer Res 2010;16(18):4583–94.

[71] Denardo DG, Brennan DJ, Rexhepaj E, Ruffell B, Shiao SL, Madden SF, et al. Leukocyte Complexity Predicts Breast Cancer Survival and Functionally Regulates Response to Chemotherapy. Cancer discovery 2011;1:54–67.

[72] Matzinger P, Kamala T. Tissue-based class control: the other side of tolerance. Nat Rev Immunol 2011;11(3):221–30.

[73] Hodi FS, O'Day SJ, McDermott DF, Weber RW, Sosman JA, Haanen JB, et al. Improved survival with ipilimumab in patients with metastatic melanoma. N Engl J Med 2010;363(8):711–23.

[74] Robert C, Thomas L, Bondarenko I, O'Day S, M DJ, Garbe C, et al. Ipilimumab plus Dacarbazine for Previously Untreated Metastatic Melanoma. N Engl J Med 2011.

[75] Brahmer JR, Drake CG, Wollner I, Powderly JD, Picus J, Sharfman WH, et al. Phase I study of single-agent anti-programmed death-1 (MDX-1106) in refractory solid tumors: safety, clinical activity, pharmacodynamics, and immunologic correlates. J Clin Oncol 2010;28(19):3167–75.

[76] Guiter C, Dusanter-Fourt I, Copie-Bergman C, Boulland ML, Le Gouvello S, Gaulard P, et al. Constitutive STAT6 activation in primary mediastinal large B-cell lymphoma. Blood 2004;104(2):543–9.

[77] Aspord C, Pedroza-Gonzalez A, Gallegos M, Tindle S, Burton EC, Su D, et al. Breast cancer instructs dendritic cells to prime interleukin 13-secreting CD4+ T cells that facilitate tumor development. J Exp Med 2007;204(5):1037–47.

[78] Hato SV, De Vries IJ, Lesterhuis WJ. STATing the importance of immune modulation by platinum chemotherapeutics. OncoImmunology 2012. In Press.

[79] Tel J, Hato SV, Torensma R, Buschow SI, Figdor CG, Lesterhuis WJ, et al. The chemotherapeutic drug oxaliplatin differentially affects blood DC function dependent on environmental cues. Cancer Immunol Immunother 2011.

[80] Zitvogel L, Kepp O, Kroemer G. Immune parameters affecting the efficacy of chemotherapeutic regimens. Nat Rev Clin Oncol 2011;8(3):151−60.

[81] Taniguchi K, Nishiura H, Yamamoto T. Requirement of the acquired immune system in successful cancer chemotherapy with cis-diamminedichloroplatinum (II) in a syngeneic mouse tumor transplantation model. J Immunother 2011;34(6):480−9.

[82] Mundy-Bosse BL, Lesinski GB, Jaime-Ramirez AC, Benninger K, Khan M, Kuppusamy P, et al. Myeloid-derived suppressor cell inhibition of the IFN response in tumor-bearing mice. Cancer Res 2011;71(15):5101−10.

[83] Hersh EM, O'Day SJ, Powderly J, Khan KD, Pavlick AC, Cranmer LD, et al. A phase II multicenter study of ipilimumab with or without dacarbazine in chemotherapy-naive patients with advanced melanoma. Invest New Drugs 2011;29(3):489−98.

[84] Lesterhuis WJ, Salmons J, Harken JA, Robinson BW, Nowak AK, Lake RA. Synergistic effect of CTLA-4 blockade and cancer chemotherapy in the induction of anti-tumor immunity. PloS One 2013. In Press.

[85] Chakraborty M, Schlom J, Hodge JW. The combined activation of positive costimulatory signals with modulation of a negative costimulatory signal for the enhancement of vaccine-mediated T-cell responses. Cancer Immunol Immunother 2007;56(9):1471−84.

[86] Gregor PD, Wolchok JD, Ferrone CR, Buchinshky H, Guevara-Patino JA, Perales MA, et al. CTLA-4 blockade in combination with xenogeneic DNA vaccines enhances T-cell responses, tumor immunity and autoimmunity to self antigens in animal and cellular model systems. Vaccine 2004;22(13-14):1700−8.

[87] Liu M, Chien CC, Burne-Taney M, Molls RR, Racusen LC, Colvin RB, et al. A pathophysiologic role for T lymphocytes in murine acute cisplatin nephrotoxicity. J Am Soc Nephrol: JASN 2006;17(3):765−74.

[88] Rini BI, Stein M, Shannon P, Eddy S, Tyler A, Stephenson Jr JJ, et al. Phase 1 dose-escalation trial of tremelimumab plus sunitinib in patients with metastatic renal cell carcinoma. Cancer 2011;117(4):758−67.

[89] Emens LA, Asquith JM, Leatherman JM, Kobrin BJ, Petrik S, Laiko M, et al. Timed sequential treatment with cyclophosphamide, doxorubicin, and an allogeneic granulocyte-macrophage colony-stimulating factor-secreting breast tumor vaccine: a chemotherapy dose-ranging factorial study of safety and immune activation. J Clin Oncol 2009;27(35):5911−8.

[90] Arlen PM, Gulley JL, Parker C, Skarupa L, Pazdur M, Panicali D, et al. A randomized phase II study of concurrent docetaxel plus vaccine versus vaccine alone in metastatic androgen-independent prostate cancer. Clin Cancer Res 2006;12(4):1260−9.

[91] Kaufman HL, Lenz HJ, Marshall J, Singh D, Garett C, Cripps C, et al. Combination chemotherapy and ALVAC-CEA/B7.1 vaccine in patients with metastatic colorectal cancer. Clin Cancer Res 2008;14(15):4843−9.

[92] Nistico P, Capone I, Palermo B, Del Bello D, Ferraresi V, Moschella F, et al. Chemotherapy enhances vaccine-induced antitumor immunity in melanoma patients. Int J Cancer 2008;124(1):130−9.

[93] Palermo B, Del Bello D, Sottini A, Serana F, Ghidini C, Gualtieri N, et al. Dacarbazine treatment before peptide vaccination enlarges T-cell repertoire diversity of melan-a-specific, tumor-reactive CTL in melanoma patients. Cancer Res 2010;70(18):7084−92.

[94] Kyte JA, Gaudernack G, Dueland S, Trachsel S, Julsrud L, Aamdal S. Telomerase peptide vaccination combined with temozolomide: a clinical trial in stage IV melanoma patients. Clin Cancer Res 2011;17(13):4568−80.

[95] Kaida M, Morita-Hoshi Y, Soeda A, Wakeda T, Yamaki Y, Kojima Y, et al. Phase 1 trial of Wilms tumor 1 (WT1) peptide vaccine and gemcitabine combination therapy in patients with advanced pancreatic or biliary tract cancer. J Immunother 2011;34(1):92−9.

[96] Neninger E, Verdecia BG, Crombet T, Viada C, Pereda S, Leonard I, et al. Combining an EGF-based cancer vaccine with chemotherapy in advanced nonsmall cell lung cancer. J Immunother 2009;32(1):92−9.

[97] Sampson JH, Aldape KD, Archer GE, Coan A, Desjardins A, Friedman AH, et al. Greater chemotherapy-induced lymphopenia enhances tumor-specific immune responses that eliminate EGFRvIII-expressing tumor cells in patients with glioblastoma. Neuro Oncol 2011;13(3):324−33.

[98] Beatty GL, Chiorean EG, Fishman MP, Saboury B, Teitelbaum UR, Sun W, et al. CD40 agonists alter tumor stroma and show efficacy against pancreatic carcinoma in mice and humans. Science 2011;331(6024):1612−6.

[99] Lynch TJ, Bondarenko IN, Luft A, Serwatowski P, Barlesi F, Chacko RT, et al. Phase II trial of ipilimumab (IPI) and paclitaxel/carboplatin (P/C) in first-line stage IIIb/IV non-small cell lung cancer (NSCLC). J Clin Oncol 2010;28 (Suppl; abstr 7531)(15s).

413

[100] Kim TG, Kim CH, Park JS, Park SD, Kim CK, Chung DS, et al. Immunological factors relating to the antitumor effect of temozolomide chemoimmunotherapy in a murine glioma model. Clin Vaccine immunol: CVI 2010;17(1):143–53.

[101] Park SD, Kim CH, Kim CK, Park JA, Sohn HJ, Hong YK, et al. Cross-priming by temozolomide enhances antitumor immunity of dendritic cell vaccination in murine brain tumor model. Vaccine 2007;25(17):3485–91.

[102] Bracci L, Moschella F, Sestili P, La Sorsa V, Valentini M, Canini I, et al. Cyclophosphamide enhances the antitumor efficacy of adoptively transferred immune cells through the induction of cytokine expression, B-cell and T-cell homeostatic proliferation, and specific tumor infiltration. Clin Cancer Res 2007;13(2 Pt 1): 644–53.

[103] van der Most RG, Currie AJ, Cleaver AL, Salmons J, Nowak AK, Mahendran S, et al. Cyclophosphamide chemotherapy sensitizes tumor cells to TRAIL-dependent CD8 T cell-mediated immune attack resulting in suppression of tumor growth. PloS one 2009;4(9):e6982.

[104] Markasz L, Skribek H, Uhlin M, Otvos R, Flaberg E, Eksborg S, et al. Effect of frequently used chemotherapeutic drugs on cytotoxic activity of human cytotoxic T-lymphocytes. J Immunother 2008;31(3):283–93.

[105] Multhoff G, Meier T, Botzler C, Wiesnet M, Allenbacher A, Wilmanns W, et al. Differential effects of ifosfamide on the capacity of cytotoxic T lymphocytes and natural killer cells to lyse their target cells correlate with intracellular glutathione levels. Blood 1995;85(8):2124–31.

[106] Kuppner MC, Scharner A, Milani V, Von Hesler C, Tschop KE, Heinz O, et al. Ifosfamide impairs the allostimulatory capacity of human dendritic cells by intracellular glutathione depletion. Blood 2003;102(10):3668–74.

[107] Gorelik L, Prokhorova A, Mokyr MB. Low-dose melphalan-induced shift in the production of a Th2-type cytokine to a Th1-type cytokine in mice bearing a large MOPC-315 tumor. Cancer Immunol Immunother 1994;39(2):117–26.

[108] Rad AN, Pollara G, Sohaib SM, Chiang C, Chain BM, Katz DR. The differential influence of allogeneic tumor cell death via DNA damage on dendritic cell maturation and antigen presentation. Cancer Res 2003;63(16):5143–50.

[109] Mizushima Y, Sendo F, Miyake T, Kobayashi H. Augmentation of specific cell-mediated immune responses to tumor cells in tumor-bearing rats pretreated wih the antileukemia drug busulfan. J Natl Cancer Inst 1981;66(4):659–65.

[110] Markasz L, Stuber G, Vanherberghen B, Flaberg E, Olah E, Carbone E, et al. Effect of frequently used chemotherapeutic drugs on the cytotoxic activity of human natural killer cells. Mol Cancer ther 2007;6(2):644–54.

[111] Nagarkatti M, Kaplan AM. The role of suppressor T cells in BCNU-mediated rejection of a syngeneic tumor. J Immunol 1985;135(2):1510–7.

[112] Nagarkatti M, Toney DM, Nagarkatti PS. Immunomodulation by various nitrosoureas and its effect on the survival of the murine host bearing a syngeneic tumor. Cancer Res 1989;49(23):6587–92.

[113] Bergmann-Leitner ES, Abrams SI. Treatment of human colon carcinoma cell lines with anti-neoplastic agents enhances their lytic sensitivity to antigen-specific CD8+ cytotoxic T lymphocytes. Cancer Immunol Immunother 2001;50(9):445–55.

[114] Beyer M, Kochanek M, Darabi K, Popov A, Jensen M, Endl E, et al. Reduced frequencies and suppressive function of CD4+CD25hi regulatory T cells in patients with chronic lymphocytic leukemia after therapy with fludarabine. Blood 2005;106(6):2018-25.

[115] Tanaka H, Matsushima H, Nishibu A, Clausen BE, Takashima A. Dual therapeutic efficacy of vinblastine as a unique chemotherapeutic agent capable of inducing dendritic cell maturation. Cancer Res 2009;69(17):6987–94.

[116] Tanaka H, Matsushima H, Mizumoto N, Takashima A. Classification of chemotherapeutic agents based on their differential in vitro effects on dendritic cells. Cancer Res 2009;69(17):6978–86.

[117] Thomas-Schoemann A, Lemare F, Mongaret C, Bermudez E, Chereau C, Nicco C, et al. Bystander effect of vinorelbine alters antitumor immune response. Int J Cancer 2011;129(6):1511–8.

[118] Wei J, DeAngulo G, Sun W, Hussain SF, Vasquez H, Jordan J, et al. Topotecan enhances immune clearance of gliomas. Cancer Immunol Immunother 2009;58(2):259–70.

[119] Terness P, Oelert T, Ehser S, Chuang JJ, Lahdou I, Kleist C, et al. Mitomycin C-treated dendritic cells inactivate autoreactive T cells: toward the development of a tolerogenic vaccine in autoimmune diseases. Proc Natl Acad Sci U S A 2008;105(47):18442–7.

[120] Xu ZY, Hosokawa M, Morikawa K, Hatakeyama M, Kobayashi H. Overcoming suppression of antitumor immune reactivity in tumor-bearing rats by treatment with bleomycin. Cancer Res 1988;48(23):6658–63.

CHAPTER 25

Immunotherapy and Cancer Therapeutics: A Rich Partnership

Gang Chen[1], Elizabeth M. Jaffee[2], Leisha A. Emens[3]

[1]Department of Oncology, Johns Hopkins University School of Medicine, The Sidney Kimmel Cancer Center at Johns Hopkins, Baltimore, MD USA

[2]The Dana and Albert "Cubby" Broccoli Professor of Oncology, Co-Director of the Gastrointestinal Cancers Program, Co-Director of the Skip Viragh Pancreatic Cancer Center, Associate Director for Translational Research, The Sidney Kimmel Cancer Center at Johns Hopkins, Baltimore, MD USA

[3]Associate Professor of Oncology, Graduate Program in Pathobiology, Department of Oncology, Johns Hopkins University School of Medicine, The Sidney Kimmel Cancer Center at Johns Hopkins, Baltimore, MD USA

I. INTRODUCTION: WHY INTEGRATE CANCER DRUGS WITH TUMOR IMMUNOTHERAPY?

Capitalizing on the power of the immune system to fight malignancy has enormous potential for cancer therapy. Although the efficacy of immunotherapy is potentially limited by systemic and local mechanisms of immune tolerance that keep the immune response in check, rapidly accumulating data illustrates a critical role for the immune system in the response to many traditional (chemotherapy, radiation (the abscopal effect)), and novel cancer therapies (molecularly targeted small molecules). Integrating immune-based therapies strategically with established and novel cancer therapeutics should generate a robust antitumor effect that takes advantage of the strengths of their individual modes of action and also leverages potential immunologic synergies. In addition to the direct antineoplastic effect of the cancer drug, such integrative immunotherapies may have the potential to manipulate existing immunoregulatory pathways for therapeutic benefit, abrogating immune tolerance and amplifying pathways that push the immune response forward. The thoughtful combination of multiple treatment modalities should allow the full power of the immune system to be unleashed, resulting in increasing survival benefits, and ultimately in the eradication and prevention of malignant disease.

II. CHEMOTHERAPY AND TUMOR IMMUNITY

Entrenched mechanisms of immune tolerance and suppression create a pathway to functional tumor immunity that is filled with obstacles. These stumbling blocks to immune-mediated tumor rejection include a pool of suboptimal, low avidity tumor-specific T cells available for recruitment, the locoregional accumulation of $CD4^+CD25^+FoxP3^+$ regulatory T cells (Treg, Chapter 33), myeloid-derived suppressor cells (MDSC, Chapter 28), tumor-associated macrophages (TAM, Chapter 27), the intratumoral secretion of inhibitory cytokines like transforming growth factor-β (TGF-β), tumor necrosis factor (TNF), and interleukin-10 (IL-10), the expression of negative accessory molecules for T-cell activation within the tumor microenvironment (B7-H1, B7-H4), and various phenotypic alterations that result in immune escape (the downregulation of tumor antigens, MHC molecules, and other molecules essential for antigen processing and presentation, Chapters 7—11). Since multiple mechanisms of immune tolerance and suppression actively keep tumor immunity in check, it is not surprising that many clinical trials testing immunotherapies alone or randomly added to standard chemotherapy in patients with advanced, treatment-refractory malignancies have failed to show evidence of clinically relevant bioactivity. In addition, many standard and high-dose chemotherapy regimens are immunosuppressive (Chapter 12), inducing or contributing to lymphopenia and lymphocyte dysfunction. Many also require the co-administration of glucocorticoids, which are both directly lympholytic and immunosuppressive [1]. Since surgery, radiation, and chemotherapy are widely used to treat most established cancers, properly integrating immune-based therapies with these standard modalities to capitalize both on their potential synergies and on their individually unique modes of action is highly attractive. Carefully choosing the drugs, dose, and timing of administration is critical for harnessing additive and synergistic therapeutic activities and optimal therapeutic benefit [2].

Introducing immune-based therapy after optimal tumor debulking—on a pallete of minimal residual disease—can mitigate the impact of tumor burden on the antitumor immune response. Some chemotherapy drugs induce immunogenic cell death, where the chemotherapy-induced treatment effect is in part directly dependent on the host immune system. Chemotherapy-induced cell death can enhance cross priming, thereby increasing the antitumor T-cell response [3]. Reflecting this mechanism, standard neoadjuvant paclitaxel therapy for breast cancer has been associated with the development of new intratumoral immune cell infiltrates [4]. Chemotherapy can also groom the tumor microenvironment for optimal immunity in a variety of ways [2]. It can alter the balance of Treg, MDSC, and immune effectors present within the tumor mass. It can also modulate the expression of tumor antigens, molecules involved in antigen processing and presentation, and accessory molecules of T-cell activation or inhibition. Finally, chemotherapy can be used to manipulate systemic pathways of immune tolerance and regulation. These direct immune-modulating effects of chemotherapy are not only drug dependent, but also dependent on dose and schedule [2]. For example, a single low dose of cyclophosphamide given 1 to 3 days before an antigen exposure can overcome immune tolerance, augmenting both humoral and cellular immunity. Conversely, cyclophosphamide given concurrently with or subsequent to an antigen exposure induces immune tolerance, thus dampening immune responses. Finally, chemotherapy-induced lymphopenia sets the stage for homeostatic proliferation, creating an environment for rebooting the immune system [5,6]. The specific mechanisms underlying the immunomodulatory effects of a number of chemotherapy drugs have been recently reviewed elsewhere [7], and are summarized in Table 25.1.

III. CLINICAL TRIALS OF CHEMOIMMUNOTHERAPY
A. Immunotherapy with standard-dose chemotherapy

Clinical data demonstrate that standard-dose chemotherapy can impact the way that cancer patients respond to a tumor vaccine in both positive and negative ways (Table 25.2). Vaccination in close proximity to standard dose cytotoxic therapy can inhibit vaccine-induced immunity, generate levels of immunity similar to those observed in the absence of chemotherapy, or enhance tumor-specific immune responses. Interestingly, tumor-specific immune responses are sometimes enhanced when vaccination occurs in the midst of active chemotherapy, and sometimes when salvage chemotherapy is given for disease progression post vaccination.

TABLE 25.1 **The Immunomodulatory Effect of Various Chemotherapy Drugs [7]**

Immunologic Process	Drugs
Antigen uptake and processing	Doxorubicin
	Daunorubicin
	Mitoxantrone
	Oxaliplatin
	5-Fluorouracil
	5'-Aza-2'-deoxycytidine
Dendritic cell activation and maturation	Cyclophosphamide
	Paclitaxel
	Vincristine
	Vinblastine
	Methotrexate
	Mitomycin-C
	Doxorubicin
	5'-Aza-2'-deoxycytidine
T-cell co-stimulation	Melphalan
	Mitomycin-C
	Cytosine arabinoside
T-cell counterstimulation	Cytosine arabinoside
Target cell lysis	Cyclophosphamide
	Paclitaxel
	Cisplatin
	Doxorubicin
Immunologic Skew	Cyclophosphamide
	Paclitaxel
	Melphalan
	Bleomycin
$CD4^+CD25^+FoxP3^+$ regulatory T cells	Cyclophosphamide
	Cisplatin
	Paclitaxel
	Temozolomide
	Fludarabine
	Gemcitabine/FOLFOX4
Myeloid-derived suppressor cells	Gemcitabine
	5-Fluorouracil
	Cyclophosphamide
	Cyclophosphamide/Doxorubicin

417

Concurrent Standard Cancer Therapy Can Inhibit Tumor Vaccines. One clinical trial conducted in patients with advanced malignancies that express the carcinoembryonic antigen (CEA) tested the canary pox vaccine ALVAC-CEA-B7.1 as a single agent in patients previously treated with chemotherapy [8]. A retrospective analysis showed that the number of vaccine-induced CEA-specific T cells was lower in patients who had received greater numbers of prior chemotherapy regimens, and in those who had most recently received standard-dose cytotoxic therapy. Another clinical trial tested a mesothelin-expressing, granulocyte-macrophage colony-stimulating factor (GM-CSF)-secreting cell-based pancreas tumor vaccine in Stage II and III pancreas cancer patients [9]. Study participants were vaccinated once prior to standard pancreaticoduodenectomy, with augmented levels of mesothelin-specific $CD8^+$ T-cells demonstrated after one vaccination. After surgery, patients then received six months of 5-fluorouracil-based chemoradiation, after which the mesothelin-specific $CD8^+$ T-cell response was undetectable. Vaccine-induced, mesothelin-specific immunity was restored after three additional vaccination cycles were given post chemoradiation, suggesting that

TABLE 25.2 Clinical Trials of Combinatorial Chemoimmunotherapy

Patient Population	n	Vaccine	Drug	Immunologic Outcome
Standard-Dose Chemotherapy				
Stage 4 colon cancer	17	CEA peptide	Standard 5-fluorouracil, leucovorin, irinotecan	50% patients with new CEA-specific T cells
Stage 4 colon cancer	118	ALVAC-CEA-B7.1	Standard 5-fluorouracil, leucovorin, irinotecan	No inhibition of CEA- specific immunity
Stage 2/3 pancreas cancer	60	GM-CSF-secreting, mesothelin$^+$ pancreas tumor cells	Vaccine once, then 5-fluorouracil-based chemoradiation, then three more vaccines	Induction of mesothelin-specific T cells, inhibited by chemoradiation, then restored by 3 vaccines
Stage 4 prostate cancer	28	PSA vaccinia/fowl pox	Standard docetaxel and dexamethasone	No inhibition of PSA-specific immunity
Stage 4 melanoma	28	GV1001 telomerase peptide	Temozolomide 200 mg/m^2	78% GV1001 immunity
Stage 4 melanoma	10	melan-A/MART-1/gp-100 peptide	No dacarbazine vs. Dacarbazine 800 mg/m^2 (n = 5 in each group)	Enhanced peptide- specific immunity with dacarbazine
Stage 4 prostate cancer	405	GM-CSF-secreting prostate tumor cells	Docetaxel 75 mg/m^2 with vaccine vs. with dexamethasone	Not reported, study terminated
Low-Dose Immunomodulatory Chemotherapy				
Stage 4 breast cancer	1028	KLH (n = 505) KLH-STn (n = 523)	CY 300mg/m^2 each arm	Not reported, no clinical difference
Stage 4 pancreas cancer	50	GM-CSF-secreting, mesothelin$^+$ pancreas tumor cells	No CY vs. CY 300 mg/m^2	Enhanced mesothelin- specific T cells with CY 300 mg/m^2
Stage 4 breast cancer	28	GM-CSF-secreting, HER-2$^+$ breast tumor cells	CY 0, 200, 250, 350 mg/m^2 DOX 0, 15, 25, 35 mg/m^2 Factorial response surface design of various doses	Increased HER-2-specific immunity with doses of CY 200 mg/m^2 plus DOX 35 mg/m^2
Stage 2-4 ovarian cancer	11	Peptide-loaded dendritic cells: HER-2, hTERT, PADRE	No CY vs. CY 300 mg/m^2	Modest T cell responses to HER-2 and hTERT

CEA=carcinoembryonic antigen; ALVAC=canary pox virus; GM-CSF=granulocyte-macrophage colony-stimulating factor; PSA=prostate specific antigen; MART-1=melanoma antigen recognized by T cell 1; KLH=keyhole limpet hemocyanin; STn=clustered carbohydrate antigen; CY=cyclophosphamide; DOX=doxorubicin; hTERT=human telomerase reverse transcriptase; PADRE=pan DR-binding peptide

418

vaccine-induced immunity had been suppressed by adjuvant therapy. A third Phase III clinical trial tested a GM-CSF-secreting, cell-based prostate cancer vaccine with standard-dose docetaxel chemotherapy; this study was launched based on the promising immunologic activity of this vaccine given as a single agent in Phase I and II clinical trials [10]. The Phase III trial enrolled 405 chemotherapy-naïve patients with symptomatic, hormone-refractory prostate cancer and a Halabi predicted survival time of 13 months [10,11]. One patient group received vaccination given with ten cycles of docetaxel 75 mg/m^2 every three weeks without prednisone, and the other patient group received 10 cycles of docetaxel 75 mg/m^2 every three weeks plus prednisone 10 mg daily. The data safety and monitoring committee noted an imbalance of deaths prior to study completion, with a greater number of deaths on the vaccine arm; all deaths were due to disease progression and death from prostate cancer. As a result, the study was terminated prior to completion. Subsequent follow-up showed that the imbalance of deaths lessened from 20 to 9. A number of factors could account for this failure, including the use of both docetaxel and prednisone in the control arm, but only docetaxel in the vaccine arm (where prednisone was held due to concern for immunosuppression). Moreover, standard-dose docetaxel was used in combination with the vaccine. This vaccine had not been tested with chemotherapy in the early stage clinical trials that led to Phase III testing, and this dose and schedule of docetaxel could have inhibited vaccine-induced tumor immunity.

Concurrent Standard Cancer Therapy Does Not Inhibit, and May Enhance, Vaccine-Induced Immunity. The impact of chemotherapy (fluorouracil, leucovorin, and irinotecan) on immunity induced by the ALVAC-CEA-B7.1 vaccine was further evaluated in a prospective follow-up study of patients with metastatic colorectal cancer [12]. This clinical trial randomized 118 patients to receive vaccine alone for 3 cycles followed by vaccine given with chemotherapy (Group 1), vaccine with tetanus toxoid adjuvant for 3 cycles followed by vaccine given with chemotherapy (Group 2), or 4 cycles of chemotherapy followed by 4 cycles of vaccination in patients without disease progression on chemotherapy (Group 3). CEA-specific T cells increased 50%, 37%, and 30% in Groups 1, 2, and 3 respectively, suggesting that systemic chemotherapy did not impact the generation of CEA-specific T cells after vaccination. There were no significant clinical differences or differential immune responses between these groups. A second clinical trial tested a CEA-specific peptide vaccine first given concurrently with 3 cycles of high-dose 5-fluorouracil/leucovorin+standard-dose irinotecan, and then alone in patients with newly diagnosed metastatic colorectal cancer [13]. About one half of enrolled patients developed CEA-specific T-cell responses by intracellular cytokine staining. During the three cycles of chemotherapy, recall antigen-specific (EBV/CMV) $CD8^+$ T cells decreased by about 14%. There were five complete responses, one partial response, five patients with stable disease, and six patients with progressive disease. A third study tested a prime/boost strategy using vaccination first with recombinant vaccinia virus (rVV)-expressing prostate-specific antigen (PSA) admixed with rVV-expressing B7.1 followed by vaccination with recombinant fowlpox virus (rF)-expressing PSA with and without concurrent weekly docetaxel at 30 mg/m^2 in patients with metastatic hormone-refractory prostate cancer [14]. This study showed a greater than three-fold increase in PSA-specific T cells by ELISPOT over 3 months regardless of docetaxel treatment. Median progression-free survival was 6.1 months compared to 3.7 months for a historical cohort treated with weekly docetaxel at 30 mg/m^2 alone. A fourth study tested the telomerase peptide vaccine GV1001 given as 8 injections over 11 weeks, with concurrent temozolomide given at 200 mg/m^2 orally for 5 days every fourth week in 25 patients with advanced melanoma [15]. Eighteen of 23 evaluable subjects (78%) developed a GV1001-specific immune response, with survival trends comparing favorably with matched controls from a benchmark meta-analysis.

Standard Cancer Therapy Given Prior to or After Vaccination May Enhance Vaccine Activity. One study of 29 patients with extensive stage small cell lung cancer (SCLC) showed that vaccination with dendritic cells transduced with an adenoviral vector expressing wild type p53 resulted in the induction of p53-specific immunity in about 60% of vaccinated patients [16]. Despite successful immunization, all patients except one developed progressive disease. Interestingly, about 60% of patients with progressive disease were fortunate to have an objective clinical response to subsequent chemotherapy, and this clinical benefit correlated with p53-specific tumor immunity. Similar observations have been reported in patients with glioblastoma vaccinated with a dendritic cell-based vaccine who subsequently received standard chemotherapy [17]. In this study, there was improved time to disease progression throughout post-vaccination salvage chemotherapy, but no improvement in time to disease progression from the last vaccination to first salvage therapy. A distinct study of 36 patients with Stage 2–4 melanoma, all of whom had no evidence of disease, tested standard-dose dacarbazine (DTIC) at 800 mg/m^2 given one day before vaccination with melan-A/MART-1/gp-100 melanoma peptide vaccination compared with vaccination alone [18]. DTIC enhanced the numbers of peptide-specific $CD8^+$ T cells induced by vaccination, and the generation and persistence of peptide-specific memory CD8$^+$ T cells. Global transcriptional analysis revealed that DTIC induced the expression of genes involved in the immune response and leukocyte activation. Further analyses revealed a broader T-cell receptor repertoire diversity, higher T-cell avidity, and greater tumor reactivity in Melan-A-specific T-cell clones derived from patients treated with chemoimmunotherapy [19]. This was associated with a trend toward longer survival. In contrast, patients treated with vaccine alone showed a tendency toward a more narrow TCR repertoire diversity, with a decrease in tumor-specific lytic activity in one patient. Notably, one preclinical study has demonstrated that the adoptive transfer of nonspecifically activated CD4$^+$ T cells could sensitize tumors to subsequent chemotherapy treatment *in vitro* and *in vivo*, providing some preclinical support for these clinical observations [20].

B. Immunotherapy with high-dose chemotherapy

Multiple groups have tested a platform of hematopoietic cell transplantation after high-dose chemotherapy with or without radiation followed by either adoptive cellular therapy or vaccine therapy. One clinical trial of adoptive cellular therapy gave T cells specific for minor histocompatibility antigens after allogeneic stem cell transplantation in 7 patients [21]. Transferred T cells persisted for up to 21 days, and 5 of 7 patients achieved complete but transient remissions post-cellular therapy. Another study tested adoptive cellular therapy with autologous tumor infiltrating lymphocytes (TIL) and interleukin-2 (IL-2) in 50 patients with metastatic melanoma randomized to receive conditioning with cyclophosphamide and fludarabine alone, or together with either 2 or 12 Gray of total body irradiation (TBI) [22]. Nonmyeloablative chemotherapy alone resulted in a response rate of 49%, whereas the addition of 2 or 12 Gray of TBI gave response rates of 52% and 72% respectively. Lymphodepletion was associated with increased serum levels of interleukin-7 and interleukin-15, and objective responses correlated with the telomere length of the transferred lymphocytes. The use of GM-CSF-secreting, cell-based autologous vaccine in the setting of autologous stem cell transplantation for acute myelogenous leukemia (AML) has been evaluated in at least two distinct clinical trials, with both demonstrating evidence of safety and immunogenicity [23,24].

C. Immunotherapy with low-dose, immunomodulatory chemotherapy

Multiple clinical trials have now been reported that use low, immune-modulating doses of chemotherapy specifically to enhance the activity of tumor vaccines rather than to lyse cancer cells directly (Table 24.2). Multiple Phase II studies investigating the use of cyclophosphamide to mitigate the inhibitory influence of suppressor T cells as they were defined some 35 years ago first showed that patients who were treated with 300 mg/m^2 of cyclophosphamide three days prior to vaccination with a clustered carbohydrate antigen-keyhole limpet hemocyanin (KLH) vaccine developed higher antibody titers and enjoyed longer survival [25]. A Phase III trial of 1028 women with metastatic breast cancer was conducted to definitively test these findings [26]. This study randomized 505 women to receive cyclophosphamide at 300 mg/m^2 plus vaccination with KLH alone, and 523 women to receive cyclophosphamide at 300 mg/m^2 plus vaccination with clustered carbohydrate-KLH. No difference in time to disease progression or overall survival emerged, although a subset analysis suggested a trend toward benefit in time to disease progression in women on concurrent endocrine therapy.

Immune-modulating doses of cyclophosphamide have also been tested in several clinical trials. One study tested cyclophosphamide at 300 mg/m^2 given one day prior to vaccination with a GM-CSF-secreting, mesothelin-expressing, cell-based vaccine compared to vaccination alone in 50 patients with metastatic pancreas cancer [27]. This study showed a trend toward increased mesothelin-specific CD8$^+$ T-cell responses, and a corresponding trend toward increased clinical benefit with cyclophosphamide-modulated vaccination compared to vaccination alone. Similar findings of clinical benefit were reported in a small trial of a similar vaccination platform where 300 mg/m^2 cyclophosphamide was given one day prior to vaccination in patients with advanced non-small cell carcinoma [28]. In this study, a transient decrease in peripheral Treg numbers with time after cyclophosphamide was observed. Another study tested a peptide vaccine consisting of monocyte-derived dendritic cells loaded with peptide epitopes specific for HER-2, hTERT, and PADRE alone or with 300 mg/m^2 cyclophopshamide given two days prior to vaccination in 11 patients with advanced ovarian cancer in remission [29]. The 3-year overall survival was 90%, and patients who received cyclophosphamide-modulated vaccination had a trend toward improvement in survival compared to patients who received vaccination alone. Cyclophosphamide treatment resulted in a transient decrease in neutrophils, but no change in lymphocytes or Tregs. Another clinical study used an innovative factorial response surface design to test a HER-2-positive, GM-CSF-secreting, cell-based breast tumor vaccine alone, or in a timed sequence with a range of doses of cyclophosphamide (0, 200, 250, 350 mg/m^2) given one day prior to vaccination, and doxorubicin (0 15, 25, 35 mg/m^2) given seven days after vaccination [30]. Vaccination by itself induced *de novo* HER-2-specific delayed type hypersensitivity (DTH), with low levels of HER-2 antibodies by ELISA also observed. The addition of cyclophosphamide at 200 mg/m^2 maintained the DTH response and augmented HER-2-specific antibody responses, whereas doses of cyclophosphamide 250 mg/m^2 or greater abrogated vaccine-induced immunity. The chemotherapy dose combination that maximized vaccine-induced HER-2-specific antibody responses was 200 mg/m^2 cyclophosphamide and 35 mg/m^2 doxorubicin. It is notable that most clinical cancer vaccine trials have historically used cyclophosphamide at 250–300 mg/m^2 for immune modulation. These data suggest that this dose may be too high, and that the therapeutic window for the immune modulating activity of low-dose cyclophosphamide may be quite narrow.

IV. IMMUNE MODULATION WITH THERAPEUTIC MONOCLONAL ANTIBODIES

Monoclonal antibodies (MAbs) for cancer therapy can be broadly divided into three classes: those that target biologic features expressed by the tumor cell itself, those that target factors elaborated by the tumor cell or the host response to it, and those that target the immune regulatory networks responsible for shaping antitumor immune responses. Of these, tumor-specific therapeutic MAbs are particularly unique since they both partially passively reconstitute the humoral arm of the tumor antigen-specific immune response, and provide critical support in establishing the antigen-specific adaptive immune response through cross-priming. Rituximab and trastuzumab, the first MAbs to be approved for cancer therapy, exemplify this category (also discussed in Chapter 14). There are currently only two monoclonal antibodies in current clinical use that target soluble host factors involved in the antitumor response, bevacizumab (specific for vascular endothelial growth factor (VEGF) and denosumab (specific for the receptor activator of nuclear factor kappa B-ligand (RANKL)). Finally, the application of therapeutic MAbs that specifically target the nodal checkpoints for T-cell activation and effector function is an area of increasing preclinical and clinical investigation. These immune checkpoint-specific therapeutic MAbs typically either amplify the positive signals that drive T-cell activation and function, or inhibit the negative signals that keep T-cell activity in check. Ipilimumab (Yervoy), is the first in this category to be FDA approved, for the treatment of malignant melanoma. This chapter will focus on the first two categories. A more in-depth discussion of MAbs that target immune checkpoints can be found in Chapter 14.

A. MAbs that target tumor cell biology

1. TRASTUZUMAB AND PERTUZUMAB: MAbs THAT TARGET THE HER-2 PATHWAY

Trastuzumab, a humanized MAb specific for the human epidermal growth factor receptor 2 (HER-2/*neu*), is widely used to treat HER-2-overexpressing breast cancers at every stage except ductal carcinoma *in situ* (DCIS). It was also recently approved for the treatment of HER-2-overexpressing metastatic gastric cancer. Trastuzumab has been thought to function primarily by inhibiting signaling through the cell surface HER-2 receptor, but it can also modulate tumor immunity through multiple mechanisms. It recruits innate immune effectors to the tumor microenvironment in order to facilitate antibody-dependent cellular cytotoxicity (ADCC) [31–33]. Trastuzumab can induce the ubiquitination and degradation of internalized HER-2 molecules, thereby increasing proteasome-dependent antigen presentation [34,35]. Accordingly, it augments the lytic activity of MHC Class 1-restricted HER-2-specific CTLs against HER-2-expressing tumor targets [36,37]. HER-2-specific MAb therapy alone induced new CD8[+] T-cell immunity specific for HER-2 in the *neu*-N murine model of HER-2-specific immune tolerance [38]. In humans, a single dose of pre-operative trastuzumab induced apoptosis in primary breast tumors within 24 hours [39], and trastuzumab-based neoadjuvant chemotherapy is associated with the development of T-bet[+] lymphoid nodules in patients with locally advanced breast cancer [40]. Importantly, these lymphoid nodules are associated with enhanced survival. Finally, trastuzumab-based chemotherapy has been associated with the development of HER-2-specific CD4[+] T-cell responses in patients with early and metastatic breast cancer [41].

These varied immune modulating effects of HER-2-specific MAb provide strong support for combining HER-2-specific MAbs with other immunotherapies, including vaccines. HER-2-specific antibodies developing in response to HER-2-specific peptide vaccination in patients can inhibit tumor growth and signaling *in vitro* [42], and can mediate ADCC in murine models [43]. Consistent with the concept that both humoral and cellular immune effectors are required for optimal antitumor immunity, the passive administration of HER-2-specific antibodies and HER-2-specific CTL together induced a more effective antitumor response than either alone in severe combined immunodeficient (SCID) mice [44]. Taking this a step further, the passive administration of two distinct HER-2-specific MAbs in sequence with a GM-CSF-secreting, HER-2-specific cell-based vaccine resulted in a more robust tumor rejection response than either MAb or vaccination alone, curing about 40% of tumor-bearing, immune tolerant *neu*-N mice [38]. This enhanced rate of tumor clearance was associated with increased numbers of vaccine-induced, tumor necrosis factor (TNF)-secreting, HER-2-specific CTL by ELISPOT, enhanced tumor antigen processing and presentation, and enhanced lysis of HER-2-expressing tumor cells [38]. To support clinical translation, the HER-2-specific MAb 7.16.4, similar to trastuzumab, was similarly evaluated [45]. Adding 7.16.4 MAb to vaccination with a GM-CSF-secreting, HER-2-specific cell-based vaccine led to a higher HER-2-specific CD8[+] T-cell response, and the protection of about 60% of tolerant *neu*-N mice from a subsequent challenge with HER-2-expressing tumor cells. Notably, both of these endpoints were dependent on the Fc portion of 7.16.4. Mechanistically, 7.16.4 enhanced locoregional immune priming through the Fc-mediated activation of dendritic cells, resulting in higher levels of proliferation and cytokine production by vaccine-induced HER-2-specific CD8[+] T cells *in vivo* [45]. Importantly, antibody-modulated vaccination promoted the evolution of the CD44[+]CD62L[+]CD8[+] HER-2-specific central memory T-cell response. Finally, the combination of low-dose cyclophosphamide, 7.16.4, and vaccination generated the highest numbers of HER-2-specific CD8[+] T cells, and protected up to 70% of *neu*-N mice from the outgrowth of established HER-2-expressing tumors (Emens, unpublished data).

These observations together provide strong support for testing trastuzumab in combination with HER-2 targeted vaccination in patients with malignancies dependent on HER-2-signaling. Two clinical trials of trastuzumab combined with vaccination have been reported (Table 25.3). In one study, a HER-2-specific T-helper peptide vaccine was combined with standard trastuzumab therapy in 22 women with metastatic HER-2[+] breast cancer [46]. This study demonstrated the safety of the combination, with about 15% of patients displaying an asymptomatic decline in cardiac ejection fraction. Immunity specific for HER-2 and other tumor antigens was enhanced, both in magnitude and by epitope spreading. Additionally, the magnitude of the immune response was inversely correlated with serum TGF-β levels. Median

TABLE 25.3 Clinical Trials Integrating Targeted Cancer Therapies and Immunotherapy

Patient Population	n	Vaccine	Drug	Immunologic Outcome
Monoclonal Antibodies				
Stage 4 HER-2+ breast cancer	22	HER-2 helper peptides	Trastuzumab	Enhanced HER-2-specific T-cell immunity, epitope spreading, decreased serum TGF-β
Stage 4 HER-2+ breast cancer	20	GM-CSF-secreting, HER-2+ breast tumor cells	Trastuzumab	Enhanced HER-2-specific DTH in about 1/3 of patients
Stage 4 prostate cancer	22	Sipuleucel-T	Bevacizumab	New immunity specific for prostatic acid phosphatase
Targeted Small Molecules				
Chronic myelogenous leukemia	19	GM-CSF-secreting chronic myelogenous leukemia cells	Imatinib mesylate	New humoral immunity
Stage 4 HER-2+ breast cancer	12	HER-2 protein	Lapatinib	HER-2-specific antibody and T-cell responses in 100% and 8% of patients respectively

TGF-β=transforming growth factor-β; DTH=delayed type hypersensitivity

survival had not yet been reached at 36 months of follow-up. In the second study, the combination of weekly trastuzumab, low-dose cyclophosphamide 300 mg/m^2, and a GM-CSF-secreting, HER-2-expressing cell-based vaccine was tested in 20 women with HER-2+ metastatic breast cancer [47]. This clinical trial demonstrated the safety of the combination regimen (with no cardiac toxicity observed), and clinical benefit rates of 50% at 6 months, and 35% at 1 year. Seven of the 20 vaccinated patients developed new or increased immunity to HER-2 by DTH. Exploratory analyses revealed an overall survival 40 months (Emens, unpublished data) compared to the historical overall survival of 13—24 months in similar patients who received standard trastuzumab alone [48,49]. Thus, this body of preclinical and clinical data strongly argues for the development of combination immunotherapies incorporating trastuzumab with cancer vaccines and other immune modulators (cyclophosphamide and immune checkpoint modulators) in patients with HER-2-dependent cancers, including breast cancer.

2. RITUXIMAB AND MAbs THAT TARGET CD20 AND B-CELL SURFACE MARKERS

Rituximab, a chimeric, partially humanized MAb specific for the cell surface molecule CD20 expressed by normal B cells and over 95% of B-cell leukemias and lymphomas, is widely used both as a single agent and combined with chemotherapy and radiation. Although the primary mechanism of action remains unclear, it has been shown to mediate antibody-dependent cellular cytotoxicity (ADCC) [30], promote apoptosis [50], and enhance cross-priming of the adaptive immune response [49]. Rituximab modulates *src* signaling in follicular lymphoma cells, leading to less interleukin-10 secretion, lower levels of active STAT-3 and bcl-2, and greater sensitivity to chemotherapy [51,52]. Rituximab therapy is known to result in profound B-cell depletion. In preclinical models, B cells have been shown to inhibit tumor-specific CD8+ cytotoxic lymphocytes, suggesting that B-cell depletion in the setting of rituximab therapy may not inhibit, and could enhance, vaccine-induced tumor immunity [53].

Consistent with this idea, one study showed that vaccine-induced immunity to an idiotype-specific vaccine in rituximab-treated mantle cell lymphoma patients was preserved despite severe B-cell depletion [54]. More recently, the induction of T-cell immunity in association with rituximab therapy in patients with B-cell lymphoma was demonstrated as manifested by the development of T-cell lymphoid aggregates within the bone marrow [55], or lymphoma idiotype-specific T-cell responses [56]. These observations support a vaccine effect of single agent rituximab therapy, and provide further support for its use in combination with vaccines and other immunotherapeutic agents.

3. CETUXIMAB, PANITUMUMAB AND MAbs THAT TARGET THE EGFR PATHWAYS

Cetuximab is a chimeric, partially humanized MAb specific for the epidermal growth factor receptor (EGFR). It is currently approved for treating colorectal cancers and head and neck cancers. Like trastuzumab and rituximab, cetuximab inhibits signaling pathways that promote tumor growth and progression, and induces apoptosis. The antibody can promote antibody-dependent cellular cytotoxicity against lung cancer cells *in vitro* [57]. Cetuximab can synergize with paclitaxel to inhibit angiogenesis and induce tumor cell apoptosis [58]. It has also been shown to promote the cross-priming of antigen-specific CTL in response to chemo-therapy- and cetuximab-treated colon cancer cells *in vitro* [59]. There is limited data available on the immune-based effects of panitumumab, but like these other therapeutic MAbs, it can induce immunity through natural killer cell–dendritic cell cross-talk [60].

B. MAbs that target host elements of the tumor microenvironment

1. BEVACIZUMAB AND MAbs THAT TARGET THE VEGF/VEGFR PATHWAYS

Bevacizumab is a chimeric, partially humanized MAb specific for the vascular endothelial growth factor (VEGF), a cytokine critical for tumor-associated angiogenesis. It is currently approved for treating colorectal cancers, glioblastomas, non-small cell lung cancers, and renal cell carcinomas. In addition to promoting neo-vessel formation, VEGF is immunosuppressive. In preclinical models it causes thymic atrophy, inhibits T-cell development, and antagonizes dendritic cell function [61,62]. MAbs specific for VEGF can improve the numbers and function of dendritic cells in tumor-bearing mice, thereby potentiating dendritic cell-based immuno-therapy [63]. Bevacizumab therapy can increase the B- and T-cell subsets in cancer patients [64], and augment the ability of dendritic cells derived from cancer patients to stimulate alloresponses and T-cell responses to recall antigens [65]. MAbs specific for the VEGF/VEGFR pathways can decrease macrophage and myeloid-derived suppressor cell (MDSC) infiltration in orthotopic pancreatic or breast tumors in mice [66]. MAbs specific for VEGF synergistically enhanced the efficacy of adoptive cellular therapy against B16 melanomas in murine models, in part by promoting the infiltration of adoptively transferred T cells into the tumors [67]. Tumor-bearing nontolerant mice treated with a MAb specific for VEGFR2 develop HER-2-specific T cells, even in the absence of vaccination [68]. In the setting of antigen-specific immune tolerance, sequencing vaccination with cyclophosphamide and doxorubicin in the setting of treatment with VEGFR2 MAb unmasks the T-cell dependent-activity of the VEGFR2 MAb and allows the vaccine to work, resulting in a tumor-free survival rate of about 70% [68].

To date, one clinical trial combining bevacizumab and a cancer vaccine has been reported. Patients with metastatic prostate cancer in biochemical relapse (rising PSA) were treated with a combination of prostatic acid phosphatase (PAP)-pulsed antigen-presenting cells (Provenge[R]) and bevacizumab (Table 25.3). All patients developed immune responses to PAP, and almost half displayed some decrease in PSA from baseline [69].

2. DENOSUMAB

Denosumab is a MAb recently approved for the management of malignant bone disease in multiple myeloma and breast cancer; it is also used to prevent fragility fractures in osteoporosis. It is specific for the signaling pathway controlled by the interactions of the RANKL and its antagonist osteoprotegerin. The RANKL is expressed at high levels by activated

T cells, and its receptor RANK is expressed by monocytes, macrophages, and dendritic cells. To date, the immune effects of denosumab in humans remain relatively uncharacterized [70].

V. IMMUNE MODULATION WITH BIOLOGICALLY TARGETED THERAPY

A. Immune-modulating effects of bisphosphonates

Bisphosphonates are in wide use for the management of osteoporosis, and the bisphosphonates pamidronate and zolendronate are approved for the management of malignant bone disease [71]. They act by inducing apoptosis in osteoclasts, thereby decreasing bone turnover. They also have immune-modulating effects. The standard bone-modifying drug zolendronate can augment the activity of dendritic cells and NK cells, thereby promoting the activation of $\gamma\delta$ and $\alpha\beta$ T cells [72]. It may also modulate tumor-associated macrophages [73].

B. Immune-modulating effects of endocrine therapy

Breast and prostate tumors are unique among the solid tumors since endocrine manipulation is an additional therapeutic strategy. For breast cancer, endocrine manipulation includes selective estrogen receptor modulators and destroyers (SERMS and SERDS: tamoxifen, raloxifene, and fulvestrant), the aromatase inhibitors (arimidex, letrozole, and exemestane), and ovarian suppression. Androgen ablation is a common treatment for prostate cancer; additional drugs are increasingly used. Endocrine manipulation can also modulate the immune system (Table 25.4).

SERMS have been reported to promote T-helper type 2 immunity, thereby favoring cancer growth and progression rather than effective tumor immunity [74]. In addition, they inhibit the differentiation and LPS-induced maturation of DCs, antagonizing the estrogen receptor to maintain them in an immature state *in vitro* [75]. Aromatase inhibitors can sensitize tumor cells to monocyte-mediated ADCC [76]. While no immunomodulatory effects of ovarian ablation are available, androgen ablation in murine models of prostate cancer have been shown to alleviate immune tolerance [77]. Furthermore, androgen ablation in prostate cancer patients results in T-cell infiltration within the prostate [78].

C. Immune-modulating effects of tyrosine kinase inhibitors

Multiple tyrosine kinase inhibitors have been developed that target pathways indispensible for tumor growth and progression, and increasing data suggest they also have immune effects (Table 25.4). Imatinib mesylate, nilotinib, and dasatinib all inhibit the BCR-ABL tyrosine kinase and the c-kit tyrosine kinase, and are highly effective therapies for chronic myelogenous leukemia (CML), gastrointestinal stromal tumors (GIST) and other hematologic malignancies or cancers that depend on BCR-ABL or c-kit signaling. Some data suggest that imatinib inhibits tumor immunity, but other data suggests that it enhances antigen-presenting cell function

425

TABLE 25.4 Small Molecule Therapeutics with Immune-Modulating Activity

Drug Class	Agent
Endocrine Modulators	Tamoxifen, raloxifene anastrozole, letrozole, exemestane
Tyrosine Kinase Inhibitors	Imatinib mesylate, dasatinib, nilotinib vemurafenib sunitinib, sorafenib
Phosphodiesterase Inhibitors	Sildenafil, tadalafil, vardenafil
Immunomodulatory Drugs	thalidomide, lenalidomide

and overcomes tumor-induced CD4$^+$ T-cell tolerance [79]. In patients, imatinib does not inhibit, and in fact promotes, the emergence of BCR-ABL-specific CD8$^+$ T cells in the bone marrow during long-term treatment [80,81]. Imatinib has been combined with a cell-based vaccine that secretes GM-CSF in CML patients (Table 25.3). This study showed an improvement in molecular responses even in patients who have previously been on imatinib therapy for quite some time [82]. In contrast, dasatinib has been reported to markedly inhibit antigen-specific effector T-cell function [83]. The BCR-ABL tyrosine kinase inhibitors also have differential effects on NK-cell activity [84]. Finally, imatinib and dasatinib have been shown to inhibit Treg [85,86].

Lapatinib is an inhibitor of the HER-2 tyrosine kinase, and is approved for treating metastatic breast cancers that overexpress HER-2. While the immunomodulatory effects of lapatinib have not been fully characterized, synergistic antitumor activity has been observed with combined HER-2-directed vaccination and pharmacologic inhibition with lapatinib in a preclinical model [87]. A clinical trial building on this model combined vaccination with a HER-2 protein vaccine given with concurrent lapatinib therapy in twelve patients with trastzumab-refractory metastatic breast cancer (Table 25.3). This regimen was safe and immunogenic, with promising trends in survival [88].

Vemurafenib is a selective BRAF inhibitor approved for the treatment of metastatic melanoma; GSK2118436 is another selective BRAF inhibitor under development. Two studies have demonstrated that selective inhibition of BRAF does not impair T-cell function, and may reverse immune evasion in melanomas to allow the T-cell response specific for melanoma to unfold [89,90]. In another study, tumor biopsies taken from 15 patients treated with one of the BRAF inhibitors demonstrated a striking increase in tumor infiltration by CD4$^+$ and CD8$^+$ lymphocytes following BRAF inhibitor treatment [91]. There was a significant correlation between intratumoral CD8$^+$ T cells, granzyme B expression, and reduction in tumor size. These observations provide strong rationale for combining BRAF inhibitors with immunotherapy for melanoma.

Sunitinib and sorafinib are multikinase inhibitors that inhibit tumor neo-vessel formation, thereby disrupting the supportive tumor microenvironment. These drugs have pleiotropic effects on tumor immunity. Sorafenib, but not sunitinib, inhibits DC- and NK-cell function, and can block the induction of primary antigen-specific T-cell responses [92]. Conversely, it can shift the macrophage cytokine profile from the M2 phenotype to the antitumor M1 phenotype [93]. In contrast, sunitinib preserves DC-, NK-, and effector T-cell function, but depletes Treg and MDSC and decreases expression of CTLA-4 and PD-1 [94]. Thus, it promotes T-helper type 1-driven CD8$^+$ T-cell responses within tumor infiltrating lymphocytes. A preclinical study demonstrated that sunitinib can facilitate the activation and recruitment of therapeutically active T cells in response to antigen-specific vaccination [95]. In patients with metastatic renal cell carcinoma, sunitinib treatment also reduced both MDSC and Treg, and restored the antitumor T-helper type 1 cytokine profile [96].

D. Immune-modulating effects of targeted small molecules

Sildafenil, tadalafil, and vardenafil are phosphodiesterase inhibitors approved for the management of erectile dysfunction and the symptoms of benign prostatic hyperplasia in men. Preclinical studies have shown that this drug class can augment endogenous antitumor immune responses in preclinical models through mitigating the suppressive influence of MDSC [93]. In addition, these drugs enhance the proliferation of T cells from patients with multiple myeloma or head and neck cancer *in vitro* [97]. Clinical trials to test these effects in cancer patients are ongoing, and similar findings have been reported in a murine model of melanoma [98].

Lenalidomide is an immunomodulatory agent approved for the treatment of multiple myeloma. It augments NK-cell numbers and function, and promotes T-cell activity by enhancing cytokine production, cell proliferation, and possibly inhibiting CTLA-4 signaling and Tregs [99]. A recent study demonstrated that humoral and cellular immune responses to a pneumococcal vaccine in patients with multiple myeloma treated with lenalidomide were increased, and that patients with a clinical myeloma response developed tumor-specific immunity with increases in myeloma-specific IFN-γ-secreting T cells and a reduction in T-helper type 17 cells [100].

Finally, epigenetic therapy is now the subject of intense clinical investigation, and exploration of the role of epigenetic modulation on tumor immunity is just beginning [101]. Recent studies have shown that it can induce re-expression of tumor antigens [102], and reverse immunologic skew to favor T-helper type 1 immunity [103].

VI. CONCLUSIONS

Cancer researchers have made enormous strides in understanding the immunobiology of the host–tumor interaction at the molecular and cellular levels. It is now clear that tumor-associated immune responses can either fuel tumor growth and progression, or prevent the establishment and outgrowth of nascent tumors. With these new insights, and a detailed understanding of how normal host cells and transformed tumor cells interact, our ability to maximize the bioactivity and clinical efficacy of immune-based therapies has never been greater. Strategically integrating standard and novel cancer therapies directed at the transformed tumor cell with cancer drugs that both target the transformed cell and modify the host–tumor interaction should overcome systemic immune tolerance and resculpt the tumor microenvironment to favor tumor rejection and effect clinical cure. Carefully working out the proper dose and sequencing of drugs that comprise integrative immunotherapy regimens in both relevant preclinical models and in clinical trials employing unique designs and the collection of multiple correlative samples will accelerate clinical progress. This will require new approaches to drug development, with close partnership between academia, biotechnology firms, large pharmaceutical companies, and government regulatory agencies. Novel scientific and clinical challenges to the successful implementation of routine tumor immunotherapies have already emerged, and will almost certainly continue to do so. One clear challenge is the development of strategies to dissociate the undesired autoimmune toxicities of successful immune-based tumor therapy from the desired antitumor effect. Another challenge is the emergence of novel pathways of resistance to immunotherapy, which will require the development of treatment strategies to overcome them. Clinical success will require not only the proper dose and sequencing of drugs, but also the optimal integration of the knowledge, effort, and resources of multiple stakeholders in order to make integrated cancer immuno-therapies the new standard of care.

CONFLICT OF INTEREST

Dr. Emens receives research funding from Genentech Incorporated, and has received honoraria for participating on regional advisory panels for Genentech Incorporated, Roche Incorporated, and Bristol Myers Squibb. Under a licensing agreement between Biosante Incorporated and the Johns Hopkins University, the University and Dr. Elizabeth Jaffee are entitled to milestone payments and royalty on sales of GM-CSF-secreting cancer vaccines. The terms of these arrangements are being managed by Johns Hopkins University in accordance with its conflict of interest policies.

ACKNOWLEDGMENTS

This work was supported by the Department of Defense (Clinical Translational Research Award W81XWH-07-1-0485), the American Cancer Society (RSG CCE 112685), the Specialized Programs in Research Excellence (SPORE) in Breast Cancer (P50CA88843), the Specialized

Programs in Research Excellence (SPORE) in GI Cancer (p50CA052), NCI R01 CA88058, Genentech Incorporated, the Gateway Foundation, the Avon Foundation, and the V Foundation.

References

[1] Herold MJ, McPherson KG, Reichardt HM. Glucocorticoids in T cell apoptosis and function. Cell Mol Life Sci 2006;63:60−72.

[2] Emens LA, Machiels JP, Reilly RT, Jaffee EM. Chemotherapy: friend or foe to cancer vaccines? Curr Opin Mol Ther 2001;3:77−84.

[3] Casares N, Pequignot NO, Tesniere A, Ghiringhelli F, Roux S, Chaput N, et al. Caspase-dependent immunogenicity of doxorubicin-induced tumor cell death. J Exp Med 2005;202:1691−701.

[4] Demaria S, Volm MD, Shapiro RL, Yee HT, Oratz R, Formenti S, et al. Development of tumor-infiltrating lymphocytes in breast cancer after neoadjuvant paclitaxel chemotherapy. Clin Cancer Res 2001;7:3025−303.

[5] Cho BK, Rao VP, Ge Q, Eisen HN, Chen J. Homeostasis-stimulated proliferation drives naïve T cells to differentiate directly into memory T cells. J Exp Med 2000;192:549−56.

[6] Goldrath AW, Bogatzki LY, Bevan MJ. Naïve T cells transiently acquire a memory-like phenotype during homeostasis-driven proliferation. J Exp Med 2000;192:557−64.

[7] Emens LA. Chemoimmunotherapy Cancer J 2010;16:295−303.

[8] Von Mehren M, Arlen P, Gulley J, Rogatko A, Cooper HS, Meropol NJ, et al. The influence of granulocyte-macrophage colony-sitmulating factor and prior chemotherapy on the immunological response to avaccine (ALVAC-CEA-B7.1) in patients with metastatic carcinoma. Clin Cancer Res 2001;7:1181−91.

[9] Lutz E, Yeo CJ, Lillemoe KD, Biedrzycki B, Kobrin B, Herman J, et al. A lethally irradiated allogeneic granulocyte-macrophage colony stimulating factor-secreting tumor vaccine for pancreatic adenocarcinoma: a phase II trial of safety, efficacy, and immune activation. Ann Surg 2011;253:328−35.

[10] Emens LA. GM-CSF-secreting vaccines for solid tumors. Curr Opin Invest Drugs 2009;10:1315−24.

[11] Small E, Demkow T, Gerritson W, et al. A Phase III trial of GVAX immunotherapy for prostate cancer in combination with docetaxel vs. docetaxel plus prednisone in symptomatic, castration-resistant prostate cancer (CRPC). GU ASCO 2009.

[12] Kaufman HL, Lenz HJ, Marshall J, Singh D, Garett C, Cripps C, et al. Combination chemotherapy and ALVAC-CEA/B7.1 vaccine in patients with metastatic colorectal cancer. Clin Cancer Res 2008;14:4843−9.

[13] Weihrauch MR, Ansen S, Jurkiewicz E, Geisen C, Xia Z, Anderson KS, et al. Phase I/II combined chemo-immunotherapy with carcinoembryonic antigen-derived HLA-A2-restricted CAP-1 peptide and irinotecan, 5-fluorouracil, and leucovorin in patients with primary metastatic colorectal cancer. Clin Cancer Res 2005;11:5993−6001.

[14] Arlen PM, Gulley JL, Parker C, Skarupa L, Pazdur M, Panicali D, et al. A randomized phase II study of concurrent docetaxel plus vaccine versus vaccine alone in metastatic androgen-independent prostate cancer. Clin Cancer Res 2006;12:1260−9.

[15] Kyte JA, Gaudernack G, Dueland S, Trachsel S, Julsrud L, Aamdal S. Telomerase peptide vaccination combined with temezolomide: a clinical trial in stage IV melanoma patients. Clin Cancer Res 2011;17:4568−80.

[16] Antonia SJ, Mirza N, Fricke I, Chiappori A, Thompson P, Williams N, et al. Combination of p53 cancer vaccine with chemotherapy in patients with extensive stage small cell lung cancer. Clin Cancer Res 2006;12:878−87.

[17] Wheeler CJ, Black KL, Liu G, Mazer M, Zhang XX, Pepkowitz S, et al. Vaccination elicits correlated immune and clinical responses in glioblastoma multiforme patients. Cancer Res 2008;68:5955−64.

[18] Nistico P, Capone I, Palermo B, Del Bello D, Ferraresi V, Moschella F, et al. Chemotherapy enhances vaccine-induced antitumor immunity in melanoma patients. Int J Cancer 2009;124:130−9.

[19] Palermo B, Del Bello D, Sottini A, Serana F, Ghidini C, Gualtieri N, et al. Dacarbazine treatment before peptide vaccination enlarges T cell repertoire diversity of melan-a-specific, tumor-reactive CTL in melanoma patients. Cancer Res 2010;70:7084−92.

[20] Radfar S, Wang Y, Khong HT. Activated CD4$^+$ T cells dramatically enhance chemotherapeutic tumor responses in vitro and in vivo. J Immmuol 2009;183:6800−7.

[21] Warren EH, Fujii N, Akatsuka Y, Chaney CN, Mito JK, Loeb KR, et al. Therapy of relapsed leukemia after allogeneic hematopoietic cell transplantation with T cells specific for minor histocompatibility antigens. Blood 2010;115:3869−78.

[22] Dudley ME, Yang JC, Sherry R, Hughes MS, Royal R, Kammula U, et al. Adoptive cell therapy for patients with metastatic melanoma: evaluation of intensive myeloablative chemoradiation preparative regimens. J Clin Oncol 2008;26:5233−9.

[23] Borrello IM, Levitsky HI, Stock W, Sher D, Qin L, DeAngelo DJ, et al. Granulocyte-macrophage colony-stimulating factor (GM-CSF)-secreting celluilar immunotherapy in combination with autologous stem cell transplantation (ASCT) as postremission therapy for acute myeloid leukemia (AML). Blood 2009;114:1736–45.

[24] Ho VT, Vanneman M, Kim H, Sasada T, Kang YJ, Pasek M, et al. Biologic activity of irradiated, autologous, GM-CSF-secreting leukemia cell vaccines early after allogeneic stem cell transplantation. Proc Natl Acad Sci USA 2009;106:15825–30.

[25] Emens LA, Jaffee EM. Toward a breast cancer vaccine: work in progress. Oncology 2003;17:1200–11.

[26] Miles D, Roche H, Martin M, Perren TJ, Cameron DA, Glaspy J, et al. Phase III multicenter clinical trial of the sialyl-TN (STn)-keyhole limpet hemocyanin (KLH) vaccine for metastatic breast cancer. Oncologist 2011;16:1092–100.

[27] Laheru D, Lutz E, Burke J, Biedrzycki B, Solt S, Onners B, et al. Allogeneic granulocyte macrophage colony-stimulating factor tumor immunotherapy alone or in sequence with cyclophosphamide for metastatic pancreatic cancer: a pilot study of safety, feasibility, and immune activation. Clin Cancer Res 2008;14:1455–63.

[28] Schiller J, Nemunaitis J, Ross H, et al. A phase 2 randomized study of GM-CSF gene-modified autologous tumor vaccine (CG8123) with and without low dose cyclophosphamide in advanced stage non-small cell lung cancer (NSCLC). Presented at the International Associated for Stud of Lung Cancer 2005.

[29] Chu CS, Boyer J, Schullery DS, Gimotty PA, Gamerman V, Bender J, et al. Phase I/II randomized trial of dendritic cell vaccination with or without cyclophosphamide for consolidation therapy of advanced ovarian cancer in first or second remission. Cancer Immunol Immunother 2011; http://dx.doi.org/10.1007/s00262-011-1081-8.

[30] Emens LA, Asquith JM, Leatherman JM, Kobrin BJ, Petrik S, Laiko M, et al. Timed sequential treatment with cyclophosphamide, doxorubicin, and an allogeneic granulocyte-macrophage colony-stimulating factor-secreting breast tumor vaccine: a chemotherapy dose-ranging factorial study of safety and immune activation. J Clin Oncol 2009;27:5911–8.

[31] Clynes RA, Towers TL, Presta LG, Ravetch JV. Inhibitory Fc receptors modulate in vivo cytotoxicity against tumor targets. Nature Med 2000;6:443–6.

[32] Gennari R, Menard S, Fagnoni F, Ponchio L, Scelsi M, Tagliabue E, et al. Pilot study of the mechanism of action of preoperative trastuzumab in patients with primary operable breast tumors overexpressing HER-2. Clin Cancer Res 2004;10:5650–5.

[33] Arnould L, Gelly M, Penault-Llorca F, Benoit L, Bonnetain F, Migeon C, et al. Trastuzumab-based treatment of HER-2-positive breast cancer: an antibody-dependent cellular cytotoxicity mechanism? Br J Cancer 2006;94:259–67.

[34] Klapper LN, Waterman H, Sela M, Yarden Y. Tumor-inhibitory antibodies to HER-2/ErbB-2 may act by recruiting c-Cbl and enhancing ubiquitination of HER-2. Cancer Res 2000;60:3384–8.

[35] Castilleja A, Ward NE, O'Brian CA, Swearingen 2nd B, Swan E, Gillogly MA, et al. Accelerated HER-2 degradation enhances ovarian tumor recognition by CTL. Implications for tumor immunogenicity. Mol Cell Biochem 2001;217:21–33.

[36] Zum Buschenfelde CM, Hermann C, Schmidt B, Peschel C, Bernhard H. Antihuman epidermal growth factor receptor 2 (HER-2) monoclonal antibody trastuzumab enhances cytolytic activity of class I-restricted HER-2-specific T lymphocytes against HER-2-overexpressing tumor cells. Cancer Res 2002;62:2244–7.

[37] Kono K, Sato E, Naganuma H, Takahasi A, Mimura K, Nukui H, Fujii H. Trastuzumab (Herceptin) enhances class I-restricted antigen presentation recognized by HER-2-neu-specific T cytotoxic lymphocytes. Clin Cancer Res 2004;10:2538–44.

[38] Wolpoe ME, Lutz ER, Ercolini AM, Murata S, Ivie SE, et al. HER-2/*neu*-specific monoclonal antibodies collaborate with HER-2/*neu*-targeted granulocyte macrophage colony-stimulating factor-secreting whole cell vaccination to augment CD8$^+$ T cell effector function and tumor-free surivival in HER-2/*neu* transgenic mice. J Immunol 2003;171:2161–9.

[39] Mohsin SK, Weiss HL, Gutierrez MC, Chamness GC, Schiff R, Digiovanna MP, et al. Neoadjuvant trastuzumab induces apoptosis in primary breast cancers. J Clin Oncol 2005;23:2460–8.

[40] Ladoire S, Arnould L, Mignot G, Apetoh L, Rebe C, Martin F, et al. T-bet expression in intratumoral lymphoid structures after neoadjuvant trastuzumab plus docetaxel for HER-2-overexpressing breast carcinoma predicts survival. Br J Cancer 2011;105:366–71.

[41] Taylor C, Hershman D, Shah N, Suciu-Foca N, Petrylak DP, Taub R, et al. Augmented HER-2-specific immunity during treatment with trastuzumab and chemotherapy. Clin Cancer Res 2007;13:5133–43.

[42] Montgomery RB, Makary E, Schiffman K, Goodell V, Disis ML. Endogenous anti-HER-2 antibodies block HER-2 phosphorylation and signaling through extracellular signal-regulated kinase. Cancer Res 2005;65:650–6.

429

[43] Jasinska J, Wagner S, Radauer C, Sedivy R, Brodowicz T, Wiltschke C, et al. Inhibition of tumor cell growth by antibodies induced after vaccination with peptides derived from the extracellular domain of HER-2/*neu*. Int J Cancer 2003;107:976—83.

[44] Reilly RT, Machiels JP, Emens LA, Ercolini AM, Okoye FI, Lei RY, et al. The collaboration of both humoral and cellular HER-2/*neu*-targeted immune responses is required for the complete eradication of HER-2/*neu*-expressing tumors. Cancer Res 2001;61:880—3.

[45] Kim PS, Armstrong TD, Song H, Wolpoe ME, Weiss V, Manning EA, et al. Antibody association with HER-2/*neu*-targeted vaccine enhances CD8$^+$ T cell responses in mice through Fc-mediated activation of DCs. J Clin Invest 2008;118:1700—11.

[46] Disis ML, Wallace DR, Gooley TA, Dang Y, Slota M, Lu H, et al. Concurrent trastuzumab and HER-2/*neu*-specific vaccination in patients with metastatic breast cancer. J Clin Oncol 2009;27:4685—92.

[47] Emens LA, Gupta R, Petrik S, Laiko M, Levi J, Leatherman JM, et al. A feasibility study of combination therapy with trastuzumab (T), cyclophosphamide (CY), and an allogeneic GM-CSF-secreting breast tumor vaccine for the treatment of HER-2$^+$ breast cancer. Proc Am Soc Clin Oncol 2011. abstr 2535.

[48] Cobleigh MA, Vogel CL, Tripathy D, Robert NJ, Scholl S, Fehrenbacher L, et al. Multinational study of the efficacy and safety of humanized anti-HER-2 monoclonal antibody in women who have HER-2-overexpressing metastatic breast cancer that progressed after chemotherapy for metastatic disease. J Clin Oncol 1999;17:2639—48.

[49] Vogel CL, Cobleigh MA, Tripathy D, Gutheil JC, Harris LN, Fehrenbacher L, et al. Efficacy and safety of trastuzumab as a single agent in first-line treatment of HER-2-overexpressing metastatic breast cancer. J Clin Oncol 2002;20:719—26.

[50] Selenko N, Maidic O, Draxier S, Berer A, Jager U, Knapp W, Stockl J. CD20 antibody (C2B8)-induced apoptosis of lymphoma cells promotes phagocytosis by dendritic cells and cross-priming of CD8$^+$ cytotoxic T cells. Leukemia 2001;15:1619—26.

[51] Vega MI, Huerta-Yepaz S, Garban H, Jazirehi A, Emmanouilides C, Bonavida B. Rituximab inhibits p38 MAPK activity in 2F7 B NHL and decreases IL-10 transcription: pivotal role of p38 MAPK in drug resistance. Oncogene 2004;23:3530—40.

[52] Jazirehi AR, Vega MI, Chatterjee D, Goodglick L, Bonavida B. Inhibition of the Raf-MEK1/2-ERK1/2 signaling pathway, Bcl-XL down-regulation, and chemosensitization of non-Hodgkin's lymphoma B cells by rituximab. Cancer Res 2004;64:7117—26.

[53] Inoue S, Leitner WW, Golding B, Scott D. Inhibitory effects of B cells on antitumor immunity. Cancer Res 2006;66:7741—7.

[54] Neelapu SS, Kwak LW, Kobrin CB, Reynolds CW, Janik JE, Dunleavy K, et al. Vaccine-induced tumor-specific immunity despite severe B-cell depletion in mantle cell lymphoma. Nat Med 2005;11:986—91.

[55] Raynaud P, Caulet-Maugendre S, Foussard C, Salles G, Moreau A, Rossi JF, et al. T-cell lymphoid aggregates in bone marrow after rituximab therapy for B-cell follicular lymphoma: a marker of therapeutic efficacy? Hum Pathol 2008;39:194—200.

[56] Hilchey SP, Hyrien O, Mosmann TR, Livingstone AM, Friedberg JW, Young F, et al. Rituximab immunotherapy results in the induction of a lymphoma idiotype-specific T-cell response in patients with follicular lymphoma: support for a "vaccinal effect" of rituximab. Blood 2009;113:3809—12.

[57] Kurai J, Chikumi H, Hashimoto K, Yamaguchi K, Yamasaki A, Sako T, et al. Antibody-dependent cellular cytotoxicity mediated by cetuximab against lung cancer cell lines. Clin Cancer Res 2007;13:1552—61.

[58] Inoue K, Slaton JW, Perrotte P, Davis DW, Bruns CJ, Hicklin DJ, et al. Paclitaxel enhances the effects of the anti-epidermal growth factor receptor monoclonal antibody ImClone C225 in mice with metastatic human bladder transitional cell carcinoma. Clin Cancer Res 2000;6:4874—84.

[59] Correale P, Botta C, Cusi MG, Del Vecchio MT, De Santi MM, Gori Savellini G, et al. Cetuximab +/− chemotherapy enhances dendritic cell-mediated phagocytosis of colon cancer cells and ignites a highly efficient colon cancer antigen-specific cytotoxic T-cell response in vitro. Int J Cancer 2012;130:1577—89.

[60] Lee SC, Srivastava RM, Lopez-Albaitero A, Ferrone S, Ferris RL. Natural killer (NK): dendritic cell (DC) cross talk induced by therapeutic monoclonal antibody triggers tumor antigen-specific T cell immunity. Immunol Res 2011;50:248—54.

[61] Almand B, Resser JR, Lindman B, Nadaf S, Clark JI, Kwon ED et al. Clinical significance of defective dendritic cell differentiation in cancer. Clin Cancer Res 6:1755—66

[62] Ohm JE, Gabrilovitch DI, Sempowski GD, Kisseleva E, Parman KS, Nadaf S, Carbone DP. VEGF inhibits T-cell development and may contribute to tumor-induced immune suppression. Blood 2003;101:4878—86.

[63] Gabrilovich DI, Ishida T, Nadaf S, Ohm JE, Carbone DP. Antibodies to vascular endothelial growth factor enhance the efficacy of cancer immunotherapy by improving endogenous dendritic cell function. Clin Cancer Res 1999;5:2963—70.

430

[64] Manzoni M, Rovati B, Ronzoni M, Loupakis F, Mariucci S, Ricci V, et al. Immunological effects of bevacizumab-based treatment in metastatic colorectal cancer. Oncology 2010;79:187—96.

[65] Osada T, Chong G, Tansik R, Hong T, Spector N, Kumar R, et al. The effect of anti-VEGF therapy on immature myeloid cell and dendritic cells in cancer patients. Cancer Immunol Immunother 2008;57:1115—24.

[66] Roland CL, Dineen SP, Lynn KD, Sullivan LA, Dellinger MT, Sadegh L, et al. Inhibition of vascular endothelial growth factor reduces angiogenesis and modulates immune cell infiltration of orthotopic breast cancer xenografts. Mol Cancer Ther 2009;8:1761—71.

[67] Shrimali RK, Yu Z, Theoret MR, Chinnasamy D, Restifo N, Rosenberg SA. Antiangiogenic agents can increase lymphocyte infiltration into tumor and enhance the effectiveness of adoptive immunotherapy of cancer. Cancer Res 2010;70:6171—80.

[68] Manning EA, Ullman JG, Leatherman JM, Asquith JM, Hansen TR, Armstrong TD, et al. A vascular endothelial growth factor receptor-2 inhibitor enhances antitumor immunity through an immune-based mechanism. Clin Cancer Res 2007;13:3951—9.

[69] Rini BI, Weinberg V, Fong L, Conry S, Hershberg RM, Small EJ. Combination immunotherapy with prostatic acid phosphatase pulsed antigen-presenting cells (provenge) plus bevacizumab in patients with serologic progression of prostate cancer after definitive local therapy. Cancer 2006;107:67—74.

[70] Ferrari-Lacraz S, Ferrari S. Do RANKL inhibitors (denosumab) affect inflammation and immunity? Osteoporos Int 2011;22:435—46.

[71] Loftus LS, Edwards-Bennett S, Sokol GH. Systemic therapy for bone metastases. Cancer Control 2012;19:145—53.

[72] Castella B, Riganti C, Fiore F, Pantaleoni F, Canepari ME, et al. Immune modulation by zolendroic acid in human myeloma: an advantageous cross-talk between Vγ9Vδ2 T cells, αβ CD8$^+$ T cells, regulatory T cells, and dendritic cells. J Immunol 2011;187:1578—90.

[73] Rogers TL, Holen I. Tumour macrophages as potential targets of bisphosphonates. J Transl Med 2011;9:177—80.

[74] Behjati S, Frank MH. The effects of tamoxifen on immunity. Curr Med Chem 2009;16:3076—80.

[75] Nalbandian G, Paharkova-Vatchkova V, Mao A, Nale S, Kovats S. The selective estrogen receptor modulators, tamoxifen and raloxifene, impair dendritic cell differentiation and activation. J Immunol 2005;175:2666—75.

[76] Braun DP, Crist KA, Shaheen F, Staren ED, Andrews S, Parker J. Aromatase inhibitors increase the sensitivity of human tumor cells to monocyte-mediated, antibody-dependent cellular cytotoxicity. Am J Surg 2005;190:570—1.

[77] Drake CG, Doody AD, Mihalyo MA, Huang CT, Kelleher E, Ravi S, et al. Androgen ablation mitigates tolerance to a prostate-prostate cancer-restricted antigen. Cancer Cell 2005;7:239—49.

[78] Mercader M, Bodner BK, Moser MT, Kwon PS, Park ES, Manecke RG, et al. T cell infiltration of the prostate induced by androgen withdrawal in patients with prostate cancer. Proc Natl Acad Sci USA 2001;98:4565—70.

[79] Wang H, Cheng F, Cuenca A, Horna P, Zheng Z, Bhalla K, Sotomayor EM. Imatinib mesylate (STI-571) enhances antigen-presenting cell function and overcomes tumor-induced CD4$^+$ T cell tolerance. Blood 2005;105:1135—43.

[80] Bocchia M, Abruzzese E, Forconi F, Ippoliti M, Trawinska MM, Pirrotta MT, et al. Imatinib does not impair specific antitumor T cell immunity in patients with chronic myeloid leukemia. Leukemia 2006;20:142—3.

[81] Riva G, Luppi M, Barozzi P, Quadrelli C, Basso S, Vallerini D, et al. Emergence of BCR-ABL-specific cytotoxic T cells in the bone marrow of patients with Ph$^+$ acute lymphoblasic leukemia during long-term imatinib mesylate treatment. Blood 2010;115:1512—8.

[82] Smith BD, Kasamon YL, Kowalski J, Gocke C, Murphy K, Miller CB, et al. K562/GM-CSF immunotherapy reduces tumor burden in chronic myeloid leukemia patients with residual disease on imatinib mesylate. Clin Cancer Res 2010;16:338—47.

[83] Weichsel R, Dix C, Wooldridge L, Clement M, Fenton-May A, Sewell AK, et al. Profound inhibition of antigen-specific T cell effector functions by dasatinib. Clin Cancer Res 2008;14:2484—91.

[84] Salih J, Hilpert J, Placke T, Grunebach F, Steinle A, Salih HR, Krusch M. The BCR/ABL-inhibitors imatinib, nilotinib, and dasatnib differentially affect NK cell reactivity. Int J Cancer 2010;127:2119—28.

[85] Larmonier N, Janikashvili N, LaCasse CJ, Larmonier CB, Cantrell J, Situ E, et al. Imatinib mesylate inhibits CD4$^+$ CD25$^+$ regulatory T cell activity and enhances active immunotherapy against BCR-ABL tumors. J Immunol 2008;181:6955—63.

[86] Fei F, Yu Y, Schmidt A, Rojewski MT, Chen B, Gotz M, et al. Dasatinib inhibits the proliferation and function of CD4$^+$CD25$^+$ regulatory T cells. Br J Haematol 2009;144:195—205.

[87] Morse MA, Wei J, Hartman Z, Xia W, Ren XR, Lei G, et al. Synergism from combined immunologic and pharmacologic inhibition of HER-2 in vivo. Int J Cancer 2010;126:2893—903.

[88] Hamilton E, Blackwell K, Hobeika AC, Clay TM, Broadwater G, Ren XR, et al. Phase I clinical trial of HER-2-specific immunotherapy with concomitant HER-2 kinase inhibition. J Transl Med 2012;10:28—34.

431

[89] Boni A, Cogdill AP, Dang P, Udayakumar D, Njauw CN, Sloss CM, et al. Selective BRAFV600E inhibition enhances T-cell recognition of melanoma without affecting lymphocyte function. Cancer Res 2010;70:5213—9.

[90] Hong DS, Vence LM, Falchook GS, Radvanyi LG, Liu C, Goodman VL, et al. BRAF(V600) inhibitor GSK2118436 targeted inhibition of mutant BRAF in cancer patients does not impair overall immune competency. Clin Cancer Res 2012; http://dx.doi.org/10.1158/1078-0432.CCR-11-2515.

[91] Wilmott JS, Long GV, Howle JR, Haydu LE, Sharma RN, Thompson JF, et al. Selective BRAF inhibitors induce marked T cell infiltration into human metastatic melanoma. Clin Cancer Res 2012;18:1386—894.

[92] Hipp MM, Hilf N, Walter S, Werth D, Brauer KM, Radsak MP, et al. Sorafenib, but not sunitinib, affects function of dendritic cells and induction of primary immune responses. Blood 2008;111:5610—20.

[93] Edwards JP, Emens LA. The multikinase inhibitor sorfenib reverses the suppression of IL-12 and enhancement of IL-10 by PGE_2 in murine macrophages. Int Immunopharmacol 2010;10:1220—8.

[94] Ozao-Choy J, Ma G, Kao J, Wang GX, Meseck M, Sung M, et al. The novel role of tyrosine kinase inhibitor in the reversal of immune suppression and modulation of tumor microenvironment for immune-based cancer therapies. Cancer Res 2009;69:2514—22.

[95] Bose A, Taylor JL, Alber S, Watkins SC, Garcia JA, Rini BI, et al. Sunitinib facilitates the activation and recruitment of therapeutic anti-tumor immunity in concert with specific vaccination. Int J Cancer 2010;129:2158—70.

[96] Ko JS, Zea AH, Rini BH, Ireland JL, Elson P, Cohen P, et al. Sunitinib mediates reversal of myeloid-derived suppressor cell accumulation in renal cell carcinoma patients. Clin Cancer Res 2009;15:2148—57.

[97] Serafini P, Meckel K, Kelso M, Noonan K, Califano J, Koch W, Dolcetti L, Bronte V, Borrello I. Phosphodiesterase-5 inhibition augments endogenous antitumor immunity by reducing myeloid-derived suppressor cell function. J Exp Med 2006;203:2691—702.

[98] Meyer C, Sevko A, Ramacher M, Bazhin AV, Falk CS, Borrello I, et al. Chronic inflammation promotes myeloid-derived suppressor cell activation blocking antitumor immunity in transgenic mouse melanoma model. Proc Natl Acad Sci USA 2011;108:17111—6.

[99] Quach H, Ritchie D, Stewart AK, Neeson P, Harrison S, Smyth MJ, Prince HM. Mechanism of action of immunomodulatory drugs (IMiDS) in multiple myeloma. Leukemia 2010;24:22—32.

[100] Noonan K, Rudraraju L, Ferguson A, Emerling A, Pasetti MF, Huff CA, Borrello I. Lenalidomide-induced immunomodulation in multiple myeloma: impact on vaccines and antitumor responses. Clin Cancer Res 2012;18:1426—34.

[101] Dubovsky JA, Villagra A, Powers JJ, Wang HW, Pinilla-Ibarz J, Sotomayor EM. Circumventing immune tolerance through epigenetic modification. Curr Pharm Des 2010;16:268—76.

[102] Dubovsky JA, Wang D, Powers JJ, Berchmans E, Smith MA, Wright KL, Sotomayor EM, Pinilla-Ibarz JA. Restoring the functional immunogenicity of chronic lymphocytic leukemia using epigenetic modifiers. Leuk Res 2011;35:394—404.

[103] Dubovsky JA, Powers JJ, Gao Y, Mariusso LF, Sotomayor EM, Pinilla-Ibarz JA. Epigenetic repolarization of T lymphocytes from chronic leukemia patients using 5-aza-2'deoxy-cytidine. Leuk Res 2011;35:1193—9.

Targeting Strategies to Defeat Immune Suppression

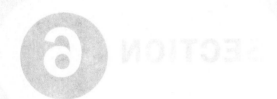

CHAPTER 26

JAK/STAT Signaling in Myeloid Cells: Targets for Cancer Immunotherapy

Saul J. Priceman[1], Jiehui Deng[1], Richard Jove[2], Hua Yu[1]
[1]Department of Cancer Immunotherapeutics & Tumor Immunology, Beckman Research Institute and City of Hope Comprehensive Cancer Center, Duarte, CA USA
[2]Molecular Medicine, Beckman Research Institute and City of Hope Comprehensive Cancer Center, Duarte, CA USA

I. INTRODUCTION

Compelling evidence over the last 20 years has established myeloid cells as critical players in suppressing antitumor immune responses and promoting cancer progression [1–11]. Myeloid cell infiltration is prominent in many human cancers, including breast cancer, lung cancer, renal cell carcinoma, melanoma, and prostate cancer, where it is uniformly and positively correlated with stage progression [12–16]. Myeloid cells modulate various critical steps required for cancer development, including suppressing antitumor immunity, promoting tumor angiogenesis, and driving cancer metastasis. Along with the vast literature basis for their impact on tumor-induced immunosuppression in mice, recent clinical evidence reinforces the immunomodulatory role of myeloid cells in the tumor microenvironment and in systemic compartments, along with their ability to suppress antitumor T-cell responses [10,17–20]. The heterogeneity and distinct functions of numerous subpopulations of myeloid cells have been delineated, uncovering valuable targets for modulating their immunosuppressive and procancer functions in the tumor microenvironment [3,6,21–26].

Among signaling mediators that may influence myeloid cell-mediated cancer progression, JAK/STATs are highlighted for their ability to transmit numerous pathways to regulate immunosuppression, tumor growth and metastasis [27–32]. Indeed, JAK/STAT signaling, and in particular the STAT3 axis is a central pathway utilized by myeloid cells to suppress antitumor immunity [27,28,33]. Genetic studies with STAT3 ablation in the myeloid compartment have established that antitumor immunity is severely constrained by STAT3, via inhibition of Th1 immunostimulatory molecules and induced expression of multiple immunosuppressive and pro-metastatic factors [33–36]. Recent preclinical studies have established JAK/STAT3 signaling blockade as a promising therapeutic strategy to promote antitumor immunity and inhibit cancer progression. This chapter will concentrate on the central role of JAK/STAT signaling in shaping the dynamic tumor-promoting and immunosuppressive phenotypes of myeloid cells, and how targeting this pathway may be widely effective in promoting antitumor immunity and enhancing immune-based therapies for human cancers.

Cancer Immunotherapy. http://dx.doi.org/10.1016/B978-0-12-394296-8.00026-9

II. OVERVIEW OF JAK/STAT SIGNALING

Owing to its direct involvement in cytokine and growth factor receptor-mediated signal transduction and gene regulation, the Janus kinase (JAK)/signaling transducers and activators of transcription (STAT) pathway is critical for immune responses, cell differentiation, migration, proliferation, and survival [37,38]. The family of STAT proteins consists of seven members: STAT1, STAT2, STAT3, STAT4, STAT5A, STAT5B, and STAT6. STATs were originally identified through their critical role in transducing signals from receptors for the interferons (IFN) and interleukin-6 (IL-6) [37,39–41]. Following ligand-dependent stimulation, receptor-associated JAKs (JAK1, JAK2, JAK3, and Tyk2) cause phosphorylation of specific tyrosine residues on cytoplasmic domains of receptors, which serve as docking sites for the STAT proteins [40,41]. Tyrosine phosphorylation of STATs results in homodimers and heterodimers with other STATs through reciprocal interactions with their Src-homology 2 (SH2) domains. STATs can also be phosphorylated by nonreceptor tyrosine kinases, such as SRC and ABL [42–45]. In addition to tyrosine phosphorylation of STATs, serine phosphorylation by serine kinases also affects their transcriptional activity. STAT dimers then translocate to the nucleus where they bind consensus DNA sequences to regulate the expression of a wide range of genes encoding cytokines, immune-modulating factors, growth factors, survival/anti-apoptotic and oncogenic proteins [27,32].

STATs control gene expression through interactions with other non-STAT transcription factors and cofactors, including IRFs, c-Fos, GR, and NF-κB. For example, NF-κB (RelA subunit) and STAT3 are found at the promoters of many of the same inflammatory genes, modulating their expression in various cancer-associated cell types [28,46,47]. STAT3 also physically interacts with the NF-κB subunit RelA in the nucleus to maintain constitutive NF-κB activation in tumors [46]. STAT5 can physically interact with the glucocorticoid receptor (GR) to control nuclear hormone receptor-dependent gene regulation [48,49]. Although tyrosine phosphorylation is classically required for STAT3 DNA binding, recent studies have also revealed unphosphorylated STAT3-mediated expression of specific genes, in part by interacting with NF-κB and regulating its nuclear import and retention [50–52]. STAT1, STAT2, and STAT3 also interact with transcriptional co-activator p300/cAMP response element-binding protein (CBP) to directly modulate gene transcription or to regulate other transcription factors, such as NF-κB [53–56]. STATs also have functional roles independent of their transcriptional regulation, which continue to be elucidated for their impact on migration and invasion. For instance, STATs have been shown to interact with focal adhesion kinase (FAK) and βPIX, a Rac1 activator, to regulate directional migration and the actin cytoskeleton [57–59], and with stathmin to regulate microtubule dynamics [60,61].

Roles for STATs in development have been explored using targeted gene knockout systems, and more recently, with tissue-specific deletion of specific STATs. For instance, global STAT1 deletion in mice resulted in dysfunctional IFN signaling and increased susceptibility to pathogenic infection [62,63]. STAT2 deletion led to defects in Type I IFN signaling and immune responses [64]. Deletion of STAT3 resulted in embryonic lethality demonstrating its critical roles during early development, and targeted deletion studies have revealed its important role in a variety of cell types [65,66]. Targeted deletion of STAT4 or STAT6 has identified their key roles in cytokine-mediated proliferation and activation of adaptive immune cells [67–69]. STAT5A and STAT5B deletion studies have demonstrated their regulation of organ development, tissue-specific gene expression, and immune responses [70,71]. Thus, STATs impact various cell types and play pivotal roles during normal and pathological development.

Several molecular mechanisms exist to negatively regulate JAK/STAT signaling, namely through interactions with suppressor of cytokine signaling (SOCS), protein inhibitor of activated STATs (PIAS), and protein tyrosine phosphatases (PTP) [72,73]. The well-described SOCS proteins inhibit JAK/STAT signaling in three primary ways, by binding and inhibiting

JAK activity, by blocking binding of STATs to receptors, and by promoting proteosomal degradation of JAK2 [74,75]. SOCS proteins are rapidly induced transcriptionally by STATs, for example, for SOCS1 by STAT1 and for SOCS3 by STAT3(74). PIAS proteins act by blocking DNA binding of STATs, or as co-repressor proteins to inhibit transcription of STAT-regulated genes [73], and PTPs dephosphorylate JAKs and block STAT activation [76]. In this manner, negative feedback mechanisms in JAK/STAT signaling tightly control their signaling output in normal cells.

III. JAK/STAT3 SIGNALING IN MYELOID CELL-MEDIATED IMMUNOSUPPRESSION

Although STATs were originally discovered for their important and highly regulated physiological roles in cytokine signaling, it is now well established that STAT3 activation is also central for cancer initiation and progression [27,28,77]. STAT3 is found aberrantly activated in the majority of solid cancers including breast cancer, colon cancer, ovarian cancer, prostate cancer and melanoma, and in some blood malignancies, including leukemia, multiple myeloma and lymphoma [27,28]. Persistent activation of STAT3 in cancer cells regulates their production of anti-apoptotic, pro-angiogenic, pro-metastatic and anti-inflammatory factors. STAT3 is activated by various cytokines and growth factors including IL-6, IL-10, IL-17, IL-23, LIF, VEGF, and many others [27,28]. Activated STAT3 can induce expression of these and other cancer-promoting factors, which leads to persistent STAT3 activation in the tumor microenvironment through a feed-forward loop. In this setting, STAT3 expression in cancer cells results in STAT3 activation in other tumor-associated stromal cells, including endothelial cells, fibroblasts, and infiltrating immune cells [27,28,30] (Figure 25.1). The first definitive study implicating STAT3 activation in cancer-associated inflammation showed that inhibition of STAT3 in cancer cells induced expression of pro-inflammatory factors such as IL-6, RANTES, and CXCL10, leading to potent antitumor immune responses by modulating innate and adaptive immunity [34]. Persistent STAT3 activation in cancer cells allowed for crosstalk with tumor-associated myeloid cells, thereby forming an immunosuppressive tumor microenvironment [34]. Thus, reciprocal upregulation of persistent JAK/STAT3 signaling in both cancer cells and myeloid cells generates a potent anti-inflammatory microenvironment that fuels cancer progression [27,28,30].

"Tumor-associated myeloid cells" is an umbrella phrase that covers several distinct subsets of immune cells with distinct modes of tumor recruitment and function. They include, but are not limited to, tumor-associated macrophages (TAMs), myeloid-derived suppressor cells (MDSCs), dendritic cells (DCs), neutrophils, mast cells, and eosinophils [1,3,78,79]. Suppressive myeloid cells are recognized for their crucial role in regulating tumor evasion of immune responses and promoting tumor growth and metastasis [3,7,9,80]. JAK/STAT signaling has recently been established as a crucial mediator of myeloid cell-mediated immunosuppression [27,28]. As one of the most abundant immune cell subset in many solid cancers, TAM recruitment is mediated by several STAT3-regulated cytokines and chemokines, including macrophage-colony stimulating factor (M-CSF), chemokine (C-C motif) ligand-2 (CCL2), IL-1β, chemokine (C-X-C motif) ligand-12 (CXCL12), and others [1,81,82]. TAMs have been typically classified as either tumoricidal (M1) or protumorigenic (M2) based on distinct gene expression profiles and key mechanisms that regulate M1/M2 skewing in tumors [78]. JAK/STAT signaling, and in particular the STAT3, STAT6, and STAT1 pathways, critically regulate myeloid cell phenotype [28,83–85]. M2 TAMs express an array of STAT3-regulated genes, including pro-angiogenic and pro-metastatic factors such as vascular endothelial growth factor (VEGF), HIF1α and matrix metalloproteinase (MMP)-2 and -9, and as well as IL-10 and PGE2 which inhibit cytotoxic T-cell responses [1,24,27,28]. M2 marker DC-SIGN is also regulated by M-CSF, IL-6 and IL-10 in a STAT3-dependent manner, contributing to the immunosuppressive properties of TAMs [86].

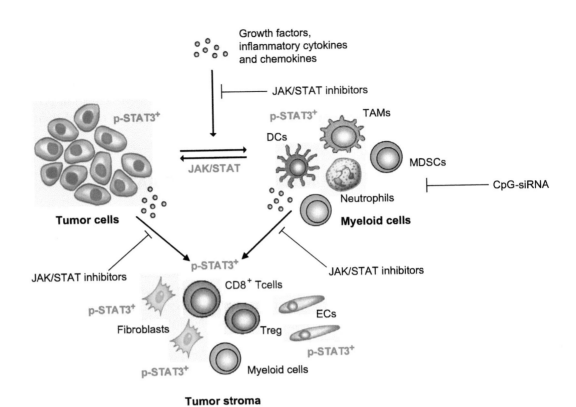

FIGURE 25.1

Persistent STAT3 activation in the tumor microenvironment fuels cancer progression. Growth factors, inflammatory cytokines and chemokines produced in the tumor microenvironment activate JAK/STAT signaling in tumor cells and in tumor-associated myeloid cells (including, but not limited to, tumor-associated macrophages (TAMs), myeloid-derived suppressor cells (MDSCs), dendritic cells (DCs), and neutrophils). Crosstalk between tumor cells, myeloid cells, and numerous stromal cell types (i.e., fibroblasts, endothelial cells, and other tumor-associated immune cells) generates persistent STAT3 activation and immunosuppression in the tumor microenvironment. Therapeutic strategies have emerged to inhibit JAK/STAT signaling by targeting tumor cells and tumor-associated stromal cells, in particular targeting STAT3 signaling specifically in myeloid cells using CpG-siRNA, producing potent anticancer effects and antitumor immunity.

Direct evidence for the impact of myeloid cell-specific STAT3 on the immunosuppressive tumor microenvironment originated from studies using conditional genetic inactivation of STAT3 in the hematopoietic compartment [33,87]. Strikingly, STAT3 inhibition improved the antitumor functions of various myeloid cell subsets, also increasing cytotoxic T cells to inhibit tumor growth through multiple mechanisms [33]. Myeloid cell-specific STAT3 deletion also enhanced DC maturation and function, induced cytolytic neutrophil and natural killer (NK) cells and inhibited tumor-infiltration of FoxP3$^+$ regulatory T cells (Tregs). Notably, STAT3 induced the TAM-mediated expression of the important pro-tumorigenic cytokine IL-23 to promote Treg populations, and also inhibited the NF-κB-dependent production of the pivotal pro-inflammatory factor IL-12 production in tumor-associated DCs to suppress antitumor immunity [36]. In a more recent study, STAT3 activation in cancer cells and tumor-associated myeloid cells was shown to regulate the expression of lipid mediator sphingosine-1 phosphate receptor-1 (S1PR1), which is required for persistent STAT3 activation in tumors [88]. S1PR1 inhibition in myeloid cells promoted antitumor immune responses with elevated expression of pro-inflammatory cytokine IFNγ, inhibiting tumor growth and metastasis [88]. Together, these studies clearly illustrate the multifactorial control of antitumor immunity in solid cancers that can be elicited by targeting the STAT3 signaling axis in tumor-associated myeloid cells.

Myeloid cell-mediated immunosuppression is primarily controlled by MDSCs, a heterogeneous immature myeloid cell population consisting of both mononuclear

(MO-MDSC) and polymorphonuclear (PMN-MDSC) cells [4,10,79, 89—91]. MDSCs expand and mobilize from the bone marrow (BM), accumulating to aberrant levels in blood, spleen, and tumors in both humans and in mouse models [10,92,93]. MDSCs have potent suppressive effects on the activation and proliferation of T cells in lymphoid tissue and at the tumor site by increasing expression of Arginase-1 (Arg1), inducible nitric oxide (iNOS), reactive oxygen species (ROS), and other immunosuppressive factors [4,5,10,17]. JAK/STAT signaling has been shown recently to regulate the expansion and suppressive properties of MDSCs in tumors [28,33,94]. Importantly, circulating MDSCs from patients with malignant melanoma or renal cell carcinoma showed higher STAT3 activity and required JAK/STAT3 signaling for their immunosuppressive properties [95,96]. Key signaling mediators are involved in systemic accumulation and recruitment of MDSCs to tumors, including stem cell factor (SCF, KIT ligand), M-CSF, CCL2, COX-2 and CXCL12, many of which are STAT3 target genes [97—101]. STAT3 also regulates expression of the myeloid-related proteins S100A8 and S100A9 in MDSCs, key pro-inflammatory factors for the recruitment and suppressive activity of MDSC in tumor-bearing mice [102,103]. Notably, overexpression of S100A9 in hematopoietic cells phenocopied the effects of STAT3 inhibition in causing defective DC differentiation and function, superior MDSC expansion and ROS-mediated suppressive activity in tumor-bearing mice [103]. Further studies also have indicated that STAT3 directly controls transcriptional activity of NADPH oxidase (NOX2), which may be responsible for ROS production in MDSCs [104].

Additional key pathways have been implicated in regulating the immunosuppressive properties of tumor-associated MDSCs. For example, HIF1α, which is transcriptionally and post-translationally regulated by STAT3 [105,106], has emerged as an important regulator of myeloid cell function in the tumor microenvironment by increasing Arg1 and iNOS expression in MDSCs [107]. Intriguingly, recent evidence suggested that tumor-derived exosomes, small microvesicles secreted by tumor cells through an exocytosis pathway for signaling turnover and cell-to-cell crosstalk, also regulate the suppressive properties of MDSCs [108]. Indeed, exosome-associated heat shock protein-72 (Hsp72), signaling through TLR2, led to activation of STAT3 in MDSCs via autocrine IL-6 signaling. Recent investigations on microRNA (miRNA)-mediated immune regulation have implicated specific miRNAs in controlling STAT3-regulated MDSC functions. miR-17-5p and miR-20a, whose expression was down-regulated in tumor-infiltrating MDSCs, blocked STAT3 expression, STAT3-induced ROS and hydrogen peroxide (H_2O_2), and concomitant suppressive properties of MDSCs [109]. Collectively, these studies demonstrate the integration of several important signaling pathways that converge upon STAT3 to regulate myeloid cell-mediated immunosuppression.

Myeloid cells have been shown to contribute to cancer progression by aberrantly accumulating at sites of future metastasis, or premetastatic niches, and facilitating the arrival of disseminated tumor cells [110—112]. These myeloid cells form clusters in specific regions of future metastasis (i.e., lungs), and interact with other cell types including fibroblasts, endothelial cells, and other immune cells [113,114]. Myeloid cells are recruited to these sites through several known tumor-induced pathways, including S100A8/A9, lysyl oxidase (LOX), Fibronectin (Fn), and MMP-9 [112,115,116]. Recent studies demonstrated that persistent STAT3 activation in myeloid cells fostered the future arrival of disseminated tumor cells by regulating prosurvival, anti-apoptotic, and prometastatic factors. In addition, tumor-associated myeloid cells required STAT3 for their expression of IL-10, Fn, COX-2 and Arg1, all of which have been implicated previously in immunosuppression [10]. Thus, STAT3 in myeloid cells may hamper antitumor immunity even prior to the arrival of tumor cells [117]. However, further investigation is warranted to better unravel the contributions of myeloid cell-mediated immunosuppression on survival and establishment of tumor cells in hostile microenvironments, such as the blood or lymph circulation or in future metastatic sites.

DCs are potent antigen-presenting cells (APCs), and lie at the intersection of innate and adaptive cellular responses for effective tumor recognition and antitumor immunity [118,119].

439

Defects in DC function are widely accepted in cancers as a major mechanism of tumor escape from immunity, marked with deficient maturation of tumor-infiltrating DCs and their inability to activate T cells [120–123]. Several members of the JAK/STAT signaling pathway are required for normal DC development and function through distinct molecular mechanisms [120]. For instance, IL-6 signaling through STAT3 is required for normal DC differentiation, and inhibition of STAT3 improved antigen-specific T-cell responses [124]. Recent evidence has also implicated STAT3 signaling in the tumor recruitment and function of DCs, which are recruited to tumors by several STAT3-regulated genes, including CXCL12, VEGF, hepatocyte growth factor (HGF), and CXCL8 [120]. Although STAT3 is downregulated during normal DC differentiation, STAT3 activity remained elevated and thereby blocked DC maturation in tumors [94,125]. DCs with highly elevated STAT3 activation display a predominantly immature phenotype, with reduced expression of co-stimulatory molecules (i.e., CD80 and CD86) and defective antigen presentation capabilities as a result of downregulated MHC Class II expression [125]. Later studies deepened support for the impact of STAT3 in DC function in solid cancers, where ablation of STAT3 effectively induced maturation of DCs and improved antigen-presentation for T-cell mediated antitumor immunity [33,34,126].

Like STAT3, other STAT proteins have important roles in various myeloid cell subsets through diverse mechanisms. For instance, the Th2 cytokines IL-4 and IL-13, signaling through STAT6, potently regulated the expression of immunosuppressive markers Retnla, Chi3l3 and Arg1 in TAMs [127–129]. IL-4/STAT6 signaling was also implicated in the epigenetic changes that shape M1/M2 macrophage phenotype, by regulating expression of H3K27 demethylase Jumonji domain containing 3 (Jmjd3) [130]. Jmjd3 expression resulted in demethylation at the promoter sites of Retnla, Chi3l3 and Arg1, thereby increasing their expression in macrophages. STAT6 activation was also required for MDSC survival and their suppressive properties through regulation of immunosuppressive factors TGFβ, Arg1 and iNOS [10,131,132]. By comparison, M1 macrophages express high levels of pro-inflammatory cytokines such as TNFα and IL-12, which promote antitumor adaptive immunity. M1 macrophages depend heavily on NF-κB and STAT1 signaling to regulate IFNγ, iNOS and pro-inflammatory cytokine production, opposing the negative regulation of pro-inflammatory gene expression by STAT3 [79]. Conversely, some studies also suggested an important role for STAT1 in M2 macrophage phenotype and inhibition of myeloid cell-mediated T-cell responses [84]. Therefore, understanding the complexity of JAK/STAT signaling in various stages of myeloid cell differentiation will elucidate new mechanistic regulation of cancer-associated immune responses by JAK/STATs, with direct implications on the development of future anticancer therapies.

IV. TARGETING JAK/STAT3 SIGNALING IN MYELOID CELLS

Therapeutic strategies to modulate the microenvironment have recently highlighted the JAK/STAT3 signaling pathway as important targets for cancer immunotherapy. Genetic ablation studies demonstrated a critical role for STAT3 in modulating inflammatory cytokines and immunosuppressive factors that effectively blocked antitumor immune responses [27,28,33]. However, lacking its own enzymatic activity, STAT3 has been difficult to target directly, and thus a large body of research has focused on inhibiting upstream signaling activators of STAT3. Because STAT3 is a point of convergence for many receptor tyrosine kinases that are activated in cancers, multitargeted small molecule receptor tyrosine kinase (RTK) inhibitors have been shown to inhibit STAT3 activity and boost immune responses. For example, the RTK inhibitor sunitinib, which inhibited tumor cell proliferation via STAT3 inhibition, also potently blocked MDSC expansion along with their reduced STAT3 activity and STAT3-regulated gene expression [133]. Treatment of metastatic renal cell carcinoma (RCC) patients with sunitinib effectively blocked systemic MDSC accumulation, associated with decreased Tregs and enhanced pro-inflammatory IFNγ production [134]. Other RTK inhibitors that have been shown to inhibit STAT3 activation, including sorafenib and imatinib, also inhibit MDSC and Treg populations [11,135–137], but whether these compounds inhibit MDSC accumulation and suppressive functions through STAT3 blockade remains to be explored. Although these RTK inhibitors target STAT3 via upstream receptor inhibition, the promiscuous nature of these drugs has attracted the development of more targeted strategies to specifically block JAK/STAT signaling in cancers.

JAK inhibitors have emerged over the past decade with effective anticancer effects and have recently been shown to modulate the tumor microenvironment in favor of antitumor immunity. The originally described JAK inhibitor, AG490, has been combined with IL-12-based immunotherapy to enhance antitumor immunity [138]. The AG490-related analog, WP1066, has also demonstrated significant antitumor effects in several cancers, resulting in enhanced cytotoxic T cells [139–141]. Although the precise immunomodulatory effects of AG490 on JAK/STAT activation in myeloid cells has yet to be determined, preclinical studies have shown that STAT3 regulates several overlapping pathways that may be major targets of AG490 [139–141]. It is also noteworthy to point out that AG490 inhibits other STATs, including STAT1 and STAT5, perhaps further explaining the overall therapeutic efficacy of this compound.

More specific inhibitors of JAK/STAT3 signaling have been evaluated recently in preclinical models. JSI-124 is a member of the cucurbitacin family of compounds that blocks JAK2/STAT3 activation and inhibits tumor growth [142]. Although the precise molecular mechanisms by which JSI-124 inhibits JAK2/STAT3 have been debated, as this compound also promotes SHP-1 and SHP-2 protein tyrosine phosphatase activities [120]. JSI-124 displays strong immunomodulatory effects, with enhanced tumor-associated DC differentiation, improved MHC class II expression and activation of antigen-specific T cells [94,126]. In addition to its effects on DC functions, JSI-124 also inhibited tumor-associated MDSCs *in vivo*, exhibiting potent antitumor effects alone or in combination with DC-based immunotherapy [94]. In an orthotopic model of glioma, JSI-124 enhanced adoptive T-cell therapy by accentuating DC maturation and promoting migration of tumor-specific T cells [143]. In melanoma models, JSI-124 enhanced the anticancer effects of the immunostimulatory molecule CpG, which signals through TLR9 to boost antitumor immunity [144]. Curcumin, a major component of the spice turmeric, has potent antitumor activity by targeting JAK/STAT3 signaling in cancer cells, thereby promoting apoptosis and inhibiting migration [145,146]. A recent study showed that curcumin blocked MDSC accumulation in tumor and spleens and promoted an M1 phenotype through STAT3 inhibition [147]. These findings deepen the evidence that JAK targeting can limit STAT3 function and de-repress antitumor immunity.

Clinical studies are now underway for the recently described novel and selective JAK inhibitor AZD1480, which has shown significant antitumor effects in preclinical models by inhibiting JAK/STAT3 signaling [148]. In immune competent tumor-bearing mice, AZD1480 inhibited accumulation of tumor-associated myeloid cells, including MDSCs, blocking the expression of several procancer factors including VEGF and IL-1β [149]. However, whether AZD1480 abrogates MDSC function and boosts antitumor immune responses remains to be fully assessed. AZD1480 is currently being evaluated in clinical trials alone or in combination with chemotherapy and it is the first specific JAK/STAT inhibitor to be tested for *in vivo* treatment of human tumors. In this setting, it will be important to further characterize the impact of JAK/STAT inhibitors on myeloid cell-mediated immunosuppression as well as determine the extent of therapeutic effects in combination approaches with other immune-based or conventional therapies.

With translational progress, there is beginning to be some shift in focus toward studies of immune-based therapy for long-term blockade of cancer cell growth and metastasis. STAT3 activation in myeloid cells makes a tremendous contribution to adaptive immune responses in tumors, and therefore promote an immunosuppressive microenvironment can have adverse effects on successes with adoptive T-cell therapy approaches. Recent studies demonstrated that STAT3 in myeloid cells constrained antitumor adaptive immunity, and that genetic ablation of

STAT3 improved effector functions of transferred T cells in a T-cell therapy melanoma model [150]. Inhibition of STAT3 expression in DCs prior to cellular transfer also led to an enhanced antitumor immune response in a mouse model of DC-based immunotherapy [151]. HER-2 DNA vaccine therapy against HER-2$^+$ breast cancers was improved in combination with inhibition of STAT3 [152]. In the latter report, a novel liposome nanoparticle approach to encapsulate the STAT3 inhibitor CDDO-Im was used to target it specifically to the tumor microenvironment and to combine this strategy with a HER-2 DNA vaccine, which prolonged tumor-free survival associated with improved myeloid cell and T-cell antitumor functions.

Unraveling the complexity of antitumor immune responses will ultimately drive successful immunotherapeutic approaches. For instance, the TLR9 agonist CpG has been shown to induce a cascade of innate and adaptive immune mediators, and it has been preclinically and clinically evaluated showing promising antitumor immunity [153,154]. However, TLR9 activation also activates STAT3, thus hampering the full potential of an agonist-based immunotherapeutic approach directed to TLR9 [155]. Recently, a novel siRNA-delivery strategy was developed based on CpG targeting of TLR9-expressing immune cells, including myeloid cells, leading to potent antitumor immune responses [156]. Treatment of tumor-bearing animals with CpG-*STAT3* siRNA conjugates resulted in potent inhibition of STAT3 activation in TAMs and DCs, along with increased pro-inflammatory cytokine production by DCs, increased functional neutrophils, and marked elevation in antitumor adaptive immunity. CpG-*STAT3* siRNA therapy was also used in combination with adoptive T-cell therapy approaches in mouse models of melanoma, where it demonstrated improved cytotoxic T-cell function and reduced Treg infiltration [150].

This technology has been expanded to inhibit critical mediators of persistent STAT3 activation, including S1PR1 [88]. CpG-*S1PR1* siRNA demonstrated significant inhibition of tumor growth and metastasis by inhibiting S1PR1-induced STAT3 activation in tumor-associated myeloid cells, associated with increased pro-inflammatory mediators such as IFN-γ and reductions in the protumor factors IL-6 and IL-1β. Myeloid clustering and the expression of immunosuppressive factors in the premetastatic niche are also potently inhibited by CpG-*S1PR1* siRNA, suggesting that blockade of S1PR1-STAT3 signaling can be targeted directly in myeloid cells to block immunosuppression, tumor growth, premetastatic niches and metastasis [117]. The CpG-siRNA delivery technology can be developed readily for other JAK/STAT family members as well as newly identified JAK/STAT-regulated signaling molecules that contribute to tumor-induced immunosuppression. Here it is noteworthy to mention that these studies have been performed in the context of mouse models, and much work remains to optimize this technology for human use. Nevertheless, the preclinical therapeutic evaluation of inhibitors of JAK/STAT3 activation has collectively demonstrated remarkable promise for the treatment of solid cancers, by reverting immunosuppression and mounting a robust antitumor immune response.

V. CONCLUDING REMARKS

Although the full spectrum of molecular mediators that drive cancer-promoting inflammation and defects in antitumor immunity remain to be uncovered, it is well established that tumor-associated myeloid cells are central cellular players in shaping the immunosuppressive tumor microenvironment and promoting cancer development. JAK/STAT signaling, and especially STAT3, has recently been linked with suppression of antitumor immunity, and with the protumor functions of various immune cells. STAT3 is highly activated in tumor-associated myeloid cells, and elevated STAT3 induces the expression of many immunosuppressive and prometastatic factors that suppress antitumor immunity, support tumor growth, and promote metastatic spread. Although further mechanistic studies are required to fully appreciate the impact of JAK/STAT3 in regulating antitumor immune responses in specific cancers, therapeutic approaches that effectively inhibit this pathway in myeloid cells may have a profound impact for cancer immunotherapy.

References

[1] Mantovani A, Schioppa T, Porta C, Allavena P, Sica A. Role of tumor-associated macrophages in tumor progression and invasion. Cancer Metastasis Rev 2006 Sep;25(3):315—22.

[2] Marigo I, Dolcetti L, Serafini P, Zanovello P, Bronte V. Tumor-induced tolerance and immune suppression by myeloid derived suppressor cells. Immunol Rev 2008 Apr;222:162—79.

[3] Murdoch C, Muthana M, Coffelt SB, Lewis CE. The role of myeloid cells in the promotion of tumour angiogenesis. Nat Rev 2008 Aug;8(8):618—31.

[4] Ostrand-Rosenberg S. Myeloid-derived suppressor cells: more mechanisms for inhibiting antitumor immunity. Cancer Immunol Immunother 2010 Oct;59(10):1593—600.

[5] Serafini P, Borrello I, Bronte V. Myeloid suppressor cells in cancer: recruitment, phenotype, properties, and mechanisms of immune suppression. Semin Cancer Biol 2006 Feb;16(1):53—65.

[6] Solinas G, Germano G, Mantovani A, Allavena P. Tumor-associated macrophages (TAM) as major players of the cancer-related inflammation. J Leukoc Biol 2009 Nov;86(5):1065—73.

[7] Condeelis J, Pollard JW. Macrophages: obligate partners for tumor cell migration, invasion, and metastasis. Cell 2006 Jan 27;124(2):263—6.

[8] Joyce JA, Pollard JW. Microenvironmental regulation of metastasis. Nat Rev 2009 Apr;9(4):239—52.

[9] Qian BZ, Pollard JW. Macrophage diversity enhances tumor progression and metastasis. Cell Apr 2;141(1):39—51.

[10] Gabrilovich DI, Nagaraj S. Myeloid-derived suppressor cells as regulators of the immune system. Nat Rev Immunol 2009 Mar;9(3):162—74.

[11] Lee H, Pal SK, Reckamp K, Figlin RA, Yu H. STAT3: a target to enhance antitumor immune response. Curr Top Microbiol Immunol 2012;344:41—59.

[12] Leek RD, Lewis CE, Whitehouse R, Greenall M, Clarke J, Harris AL. Association of macrophage infiltration with angiogenesis and prognosis in invasive breast carcinoma. Cancer Res 1996 Oct 15;56(20):4625—9.

[13] Takanami I, Takeuchi K, Kodaira S. Tumor-associated macrophage infiltration in pulmonary adenocarcinoma: association with angiogenesis and poor prognosis. Oncology 1999;57(2):138—42.

[14] Ikemoto S, Yoshida N, Narita K, Wada S, Kishimoto T, Sugimura K, et al. Role of tumor-associated macrophages in renal cell carcinoma. Oncol Rep 2003 Nov-Dec;10(6):1843—9.

[15] Jensen TO, Schmidt H, Moller HJ, Hoyer M, Maniecki MB, Sjoegren P, et al. Macrophage markers in serum and tumor have prognostic impact in American Joint Committee on Cancer stage I/II melanoma. J Clin Oncol 2009 Jul 10;27(20):3330—7.

[16] Bigotti G, Coli A, Castagnola D. Distribution of Langerhans cells and HLA class II molecules in prostatic carcinomas of different histopathological grade. Prostate 1991;19(1):73—87.

[17] Ostrand-Rosenberg S, Sinha P. Myeloid-derived suppressor cells: linking inflammation and cancer. J Immunol 2009 Apr 15;182(8):4499—506.

[18] Filipazzi P, Huber V, Rivoltini L. Phenotype, function and clinical implications of myeloid-derived suppressor cells in cancer patients. Cancer Immunol Immunother. Feb;61(2):255—63.

[19] Filipazzi P, Valenti R, Huber V, Pilla L, Canese P, Iero M, et al. Identification of a new subset of myeloid suppressor cells in peripheral blood of melanoma patients with modulation by a granulocyte-macrophage colony-stimulation factor-based antitumor vaccine. J Clin Oncol 2007 Jun 20;25(18):2546—53.

[20] Montero AJ, Diaz-Montero CM, Kyriakopoulos CE, Bronte V, Mandruzzato S. Myeloid-derived suppressor cells in cancer patients: a clinical perspective. J Immunother. Feb-Mar;35(2):107—15.

[21] Nardin A, Abastado JP. Macrophages and cancer. Front Biosci 2008;13:3494—505.

[22] Noonan DM, De Lerma Barbaro A, Vannini N, Mortara L, Albini A. Inflammation, inflammatory cells and angiogenesis: decisions and indecisions. Cancer Metastasis Rev 2008 Mar;27(1):31—40.

[23] Pollard JW. Trophic macrophages in development and disease. Nat Rev Immunol 2009 Apr;9(4):259—70.

[24] Sica A, Mantovani A, Allavena P. Tumour-associated macrophages are a distinct M2 polarised population promoting tumour progression: potential targets of anti-cancer therapy. Eur J Cancer 2006 Apr;42(6):717—27.

[25] Sinha P, Clements VK, Miller S, Ostrand-Rosenberg S. Tumor immunity: a balancing act between T cell activation, macrophage activation and tumor-induced immune suppression. Cancer Immunol Immunother 2005 Nov;54(11):1137—42.

[26] Movahedi K, Guilliams M, Van den Bossche J, Van den Bergh R, Gysemans C, Beschin A, et al. Identification of discrete tumor-induced myeloid-derived suppressor cell subpopulations with distinct T cell-suppressive activity. Blood 2008 Apr 15;111(8):4233—44.

[27] Yu H, Kortylewski M, Pardoll D. Crosstalk between cancer and immune cells: role of STAT3 in the tumour microenvironment. Nat Rev Immunol 2007 Jan;7(1):41—51.

[28] Yu H, Pardoll D, Jove R. STATs in cancer inflammation and immunity: a leading role for STAT3. Nat Rev 2009 Nov;9(11):798–809.

[29] Aggarwal BB, Kunnumakkara AB, Harikumar KB, Gupta SR, Tharakan ST, Koca C, et al. Signal transducer and activator of transcription-3, inflammation, and cancer: how intimate is the relationship? Ann NY Acad Sci 2009 Aug;1171:59–76.

[30] Kortylewski M, Yu H. Role of Stat3 in suppressing anti-tumor immunity. Curr Opin Immunol 2008 Apr;20(2):228–33.

[31] Kortylewski M, Yu H. Stat3 as a potential target for cancer immunotherapy. J Immunother 2007 Feb-Mar; 30(2):131–9.

[32] Shuai K, Liu B. Regulation of JAK-STAT signalling in the immune system. Nat Rev Immunol 2003 Nov;3(11):900–11.

[33] Kortylewski M, Kujawski M, Wang T, Wei S, Zhang S, Pilon-Thomas S, et al. Inhibiting Stat3 signaling in the hematopoietic system elicits multicomponent antitumor immunity. Nat Med 2005 Dec;11(12):1314–21.

[34] Wang T, Niu G, Kortylewski M, Burdelya L, Shain K, Zhang S, et al. Regulation of the innate and adaptive immune responses by Stat-3 signaling in tumor cells. Nat Med 2004 Jan;10(1):48–54.

[35] Kujawski M, Kortylewski M, Lee H, Herrmann A, Kay H, Yu H. Stat3 mediates myeloid cell-dependent tumor angiogenesis in mice. J Clin Invest 2008 Oct;118(10):3367–77.

[36] Kortylewski M, Xin H, Kujawski M, Lee H, Liu Y, Harris T, et al. Regulation of the IL-23 and IL-12 balance by Stat3 signaling in the tumor microenvironment. Cancer cell 2009 Feb 3;15(2):114–23.

[37] Darnell Jr JE, Kerr IM, Stark GR. Jak-STAT pathways and transcriptional activation in response to IFNs and other extracellular signaling proteins. Science (New York, NY) 1994 Jun 3;264(5164):1415–21.

[38] Bromberg J, Darnell Jr JE. The role of STATs in transcriptional control and their impact on cellular function. Oncogene 2000 May 15;19(21):2468–73.

[39] Shuai K, Stark GR, Kerr IM, Darnell Jr JE. A single phosphotyrosine residue of Stat91 required for gene activation by interferon-gamma. Science (New York, NY) 1993 Sep 24;261(5129):1744–6.

[40] Darnell Jr JE. STATs and gene regulation. Science (New York, NY) 1997 Sep 12;277(5332):1630–5.

[41] Levy DE, Darnell Jr JE. Stats: transcriptional control and biological impact. Nat Rev Mol Cell Biol 2002 Sep;3(9):651–62.

[42] Yu CL, Meyer DJ, Campbell GS, Larner AC, Carter-Su C, Schwartz J, et al. Enhanced DNA-binding activity of a Stat3-related protein in cells transformed by the Src oncoprotein. Science (New York, NY) 1995 Jul 7;269(5220):81–3.

[43] Turkson J, Bowman T, Garcia R, Caldenhoven E, De Groot RP, Jove R. Stat3 activation by Src induces specific gene regulation and is required for cell transformation. Mol Cell Biol 1998 May;18(5):2545–52.

[44] de Groot RP, Raaijmakers JA, Lammers JW, Jove R, Koenderman L. STAT5 activation by BCR-Abl contributes to transformation of K562 leukemia cells. Blood 1999 Aug 1;94(3):1108–12.

[45] Hilbert DM, Migone TS, Kopf M, Leonard WJ, Rudikoff S. Distinct tumorigenic potential of abl and raf in B cell neoplasia: abl activates the IL-6 signaling pathway. Immunity 1996 Jul;5(1):81–9.

[46] Lee H, Deng J, Xin H, Liu Y, Pardoll D, Yu H. A requirement of STAT3 DNA binding precludes Th-1 immunostimulatory gene expression by NF-kappaB in tumors. Cancer Res 2011 Jun 1;71(11):3772–80.

[47] Grivennikov SI, Karin M. Dangerous liaisons: STAT3 and NF-kappaB collaboration and crosstalk in cancer. Cytokine Growth Factor Rev 2010 Feb;21(1):11–9.

[48] Cella N, Groner B, Hynes NE. Characterization of Stat5a and Stat5b homodimers and heterodimers and their association with the glucocortiocoid receptor in mammary cells. Mol Cell Biol 1998 Apr;18(4):1783–92.

[49] Stocklin E, Wissler M, Gouilleux F, Groner B. Functional interactions between Stat5 and the glucocorticoid receptor. Nature 1996 Oct 24;383(6602):726–8.

[50] Yang J, Stark GR. Roles of unphosphorylated STATs in signaling. Cell Res 2008 Apr;18(4):443–51.

[51] Yang J, Liao X, Agarwal MK, Barnes L, Auron PE, Stark GR. Unphosphorylated STAT3 accumulates in response to IL-6 and activates transcription by binding to NFkappaB. Genes Dev 2007 Jun 1;21(11):1396–408.

[52] Yang J, Chatterjee-Kishore M, Staugaitis SM, Nguyen H, Schlessinger K, Levy DE, et al. Novel roles of unphosphorylated STAT3 in oncogenesis and transcriptional regulation. Cancer Res 2005 Feb 1;65(3):939–47.

[53] Yuan ZL, Guan YJ, Chatterjee D, Chin YE. Stat3 dimerization regulated by reversible acetylation of a single lysine residue. Science (New York, NY) 2005 Jan 14;307(5707):269–73.

[54] Zhang JJ, U.Vinkemeier, Gu W, Chakravarti D, Horvath CM, Darnell Jr JE. Two contact regions between Stat1 and CBP/p300 in interferon gamma signaling. Proceedings of the National Academy of Sciences of the United States of America 1996 Dec 24;93(26):15092–6.

[55] Bhattacharya S, Eckner R, Grossman S, Oldread E, Arany Z, D'Andrea A, et al. Cooperation of Stat2 and p300/ CBP in signalling induced by interferon-alpha. Nature 1996 Sep 26;383(6598):344–7.

[56] Lee H, Herrmann A, Deng JH, Kujawski M, Niu G, Li Z, et al. Persistently activated Stat3 maintains constitutive NF-kappaB activity in tumors. Cancer cell 2009 Apr 7;15(4):283—93.

[57] Teng TS, Lin B, Manser E, Ng DC, Cao X. Stat3 promotes directional cell migration by regulating Rac1 activity via its activator betaPIX. J Cell Sci 2009 Nov 15;122(Pt 22):4150—9.

[58] Xie B, Zhao J, Kitagawa M, Durbin J, Madri JA, Guan JL, et al. Focal adhesion kinase activates Stat1 in integrin-mediated cell migration and adhesion. J Biol Chem 2001 Jun 1;276(22):19512—23.

[59] Silver DL, Naora H, Liu J, Cheng W, Montell DJ. Activated signal transducer and activator of transcription (STAT) 3: localization in focal adhesions and function in ovarian cancer cell motility. Cancer Res 2004 May 15;64(10):3550—8.

[60] Ng DC, Lin BH, Lim CP, Huang G, Zhang T, Poli V, et al. Stat3 regulates microtubules by antagonizing the depolymerization activity of stathmin. J Cell Biol 2006 Jan 16;172(2):245—57.

[61] Verma NK, Dourlat J, Davies AM, Long A, Liu WQ, Garbay C, et al. STAT3-stathmin interactions control microtubule dynamics in migrating T-cells. J Biol Chem 2009 May 1;284(18):12349—62.

[62] Meraz MA, White JM, Sheehan KC, Bach EA, Rodig SJ, Dighe AS, et al. Targeted disruption of the Stat1 gene in mice reveals unexpected physiologic specificity in the JAK-STAT signaling pathway. Cell 1996 Feb 9;84(3):431—42.

[63] Durbin JE, Hackenmiller R, Simon MC, Levy DE. Targeted disruption of the mouse Stat1 gene results in compromised innate immunity to viral disease. Cell 1996 Feb 9;84(3):443—50.

[64] Park C, Li S, Cha E, Schindler C. Immune response in Stat2 knockout mice. Immunity 2000 Dec;13(6):795—804.

[65] Takeda K, Noguchi K, Shi W, Tanaka T, Matsumoto M, Yoshida N, et al. Targeted disruption of the mouse Stat3 gene leads to early embryonic lethality. Proceedings of the National Academy of Sciences of the United States of America 1997 Apr 15;94(8):3801—4.

[66] Levy DE, Lee CK. What does Stat3 do? J Clin Invest 2002 May;109(9):1143—8.

[67] Takeda K, Tanaka T, Shi W, Matsumoto M, Minami M, Kashiwamura S, et al. Essential role of Stat6 in IL-4 signalling. Nature 1996 Apr 18;380(6575):627—30.

[68] Kaplan MH, Schindler U, Smiley ST, Grusby MJ. Stat6 is required for mediating responses to IL-4 and for development of Th2 cells. Immunity 1996 Mar;4(3):313—9.

[69] Kaplan MH, Sun YL, Hoey T, Grusby MJ. Impaired IL-12 responses and enhanced development of Th2 cells in Stat4-deficient mice. Nature 1996 Jul 11;382(6587):174—7.

[70] Teglund S, McKay C, Schuetz E, van Deursen JM, Stravopodis D, Wang D, et al. Stat5a and Stat5b proteins have essential and nonessential, or redundant, roles in cytokine responses. Cell 1998 May 29;93(5):841—50.

[71] Wei L, Laurence A, O'Shea JJ. New insights into the roles of Stat5a/b and Stat3 in T cell development and differentiation. Semin Cell Dev Biol 2008 Aug;19(4):394—400.

[72] Shuai K. Modulation of STAT signaling by STAT-interacting proteins. Oncogene 2000 May 15;19(21):2638—44.

[73] Shuai K. Regulation of cytokine signaling pathways by PIAS proteins. Cell Res 2006 Feb;16(2):196—202.

[74] Yoshimura A, Naka T, Kubo M. SOCS proteins, cytokine signalling and immune regulation. Nat Rev Immunol 2007 Jun;7(6):454—65.

[75] Kubo M, Hanada T, Yoshimura A. Suppressors of cytokine signaling and immunity. Nat Immunol 2003 Dec;4(12):1169—76.

[76] Xu D, Qu CK. Protein tyrosine phosphatases in the JAK/STAT pathway. Front Biosci 2008;13:4925—32.

[77] Bromberg J. Stat proteins and oncogenesis. J Clin Invest 2002 May;109(9):1139—42.

[78] Gordon S, Martinez FO. Alternative activation of macrophages: mechanism and functions. Immunity 2010 May 28;32(5):593—604.

[79] Sica A, Bronte V. Altered macrophage differentiation and immune dysfunction in tumor development. J Clin Invest 2007 May;117(5):1155—66.

[80] Solinas G, Marchesi F, Garlanda C, Mantovani A, Allavena P. Inflammation-mediated promotion of invasion and metastasis. Cancer Metastasis Rev. Jun;29(2):243—8.

[81] Mantovani A, Savino B, Locati M, Zammataro L, Allavena P, Bonecchi R. The chemokine system in cancer biology and therapy. Cytokine Growth Factor Rev Feb;21(1):27—39.

[82] Murdoch C, Giannoudis A, Lewis CE. Mechanisms regulating the recruitment of macrophages into hypoxic areas of tumors and other ischemic tissues. Blood 2004 Oct 15;104(8):2224—34.

[83] Biswas SK, Gangi L, Paul S, Schioppa T, Saccani A, Sironi M, et al. A distinct and unique transcriptional program expressed by tumor-associated macrophages (defective NF-kappaB and enhanced IRF-3/STAT1 activation). Blood 2006 Mar 1;107(5):2112—22.

[84] Kusmartsev S, Gabrilovich DI. STAT1 signaling regulates tumor-associated macrophage-mediated T cell deletion. J Immunol 2005 Apr 15;174(8):4880—91.

445

[85] Bronte V, Serafini P, De Santo C, Marigo I, Tosello V, Mazzoni A, et al. IL-4-induced arginase 1 suppresses alloreactive T cells in tumor-bearing mice. J Immunol 2003 Jan 1;170(1):270–8.

[86] Dominguez-Soto A, Sierra-Filardi E, Puig-Kroger A, Perez-Maceda B, Gomez-Aguado F, Corcuera MT, et al. Dendritic cell-specific ICAM-3-grabbing nonintegrin expression on M2-polarized and tumor-associated macrophages is macrophage-CSF dependent and enhanced by tumor-derived IL-6 and IL-10. J Immunol 2011 Feb 15;186(4):2192–200.

[87] Cheng F, Wang HW, Cuenca A, Huang M, Ghansah T, Brayer J, et al. A critical role for Stat3 signaling in immune tolerance. Immunity 2003 Sep;19(3):425–36.

[88] Lee H, Deng J, Kujawski M, Yang C, Liu Y, Herrmann A, et al. STAT3-induced S1PR1 expression is crucial for persistent STAT3 activation in tumors. Nat Med 2010 Dec;16(12):1421–8.

[89] Bronte V, Apolloni E, Cabrelle A, Ronca R, Serafini P, Zamboni P, et al. Identification of a CD11b(+)/Gr-1(+)/CD31(+) myeloid progenitor capable of activating or suppressing CD8(+) T cells. Blood 2000 Dec 1;96(12):3838–46.

[90] Gallina G, Dolcetti L, Serafini P, De Santo C, Marigo I, Colombo MP, et al. Tumors induce a subset of inflammatory monocytes with immunosuppressive activity on CD8+ T cells. J Clin Invest 2006 Oct;116(10):2777–90.

[91] Condamine T, Gabrilovich DI. Molecular mechanisms regulating myeloid-derived suppressor cell differentiation and function. Trends Immunol 2011 Jan;32(1):19–25.

[92] Youn JI, Nagaraj S, Collazo M, Gabrilovich DI. Subsets of myeloid-derived suppressor cells in tumor-bearing mice. J Immunol 2008 Oct 15;181(8):5791–802.

[93] Almand B, Clark JI, Nikitina E, van Beynen J, English NR, Knight SC, et al. Increased production of immature myeloid cells in cancer patients: a mechanism of immunosuppression in cancer. J Immunol 2001 Jan 1;166(1):678–89.

[94] Nefedova Y, Nagaraj S, Rosenbauer A, Muro-Cacho C, Sebti SM, Gabrilovich DI. Regulation of dendritic cell differentiation and antitumor immune response in cancer by pharmacologic-selective inhibition of the janus-activated kinase 2/signal transducers and activators of transcription 3 pathway. Cancer Res 2005 Oct 15;65(20):9525–35.

[95] Poschke I, Mougiakakos D, Hansson J, Masucci GV, Kiessling R. Immature immunosuppressive CD14+HLA-DR-/low cells in melanoma patients are Stat3hi and overexpress CD80, CD83, and DC-sign. Cancer Res Jun 1;70(11):4335–45.

[96] Lechner MG, Megiel C, Russell SM, Bingham B, Arger N, Woo T, et al. Functional characterization of human Cd33+ and Cd11b+ myeloid-derived suppressor cell subsets induced from peripheral blood mononuclear cells co-cultured with a diverse set of human tumor cell lines. J Transl Med 2011;9:90.

[97] Pan PY, Wang GX, Yin B, Ozao J, Ku T, Divino CM, et al. Reversion of immune tolerance in advanced malignancy: modulation of myeloid-derived suppressor cell development by blockade of stem-cell factor function. Blood 2008 Jan 1;111(1):219–28.

[98] Priceman SJ, Sung JL, Shaposhnik Z, Burton JB, Torres-Collado AX, Moughon DL, et al. Targeting distinct tumor-infiltrating myeloid cells by inhibiting CSF-1 receptor: combating tumor evasion of antiangiogenic therapy. Blood 2010 Feb 18;115(7):1461–71.

[99] Huang B, Lei Z, Zhao J, Gong W, Liu J, Chen Z, et al. CCL2/CCR2 pathway mediates recruitment of myeloid suppressor cells to cancers. Cancer Lett 2007 Jul 8;252(1):86–92.

[100] Sinha P, Clements VK, Fulton AM, Ostrand-Rosenberg S. Prostaglandin E2 promotes tumor progression by inducing myeloid-derived suppressor cells. Cancer Res 2007 May 1;67(9):4507–13.

[101] Williams SA, Harata-Lee Y, Comerford I, Anderson RL, Smyth MJ, McColl SR. Multiple functions of CXCL12 in a syngeneic model of breast cancer. Mol Cancer 2010;9:250.

[102] Sinha P, Okoro C, Foell D, Freeze HH, Ostrand-Rosenberg S, Srikrishna G. Proinflammatory S100 proteins regulate the accumulation of myeloid-derived suppressor cells. J Immunol 2008 Oct 1;181(7):4666–75.

[103] Cheng P, Corzo CA, Luetteke N, Yu B, Nagaraj S, Bui MM, et al. Inhibition of dendritic cell differentiation and accumulation of myeloid-derived suppressor cells in cancer is regulated by S100A9 protein. J Exp Med 2008 Sep 29;205(10):2235–49.

[104] Corzo CA, Cotter MJ, Cheng P, Cheng F, Kusmartsev S, Sotomayor E, et al. Mechanism regulating reactive oxygen species in tumor-induced myeloid-derived suppressor cells. J Immunol 2009 May 1;182(9):5693–701.

[105] Xu Q, Briggs J, Park S, Niu G, Kortylewski M, Zhang S, et al. Targeting Stat3 blocks both HIF-1 and VEGF expression induced by multiple oncogenic growth signaling pathways. Oncogene 2005 Aug 25;24(36):5552–60.

[106] Jung JE, Lee HG, Cho IH, Chung DH, Yoon SH, Yang YM, et al. STAT3 is a potential modulator of HIF-1-mediated VEGF expression in human renal carcinoma cells. Faseb J 2005 Aug;19(10):1296–8.

[107] Corzo CA, Condamine T, Lu L, Cotter MJ, Youn JI, Cheng P, et al. HIF-1alpha regulates function and differentiation of myeloid-derived suppressor cells in the tumor microenvironment. J Exp Med 2010 Oct 25;207(11):2439–53.

[108] Chalmin F, Ladoire S, Mignot G, Vincent J, Bruchard M, Remy-Martin JP, et al. Membrane-associated Hsp72 from tumor-derived exosomes mediates STAT3-dependent immunosuppressive function of mouse and human myeloid-derived suppressor cells. J Clin Invest 2010 Feb;120(2):457–71.

[109] Zhang M, Liu Q, Mi S, Liang X, Zhang Z, Su X, et al. Both miR-17-5p and miR-20a alleviate suppressive potential of myeloid-derived suppressor cells by modulating STAT3 expression. J Immunol 2011 Apr 15;186(8):4716–24.

[110] Kaplan RN, Psaila B, Lyden D. Bone marrow cells in the 'pre-metastatic niche': within bone and beyond. Cancer Metastasis Rev 2006 Dec;25(4):521–9.

[111] Peinado H, Lavotshkin S, Lyden D. The secreted factors responsible for pre-metastatic niche formation: old sayings and new thoughts. Semin Cancer Biol 2011 Apr;21(2):139–46.

[112] Kaplan RN, Riba RD, Zacharoulis S, A.H.Bramley, Vincent L, Costa C, et al. VEGFR1-positive haematopoietic bone marrow progenitors initiate the pre-metastatic niche. Nature 2005 Dec 8;438(7069):820–7.

[113] Kaplan RN, Rafii S, Lyden D. Preparing the "soil": the premetastatic niche. Cancer Res 2006 Dec 1;66(23):11089–93.

[114] Psaila B, Lyden D. The metastatic niche: adapting the foreign soil. Nat Rev 2009 Apr;9(4):285–93.

[115] Rafii S, Lyden D. S100 chemokines mediate bookmarking of premetastatic niches. Nat Cell Biol 2006 Dec;8(12):1321–3.

[116] Erler JT, Bennewith KL, Cox TR, Lang G, Bird D, Koong A, et al. Hypoxia-induced lysyl oxidase is a critical mediator of bone marrow cell recruitment to form the premetastatic niche. Cancer cell 2009 Jan 6;15(1):35–44.

[117] Deng J, Liu Y, Lee H, Herrmann A, Zhang W, Zhang C, et al. S1PR1-STAT3 signaling is crucial for myeloid cell colonization at future metastatic sites. Cancer cell 2012; in press.

[118] Gabrilovich D. Mechanisms and functional significance of tumour-induced dendritic-cell defects. Nat Rev Immunol 2004 Dec;4(12):941–52.

[119] Kusmartsev S, Gabrilovich DI. Immature myeloid cells and cancer-associated immune suppression. Cancer Immunol Immunother 2002 Aug;51(6):293–8.

[120] Nefedova Y, Gabrilovich DI. Targeting of Jak/STAT pathway in antigen presenting cells in cancer. Curr Cancer Drug Targets 2007 Feb;7(1):71–7.

[121] Bergeron A, El-Hage F, Kambouchner M, Lecossier D, Tazi A. Characterisation of dendritic cell subsets in lung cancer micro-environments. Eur Respir J 2006 Dec;28(6):1170–7.

[122] Troy AJ, Summers KL, Davidson PJ, Atkinson CH, Hart DN. Minimal recruitment and activation of dendritic cells within renal cell carcinoma. Clin Cancer Res 1998 Mar;4(3):585–93.

[123] Della Bella S, Gennaro M, Vaccari M, Ferraris C, Nicola S, Riva A, et al. Altered maturation of peripheral blood dendritic cells in patients with breast cancer. Br J Cancer 2003 Oct 20;89(8):1463–72.

[124] Laouar Y, Welte T, Fu XY, Flavell RA. STAT3 is required for Flt3L-dependent dendritic cell differentiation. Immunity 2003 Dec;19(6):903–12.

[125] Nefedova Y, Huang M, Kusmartsev S, Bhattacharya R, Cheng P, Salup R, et al. Hyperactivation of STAT3 is involved in abnormal differentiation of dendritic cells in cancer. J Immunol 2004 Jan 1;172(1):464–74.

[126] Nefedova Y, Cheng P, Gilkes D, Blaskovich M, Beg AA, Sebti SM, et al. Activation of dendritic cells via inhibition of Jak2/STAT3 signaling. J Immunol 2005 Oct 1;175(7):4338–46.

[127] Kuroda E, Ho V, Ruschmann J, Antignano F, Hamilton M, Rauh MJ, et al. SHIP represses the generation of IL-3-induced M2 macrophages by inhibiting IL-4 production from basophils. J Immunol 2009 Sep 15;183(6):3652–60.

[128] Sinha P, Clements VK, Ostrand-Rosenberg S. Interleukin-13-regulated M2 macrophages in combination with myeloid suppressor cells block immune surveillance against metastasis. Cancer Res 2005 Dec 15;65(24):11743–51.

[129] Ostrand-Rosenberg S, Grusby MJ, Clements VK. Cutting edge: STAT6-deficient mice have enhanced tumor immunity to primary and metastatic mammary carcinoma. J Immunol 2000 Dec 1;165(11):6015–9.

[130] Ishii M, Wen H, Corsa CA, Liu T, Coelho AL, Allen RM, et al. Epigenetic regulation of the alternatively activated macrophage phenotype. Blood 2009 Oct 8;114(15):3244–54.

[131] Takaku S, Terabe M, Ambrosino E, Peng J, Lonning S, McPherson JM, et al. Blockade of TGF-beta enhances tumor vaccine efficacy mediated by CD8(+) T cells. Int J Cancer 2010 Apr 1;126(7):1666–74.

[132] Roth F, A.C.De La Fuente, Vella JL, Zoso A, Inverardi L, Serafini P. Aptamer-Mediated Blockade of IL4Ralpha Triggers Apoptosis of MDSCs and Limits Tumor Progression. Cancer Res 2012 Mar 6.

447

[133] Xin H, Zhang C, Herrmann A, Du Y, Figlin R, Yu H. Sunitinib inhibition of Stat3 induces renal cell carcinoma tumor cell apoptosis and reduces immunosuppressive cells. Cancer Res 2009 Mar 15;69(6):2506–13.

[134] Ko JS, Rayman P, Ireland J, Swaidani S, Li G, Bunting KD, et al. Direct and differential suppression of myeloid-derived suppressor cell subsets by sunitinib is compartmentally constrained. Cancer Res 2009 May 1;70(9):3526–36.

[135] Cao M, Xu Y, Youn JI, Cabrera R, Zhang X, Gabrilovich D, et al. Kinase inhibitor Sorafenib modulates immunosuppressive cell populations in a murine liver cancer model. Lab Invest 2011 Apr;91(4):598–608.

[136] Larmonier N, Janikashvili N, LaCasse CJ, Larmonier CB, Cantrell J, Situ E, et al. Imatinib mesylate inhibits CD4+ CD25+ regulatory T cell activity and enhances active immunotherapy against BCR-ABL- tumors. J Immunol 2008 Nov 15;181(10):6955–63.

[137] Yang F, Jove V, Xin H, Hedvat M, Van Meter TE, Yu H. Sunitinib induces apoptosis and growth arrest of medulloblastoma tumor cells by inhibiting STAT3 and AKT signaling pathways. Mol Cancer Res 2008 Jan;8(1):35–45.

[138] Burdelya L, Catlett-Falcone R, Levitzki A, Cheng F, Mora LB, Sotomayor E, et al. Combination therapy with AG-490 and interleukin 12 achieves greater antitumor effects than either agent alone. Mol Cancer Ther 2002 Sep;1(11):893–9.

[139] Hussain SF, Kong LY, Jordan J, Conrad C, Madden T, Fokt I, et al. A novel small molecule inhibitor of signal transducers and activators of transcription 3 reverses immune tolerance in malignant glioma patients. Cancer Res 2007 Oct 15;67(20):9630–6.

[140] Kong LY, Wu AS, Doucette T, Wei J, Priebe W, Fuller GN, et al. Intratumoral mediated immunosuppression is prognostic in genetically engineered murine models of glioma and correlates to immunotherapeutic responses. Clin Cancer Res 2008 Dec 1;16(23):5722–33.

[141] Kong LY, Wei J, Sharma AK, Barr J, Abou-Ghazal MK, Fokt I, et al. A novel phosphorylated STAT3 inhibitor enhances T cell cytotoxicity against melanoma through inhibition of regulatory T cells. Cancer Immunol Immunother 2009 Jul;58(7):1023–32.

[142] Blaskovich MA, Sun J, Cantor A, Turkson J, Jove R, Sebti SM. Discovery of JSI-124 (cucurbitacin I), a selective Janus kinase/signal transducer and activator of transcription 3 signaling pathway inhibitor with potent antitumor activity against human and murine cancer cells in mice. Cancer Res 2003 Mar 15;63(6):1270–9.

[143] Fujita M, Zhu X, Sasaki K, Ueda R, Low KL, Pollack IF, et al. Inhibition of STAT3 promotes the efficacy of adoptive transfer therapy using type-1 CTLs by modulation of the immunological microenvironment in a murine intracranial glioma. J Immunol 2008 Feb 15;180(4):2089–98.

[144] Molavi O, Ma Z, Hamdy S, Lai R, Lavasanifar A, Samuel J. Synergistic antitumor effects of CpG oligodeoxynucleotide and STAT3 inhibitory agent JSI-124 in a mouse melanoma tumor model. Immunol Cell Biol 2008 Aug-Sep;86(6):506–14.

[145] Bharti AC, Donato N, Aggarwal BB. Curcumin (diferuloylmethane) inhibits constitutive and IL-6-inducible STAT3 phosphorylation in human multiple myeloma cells. J Immunol 2003 Oct 1;171(7):3863–71.

[146] Friedman L, Lin L, Ball S, Bekaii-Saab T, Fuchs J, Li PK, et al. Curcumin analogues exhibit enhanced growth suppressive activity in human pancreatic cancer cells. Anticancer Drugs 2009 Jul;20(6):444–9.

[147] Tu SP, Jin H, Shi JD, Zhu LM, Suo Y, Lu G, et al. Curcumin induces the differentiation of myeloid-derived suppressor cells and inhibits their interaction with cancer cells and related tumor growth. Cancer Prev Res (Philadelphia, Pa 2012 Feb;5(2):205–15.

[148] Hedvat M, Huszar D, Herrmann A, Gozgit JM, Schroeder A, Sheehy A, et al. The JAK2 inhibitor AZD1480 potently blocks Stat3 signaling and oncogenesis in solid tumors. Cancer cell 2009 Dec 8;16(6):487–97.

[149] Xin H, Herrmann A, Reckamp K, Zhang W, Pal S, Hedvat M, et al. Antiangiogenic and antimetastatic activity of JAK inhibitor AZD1480. Cancer Res 2011 Nov 1;71(21):6601–10.

[150] Herrmann A, Kortylewski M, Kujawski M, Zhang C, Reckamp K, Armstrong B, et al. Targeting Stat3 in the myeloid compartment drastically improves the in vivo antitumor functions of adoptively transferred T cells. Cancer Res 2010 Oct 1;70(19):7455–64.

[151] Iwata-Kajihara T, Sumimoto H, Kawamura N, Ueda R, Takahashi T, Mizuguchi H, et al. Enhanced cancer immunotherapy using STAT3-depleted dendritic cells with high Th1-inducing ability and resistance to cancer cell-derived inhibitory factors. J Immunol 2011 Jul 1;187(1):27–36.

[152] Liao D, Liu Z, Wrasidlo WJ, Luo Y, Nguyen G, Chen T, et al. Targeted therapeutic remodeling of the tumor microenvironment improves an HER-2 DNA vaccine and prevents recurrence in a murine breast cancer model. Cancer Res 2011 Sep 1;71(17):5688–96.

[153] Jahrsdorfer B, Weiner GJ. CpG oligodeoxynucleotides for immune stimulation in cancer immunotherapy. Curr Opin Investig Drugs 2003 Jun;4(6):686–90.

[154] Jahrsdorfer B, Weiner GJ. CpG oligodeoxynucleotides as immunotherapy in cancer. Cancer Ther 2008 Mar;3(1):27–32.

448

[155] Kortylewski M, Kujawski M, Herrmann A, Yang C, Wang L, Liu Y, et al. Toll-like receptor 9 activation of signal transducer and activator of transcription 3 constrains its agonist-based immunotherapy. Cancer Res 2009 Mar 15;69(6):2497—505.

[156] Kortylewski M, Swiderski P, Herrmann A, Wang L, Kowolik C, Kujawski M, et al. In vivo delivery of siRNA to immune cells by conjugation to a TLR9 agonist enhances antitumor immune responses. Nat Biotechnol 2009 Oct;27(10):925—32.

CHAPTER 27

Tumor-associated Macrophages in Cancer Growth and Progression

Alberto Mantovani[1,2], Maria Rosaria Galdiero[1,3], Paola Allavena[1], Antonio Sica[1,4]
[1]Humanitas Clinical and Research Center, Rozzano, Milan, Italy
[2]Department of Biotechnology and Translational Medicine, University of Milan, Rozzano, Milan, Italy
[3]Division of Allergy and Clinical Immunology, University of Naples, Naples, Italy
[4]DiSCAFF, University of Piemonte Orientale A. Avogadro, Novara, Italy

I. INTRODUCTION

Links between inflammation and cancer were first made in the nineteenth century, on the basis of observations that tumors often originated at sites of chronic inflammation and that inflammatory cells were present in biopsied samples from tumors [12]. The idea that these processes are connected waned for more than a century, but there has been a recent resurgence in interest.

Epidemiological studies have revealed that chronic inflammation predisposes individuals to different forms of cancer, such as colon, prostate, and liver cancer, and that usage of nonsteroidal anti-inflammatory agents can protect against the emergence of various tumors. An inflammatory component is present in the microenvironment of most neoplastic tissues, including those not causally related to an obvious inflammatory process. Thus, several lines of evidence have led to a generally accepted paradigm that inflammation and cancer are linked [14,92].

Hallmarks of cancer-associated inflammation include the infiltration of leukocytes, the presence of soluble mediators (cytokines and chemokines), tissue remodeling and angiogenesis.

Strong evidence suggests that cancer-associated inflammation promotes tumor growth and progression [12,14,36,91]. By the late 1970s it was found that tumor growth is promoted by tumor-associated macrophages (TAM), an important component of the leukocyte infiltrate in tumors [12,14,36,88,91]. Accordingly, in many but not all human tumors, a high frequency of infiltrating TAM is associated with poor prognosis [120]. Interestingly, this pathological finding has reemerged in the postgenomic era: genes associated with leukocyte or macrophage infiltration (e.g., CD68) are part of the molecular signatures that herald poor prognosis in lymphomas and breast carcinomas [110]. Gene-modified mice and cell transfer have provided direct evidence for the protumor function of myeloid cells and their effector molecules. These results raise the interesting possibility of targeting myelomonocytic cells associated with cancer as an innovative therapeutic strategy. Here, we will review key properties of TAM emphasizing recent genetic evidence and emerging targets for therapeutic intervention.

451

II. MACROPHAGE POLARIZATION

Heterogeneity and plasticity are hallmarks of mononuclear phagocytes [53,88,89,146]. Lineage-defined populations of mononuclear phagocytes have not been identified but already at the short-lived stage of circulating precursor monocyte subsets characterized by differential expression of the FcγRIII receptor (CD16) or of chemokine receptors (CCR2, CX3CR1 and CCR8) and by different functional properties have been described. Once in tissues macrophages acquire distinct morphological and functional properties directed by the tissue (e.g., the lung alveolar macrophage) and immunological microenvironment.

In response to signals derived from microbes, damaged tissues or activated lymphocytes [20], monocytes/macrophages undergo a reprogramming which leads to the emergence of a spectrum of distinct functional phenotypes. In more detail, mirroring the Th1/Th2 nomenclature, macrophages undergo two different polarization states: classically activated M1 phenotype and alternatively activated M2 phenotype [54,88]. Classically activated M1 macrophages have long been known to be induced by IFN-γ alone or in concert with microbial stimuli (e.g., LPS) or cytokines (e.g., TNF and GM-CSF). IL-4 and IL-13 were subsequently found to be more than simple inhibitors of macrophage activation and to induce an alternative M2 form of macrophage activation [53]. It is now known that many other cytokines can govern M2 polarization. IL-33 is a cytokine of the IL-1 family associated with Th2 and M2 polarization [65,78]. IL-33 amplifies IL-13-induced polarization of alveolar macrophages to an M2 phenotype characterized by the upregulation of YM1, arginase 1, CCL24 and CCL17, which mediate lung eosinophilia and inflammation [78]. IL-21 is another Th2-associated cytokine shown to drive M2 activation of macrophages [113].

Macrophages can also be polarized into an "M2-like" state, which shares some but not all the signature features of M2 cells. In fact, various stimuli, such as antibody immune complexes together with LPS or IL-1, glucocorticoids, transforming growth factor-β (TGF-β) and IL-10, result in M2-like functional phenotypes that share properties with IL-4- or IL-13-activated macrophages (such as high expression of mannose receptor, IL-10 and angiogenic factors) [89]. Variations on the theme of M2 polarization are also found *in vivo* (for example, in the placenta and embryo, and during helminth infection, *Listeria* infection, obesity and cancer) [9,58,109,122,123]. M1 and M2 or M2-like polarized macrophages represent extremes of a continuum in a spectrum of functional states [88,20,103].

In general, M1 cells have an IL-12 [high], IL-23 [high], IL-10 [low] phenotype; are efficient producers of effector molecules (reactive oxygen and nitrogen intermediates) and inflammatory cytokines (IL-1β, TNF, IL-6); participate as inducer and effector cells in polarized Th1 responses; mediate resistance against intracellular parasites and tumors. In contrast, the various forms of M2 macrophages share an IL-12 [low], IL-23 [low], IL-10 [high] phenotype with variable capacity to produce inflammatory cytokines depending on the signal utilized. M2 cells generally have high levels of scavenger, mannose and galactose-type receptors, and the arginine metabolism is shifted to ornithine and polyamines. Polarized macrophages present also differential regulation of components of the IL-1 system [41] with low IL-1β and low caspase I, high IL-1ra and high decoy type II receptor in M2 cells.

In general, M2 cells take part in polarized Th2 responses, parasite clearance [108], dampening of inflammation, tissue remodeling [166], angiogensis, tumor progression and immunoregulatory functions [20].

Immature myeloid suppressor cells have functional properties and a transcriptional profile related to M2 cells [19]. Moreover, polarization of neutrophil functions has also been reported [47,155].

M1 and M2 macrophages have distinct chemokinome profiles, with M1 macrophages expressing Th1-cell-attracting chemokines such as CXCL9 and CXCL10 and M2 macrophages expressing the chemokines CCL17, CCL22 and CCL24 [91,98]. Chemokines can also influence macrophage polarization, with CCL2 and CXCL4 driving macrophages to an M2-like phenotype [52,127]. Moreover, M1- and M2-polarized macrophages have distinct features in terms of the metabolism of iron, folate and glucose [118,125,128].

Recent evidence shows the importance of metabolism in shaping the functional phenotype of macrophages in response to distinct polarizing stimuli in the tissue microenvironment, under normal as well as pathological settings. There is a bidirectional crosstalk between metabolism and macrophages: macrophages not only exert "extrinsic" effects to regulate metabolism (via release of soluble mediators such as inflammatory cytokines), but also exhibit "intrinsic" effects wherein the metabolic status of these cells shape their functional phenotype. Indeed, recent data suggest macrophages possess distinct metabolic features that regulate their functional polarization [21].

First of all, polarized macrophages show a distinct regulation of glucose metabolism. Macrophages in response to M1 stimuli display a metabolic shift towards the anaerobic glycolytic pathway, while exposure to M2 stimuli like IL-4 shows a minor effect [128]. The use of specific metabolic pathways can be functionally related to different purposes. M1-activated macrophages are often associated with acute infection: these cells need to quickly trigger microbicidal activity as well as keep up with the hypoxic tissue microenvironment [107]. In this context, an anaerobic process like glycolysis is best-suited to meet their rapid energy requirements. In contrast, M2 polarization-related functions like tissue remodeling, repair and healing require a sustained supply of energy. This request is fulfilled by oxidative glucose metabolism (fatty acid oxidation) which is believed to be the metabolic pathway of choice in M2 macrophages [159].

Also the amino acid metabolism is closely linked to the functional phenotype of myelomonocytic cells. M1 macrophages are characterized by the expression of NOS2 and production of NO, which is an important effector for their microbicidal activity [84]. In contrast, M2 macrophages do not produce NO, but express high levels of Arg I, which catalyzes polyamines production, which is necessary for collagen synthesis, cell proliferation, fibrosis and other tissue remodeling functions [114].

Furthermore, recent studies in mouse as well as human macrophages show striking differences in iron metabolism between M1 and M2 polarized cells [34,125]. M1 macrophages express high levels of proteins involved in iron storage, such as Ferritin, while expressing low levels of Ferroportin, an iron exporter. In contrast, M2 macrophages show low levels of Ferritin but high levels of Ferroportin. This divergent iron metabolism can be related to clear functional outcomes. Sequestration of iron by M1 cells would have a bacteriostatic effect (since iron is essential for supporting growth) and thus support host protection to infection. Conversely, iron release from M2 cells would favor tissue repair as well as tumor growth, consistent with the functional phenotype of these cells. Based on the facts presented above, it is clear that divergent iron management seems to be an important metabolic signature in polarized macrophages [28].

Collectively, these facts highlight that metabolic adaptation is an integral aspect of macrophage polarization and their functional diversity.

Moreover, in the last ten years, profiling techniques and genetic approaches have put to a test and shed new light on the M1/M2 paradigm. Transcriptional profiling has offered a comprehensive picture of the genetic programs activated in polarized macrophages, led to the discovery of new polarization-associated genes (e.g., Fizz and YM-1), tested the validity of the paradigm *in vivo* in selected diseases [19,38,151], and questioned the generality of some assumptions. For instance, unexpectedly arginase is not expressed prominently in human IL-4-induced M2 cells [142]. M2 cells express high levels of the chitinase-like YM-1. Chitinases represent an antiparasite strategy conserved in evolution and there is now evidence that acidic mammalian chitinase induced by IL-13 in macrophages is an important mediator of type II inflammation [172].

III. MACROPHAGE RECRUITMENT AT THE TUMOR SITE

Since the first observation by Rudolf Virchow, who suggested that cancers arise at regions of chronic inflammation, the origin of TAM has been studied in terms of recruitment, survival and proliferation. TAM derive from circulating monocytes and are recruited at the tumor site by a tumor-derived chemotactic factor for monocytes, originally described by this group [24] and later identified as the chemokine CCL2/MCP-1 [99,169] (Figure 27.1).

Chemokines produced by malignant and stromal cells contribute to the extent and phenotype of the tumor-associated leukocyte component, to angiogenesis and to the generation of the fibroblast stroma [6,87,95]. CC chemokines, especially CCL2 and CCL5, are major attractants of monocyte and macrophage precursors to the tumor microenvironment and levels of these correlate with the extent of the myeloid cell infiltrate [8,120,121,161].

CCL2 is probably the most frequently found CC chemokine in tumors. Most human carcinomas produce CCL2 (Table 27.1) and its levels of expression correlate with the increased infiltration of macrophages [13,33,88]. Interestingly, CCL2 production has also been detected in TAM, indicating the existence of an amplification loop for their recruitment [88]. Moreover, this chemokine also enhances survival of TAM once they are in the tumor microenvironment [171]. Other CC chemokines related to CCL2, such as CCL7 and CCL8, are also produced by tumors and shown to recruit monocytes [15].

Along with the supposed protumoral role of TAM, the local production of chemokines and the extent of TAM infiltration have been studied as prognostic factors. For example, in human breast and esophagus cancers, CCL2 levels correlated with the extent of macrophage

454

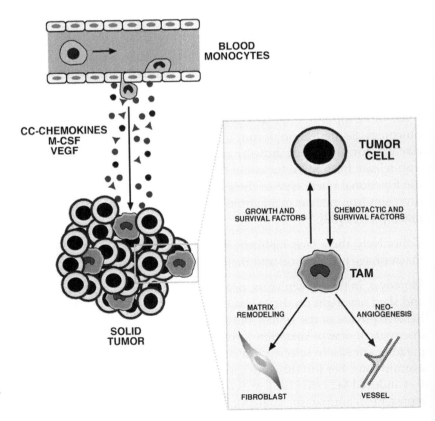

FIGURE 27.1

Tumor-derived chemotactic factors (CC-chemokines, e.g., CCL2, Macrophage Colony Stimulating Factor (M-CSF) and Vascular Endothelial Growth Factor (VEGF), actively recruit circulating blood monocytes at the tumor site. In the tumor micro-environment monocytes differentiate into Tumor-Associated Macrophages (TAM), which establish a symbiotic relationship with tumor cells. The above tumor-derived factors positively modulate TAM survival. From their own, TAM secrete growth factors which promote tumor cell proliferation and survival, regulate matrix deposition and remodeling and activate neo-angiogenesis. *Modified from Sica et al. Eur J Cancer 2006.*

TABLE 27.1 Tumor- and/or Stroma-derived Chemokines

Ligand	Producing tumor
CXC family	
CXCL1/Groa	Colon carcinoma [80]
CXCL8/IL-8	Melanoma [61], breast [11]
CXCL9/Mig	Hodgkin's disease [153]
CXCL10/IP-10	Hodgkin lymphoma and nasopharygeal carcinoma [152]
CXCL12/SDF-1	Melanoma [136]; prostate, breast, ovary [130]; pancreas [97]
CXCL13/BCA1	Non-Hodgkin B-cell lymphoma [149]
CC family	
CCL1/I-309	Adult T-cell leucemia [131]
CCL2/MCP-1	Pancreas [132]; sarcomas, gliomas, lung, breast, cervix, ovary, melanoma [87]
CCL3/MIP-1a	Schwann cell tumors [102]
CCL3LI/LD78b	Glioblastoma [75]
CCL5/RANTES	Breast [156]; melanoma [112]
CCL6	NSLC [168]
CCL7/MCP-3	Osteosarcoma [33]
CCL8/MCP-2	Osteosarcoma [33]
CCL11/eotaxin	T-cell lymphoma [72]
CCL17/TARC	Lymphoma [160]
CCL18/PARC	Ovary [141]
CCL22/MDC	Ovary [133]
CCL28/MEC	Hodgkin's disease [64]

infiltration, lymph-node metastasis and clinical aggressiveness [10,132]. In an experimental model of nontumorigenic melanoma, low levels of CCL2 secretion, with "physiological" accumulation of TAM, promoted tumor formation, while high CCL2 secretion resulted in massive macrophage infiltration into the tumor mass and in its destruction [106]. In pancreatic cancer patients, high serum levels of CCL2 were associated with more favorable prognosis and with a lower proliferative index of tumor cells [101]. These biphasic effects of CCL2 are consistent with the "macrophage balance" hypothesis [86] and emphasize the concept that levels of macrophage infiltration similar to those observed in human malignant lesions express protumor activity [18].

A variety of other chemokines have been detected in neoplastic tissues as products of either tumor cells or stromal elements (Table 27.1).

These molecules play an important role in tumor progression by direct stimulation of neoplastic growth, promotion of inflammation and induction of angiogenesis. In spite of constitutive production of neutrophil chemotactic proteins by tumor cells, CXCL8 and related chemokines, neutrophils are not an obvious constituent of the leukocyte infiltrate. However, in the context of cancer-related inflammation, neutrophils appear as a source of inflammatory mediators and therefore have emerged as a candidate that may modulate and promote the tumorogenic process [93]. Moreover, tumor-associated neutrophils have also been proposed as key mediators of malignant transformation, tumor progression and angiogenesis and in the modulation of antitumor immunity [96]. Macrophages are also recruited by molecules other than chemokines. In particular, tumor-derived cytokines interacting with tyrosine kinase receptors, such as vascular endothelial growth factor (VEGF) and macrophage colony stimulating factor (M-CSF) [43] promote macrophage recruitment, as well as macrophage survival and proliferation, the latter generally limited to murine TAM [43,88] (Figure 27.1). Using genetic approaches, it has been demonstrated that depletion of M-CSF markedly decreases the infiltration of macrophages at the tumor site, and this correlates with a significant delay in tumor progression. By contrast, overexpression of M-CSF by tumor cells dramatically increased macrophage recruitment and this was correlated with accelerated tumor growth [3]. M-CSF overexpression is common among tumors of the reproductive system, including ovarian, uterine, breast and prostate, and correlates with poor prognosis [116]. Moreover, placenta-derived growth factor (PlGF), a molecule related to VEGF in terms of structure and receptor usage, has been reported to promote the survival of TAM [2].

IV. TAM EXPRESS SELECTED M2 PROTUMORAL FUNCTIONS

Cancer-related inflammation is characterized by the recruitment of cells of the monocyte-macrophage lineage to tumor tissues [20,92,116], which also home and condition the premetastatic niche, to favor secondary localization of cancer [45,70,165].

TAM generally express an M2-like phenotype [20], with low interleukin-12 (IL-12) expression, high IL-10 expression and low tumoricidal activity, and promote tumor-cell proliferation, tissue remodeling and angiogenesis.

A significant amount of evidence indicates that tumor cell products, including extracellular matrix components, IL-10, CSF-1 and chemokines (e.g., CCL17 and CXCL4) activate macrophages and set them in an M2-like, cancer-promoting mode [45,52,71,76,92,127].

The immunosuppressive cytokines IL-10 and TGFβ are produced by both cancer cells (ovary) and TAM [88]. IL-10 promotes the differentiation of monocytes to mature macrophages and blocks their differentiation to DC [6]. Thus, a gradient of tumor-derived IL-10 may account for differentiation along the DC versus the macrophage pathway in different microanatomical localizations in a tumor. Such a situation was observed in papillary carcinoma of the thyroid, where TAM are evenly distributed throughout the tissue, in contrast to DC which are present in the periphery [137]. Interestingly, it was shown that Stat3 is constitutively activated in tumor cells [164] and in diverse tumor-infiltrating immune cells [74], leading to inhibition of the production of several pro-inflammatory cytokines and chemokines and to the release of factors that suppress dendritic cell maturation. Noteworthy, ablating Stat3 in hematopoietic cells triggers an intrinsic immune-surveillance system that inhibits tumor growth and metastasis [74].

As previously discussed, IL-10 promotes an M2-like alternative pathway of macrophage activation and induces TAM to express M2-related functions. Indeed, under many aspects TAM summarize a number of functions expressed by M2 macrophages, involved in tuning inflammatory responses and adaptive immunity, scavenging debris, promoting angiogenesis, tissue remodeling and repair. The production of IL-10, TGFβ and PGE2 by cancer cells and TAM [88] contributes to a general suppression of antitumor activities (Figure 27.2).

TAM are poor producers of NO [40] and, *in situ* in ovarian cancer, only a minority of tumors and, in these, a minority of macrophages localized at the periphery scored positive for iNOS [73]. Moreover, in contrast to M1 polarized macrophages, TAM have been shown to be poor producers of reactive oxygen intermediates (ROIs), consistent with the hypothesis that these cells represent a skewed M2 population [73].

Moreover, TAM were reported to express low levels of inflammatory cytokines (e.g., IL-12, IL-1β, TNFα, IL-6) [88]. Activation of NF-κB is a necessary event promoting transcription of several pro-inflammatory genes. Our previous studies [144] indicated that TAM display defective NF-κB activation in response to the M1 polarizing signal LPS and we observed similar results in response to the proinflammatory cytokines TNFα and IL-1β (Biswas et al., Blood 2006 and unpublished observation). Thus, in terms of cytotoxicity and expression of inflammatory cytokines TAM resemble the M2 macrophages. Unexpectedly, TAM display high

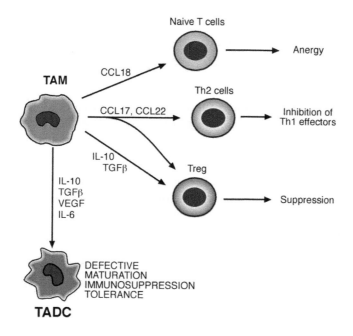

FIGURE 27.2
Suppressive effects of TAM on adaptive immunity. TAM produce cytokines negatively modulating the outcome of a potential antitumor response. IL-10, IL-6,VEGF and TGFβ inhibit the maturation and activation of Tumor-Associated Dendritic Cells (TADC). IL-10, TGFβ and selected chemokines act on T-helper 2 (Th2)-polarized lymphocytes and T-regulatory cells which are ineffective in antitumor immunity and suppress antitumor responses.
Modified from Sica et al. Eur J Cancer 2006.

levels of IRF-3/STAT-1 activation, which may be part of the molecular events promoting TAM-mediated T-cell deletion [79].

In agreement with the M2 signature, TAM also express high levels of both the scavenger receptor-A (SR-A) [19] and the mannose receptor (MR) [7a]. Further, TAM are poor antigen-presenting cells [88].

It has been proposed that the carbohydrate-binding protein galectin-1, which is abundantly expressed by ovarian cancer [157] and shows specific anti-inflammatory effects, tunes the classic pathway of L-arginine, resulting in a strong inhibition of the nitric oxide production by lipopolysaccharide-activated macrophages.

Myelomonocytic cells influence nearly all steps of carcinogenesis and tumor progression [92,117,147]. These include the following: contribution to genetic alterations and instability; regulation of senescence [126] promotion of angiogenesis and lymphangiogenesis [30,81,105]; suppression of adaptive immunity [77] interaction with and remodeling of the extracellular matrix; and promotion of invasion and metastasis [81].

Angiogenesis represents a key event in tumor growth and progression. In several studies in human cancer, TAM accumulation has been associated with angiogenesis and with the production of angiogenic factors such as VEGF and platelet-derived endothelial cell growth factor [88]. M2 macrophages support angiogenesis and lymphangiogenesis by releasing pro-angiogenic growth factors such as IL-8, VEGFA, VEGFC and EGF [81,88,105,139]. Macrophages act as "bridge cells" or "cellular chaperones" that guide the fusion of endothelial tip cells (vascular anastomosis) and facilitate vascular sprouting [46,139].

In human cervical cancer, VEGF-C production by TAMs plays a role in peritumoral lymphoangiogenesis and subsequent dissemination of cancer cells with formation of lymphatic metastasis [140]. Additionally, TAM participate in the pro-angiogenic process by producing the angiogenic factor thymidine phosporylase (TP), which promotes endothelial cell migration *in vitro* and whose levels of expression are associated with tumor neovascularization [66]. TAM contribute to tumor progression also by producing pro-angiogenic and tumor-inducing chemokines, such as CCL2 [162]. Moreover, TAM accumulate in hypoxic regions of tumors and hypoxia triggers a pro-angiogenic program in these cells (see below). Therefore, macrophages recruited *in situ* represent an indirect pathway of amplification of angiogenesis, in concert with angiogenic molecules directly produced by tumor cells. On the anti-angiogenic side, in a murine model, GM-CSF released from a primary tumor upregulated TAM-derived metalloelastase and angiostatin production, thus suppressing tumor growth of metastases [42].

Finally TAM express molecules that affect tumor cell proliferation, angiogenesis and tissue remodeling. These include epidermal growth factor (EGF), members of the FGF family, TGFβ, VEGF, chemokines. In lung cancer, TAM may favor tumor progression by contributing to stroma formation and angiogenesis through their release of PDGF, in conjunction with TGF-β1 production by cancer cells [88]. Macrophages can produce enzymes and inhibitors that regulate the digestion of the extracellular matrix, such as MMPs, plasmin, urokinase-type plasminogen activator (uPA) and the uPA receptor. Direct evidence has been presented that MMP-9 derived from hematopoietic cells of host origin contributes to skin carcinogenesis [35]. Chemokines have been shown to induce gene expression of various MMPs and, in particular, MMP-9 production, along with the uPA receptor [83]. Evidence suggests that MMP-9 has complex effects beyond matrix degradation, including promotion of the angiogenesis switch and release of growth factors [35].

Moreover, IL-4-activated macrophages, as well as cells exposed to IL-10, TGF-β and tumor supernatants, selectively express the fibronectin isoform MSF (migration-stimulating factor) [150]. MSF lacks a typical RGD (Arg-Gly-Asp) motif and is a potent motogen for monocytes; however, its role in ontogeny and immunopathology remains to be defined.

The mechanisms responsible for the M2 polarization of TAM have not been completely defined yet. Recent data point to tumor (ovarian, pancreatic) derived signals that promote M2 differentiation of mononuclear phagocytes (Marchesi, unpublished data) [59].

V. MODULATION OF ADAPTIVE IMMUNITY BY TAM

It has long been known that TAM have poor antigen-presenting capacity and can actually suppress T-cell activation and proliferation [88]. The suppressive mediators produced by TAM include prostaglandins, IL-10 and TGFβ and indoleamine dioxigenase (IDO) metabolites [89]. Moreover, TAM are unable to produce IL-12, even upon stimulation by IFN-γ and lipopolysaccharide (LPS) [144]. With this cytokine profile, which is characteristic of M2 macrophages, TAM are unable to trigger Th1 polarized immune responses, but rather induce T-regulatory cells (Treg) (Figure 27.2). Treg cells possess a characteristic anergic phenotype and strongly suppress the activity of effector T cells and other inflammatory cells, such as monocytes. Infiltrating Treg cells strongly affect the tumor microenvironment by producing high levels of immunosuppressive cytokines (IL-10, TGFβ) [68].

Suppression of T-cell mediated antitumor activity by Treg cells is associated with increased tumor growth and, hence, decreased survival [133]. For instance, in patients with advanced ovarian cancer, an increase in the number of functionally active Treg cells present in the ascites was predictive of reduced survival [37]. M2-polarized macrophages not only drive the differentiation of CD25+GITR+Foxp3+ Treg cells [135] but also regulate their recruitment by releasing CCL22 [37].

Immature myeloid suppressor cells present in the neoplastic tissue of some tumors have been shown to potently inhibit T-cell responses [25]. The relationship if any, of immature myeloid suppressor cells with TAM remains to be defined.

The complex network of chemokines present at the tumor site can play a role also in the induction of the adaptive immunity. Chemokines also regulate the amplification of polarized T-cell responses (Figure 27.2). Some chemokines may enhance specific host immunity against tumors, but on the other hand other chemokines may contribute to escape from the immune system, by recruiting Th2 effectors and Treg cells [89]. As mentioned above, in addition to being a target for chemokines, TAM are a source of a selected set of these mediators (CCL2, CCL17, CCL18, CCL22). CCL18 was recently identified as the most abundant chemokine in human ovarian ascites fluid. When the source of CCL18 was investigated, it was tracked to TAM, with no production by ovarian carcinoma cells [141]. CCL18 is a CC chemokine produced constitutively by immature DC and inducible in macrophages by IL-4, IL-13 and IL-10. Since IL-4 and IL-13 are not expressed in substantial amounts in ovarian cancer, it is likely that IL-10, produced by tumor cells and macrophages themselves, accounts for CCL18 production by TAM. CCL18 is an attractant for naive T cells [1]. Attraction of naive T cells in a peripheral microenvironment dominated by M2 macrophages and immature DC is likely to induce T-cell anergy.

Work in gene-modified mice has shown that CCL2 can orient specific immunity in a Th2 direction. Although the exact mechanism for this action has not been defined, it may include stimulation of IL-10 production in macrophages [56]. Overall, TAM-derived chemokines most frequently recruit effector T cells inefficient to mount a protective antitumor immunity. TAM also produce chemokines specifically attracting T cells with immunosuppressive functions.

VI. TARGETING TAM

Specific macrophage-targeted therapies are moving the first steps in the clinical field. However, therapeutic approaches not originally designed as macrophage oriented or specific, turn out to affect macrophage activation and polarization. These off-target settings provide insights and lessons for the development of more specifically directed approaches [146]. Figure 27.3 provides a summary of selected macrophage-specific and off-target macrophage modifying therapeutic approaches.

A. Activation

There is evidence from experimental cancer models that it may be possible to "re-educate" tumor-promoting TAM to reject malignant cells [17,44,60,144]. In proof of concept and in a large clinical study in ovarian cancer patients, IFN-γ was found to activate TAM with unequivocal evidence of clinical responses [7]. In a model of pancreatic ductal adenocarcinoma, CD40 agonist antibodies promoted a remarkable antitumor effect and induced high expression of M1 markers (MHC class II and CD86) in macrophages [17].

Defective NF-κB activation in TAM correlates with impaired expression of NF-κB-dependent inflammatory functions (e.g., expression of cytotoxic mediators, NO) and cytokines, including Tumor-Necrosis Factor (TNFα), IL-1 and IL-12 [88,144,154]. Restoration of NF-κB activity in TAM is therefore a potential strategy to restore M1 inflammation and intratumoral cytotoxicity. In agreement, recent evidence indicates that restoration of an M1 phenotype in TAM may provide therapeutic benefit in tumor-bearing mice. In particular, combination of CpG plus an anti-IL-10 receptor antibody switched infiltrating macrophages from M2 to M1 and triggered innate response debulking large tumors within 16 hours [57]. It is likely that this treatment may restore NF-κB activation and inflammatory functions by TAM. Moreover, TAM from STAT6$^{-/-}$ tumor-bearing mice display an M1 phenotype, with low levels of arginase and high levels of NO. As a result, these mice immunologically rejected spontaneous mammary carcinoma [148]. The SHIP1 phosphatase was shown to play a critical role in programming macrophage M1 versus M2 functions. Mice deficient for SHIP1 display a skewed development away from M1 macrophages (which have high inducible nitric oxide synthase levels and produce NO), towards M2 macrophages (which have high arginase levels and

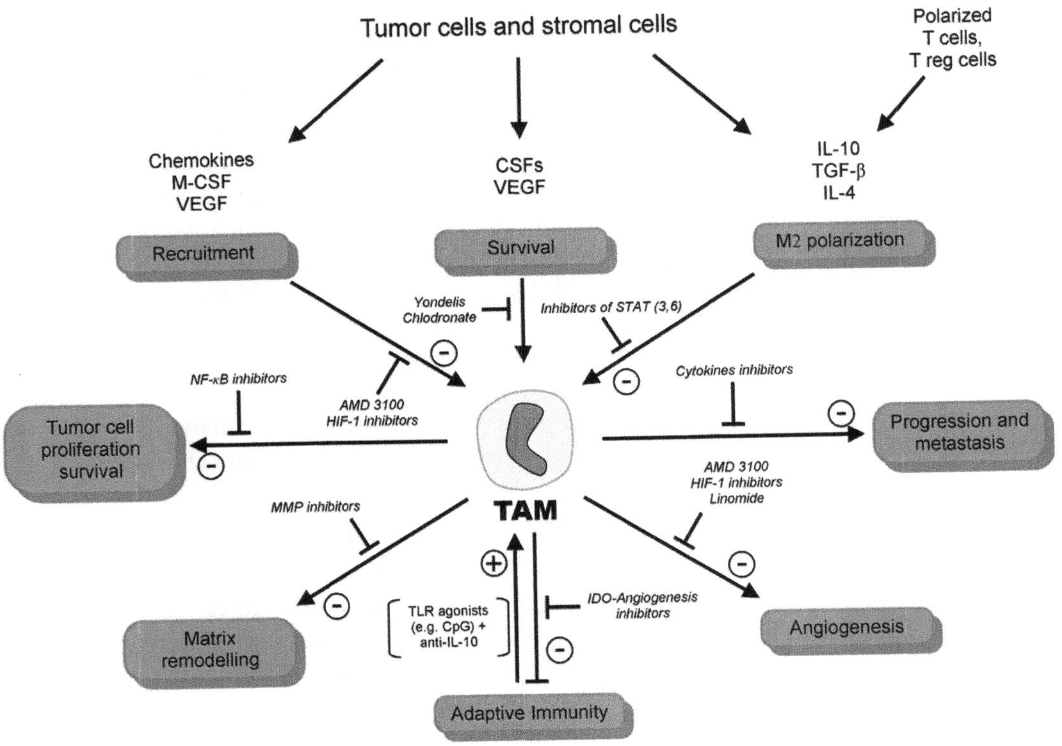

FIGURE 27.3

Multifaced therapeutic approaches to prevent TAM protumoral functions. TAM promote tumor progression by favoring angiogenesis, suppression of adaptive immunity, matrix remodeling, tumor progression and metastasis. The figure summarizes strategies impairing selective TAM protumoral functions (−) or restoring antitumor activities (+). Cytotoxic drugs (e.g., Yondelis) may decrease TAM number and prevent protumoral functions. A similar result may be obtained by limiting TAM recruitment (Linomide, HIF-1 inhibitors, AMD3100). Restoration of M1 immunity (STAT-3 and -6 inhibitors; anti-IL-10 plus CpG; IDO inhibitors) would provide cytotoxic activity and re-activation of Th1 specific antitumor immunity. Inhibition of both pro-inflammatory cytokines and growth factors expression (NF-κB inhibitors) may disrupt inflammatory circuits supporting tumor growth and progression. MMPs inhibitors would prevent cancer cells' spread and metastasis. Finally, inhibitors of TAM-mediated angiogenesis (Linomide, HIF-1 inhibitors, AMD3100) would restrain blood supply and inhibit tumor growth. M-CSF (Macrophage-Colony Stimulating Factor); VEGF (Vascular Endothelial Growth Factor); CSFs (Colony-Stimulating Factors); IL- (Interleukin-); TGF-β (Transforming Growth Factor-β); IDO (indoleamine 2,3-dioxygenase); MMP inhibitors (Matrix metalloproteinase inhibitors); TLR agonists (Toll-Like Receptor agonists); STAT (signal transducer and activator of transcription); NF-κB (nuclear factor-kappaB).

produce ornithine) [124]. Finally, some reports have identified a myeloid M2-biased cell population in lymphoid organs and peripheral tissues of tumor-bearing hosts, referred to as the myeloid suppressor cells (MSC), which are suggested to contribute to the immunosuppressive phenotype [26]. These cells are phenotypically distinct from TAM and are characterized by the expression of the Gr-1 and CD11b markers. MSC use two enzymes involved in the arginine metabolism to control T-cell response: inducible nitric oxide synthase and arginase 1, which deplete the milieau of arginine, causing peroxinitrite generation, as well as lack of CD3ζ chain expression and T-cell apoptosis. In prostate cancer, selective antagonists of these two enzymes were proved beneficial in restoring T-cell-mediated cytotoxicity [27]. Based on the observation that constitutively activated STAT-3 plays a pivotal role in human tumor malignancy, the discovery of selective inhibitors of this pathway appears a promising strategy with antitumor activity against human and murine cancer cells in mice [22].

B. Recruitment

Monocyte attractants are diverse and include members of the chemokine superfamily, CCL2/ MCP-1 in particular, and growth factors interacting with tyrosine kinase receptors, CSF-1 and VEGF [16,121,163]. In more detail, some results in MCP-1/CCL2 gene targeted mice suggest that this chemokine can indeed promote progression in a Her2/neu-driven spontaneous mammary carcinoma model [33]. CCL2 has been shown to play a role not only in attracting tumor-promoting macrophages in carcinoma of the prostate but also in promoting their survival and M2 polarization [127]. Antibodies directed against CCL2/CCR2 have been generated and have proven active in prostate and breast cancer [82,121] and they are currently being evaluated in humans in prostate and ovarian cancers [48,67]. A CCL2 inhibitor (bindarit) has proven active in preclinical models of cancer and vascular pathology, resulting in inhibition of monocyte recruitment [49]. This agent is undergoing clinical evaluation. Thus, available information suggests that chemokines represent a valuable therapeutic target in neoplasia. CSF-1 was identified as an important regulator of mammary tumor progression to metastasis, by regulating infiltration, survival and proliferation of TAM. Transgenic expression of CSF-1 in mammary epithelium led to the acceleration of the late stages of carcinoma and increased lung metastasis, suggesting that agents directed at CSF-1/CSF-1R activity could have important therapeutic effects [116,3]. CSF-1 receptor (c-fms) kinase inhibitors have been generated, with anti-angiogenic and anti-metastatic activity in acute myeloid leukemia and melanoma models [85]. Anti-CSF-1 antibodies and antisense oligonucleotides suppressed macrophage infiltration and xenografts mammary tumor growth in mice [4,111].

Goswami et al. [55] described a role of TAM in promoting invasion of breast carcinoma cells via a CSF-1/EGF paracrine loop. Thus, disruption of this circuit by blockade of either EGF receptor or CSF-1 receptor signaling may represent a new therapeutic strategy to inhibit both macrophage and tumor cell migration and invasion.

Moreover, it was found that anti-M-CSF antibodies, which interferes with TAM recruitment in different mammary carcinoma models, restored susceptibility *in vivo* to combination chemotherapy, implying a role of TAM in chemoresistance of tumors [111].

Genes of the Wnt family play a crucial role in cellular proliferation, migration and tissue patterning during embryonic development. Activation of Wnt 5a member in macrophages co-cultured with breast cancer cells was recently shown to induce cancer cell invasion through a TNF-a-mediated induction of the MMP-7 metalloprotease. This novel circuit links the migration-regulating Wnt pathway with the proteolitic cascade, both mechanisms being indispensable for successful invasion and the Wnt antagonist dickkopf-1, inhibited cancer cell invasiveness [119].

Several results have shed new light on the links between certain TAM chemokines and genetic events that cause cancer. The CXCR4 receptor lies downstream of the vonHippel/Lindau/ hypoxiainducible factor (HIF) axis. Transfer of activated *ras* into a cervical carcinoma line, HeLa, induces IL-8/CXCL8 production that is sufficient to promote angiogenesis and progression. Moreover, a frequent early and sufficient gene rearrangement that causes papillary thyroid carcinoma (Ret-PTC) activates an inflammatory genetic program that includes CXCR4 and inflammatory chemokines in primary human thyrocytes [23]. The emerging direct connections between oncogenes, inflammatory mediators and the chemokine system provide a strong impetus for exploration of the anticancer potential of anti-inflammatory strategies. It was further demonstrated in non-small cell lung cancer (NSCLC) that mutation of the tumor suppressor gene PTEN results in upregulation of HIF-1 activity and ultimately in HIF-1-dependent transcription of the CXCR4 gene, which provides a mechanistic basis for the upregulation of CXCR4 expression and promotion of metastasis formation [115]. It appears therefore that targeting HIF-1 activity may disrupt the HIF-1/CXCR4 pathway and affect TAM accumulation, as well as cancer cell spreading and survival. The HIF-1-inducible vascular endothelial growth factor (VEGF) is commonly produced by tumors and elicits monocyte migration.

As mentioned above, there is evidence that VEGF can significantly contribute to macrophage recruitment in tumors. Along with CSF-1, this molecule also promotes macrophage survival and proliferation. Due to the localization of TAM into the hypoxic regions of tumors, viral vectors were used to transduce macrophages with therapeutic genes, such as IFN-γ, that were

461

activated only in low oxygen conditions [29]. These works present promising approaches which use macrophages as vehicles to deliver gene therapy in regions of tumor hypoxia.

C. Angiogenesis

VEGF is a potent angiogenic factor as well as a monocyte attractant that contributes to TAM recruitment. TAM promote angiogenesis and there is evidence that inhibition of TAM recruitment plays an important role in anti-angiogenic strategies. We found that, in addition to VEGF, the angiogenic program established by hypoxia may rely also on the increased expression of CXCR4 by TAM and endothelial cells [138]. Intratumoral injection of CXCR4 antagonists, such as the bicyclam AMD3100, may potentially work as *in vivo* inhibitors of tumor angiogenesis. Linomide, an anti-angiogenic agent, caused significant reduction of the tumor volume, in a murine prostate cancer model, by inhibiting the stimulatory effects of TAM on tumor angiogenesis [69]. Based on this, the effects of linomide, or other anti-angiogenic drugs, on the expression of pro- and anti-angiogenic molecules by TAM may be considered valuable targets for anticancer therapy.

D. Survival

Antitumor agents with selective cytotoxic activity on monocyte-macrophages would be ideal therapeutic tools for their combined action on tumor cells and TAM. We reported that Yondelis (Trabectedin), a natural product derived from the marine organism *Ecteinascidia turbinata*, with potent antitumor activity [143] is specifically cytotoxic to macrophages and TAM, while sparing the lymphocyte subset. This compound inhibits NF-Y, a transcription factor of major importance for mononuclear phagocyte differentiation. In addition, Yondelis inhibits the production of CCL2 and IL-6 both by TAM and tumor cells [5]. These anti-inflammatory properties of Yondelis may be an extended mechanism of its antitumor activity. The EMEA-approved anticancer agent Trabectedin has a remarkably selective cytotoxic action for mononuclear phagocytes *in vitro* and *in vivo*, in mice and in humans [50]. Evidence suggests that the antitumor activity of this agent is to a large extent mediated by macrophage depletion [50a]. Finally, pro-inflammatory cytokines (e.g., IL-1 and TNF), expressed by infiltrating leukocytes, can activate NF-κB in cancer cells and contribute to their proliferation, survival and metastasis [12,14], thus representing potential anticancer targets.

E. Matrix remodeling

Macrophages are a major source of proteases and, interestingly, MMP-9 has been found to be preferentially expressed in M2 versus M1 cells [98].

TAM produce several matrix-metalloproteases (e.g., MMP2, MMP9) which degrade proteins of the extracellular matrix, and also produce activators of MMPs, such as chemokines [39]. Inhibition of this molecular pattern may prevent degradation of extracellular matrix, as well as tumor cell invasion and migration. TAM or neutrophil-derived proteases (e.g., MMP-9 or cathepsin B) stimulate cancer invasion and metastasis [32,63,158].

The biphosphonate zoledronic acid is a prototypical MMP inhibitor. In cervical cancer this compound suppressed MMP-9 expression by infiltrating macrophages and inhibited metalloprotease activity, reducing angiogenesis and cervical carcinogenesis [51]. Most recent evidence showed that it can trigger the reversal of the TAM phenotype from protumoral M2 to tumoricidal M1 [129]. The halogenated bisphosphonate derivative chlodronate is a macrophage toxin that depletes selected macrophage populations. Given the current clinical usage of this and similar agents it is important to assess whether they have potential as TAM toxins. In support of this hypothesis, clodronate encapsulated in liposomes efficiently depleted TAM in murine teratocarcinoma and human rhabdomyosarcoma mouse tumor models, resulting in significant inhibition of tumor growth [170].

The secreted protein acidic and rich in cysteine (SPARC) has gained much interest in cancer, being either upregulated or downregulated in progressing tumors. SPARC produced by macrophages present in tumor stroma can modulate collagen density, leukocyte, and blood vessel infiltration [134].

F. Effector molecules

Cyclooxygenase (COX) is a key enzyme in the prostanoid biosynthetic pathway. COX-2 is upregulated by activated oncogenes (i.e., ß-catenin, MET) but is also produced by TAM in response to tumor-derived factors like mucin in the case of colon cancer. The usage of COX-2 inhibitors in the form of nonsteroidal anti-inflammatory drugs is associated with reduced risk of diverse tumors (colorectal, esophagus, lung, stomach, and ovary). Selective COX-2 inhibitors are now thought as part of combination therapy [31].

SOCS-1 deficiency is associated to IFN-γ-dependent spontaneous development of colorectal carcinomas. Under these conditions accumulation of aberrantly activated TAM *in situ* is observed and these cells account for expression of carcinogenesis related enzymes (COX2, iNOS) [62].

The IFN-γ-inducible enzyme indoleamine 2,3-dioxygenase is a well-known suppressor of T-cell activation. It catalyzes the initial rate-limiting step in tryptophan catabolism, which leads to the biosynthesis of nicotinamide adenine dinucleotide. By depleting tryptophan from local microenvironment, indoleamine 2,3-dioxygenase (IDO) blocks activation of T lymphocytes.

Ectopic expression of IDO in tumor cells has been shown to inhibit T-cell responses [100]. Recently it was shown that inhibition of IDO may cooperate with cytotoxic agents to elicit regression of established tumors and may increase the efficacy of cancer immunotherapy [104].

Prostate cancer is strongly linked to inflammation based on epidemiological and molecular analysis [14]. TAM mediate hormone resistance in prostate cancer by a nuclear receptor derepression pathway. TAM in prostate cancer, via IL-1, convert selective androgen receptor antagonists/modulators into agonists [173].

TNF promotes asbestos carcinogenesis by blocking death of mesothelial cells via the NF-κB pathway [167]. Figure 27.3 summarizes therapeutic approaches to prevent TAM protumoral functions.

463

VII. CONCLUDING REMARKS

Inflammatory reactions, and macrophages in particular, can exert a dual role on tumor growth and progression [86]. Though the presence of TAM has been long considered as evidence for a host response against the growing tumor, it has become increasingly clear that TAM are redirected by the neoplastic environment and play active roles in the process of tumor progression and invasion. Molecular and biological studies have been supported by a large number of clinical studies that found a significant correlation between the high macrophage content of tumors and poor patient prognosis. TAM share many similarities with the prototypic polarized M2 mononuclear phagocyte population, in terms of gene expression and functions. In line with known properties of M2 macrophage populations, several evidence suggests that TAM promote tumor progression and metastasis by activating circuits that regulate tumor growth, adaptive immunity, stroma formation and angiogenesis. In this context, metabolic adaptation is an integral aspect of macrophage polarization and their functional diversity. Analysis of the mechanisms mediating this phenotype involve defective NF-κB activation [144], an event likely responsible for the inability of TAM to mount effective M1 inflammatory responses [19,88]. Much progress has been made in defining the molecular mechanisms driving macrophage polarization. However, further clarification of mechanisms promoting functional diversion of macrophages towards an M2 direction is expected to disclose new valuable therapeutic targets against tumors.

Several studies have displayed key molecules and pathways driving recruitment and activation of TAM and the TAM transcriptome was provided in a murine fibrosarcoma [19]. Despite these efforts, TAM functions have been significantly characterized only in animal models, and even today their phenotypic characterization remains only partial in human cancers. Moreover, it is still unknown whether different tumor microenvironments, likely established by different tumor types, may drive different functional phenotypes of TAM and contribute to specific pro- or antitumor activities. As new inflammatory players, recent findings suggest a general protumoral function of Toll-like receptors (TLR) in the cancer microenvironment [90].

Along with TAM recruitment, activation and polarization mechanisms, the functional hetereogenicity of TAM should be viewed as an additional level of investigation in developing innovative anticancer strategies.

ACKNOWLEDGMENTS

This work was supported by Associazione Italiana Ricerca sul Cancro (AIRC), Italy; by European Community and by Ministero Istruzione Università Ricerca (MIUR), Italy; Istituto Superiore Sanità (ISS).

References

[1] Adema GJ, Hartgers F, Verstraten R, de Vries E, Marland G, Menon S, et al. A dendritic-cell-derived C-C chemokine that preferentially attracts naive T cells. Nature 1997;387:713−7.

[2] Adini T, Kornaga F, Firoozbakht Benjamin LE. Placental growth factor is a survival factor for tumor endothelial cells and macrophages. Cancer Res 2002;62:2749−52.

[3] Aharinejad S, Abraham D, Paulus P, Abri H, Hofmann M, Grossschmidt K, et al. Colony-stimulating factor-1 antisense treatment suppresses growth of human tumor xenografts in mice. Cancer Res 2002;62:5317−24.

[4] Aharinejad S, Paulus P, Sioud M, Hofmann M, Zins K, Schafer R, et al. Colony-stimulating factor-1 blockade by antisense oligonucleotides and small interfering RNAs suppresses growth of human mammary tumor xenografts in mice. Cancer Res 2004;64:5378−84.

[5] Allavena P, Peccatori F, Maggioni D, Erroi A, Sironi M, Colombo N, et al. Intraperitoneal recombinant gamma-interferon in patients with recurrent ascitic ovarian carcinoma: modulation of cytotoxicity and cytokine production in tumor-associated effectors and of major histocompatibility antigen expression on tumor cells. Cancer Res 1990;50:7318−23.

[6] Allavena P, Sica A, Vecchi A, Locati M, Sozzani S, Mantovani A. The chemokine receptor switch paradigm and dendritic cell migration: its significance in tumor tissues. Immunol Rev 2000;177:141−9.

[7] Allavena P, Signorelli M, Chieppa M, Erba E, Bianchi G, Marchesi F, et al. Anti-inflammatory properties of the novel antitumor agent Yondelis (trabectedin) inhibition of macrophage differentiation and cytokine production. Cancer Res 2005;65:2964−71.

[7a] Allavena P, Chieppa M, Bianchi G, Solinas G, Fabbri M, Laskarin G, et al. Engagement of the mannose receptor by tumoral mucins activates an immune suppressive phenotype in human tumor-associated macrophages. Clin Dev Immunol 2010;2010:547179.

[8] Allavena P, Germano G, Marchesi F, Mantovani A. Chemokines in cancer related inflammation. Exp Cell Res 2011;317:664−73.

[9] Auffray C, Fogg D, Garfa M, Elain G, Join-Lambert O, Kayal S, et al. Monitoring of blood vessels and tissues by a population of monocytes with patrolling behavior. Science 2007;317:666−70.

[10] Azenshtein E, Luboshits G, Shina S, Neumark E, Shahbazian D, Weil M, et al. The CC chemokine RANTES in breast carcinoma progression: regulation of expression and potential mechanisms of promalignant activity. Cancer Res 2002;62:1093−102.

[11] Azenshtein E, Meshel T, Shina S, Barak N, Keydar I, Ben-Baruch A. The angiogenic factors CXCL8 and VEGF in breast cancer: regulation by an array of pro-malignancy factors. Cancer Lett 2005;217:73−86.

[12] Balkwill F, Mantovani A. Inflammation and cancer: back to Virchow? Lancet 2001;357:539−45.

[13] Balkwill F. Cancer and the chemokine network. Nat Rev Cancer 2004;4:540−50.

[14] Balkwill F, Charles KA, Mantovani A. Smoldering and polarized inflammation in the initiation and promotion of malignant disease. Cancer Cell 2005;7:211–7.

[15] Balkwill FR. The chemokine system and cancer. J Pathol 2012;226:148–57.

[16] Barleon B, Sozzani S, Zhou D, Weich HA, Mantovani A, Marme D. Migration of human monocytes in response to vascular endothelial growth factor (VEGF) is mediated via the VEGF receptor flt-1. Blood 1996;87:3336–43.

[17] Beatty GL, Chiorean EG, Fishman MP, Saboury B, Teitelbaum UR, Sun W, et al. CD40 agonists alter tumor stroma and show efficacy against pancreatic carcinoma in mice and humans. Science 2011;331:1612–6.

[18] Bingle L, Brown NJ, Lewis CE. The role of tumor-associated macrophages in tumor progression: implications for new anticancer therapies. J Pathol 2000;196:254–65.

[19] Biswas SK, Gangi L, Paul S, Schioppa T, Saccani A, Sironi M, et al. A distinct and unique transcriptional program expressed by tumor-associated macrophages (defective NF-kappaB and enhanced IRF-3/STAT1 activation). Blood 2006;107:2112–22.

[20] Biswas SK, Mantovani A. Macrophage plasticity and interaction with lymphocyte subsets: cancer as a paradigm. Nat Immunol 2010;11:889–96.

[21] Biswas SK, Mantovani A. Orchestration of metabolism by macrophages. Cell Metab 2012;15:432–7.

[22] Blaskovich MA, Sun J, Cantor A, Turkson J, Jove R, Sebti SM. Discovery of JSI-124 (cucurbitacin I), a selective Janus kinase/signal transducer and activator of transcription 3 signaling pathway inhibitor with potent antitumor activity against human and murine cancer cells in mice. Cancer Res 2003;63:1270–9.

[23] Borrello MG, Alberti L, Fischer A, Degl'innocenti D, Ferrario C, Gariboldi M, et al. Induction of a proinflammatory program in normal human thyrocytes by the RET/PTC1 oncogene. Proc Natl Acad Sci U S A 2005;102:14825–30.

[24] Bottazzi B, Polentarutti N, Acero R, Balsari A, Boraschi D, Ghezzi P, et al. Regulation of the macrophage content of neoplasms by chemoattractants. Science 1983;220:210–2.

[25] Bronte V, Serafini P, Mazzoni A, Segal DM, Zanovello P. L-arginine metabolism in myeloid cells controls T-lymphocyte functions. Trends Immunol 2003;24:302–6.

[26] Bronte V, Zanovello P. Regulation of immune responses by L-arginine metabolism. Nat Rev Immunol 2005A;5:641–54.

[27] Bronte V, Kasic T, Gri G, Gallana K, Borsellino G, Marigo I, et al. Boosting antitumor responses of T lymphocytes infiltrating human prostate cancers. J Exp Med 2005B;201:1257–68.

[28] Cairo G, Recalcati S, Mantovani A, Locati M. Iron trafficking and metabolism in macrophages: contribution to the polarized phenotype. Trends Immunol 2011;32:241–7.

[29] Carta L, Pastorino S, Melillo G, Bosco MC, Massazza S, Varesio L. Engineering of macrophages to produce IFN-gamma in response to hypoxia. J Immunol 2001;166:5374–80.

[30] Clear AJ, Lee AM, Calaminici M, Ramsay AG, Morris KJ, Hallam S, et al. Increased angiogenic sprouting in poor prognosis FL is associated with elevated numbers of CD163+ macrophages within the immediate sprouting microenvironment. Blood 2010;115:5053–6.

[31] Colombo MP, Mantovani A. Targeting myelomonocytic cells to revert inflammation-dependent cancer promotion. Cancer Res 2005;65:9113–6.

[32] Condeelis J, Pollard JW. Macrophages: obligate partners for tumor cell migration, invasion, and metastasis. Cell 2006;124:263–6.

[33] Conti I, Rollins BJ. CCL2 (monocyte chemoattractant protein-1) and cancer. Semin Cancer Biol 2004;14:149–54.

[34] Corna G, Campana L, Pignatti E, Castiglioni A, Tagliafico E, Bosurgi L, et al. Polarization dictates iron handling by inflammatory and alternatively activated macrophages. Haematologica 2010;95:1814–22.

[35] Coussens LM, Tinkle CL, Hanahan D, Werb Z. MMP-9 supplied by bone marrow-derived cells contributes to skin carcinogenesis. Cell 2000;103:481–90.

[36] Coussens LM, Werb Z. Inflammation and cancer. Nature 2002;420:860–7.

[37] Curiel TJ, Coukos G, Zou L, Alvarez X, Cheng P, Mottram P, et al. Specific recruitment of regulatory T cells in ovarian carcinoma fosters immune privilege and predicts reduced survival. Nat Med 2004;10:942–9.

[38] Desnues B, Lepidi H, Raoult D, Mege JL. Whipple disease: intestinal infiltrating cells exhibit a transcriptional pattern of M2/alternatively activated macrophages. J Infect Dis 2005;192:1642–6.

[39] de Visser KE, Eichten A, Coussens LM. Paradoxical roles of the immune system during cancer development. Nat Rev Cancer 2006;6:24–37.

[40] DiNapoli MR, Calderon CL, Lopez DM. The altered tumoricidal capacity of macrophages isolated from tumor-bearing mice is related to reduced expression of the inducible nitric oxide synthase gene. J Exp Med 1996;183:1323–9.

[41] Dinarello CA. Blocking IL-1 in systemic inflammation. J Exp Med 2005;201:1355–9.

465

[42] Dong Z, Yoneda J, Kumar R, Fidler IJ. Angiostatin-mediated suppression of cancer metastases by primary neoplasms engineered to produce granulocyte/macrophage colony-stimulating factor. J Exp Med 1998;188:755–63.

[43] Duyndam MC, Hilhorst MC, Schlüper HM, Verheul HM, van Diest PJ, Kraal G, et al. Vascular endothelial growth factor-165 overexpression stimulates angiogenesis and induces cyst formation and macrophage infiltration in human ovarian cancer xenografts. Am J Pathol 2002;160:537–48.

[44] Duluc D, Corvaisier M, Blanchard S, Catala L, Descamps P, Gamelin E, et al. Interferon-gamma reverses the immunosuppressive and protumoral properties and prevents the generation of human tumor-associated macrophages. Int J Cancer 2009;125:367–73.

[45] Erler JT, Bennewith KL, Cox TR, Lang G, Bird D, Koong A, et al. Hypoxia-induced lysyl oxidase is a critical mediator of bone marrow cell recruitment to form the premetastatic niche. Cancer Cell 2009;15:35–44.

[46] Fantin A, Vieira JM, Gestri G, Denti L, Schwarz Q, Prykhozhij S, et al. Tissue macrophages act as cellular chaperones for vascular anastomosis downstream of VEGF-mediated endothelial tip cell induction. Blood 2010;116:829–40.

[47] Fridlender ZG, Sun J, Kim S, Kapoor V, Cheng G, Ling L, et al. Polarization of tumor-associated neutrophil phenotype by TGF-beta: "N1" versus "N2" TAN. Cancer Cell 2009;16:183–94.

[48] Garber K. First results for agents targeting cancer-related inflammation. J Natl Cancer Inst 2009;101:1110–2.

[49] Gazzaniga S, Bravo AI, Guglielmotti A, van Rooijen N, Maschi F, Vecchi A, et al. Targeting tumor-associated macrophages and inhibition of MCP-1 reduce angiogenesis and tumor growth in a human melanoma xenograft. J Invest Dermatol 2007;127:2031–41.

[50] Germano G, Frapolli R, Simone M, Tavecchio M, Erba E, Pesce S, et al. Antitumor and anti-inflammatory effects of trabectedin on human myxoid liposarcoma cells. Cancer Res 2010;70:2235–44.

[50a] Germano G, Frappolli R, Belgiovine C, Anselmo A, Pesce S, Liguori M, Erba E, et al. Role of macrophage targeting in the antitumor activity of trabectedin. Cancer Cell. 2013;23:249–62.

[51] Giraudo E, Inoue M, Hanahan D. An amino-bisphosphonate targets MMP-9-expressing macrophages and angiogenesis to impair cervical carcinogenesis. J Clin Invest 2004;114:623–33.

[52] Gleissner CA, Shaked I, Little KM, Ley K. CXC chemokine ligand 4 induces a unique transcriptome in monocyte-derived macrophages. J Immunol 2010;184:4810–8.

[53] Gordon S. Alternative activation of macrophages. Nat Rev Immunol 2003;3:23–35.

[54] Gordon S, Taylor PR. Monocyte and macrophage heterogeneity. Nat Rev Immunol 2005;5:953–64.

[55] Goswami S, Sahai E, Wyckoff JB, Cammer M, Cox D, Pixley FJ, et al. Macrophages promote the invasion of breast carcinoma cells via a colony-stimulating factor-1/epidermal growth factor paracrine loop. Cancer Res 2005;65:5278–83.

[56] Gu L, Tseng S, Horner RM, Tam C, Loda M, Rollins BJ. Control of TH2 polarization by the chemokine monocyte chemoattractant protein-1. Nature 2000;404:407–11.

[57] Guiducci C, Vicari AP, Sangaletti S, Trinchieri G, Colombo MP. Redirecting in vivo elicited tumor infiltrating macrophages and dendritic cells towards tumor rejection. Cancer Res 2005;65:3437–46.

[58] Gustafsson C, Mjösberg J, Matussek A, Geffers R, Matthiesen L, Berg G, et al. Gene expression profiling of human decidual macrophages: evidence for immunosuppressive phenotype. PLoS One 2008;3:e2078.

[59] Hagemann T, Wilson J, Burke F, Kulbe H, Li NF, Pluddemann A, et al. Ovarian cancer cells polarize macrophages toward a tumor-associated phenotype. J Immunol 2006;176:5023–32.

[60] Hagemann T, Lawrence T, McNeish I, Charles KA, Kulbe H, Thompson RG, et al. Re-educating tumor-associated macrophages by targeting NF-kappaB. J Exp Med 2008;205:1261–8.

[61] Haghnegahdar H, Du J, Wang D, Strieter RM, Burdick MD, Nanney LB, et al. The tumorigenic and angiogenic effects of MGSA/GRO proteins in melanoma. J Leukoc Biol 2000;67:53–62.

[62] Hanada T, Kobayashi T, Chinen T, Saeki K, Takaki H, Koga K, et al. IFNgamma-dependent, spontaneous development of colorectal carcinomas in SOCS1-deficient mice. J Exp Med 2006;203:1391–7.

[63] Hanahan D, Weinberg RA. The hallmarks of cancer. Cell 2000;100:57–70.

[64] Hanamoto H, Nakayama T, Miyazato H, Takegawa S, Hieshima K, Tatsumi Y, et al. Expression of CCL28 by Reed-Sternberg cells defines a major subtype of classical Hodgkin's disease with frequent infiltration of eosinophils and/or plasma cells. Am J Pathol 2004;164:997–1006.

[65] Hazlett LD, McClellan SA, Barrett RP, Huang X, Zhang Y, Wu M, et al. IL-33 shifts macrophage polarization, promoting resistance against Pseudomonas aeruginosa keratitis. Invest Ophthalmol Vis Sci 2010;51:1524–32.

[66] Hotchkiss A, Ashton AW, Klein RS, Lenzi ML, Zhu GH, Schwartz EL. Mechanisms by which tumor cells and monocytes expressing the angiogenic factor thymidine phosphorylase mediate human endothelial cell migration. Cancer Res 2003;63:527–33.

[67] Izhak L, Wildbaum G, Weinberg U, Shaked Y, Alami J, Dumont D, et al. Predominant expression of CCL2 at the tumor site of prostate cancer patients directs a selective loss of immunological tolerance to CCL2 that could be amplified in a beneficial manner. J Immunol 2010;184:1092—101.

[68] Jarnicki AG, Lysaght J, Todryk S, Mills KH. Suppression of antitumor immunity by IL-10 and TGF-beta-producing T cells infiltrating the growing tumor: influence of tumor environment on the induction of CD4+ and CD8+ regulatory T cells. J Immunol 2006;177:896—904.

[69] Joseph IB, Isaacs JT. Macrophage role in the anti-prostate cancer response to one class of antiangiogenic agents. J Natl Cancer Inst 1998;90:1648—53.

[70] Kaplan RN, Riba RD, Zacharoulis S, Bramley AH, Vincent L, Costa C, et al. VEGFR1-positive haematopoietic bone marrow progenitors initiate the pre-metastatic niche. Nature 2005;438:820—7.

[71] Kim S, Takahashi H, Lin WW, Descargues P, Grivennikov S, Kim Y, et al. Carcinoma-produced factors activate myeloid cells through TLR2 to stimulate metastasis. Nature 2009;457:102—6.

[72] Kleinhans M, Tun-Kyi A, Gilliet M, Kadin ME, Dummer R, Burg G, et al. Functional expression of the eotaxin receptor CCR3 in CD30+ cutaneous T-cell lymphoma. Blood 2003;101:1487—93.

[73] Klimp AH, Hollema H, Kempinga C, van der Zee AG, de Vries EG, Daemen T. Expression of cyclooxygenase-2 and inducible nitric oxide synthase in human ovarian tumors and tumor-associated macrophages. Cancer Res 2001;61:7305—9.

[74] Kortylewski M, Kujawski M, Wang T, Wei S, Zhang S, Pilon-Thomas S, et al. Inhibiting Stat3 signaling in the hematopoietic system elicits multicomponent antitumor immunity. Nat Med 2005;11:1314—21.

[75] Kouno J, Nagai H, Nagahata T, Onda M, Yamaguchi H, Adachi K, et al. Up-regulation of CC chemokine, CCL3L1, and receptors, CCR3, CCR5 in human glioblastoma that promotes cell growth. J Neurooncol 2004;70:301—7.

[76] Kuang DM, Wu Y, Chen N, Cheng J, Zhuang SM, Zheng L. Tumor-derived hyaluronan induces formation of immunosuppressive macrophages through transient early activation of monocytes. Blood 2007;110: 587—95.

[77] Kuang DM, Zhao Q, Peng C, Xu J, Zhang JP, Wu C, et al. Activated monocytes in peritumoral stroma of hepatocellular carcinoma foster immune privilege and disease progression through PD-L1. J Exp Med 2009;206:1327—37.

[78] Kurowska-Stolarska M, Stolarski B, Kewin P, Murphy G, Corrigan CJ, Ying S, et al. IL-33 amplifies the polarization of alternatively activated macrophages that contribute to airway inflammation. J Immunol 2009;183:6469—77.

[79] Kusmartsev S, Gabrilovich DI. STAT1 signaling regulates tumor-associated macrophage-mediated T cell deletion. J Immunol 2005;174:4880—91.

[80] Li A, Varney ML, Singh RK. Constitutive expression of growth regulated oncogene (gro) in human colon carcinoma cells with different metastatic potential and its role in regulating their metastatic phenotype. Clin Exp Metastasis 2004;21:571—9.

[81] Lin EY, Li JF, Gnatovskiy L, Deng Y, Zhu L, Grzesik DA, et al. Macrophages regulate the angiogenic switch in a mouse model of breast cancer. Cancer Res 2006;66:11238—46.

[82] Loberg RD, Ying C, Craig M, Day LL, Sargent E, Neeley C, et al. Targeting CCL2 with systemic delivery of neutralizing antibodies induces prostate cancer tumor regression in vivo. Cancer Res 2007;67:9417—24.

[83] Locati M, Deuschle U, Massardi ML, Martinez FO, Sironi M, Sozzani S, et al. Analysis of the gene expression profile activated by the CC chemokine ligand 5/RANTES and by lipopolysaccharide in human monocytes. J Immunol 2002;168:3557—62.

[84] MacMicking J, Xie QW, Nathan C. Nitric oxide and macrophage function. Annu Rev Immunol 1997;15:323—50.

[85] Manthey CL, Johnson DL, Illig CR, Tuman RW, Zhou Z, Baker JF, et al. JNJ-28312141, a novel orally active colony-stimulating factor-1 receptor/FMS-related receptor tyrosine kinase-3 receptor tyrosine kinase inhibitor with potential utility in solid tumors, bone metastases, and acute myeloid leukemia. Mol Cancer Ther 2009;8:3151—61.

[86] Mantovani A, Bottazzi B, Colotta F, Sozzani S, Ruco L. The origin and function of tumor-associated macrophages. Immunol Today 1992;13:265—70.

[87] Mantovani A. The chemokine system: redundancy for robust outputs. Immunol Today 1999;20:254—7.

[88] Mantovani A, Sozzani S, Locati M, Allavena P, Sica A. Macrophage polarization: tumor-associated macrophages as a paradigm for polarized M2 mononuclear phagocytes. Trends Immunol 2002;23:549—55.

[89] Mantovani A, Sica A, Sozzani S, Allavena P, Vecchi A, Locati M. The chemokine system in diverse forms of macrophage activation and polarization. Trends Immunol 2004;25:677—86.

[90] Mantovani A, Garlanda C. Inflammation and multiple myeloma: the Toll connection. Leukemia 2006;20:937—8.

[91] Mantovani A. From phagocyte diversity and activation to probiotics: back to Metchnikoff. Eur J Immunol 2008;38:3269—73.

[92] Mantovani A, Allavena P, Sica A, Balkwill F. Cancer-related inflammation. Nature 2008;454:436—44.

[93] Mantovani A. The yin-yang of tumor-associated neutrophils. Cancer Cell 2009;16:173—4.

[94] Mantovani A, Sica A. Macrophages, innate immunity and cancer: balance, tolerance, and diversity. Curr Opin Immunol 2010;22:231—7.

[95] Mantovani A, Savino B, Locati M, Zammataro L, Allavena P, Bonecchi R. The chemokine system in cancer biology and therapy. Cytokine Growth Factor Rev 2010;21:27—39.

[96] Mantovani A, Cassatella MA, Costantini C, Jaillon S. Neutrophils in the activation and regulation of innate and adaptive immunity. Nat Rev Immunol 2011;11:519—31.

[97] Marchesi F, Monti P, Leone BE, Zerbi A, Vecchi A, Piemonti L, et al. Increased survival, proliferation, and migration in metastatic human pancreatic tumor cells expressing functional CXCR4. Cancer Res 2004;64:8420—7.

[98] Martinez FO, Gordon S, Locati M, Mantovani A. Transcriptional profiling of the human monocyte-macrophage differentiation and polarization: new molecules and patterns of gene expression. J Immunol 2006;177:7303—11.

[99] Matsushima K, Larsen CG, DuBois GC, Oppenheim JJ. Purification and characterization of a novel monocyte chemotactic and activating factor produced by a human myelomonocytic cell line. J Exp Med 1999;169:1485—90.

[100] Mellor AL, Keskin DB, Johnson T, Chandler P, Munn DH. Cells expressing indoleamine 2,3-dioxygenase inhibit T cell responses. J Immunol 2002;168:3771—6.

[101] Monti P, Leone BE, Marchesi F, Balzano G, Zerbi A, Scaltrini F, et al. The CC chemokine MCP-1/CCL2 in pancreatic cancer progression: regulation of expression and potential mechanisms of antimalignant activity. Cancer Res 2003;63:7451—61.

[102] Mori K, Chano T, Yamamoto K, Matsusue Y, Okabe H. Expression of macrophage inflammatory protein-1alpha in Schwann cell tumors. Neuropathology 2004;24:131—5.

[103] Mosser DM, Edwards JP. Exploring the full spectrum of macrophage activation. Nat Rev Immunol 2008;8:958—69.

[104] Muller AJ, DuHadaway JB, Donover PS, Sutanto-Ward E, Prendergast GC. Inhibition of indoleamine 2,3-dioxygenase, an immunoregulatory target of the cancer suppression gene Bin1, potentiates cancer chemotherapy. Nat Med 2005;11:312—9.

[105] Murdoch C, Muthana M, Coffelt SB, Lewis CE. The role of myeloid cells in the promotion of tumor angiogenesis. Nat Rev Cancer 2008;8:618—31.

[106] Nesbit M, Schaider H, Miller TH, Herlyn M. Low-level monocyte chemoattractant protein-1 stimulation of monocytes leads to tumor formation in nontumorigenic melanoma cells. J Immunol 2001;166:6483—90.

[107] Nizet V, Johnson RS. Interdependence of hypoxic and innate immune responses. Nat Rev Immunol 2009;9:609—17.

[108] Noel W, Raes G, Hassanzadeh Ghassabeh G, De Baetselier P, Beschin A. Alternatively activated macrophages during parasite infections. Trends Parasitol 2004;20:126—33.

[109] Odegaard JI, Ricardo-Gonzalez RR, Goforth MH, Morel CR, Subramanian V, Mukundan L, et al. Macrophage-specific PPARgamma controls alternative activation and improves insulin resistance. Nature 2007;447:1116—20.

[110] Paik S, Shak S, Tang G, Kim C, Baker J, Cronin M, et al. A multigene assay to predict recurrence of tamoxifen-treated, node-negative breast cancer. N Engl J Med 2004;351:2817—26.

[111] Paulus P, Stanley ER, Schafer R, Abraham D, Aharinejad S. Colony-stimulating factor-1 antibody reverses chemoresistance in human MCF-7 breast cancer xenografts. Cancer Res 2006;66:4349—56.

[112] Payne AS, Cornelius LA. The role of chemokines in melanoma tumor growth and metastasis. J Invest Dermatol 2002;118:915—22.

[113] Pesce J, Kaviratne M, Ramalingam TR, Thompson RW, Urban Jr JF, Cheever AW, et al. The IL-21 receptor augments Th2 effector function and alternative macrophage activation. J Clin Invest 2006;116:2044—55.

[114] Pesce JT, Ramalingam TR, Mentink-Kane MM, Wilson MS, El Kasmi KC, Smith AM, et al. Arginase-1-expressing macrophages suppress Th2 cytokine-driven inflammation and fibrosis. PLoS pathogens 2009;5:e1000371.

[115] Phillips RJ, Mestas J, Gharaee-Kermani M, Burdick MD, Sica A, Belperio JA, et al. Epidermal growth factor and hypoxia-induced expression of CXC chemokine receptor 4 on non-small cell lung cancer cells is regulated by the phosphatidylinositol 3-kinase/PTEN/AKT/mammalian target of rapamycin signaling pathway and activation of hypoxia inducible factor-1alpha. J Biol Chem 2005;280:22473—81.

[116] Pollard JW. Tumor-educated macrophages promote tumor progression and metastasis. Nat Rev Cancer 2004;4:71—8.

468

[117] Pollard JW. Trophic macrophages in development and disease. Nat Rev Immunol 2009;9:259—70.

[118] Puig-Kröger A, Sierra-Filardi E, Domínguez-Soto A, Samaniego R, Corcuera MT, Gómez-Aguado F, et al. Folate receptor beta is expressed by tumor-associated macrophages and constitutes a marker for M2 anti-inflammatory/regulatory macrophages. Cancer Res 2009;69:9395—403.

[119] Pukrop T, Klemm F, Hagemann T, Gradl D, Schulz M, Siemes S, et al. Wnt 5a signaling is critical for macrophage-induced invasion of breast cancer cell lines. Proc Natl Acad Sci U S A 2006;103:5454—9.

[120] Qian BZ, Pollard JW. Macrophage diversity enhances tumor progression and metastasis. Cell 2010;141:39—51.

[121] Qian BZ, Li J, Zhang H, Kitamura T, Zhang J, Campion LR, et al. CCL2 recruits inflammatory monocytes to facilitate breast-tumor metastasis. Nature 2011;475:222—5.

[122] Rae F, Woods K, Sasmono T, Campanale N, Taylor D, Ovchinnikov DA, et al. Characterisation and trophic functions of murine embryonic macrophages based upon the use of a Csf1r-EGFP transgene reporter. Dev Biol 2007;308:232—46.

[123] Raes G, Brys L, Dahal BK, Brandt J, Grooten J, Brombacher F, et al. Macrophage galactose-type C-type lectins as novel markers for alternatively activated macrophages elicited by parasitic infections and allergic airway inflammation. J Leukoc Biol 2005;77:321—7.

[124] Rauh MJ, Sly LM, Kalesnikoff J, Hughes MR, Cao LP, Lam V, et al. The role of SHIP1 in macrophage programming and activation. Biochem Soc Trans 2004;32:785—8.

[125] Recalcati S, Locati M, Marini A, Santambrogio P, Zaninotto F, De Pizzol M, et al. Differential regulation of iron homeostasis during human macrophage polarized activation. Eur J Immunol 2010;40:824—35.

[126] Reimann M, Lee S, Loddenkemper C, Dörr JR, Tabor V, Aichele P, et al. Tumor stroma-derived TGF-beta limits myc-driven lymphomagenesis via Suv39h1-dependent senescence. Cancer Cell 2010;17:262—72.

[127] Roca H, Varsos ZS, Sud S, Craig MJ, Ying C, Pienta KJ. CCL2 and interleukin-6 promote survival of human CD11b+ peripheral blood mononuclear cells and induce M2-type macrophage polarization. J Biol Chem 2009;284:34342—54.

[128] Rodríguez-Prados JC, Través PG, Cuenca J, Rico D, Aragonés J, Martín-Sanz P, et al. Substrate fate in activated macrophages: a comparison between innate, classic, and alternative activation. J Immunol 2010;185:605—14.

[129] Rogers TL, Holen I. Tumor macrophages as potential targets of bisphosphonates. J Transl Med 2011;9:177.

[130] Rollins B. Chemokines and Cancer. Totowa, NJ: Humana Press; 1999.

[131] Ruckes T, Saul D, Van Snick J, Hermine O, Grassmann R. Autocrine antiapoptotic stimulation of cultured adult T-cell leukemia cells by overexpression of the chemokine I-309. Blood 2001;98:1150—9.

[132] Saji H, Koike M, Yamori T, Saji S, Seiki M, Matsushima K, et al. Significant correlation of monocyte chemoattractant protein-1 expression with neovascularization and progression of breast carcinoma. Cancer 2001;92:1085—91.

[133] Sakaguchi S. Naturally arising Foxp3-expressing CD25+CD4+ regulatory T cells in immunological tolerance to self and non-self. Nat Immunol 2005;6:345—52.

[134] Sangaletti S, Stoppacciaro A, Guiducci C, Torrisi MR, Colombo MP. Leukocyte, rather than tumor-produced SPARC, determines stroma and collagen type IV deposition in mammary carcinoma. J Exp Med 2003;198:1475—85.

[135] Savage ND, de Boer T, Walburg KV, Joosten SA, van Meijgaarden K, Geluk A, et al. Human anti-inflammatory macrophages induce Foxp3+ GITR+ CD25+ regulatory T cells, which suppress via membrane-bound TGFbeta-1. J Immunol 2008;181:2220—6.

[136] Scala S, Ottaiano A, Ascierto PA, Cavalli M, Simeone E, Giuliano P, et al. Expression of CXCR4 predicts poor prognosis in patients with malignant melanoma. Clin Cancer Res 2005;11:1835—41.

[137] Scarpino S, Stoppacciaro A, Ballerini F, Marchesi M, Prat M, Stella MC, et al. Papillary carcinoma of the thyroid: hepatocyte growth factor (HGF) stimulates tumor cells to release chemokines active in recruiting dendritic cells. Am J Pathol 2000;156:831—7.

[138] Schioppa T, Uranchimeg B, Saccani A, Biswas SK, Doni A, Rapisarda A, et al. Regulation of the chemokine receptor CXCR4 by hypoxia. J Exp Med 2003;198:1391—402.

[139] Schmidt T, Carmeliet P. Blood-vessel formation: Bridges that guide and unite. Nature 2010;465:697—9.

[140] Schoppmann SF, Birner P, Stockl J, Kalt R, Ullrich R, Caucig C, et al. Tumor-associated macrophages express lymphatic endothelial growth factors and are related to peritumoral lymphoangiogenesis. Am J Pathol 2002;161:947—56.

[141] Schutyser E, Struyf S, Proost P, Opdenakker G, Laureys G, Verhasselt B, et al. Identification of biologically active chemokine isoforms from ascitic fluid and elevated levels of CCL18/pulmonary and activation-regulated chemokine in ovarian carcinoma. J Biol Chem 2002;277:24584—93.

[142] Scotton CJ, Martinez FO, Smelt MJ, Sironi M, Locati M, Mantovani A, et al. Transcriptional profiling reveals complex regulation of the monocyte IL-1 beta system by IL-13. J Immunol 2005;174:834—45.

[143] Sessa C, De Braud F, Perotti A, Bauer J, Curigliano G, Noberasco C, et al. Trabectedin for women with ovarian carcinoma after treatment with platinum and taxanes fails. J Clin Oncol 2005;23:1867—74.

[144] Sica A, Saccani A, Bottazzi B, Polentarutti N, Vecchi A, van Damme J, et al. Autocrine production of IL-10 mediates defective IL-12 production and NF-kappa B activation in tumor-associated macrophages. J Immunol 2000;164:762—7.

[145] Sica A, Schioppa T, Mantovani A, Allavena P. Tumor-associated macrophages are a distinct M2 polarised population promoting tumor progression: potential targets of anti-cancer therapy. Eur J Cancer 2006;42:717—27.

[146] Sica A, Mantovani A. Macrophage plasticity and polarization: in vivo veritas. J Clin Invest 2012;122: 787—95.

[147] Sierra JR, Corso S, Caione L, Cepero V, Conrotto P, Cignetti A, et al. Tumor angiogenesis and progression are enhanced by Sema4D produced by tumor-associated macrophages. J Exp Med 2008;205:1673—85.

[148] Sinha P, Clements VK, Ostrand-Rosenberg S. Reduction of myeloid-derived suppressor cells and induction of M1 macrophages facilitate the rejection of established metastatic disease. J Immunol 2005; 174:636—45.

[149] Smith JR, Braziel RM, Paoletti S, Lipp M, Uguccioni M, Rosenbaum JT. Expression of B-cell-attracting chemokine 1 (CXCL13) by malignant lymphocytes and vascular endothelium in primary central nervous system lymphoma. Blood 2003;101:815—21.

[150] Solinas G, Schiarea S, Liguori M, Fabbri M, Pesce S, Zammataro L, et al. Tumor-conditioned macrophages secrete migration-stimulating factor: a new marker for M2-polarization, influencing tumor cell motility. J Immunol 2010;185:642—52.

[151] Takahashi H, Tsuda Y, Takeuchi D, Kobayashi M, Herndon DN, Suzuki F. Influence of systemic inflammatory response syndrome on host resistance against bacterial infections. Crit Care Med 2004;32:1879—85.

[152] Teichmann M, Meyer B, Beck A, Niedobitek G. Expression of the interferon-inducible chemokine IP-10 (CXCL10), a chemokine with proposed anti-neoplastic functions, in Hodgkin lymphoma and nasopharyngeal carcinoma. J Pathol 2005;20:68—75.

[153] Teruya-Feldstein J, Tosato G, Jaffe ES. The role of chemokines in Hodgkin's disease. Leuk Lymphoma 2000;38:363—71.

[154] Torroella-Kouri M, Ma X, Perry G, Ivanova M, Cejas PJ, Owen JL, et al. Diminished expression of transcription factors nuclear factor kappaB and CCAAT/enhancer binding protein underlies a novel tumor evasion mechanism affecting macrophages of mammary tumor-bearing mice. Cancer Res 2005;65: 10578—84.

[155] Tsuda Y, Takahashi H, Kobayashi M, Hanafusa T, Herndon DN, Suzuki F. Three different neutrophil subsets exhibited in mice with different susceptibilities to infection by methicillin-resistant Staphylococcus aureus. Immunity 2004;21:215—26.

[156] Ueno T, Toi M, Saji H, Muta M, Bando H, Kuroi K, et al. Significance of macrophage chemoattractant protein-1 in macrophage recruitment, angiogenesis, and survival in human breast cancer. Clin Cancer Res 2000;6:3282—389.

[157] Van den Brule F, Califice S, Garnier F, Fernandez PL, Berchuck A, Castronovo V. Galectin-1 accumulation in the ovary carcinoma peritumoral stroma is induced by ovary carcinoma cells and affects both cancer cell proliferation and adhesion to laminin-1 and fibronectin. Lab Invest 2003;83:377—86.

[158] Vasiljeva O, Papazoglou A, Kruger A, Brodoefel H, Korovin M, Deussing J, et al. Tumor cell-derived and macrophage-derived cathepsin B promotes progression and lung metastasis of mammary cancer. Cancer Res 2006;66:5242—50.

[159] Vats D, Mukundan L, Odegaard JI, Zhang L, Smith KL, Morel CR, et al. Oxidative metabolism and PGC-1beta attenuate macrophage-mediated inflammation. Cell Metab 2006;4:13—24.

[160] Vermeer MH, Dukers DF, ten Berge RL, Bloemena E, Wu L, Vos W, et al. Differential expression of thymus and activation regulated chemokine and its receptor CCR4 in nodal and cutaneous anaplastic large-cell lymphomas and Hodgkin's disease. Mod Pathol 2002;15:838—44.

[161] Vetrano S, Borroni EM, Sarukhan A, Savino B, Bonecchi R, Correale C, et al. The lymphatic system controls intestinal inflammation and inflammation-associated Colon Cancer through the chemokine decoy receptor D6. Gut 2009;59:197—206.

[162] Vicari AP, Caux C. Chemokines in cancer. Cytokine Growth Factor Rev 2002;13:143—54.

[163] Wang JM, Sherry B, Fivash MJ, Kelvin DJ, Oppenheim JJ. Human recombinant macrophage inflammatory protein-1 alpha and -beta and monocyte chemotactic and activating factor utilize common and unique receptors on human monocytes. J Immunol 1993;150:3022—9.

[164] Wang T, Niu G, Kortylewski M, Burdelya L, Shain K, Zhang S, et al. Regulation of the innate and adaptive immune responses by Stat-3 signaling in tumor cells. Nat Med 2004;10:48—54.

[165] Wels J, Kaplan RN, Rafii S, Lyden D. Migratory neighbors and distant invaders: tumor-associated niche cells. Genes Dev 2008;22:559—74.

[166] Wynn TA. Fibrotic disease and the T(H)1/T(H)2 paradigm. Nat Rev Immunol 2004;4:583—94.

[167] Yang H, Bocchetta M, Kroczynska B, Elmishad AG, Chen Y, Liu Z, et al. TNF-alpha inhibits asbestos-induced cytotoxicity via a NF-kappaB-dependent pathway, a possible mechanism for asbestos-induced oncogenesis. Proc Natl Acad Sci U S A 2006;103:10397—402.

[168] Yi F, Jaffe R, Prochownik EV. The CCL6 chemokine is differentially regulated by c-Myc and L-Myc, and promotes tumorigenesis and metastasis,. Cancer Res 2003;63:2923—32.

[169] Yoshimura T, Robinson EA, Tanaka S, Appella E, Kuratsu J, Leonard EJ. Purification and aminoacid analysis of two human glioma-derived monocyte chemoattractants. J Exp Med 1989;169:1449—59.

[170] Zeisberger SM, Odermatt B, Marty C, Zehnder-Fjallman AH, Ballmer-Hofer K, Schwendener RA. Clodronate-liposome-mediated depletion of tumor-associated macrophages: a new and highly effective antiangiogenic therapy approach. Br J Cancer 2006;95:272—81.

[171] Zhang J, Patel L, Pienta KJ. CC chemokine ligand 2 (CCL2) promotes prostate cancer tumorigenesis and metastasis. Cytokine Growth Factor Rev 2010;21:41—8.

[172] Zhu Z, Zheng T, Homer RJ, Kim YK, Chen NY, Cohn L, et al. Acidic mammalian chitinase in asthmatic Th2 inflammation and IL-13 pathway activation. Science 2004;304:1678—82.

[173] Zhu P, Baek SH, Bourk EM, Ohgi KA, Garcia-Bassets I, Sanjo H, et al. Macrophage/cancer cell interactions mediate hormone resistance by a nuclear receptor derepression pathway. Cell 2006;124:615—29.

CHAPTER 28

Tumor-induced Myeloid-derived Suppressor Cells

Suzanne Ostrand-Rosenberg, Pratima Sinha, Daniel W. Beury, Olesya Chornoguz, Katherine H. Parker
Dept. Biological Sciences, University of Maryland Baltimore County (UMBC), Baltimore, MD USA

I. INTRODUCTION

A. Early history of MDSC

The development of innovative immune-based cancer therapies that started in the early 1990s was viewed with extensive optimism and excitement, although it was tempered with the knowledge that patients with advanced cancer were frequently immune suppressed.

"Natural suppressor" cells were first identified in the mid 1980s in tumor-free mice where they inhibited T-cell proliferation and cytotoxic T lymphocytes (CTL) in an antigen- and MHC-independent manner [1], and reduced the growth of several tumor cell lines [2]. Studies on these cells were minimal until the late 1990s, when $CD34^+$ granulocytic/monocytic suppressor cells with the capacity to differentiate into dendritic cells (DC) were identified in patients with head and neck cancer [3–5]. These cells displayed diverse phenotypes and lacked markers for mature T, B, NK cells and macrophages, but expressed monocyte-myeloid markers. Similar suppressor cells were found in patients with other types of cancers. These cells prevented the activation of T lymphocytes within the tumor microenvironment [6] and in *in vitro* assays [7], and were chemoattracted by tumor-produced vascular endothelial growth factor (VEGF).

Suppressive myeloid cells were also observed in mice with transplanted [8–10] or spontaneous [11] tumors. The mouse cells displayed the granulocytic and macrophage markers Gr1 and CD11b/Mac1, and their accumulation *in vivo* and *in vitro* correlated with tumor-produced granulocyte/monocyte-colony stimulating factor (GM-CSF). These cells inhibited antigen-specific activation of $CD8^+$ T cells and required cell-to-cell contact to mediate their effects [9,10,12].

The first hint of how these cells suppressed came from studies in which patients' decreased T-cell production of cytokines was observed to correlate with high levels of granulocytes and reduced expression of T-cell receptor (TcR) ζ chain [13]. Cytokine production was restored by the addition of catalase, a hydrogen peroxide scavenger, suggesting that reactive oxygen species (ROS), such as H_2O_2, mediated suppression [14]. In early reports the suppressive cells were referred to by various names including immature myeloid cells (ImC), myeloid suppressor cells (MSC), immature macrophages (iMacs), etc. The lack of a uniform nomenclature was confusing, and the term "myeloid-derived suppressor cells" (MDSC) was adapted in 2007 [15].

473

B. MDSC regulate tumor progression through multiple immune and nonimmune mechanisms

Studies in mice demonstrated that MDSC are a key cell population that facilitates primary tumor progression and metastasis, and that reducing MDSC in combination with adoptive T-cell transfer or active T-cell-targeted immunotherapy results in rejection of primary tumor and/or metastatic disease [11,16–22]. Studies with cancer patients demonstrated that levels of circulating MDSC are correlated with clinical cancer stage and metastatic tumor burden [23], and are a prognostic indicator of tumor progression [24]. Treatment of cancer patients with drugs that reduce MDSC levels as well as *in vitro* studies with patients' peripheral blood mononuclear cells (PBMC) demonstrated that much of the immune suppression in cancer patients is due to MDSC and that removal or inactivation of MDSC restores immune competence [25–28]. MDSC impair antitumor immunity through their suppression of adaptive and innate immune cells (CD4+ T, CD8+ T, NK, M1 macrophages, and dendritic cells (DC)), and by facilitating the development of cells that promote tumor progression (M2 macrophages, T-regulatory cells (T regs)) (Figure 28.1).

MDSC also promote tumor progression through non-immune mechanisms. Their production of matrix metalloprotease-9 (MMP-9) drives VEGF release and subsequent tumor neovascularization [29–31], and they facilitate tumor cell invasion and metastasis [32]. MDSC also induce epithelial mesenchymal transition (EMT) thus promoting cancer dissemination [33]. Because they promote tumor growth through multiple mechanisms, MDSC are a significant obstacle to active T-cell-based cancer immunotherapies and the development of adaptive and innate antitumor immunity.

C. MDSC are also present in noncancerous settings

MDSC are also induced in noncancerous disease settings. Infection increases MDSC levels in individuals with sepsis [34,35], toxoplasmosis [36], candidiasis [37], Leishmaniasis [38], or infected with Trypanosoma cruzi [39]. MDSC also accumulate in stressed [40,41] and aging individuals [42], and during autoimmune disease including inflammatory bowel disease [43], mouse models of experimental autoimmune encephalomyelitis (EAE) [44], and uveoretinitis [45]. Because they suppress immunity, MDSC are being used to combat undesirable

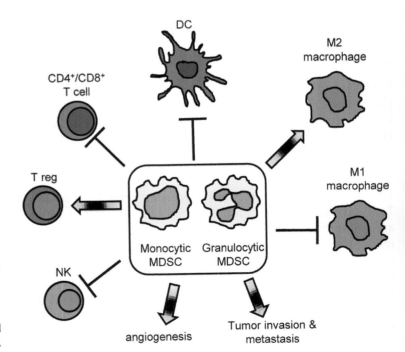

FIGURE 28.1

MDSC promote tumor progression and metastasis through multiple mechanisms. MDSC inhibit antitumor immunity by suppressing the development of dendritic cells (DC), blocking the activation and trafficking of CD4+ and CD8+ T cells, blocking the cytotoxic activity of natural killer (NK) cells, polarizing macrophages from an M1 to M2 phenotype, promoting the development of T-regulatory cells (Tregs), and promoting angiogenesis and tumor invasion and metastasis.

autoimmunity. A few examples include retention of allogeneic islet grafts [46], induction of Tregs to protect against type I diabetes [47], inhibition of graft-vs-host-disease [48], and reduction of autoimmunity in multiple sclerosis patients [49].

This chapter describes the role of MDSC in mediating immune suppression in individuals with cancer. Other chapters discuss the role of additional tumor-promoting immune cell populations including DC (Chapter 18) and tumor-associated macrophages (Chapter 27).

II. MOUSE AND HUMAN MDSC ARE A HETEROGENEOUS MIXTURE OF IMMATURE MYELOID CELLS

Mouse and human tumor-induced MDSC are a heterogeneous population of cells derived from myeloid progenitors. Based on their phenotype and morphology, MDSC are immature cells at different stages of myelopoiesis. The heterogeneity encompasses differences in expression of cell surface markers, molecules responsible for suppressive activity, stage of differentiation within myelopoiesis, and nuclear morphology. The variation in MDSC populations is partially due to the unique *in vivo* microenvironment in which MDSC arise, as a result of different tumors producing different combinations of factors that drive MDSC development. MDSC phenotype may also vary with the growth kinetics and stage of cancer because tumors evolve and change through the process of immunoediting [50,51]. Despite this potential for variation, mouse and human MDSC have been divided into two major subpopulations: monocytic (MO-MDSC) and granulocytic (PMN-MDSC) MDSC. Since mouse and human MDSC are phenotypically distinct, they will be described separately.

A. Mouse MDSC phenotype

Mouse MDSC are identified in the liver [52], spleen, blood, and at the tumor site of tumor-bearing mice based on their expression of particular cell surface makers (see Table 28.1 for a comparison of the phenotype of mouse and human MDSC and their ability to suppress T-cell activation). All mouse MDSC express the granulocytic cell surface marker Gr1, and the monocyte/macrophage cell surface marker CD11b. Gr1 includes the Ly6C and Ly6G moieties which are the markers that distinguish MO-MDSC from PMN-MDSC, with PMN-MDSC being $Gr1^{hi/med}CD11b^+Ly6C^-Ly6G^+$ and MO-MDSC being $Gr1^{med}CD11b^+Ly6C^+Ly6G^{low/-}$. PMN-MDSC are polymorphonuclear, while MO-MDSC are mononuclear. MO-MDSC are side scatter low (SSC^{low}), while PMN-MDSC are SSC^{hi}. The two subpopulations also differ in the effector molecules they use to suppress T-cell activation. PMN-MDSC contain Arg1 and ROS, while MO-MDSC also contain iNOS (NOS2). MO-MDSC usually express higher levels of F4/80 (macrophage marker), CD115 (c-fms the receptor for M-CSF/CSF-1), and CCR2 (receptor for MCP-1), although these markers are not uniformly expressed by MDSC induced by all tumors [53–57]. A small percentage of mouse MDSC also express the co-inhibitory molecule programmed death ligand-1 (PD-L1), although PD-L1 expression does not contribute to MDSC suppression [54]. MO-MDSC, but not PMN-MDSC, mature in vitro and acquire markers of macrophages (F4/80) and DC (CD11c) when cultured with GM-CSF [54].

The phenotypes described in the previous paragraph are for MDSC obtained from either the spleen and/or blood of tumor-bearing mice. Splenic and blood MDSC from the same tumor-bearing mouse are similar in phenotype [56]. Tumor-infiltrating MDSC also have a similar phenotype as blood and splenic MDSC from the same tumor-bearing mouse, although they are more suppressive on a per-cell basis [58]. The increased potency is likely due to the increased production of Arg1 and NO that occurs when MDSC are in the immediate tumor microenvironment [59]. Low levels of $Gr1^+CD11b^+$ cells are also present in the blood and spleen of tumor-free mice and have a phenotype similar to $Gr1^+CD11b^+$ cells of tumor-bearing mice [56].

TABLE 28.1 Phenotypes Of Mouse and Human MDSC

Species	MDSC population	Markers	References
Mouse	All MDSC	Gr1$^+$CD11b$^+$	[9,11,12,16,53,54,189]
		Arg1$^+$	[16,54,93,94]
	Monocytic	Ly6G$^{-/low}$	[53,190]
		CD11b$^+$SSC^{low}	
		Ly6C^{high}Ly6G$^-$	[53,54]
		mononuclear	[53,190]
		iNOS$^+$ (NOS2)	[54]
		ROS$^+$	[54]
		F4/80$^{med/hi}$	[53,54,166,191]
		CD115$^{med/hi}$	[53,55]
		CCR2$^{med/hi}$	[53,112]
		IL-4Rα^+ (CD124)	[53,57,166,191]
	Granulocytic	Ly6G$^+$CD11b$^+$SSC^{high}	[53]
		Ly6C$^{low/-}$Ly6G$^+$	[53,54]
		polymorphonuclear	[53,190]
		iNOS$^-$ (NOS2)	[54]
		ROS$^+$	[54]
		F4/80$^{low/-}$	[53,54,166]
		CD115$^-$	[53]
		CCR2^{low}	[53]
		IL-4R$\alpha^{+/-}$ (CD124)	[53,166]
Human	Not associated with a specific subpopulation	CD33	[7,23,25,70,192−194]
		CD3$^-$	[7]
		CD16$^-$	
		CD19$^-$	
		CD20$^-$	
		CD56$^-$	
		HLA-DR$^{low/-}$	[7,23,75,192]
		CD11b$^+$	[23]
		Arg1	[72,73]
		S100A9	[155]
	Monocytic	CD14$^+$	[64,75]
		CD15$^{low/-}$	[64]
		IL-4Rα^+	[76]
	Granulocytic	CD14$^-$	[64,73]
		CD15$^+$	[64,73]

The Gr1$^+$CD11b$^+$ phenotype and polymorphonuclear morphology of PMN-MDSC are also characteristic of neutrophils, and have raised the question of whether MDSC are a distinct population from neutrophils. MDSC are not neutrophils, but are progenitor cells with the capacity to differentiate into neutrophils. In contrast to neutrophils, PMN-MDSC do not express CD244.1 or M-CSF receptor. Neutrophils are more phagocytic and express higher levels of TNFα and lysosomal proteins as compared to PMN-MDSC. Most importantly, PMN-MDSC, but not neutrophils, suppress T-cell activation [60].

B. Human MDSC phenotype

Human MDSC have been studied most extensively in patients with solid tumors where virtually all patients have elevated levels of MDSC that directly correlate with clinical cancer stage and metastatic tumor burden [23] (reviewed in [61−66]). Specifically, MDSC have been identified in patients with head and neck squamous cell carcinoma [7,67−69], breast cancer [7,14,23,27], non-small cell lung cancer [7,23,28,67,70,71], renal cell carcinoma [72,73], melanoma [23,74−77], colon and colorectal cancer [14,23,27,76], gastrointestinal cancer [78], bladder cancer [79], pancreatic adenocarcinoma [14,23,24,80,81], esophageal cancer [24], urothelial tract cancer [67], prostate cancer [23,82], gastric cancer [24], and sarcoma, carcinoid, gall bladder, adrenocortical, thyroid, and hepatocellular carcinoma [23,83]. Elevated MDSC levels are also in the blood of patients with hematological malignancies, including multiple myeloma [69,84] and non-Hodgkin's lymphoma [85].

There is extensive heterogeneity with respect to the expression and level of cell surface markers in human MDSC. Therefore, the phenotype of human MDSC is not as clearly defined as the phenotype of mouse MDSC (Table 28.1). Much of the confusion is due to the lack of a human analog for mouse Gr1. The marker used to identify human "natural suppressor" cells in early studies (CD34) is no longer widely used [4,6,86]. Instead, the monocyte/macrophage marker CD11b, the monocyte differentiation antigen CD14, and the mature monocyte marker CD15 are used, in addition to IL-4Rα, and the myeloid lineage marker CD33. Human MDSC also lack HLA-DR and the lineage markers characteristic of lymphocytes and natural killer cells. The variation in expression of these markers makes it difficult to provide a definitive phenotype for human MDSC. This heterogeneity also underscores the necessity to demonstrate that the putative MDSC population is functionally suppressive. The uncertainty in phenotype may be resolved in the future if additional MDSC subpopulations are characterized.

Despite this lack of consensus, human MDSC are categorized as either MO-MDSC or PMN-MDSC based on their expression of CD14 vs. CD15. Human MO-MDSC are typically CD11b$^+$CD14$^+$CD15$^-$IL-4Rα$^+$, while human PMN-MDSC are CD11b$^+$CD14$^-$CD15$^+$ [64].

Recent reviews summarize the markers of human MDSC [61−65].

III. MDSC USE DIVERSE SUPPRESSIVE MECHANISMS TO INHIBIT ANTITUMOR IMMUNITY

MDSC act on multiple target cells and are exceptionally multifaceted in the mechanisms they use to suppress antitumor immunity.

A. MDSC effects on T-cell activation

Suppression of T-cell activation is a hallmark of mouse and human MDSC function. Mouse MDSC suppress anti-CD3/CD28-activated T cells and TcR transgenic T cells activated *in vitro* with cognate peptide [16,17]. Adoptive transfer of MDSC into tumor-free mice prevents antigen-driven T-cell activation [81,87]. Studies with PBMC from cancer patients demonstrated that depletion of MDSC significantly increased T-cell activation *in vitro* [28].

MDSC suppression of CD8$^+$ T cells is considered antigen-specific since mouse MDSC consistently express MHC class I molecules and antibody blocking of MHC class I abrogates suppression (reviewed in [88,89]). It is controversial whether suppression of CD4$^+$ T cells is antigen-specific or nonspecific. Most mouse and human MDSC do not express MHC class II or express very low levels of MHC II, suggesting it is unlikely that CD4$^+$ T-cell suppression involves presentation of MHC II/peptide complexes. The finding that MHC class II$^-$ MDSC suppress both syngeneic and allogeneic cognate antigen-activated TcR transgenic CD4$^+$ T cells argues that suppression is not antigen-specific [16]. MDSC from tumor-bearing MHC II-deficient mice have similar suppressive activity as MDSC from wild type mice further supporting a nonspecific mechanism (Clements and Ostrand-Rosenberg, unpublished results). A recent study using the same MHC class II-deficient mice concludes that CD4 suppression is antigen-specific provided MDSC express a sufficient level of MHC class II [90]. However, most MDSC have no or very low levels of MHC II so most suppression of CD4$^+$ T cells is probably not antigen-specific.

In vitro studies demonstrated that MDSC-mediated suppression is significantly decreased if MDSC and T cells are separated by a semipermeable membrane, indicating that either cell-to-cell contact or very close proximity is required. These findings are in agreement with the identification of Arg1, nitric oxide (NO), ROS, and peroxynitrite (ONOO⁻) as secreted MDSC products that mediate T-cell suppression. Since Arg1, NO, and ROS are themselves not antigen-specific, it is likely that they are released in an antigen-specific fashion, but once released, act on any target cell in their local environment. Since these molecules diffuse and turn over rapidly, they are likely to be effective only for a short time in the region of their immediate release. Suppressive mechanisms used by MDSC have been recently reviewed [69,88,91,92].

1. ARGINASE AND NITRIC OXIDE

Arg1 and inducible nitric oxide synthase (iNOS or NOS2) degrade L-arginine and generate NO, respectively (Figure 28.2A). Studies with both mouse and human MDSC showed that inhibition of Arg1 restores T-cell activation in the presence of MDSC, demonstrating that Arg1 is an important immune suppressive molecule of MDSC [73,93,94]. Arg1 suppresses T-cell activation by depriving T cells of the amino acid L-arginine. This deprivation downregulates the TcR-associated ζ chain [13,95] which is essential for T-cell activation because it activates cyclin D3 and cyclin-dependent kinase 4 which initiate cell proliferation [96]. NO suppresses T-cell activation by destabilizing IL-2 mRNA and blocking the phosphorylation of JAK1, JAK3, STAT5, ERK, and AKT. These molecules are downstream of the IL-2 receptor and their activation and IL-2 synthesis are essential for T-cell proliferation [97]. MDSC within the hypoxic microenvironment of solid tumors have elevated levels of Arg1 and iNOS caused by activation of hypoxia-inducible factor-1α (HIF-1α). Under the influence of HIF-1α, tumor-infiltrating MDSC differentiate into macrophages, demonstrating the plasticity of MDSC and the impact of their environment [98]. L-arginine metabolism by MDSC and the immune suppressive effects of Arg1 and NO are reviewed in Chapter 34 [97,99].

2. REACTIVE OXYGEN SPECIES

ROS are well-established products of MDSC that block T-cell activation since inhibition of ROS decreases the suppressive potency of both mouse [100] and human MDSC (Figure 28.2B)

FIGURE 28.2
MDSC suppress T-cell activation by the production of arginase, NO, and reactive oxygen species (ROS). (A) Suppressive effects of arginase. L-arginine is the substrate for arginase 1 (arg) and inducible nitric oxide synthase (iNOS) which degrade L-arginine to urea, ornithine, NO, and other L-arginine metabolites. Arginase released from MDSC depletes T cells of arginine which downregulates the TcRζ chain and prevents T cells from proliferating by inhibiting cyclin D3 and cdk4. NO released by MDSC blocks T-cell activation by destabilizing IL-2 mRNA and preventing signaling through the transcription factors JAK1, JAK3, STAT5, ERK, and AKT which are downstream of the IL-2 receptor. (B) Suppressive effects of ROS. Tumor cell-produced factors activate (green arrow) STAT3 which activates the heterodimeric enzyme NADPH oxidase (NOX2). Activated NOX2 increases intracellular levels of ROS, including NO and superoxide (O₂⁻). NO + O₂⁻ react to form peroxynitrite (ONOO⁻) which inhibits T cell-mediated killing by nitrating and nitrosylating the TcR of CD8⁺ T cells and the MHC class I/peptide complex of tumor cells.

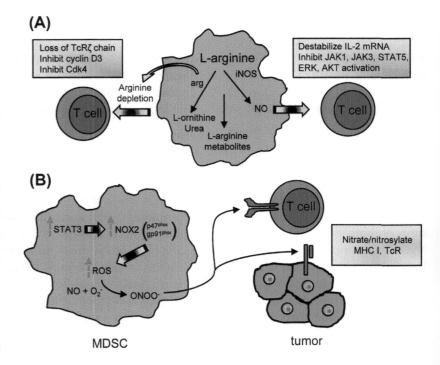

[68,101]. Treatment of MDSC with catalase or uric acid reduced suppressive potency, indicating that hydrogen peroxide and peroxynitrite are partially responsible for suppression. Treatment with an arginase inhibitor reduced suppressive activity and ROS content, demonstrating that arginine metabolites probably contribute to the generation of ROS [100]. Intracellular levels of ROS are regulated by the enzyme NADPH oxidase (NOX2) which produces superoxide (O_2^-) via oxidation of NADPH and subsequent reduction of O_2. NOX2 consists of six subunits, two of which are implicated in MDSC suppression: p47^{phox} and gp91^{phox}. MDSC deficient for gp91^{phox} have limited suppressive activity and rapidly differentiate into macrophages and DC, confirming the role of ROS in MDSC function [68]. Expression of the p47^{phox} and gp91^{phox} subunits is regulated by the transcription factor STAT3. Tumor cell-conditioned medium activated the JAK2/STAT3 pathway, induced proliferation of immature myeloid cells, and prevented their differentiation into DC. STAT3-deficient progenitor cells were nonresponsive to conditioned medium and STAT3 inhibitors prevented proliferation [102]. STAT3 activation in MDSC also regulates MDSC production of VEGF and tumor angiogenesis [103]. Therefore, phosphorylation of STAT3 is a key regulatory step driving the accumulation of MDSC, maintaining MDSC as immature cells, enhancing MDSC suppression, and facilitating MDSC-mediated angiogenesis.

Peroxynitrite is among the most powerful oxidants activated by STAT3. It arises from the spontaneous interaction of NO and superoxide, and nitrates and nitrosylates amino acids. MDSC-generated peroxynitrite disarms tumor-reactive T cells and protects tumor cells against CD8-mediated T-cell lysis. Peroxynitrite nitrates the TcR of T cells, thereby altering TcR structure and preventing T-cell recognition of MHC/class I-peptide complexes [104]. Peroxynitrite also nitrates MHC class I molecules, thereby altering their structure so they cannot be recognized by T cells [105]. The short half-life and rapid diffusion rate of ROS are likely the reasons that MDSC-mediated suppression requires close proximity of MDSC and target cells. Given that MDSC, tumor cells, and T cells are closely associated within the tumor microenvironment, these mechanisms are probably major contributors to MDSC-mediated immune suppression.

3. CYSTINE/CYSTEINE DEPRIVATION

MDSC also sequester cysteine, which is an essential amino acid for T cells (Figure 28.3). Most cells generate cysteine by importing extracellular cystine (oxidized form) and reducing it to cysteine in their intracellular reducing environment, or by converting intracellular methionine to cysteine. Import of cystine requires the heterodimeric x_c^- transporter and conversion of methionine requires cystathionase. T cells lack cystathionase and the xCT chain of the x_c^- transporter and therefore cannot generate cysteine either by importing cystine or conversion of methionine [106–108]. Because cysteine is essential for proliferation and protein synthesis, T cells must obtain their cysteine from exogenous sources. For this reason, the reducing agent, 2-mercaptoethanol, is typically included in *in vitro* T-cell studies so that cystine is reduced extracellularly and free cysteine is available for T-cell utilization. *In vivo*, T cells obtain their cysteine during antigen processing and presentation, when antigen-presenting cells (APC; macrophages and/or DC) complex with T cells. APC then release excess cysteine which is imported by T cells through their neutral amino acid transporter, ASC. APC also release thioredoxin which reduces cystine to cysteine, making additional cysteine available to T cells [109]. Because cysteine is rapidly oxidized to cystine in the extracellular environment, T-cell uptake of exogenous cysteine is only efficient when T cells and antigen-presenting cells are in very close proximity during the antigen presentation process [108].

MDSC lack cystathionase, do not express the ASC transporter, and do not export cysteine [108]. Radioactive uptake studies demonstrated that MDSC compete with macrophages and DC for extracellular cystine, and that as MDSC levels increase, cystine is depleted in the extracellular environment. Increasing levels of MDSC in tumor-bearing mice correlated with decreased levels of cystine in serum, demonstrating that MDSC decrease cystine availability

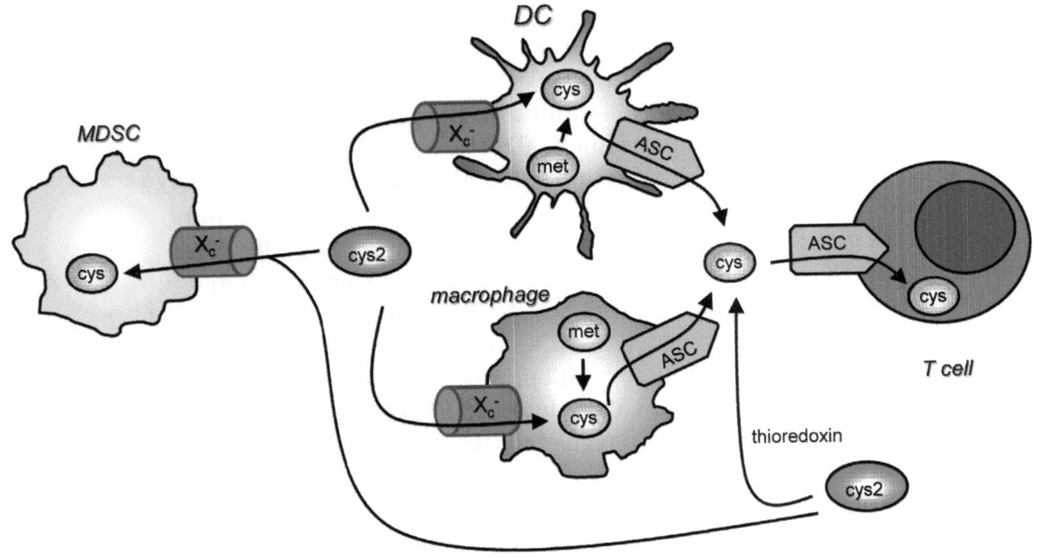

FIGURE 28.3

MDSC suppress T-cell activation by sequestering cystine/cysteine. Macrophages and DC generate cysteine (cys) by importing cystine (cys2) through the X_c^- transporter (xcT+4F2 heterodimer), and reducing it intracellularly to cysteine (cys), or by cystathionase-mediated conversion of intracellular methionine to cysteine. DC and macrophages export excess cysteine through the ASC neutral amino acid transporter. Macrophages and DC also release thioredoxin which reduces extracellular cystine to cysteine. T cells do not produce cystathionase or xcT and therefore must obtain their cysteine from macrophages and DC during antigen processing and presentation when these cells are in close proximity. MDSC also do not produce cystathionase so they generate cysteine exclusively by importing cystine through their X_c^- transporter. MDSC do not express ASC transporter so they do not export cysteine. MDSC compete with DC and macrophages for cystine, and as MDSC levels increase they deplete their environment of cystine. In the absence of extracellular cystine, there is no substrate for thioredoxin and DC and macrophages do not produce excess cysteine, resulting in inhibition of T-cell activation and proliferation.

in vivo. The diminished supply of extracellular cystine limits the amount of cysteine available to T cells because (i) cystine is unavailable for reduction by thioredoxin; and (ii) APC must generate their cysteine exclusively from methionine and therefore do not produce excess cysteine for export. As a result, T-cell activation is arrested due to insufficient cysteine [108]. Provision of a stabilized extracellular form of cysteine (N-acetylated cysteine) restores T-cell activation *in vitro* [108], and improves T-cell activation *in vivo* (Srivastava and Ostrand-Rosenberg, unpublished results).

4. MDSC FACILITATE THE DEVELOPMENT OF T-REGULATORY CELLS

MDSC also induce forkhead box P3$^+$ (Foxp3) CD4$^+$ T regs. In mouse tumor systems Treg induction requires IFN-γ and IL-10, is independent of NO [55], TGFβ, and IL-13, but is Arg1-dependent[110] as shown *in vitro* using Arg1 and iNOS inhibitors, antibodies to IFN-γ and IL-10, and *in vivo* using IL-10 receptor-deficient mice. CD40-deficient MO-MDSC do not induce Tregs, demonstrating that CD40 is required for mouse MDSC induction of Tregs [111]. Monocytic MDSC from hepatocellular carcinoma patients (CD14$^+$HLA-DR$^{low/-}$) also induce CD4$^+$CD25$^+$Foxp3$^+$ Tregs following co-culture with T cells isolated from autologous PBMC [83].

B. MDSC disrupt T-cell trafficking

T-cell activation and effector function require trafficking of T cells to lymph nodes and tumor sites. Both of these trafficking processes are disrupted by MDSC. MDSC from mice carrying tumors secreting high levels of GM-CSF are MO-MDSC that express the chemokine receptor CCR2 [112]. CCL2, the ligand for CCR2, is present in the tumor microenvironment and is a chemoattractant for CCR2$^+$ MDSC [113]. Tumors secreting GM-CSF contain few CD8$^+$

T cells. Depletion of intratumoral CCR2$^+$ MDSC produces an infusion of CD8$^+$ T cells that facilitates the therapeutic efficacy of adoptive T-cell transfer [112].

L-selectin (CD62L) is a homing receptor for T cells and is critical for directing naïve T cells to lymph nodes and areas of inflammation. Peripheral blood T cells in tumor-bearing mice have reduced expression of CD62L. CD62L decrease is driven by MDSC since (i) co-culture of naïve T cells with MDSC reduces T-cell CD62L; (ii) aged tumor-free mice have elevated MDSC and reduced CD62L; and (iii) tumor-free mice treated with the MDSC inducing agent plasminogen activator urokinase contain T cells with reduced CD62L. MDSC downregulate CD62L by translocating ADAM 17 (disintegrin and metalloproteinase 17), an enzyme that cleaves cell surface CD62L, from their cytosol to their plasma membrane [114].

C. MDSC promote tumor progression through cross-talk with macrophages

MDSC also drive suppression of macrophages, and macrophages reciprocally increase the potency of MDSC. Macrophages within the tumor microenvironment facilitate tumor invasion and metastasis through multiple immune and non-immune mechanisms [115—118], and display extensive plasticity with M1 and M2 phenotypes representing the extremes. M1-type macrophages are cytotoxic for tumor cells, function as APC to activate tumor-reactive cytotoxic T cells for a type 1 immune response, and produce IL-12 which activates natural killer (NK) cells (reviewed in Chapter 9 [119]). Tumor associated macrophages (TAMs), however, are M2-type cells (also known as "alternatively activated macrophages") that are IL-12^{low}IL-10^{high}. The loss of IL-12 and increase in IL-10 inhibits NK development, and polarizes immunity towards a tumor-promoting type 2 phenotype. M2 polarization is driven by multiple cell populations, including type 2 CD4$^+$ T cells [120], T regs [121], B cells [122,123], tumor cells [124], and MDSC. MDSC polarize through their production of IL-10 which downregulates macrophage production of IL-12. Macrophages, in turn, increase MDSC production of IL-10, thereby exacerbating their own polarization. This process requires cell-to-cell contact, probably for maintenance of a high local concentration of IL-10, and is amplified by inflammation [125].

D. MDSC inhibit NK- and NKT-mediated antitumor immunity

MDSC suppress NK cytotoxic function and inhibit NK production of IFNγ through a mechanism that is cell-contact dependent [126—128]. Mouse hepatocellular carcinoma-induced MDSC mediate this effect by plasma membrane-bound TGFβ [126]. MDSC recognize NK cells via the NK receptor NKp30 [129] and downregulate expression of the NKG2D receptor [126]. Heightened inflammation in the tumor microenvironment induces a subpopulation of Ly6C^{low} granulocytic MDSC that are particularly effective in inhibiting NK function [130].

Similar to M1 and M2 macrophages, NKT I cells facilitate tumor rejection, while NKT II cells enhance tumor growth. NKT II-produced IL-13 increased the accumulation of MDSC in a CD1d-specific fashion in fibrosarcoma-bearing mice. These MDSC produced high levels of TGFβ which blocked immune surveillance and facilitated the recurrence of primary fibrosarcomas [131].

IV. INFLAMMATION DRIVES MDSC ACCUMULATION AND SUPPRESSION

A causative relationship between chronic inflammation and increased risk of cancer was first postulated more than 140 years ago [132]. Epidemiological studies, evaluation of patients on long-term nonsteroidal anti-inflammatory drugs (NSAIDS), and experimental studies blocking inflammation have confirmed the connection [133—135]. Chronic inflammation promotes tumor progression through nonimmune and immune mechanisms, with MDSC

481

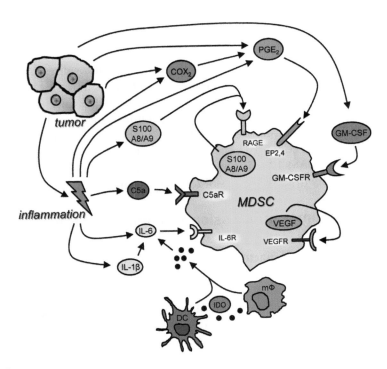

FIGURE 28.4
Pro-inflammatory mediators and growth factors drive the development of MDSC. Chronic inflammation includes the production of pro-inflammatory mediators such as PGE2, COX2, IL-6, S100A8/A9, and complement component C5a which bind to their respective receptors on MDSC and drive the accumulation of MDSC. Chronic inflammation also includes the production of IL-1β; however, MDSC do not express the IL-1 receptor, so IL-1β drives MDSC indirectly through its downstream effector IL-6. Many tumor cells also produce COX2, PGE2, IL-6, and/or GM-CSF. Macrophage and DC production of IDO drive MDSC accumulation by upregulating IL-6. MDSC production of S100A8/A9 and VEGF provide for autocrine growth regulation.

induction being a dominant immune mechanism. Pro-inflammatory mediators play an essential role in the accumulation and suppressive potency of MDSC, and chronic inflammation probably facilitates tumor development by inducing MDSC that inhibit immune surveillance and adaptive T-cell-mediated immunity [133,136,137]. Inflammation-induced MDSC development is reviewed in [133,136] and described below. Figure 28.4 illustrates pro-inflammatory mediators that induce MDSC development.

A. Prostaglandin E2 (PGE$_2$) and cyclooxygenase 2 (COX$_2$)

Inflammatory PGE$_2$ is generated from arachidonic acid through the action of the enzyme COX$_2$. PGE$_2$ mediates its effects through four prostanoid receptors (EP1, 2, 3 and 4), and many mouse and human tumors, as well as MDSC, produce PGE$_2$ and COX$_2$. Regular use of NSAIDS, including COX$_2$ inhibitors, protects high-risk individuals from developing cancer and delays tumor growth [138]. The protumor effects of PGE$_2$ and COX$_2$ are partially mediated by their induction of MDSC as shown by studies in which treatment with COX$_2$ inhibitors or NSAIDS delayed tumor progression, reduced MDSC levels, and/or improved antitumor immunity [139–143]. *In vivo* or *in vitro* treatment of tumor-bearing mice with antibodies to PGE$_2$ or with an EP-4 antagonist reduced MDSC expression of Arg1 [140], while treatment with celecoxib reduced intratumor levels of the MDSC chemoattractant CCL2 [139]. EP-2-deficiency delays tumor progression and reduces MDSC levels [141].

PGE$_2$ induces MDSC by expanding mouse bone marrow progenitor cells at the expense of DC [141], while COX$_2$ inhibitors and PGE$_2$ antagonists prevent MDSC differentiation [141,144]. PGE$_2$ similarly drives human peripheral blood progenitor cells to differentiate into CD11b$^+$CD33$^+$ cells that express high levels of NOS2, IL-10, Arg1, and IL-4Rα [145].

B. IL-1β and IL-6

IL-1β is a potent driver of MDSC accumulation and suppression. Mouse mammary carcinoma or fibrosarcoma cells transfected with a secreted form of IL-1β produce a highly inflammatory tumor microenvironment and are more aggressive than their non-IL-1β-expressing counterparts. IL-1β-transfected tumors also induce higher levels of MDSC that are more suppressive for both T cells and NK cells [130,146,147]. Similarly, transgenic mice overexpressing IL-1β in the stomach develop inflammation and gastric cancer, and mobilize MDSC [148]. Mice deficient for IL-1 receptor antagonist (IL-1Ra), the natural inhibitor of IL-1β, developed high levels of MDSC with elevated suppressive potency [149]. Conversely, tumor-bearing IL-1-receptor-deficient mice [149] and wild type mice treated with soluble IL-1Ra [147] had slower growing tumors and less suppressive MDSC. IL-1β extends the half-life of MDSC [146] by increasing MDSC resistance to Fas-FasL mediated apoptosis [150].

As described in Section IIIC, MDSC-produced IL-10 downregulates macrophage production of IL-12. IL-1β drives this effect by increasing MDSC production of IL-10, which decreases macrophage production of IL-12, and polarizes immunity towards a tumor-promoting type 2 response. Alteration of MDSC phenotype occurs by signaling through the TLR4 pathway and involves an increase in MDSC expression of the LPS receptor CD14 [151].

IL-6-transfected tumor cells also increase MDSC levels [149], and IL-6 in combination with GM-CSF drives differentiation of MDSC from mouse bone marrow progenitor cells *in vitro*. When adoptively transferred into syngeneic mice these MDSC sustain survival of allogeneic islet transplants by tolerizing T cells. The tolerogenic function of *in vitro* generated MDSC and tumor-induced MDSC required expression of the C/EBPβ transcription factor that regulates "emergency" granulopoiesis [87].

IL-6 induction of MDSC is also likely to contribute to the tolerogenic activity of indoleamine 2,3 dioxygenase (IDO) (see Chapters 32 and 33 for a discussion of IDO). IDO1 nullizygous mice are resistant to oncogenic Kras-induced lung tumor formation and metastatic mammary carcinoma, and have reduced levels of IL-6 in their tumor tissue. MDSC from the IDO1-deficient mice are less suppressive than MDSC from IDO1-sufficient mice and provision of IL-6 restores MDSC function, consistent with the concept that IDO1 induction of IL-6 drives MDSC potency [152].

IL-6 is considered to be downstream of IL-1β in the inflammatory cascade. The finding that provision of IL-6 to IL-1 receptor-deficient mice restores MDSC levels supports this order [149], and suggests that IL-1β and IL-6 induce MDSC through a common induction pathway.

C. S100A8/A9

Heterodimeric S100A8/A9 is present in most inflammatory conditions where it amplifies inflammation by chemoattracting leukocytes that release additional inflammatory molecules. S100A9-deficient mice immunologically reject transplanted tumors, an effect that is reversed by adoptive transfer of wild type tumor-induced MDSC. Tumor-free transgenic mice over-expressing S100A9 have reduced levels of DC and macrophages, and accumulate MDSC. Overexpression of S100A9 in embryonic stem cells results in defective DC development and excess differentiation of MDSC [153]. S100A8/A9 also chemoattracts MDSC by binding to N-glycan-tagged plasma membrane receptors, including Receptor for Advanced Glycation Endproducts (RAGE). Receptor binding initiates signaling through STAT3 and NF-κB [56,153]. MDSC themselves synthesize S100A8/A9, thereby facilitating an autocrine feedback loop that amplifies MDSC accumulation [56,154]. S100A9 has recently been identified as a marker for CD14$^+$HLA-DR$^-$ human MDSC [155].

D. Complement component C5a

C5a (also known as anaphylatoxin), a pro-inflammatory product of the classical and lectin complement pathways, protects and enhances the growth of established tumors. MDSC express the receptor for C5a, and are chemoattracted to C5a that accumulates within tumor vasculature. In addition to recruiting MDSC to the tumor microenvironment, C5a also upregulates ROS, reactive nitrogen species, and Arg1, thereby amplifying MDSC suppression [156–159].

E. Vascular endothelial growth factor

Early studies demonstrated that in addition to its function in angiogenesis, VEGF drives the accumulation of MDSC by perturbing myelopoiesis. High levels of VEGF block DC development, reduce T-cell activation, and increase the numbers of $Gr1^+$ cells [160], while treatment with antibodies to VEGF improves T-cell-based immunotherapy and delays tumor progression [161]. Oxidative stress, which is characteristic of solid tumors, increases VEGF receptor expression on MDSC [162]. VEGF is also a chemoattractant for MDSC [86,163] and since MDSC synthesize VEGF, they support their own progression through an autocrine pathway. In addition to promoting immunosuppressive functions of MDSC, MDSC-produced VEGF also supports tumor angiogenesis and neovascularization [29].

F. Granulocyte-macrophage colony stimulating factor and granulocyte colony stimulating factor (G-CSF)

GM-CSF is a required cytokine for the differentiation of DC, and administration of GM-CSF in mouse tumor models has antitumor efficacy. In the clinic, GM-CSF has been used as an adjuvant, to expand DC *ex vivo*, and as the transfected component of cell-based vaccines. However, high doses of GM-CSF induce the accumulation of MDSC in mouse systems [164,165], and studies in which tumor production of GM-CSF was knocked down by RNA interference demonstrated that GM-CSF expands MDSC [166]. A recent clinical trial in stage IV metastatic melanoma patients demonstrated that a GM-CSF-based vaccine induced $CD14^+HLA-DR^{-/low}$ MDSC that suppressed immunity by producing TGFβ [75]. Therefore, although GM-CSF matures DC, it also induces MDSC. Whether GM-CSF can be adequately dosed in patients to promote DC function without inducing immune suppression remains to be determined.

There are contradictory findings as to whether G-CSF induces MDSC. G-CSF has preferentially induced $Gr1^{high}CD11b^+$MDSC that are less suppressive than $Gr1^{int}CD11b^+$ cells, suggesting that G-CSF does not regulate the development of immune suppressive myeloid cells [166]. In another mouse tumor system, G-CSF expanded and chemoattracted $CD11b^+Ly6G^+Ly6C^+$ myeloid cells to the lungs even before tumor cells metastasized to this site. The $Ly6G^+Ly6C^+$ cells secreted Bv8, a pro-angiogenic protein that is an endocrine analog of VEGF and also an inducer of hematopoiesis [167]. These results suggest that G-CSF favors the differentiation of myeloid cells that promote angiogenesis and are not immune suppressive, while GM-CSF drives the accumulation of MDSC that suppress T-cell activation. However, the $CD11b^+Ly6G^+Ly6C^+$ cells were not tested for immune suppressive activity and the $Gr1^{high}CD11b^+$ cells were not tested for production of Bv8, so additional studies are necessary to clarify the function(s) of MDSC induced by G-CSF.

V. MDSC TURNOVER

In contrast to MDSC induction, much less is known about the regulation of MDSC half-life. MDSC are present within the tumor microenvironment where a subset differentiates into macrophages [98]. However, the fate of MDSC in the blood, spleen, and bone marrow is unclear. Given that nontumor sites contain more MDSC than tumor sites, it is unlikely that all MDSC eventually migrate to the tumor site and differentiate. Using BrdU *in vivo* labeling in mice, MDSC were shown to originate in the bone marrow. Parabiosis studies of tumor-bearing mice demonstrated that MDSC circulating in the blood have a half-life of <24 hrs [168]. This rapid *in vivo* turnover agrees with the short survival time of MDSC in culture (~24 hrs), and suggests that most MDSC do not migrate into tumors. Because IL-1β increases MDSC half-life [146], IL-1β-induced and conventionally induced MDSC were screened by mass spectrometry to identify proteins and signaling pathways that regulate MDSC survival. These studies identified the Fas-FasL apoptotic pathway and caspase 3 and 8 proteins as likely candidates [150]. Flow cytometry, western blotting, confocal microscopy, and viability studies demonstrated that the half-life of Fas$^+$ MDSC was regulated by susceptibility to Fas-FasL-mediated apoptosis, and that inflammation decreases susceptibility to apoptosis [58,150]. *In vivo* mouse studies confirmed that MDSC levels in tumor-free mice were regulated by FasL$^+$ T cells through Fas-FasL-mediated apoptosis [58]. Activated FasL$^+$ T cells are continuously present in healthy individuals due to activation by environmental antigens. However, T cells are frequently tolerized/anergized in individuals with advanced cancer. Therefore, although T-cell Fas-FasL-mediated apoptosis may regulate MDSC levels in tumor-free individuals, it is unlikely to regulate MDSC half-life in tumor-bearing individuals with high levels of MDSC.

VI. THERAPEUTIC APPROACHES FOR REDUCING MDSC-MEDIATED IMMUNE SUPPRESSION

There has been intense interest in identifying reagents that decrease MDSC levels or limit MDSC suppression. Table 28.2 lists these reagents and therapeutic strategies, which are discussed in the following paragraphs. This topic has been reviewed recently [169].

One of the first drugs shown to reduce MDSC levels was all-trans retinoic acid (ATRA). Treatment of tumor-bearing mice with ATRA decreased the accumulation of Gr1$^+$CD11b$^+$ cells in the spleen by inducing MDSC to mature to DC, macrophages and/or granulocytes [21]. Studies with renal cell carcinoma patients confirmed that ATRA treatment reduced levels of MDSC, and further demonstrated that ATRA improved antigen presentation by monocytes and improved T-cell activation [25,26].

As discussed in section IVA, nonsteroidal anti-inflammatory drugs (NSAIDS), as well as COX$_2$ inhibitors such as celecoxib, significantly reduce the risk of breast cancer [138,170], and have proved to be useful therapeutic and chemopreventative agents for colorectal cancer [171]. Since COX$_2$ inhibitors reduce MDSC accumulation and suppressive activity in mice with tumors [172], their therapeutic efficacy may be partially due to their effects on MDSC.

Several chemotherapeutic drugs that impair cell proliferation and are used to treat cancer patients also reduce MDSC levels. The DNA synthesis inhibitor gemcitabine (GEMZAR) reduced MDSC levels in the spleen and increased the tumoricidal activity of NK cells and CD8$^+$ T cells in tumor-bearing mice, without impacting other immune effector cells [128,125,173,174]. The DNA synthesis inhibitor 5-fluorouracil also induces MDSC apoptosis and may be more effective than gemcitabine [173]. Docetaxel, an antimicrotubule agent that inhibits mitosis, similarly reduces MDSC in tumor-bearing mice, but mediates its effects by maturing MDSC to M1-like macrophages [175]. Paclitaxel, another chemotherapeutic drug that interferes with microtubule formation and mitosis, also limits MDSC accumulation by promoting MDSC differentiation [176].

Other compounds also reduce MDSC-mediated immune suppression by maturing MDSC. IL-12 matures not only MDSC, but also macrophages and DC to enhance cross presentation of tumor antigens and thereby facilitate antitumor immunity [177]. Curcumin, a natural phenol that gives the spice turmeric its distinctive color and flavor, converts MDSC into M1-like macrophages by reducing MDSC production of IL-6 and inhibiting activation of STAT3

485

TABLE 28.2 Therapeutic Inhibition of MDSC

Agent	Species	Mechanism/Effect	References
All trans retinoic acid (ATRA)	Mouse DA-3, C3, MethA tumors; renal cell carcinoma patients	Matures MDSC into antigen presenting cells	[25,26,195]
Amino bisphosphonate	BALB/c neuT transgenic mice	Reduces MMP9, VEGF, myelopoiesis, and tumor stroma	[196]
COX$_2$/PGE$_2$ inhibitors,	Mouse 4T1, 3LL, mesothelioma, chemically-induced tumors; glioma induction by DNA injection; colorectal cancer chemoprevention & treatment	Blocks PGE2; reduces CCL2	[139–143,171]
CpG	Mouse CT26 tumor; CEA transgenic mice	Binds MDSC-expressed TLR9 and matures MDSC to non-suppressive cells	[185,186]
Curcumin	Mouse CT26; human MKN-45 tumor	Matures MDSC to M1-like cells; decreases MDSC production of IL-6; inhibits activation of STAT3 and NFκB	[178]
Dimethyl amiloride	Mouse CT26, TS/A EL4 tumors; breast, colon, prostate cancer patients	Blocks exosome release by tumor cells	[187]
Docetaxel	Mouse 4T1 tumor	Matures MDSC to M1-like macrophages	[175]
5-fluorouracil	Mouse EL-4 tumor	Reduces MDSC levels	[173]
Gemcitabine	Mouse TC-1, AB12, AE-17, EL-4, 3LL, 4T1 tumors	Reduces MDSC levels	[125,126,128,173]
Icariin	Mouse 4T1 tumor	Decreases ROS, NO, IL-6, IL-10, & S100A8/A9 in MDSC	[188]
IL-12	Mouse B16, S91 tumors	Matures myeloid-derived cells to cells that facilitate cross-presentation of tumor antigens	[177]
NSAIDS, nitroaspirin	Mouse MuLV-induced lymphoma; mouse CT26, MBL-2, P815 tumors	Inhibit NOS2 and Arg1 in MDSC	[22]
Paclitaxel	In vitro cytokine-induced bone marrow progenitors	Matures MDSC into DC	[176]
Phosphodiesterase-5 (PDE5) inhibitors	Mouse CT26, TS/A, MCA2-3, B16, 4T1 tumors; multiple myeloma, head & neck cancer patients	Reduce MDSC levels of arg 1 and NOS2	[69]
Sunitinib (sutent)	Renal cell carcinoma patients; mouse RENCA, CT26, MCA26, 3LL tumors	Inhibits STAT3 activation in MDSC	[181–184]
Triterpenoid CDDO-Me	Mouse 3LL, EL-4 tumors; renal cell carcinoma, sarcoma, pancreatic cancer patients	Reduces ROS levels in MDSC	[81]
Very small size proteoliposomes (VSSP)	Mouse MCA203, EG.7 tumors	Mature MDSC to antigen presenting cells	[179]
Vitamin D3	Mouse 3LL tumor	Reduces level of CD34$^+$ cells	[18]
Block c-kit	Mouse MCA26 tumor	Blocks stem cell factor receptor on MDSC	[180]

and NF-κB [178]. MDSC are also matured by the recently developed nanoparticulated adjuvant called "very small-sized proteoliposomes" (VSSP). VSSPs increase myelopoiesis and generate MDSC; however, the MDSC quickly develop into functional antigen-presenting cells that promote antitumor immunity [179].

Amino bisphosphonate drugs are used to treat bone marrow metastases and inhibit tumor stromal cells from producing MMP-9 and VEGF. These drugs reduced MDSC levels in transgenic mice with spontaneously developing mammary carcinoma, identifying amino-bisphosphonates as potential MDSC-reducing agents [11].

Receptor tyrosine kinase inhibitors (RTKI) are increasingly being used clinically to perturb signal transduction pathways regulating malignant cell growth. Sunitinib (Sutent) is a RTKI that inhibits signaling through the receptors for VEGF, platelet-derived growth factor, stem cell factor (c-kit), flt3 ligand, and colony-stimulating factor (CSF-1). It is used in the treatment of renal cell carcinoma. VEGF and CSF-1 contribute to the accumulation of MDSC, and inhibition of c-kit by RNA interference decreases MDSC levels and improves T-cell activation [180]. Based on these observations, several groups assessed MDSC levels in Sunitinib-treated experimental animals [181–183] and renal cell carcinoma patients [181–184], and found significant reductions of both MO-MDSC and PMN-MDSC. Sunitinib acts at least partially by reducing STAT3 activation [183], however, high levels of GM-CSF confer resistance to the drug [181].

Phosphodiesterase-5 (PDE5) inhibitors such as sildenafil (Viagra) downregulate Arg1 and NOS2, two of the effector molecules used by MDSC to suppress T-cell activation. In addition to their therapeutic effects for erectile dysfunction, pulmonary hypertension, and cardiac hypertrophy, PDE5 inhibitors also impact tumor growth. In mouse tumor systems PDE5 inhibitors delayed tumor progression and increased intratumoral T-cell activation and infiltration. They also restored *in vitro* activation of T cells from patients with multiple myeloma and with head and neck cancer, presumably by inhibiting Arg1 and NOS2 in MO-MDSC [69].

Several Toll-like receptor (TLR) agonists are showing promise as immune adjuvants. Unmethylated CpG dinucleotides, which bind to TLR9, induce the differentiation of DC and CD4[+] Th1 cells. They also reduces MO-MDSC and TLR9[+] PMN-MDSC by maturing them to M1-like macrophages [185]. Mouse PMN-MDSC also lose their suppressive activity in response to IFNα released by TLR9[+] plasmacytoid DC following activation by CpG [186].

Tumor-derived exosomes (TDE) contribute to the accumulation and suppressive activity of MDSC through their expression of Hsp-72, which activates STAT3 and the ERK signal transduction pathways in MDSC. The drug amiloride reduces TDE effects by preventing exosome formation [187].

In vitro treatment with the anti-inflammatory triterpenoid C-28 methyl ester of 2-cyano-3,12-dioxooleana-1,9,-dien-28-oic acid (CDDO-Me) eliminated MDSC-mediated T-cell suppression without affecting Arg1 or NO levels. Mice treated with CDDO-Me had delayed tumor growth due to improved antitumor immunity and developed less suppressive MDSC, although the proportion of MDSC in the spleen was not altered. Treatment of pancreatic cancer patients with CDDO-Me plus gemcitabine did not impact blood levels of MDSC; however, T-cell responses to tetanous toxoid were increased, consistent with the concept that CDDO-Me restores T-cell activation by inhibiting MDSC function [81].

ICT (3,5,7-trihydroxy-4'-methoxy-8-(3-hydroxy-3methylbutyl)-flavone), a derivative of Icariin, and the major component of the traditional Chinese medicine Herba Epimedii, also inhibited tumor growth. Treatment of tumor-bearing mice with ICT decreased MDSC levels in spleen, increased levels of DC and macrophages, and improved CD8[+] T-cell production of IFN-γ. These effects accompanied a decrease in MDSC levels of ROS and NO, as well as downregulation of IL-10 and IL-6, suggesting that the effects of ICT are due to altering the phenotype of MDSC [188].

VII. CONCLUSIONS

The last ~10 years have seen a growing awareness of the role of tumor-induced immune suppression in preventing the efficacy of cancer immunotherapies. Due to their suppressive potency and presence in most experimental animals and patients with cancer, MDSC are recognized as a major cause of immune suppression. The identification of pro-inflammatory mediators as inducers of MDSC has revealed new pathways and targets to prevent MDSC accumulation, and these findings could lead to the development of therapeutic and prophylactic cancer drugs. Advances in understanding the mechanisms used by MDSC to suppress adaptive and innate immunity are revealing signal transduction pathways operative in MDSC, and the regulatory molecules within these pathways are also potential drug targets.

Although the last ~10 years have seen exceptional progress in understanding MDSC biology, there remain significant issues. A better understanding of the regulation of MDSC phenotype and more precise phenotype identification are essential so therapies can be tailored and customized to the specific MDSC population present in individual patients. The heterogeneity and diversity of MDSC make this goal especially challenging. Little is known about the regulation of MDSC half-life, and studies in this area could reveal strategies for hastening rates of turnover. Many suppressive mechanisms used by MDSC have already been identified; however, it is likely that these multitasking cells use additional mechanisms that have not as yet been identified. It is imperative to identify all of the suppressive mechanisms employed by MDSC, so potential therapies can be fully evaluated for their efficacy.

ACKNOWLEDGMENTS

Studies from the authors' lab were supported by NIH RO1CA115880, RO1CA8432, RO1GM021248, and American Cancer Society grant IRG-97-153-07. OC and DB were supported by DOD Breast Cancer Program predoctoral fellowships W81XWH-10-1-0027 and W81XWH-11-1-0115, respectively. KP was supported by US Department of Education grant P200A090094-11.

References

[1] Strober S. Natural suppressor (NS) cells, neonatal tolerance, and total lymphoid irradiation: exploring obscure relationships. Annu Rev Immunol 1984;2:219—37.

[2] Sugiura K, Inaba M, Ogata H, Yasumuzu R, Sardina EE, Inaba K, et al. Inhibition of tumor cell proliferation by natural suppressor cells present in murine bone marrow. Cancer Res 1990;50(9):2582—6.

[3] Young MR, Wright MA, Lozano Y, Prechel MM, Benefield J, Leonetti JP, et al. Increased recurrence and metastasis in patients whose primary head and neck squamous cell carcinomas secreted granulocyte-macrophage colony-stimulating factor and contained CD34+ natural suppressor cells. Int J Cancer 1997;74(1):69—74.

[4] Young MR, Wright MA, Lozano Y, Matthews JP, Benefield J, Prechel MM. Mechanisms of immune suppression in patients with head and neck cancer: influence on the immune infiltrate of the cancer. Int J Cancer 1996;67(3):333—8.

[5] Garrity T, Pandit R, Wright MA, Benefield J, Keni S, Young MR. Increased presence of CD34+ cells in the peripheral blood of head and neck cancer patients and their differentiation into dendritic cells. Int J Cancer 1997;73(5):663—9.

[6] Young MR, Petruzzelli GJ, Kolesiak K, Achille N, Lathers DM, Gabrilovich DI. Human squamous cell carcinomas of the head and neck chemoattract immune suppressive CD34(+) progenitor cells. Hum Immunol 2001;62(4):332—41.

[7] Almand B, Clark JI, Nikitina E, van Beynen J, English NR, Knight SC, et al. Increased production of immature myeloid cells in cancer patients: a mechanism of immunosuppression in cancer. J Immunol 2001;166(1):678—89.

[8] Bronte V, Wang M, Overwijk WW, Surman DR, Pericle F, Rosenberg SA, et al. Apoptotic death of CD8+ T lymphocytes after immunization: induction of a suppressive population of Mac-1+/Gr-1+ cells. J Immunol 1998;161(10):5313—20.

[9] Bronte V, Chappell DB, Apolloni E, Cabrelle A, Wang M, Hwu P, et al. Unopposed production of granulocyte-macrophage colony-stimulating factor by tumors inhibits CD8+ T cell responses by dysregulating antigen-presenting cell maturation. J Immunol 1999;162(10):5728–37.

[10] Gabrilovich DI, Velders MP, Sotomayor EM, Kast WM. Mechanism of immune dysfunction in cancer mediated by immature Gr-1+ myeloid cells. J Immunol 2001;166(9):5398–406.

[11] Melani C, Chiodoni C, Forni G, Colombo MP. Myeloid cell expansion elicited by the progression of spontaneous mammary carcinomas in c-erbB-2 transgenic BALB/c mice suppresses immune reactivity. Blood 2003;102(6):2138–45.

[12] Bronte V, Apolloni E, Cabrelle A, Ronca R, Serafini P, Zamboni P, et al. Identification of a CD11b(+)/Gr-1(+)/CD31(+) myeloid progenitor capable of activating or suppressing CD8(+) T cells. Blood 2000;96(12):3838–46.

[13] Ezernitchi AV, Vaknin I, Cohen-Daniel L, Levy O, Manaster E, Halabi A, et al. TCR zeta down-regulation under chronic inflammation is mediated by myeloid suppressor cells differentially distributed between various lymphatic organs. J Immunol 2006;177(7):4763–72.

[14] Schmielau J, Finn OJ. Activated granulocytes and granulocyte-derived hydrogen peroxide are the underlying mechanism of suppression of t-cell function in advanced cancer patients. Cancer Res 2001;61(12):4756–60.

[15] Gabrilovich DI, Bronte V, Chen SH, Colombo MP, Ochoa A, Ostrand-Rosenberg S, et al. The terminology issue for myeloid-derived suppressor cells. Cancer Res 2007;67(1): 425; author reply 6.

[16] Sinha P, Clements VK, Ostrand-Rosenberg S. Reduction of myeloid-derived suppressor cells and induction of M1 macrophages facilitate the rejection of established metastatic disease. J Immunol 2005;174(2):636–45.

[17] Sinha P, Clements VK, Ostrand-Rosenberg S. Interleukin-13-regulated M2 macrophages in combination with myeloid suppressor cells block immune surveillance against metastasis. Cancer Res 2005;65(24):11743–51.

[18] Wiers KM, Lathers DM, Wright MA, Young MR. Vitamin D3 treatment to diminish the levels of immune suppressive CD34+ cells increases the effectiveness of adoptive immunotherapy. J Immunother 2000;23(1):115–24.

[19] Young MR, Ihm J, Lozano Y, Wright MA, Prechel MM. Treating tumor-bearing mice with vitamin D3 diminishes tumor-induced myelopoiesis and associated immunosuppression, and reduces tumor metastasis and recurrence. Cancer Immunol Immunother 1995;41(1):37–45.

[20] Li Q, Pan PY, Gu P, Xu D, Chen SH. Role of immature myeloid Gr-1+ cells in the development of antitumor immunity. Cancer Res 2004;64(3):1130–9.

[21] Kusmartsev S, Cheng F, Yu B, Nefedova Y, Sotomayor E, Lush R, et al. All-trans-retinoic acid eliminates immature myeloid cells from tumor-bearing mice and improves the effect of vaccination. Cancer Res 2003;63(15):4441–9.

[22] De Santo C, Serafini P, Marigo I, Dolcetti L, Bolla M, Del Soldato P, et al. Nitroaspirin corrects immune dysfunction in tumor-bearing hosts and promotes tumor eradication by cancer vaccination. Proc Natl Acad Sci U S A 2005;102(11):4185–90.

[23] Diaz-Montero CM, Salem ML, Nishimura MI, Garrett-Mayer E, Cole DJ, Montero AJ. Increased circulating myeloid-derived suppressor cells correlate with clinical cancer stage, metastatic tumor burden, and doxorubicin-cyclophosphamide chemotherapy. Cancer Immunol Immunother 2008.

[24] Gabitass RF, Annels NE, Stocken DD, Pandha HA, Middleton GW. Elevated myeloid-derived suppressor cells in pancreatic, esophageal and gastric cancer are an independent prognostic factor and are associated with significant elevation of the Th2 cytokine interleukin-13. Cancer Immunol Immunother 2011;60(10):1419–30.

[25] Kusmartsev S, Su Z, Heiser A, Dannull J, Eruslanov E, Kubler H, et al. Reversal of myeloid cell-mediated immunosuppression in patients with metastatic renal cell carcinoma. Clin Cancer Res 2008;14(24):8270–8.

[26] Mirza N, Fishman M, Fricke I, Dunn M, Neuger AM, Frost TJ, et al. All-trans-retinoic acid improves differentiation of myeloid cells and immune response in cancer patients. Cancer Res 2006;66(18):9299–307.

[27] Solito S, Falisi E, Diaz-Montero CM, Doni A, Pinton L, Rosato A, et al. A human promyelocytic-like population is responsible for the immune suppression mediated by myeloid-derived suppressor cells. Blood 2011;118(8):2254–65.

[28] Srivastava MK, Bosch JJ, Wilson AL, Edelman MJ, Ostrand-Rosenberg S. MHC II lung cancer vaccines prime and boost tumor-specific CD4+ T cells that cross-react with multiple histologic subtypes of nonsmall cell lung cancer cells. Int J Cancer 2010;127(11):2612–21.

[29] Yang L, DeBusk LM, Fukuda K, Fingleton B, Green-Jarvis B, Shyr Y, et al. Expansion of myeloid immune suppressor Gr+CD11b+ cells in tumor-bearing host directly promotes tumor angiogenesis. Cancer Cell 2004;6(4):409–21.

[30] Shojaei F, Zhong C, Wu X, Yu L, Ferrara N. Role of myeloid cells in tumor angiogenesis and growth. Trends Cell Biol 2008;18(8):372–8.

[31] Boelte KC, Gordy LE, Joyce S, Thompson MA, Yang L, Lin PC. Rgs2 mediates pro-angiogenic function of myeloid derived suppressor cells in the tumor microenvironment via upregulation of MCP-1. PLoS One 2011;6(4):e18534.

[32] Yang L, Huang J, Ren X, Gorska AE, Chytil A, Aakre M, et al. Abrogation of TGF beta signaling in mammary carcinomas recruits Gr-1+CD11b+ myeloid cells that promote metastasis. Cancer Cell 2008;13(1):23–35.

[33] Toh B, Wang X, Keeble J, Sim WJ, Khoo K, Wong WC, et al. Mesenchymal transition and dissemination of cancer cells is driven by myeloid-derived suppressor cells infiltrating the primary tumor. PLoS Biol 2011;9(9):e1001162.

[34] Delano MJ, Scumpia PO, Weinstein JS, Coco D, Nagaraj S, Kelly-Scumpia KM, et al. MyD88-dependent expansion of an immature GR-1(+)CD11b(+) population induces T cell suppression and Th2 polarization in sepsis. J Exp Med 2007;204(6):1463–74.

[35] Sander LE, Sackett SD, Dierssen U, Beraza N, Linke RP, Muller M, et al. Hepatic acute-phase proteins control innate immune responses during infection by promoting myeloid-derived suppressor cell function. J Exp Med 2010;207(7):1453–64.

[36] Voisin MB, Buzoni-Gatel D, Bout D, Velge-Roussel F. Both expansion of regulatory GR1+ CD11b+ myeloid cells and anergy of T lymphocytes participate in hyporesponsiveness of the lung-associated immune system during acute toxoplasmosis. Infect Immun 2004;72(9):5487–92.

[37] Mencacci A, Montagnoli C, Bacci A, Cenci E, Pitzurra L, Spreca A, et al. CD80+Gr-1+ myeloid cells inhibit development of antifungal Th1 immunity in mice with candidiasis. J Immunol 2002;169(6):3180–90.

[38] Sunderkotter C, Nikolic T, Dillon MJ, Van Rooijen N, Stehling M, Drevets DA, et al. Subpopulations of mouse blood monocytes differ in maturation stage and inflammatory response. J Immunol 2004;172(7):4410–7.

[39] Goni O, Alcaide P, Fresno M. Immunosuppression during acute Trypanosoma cruzi infection: involvement of Ly6G (Gr1(+))CD11b(+)immature myeloid suppressor cells. Int Immunol 2002;14(10):1125–34.

[40] Makarenkova VP, Bansal V, Matta BM, Perez LA, Ochoa JB. CD11b+/Gr-1+ myeloid suppressor cells cause T cell dysfunction after traumatic stress. J Immunol 2006;176(4):2085–94.

[41] Mundy-Bosse BL, Thornton LM, Yang HC, Andersen BL, Carson WE. Psychological stress is associated with altered levels of myeloid-derived suppressor cells in breast cancer patients. Cell Immunol 2011;270(1):80–7.

[42] Grizzle WE, Xu X, Zhang S, Stockard CR, Liu C, Yu S, et al. Age-related increase of tumor susceptibility is associated with myeloid-derived suppressor cell mediated suppression of T cell cytotoxicity in recombinant inbred BXD12 mice. Mech Ageing Dev 2007;128(11-12):672–80.

[43] Haile LA, von Wasielewski R, Gamrekelashvili J, Kruger C, Bachmann O, Westendorf AM, et al. Myeloid-derived suppressor cells in inflammatory bowel disease: a new immunoregulatory pathway. Gastroenterology 2008;135(3):871–81, 81 e1–5.

[44] Zhu B, Bando Y, Xiao S, Yang K, Anderson AC, Kuchroo VK, et al. CD11b+Ly-6C(hi) suppressive monocytes in experimental autoimmune encephalomyelitis. J Immunol 2007;179(8):5228–37.

[45] Kerr EC, Raveney BJ, Copland DA, Dick AD, Nicholson LB. Analysis of retinal cellular infiltrate in experimental autoimmune uveoretinitis reveals multiple regulatory cell populations. J Autoimmun 2008;31(4):354–61.

[46] Chou HS, Hsieh CC, Charles R, Wang L, Wagner T, Fung JJ, et al. Myeloid-derived suppressor cells protect islet transplants by b7-h1 mediated enhancement of T regulatory cells. Transplantation 2012;93(3):272–82.

[47] Yin B, Ma G, Yen CY, Zhou Z, Wang GX, Divino CM, et al. Myeloid-derived suppressor cells prevent type 1 diabetes in murine models. J Immunol 2010;185(10):5828–34.

[48] Highfill SL, Rodriguez PC, Zhou Q, Goetz CA, Koehn BH, Veenstra R, et al. Bone marrow myeloid-derived suppressor cells (MDSCs) inhibit graft-versus-host disease (GVHD) via an arginase-1-dependent mechanism that is up-regulated by interleukin-13. Blood 2010;116(25):5738–47.

[49] Ioannou M, Alissafi T, Lazaridis I, Deraos G, Matsoukas J, Gravanis A, et al. Crucial role of granulocytic myeloid-derived suppressor cells in the regulation of central nervous system autoimmune disease. J Immunol 2012;188(3):1136–46.

[50] DuPage M, Mazumdar C, Schmidt LM, Cheung AF, Jacks T. Expression of tumour-specific antigens underlies cancer immunoediting. Nature 2012;482(7385):405–9.

[51] Matsushita H, Vesely MD, Koboldt DC, Rickert CG, Uppaluri R, Magrini VJ, et al. Cancer exome analysis reveals a T-cell-dependent mechanism of cancer immunoediting. Nature 2012;482(7385):400–4.

[52] Ilkovitch D, Lopez DM. The liver is a site for tumor-induced myeloid-derived suppressor cell accumulation and immunosuppression. Cancer Res 2009;69(13):5514–21.

[53] Movahedi K, Guilliams M, Van den Bossche J, Van den Bergh R, Gysemans C, Beschin A, et al. Identification of discrete tumor-induced myeloid-derived suppressor cell subpopulations with distinct T cell-suppressive activity. Blood 2008;111(8):4233–44.

[54] Youn JI, Nagaraj S, Collazo M, Gabrilovich DI. Subsets of myeloid-derived suppressor cells in tumor-bearing mice. J Immunol 2008;181(8):5791–802.

[55] Huang B, Pan PY, Li Q, Sato AI, Levy DE, Bromberg J, et al. Gr-1+CD115+ Immature Myeloid Suppressor Cells Mediate the Development of Tumor-Induced T Regulatory Cells and T-Cell Anergy in Tumor-Bearing Host. Cancer Res 2006;66(2):1123–31.

[56] Sinha P, Okoro C, Foell D, Freeze HH, Ostrand-Rosenberg S, Srikrishna G. Proinflammatory S100 proteins regulate the accumulation of myeloid-derived suppressor cells. J Immunol 2008;181(7):4666–75.

[57] Gallina G, Dolcetti L, Serafini P, De Santo C, Marigo I, Colombo MP, et al. Tumors induce a subset of inflammatory monocytes with immunosuppressive activity on CD8+ T cells. J Clin Invest 2006;116(10):2777–90.

[58] Sinha P, Chornoguz O, Clements VK, Artemenko KA, Zubarev RA, Ostrand-Rosenberg S. Myeloid-derived suppressor cells express the death receptor Fas and apoptose in response to T cell-expressed FasL. Blood 2011;117(20):5381–90.

[59] Jia W, Jackson-Cook C, Graf MR. Tumor-infiltrating, myeloid-derived suppressor cells inhibit T cell activity by nitric oxide production in an intracranial rat glioma + vaccination model. J Neuroimmunol 2010;223(1-2):20–30.

[60] Youn JI, Collazo M, Shalova IN, Biswas SK, Gabrilovich DI. Characterization of the nature of granulocytic myeloid-derived suppressor cells in tumor-bearing mice. J Leukoc Biol 2012;91(1):167–81.

[61] Chioda M, Peranzoni E, Desantis G, Papalini F, Falisi E, Solito S, et al. Myeloid cell diversification and complexity: an old concept with new turns in oncology. Cancer Metastasis Rev 2011;30(1):27–43.

[62] Filipazzi P, Huber V, Rivoltini L. Phenotype, function and clinical implications of myeloid-derived suppressor cells in cancer patients. Cancer Immunol Immunother 2012;61(2):255–63.

[63] Greten TF, Manns MP, Korangy F. Myeloid derived suppressor cells in human diseases. Int Immunopharmacol 2011;11(7):802–7.

[64] Montero AJ, Diaz-Montero CM, Kyriakopoulos CE, Bronte V, Mandruzzato S. Myeloid-derived Suppressor Cells in Cancer Patients: A Clinical Perspective. J Immunother 2012;35(2):107–15.

[65] Peranzoni E, Zilio S, Marigo I, Dolcetti L, Zanovello P, Mandruzzato S, et al. Myeloid-derived suppressor cell heterogeneity and subset definition. Curr Opin Immunol 2010;22(2):238–44.

[66] Tadmor T, Attias D, Polliack A. Myeloid-derived suppressor cells—their role in haemato-oncological malignancies and other cancers and possible implications for therapy. Br J Haematol 2011;153(5):557–67.

[67] Brandau S, Trellakis S, Bruderek K, Schmaltz D, Steller G, Elian M, et al. Myeloid-derived suppressor cells in the peripheral blood of cancer patients contain a subset of immature neutrophils with impaired migratory properties. J Leukoc Biol 2011;89(2):311–7.

[68] Corzo CA, Cotter MJ, Cheng P, Cheng F, Kusmartsev S, Sotomayor E, et al. Mechanism regulating reactive oxygen species in tumor-induced myeloid-derived suppressor cells. J Immunol 2009;182(9):5693–701.

[69] Serafini P, Meckel K, Kelso M, Noonan K, Califano J, Koch W, et al. Phosphodiesterase-5 inhibition augments endogenous antitumor immunity by reducing myeloid-derived suppressor cell function. J Exp Med 2006;203(12):2691–702.

[70] Srivastava MK, Bosch JJ, Thompson JA, Ksander BR, Edelman MJ, Ostrand-Rosenberg S. Lung cancer patients' CD4(+) T cells are activated in vitro by MHC II cell-based vaccines despite the presence of myeloid-derived suppressor cells. Cancer Immunol Immunother 2008;57(10):1493–504.

[71] Liu CY, Wang YM, Wang CL, Feng PH, Ko HW, Liu YH, et al. Population alterations of L-arginase- and inducible nitric oxide synthase-expressed CD11b+/CD14/CD15+/CD33+ myeloid-derived suppressor cells and CD8+ T lymphocytes in patients with advanced-stage non-small cell lung cancer. J Cancer Res Clin Oncol 2010;136(1):35–45.

[72] Rodriguez PC, Ernstoff MS, Hernandez C, Atkins M, Zabaleta J, Sierra R, et al. Arginase I-producing myeloid-derived suppressor cells in renal cell carcinoma are a subpopulation of activated granulocytes. Cancer Res 2009;69(4):1553–60.

[73] Zea AH, Rodriguez PC, Atkins MB, Hernandez C, Signoretti S, Zabaleta J, et al. Arginase-producing myeloid suppressor cells in renal cell carcinoma patients: a mechanism of tumor evasion. Cancer Res 2005;65(8):3044–8.

[74] Daud AI, Mirza N, Lenox B, Andrews S, Urbas P, Gao GX, et al. Phenotypic and functional analysis of dendritic cells and clinical outcome in patients with high-risk melanoma treated with adjuvant granulocyte macrophage colony-stimulating factor. J Clin Oncol 2008;26(19):3235–41.

[75] Filipazzi P, Valenti R, Huber V, Pilla L, Canese P, Iero M, et al. Identification of a new subset of myeloid suppressor cells in peripheral blood of melanoma patients with modulation by a granulocyte-macrophage colony-stimulation factor-based antitumor vaccine. J Clin Oncol 2007;25(18):2546–53.

[76] Mandruzzato S, Solito S, Falisi E, Francescato S, Chiarion-Sileni V, Mocellin S, et al. IL4Ralpha+ myeloid-derived suppressor cell expansion in cancer patients. J Immunol 2009;182(10):6562–8.

[77] Poschke I, Mougiakakos D, Hansson J, Masucci GV, Kiessling R. Immature immunosuppressive CD14+HLA-DR-/low cells in melanoma patients are Stat3hi and overexpress CD80, CD83, and DC-sign. Cancer Res 2010;70(11):4335–45.

[78] Choi J, Suh B, Ahn YO, Kim TM, Lee JO, Lee SH, et al. CD15+/CD16low human granulocytes from terminal cancer patients: granulocytic myeloid-derived suppressor cells that have suppressive function. Tumour Biol 2012;33(1):121–9.

[79] Eruslanov E, Neuberger M, Daurkin I, Perrin GQ, Algood C, Dahm P, et al. Circulating and tumor-infiltrating myeloid cell subsets in patients with bladder cancer. Int J Cancer 2012;130(5):1109–19.

[80] Porembka MR, Mitchem JB, Belt BA, Hsieh CS, Lee HM, Herndon J, et al. Pancreatic adenocarcinoma induces bone marrow mobilization of myeloid-derived suppressor cells which promote primary tumor growth. Cancer Immunol Immunother 2012.

[81] Nagaraj S, Youn JI, Weber H, Iclozan C, Lu L, Cotter MJ, et al. Anti-inflammatory triterpenoid blocks immune suppressive function of MDSCs and improves immune response in cancer. Clin Cancer Res 2010;16(6):1812–23.

[82] Vuk-Pavlovic S, Bulur PA, Lin Y, Qin R, Szumlanski CL, Zhao X, et al. Immunosuppressive CD14+HLA–DRlow/- monocytes in prostate cancer. Prostate 2010;70(4):443–55.

[83] Hoechst B, Ormandy LA, Ballmaier M, Lehner F, Kruger C, Manns MP, et al. A new population of myeloid-derived suppressor cells in hepatocellular carcinoma patients induces CD4(+)CD25(+)Foxp3(+) T cells. Gastroenterology 2008;135(1):234–43.

[84] Brimnes MK, Vangsted AJ, Knudsen LM, Gimsing P, Gang AO, Johnsen HE, et al. Increased level of both CD4+FOXP3+ regulatory T cells and CD14+HLA-DR/low myeloid-derived suppressor cells and decreased level of dendritic cells in patients with multiple myeloma. Scand J Immunol 2010;72(6):540–7.

[85] Lin Y, Gustafson MP, Bulur PA, Gastineau DA, Witzig TE, Dietz AB. Immunosuppressive CD14+HLA–DR(low)/- monocytes in B-cell non-Hodgkin lymphoma. Blood 2011;117(3):872–81.

[86] Young MR, Kolesiak K, Wright MA, Gabrilovich DI. Chemoattraction of femoral CD34+ progenitor cells by tumor-derived vascular endothelial cell growth factor. Clin Exp Metastasis 1999;17(10):881–8.

[87] Marigo I, Bosio E, Solito S, Mesa C, Fernandez A, Dolcetti L, et al. Tumor-induced tolerance and immune suppression depend on the C/EBPbeta transcription factor. Immunity 2010;32(6):790–802.

[88] Gabrilovich DI, Nagaraj S. Myeloid-derived suppressor cells as regulators of the immune system. Nat Rev Immunol 2009;9(3):162–74.

[89] Solito S, Bronte V, Mandruzzato S. Antigen specificity of immune suppression by myeloid-derived suppressor cells. J Leukoc Biol 2011;90(1):31–6.

[90] Nagaraj S, Nelson A, Youn JI, Cheng P, Quiceno D, Gabrilovich DI. Antigen-Specific CD4+ T Cells Regulate Function of Myeloid-Derived Suppressor Cells in Cancer via Retrograde MHC Class II Signaling. Cancer Res 2012;72(4):928–38.

[91] Condamine T, Gabrilovich DI. Molecular mechanisms regulating myeloid-derived suppressor cell differentiation and function. Trends Immunol 2011;32(1):19–25.

[92] Ostrand-Rosenberg S. Myeloid-derived suppressor cells: more mechanisms for inhibiting antitumor immunity. Cancer Immunol Immunother 2010;59(10):1593–600.

[93] Bronte V, Serafini P, De Santo C, Marigo I, Tosello V, Mazzoni A, et al. IL-4-induced arginase 1 suppresses alloreactive T cells in tumor-bearing mice. J Immunol 2003;170(1):270–8.

[94] Rodriguez PC, Quiceno DG, Zabaleta J, Ortiz B, Zea AH, Piazuelo MB, et al. Arginase I production in the tumor microenvironment by mature myeloid cells inhibits T-cell receptor expression and antigen-specific T-cell responses. Cancer Res 2004;64(16):5839–49.

[95] Rodriguez PC, Zea AH, Culotta KS, Zabaleta J, Ochoa JB, Ochoa AC. Regulation of T cell receptor CD3zeta chain expression by L-arginine. J Biol Chem 2002;277(24):21123–9.

[96] Rodriguez PC, Quiceno DG, Ochoa AC. L-arginine availability regulates T-lymphocyte cell-cycle progression. Blood 2007;109(4):1568–73.

[97] Bronte V, Zanovello P. Regulation of immune responses by L-arginine metabolism. Nat Rev Immunol 2005;5(8):641–54.

[98] Corzo CA, Condamine T, Lu L, Cotter MJ, Youn JI, Cheng P, et al. HIF-1alpha regulates function and differentiation of myeloid-derived suppressor cells in the tumor microenvironment. J Exp Med 2010;207(11):2439–53.

[99] Rodriguez PC, Ochoa AC. Arginine regulation by myeloid derived suppressor cells and tolerance in cancer: mechanisms and therapeutic perspectives. Immunol Rev 2008;222:180–91.

[100] Kusmartsev S, Nefedova Y, Yoder D, Gabrilovich DI. Antigen-specific inhibition of CD8+ T cell response by immature myeloid cells in cancer is mediated by reactive oxygen species. J Immunol 2004;172(2):989–99.

[101] Tacke RS, Lee HC, Goh C, Courtney J, Polyak SJ, Rosen HR, et al. Myeloid suppressor cells induced by hepatitis C virus suppress T-cell responses through the production of reactive oxygen species. Hepatology 2012;55(2):343–53.

[102] Nefedova Y, Huang M, Kusmartsev S, Bhattacharya R, Cheng P, Salup R, et al. Hyperactivation of STAT3 is involved in abnormal differentiation of dendritic cells in cancer. J Immunol 2004;172(1):464–74.

[103] Kujawski M, Kortylewski M, Lee H, Herrmann A, Kay H, Yu H. Stat3 mediates myeloid cell-dependent tumor angiogenesis in mice. J Clin Invest 2008;118(10):3367–77.

[104] Nagaraj S, Gupta K, Pisarev V, Kinarsky L, Sherman S, Kang L, et al. Altered recognition of antigen is a mechanism of CD8+ T cell tolerance in cancer. Nat Med 2007;13(7):828–35.

[105] Lu T, Ramakrishnan R, Altiok S, Youn JI, Cheng P, Celis E, et al. Tumor-infiltrating myeloid cells induce tumor cell resistance to cytotoxic T cells in mice. J Clin Invest 2011;121(10):4015–29.

[106] Bannai S. Transport of cystine and cysteine in mammalian cells. Biochim Biophys Acta 1984;779(3): 289–306.

[107] Gmunder H, Eck HP, Droge W. Low membrane transport activity for cystine in resting and mitogenically stimulated human lymphocyte preparations and human T cell clones. Eur J Biochem 1991;201(1):113–7.

[108] Srivastava MK, Sinha P, Clements VK, Rodriguez P, Ostrand-Rosenberg S. Myeloid-derived suppressor cells inhibit T-cell activation by depleting cystine and cysteine. Cancer Res 2010;70(1):68–77.

[109] Angelini G, Gardella S, Ardy M, Ciriolo MR, Filomeni G, Di Trapani G, et al. Antigen-presenting dendritic cells provide the reducing extracellular microenvironment required for T lymphocyte activation. Proc Natl Acad Sci U S A 2002;99(3):1491–6.

[110] Serafini P, Mgebroff S, Noonan K, Borrello I. Myeloid-derived suppressor cells promote cross-tolerance in B-cell lymphoma by expanding regulatory T cells. Cancer Res 2008;68(13):5439–49.

[111] Pan PY, Ma G, Weber KJ, Ozao-Choy J, Wang G, Yin B, et al. Immune stimulatory receptor CD40 is required for T-cell suppression and T regulatory cell activation mediated by myeloid-derived suppressor cells in cancer. Cancer Res 2010;70(1):99–108.

[112] Lesokhin AM, Hohl TM, Kitano S, Cortez C, Hirschhorn-Cymerman D, Avogadri F, et al. Monocytic CCR2+ Myeloid-Derived Suppressor Cells Promote Immune Escape by Limiting Activated CD8 T-cell Infiltration into the Tumor Microenvironment. Cancer Res 2012.

[113] Huang B, Lei Z, Zhao J, Gong W, Liu J, Chen Z, et al. CCL2/CCR2 pathway mediates recruitment of myeloid suppressor cells to cancers. Cancer Lett 2007;252(1):86–92.

[114] Hanson EM, Clements VK, Sinha P, Ilkovitch D, Ostrand-Rosenberg S. Myeloid-derived suppressor cells down-regulate L-selectin expression on CD4+ and CD8+ T cells. J Immunol 2009;183(2):937–44.

[115] Mantovani A, Allavena P, Sica A, Balkwill F. Cancer-related inflammation. Nature 2008;454(7203):436–44.

[116] Mantovani A, Sica A. Macrophages, innate immunity and cancer: balance, tolerance, and diversity. Curr Opin Immunol 2010;22(2):231–7.

[117] Qian BZ, Pollard JW. Macrophage diversity enhances tumor progression and metastasis. Cell 2010;141(1):39–51.

[118] Gabrilovich D, Ostrand-Rosenberg S, Bronte V. Coordinated regulation of meyloid cells by tumours. Nat Rev Immunol 2012 (in press).

[119] Biswas SK, Mantovani A. Macrophage plasticity and interaction with lymphocyte subsets: cancer as a paradigm. Nat Immunol 2010;11(10):889–96.

[120] DeNardo DG, Barreto JB, Andreu P, Vasquez L, Tawfik D, Kolhatkar N, et al. CD4(+) T cells regulate pulmonary metastasis of mammary carcinomas by enhancing protumor properties of macrophages. Cancer Cell 2009;16(2):91–102.

[121] Tiemessen MM, Jagger AL, Evans HG, van Herwijnen MJ, John S, Taams LS. CD4+CD25+Foxp3+ regulatory T cells induce alternative activation of human monocytes/macrophages. Proc Natl Acad Sci U S A 2007;104(49):19446–51.

[122] de Visser KE, Korets LV, Coussens LM. De novo carcinogenesis promoted by chronic inflammation is B lymphocyte dependent. Cancer Cell 2005;7(5):411–23.

[123] Wong SC, Puaux AL, Chittezhath M, Shalova I, Kajiji TS, Wang X, et al. Macrophage polarization to a unique phenotype driven by B cells. Eur J Immunol 2010;40(8):2296–307.

[124] Hagemann T, Wilson J, Burke F, Kulbe H, Li NF, Pluddemann A, et al. Ovarian cancer cells polarize macrophages toward a tumor-associated phenotype. J Immunol 2006;176(8):5023–32.

[125] Sinha P, Clements VK, Bunt SK, Albelda SM, Ostrand-Rosenberg S. Cross-talk between myeloid-derived suppressor cells and macrophages subverts tumor immunity toward a type 2 response. J Immunol 2007;179(2):977–83.

[126] Li H, Han Y, Guo Q, Zhang M, Cao X. Cancer-expanded myeloid-derived suppressor cells induce anergy of NK cells through membrane-bound TGF-beta 1. J Immunol 2009;182(1):240–9.

[127] Liu C, Yu S, Kappes J, Wang J, Grizzle WE, Zinn KR, et al. Expansion of spleen myeloid suppressor cells represses NK cell cytotoxicity in tumor-bearing host. Blood 2007;109(10):4336–42.

[128] Suzuki E, Kapoor V, Jassar AS, Kaiser LR, Albelda SM. Gemcitabine selectively eliminates splenic Gr-1+/CD11b+ myeloid suppressor cells in tumor-bearing animals and enhances antitumor immune activity. Clin Cancer Res 2005;11(18):6713–21.

[129] Hoechst B, Voigtlaender T, Ormandy L, Gamrekelashvili J, Zhao F, Wedemeyer H, et al. Myeloid derived suppressor cells inhibit natural killer cells in patients with hepatocellular carcinoma via the NKp30 receptor. Hepatology 2009;50(3):799–807.

493

[130] Elkabets M, Ribeiro VS, Dinarello CA, Ostrand-Rosenberg S, Di Santo JP, Apte RN, et al. IL-1beta regulates a novel myeloid-derived suppressor cell subset that impairs NK cell development and function. Eur J Immunol 2010;40(12):3347−57.

[131] Terabe M, Matsui S, Park JM, Mamura M, Noben-Trauth N, Donaldson DD, et al. Transforming growth factor-beta production and myeloid cells are an effector mechanism through which CD1d-restricted T cells block cytotoxic T lymphocyte-mediated tumor immunosurveillance: abrogation prevents tumor recurrence. J Exp Med 2003;198(11):1741−52.

[132] Balkwill F, Mantovani A. Inflammation and cancer: back to Virchow? Lancet 2001;357(9255):539−45.

[133] Ostrand-Rosenberg S, Sinha P. Myeloid-derived suppressor cells: linking inflammation and cancer. J Immunol 2009;182(8):4499−506.

[134] Baniyash M. Chronic inflammation, immunosuppression and cancer: new insights and outlook. Semin Cancer Biol 2006;16(1):80−8.

[135] Tan TT, Coussens LM. Humoral immunity, inflammation and cancer. Curr Opin Immunol 2007;19(2):209−16.

[136] Bronte V. Myeloid-derived suppressor cells in inflammation: uncovering cell subsets with enhanced immunosuppressive functions. Eur J Immunol 2009;39(10):2670−2.

[137] Meyer C, Sevko A, Ramacher M, Bazhin AV, Falk CS, Osen W, et al. Chronic inflammation promotes myeloid-derived suppressor cell activation blocking antitumor immunity in transgenic mouse melanoma model. Proc Natl Acad Sci USA 2011;108(41):17111−6.

[138] Harris RE, Beebe-Donk J, Alshafie GA. Reduction in the risk of human breast cancer by selective cyclooxygenase-2 (COX-2) inhibitors. BMC Cancer 2006;6:27.

[139] Fujita M, Kohanbash G, Fellows-Mayle W, Hamilton RL, Komohara Y, Decker SA, et al. COX-2 blockade suppresses gliomagenesis by inhibiting myeloid-derived suppressor cells. Cancer Res 2011;71(7):2664−74.

[140] Rodriguez PC, Hernandez CP, Quiceno D, Dubinett SM, Zabaleta J, Ochoa JB, et al. Arginase I in myeloid suppressor cells is induced by COX-2 in lung carcinoma. J Exp Med 2005;202(7):931−9.

[141] Sinha P, Clements VK, Fulton AM, Ostrand-Rosenberg S. Prostaglandin E2 promotes tumor progression by inducing myeloid-derived suppressor cells. Cancer Res 2007;67(9):4507−13.

[142] Talmadge JE, Hood KC, Zobel LC, Shafer LR, Coles M, Toth B. Chemoprevention by cyclooxygenase-2 inhibition reduces immature myeloid suppressor cell expansion. Int Immunopharmacol 2007;7(2):140−51.

[143] Veltman JD, Lambers ME, van Nimwegen M, Hendriks RW, Hoogsteden HC, Aerts JG, et al. COX-2 inhibition improves immunotherapy and is associated with decreased numbers of myeloid-derived suppressor cells in mesothelioma. Celecoxib influences MDSC function. BMC Cancer 2010;10:464.

[144] Eruslanov E, Daurkin I, Ortiz J, Vieweg J, Kusmartsev S. Pivotal Advance: Tumor-mediated induction of myeloid-derived suppressor cells and M2-polarized macrophages by altering intracellular PGE catabolism in myeloid cells. J Leukoc Biol 2010;88(5):839−48.

[145] Obermajer N, Muthuswamy R, Lesnock J, Edwards RP, Kalinski P. Positive feedback between PGE2 and COX2 redirects the differentiation of human dendritic cells toward stable myeloid-derived suppressor cells. Blood 2011;118(20):5498−505.

[146] Bunt SK, Sinha P, Clements VK, Leips J, Ostrand-Rosenberg S. Inflammation Induces Myeloid-Derived Suppressor Cells that Facilitate Tumor Progression. J Immunol 2006;176(1):284−90.

[147] Song X, Krelin Y, Dvorkin T, Bjorkdahl O, Segal S, Dinarello CA, et al. CD11b+/Gr-1+ immature myeloid cells mediate suppression of T cells in mice bearing tumors of IL-1beta-secreting cells. J Immunol 2005;175(12):8200−8.

[148] Tu S, Bhagat G, Cui G, Takaishi S, Kurt-Jones EA, Rickman B, et al. Overexpression of interleukin-1beta induces gastric inflammation and cancer and mobilizes myeloid-derived suppressor cells in mice. Cancer Cell 2008;14(5):408−19.

[149] Bunt SK, Yang L, Sinha P, Clements VK, Leips J, Ostrand-Rosenberg S. Reduced inflammation in the tumor microenvironment delays the accumulation of myeloid-derived suppressor cells and limits tumor progression. Cancer Res 2007;67(20):10019−26.

[150] Chornoguz O, Grmai L, Sinha P, Artemenko KA, Zubarev RA, Ostrand-Rosenberg S. Proteomic pathway analysis reveals inflammation increases myeloid-derived suppressor cell resistance to apoptosis. Molecular & cellular proteomics: MCP 2011;10(3):M110 002980.

[151] Bunt SK, Clements VK, Hanson EM, Sinha P, Ostrand-Rosenberg S. Inflammation enhances myeloid-derived suppressor cell cross-talk by signaling through Toll-like receptor 4. J Leukoc Biol 2009;85(6):996−1004.

[152] Smith C, Chang M, Parker K, Beury D, DuHadaway J, Flick H, et al. IDO is a nodal pathogenic driver of lung cancer and metastasis development. submitted 2012.

[153] Cheng P, Corzo CA, Luetteke N, Yu B, Nagaraj S, Bui MM, et al. Inhibition of dendritic cell differentiation and accumulation of myeloid-derived suppressor cells in cancer is regulated by S100A9 protein. J Exp Med 2008;205(10):2235−49.

494

[154] Turovskaya O, Foell D, Sinha P, Vogl T, Newlin R, Nayak J, et al. RAGE, carboxylated glycans and S100A8/A9 play essential roles in colitis-associated carcinogenesis. Carcinogenesis 2008;29(10):2035—43.

[155] Zhao F, Hoechst B, Duffy A, Gamrekelashvili J, Fioravanti S, Manns MP, et al. S100A9 a new marker for monocytic human myeloid derived suppressor cells. Immunology 2012.

[156] Markiewski MM, DeAngelis RA, Benencia F, Ricklin-Lichtsteiner SK, Koutoulaki A, Gerard C, et al. Modulation of the antitumor immune response by complement. Nat Immunol 2008;9(11):1225—35.

[157] Markiewski MM, Lambris JD. Is complement good or bad for cancer patients? A new perspective on an old dilemma. Trends Immunol 2009;30(6):286—92.

[158] Markiewski MM, Lambris JD. Unwelcome complement. Cancer Res 2009;69(16):6367—70.

[159] Ostrand-Rosenberg S. Cancer and complement. Nature biotechnol 2008;26(12):1348—9.

[160] Gabrilovich D, Ishida T, Oyama T, Ran S, Kravtsov V, Nadaf S, et al. Vascular endothelial growth factor inhibits the development of dendritic cells and dramatically affects the differentiation of multiple hematopoietic lineages in vivo. Blood 1998;92(11):4150—66.

[161] Gabrilovich DI, Ishida T, Nadaf S, Ohm JE, Carbone DP. Antibodies to vascular endothelial growth factor enhance the efficacy of cancer immunotherapy by improving endogenous dendritic cell function. Clin Cancer Res 1999;5(10):2963—70.

[162] Kusmartsev S, Eruslanov E, Kubler H, Tseng T, Sakai Y, Su Z, et al. Oxidative stress regulates expression of VEGFR1 in myeloid cells: link to tumor-induced immune suppression in renal cell carcinoma. J Immunol 2008;181(1):346—53.

[163] Gabrilovich DI, Chen HL, Girgis KR, Cunningham HT, Meny GM, Nadaf S, et al. Production of vascular endothelial growth factor by human tumors inhibits the functional maturation of dendritic cells. Nat Med 1996;2(10):1096—103.

[164] Serafini P, Carbley R, Noonan KA, Tan G, Bronte V, Borrello I. High-dose granulocyte-macrophage colony-stimulating factor-producing vaccines impair the immune response through the recruitment of myeloid suppressor cells. Cancer Res 2004;64(17):6337—43.

[165] Morales JK, Kmieciak M, Knutson KL, Bear HD, Manjili MH. GM-CSF is one of the main breast tumor-derived soluble factors involved in the differentiation of CD11b-Gr1- bone marrow progenitor cells into myeloid-derived suppressor cells. Breast Cancer Res Treat 2010;123(1):39—49.

[166] Dolcetti L, Peranzoni E, Ugel S, Marigo I, Fernandez Gomez A, Mesa C, et al. Hierarchy of immunosuppressive strength among myeloid-derived suppressor cell subsets is determined by GM-CSF. Eur J Immunol 2010;40(1):22—35.

[167] Kowanetz M, Wu X, Lee J, Tan M, Hagenbeek T, Qu X, et al. Granulocyte-colony stimulating factor promotes lung metastasis through mobilization of Ly6G+Ly6C+ granulocytes. Proc Natl Acad Sci USA 2010;107(50):21248—55.

[168] Sawanobori Y, Ueha S, Kurachi M, Shimaoka T, Talmadge JE, Abe J, et al. Chemokine-mediated rapid turnover of myeloid-derived suppressor cells in tumor-bearing mice. Blood 2008;111(12):5457—66.

[169] Ugel S, Delpozzo F, Desantis G, Papalini F, Simonato F, Sonda N, et al. Therapeutic targeting of myeloid-derived suppressor cells. Curr Opin Pharmacol 2009;9(4):470—81.

[170] Ashok V, Dash C, Rohan TE, Sprafka JM, Terry PD. Selective cyclooxygenase-2 (COX-2) inhibitors and breast cancer risk. Breast 2011;20(1):66—70.

[171] Wang D, Dubois RN. The role of COX-2 in intestinal inflammation and colorectal cancer. Oncogene 2010;29(6):781—8.

[172] Sinha P, Clements VK, Miller S, Ostrand-Rosenberg S. Tumor immunity: a balancing act between T cell activation, macrophage activation and tumor-induced immune suppression. Cancer Immunol Immunother 2005;54(11):1137—42.

[173] Vincent J, Mignot G, Chalmin F, Ladoire S, Bruchard M, Chevriaux A, et al. 5-Fluorouracil selectively kills tumor-associated myeloid-derived suppressor cells resulting in enhanced T cell-dependent antitumor immunity. Cancer Res 2010;70(8):3052—61.

[174] Le HK, Graham L, Cha E, Morales JK, Manjili MH, Bear HD. Gemcitabine directly inhibits myeloid derived suppressor cells in BALB/c mice bearing 4T1 mammary carcinoma and augments expansion of T cells from tumor-bearing mice. Int Immunopharmacol 2009;9(7-8):900—9.

[175] Kodumudi KN, Woan K, Gilvary DL, Sahakian E, Wei S, Djeu JY. A novel chemoimmunomodulating property of docetaxel: suppression of myeloid-derived suppressor cells in tumor bearers. Clin Cancer Res 2010;16(18):4583—94.

[176] Michels T, Shurin GV, Naiditch H, Sevko A, Umansky V, Shurin MR. Paclitaxel promotes differentiation of myeloid-derived suppressor cells into dendritic cells in vitro in a TLR4-independent manner. J Immunotoxicol 2012.

[177] Kerkar SP, Goldszmid RS, Muranski P, Chinnasamy D, Yu Z, Reger RN, et al. IL-12 triggers a programmatic change in dysfunctional myeloid-derived cells within mouse tumors. J Clin Invest 2011;121(12):4746—57.

[178] Tu SP, Jin H, Shi JD, Zhu LM, Suo Y, Lu G, et al. Curcumin induces the differentiation of myeloid-derived suppressor cells and inhibits their interaction with cancer cells and related tumor growth. Cancer Prev Res (Phila) 2012;5(2):205—15.

[179] Fernandez A, Mesa C, Marigo I, Dolcetti L, Clavell M, Oliver L, et al. Inhibition of tumor-induced myeloid-derived suppressor cell function by a nanoparticulated adjuvant. J Immunol 2011;186(1):264—74.

[180] Pan PY, Wang GX, Yin B, Ozao J, Ku T, Divino CM, et al. Reversion of immune tolerance in advanced malignancy: modulation of myeloid-derived suppressor cell development by blockade of stem-cell factor function. Blood 2008;111(1):219—28.

[181] Ko JS, Rayman P, Ireland J, Swaidani S, Li G, Bunting KD, et al. Direct and differential suppression of myeloid-derived suppressor cell subsets by sunitinib is compartmentally constrained. Cancer Res 2010;70(9):3526—36.

[182] Ozao-Choy J, Ma G, Kao J, Wang GX, Meseck M, Sung M, et al. The novel role of tyrosine kinase inhibitor in the reversal of immune suppression and modulation of tumor microenvironment for immune-based cancer therapies. Cancer Res 2009;69(6):2514—22.

[183] Xin H, Zhang C, Herrmann A, Du Y, Figlin R, Yu H. Sunitinib inhibition of Stat3 induces renal cell carcinoma tumor cell apoptosis and reduces immunosuppressive cells. Cancer Res 2009;69(6):2506—13.

[184] Ko JS, Zea AH, Rini BI, Ireland JL, Elson P, Cohen P, et al. Sunitinib mediates reversal of myeloid-derived suppressor cell accumulation in renal cell carcinoma patients. Clin Cancer Res 2009;15(6):2148—57.

[185] Shirota Y, Shirota H, Klinman DM. Intratumoral injection of CpG oligonucleotides induces the differentiation and reduces the immunosuppressive activity of myeloid-derived suppressor cells. J Immunol 2012;188(4):1592—9.

[186] Zoglmeier C, Bauer H, Norenberg D, Wedekind G, Bittner P, Sandholzer N, et al. CpG blocks immunosuppression by myeloid-derived suppressor cells in tumor-bearing mice. Clin Cancer Res 2011;17(7):1765—75.

[187] Chalmin F, Ladoire S, Mignot G, Vincent J, Bruchard M, Remy-Martin JP, et al. Membrane-associated Hsp72 from tumor-derived exosomes mediates STAT3-dependent immunosuppressive function of mouse and human myeloid-derived suppressor cells. J Clin Invest 2010;120(2):457—71.

[188] Zhou J, Wu J, Chen X, Fortenbery N, Eksioglu E, Kodumudi KN, et al. Icariin and its derivative, ICT, exert anti-inflammatory, anti-tumor effects, and modulate myeloid derived suppressive cells (MDSCs) functions. Int Immunopharmacol 2011;11(7):890—8.

[189] Kusmartsev S, Gabrilovich DI. Immature myeloid cells and cancer-associated immune suppression. Cancer Immunol Immunother 2002;51(6):293—8.

[190] Greifenberg V, Ribechini E, Rossner S, Lutz MB. Myeloid-derived suppressor cell activation by combined LPS and IFN-gamma treatment impairs DC development. Eur J Immunol 2009;39(10):2865—76.

[191] Umemura N, Saio M, Suwa T, Kitoh Y, Bai J, Nonaka K, et al. Tumor-infiltrating myeloid-derived suppressor cells are pleiotropic-inflamed monocytes/macrophages that bear M1- and M2-type characteristics. J Leukoc Biol 2008;83(5):1136—44.

[192] Finke J, Ko J, Rini B, Rayman P, Ireland J, Cohen P. MDSC as a mechanism of tumor escape from sunitinib mediated anti-angiogenic therapy. Int Immunopharmacol 2011;11(7):856—61.

[193] Lechner MG, Liebertz DJ, Epstein AL. Characterization of cytokine-induced myeloid-derived suppressor cells from normal human peripheral blood mononuclear cells. J Immunol 2010;185(4):2273—84.

[194] Lechner MG, Megiel C, Russell SM, Bingham B, Arger N, Woo T, et al. Functional characterization of human Cd33+ and Cd11b+ myeloid-derived suppressor cell subsets induced from peripheral blood mononuclear cells co-cultured with a diverse set of human tumor cell lines. J Transl Med 2011;9:90.

[195] Kusmartsev S, Gabrilovich DI. Inhibition of myeloid cell differentiation in cancer: the role of reactive oxygen species. J Leukoc Biol 2003;74(2):186—96.

[196] Melani C, Sangaletti S, Barazzetta FM, Werb Z, Colombo MP. Amino-biphosphonate-mediated MMP-9 inhibition breaks the tumor-bone marrow axis responsible for myeloid-derived suppressor cell expansion and macrophage infiltration in tumor stroma. Cancer Res 2007;67(23):11438—46.

CHAPTER 29

HyperAcute Vaccines: A Novel Cancer Immunotherapy

Gabriela R. Rossi, Nicholas N. Vahanian, W. Jay Ramsey, Charles J. Link
NewLink Genetic Corporation, Ames, Iowa USA

I. BACKGROUND AND HISTORICAL PERSPECTIVE

The development of HyperAcute® cancer vaccines was inspired by observations taken from the fields of cancer gene therapy and xenotransplantation. The first observation was made in a gene therapy cancer clinical trial treating patients with recurrent ovarian or fallopian tube cancers. The original goal of this trial was gene transfer of the Herpes Simplex virus thymidine kinase (HSVtk) gene into tumor cells followed by administration of the cytotoxic prodrug Gancyclovir (GCV) to destroy the tumor. The procedure consisted of infusing murine retroviral producer cells (VPCs) into the peritoneal cavity of patients followed by administration of GCV. The vector producer cells were engineered to propagate retroviral vectors encoding the HSVtk gene that could transduce tumor cells *in situ*. A Phase I trial of 10 patients was conducted, using intraperitoneal (IP) injections of 10^6-10^8 murine vector producer cells cells/kg. Four weeks following the IP infusions, patients were treated with GCV for 2 weeks.

Viable VPCs were recovered from peritoneal washes on day 3 and/or day 7 after infusion at the two highest dose levels, but none were detected at day 14. Quantitative PCR analysis of intraperitoneal tumor biopsies demonstrated <1% gene transfer, which was insufficient to mediate an antitumor effect. Yet, surprisingly, 4/10 evaluable patients had objective antitumor responses despite the very poor gene transfer efficiency. One patient had a complete resolution of a 2 cm mass on CT scan and a 70% reduction of CA125 antigen. A second patient had a partial response, the third patient had a minor response, and the fourth patient showed a mixed response to the treatment in the form of resolved malignant ascites occurring prior to GCV infusion. Interestingly, these patients developed peripheral blood and peritoneal eosinophilia in the period after the IP xenograft infusions consistent with the apparent role of eosinophils as important immune effector cells against xenogeneic cells, e.g., parasites [1–5].

These results suggested that the presence of $\alpha Gal^{(+)}$ xenogeneic cells in the vicinity of the tumor might have triggered a hyperacute rejection process, characterized by complement activation and inflammation that resulted in antitumor immunization. Consistent with this hypothesis, investigation of the patient's sera drawn before and after the treatment demonstrated a potent increase in their anti-αGal antibody titers. Furthermore, the patient's serum was able to mediate *in vitro* complement-mediated cell destruction of the murine VPCs injected into the patient. These observations concerning the immune physiology of the peritoneal cavity during a hyperacute rejection of xenografted cells ultimately led to a hyperacute-based mechanistic hypothesis of immune mediated destruction of ovarian cancer seen in this group of patients [2].

497

Cancer Immunotherapy. http://dx.doi.org/10.1016/B978-0-12-394296-8.00029-4

The phenomena of hyperacute rejection is typical in xenotransplantation scenarios that involve organ transfer where the donor is a lower mammal and the recipient is an old world primate. Typical of such cases, the graft vasculature of the donor organ is effectively destroyed within minutes of exposure to the host circulation [6]. The rejection mechanism involves recognition of donor vascular endothelial cells which have αGal epitopes on their surface that are rapidly bound by high-titer host circulating anti-αGal antibodies. These antibodies are complement fixing and the αGal$^{(+)}$ cells are rapidly lysed with high efficiency. The universality and robustness of the response creates an absolute block to successful xenotransplantation. The hyperacute rejection mainly occurs after binding of natural antibodies of the recipient to the αGal containing xenoantigens expressed on endothelial cells in the graft, leading to rapid complement activation and complete destruction of the graft. Additionally, non-complement fixing natural anti-αGal Ab induces Ab-dependent cell-mediated cytotoxicity (ADCC) that initiates tissue damage in xenotransplants mediated by NK cells [7–10].

The synthesis of αGal epitopes in various nonhuman mammals is catalyzed by the enzyme α [1,3] galactosyltransferase (αGT) in the Golgi apparatus of cells by the following reaction:

$$\text{Gal}\alpha(1,4)\text{GlcNAc-R} + \text{UDP-Gal} \rightarrow \text{Gal}\alpha(1\text{-}3)\text{Gal}\alpha(1,4)\text{GlcNAc} - \text{R}$$

This enzyme is active in New World monkeys but not in Old World monkeys and humans. Interestingly, the αGT gene is present in the human genome, but it is not transcribed. Moreover, two frame shift mutations are present (deletions generating premature stop codons) in human exons encoding the enzyme [11]. As a consequence, humans lack the αGal epitope in glycoproteins and glycolipids and will develop antibodies against it if exposed to naturally occurring αGal-containing proteins [12,13]. Production of this natural anti-αGal antibody in humans is constantly stimulated by the presence of αGal carbohydrate residues on intestinal and pulmonary microorganism flora [14]. These antibodies are typically acquired in the first six months of life in parallel with the transition to a more adult diet and/or colonization with adult colonic flora. The resulting antibody titers against the αGal epitope are among the highest recorded in humans, and anti-αGal antibodies can comprise >1% of the entire circulating antibody repertoire [15].

Based on the observations above, it was hypothesized that αGal epitope-mediated hyperacute rejection could be exploited as a therapeutic approach to treat human malignancies [2,16–18], and thus, a novel immunotherapy was developed. This immunotherapy leverages the power of the hyperacute rejection of αGal xenoepitopes expressed by vaccinating cells. Allogeneic human cancer cell lines, naturally αGal$^{(-)}$, are genetically engineered to express αGal epitopes, creating partially xenogeneic HyperAcute cells that are used to induce immunity that is cross-reactive with patient tumors. The construction, characterization and clinical application of this new immunotherapy are presented here. Sections below expand on preclinical studies, immunological mechanisms and human clinical trials currently underway.

II. PRECLINICAL DEVELOPMENT OF HYPERACUTE® IMMUNOTHERAPY

A. *In Vitro* experiments using human cells

Different types of viral vectors expressing the murine αGT gene were developed and used to transduce human αGal$^{(-)}$ cells. *In vitro* experiments demonstrated the efficient transduction of human cells leading to expression αGal epitopes (Figure 29.1A,B). Independent of the vector system, genetically modified cells expressing αGal are readily lysed by normal human serum in the presence of complement, whereas parental cells lacking αGal expression are not lysed under the same conditions (Figure 29.1C,D), confirming published data [19].

Typical of human tumor cell lines the parental CL1 cells are not lysed by autologous human serum. After transfer of the αGT gene to the CL1 parental cells (HyperAcute cells), addition of human sera and complement results in rapid and near complete destruction of these cells.

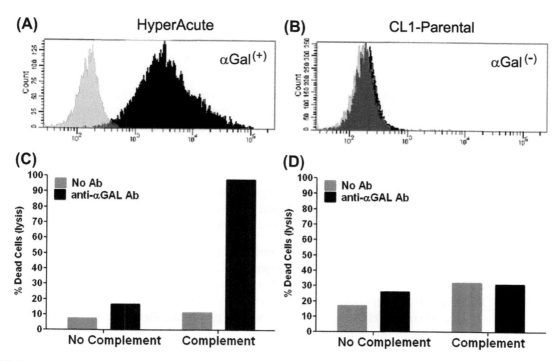

FIGURE 29.1

Lysis mediated by complement and anti-αGal Ab of HyperAcute cells. (A) Human cells are genetically modified to express αGal epitopes to constitute the HyperAcute cells. (B) Parental human cell lines lack the expression of αGal epitopes. (C) Lysis mediated by complement and anti-αGal Ab observed in HyperAcute cells. (D) Lysis is not observed in parental human cell lines.

B. Antitumor studies in animal models

499

The effectiveness of HyperAcute vaccines at inducing antitumor immunity has been verified in animal models using genetically modified mice. The mice used in these studies lack a functional αGT gene and have insignificant (often undetectable) anti-αGal antibody [20,21]. The animals can be immunized with αGal$^{(+)}$ cells, such as rabbit red blood cells, to induce anti-αGal antibody in titers similar to that found in human serum. The murine melanoma tumor cell line B16F0, was identified as negative for αGal and thereby to offer a well-characterized animal model that mimics the human scenario where both the tumor and the host are αGal$^{(-)}$.

1. REDUCED TUMORIGENICITY OF αGAL$^{(+)}$ MURINE MELANOMA CELLS

The first proof of principle experiment established whether tumor cells that express αGal epitopes would be susceptible to complement-dependent lysis mediated by anti-αGal antibodies *in vivo*, reducing tumorigenicity of these cells. To test this concept, αGT deficient mice were challenged with B16 melanoma cells genetically modified to express the αGal epitope. This series of experiments provided data highlighting effects of αGal expression on tumor cells in αGT deficient mice (αGT KO):

1. The presence of anti-αGal antibodies is necessary to observe reduced tumorigenicity of αGal$^{(+)}$ tumors. When wild type mice (immune tolerant to αGal) are challenged with an αGal$^{(+)}$ tumor, the tumor grows showing no reduction in tumorigenicity.
2. αGal$^{(+)}$ tumor cells are rejected *in vivo* when administered both subcutaneously and intravenously in αGT KO mice, preventing tumor development in about half of the animals challenged.
3. αGal$^{(+)}$ tumors that do grow in αGT KO mice are smaller when compared to αGal$^{(-)}$ tumors.
4. The kinetics of tumor growth suggests that immune mechanisms restrain growth of αGal-expressing tumors.

5. Long-term survival was observed in mice challenged with $\alpha Gal^{(+)}$ melanoma cells, whereas no long-term survivors are seen in animals engrafted with $\alpha Gal^{(-)}$ tumors.

6. Mice surviving challenge with $\alpha Gal^{(+)}$ melanoma cells are protected against a subsequent challenge with $\alpha Gal^{(-)}$ tumor.

Together, these results indicated that mice receiving $\alpha Gal^{(+)}$ tumor cells could develop immunity against $\alpha Gal^{(-)}$ tumor, suggesting that $\alpha Gal^{(+)}$ cells could be used as vaccines to immunize mice with pre-established $\alpha Gal^{(-)}$ tumors [17,22,23].

2. ANTITUMOR EFFECT OF $\alpha GAL^{(+)}$ MURINE MELANOMA VACCINE CELLS

Subsequent studies determined whether genetically modified and irradiated $\alpha Gal^{(+)}$ murine melanoma cells, comprising either syngeneic or allogeneic vaccines, would induce antitumor immunity in mice that were challenged subsequently with $\alpha Gal^{(-)}$ melanoma tumors. The following is a summary of the observed results:

1. Treatment of established subcutaneous and pulmonary tumors was successfully achieved by vaccination with syngeneic or allogeneic $\alpha Gal^{(+)}$ melanoma cell vaccine (HyperAcute).

2. T cells specific for $\alpha Gal^{(-)}$ melanoma cells were induced after vaccination with HyperAcute.

3. Strong T-cell-dependent immunity could be transferred from mice receiving the HyperAcute vaccine, preventing growth of pre-established lung melanoma metastases in recipients of the immune graft.

4. Classic mononuclear cell infiltrates were found in subcutaneous tumor from mice receiving HyperAcute vaccine, indicating that melanoma-specific T cells migrated into the tumor.

5. Non-classical cell infiltrates were found inside subcutaneous tumors from mice receiving HyperAcute vaccination. Interestingly, mast cells, eosinophils, plasma B cells and other leukocytes were found inside the tumors, suggestive of a broad immunological response.

6. No toxicity was observed in mice receiving syngeneic HyperAcute vaccines and allogeneic HyperAcute vaccines.

These experimental results demonstrate that allogeneic HyperAcute melanoma vaccines can induce strong cellular immunity against syngeneic $\alpha Gal^{(-)}$ melanoma leading to rejection of established tumors in mouse models [23–25]. These findings were the most suggestive that treatment strategies using HyperAcute technology were potentially useful for the treatment of human malignancies.

The following figures present only a few examples of the supporting evidence for the most relevant preclinical data.

HyperAcute allogeneic vaccines are effective at inhibiting the growth of pre-existing B16 tumors, significantly increasing the percent of animals that survive a lethal challenge with B16 melanoma (Figure 29.2, 55% vs. 5% $p < 0.001$). The HyperAcute vaccine treatment was effective since ~50% of mice survived and remained tumor free.

HyperAcute allogeneic vaccines are also effective at inhibiting growth of pre-existing disseminated tumors, as shown in examinations of the pulmonary burden of models exhibiting lung metastasis (Figure 29.3).

In adoptive transfer experiments, a significant decrease in the lung melanoma burden of recipient mice receiving T cells from mice vaccinated with HyperAcute allogeneic vaccine was observed. No reduction of lung melanoma metastases was observed in mice receiving T cells from control mice vaccinated with $\alpha Gal^{(-)}$ S91M3. A stronger protective T-cell-mediated antitumor immunity is generated by vaccination with HyperAcute allogeneic vaccines than with $\alpha Gal^{(-)}$ vaccines (Figure 29.4).

C. Immunological mechanism proposed

The experimental data shown above indicated that vaccination with $\alpha Gal^{(+)}$ allogeneic or autologous whole cell vaccines exerted a potent antitumor response in a therapeutic setting,

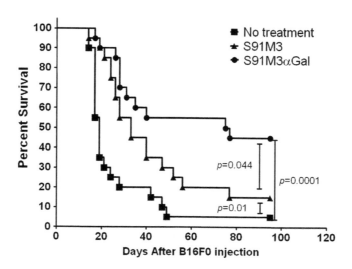

FIGURE 29.2

Treatment of pre-existing subcutaneous melanoma tumors with HyperAcute cells. Mice were challenged subcutaneously with B16F0. On days 5, 12, and 19 they received control vaccines S91M3 (αGal$^{(-)}$) or S91M3αGal (HyperAcute) vaccine cells. Survival analysis was performed using log-rank test. The difference in the mean survival using log-rank test is indicated.

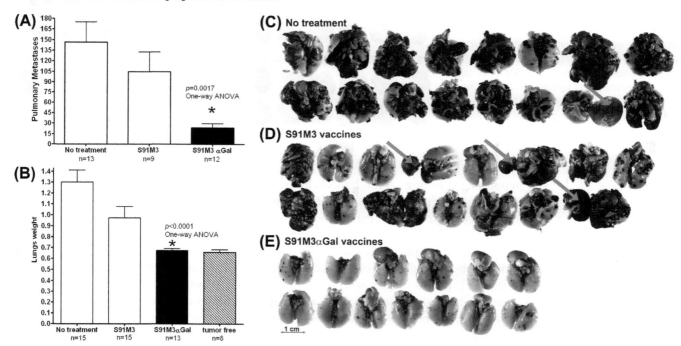

501

FIGURE 29.3

Treatment of pre-existing pulmonary melanoma tumors with HyperAcute vaccines. Pulmonary metastases were established by intravenous injection of B16F0 cells. Mice received either S91M3 (αGal$^{(-)}$) or S91M3αGal (HyperAcute) vaccine cells or no treatment on days 4, 12, and 19 after tumor inoculation. On day 28 after tumor inoculation, mice were humanely euthanized and lungs were collected. Pulmonary tumors were enumerated in a blinded manner. Results from two experiments are shown and express the mean of tumors burden in each group and errors are the SEM (A, B). The number of animals in each group is indicated. The lung weight of tumor-free animals is included. Lungs pictures from animals in panel B are shown for nonvaccinated animals (C) or from animals vaccinated with S91M3 (αGal$^{(-)}$) (D) or S91M3αGal HyperAcute (E). Arrows show tumors localized in distal sites (peritoneal cavity and liver metastasis) in control groups.

against localized or disseminated tumors. This antitumor response requires the presence of anti-αGal antibodies. Moreover, the vaccine elicits transferable T-cell-mediated effector cells that infiltrate the endogenous αGal$^{(-)}$ tumor. In addition, nonclassical infiltrating cells such as eosinophils are observed infiltrating the tumor after vaccination with HyperAcute vaccines.

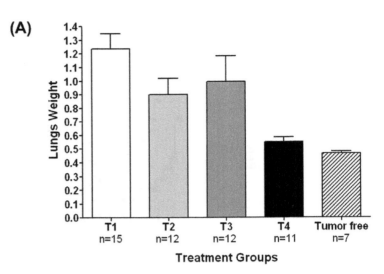

(A)

FIGURE 29.4

Adoptive T-cell transfer of melanoma-specific T cells induced by HyperAcute vaccines. (A) Donor mice received 3 weekly doses of whole cell vaccines (S91M3 or S91M3αGal). Two weeks after the last vaccination mice were humanely euthanized and spleens were collected. CD8$^+$ T cells were purified by magnetic cell sorting. Recipient mice were injected intravenously with B16F0 cells. Eight days after tumor challenge they were randomized into four different groups and subjected to the following treatments: group 1 received no T cells (T1); group 2 were inoculated intravenously with purified CD8$^+$ T cells from nonvaccinated animals (T2); group 3 received CD8$^+$ T cells from mice vaccinated with S91M3 cells (T3); and group 4 received CD8$^+$ T cells from mice vaccinated with S91M3αGal HyperAcute cells (T4). As a control, age-matched untreated, tumor-free animals were included. Four weeks after tumor inoculation mice were euthanized and lungs were collected. Lungs weight was determined and plotted. Results express the mean lungs weight. Error bars = SEM. One-way analysis of variance P = 0.0004 for all data sets. One-way analysis of variance excluding tumor-free animals P = 0.0045. (B) Lung pictures of recipient mice in each group (excluding tumor-free animals).

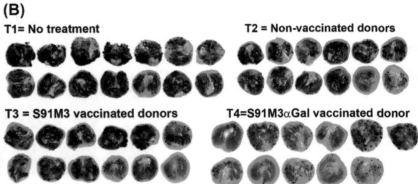

(B)

T1= No treatment   T2 = Non-vaccinated donors

T3 = S91M3 vaccinated donors   T4=S91M3αGal vaccinated donor

The hypothesized biological mechanism thought to permit successful vaccination based on αGal-mediated hyperacute rejection is shown in Figure 29.5. According to our model, allogeneic tumor vaccine cells [1] expressing αGal epitopes on their surface [2] are injected intradermally or subcutaneously in hosts with naturally acquired or induced high titers of anti-αGal Ab (humans or animal models respectively). The antitumor immune response is believed to be initiated by opsonization of the αGal$^{(+)}$ vaccine cells by anti-αGal antibody immediately after injection [3]. This triggers several mechanisms of cell destruction and antigen presentation. First, antibody opsonization of αGal epitopes facilitates complement-mediated cell lysis [4] and FcγR-mediated phagocytosis [5], an efficient mechanism of antigen uptake and processing. The anti-αGal and αGal epitope interaction activates the complement system and generates chemotactic complement cleavage peptides such as C3a and C5a, which induce an extensive recruitment of antigen-presenting cell (APC) [26,27]. In addition, complement activation and cell lysis triggers the production of pro-inflammatory "danger signals" [28], due to the cell debris that acts as an immune adjuvant by releasing heat shock proteins, toll-like receptors (TLRs), calreticulin, and other damage associated molecular pattern molecules (DAMPs) [29,30]. These molecules are potent APC activators that initiate and perpetuate immune response in a noninfectious inflammatory response that empowers APC for efficient T-cell stimulation [31–35]. In addition, NKT cells are suggested to participate in the induction of antitumor immunity by recognizing αGal-glycolipids and releasing large quantities of cytokines.

Different antigen uptake and processing pathways control the presentation of antigenic peptides, by either MHC class I molecules to cytotoxic T cells (endogenous pathway) or MHC class II molecules to helper (CD4+) T cells (exogenous pathway) [36]. To deliver exogenous

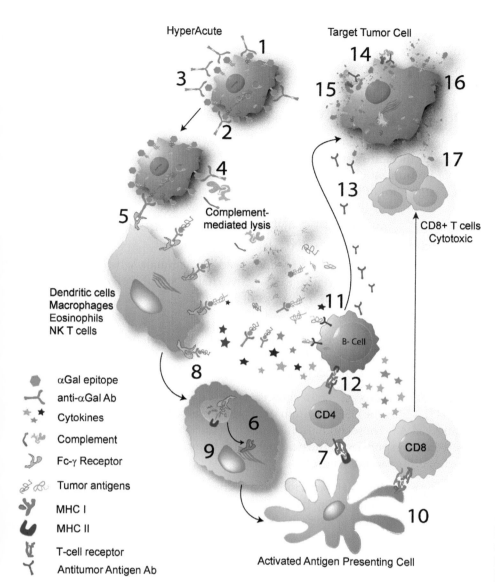

HyperAcute

Target Tumor Cell

Complement-
mediated lysis

CD8+ T cells
Cytotoxic

Dendritic cells
Macrophages
Eosinophils
NK T cells

B- Cell

αGal epitope
anti-αGal Ab
Cytokines
Complement
Fc-γ Receptor
Tumor antigens
MHC I
MHC II
T-cell receptor
Antitumor Antigen Ab

CD4

CD8

Activated Antigen Presenting Cell

FIGURE 29.5
Model proposed for induction of
cell-mediated antitumor immunity by
HyperAcute immunotherapy. Description
in the text.

503

antigen to the endogenous pathway and favor development of a cytotoxic (CD8+) T-cell
response, the engagement of the FcγR receptor to mediate antigen uptake of immunocomplexes is thought to be very important, as it stimulates the crosspresentation pathway [37–40].
Indeed, several studies indicate that, in addition to classical helper T-cell priming, antigen
acquired through endocytosis by DC via the FcγR results in the induction of T-cell effector
immunity [37,38]. Thus, engagement of the FcγR induces DC activation and maturation.
Other target cells that might be recruited to the site of immunization by FcγR engagement
include neutrophils, eosinophils and NK cells.

For HyperAcute vaccines, three mechanisms of antigen uptake are proposed to take place.
First, the exogenous pathway involving phago/pinocytosis sends antigens through the
endogenous endosomal/lysosomal pathway, resulting in the activation and proliferation of
helper T cells [6,7]. Second, FcγR-mediated antigen uptake of immunocomplexes involving
anti-αGal antibodies [8] will favor the crosspresentation pathway [9], resulting in preferential
activation of cytotoxic T cells [10]. Third, binding of tumor specific antigen molecules to
membrane-bound antibody present in naive B cells [11] will result in B-cell activation and
differentiation, and also in MHC class II antigen presentation that further stimulates

proliferation of memory (CD4+) T cells that recognize those antigens [12]. After activation and stimulation, the B cells proliferate, differentiate and produce cell surface antitumor antibodies [13], possibly facilitating killing of target tumor cell by complement-mediated cell lysis [14], antibody-dependent cell cytotoxicity [15] and FcγR-dependent phagocytosis [16]. Additionally, target cell destruction is achieved by cytotoxic CD8$^+$ T cells previously activated by differentiated dendritic and helper CD4$^+$ T cells [17].

In summary, HyperAcute vaccines achieve efficient cell destruction and antigen processing within minutes after vaccine administration. It is suggested that the strong initial immune reaction at the site of immunization induces both an effective antitumor immune response and also generates a large pool of long-lasting memory cells.

1. THE PRESENCE OF αGAL EPITOPES AND ANTI-αGAL ANTIBODIES IS NECESSARY TO ACHIEVE A STRONG ANTITUMOR RESPONSE

The requirement of anti-αGal Ab was demonstrated in wild type animals, which are immune tolerant to αGal epitopes. These animals failed to reject live challenge with B16αGal in striking contrast to αGT KO animals that develop high titers of anti-αGAL Ab, which reject a lethal challenge with B16αGal [23].

The presence of αGal epitopes in vaccine cells is also shown to be required to induce effective antitumor immunity. Both syngeneic and allogeneic vaccines lacking the expression of αGal epitopes failed to treat established tumors (Figure 29.2 and Figure 29.3 [24,25,41]).

Moreover, the efficacy of αGal expressing vaccines is abolished in wild type, αGal positive animals (Figure 29.7D). Wild type C57Bl/6 animals are immune tolerant to αGal epitopes and do not develop anti-αGal Ab. These animals, inoculated with B16 cells and vaccinated with B16αGal vaccines, were unresponsive to the treatment. This demonstrated that the presence of anti-αGal Ab is required for vaccine efficacy.

Figure 29.6 shows that precoating of HyperAcute vaccines increased the *in vivo* proliferation of lymphocytes in draining and nondraining lymph nodes, suggesting that the binding of HyperAcute cells by anti-αGal Ab is a necessary step in the induction of the antitumor

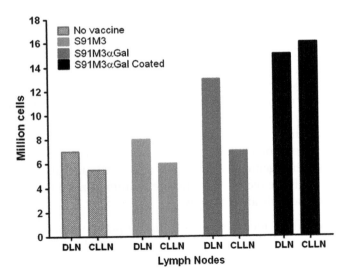

FIGURE 29.6

Precoating of HyperAcute vaccines increased the *in vivo* proliferation of lymphocytes in draining and nondraining lymph nodes. Mice received no treatment or they were immunized with S91M3, S91M3αGal or S91M3αGal precoated with polyclonal murine anti-αGal Ab. One day after immunization draining and nondraining lymph nodes were collected and cells present in the tissues were extracted and counted.

response. This result is supported by Abdel-Motal et al. [42]. The *in vivo* formation of immune complexes with anti-αGal and the effective internalization of immune complexes by APC, via Fc/FcγR interaction, resulted in effective activation of vaccine specific CD4+ and CD8+ T cells, and high cellular and humoral immune response [42].

2. BINDING OF ANTI-αGAL AB TO αGAL EPITOPES INDUCES THE RECRUITMENT OF APC, NEUTROPHILS NK AND EOSINOPHILS, AND THE ACTIVATION OF THESE CELLS PLAYS A ROLE IN ANTITUMOR IMMUNITY

Using αGal$^{(+)}$ liposomes for wound healing it was demonstrated that macrophages and neutrophils are recruited and activated accelerating wound healing in aGT KO mice [43]. Similarly, intratumor inoculation of glycolipids induced the recruitment of APC and the induction of antitumor immunity [44]. The role of αGal expressing glycolipids and NKT cells was evaluated in a double knockout animal lacking the expression of αGal epitopes and CD1-restricted T cells (αGTCD1 DKO animals). NKT cells are first responder T cells that serve as a bridge between the innate and adaptive immune system, recognizing lipid and glycolipid antigens in the context of the nonclassical class I MHC molecule CD1d. NKT cells can become involved in infectious diseases and induce allergy, or mediate a protective role in certain autoimmune diseases due to their suppressor activities, depending on their cytokine profile. In cancer, they can play opposite roles, contributing to antitumor immunity or suppressing it [45–48]. Our experiments indicate that in both the subcutaneous model and in the pulmonary model, NKT-cell ablation abolishes αGal-expressing vaccine efficacy (Figure 29.7 and Figure 29.8). These results demonstrate that NKT cells play an important role in the induction of antitumor immunity induced by HyperAcute vaccines. Further, many patients enrolled in a HyperAcute vaccine study for pancreatic cancer have shown increased eosinophils in peripheral blood counts (Figure 29.9). Thus, in accordance with previous observations in the ovarian clinical trials, increased activity of eosinophils may also be related to the biological activity of Hyper-Acute immunotherapy.

3. CELL INTEGRITY IS IMPORTANT FOR THE POTENCY OF HYPERACUTE IMMUNOTHERAPY

HyperAcute vaccines are irradiated whole tumor cell vaccines. The importance of cell integrity for the potency of the vaccine was evaluated in animal models. The conventional vaccine was prepared by rapidly thawing of cryopreserved and irradiated vaccine cells, with aliquots of this preparation lysed by two cycles of rapid freezing and thawing using liquid nitrogen. This preparation was shown to be 100% lysed (loss of cell integrity) by flow cytometry. Equal volumes of these two preparations were mixed to prepare a 50% lysed vaccine.

Vaccine preparations were confirmed by flow cytometry for each of the three injections used to treat animals with B16 melanoma tumors. Figure 29.10 shows that cell integrity is important for vaccine efficacy (potency), since complete lysis of the whole cell components abrogated antitumor efficacy. As shown previously, administration of the conventional S91M3αGal whole cell vaccine induces significant tumor retardation as previously shown [25]. However, while vaccines that lost 100% of cell integrity (100% lysis) were unable to retard tumor growth, 50% lysed vaccine preparations induced tumor retardation similar to the conventional whole cell vaccine (Figure 29.10A). Vaccines that lost cell integrity (100% lysis) were also unable to increase the survival of animals bearing melanoma tumors. On the contrary, vaccine cells that had only 50% viability were as efficient as the conventional whole cell vaccines to increase survival (Figure 29.10B). In conclusion, these results establish that the antitumor efficacy (potency) of HyperAcute vaccine preparations rely upon whole cell integrity.

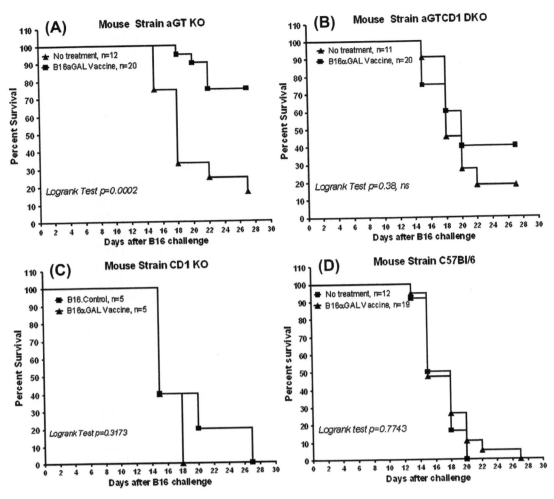

FIGURE 29.7

NKT cells are required in the mechanism for HyperAcute vaccines efficacy in the subcutaneous tumor model. The efficacy of HyperAcute vaccines was compared in 4 strains of mice. (A) αGT knockout (KO) animals; (B) αGTCD1 double knockout (DKO) animals; (C) CD1 KO animals; and (D) the wild type C57Bl/6 mice. The number of animals in each group and treatment is indicated. Mice were injected with B16F0 and 4 days later they received either no treatment or three doses of B16αGal(+) HyperAcute vaccine. (A) Significant improved survival is observed in αGT KO receiving HyperAcute vaccines. The lack of NKT cells in the αGTCD1 DKO abolished the efficacy of HyperAcute vaccines (B) as well as the expression of αGT in either CD1 KO and wild type animals (C and D, respectively). Log-rank test p values are depicted.

4. HYPERACUTE VACCINE INDUCES THE EXPANSION OF T CELLS WITH ANTITUMOR ACTIVITY IN NON-SMALL LUNG CANCER PATIENTS

B16 melanoma-bearing mice vaccinated with αGal(+) cells show greater T-cell proliferation, enhanced reactivity to melanoma peptides (as evidenced by intracellular TNFα staining) and cytotoxic T lymphocytes (detected by IFN-γ release and T-cell transfer experiments) than animals vaccinated with αGal(−) cells. These characters are transferable by T cells from these animals and capable of mediating an antitumor response [24,25].

We extended these preclinical observations in clinical trials of a HyperAcute vaccine developed for treatment of lung cancer. In the HyperAcute-Lung clinical study, 18 evaluable patients were tested for the production of interferon-gamma (IFN-γ) by peripheral blood lymphocytes by ELISPOT. Notably, 11 out of 18 tested patients responded with 10-fold increased IFN-γ after immunization. Notably, patients that responded with IFN-γ exhibited significant increased overall survival (Figure 29.11).

The human lung cancer cell lines used in this study to generate the HyperAcute-Lung vaccine were nonmodified parental (wild type) cell lines. However, in testing responses to this

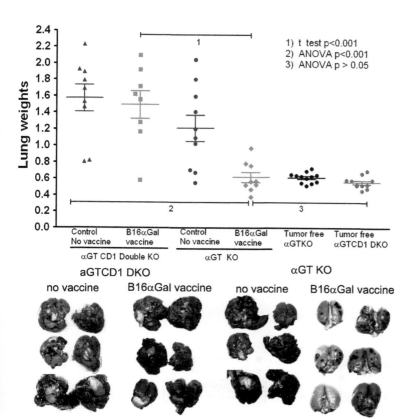

1) t test p<0.001
2) ANOVA p<0.001
3) ANOVA p > 0.05

FIGURE 29.8

NKT cells are required in the mechanism for HyperAcute vaccines efficacy in the pulmonary metastatic tumor model. The efficacy of HyperAcute vaccines was compared in αGT knockout (KO) animals and αGTCD1 double knockout (DKO) animals. Mice were injected intravenously with B16FO and subsequently they were vaccinated with of B16αGal$^{(+)}$ HyperAcute vaccines or received no vaccine. Lung pulmonary burden was determined 4 weeks later. ANOVA and t test p values are shown.

vaccine we also examined responses against a human lung adenocarcinoma cell line that was not a component of the irradiated whole cell HyperAcute-Lung vaccine that has been used for immunization of patients. Interestingly, high responder patients also developed reactivity to this noncomponent cell line, illustrating the ability of the vaccine to generate cross-reactivity to other lung cancer cell lines. This result was highly encouraging, because it supported the

507

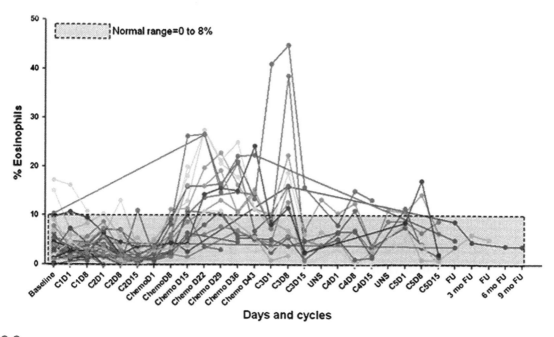

FIGURE 29.9

Increased eosinophils in patients receiving HyperAcute-Pancreas (Algenpantucel-L) vaccines. Eosinophils counts in patients enrolled in HyperAcute-Pancreas (Algenpantucel-L) clinical trial. Normal range is depicted.

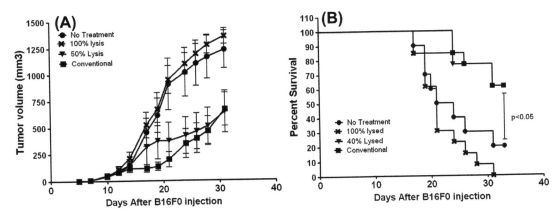

FIGURE 29.10

Cell integrity is required for potency of HyperAcute vaccine. Mice received a single subcutaneous injection with B16F0 and subsequently they were vaccinated with conventional S91M3αGal HyperAcute vaccine or with preparation of vaccines that were 40–50% or 100% lyzed. (A) Tumor kinetics of all groups; (B) Kaplan-Meir survival analysis. Lon-rank test *p* value is shown.

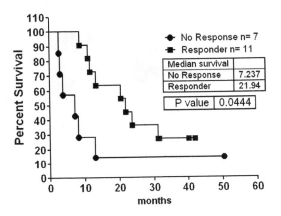

FIGURE 29.11

IFN-gamma production by peripheral blood lymphocytes after vaccination correlated with better overall survival in patients treated with HyperAcute-Lung. IFN-γ production was measured by ELISPOT. The reactivity of vaccinated patient's effector PBMC cultured with tumor-loaded autologous DC pulsed with irradiated parental cell lines was measured before and after immunization. Kaplan-Meier curve for the overall survival of responder and nonresponder patients in the IFN-γ ELISPOT assay. Responders were defined as those patients producing 10-fold or more increased IFN-γ after vaccination on half of the cell lines tested. The difference among responders and nonresponders is statistically significant ($p < 0.0444$).

notion that HyperAcute immunotherapy can induce cross-reactivity to patients' own tumor cells. In summary, these findings strongly suggested that HyperAcute immunotherapy can activate lymphocytes to eradicate tumor cells in a manner that is sufficiently effective to increase patient survival, providing a significant clinical benefit.

III. CLINICAL DEVELOPMENT OF HYPERACUTE IMMUNOTHERAPY

A. Introduction

HyperAcute immunotherapies are composed of an irradiated mixture of human allogeneic whole cancer cell lines that were genetically modified to add αGal residues to cell-surface lipids and proteins. This preparation therefore constitutes an off-the-shelf immunotherapy for cancer treatment. The αGal epitopes in this irradiated whole cell vaccine essentially function as a molecular adjuvant, harnessing the mechanism responsible for hyperacute rejection of xenotransplants. The immunostimulatory mechanism provided by the αGal is geared to break tolerance and enable longer duration of antitumor effects, while avoiding the risk of immunosuppressive counter-response posed by certain other immunoregulatory agents (e.g., GM-CSF).

HyperAcute immunotherapies now have been tested in multiple Phase 2 trials for various indications, including advanced non-small lung cancer, (Phase 1-2, n = 54), stage III/IV melanoma (Phase 1-2, n = 31), prostate (Phase 1, n = 8), pancreas (Phase 1-2, n = 86). Currently, the HyperAcute Pancreas immunotherapy is being tested in a 1:1 randomized Phase 3 study for treatment of resected pancreatic cancer. In these studies, a broad range of responses have been observed ranging from local to systemic skin reactions, objective tumor responses and immunological responses. Below is a brief description of indications, safety and efficacy data reported thus far for HyperAcute clinical trials.

B. Composition and indications

HyperAcute cancer immunotherapies are human tumor cell lines genetically modified to express αGal epitopes. After genetic modification these cells are subsequently selected for expression of αGal epitopes by fluorescence activated cell sorting. After growth HyperAcute cells are irradiated and resuspended in a pharmacologically acceptable carrier that preserves cell integrity during cryopreservation. The tumor cell lines used in the composition of vaccines of a particular cancer type are derived from cancers of the same tissue type and selected based on their expression profile of cell surface tumor-associated antigens.

HyperAcute immunotherapy is administered to human patients as a whole cell product. No specific safety precautions are necessary because administered cells have been lethally irradiated before freezing. Frozen vials of each vaccine cell line are carefully thawed, and equal amounts of each cell line component of the immunotherapy are injected into the patient intradermally at several sites in each treatment session. Dose escalation studies determined optimal dosing and scheduling for each indication for the treatment of solid tumors.

C. Safety data

The collective safety data from the four clinical studies, including a dose escalation study for the treatment of lung cancer, indicates that HyperAcute Immunotherapy has a favorable safety profile. No dose-limiting toxicities were reported and the maximum tolerated dose was not reached [49–51]. The most frequently reported adverse events were injection site reactions. Most patients responded with self-resolving skin reactions that are localized at the site of immunization. These skin manifestations vary from rapid-acute sensitization that occurs within minutes to hours after injection to delayed type of reactions that occur within days to

509

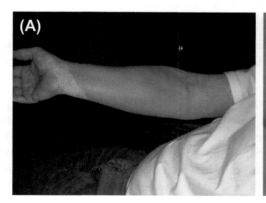
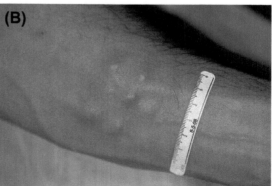

FIGURE 29.12

Skin reactions frequently observed after HyperAcute immunotherapy. Picture (A) shows a commonly observed rapid-acute inflammatory reaction at the site of immunization. Picture (B) shows a delayed-type hypersensitivity-like reaction that occurs days to weeks after immunization. These skin reactions resolve without intervention in the vast majority of the cases reported.

one week after immunization (Figure 29.12A, B respectively). Skin reactions associated with redness, swelling induration and itchiness are common adverse events attributed to the HyperAcute immunotherapy.

Interestingly, skin reactions have been described where the vaccine injection site "flared up" under random circumstances, i.e., during a common cold up to one year after immunization was completed. Furthermore, later vaccinations also have been observed to produce flare-type skin reactions at a previous vaccine site, frequently in the opposite limb. These observations are intriguing since they strongly suggest the persistence of immunological effector cells that respond upon recall at the initial vaccination site [52–56]. Further, these responses suggest that HyperAcute immunotherapy can elicit immunological memory. Memory T cells in nonlymphoid tissue, like skin, have been reported to enhance local and systemic immunity during infection [52]. Thus, flare reactions at the original injection site in patients receiving HyperAcute immunotherapy might be explained by re-induction of long-lasting antitumor memory cells. Notably, favorable clinical responses have been documented in some patients experiencing these responses. Ongoing clinical trials might provide further information about these intriguing observations.

D. Clinical responses

1. HYPERACUTE-PANCREAS (ALGENPANTUCEL-L [NLG0205])

After Phase I safety testing was completed, a Phase II, single arm, open label multicentered study was opened to enroll patients with newly diagnosed Stage 1 or 2 pancreatic carcinoma who had undergone surgical tumor resection within 6 weeks prior to enrollment (NCT00569387). Patients received a gemcitabine + chemoradiation regimen plus the HyperAcute-Pancreas (algenpantucel-L) immunotherapy for up to 14 intradermal immunizations.

The primary objective of this Phase II study was to assess disease-free survival (DFS), with DFS at one year following initiation of treatment as the primary endpoint. Since eligible patients had no evidence of disease at the time of enrollment in the study, appearance of new lesions constituted progression of disease. The one year DFS rate was calculated as the proportion of patients who show no evidence of disease 12 months from the date of study entry. This study enrolled 73 subjects with 69 evaluable patients.

This trial added HyperAcute-pancreas (algenpantucel-L) immunotherapy to the standard-of-care treatment regimen defined in RTOG 9704(57) as adjuvant 5-FU chemoradiotherapy plus gemcitabine. It also provided an opportunity to perform a dose-finding analysis of cohorts receiving biweekly algenpantucel-L injections of 100 million or 300 million cells. As of September 1, 2010, all patients had reached at least 20 months of follow-up with a median follow-up period of 26.6 months for the 69 evaluated patents.

The Kaplan-Meier estimated overall survival in this Phase 2 clinical trial, referred to as NLG0205, compares favorably to data from RTOG 97-04, a trial used to help define the current standard of care.

At 12 months after surgery overall survival for the combined 69 evaluable patient population in NLG0205 is 86%. Patients treated at both dose levels in NLG0205 compare favorably to the 63% one-year overall survival calculated by the Memorial Sloan Kettering Cancer Center nomogram for the NLG0205 patient population [58]. Furthermore, both dose levels in NLG0205 compare favorably to the 69% one-year overall survival observed for the 221 patients who received gemcitabine plus 5-FU based chemoradiotherapy in the RTOG 97-04 study [57] (Table 29.1).

The Kaplan-Meier estimate of median overall survival was 24.4 months for the combined patient population in NLG0205 versus 16.6 months predicted by the Memorial Sloan Kettering Cancer Center nomogram [58], for NLG0205 patients based on their study entry

TABLE 29.1 Comparative Results for HyperAcute-Pancreas NLG0205 at One Year

	Disease-Free Survival	Overall Survival
Brennan et al., 2005 nomogram [58]	Not Applicable	63%
RTOG 97-04 (221 ptients) [57]	<50%	69%
NLG-0205-100 million cell dose group	52%	80%
NLG-0205-300 million cell dose group	81%	96%

characteristics and 18.8 months for RTOG 97-04 patients (based on 221 patients receiving gemcitabine plus 5-FU based chemoradiotherapy).

This encouraging data prompted the initiation of a multicentered phase 3 study currently recruiting patients (NCT01072981).

2. HYPERACUTE-LUNG (NLG0101)

This study was a single-arm, open-label clinical trial conducted at the National Cancer Institute for the treatment of refractory, recurrent or metastatic non-small lung cancer (NSCLC, NCT00073398). Its primary endpoint, besides safety, was to assess tumor response rate after administration of HyperAcute-Lung, with a secondary endpoint to assess overall survival. For the Phase 1 portion of this clinical trial, in addition to safety, a positive response included stable disease for 16 weeks in patients who had enrolled after having previously shown progressive disease. A total of 17 patients in the Phase 1 portion and 37 patients in the Phase 2 portion were injected with the HyperAcute-Lung immunotherapy. Of 37 patients in the Phase 2 portion, only 28 were evaluated for clinical response. In the Phase 1 portion, four cohorts of patients each received injections of 3 million, 10 million, 30 million, or 100 million cells every four weeks for four doses, and one cohort of three patients received an initial dose of 500 million cells, followed by injections of 300 million cells every two weeks for up to seven doses. In the Phase 2 portion, the 28 patients evaluated received injections of 300 million cells every two weeks for up to eight doses.

The Phase 1 portion of this clinical trial demonstrated a favorable safety profile, with no dose-limiting toxicities at any of the five escalating dose levels. There have been no reported grade four adverse events attributed to HyperAcute-Lung. The most common treatment-related adverse reactions for HyperAcute-Lung were injection site reaction [49].

The interim results of the Phase 2 clinical trial for HyperAcute Lung were encouraging. As of 2011, results for the 28 patients evaluated in the Phase 2 clinical trial group showed a median overall survival of 11.3 months, and a one-year survival rate of 46%.

Prior Phase 3 studies showed that in the refractory, recurrent or metastatic NSCLC setting (second line therapy), the median overall survival of patients receiving best supportive care was 4.6 months and the median overall survival of patients receiving pemetrexed or docetaxel (Taxotere) therapy was approximately eight months [59,60]. Results from the Phase 2 study indicated that HyperAcute-Lung immunotherapy compared favorably to current standard-of-care cytotoxic chemotherapy. Table 29.2 summarizes comparative results for second-line treatment in advanced NSCLC with pemetrexed, docetaxel and HyperAcute-Lung, including safety data. HyperAcute-Lung immunotherapy produced an encouraging 11.3 month median overall survival in the Phase 2 study, with a favorable safety profile, prompting an ongoing evaluation of alternative designs for a Phase 2B/3 clinical trial in NSCLC.

3. HYPERACUTE-MELANOMA IN COMBINATION WITH PEG-INTRON

The HyperAcute-Melanoma immunotherapy was combined in a collaborative investigator-initiated Phase 2 clinical study for the treatment of advanced melanoma. The study treatment

TABLE 29.2 Comparative Results for the Treatment of NSCLC with HyperAcute-Lung

Therapy	Overall Survival (months)	12 month Survival	Serious Adverse Events (CTC Grade 3 or 4) Attributed to Therapy			
			Nausea	Fatigue	Anemia	Neutrope nia
Best Supportive Care [59]	4.6	11%	–	–	–	–
Docetaxel [59]	7.5	37%	1.80%	5.40%	4.30%	40.20%
Pemetrexed [60]	8.3	30%	2.60%	5.30%	4.20%	5.30%
HyperAcute-Lung	11.3	46%	0%	0%	0%	0%

consisted of 12 weekly injections of HyperAcute-Melanoma with PEG-Intron being co-administered in weeks five through 12. This was the first instance of a HyperAcute immunotherapy product tested in combination with another approved immunomodulator (PEG-Intron). The primary objective of this clinical trial was to conduct correlative scientific studies of patient tumor and peripheral blood samples to evaluate the mechanism of any observed anti-tumor effect involving the innate or cell-mediated host immune responses to HyperAcute immunotherapy when combined with PEG-Intron. In this clinical trial, 25 patients were treated.

HyperAcute Melanoma demonstrated good tolerability and a favorable safety profile, with no systemic, drug-related serious adverse events characterized by the investigators as possibly or probably attributable to the vaccine. The most common nonserious adverse events reported were injection site reactions as before [51].

HyperAcute-Melanoma appeared to produce immunologic effects that are known to impact clinical outcomes. Vitiligo is an autoimmune condition implicated in clinical trials of other immunotherapy products as correlated with a favorable response to therapy in melanoma patients [61–63]. Interestingly, vitiligo was observed in 4 out of 25 (16%) patients and correlated with clinical response. Furthermore, all patients evaluated developed autoimmune antibodies. Durable clinical responses were observed in this trial, encouraging evaluation of further clinical trial designs using HyperAcute-Melanoma alone or in combination in new settings.

E. Response evaluation in immunotherapy trials

Similar to what has been reported in other high-profile immunotherapy studies, multiple patients showed either delayed tumor responses or long-term stable disease despite initial progression by Response Evaluation Criteria in Solid Tumors (RECIST) criteria. In the HyperAcute prostate study, one patient characterized as a nonresponder according to RECIST remained alive with a stable bone metastasis for over 70 months. Likewise, similar observations have been documented in HyperAcute lung, melanoma, and pancreas clinical studies.

Recently four different response patterns have been recognized in large immunotherapy trials: (a) shrinkage in baseline lesions, without new lesions; (b) durable stable disease (which in some patients is followed by a slow, steady decline in total tumor burden); (c) response after an initial increase in total tumor burden; and (d) response in the presence of new lesions. All these patterns were associated with favorable survival [64,65]. Overall, the clinical responses patterns observed in the HyperAcute immunotherapy trials concur with the systematic criteria for Immune-Related Response Criteria as a way to measure beneficial clinical responses in immunotherapy trials [64,66,67].

Immunologic laboratory parameters have been evaluated in an attempt to find surrogate markers to evaluate efficacy in these trials. Some of these studies, briefly described below, seem to suggest that immunological parameters as well as delayed and complex clinical tumor responses might be a more accurate way to determine efficacy in immunotherapy trials.

F. Overview of immunological responses to hyperacute immunotherapy

The effects of HyperAcute immunotherapy on immunological parameters in patients on trial have been assessed using a panel of *in vitro* assays. The measurement of immune responses after immunization allows the association of immunogenicity with eventual clinical outcome. Ideally, some of such measurements may potentially be used to monitor the immunotherapy and act as supporting or surrogate endpoints for efficacy immunotherapy clinical trials.

Analysis of immunological responses in patients vaccinated with HyperAcute immunotherapy in clinical trials of lung, prostate, melanoma and pancreatic cancer showed the following.

- Baseline levels of IgG anti-αGal antibodies were quite variable. The vast majority of tested patients responded with elevated IgG anti-αGal antibody levels after immunization (2 to over 100 fold), demonstrating a clear biological effect of HyperAcute immunotherapy.
- HyperAcute immunotherapy can elicit the production of antitumor antibodies (Ab) and can overcome tolerance by inducing antibodies (IgG) recognizing peptides derived from several proteins commonly overexpressed in prostate cancer.
- Anti-Mesothelin Ab anti-CEA Ab were increased post immunization in the HyperAcute Pancreas study.
- Antitumor Ab were detected in the HyperAcute-Melanoma (anti-tyrosinase Ab) and HyperAcute-Lung trials (anti-CEA Ab).
- Importantly, the production of interferon gamma by T cells obtained from immunized patients was associated with better survival in the HyperAcute-Lung study.
- Cross-priming to nonrelated lung cell lines was demonstrated in patients receiving HyperAcute-Lung immunotherapy.
- The majority of patients tested have elevated IL-5 as measured by ELISPOT after immunization, suggesting that this cytokine may play a role in the biologic properties of HyperAcute immunotherapy.
- In the HyperAcute Pancreas study a considerable number of patients develop eosinophilia suggesting that these cells might play a role in the mechanism for this immunotherapy activity.

In summary HyperAcute immunotherapy is a novel approach that shows signs of clinical efficacy and immune activation in a number of trials and disease settings. The immunologic manifestations of HyperAcute immunizations are multifaceted, as evidenced by the provocative skin reactions and activation of both cellular and humoral arms of the immune system. Future clinical trials and combination trials will help elucidate further this novel immunotherapy.

IV. CONCLUSIONS

The hyperacute rejection of a xenotransplant is characterized by a complement mediated antibody immune response dependent on αGal epitopes. Based on these immunologic reactions, we hypothesized that the hyperacute rejection mechanism could be exploited to alter antigen processing resulting in a novel therapeutic approach to treat human malignancies. In animal models αGal epitopes expressed on genetically engineered allogeneic tumor vaccines elicit a potent T-cell dependent antitumor immunity. In clinical studies of patients with malignancies, the immunologic manifestations of HyperAcute immunization are multifaceted with activation of both cellular and humoral arms of the immune system. Ongoing studies aim to confirm the therapeutic benefit of this class of drug including laboratory studies to identify mechanisms of action and surrogate markers of activity. This innovative immunotherapy was designed to break immune tolerance of tumor and to stimulate effective antitumor immunity. The data obtained in ongoing clinical studies indicates that HyperAcute immunotherapy can use a straightforward genetic engineering approach to develop potent, cost-effective "off the shelf" human cancer vaccines with a highly tolerable toxicity profile. Continuation and expansion of clinical studies, including extension to new diseases and combinations with existing modalities, are indicated.

ACKNOWLEDGMENTS

The authors wish to acknowledge our colleagues at NewLink Genetics for their numerous contributions to the design and execution of the studies reported here. We also wish to recognize the contributions made by the numerous investigators, their institutions, and the patients participating in these clinical studies that contribute to our advancement in knowledge.

References

[1] Lee JJ, Jacobsen EA, McGarry MP, Schleimer RP, Lee NA. Eosinophils in health and disease: the LIAR hypothesis. Clin Exp Allergy 2010 Apr;40(4):563–75.

[2] Link Jr CJ, Seregina T, Atchison R, Hall A, Muldoon R, Levy JP. Eliciting hyperacute xenograft response to treat human cancer: alpha(1,3) galactosyltransferase gene therapy. Anticancer Res. 1998;18(4A):2301–8.

[3] Link Jr CJ, Seregina T, Levy JP, Martin M, Ackermann M, Moorman DW. Murine retroviral vector producer cells survival and toxicity in the dog liver. In Vivo 2000;14(5):643–9.

[4] Link CJ, Seregina T, Traynor A, Burt RK. Cellular suicide therapy of malignant disease. Stem Cells 2000;18(3):220–6.

[5] Link Jr CJ, Moorman D, Seregina T, Levy JP, Schabold KJ. A phase I trial of in vivo gene therapy with the herpes simplex thymidine kinase/ganciclovir system for the treatment of refractory or recurrent ovarian cancer. Hum Gene Ther 1996;7(9):1161–79.

[6] Joziasse DH, Oriol R. Xenotransplantation: the importance of the Galalpha1,3Gal epitope in hyperacute vascular rejection. Biochim Biophys Acta 1999;1455(2-3):403–18.

[7] Baumann BC, Forte P, Hawley RJ, Rieben R, Schneider MK, Seebach JD. Lack of galactose-alpha-1,3-galactose expression on porcine endothelial cells prevents complement-induced lysis but not direct xenogeneic NK cytotoxicity. J Immunol 2004 May 15;172(10):6460–7.

[8] Schaapherder AF, Daha MR, te Bulte MT, van der Woude FJ, Gooszen HG. Antibody-dependent cell-mediated cytotoxicity against porcine endothelium induced by a majority of human sera. Transplantation 1994 May 15;57(9):1376–82.

[9] Watier H, Guillaumin JM, Vallee I, Thibault G, Gruel Y, Lebranchu Y, et al. Human NK cell-mediated direct and IgG-dependent cytotoxicity against xenogeneic porcine endothelial cells. Transpl Immunol 1996 Dec;4(4):293–9.

[10] Watier H, Guillaumin JM, Piller F, Lacord M, Thibault G, Lebranchu Y, et al. Removal of terminal alpha-galactosyl residues from xenogeneic porcine endothelial cells. Decrease in complement-mediated cytotoxicity but persistence of IgG1-mediated antibody-dependent cell-mediated cytotoxicity. Transplantation 1996 Jul 15;62(1):105–13.

[11] Joziasse DH, Shaper JH, Jabs EW, Shaper NL. Characterization of an alpha 1—3-galactosyltransferase homologue on human chromosome 12 that is organized as a processed pseudogene. J Biol Chem 1991 Apr 15;266(11):6991–8.

[12] Larsen RD, Rivera-Marrero CA, Ernst LK, Cummings RD, Lowe JB. Frameshift and nonsense mutations in a human genomic sequence homologous to a murine UDP-Gal:beta-D-Gal(1,4)-D-GlcNAc alpha(1,3)-galactosyltransferase cDNA. J Biol Chem 1990;265(12):7055–61.

[13] Galili U, Shohet SB, Kobrin E, Stults CL, Macher BA. Man, apes, and Old World monkeys differ from other mammals in the expression of alpha-galactosyl epitopes on nucleated cells. J Biol Chem 1988;263(33):17755–62.

[14] Posekany KJ, Pittman HK, Bradfield JF, Haisch CE, Verbanac KM. Induction of cytolytic anti-Gal antibodies in alpha-1,3-galactosyltransferase gene knockout mice by oral inoculation with Escherichia coli O86:B7 bacteria. Infect Immun 2002 Nov;70(11):6215–22.

[15] Galili U, Anaraki F, Thall A, Hill-Black C, Radic M. One percent of human circulating B lymphocytes are capable of producing the natural anti-Gal antibody. Blood 1993 Oct 15;82(8):2485–93.

[16] Galili U, LaTemple DC. Natural anti-Gal antibody as a universal augmenter of autologous tumor vaccine immunogenicity. Immunol Today 1997 Jun;18(6):281–5.

[17] Posekany KJ, Pittman HK, Swanson MS, Haisch CE, Verbanac KM. Suppression of Lewis lung tumor development in alpha 1,3 galactosyltransferase knock-out mice. Anticancer Res 2004 Mar-Apr;24(2B):605—12.

[18] Galili U. Autologous tumor vaccines processed to express alpha-gal epitopes: a practical approach to immunotherapy in cancer. Cancer Immunol Immunother 2004 Nov;53(11):935—45.

[19] Jager U, Takeuchi Y, Porter C. Induction of complement attack on human cells by Gal(alpha1,3)Gal xenoantigen expression as a gene therapy approach to cancer. Gene Ther 1999 Jun;6(6):1073—83.

[20] Thall AD, Maly P, Lowe JB. Oocyte Gal alpha 1,3Gal epitopes implicated in sperm adhesion to the zona pellucida glycoprotein ZP3 are not required for fertilization in the mouse. J Biol Chem 1995;270(37):21437—40.

[21] Thall AD, Murphy HS, Lowe JB. alpha 1,3-Galactosyltransferase-deficient mice produce naturally occurring cytotoxic anti-Gal antibodies. Transplant Proc 1996;28(2):556—7.

[22] Unfer RC, Hellrung D, Link Jr CJ. Immunity to the alpha(1,3)galactosyl epitope provides protection in mice challenged with colon cancer cells expressing alpha(1,3)galactosyl-transferase: a novel suicide gene for cancer gene therapy. Cancer Res 2003 Mar 1;63(5):987—93.

[23] Rossi GR, Unfer RC, Seregina T, Link CJ. Complete protection against melanoma in absence of autoimmune depigmentation after rejection of melanoma cells expressing alpha(1,3)galactosyl epitopes. Cancer Immunol Immunother 2005 May;54:999—1009.

[24] Rossi GR, Mautino MR, Unfer RC, Seregina TM, Vahanian N, Link CJ. Effective treatment of preexisting melanoma with whole cell vaccines expressing A(1,3)-galactosyl epitopes. Cancer Res 2005;65(22):10555—61. 2005.

[25] Rossi G, Mautino MR, Awwad D, Husske K, Lejukole H, Koenigsfeld M, et al. Allogeneic melanoma vaccine expressing aGal epitopes induces antitumor immunity to autologous antigens in mice without signs of toxicity. J Immunother 2008;31(6):545—54.

[26] Stager S, Alexander J, Kirby AC, Botto M, Rooijen NV, Smith DF, et al. Natural antibodies and complement are endogenous adjuvants for vaccine-induced CD8+ T-cell responses. Nat Med 2003 Oct;9(10):1287—92.

[27] Galili U, Wigglesworth K, Abdel-Motal UM. Accelerated healing of skin burns by anti-Gal/alpha-gal liposomes interaction. Burns 2009 Mar;36(2):239—51.

[28] Matzinger P. The danger model: a renewed sense of self. Science 2002 Apr 12;296(5566):301—5.

[29] Foell D, Wittkowski H, Vogl T, Roth J. S100 proteins expressed in phagocytes: a novel group of damage-associated molecular pattern molecules. J Leukoc Biol. 2007 Jan;81(1):28—37.

[30] Bianchi ME. DAMPs, PAMPs and alarmins: all we need to know about danger. J Leukoc Biol 2007 Jan;81(1):1—5.

[31] Takeda K, Kaisho T, Akira S. Toll-like receptors. Annu Rev Immunol 2003;21:335—76.

[32] Akira S, Takeda K, Kaisho T. Toll-like receptors: critical proteins linking innate and acquired immunity. Nat Immunol 2001 Aug;2(8):675—80.

[33] Lotze MT, Zeh HJ, Rubartelli A, Sparvero LJ, Amoscato AA, Washburn NR, et al. The grateful dead: damage-associated molecular pattern molecules and reduction/oxidation regulate immunity. Immunol Rev 2007 Dec;220:60—81.

[34] Ellerman JE, Brown CK, de Vera M, Zeh HJ, Billiar T, Rubartelli A, et al. Masquerader: high mobility group box-1 and cancer. Clin Cancer Res 2007 May 15;13(10):2836—48.

[35] Lotze MT, Deisseroth A, Rubartelli A. Damage associated molecular pattern molecules. Clin Immunol 2007 Jul;124(1):1—4.

[36] Honey K, Rudensky AY. Lysosomal cysteine proteases regulate antigen presentation. Nat Rev Immunol 2003 Jun;3(6):472—82.

[37] Schuurhuis DH, Ioan-Facsinay A, Nagelkerken B, van Schip JJ, Sedlik C, Melief CJ, et al. Antigen-antibody immune complexes empower dendritic cells to efficiently prime specific CD8+ CTL responses in vivo. J Immunol 2002 Mar 1;168(5):2240—6.

[38] Heath WR, Carbone FR. Cross-presentation, dendritic cells, tolerance and immunity. Annu Rev Immunol 2001;19:47—64.

[39] Li M, Davey GM, Sutherland RM, Kurts C, Lew AM, Hirst C, et al. Cell-associated ovalbumin is cross-presented much more efficiently than soluble ovalbumin in vivo. J Immunol 2001 May 15;166(10):6099—103.

[40] Rafiq K, Bergtold A, Clynes R. Immune complex-mediated antigen presentation induces tumor immunity. J Clin Invest 2002 Jul;110(1):71—9.

[41] LaTemple DC, Abrams JT, Zhang SY, Galili U. Increased immunogenicity of tumor vaccines complexed with anti-Gal: studies in knockout mice for alpha1,3galactosyltransferase. Cancer Res 1999;59(14):3417—23.

[42] Abdel-Motal UM, Wigglesworth K, Galili U. Mechanism for increased immunogenicity of vaccines that form in vivo immune complexes with the natural anti-Gal antibody. Vaccine 2009 May 18;27(23):3072—82.

[43] Wigglesworth KM, Racki WJ, Mishra R, Szomolanyi-Tsuda E, Greiner DL, Galili U. Rapid recruitment and activation of macrophages by anti-Gal/alpha-Gal liposome interaction accelerates wound healing. J Immunol 2011 Apr 1;186(7):4422—32.

515

[44] Galili U, Wigglesworth K, Abdel-Motal UM. Intratumoral injection of alpha-gal glycolipids induces xenograft-like destruction and conversion of lesions into endogenous vaccines. J Immunol 2007 Apr 1;178(7):4676—87.

[45] Kinjo Y, Ueno K. iNKT cells in microbial immunity: recognition of microbial glycolipids. Microbiol Immunol 2011 Jul;55(7):472—82.

[46] Terabe M, Berzofsky JA. The role of NKT cells in tumor immunity. Adv Cancer Res 2008;101:277—348.

[47] Berzofsky JA, Terabe M. A novel immunoregulatory axis of NKT cell subsets regulating tumor immunity. Cancer Immunol Immunother 2008 Nov;57(11):1679—83.

[48] Berzofsky JA, Terabe M. The contrasting roles of NKT cells in tumor immunity. Curr Mol Med 2009 Aug;9(6):667—72.

[49] Morris JC, Rossi GR, Vahanian NN, Janik JE, Tennant L, Ramsey WJ, et al. Phase I/II study of antitumor vaccination using lung cancer cells expressing murine α(1,3)galactosyltransferase (αGT) in non-small cell lung cancer (NSCLC). AACR Annual Meeting abstract number 2010;2423.

[50] Hardacre JM, Mulcahy MF, Talamoni M, Obel JC, Rocha Lima CMS, Safran H, et al. Effect of hyperacute immunotherapy in addition to standard adjuvant therapy for resected pancreatic cancer on disease-free and overall survival: Preliminary analysis of phase II data. J Clin Oncol 2010;(Suppl. 4059):abstr.

[51] Riker AI, Alsfeld M, Harrison D, Foxworth Q, Lee G, Rossi R, et al. A phase II clinical trial of a novel combinatorial antitumor immunotherapy for patients with high-risk resected stage III and metastatic melanoma. J Clin Oncol 2010;(Suppl. 4059):abstr.

[52] Gebhardt T, Wakim LM, Eidsmo L, Reading PC, Heath WR, Carbone FR. Memory T cells in nonlymphoid tissue that provide enhanced local immunity during infection with herpes simplex virus. Nat Immunol 2009 May;10(5):524—30.

[53] Wakim LM, Gebhardt T, Heath WR, Carbone FR. Cutting edge: local recall responses by memory T cells newly recruited to peripheral nonlymphoid tissues. J Immunol 2008 Nov 1;181(9):5837—41.

[54] Wakim LM, Waithman J, van Rooijen N, Heath WR, Carbone FR. Dendritic cell-induced memory T cell activation in nonlymphoid tissues. Science 2008 Jan 11;319(5860):198—202.

[55] Obar JJ, Jellison ER, Sheridan BS, Blair DA, Pham QM, Zickovich JM, et al. Pathogen-induced inflammatory environment controls effector and memory CD8+ T cell differentiation. J Immunol 2011 Nov 15;187(10):4967—78.

[56] Sheridan BS, Lefrancois L. Regional and mucosal memory T cells. Nat Immunol 2011 Jun;12(6):485—91.

[57] Regine WF, Winter KA, Abrams RA, Safran H, Hoffman JP, Konski A, et al. Fluorouracil vs gemcitabine chemotherapy before and after fluorouracil-based chemoradiation following resection of pancreatic adenocarcinoma: a randomized controlled trial. JAMA 2008 Mar 5;299(9):1019—26.

[58] Brennan MF, Kattan MW, Klimstra D, Conlon K. Prognostic nomogram for patients undergoing resection for adenocarcinoma of the pancreas. Ann Surg 2004 Aug;240(2):293—8.

[59] Shepherd FA, Dancey J, Ramlau R, Mattson K, Gralla R, O'Rourke M, et al. Prospective randomized trial of docetaxel versus best supportive care in patients with non-small-cell lung cancer previously treated with platinum-based chemotherapy. J Clin Oncol 2000 May;18(10):2095—103.

[60] Hanna N, Shepherd FA, Fossella FV, Pereira JR, De Marinis F, von Pawel J, et al. Randomized phase III trial of pemetrexed versus docetaxel in patients with non-small-cell lung cancer previously treated with chemotherapy. J Clin Oncol 2004 May 1;22(9):1589—97.

[61] Byrne KT, Cote AL, Zhang P, Steinberg SM, Guo Y, Allie R, et al. Autoimmune melanocyte destruction is required for robust CD8+ memory T cell responses to mouse melanoma. J Clin Invest 2011 May 2;121(5):1797—809.

[62] Quaglino P, Marenco F, Osella-Abate S, Cappello N, Ortoncelli M, Salomone B, et al. Vitiligo is an independent favourable prognostic factor in stage III and IV metastatic melanoma patients: results from a single-institution hospital-based observational cohort study. Ann Oncol 2009 Feb;21(2):409—14.

[63] Gogas H, Ioannovich J, Dafni U, Stavropoulou-Giokas C, Frangia K, Tsoutsos D, et al. Prognostic significance of autoimmunity during treatment of melanoma with interferon. N Engl J Med 2006 Feb 16;354(7):709—18.

[64] Wolchok JD, Hoos A, O'Day S, Weber JS, Hamid O, Lebbe C, et al. Guidelines for the evaluation of immune therapy activity in solid tumors: immune-related response criteria. Clin Cancer Res 2009 Dec 1;15(23):7412—20.

[65] Small EJ, Schellhammer PF, Higano CS, Redfern CH, Nemunaitis JJ, Valone FH, et al. Placebo-controlled phase III trial of immunologic therapy with sipuleucel-T (APC8015) in patients with metastatic, asymptomatic hormone refractory prostate cancer. J Clin Oncol 2006 Jul 1;24(19):3089—94.

[66] Hoos A, Eggermont AM, Janetzki S, Hodi FS, Ibrahim R, Anderson A, et al. Improved endpoints for cancer immunotherapy trials. J Natl Cancer Inst 2010 Sep 22;102(18):1388—97.

[67] FDA, S. USDHH. Guidance for Industry. Clinical Considerations for Therapeutic Cancer Vaccines 2009.

CHAPTER 30

Tumor Exosomes and Their Impact on Immunity and Cancer Progression

Veronica Huber, Paola Filipazzi, Licia Rivoltini
Unit of Immunotherapy of Human Tumors, Fondazione IRCCS Istituto Nazionale dei Tumori, Milan, Italy

I. INTRODUCTION

Tumor immunity occurs in the initial phase of neoplastic transformation and may influence disease progression and patient prognosis. However, a complex network of mechanisms directly mediated by tumor cells or by the pro-inflammatory associated milieu progressively blunts immune reactivity, thereby ultimately silencing adaptive immunity against cancer cells. This phenomenon has been demonstrated to occur not only at the primary tumor site, but also in regional or distant immune districts, such as draining lymph nodes or the bone marrow, suggesting the presence of factors capable of molding immune responses at systemic level. An increasing interest has been focused recently on tumor exosomes as a pathophysiologically relevant pathway for delivery of defined signals from the primary tumor site to distant organs. These nanovesicular organelles are in fact hypothesized to represent an efficient tool for tumor cells to influence host responses without the need for a cell-to-cell contact.

In this chapter, we outline the main known features of tumor exosomes and their potential functions in the cancer-bearing host, including studies that have dealt with nano-organelles that have been variously named yet shared the canonical features of exosomes. In addition, as specific studies focused on biogenesis and composition have been mostly performed in nontumor cell models, data referring to these pathways are also reported, to provide a wider view on the biological nature and function of exosomes.

II. DISCOVERY AND DEFINITION OF EXOSOMES

The term *exosome* as a nonplasma membrane-derived vesicle emerged for the first time during studies about the transferrin receptor (TfR) "shedding" by reticulocytes undergoing maturation [1,3]. These vesicular structures were then investigated in different cell types, and common features in terms of size, endosomal origin [4], release mechanisms and composition, were identified. However, a cell type-specific repertoire in terms of protein content was also revealed by proteomic studies [5].

The exosomes, when analyzed by electron microscopy, appear as "cup shaped" or round, depending on the imaging procedure, presenting as membrane vesicles of about 50–100 nm diameter [6] but heterogeneous in size, with smaller vesicles often observed in the same preparation.

517

Cancer Immunotherapy. http://dx.doi.org/10.1016/B978-0-12-394296-8.00030-0

Various classifications based on standard visualization by fluorescence or transmitted light microscopy techniques, density gradient centrifugation, and purity assessment of isolated fractions, together with expression of endosomal markers such as CD63, CD81 and other exosome-associated tetraspanins, have been proposed [7,8]. The achievement of such standard requirements has greatly contributed to the reliability of exosome science.

Exosomes have been detected in several body fluids, such as plasma [9], bronchoalveolar fluid [10], urine [11], sperm [12], amniotic fluid [13], saliva [14] and bile [15], suggesting that their release is a common trait of normal cells under physiological conditions. These nano-vesicles have been also purified from *in vitro* cultures of several different cells, including cells from blood (reticulocytes, mast cells, dendritic cells (DCs), platelets, B and T lymphocytes) and nervous systems [16], as well as fibroblasts [17], keratinocytes [18], epithelial cells [19], endothelial cells and mesenchymal stem cells [20].

III. BIOGENESIS AND COMPOSITION OF EXOSOMES FROM NORMAL AND TUMOR CELLS

Exosomes are generated within a late endocytic compartment known as multivesicular body (MVB), which is formed by progressive processes of membrane invagination into the lumen, permitting subsequent release into the extracellular milieu by fusion with the plasma membrane. Through this pathway, molecules inserted into the exosome membrane are thought to maintain the same orientation displayed in the whole cell (i.e., with extracellular domains exposed to the external milieu), thereby retaining their ability to bind cognate ligands. Exosome biogenesis was initially investigated in the late 1980s by the same investigators who first reported exosomes in red cells [2]. In this initial study, they used immuno-electron microscopy to monitor the externalization of the transferrin receptor (TfR) by maturing reticulocytes, describing how TfR became enclosed in endosome-contained small vesicles ("intraluminal vesicles," now defined as MVB), followed by endosome fusion with the plasma membrane and release into the extracellular compartment. Nowadays, this is still considered the major pathway of exosome biogenesis and release in normal as well as pathological cells (Figure 30.1), although specific studies addressing this process in tumor cells are still scanty. Interestingly, there is some consensus about the evidence that the release is constitutive and more abundant in transformed cells with respect to normal counterparts, through molecular mechanisms that remain unaddressed. Nevertheless, the production can be modulated, at least *in vitro*, by microenvironment conditions [21] such as thermal and oxidative stress [22], pH variations [23], anticancer therapies [24], or cell detachment [25].

Despite the small size, the composition in terms of proteins, lipids and genetic material is rich and complex. In terms of proteins, the most comprehensive information comes from proteomic studies performed by SDS-PAGE or LC-MS/MS approaches on preparations derived from cell supernatants or biologic fluids. The first analyses were performed in nontumor cells such as DCs, human intestinal epithelial cells and EBV-transformed B lymphocytes, revealing the presence of common, as well as cell-type specific, constituents, originating from both the membrane and the intracellular compartments of the producing cells [26–30]. The common protein repertoire seen in exosomes derives mostly from the expression of endosomal markers (including molecules of the tetraspan family, such as CD63, CD9, CD81 and CD82) and transmembrane proteins like MHC molecules, adhesion molecules (ICAM1, EpCAM), integrins, surface peptidases (CD13 and CD26), and GPI-anchored molecules (CD55 and CD59) [31,32]. Some shared protein patterns derive from other vesicular compartments, including molecules associated with the internal side of vesicular membranes (clathrin, annexins, GTPases of the Rab family and raft proteins such as flotillin-1), and various cytosolic molecules, including chaperones of the Heat Shock Protein family (e.g., HSP60 and 70), cytoskeletal proteins, signal transduction molecules (protein kinases), and enzymes [33].

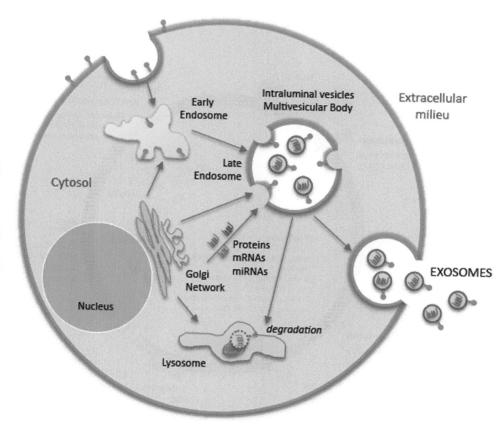

FIGURE 30.1

Exosome biogenesis. Late endosomes, which are part of the endosomal compartment, devoted to the uptake and processing of macromolecules from the extracellular milieu and plasma membrane, bud off and form intraluminal vesicles (forming a structure also known as multivesicular body, MVB). MVB can either fuse with lysosomes for degradation or with the plasma membrane, leading to the release of the inner vesicles' content (exosomes) into the extracellular space.

519

Exosomal proteins of defined cell subsets have been mostly investigated in immune cells, particularly DC and B lymphocytes, where they are related to the antigen-presenting and activating properties of these cells and include MHC class II molecules, CD86 and ICAM-1 [30,34]. In these cell subsets, exosome composition differs according to the activation state of the producing cells, implying that the protein cargo may be subjected to a dynamic regulation and be part of the functional equipment of immune cells. The protein repertoire of tumor exosomes have been also found to mirror the content of the producing cells and thus to include cancer-related molecules, like tumor antigens (e.g., MelanA/Mart-1 and gp100 in melanoma exosomes [35,36], CEA in exosomes secreted by colorectal carcinoma [37], PSA in prostate cancer [38], pro-apoptotic molecules (like FasL and TRAIL) [36,37,39], growth factor receptors (EGF-R, HER2) [21,40], pro-inflammatory and immunosuppressive cytokines (TNFα and TGFβ) [17,41], and proteins involved in oncogene-associated signaling pathways (e.g., β-catenin and Notch ligands) [42,43]. Interestingly, most of these molecules have been proven to be functionally active, charging tumor exosomes with a vast array of potential functions in cancer-bearing hosts, as detailed below.

Precise mechanisms of protein sorting are believed to guide the selective cargo of defined proteins into exosomes. A major role is played by the so-called vesicular ESCRT complex, as suggested by the presence in exosomes from immune cells of proteins involved in the ubiquitination process and in the formation of internal MVB vesicles, such as Alix/AIP1 and Tsg101 [44]. ESCRT has been also found to mediate exosome release by tumor cells [45,46], although scattered data suggest the additional involvement of alternative pathways, such as the recycling endosomal trans-Golgi network [47].

Similarly to proteins, a specific lipid enrichment, displaying both common and cell-specific features, characterizes secreted exosomes. With respect to the plasma membrane, exosome-limiting membrane is enriched in sphingomyelin, cholesterol and GM3 glycolipid. These

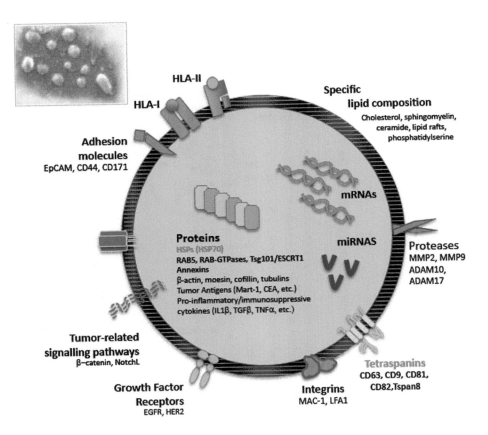

FIGURE 30.2

Composition of tumor exosomes.

A schematic summary of the protein repertoire, lipid features of the limiting membrane, and genetic material (mRNAs and miRNAs) detected so far in tumor exosomes. In red are the most abundant exosome proteins (CD63 and HSPs), according to proteomic analysis. For more detailed information, refer to the ExoCarta database at http://exocarta.org/index.html. In the inner box, exosomes form melanoma cell supernatant, as detected by scanning electron microscopy.

lipids are present as associated with raft proteins (such as flottilin, stomatin, caveolin and lyn) [48], suggesting the accumulation of lipid rafts and a potential involvement of these exosomal microdomains in cell signaling processes [27,49]. Interestingly, exosome phospholipids are subjected to more active transbilayer movements (the "flip-flop" process) with respect to plasma membrane [50], which might play a role in the ability of exosomes to fuse with other membranes and in their stability during circulation.

Notably, exosomes also carry functional mRNA and miRNA. The first evidence was brought by Valadi and collaborators, who reported that RNAs from mast cell exosomes are transferable and translated once entering target cells [51]. Small RNAs playing a role in cancer have been also found (e.g., let-7, miR-15, miR-16 and miR-375). However, profiling results for exosome miRNA are not yet conclusive. Additionally, it remains unclear whether all or only selected miRNA sequences are sorted into exosomes. Nevertheless, miRNA are abundant in tumor exosomes [52,53] and there has been an explosion of interest in exploiting the miRNA profiles of exosomes purified from serum to discover novel diagnostic/prognostic markers, as specifically discussed below.

A schematic representation of exosome composition is depicted in Figure 30.2 and a more complete and constantly updated view of the protein, lipid and RNA content of exosomes can be found online at http://exocarta.org/vesiclepedia [54] and http://evpedia.info/repositories.

IV. SEPARATION AND HANDLING OF EXOSOMES

Although novel approaches are constantly evolving for exosome visualization (such as for instance Nanoparticle Tracking Analysis, (NTA)) [55], the precise morphology of these nanovesicles can be documented fully only by electron microscopy. Because of this situation it is nearly impossible to determine the composition of exosome preparations in real time and the potential presence of contaminating vesicles is challenging to routinely rule out.

Consequently, exosome isolation from cell supernatants or biological fluids must rely on controlled protocols to reproducibly obtain relatively pure material. Indeed, the problem of contamination with other vesicular structures such as apoptotic blebs, microvesicles and organelles deriving from intracellular compartments like mitochondria, Golgi or endoplasmic reticulum, remains an open question and a limitation in the careful interpretation of exosome-related phenotypic and functional studies. Here it is worth mentioning that exosome preparations can be stored for prolonged periods at −80°C, with a significant maintenance of the organelles' structure and function, allowing stored preparations to be confirmed retrospectively. Ultracentrifuged preparations can be loaded onto sucrose gradients, with exosomes floating at their characteristic density. Some groups use slightly different protocols, such as size exclusion chromatography, followed by ultracentrifugation [56,57] or capture by antibody-coated beads [58]. However, these protocols cannot be applied for functional studies, since the elution of exosomes from the antibody could provide alterations of their surface.

Recently, a new commercial compound called ExoQuick has been proposed to rapidly precipitate exosomes from small volumes of body fluids or culture supernatants. This method, potentially reducing material loss and avoiding ultracentrifugations, sounds appealing for miRNAs studies. However, definitive information about the actual nature of the vesicles entrapped by this reagent is presently lacking.

An additional unsolved concern is the appropriate approach for exosome quantification. Besides the measurement of total protein content in purified preparations by conventional assays, ELISA-based assays for exosome-related markers (such as CD63 or caveolin) are being developed [59]. Nevertheless, standardized approaches for the selective quantification of tumor exosomes, possible through the detection of surface-expressed tumor markers, have yet to be fully defined.

V. IMMUNOSUPPRESSIVE ROLE OF TUMOR EXOSOMES

Cancer cells shape their microenvironment and affect the functionality of the immune system by pathways involving cell-to-cell contact and the release of suppressive soluble factors [60]. Exosomes have emerged recently as an important alternative mechanism through which tumors can alter their milieu at local and systemic level [61,62]. Indeed, the evidence that exosomes of potential tumor origin can be abundantly found in peripheral blood and malignant effusions of patients with different cancer histologies [37,63,64], often associated with disease stage and tumor burden [38,59,65], strongly supports the involvement of these organelles in cancer progression [66].

Although their abundant expression of tumor antigens has suggested a potential role as an acellular cancer vaccine strategy [64,67−70], as discussed below, an increasing number of studies indicates that the pathophysiological role of tumor-derived exosomes might favor a greater impact on immune suppression and tumor promotion.

Almost all immune cell subtypes have been evaluated *in vitro* and *in vivo* for their response to interaction with exosomes derived from cancer cells of different histologies. In what follows below we illustrate major findings in this regard (Figure 30.3A).

A. Effects on effector T cells

Some of the earliest evidence that tumor exosomes might contribute to blunting cancer-specific T cells, at least in defined phases of their activation state, derives from studies focused on FasL expression. Apoptosis via Fas/FasL interaction represents indeed one of the major pathways controlling T-cell homeostasis through the selective elimination of over-reactive Fas-expressing T cells [71−74]. Several years ago, tumor cells, particularly from melanoma and colorectal carcinoma, were reported to express bioactive FasL, as a novel pathway of immune

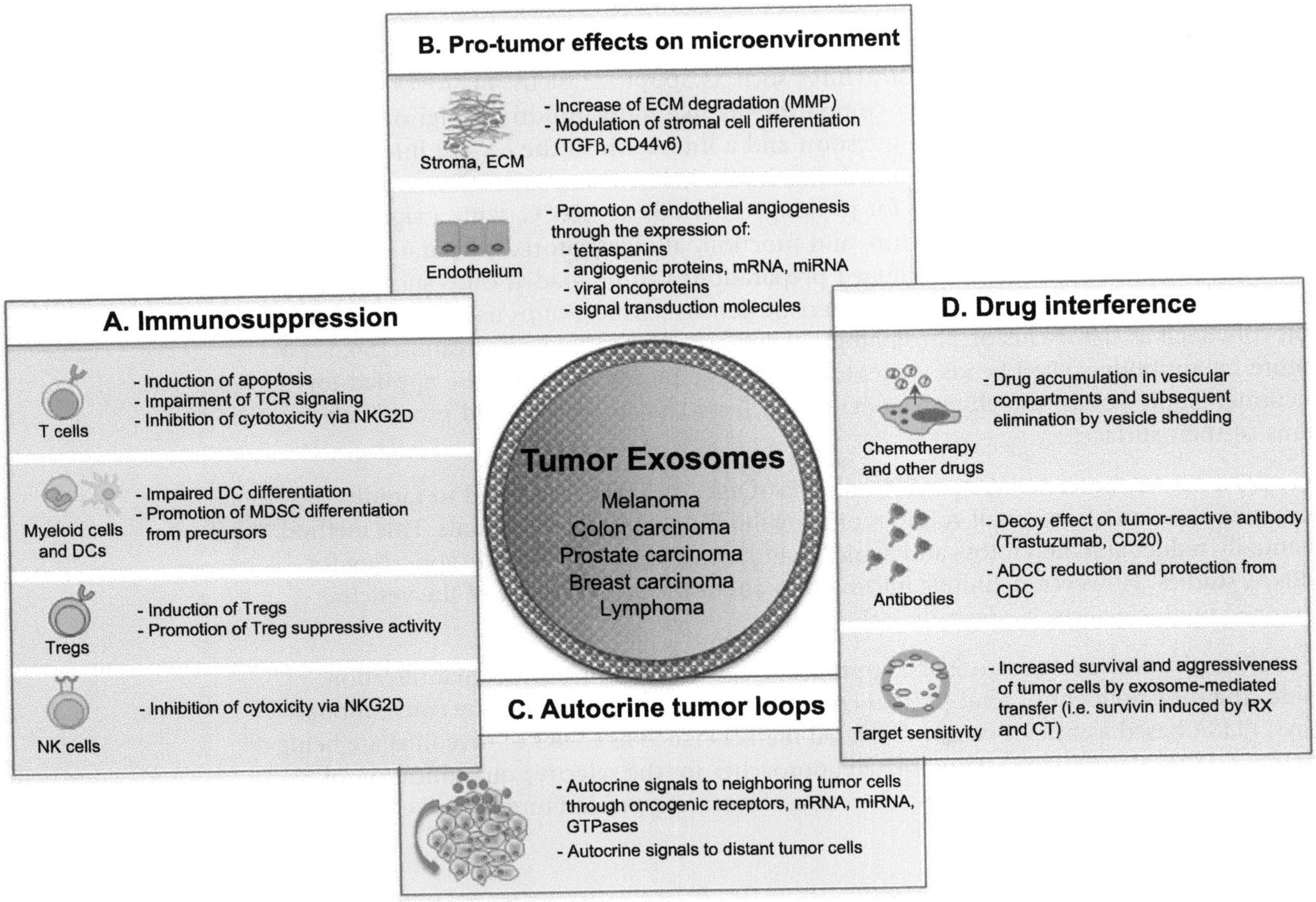

B. Pro-tumor effects on microenvironment

Stroma, ECM
- Increase of ECM degradation (MMP)
- Modulation of stromal cell differentiation (TGFβ, CD44v6)

Endothelium
- Promotion of endothelial angiogenesis through the expression of:
  - tetraspanins
  - angiogenic proteins, mRNA, miRNA
  - viral oncoproteins
  - signal transduction molecules

A. Immunosuppression

T cells
- Induction of apoptosis
- Impairment of TCR signaling
- Inhibition of cytotoxicity via NKG2D

Myeloid cells and DCs
- Impaired DC differentiation
- Promotion of MDSC differentiation from precursors

Tregs
- Induction of Tregs
- Promotion of Treg suppressive activity

NK cells
- Inhibition of cytoxicity via NKG2D

Tumor Exosomes

Melanoma
Colon carcinoma
Prostate carcinoma
Breast carcinoma
Lymphoma

D. Drug interference

Chemotherapy and other drugs
- Drug accumulation in vesicular compartments and subsequent elimination by vesicle shedding

Antibodies
- Decoy effect on tumor-reactive antibody (Trastuzumab, CD20)
- ADCC reduction and protection from CDC

Target sensitivity
- Increased survival and aggressiveness of tumor cells by exosome-mediated transfer (i.e. survivin induced by RX and CT)

C. Autocrine tumor loops
- Autocrine signals to neighboring tumor cells through oncogenic receptors, mRNA, miRNA, GTPases
- Autocrine signals to distant tumor cells

FIGURE 30.3

Pathways potentially played by tumor exosomes in cancer development and progression. Data refer to exosomes released by different tumor histotypes, including melanoma, colorectal carcinoma, prostate and breast cancers and lymphoma. As depicted, several lines of evidence attribute to these nanovesicles the ability to inhibit antitumor immunity by different pathways, to contribute to stroma remodeling and neoangiogenesis, and to promote autocrine loops that can interfere with cancer therapies.

escape [75,76]. In 2002 we found FasL in melanoma cell supernatants in association with small organelles, initially termed microvesicles, sharing with exosomes the size (50–100 nm), expression of specific markers (e.g., CD63) and presence of melanosomal proteins (e.g., gp100 and MART-1) [36]. In subsequent years, many tumor cell lines of different histologies, including prostate [77], head and neck cancer [39,80], melanoma [78], colorectal carcinoma [37], and gastric cancer [79], have been reported to release pro-apoptotic exosomes that carry FasL and TRAIL on their surface. Taken together, these findings depict the ability of tumor-released vesicles to eliminate activated T cells by a simple ligand-receptor interaction. Notably, this function could also be shown with exosomes isolated from biological fluids, such as plasma and ascites [37,57,81], ascribing this mechanism a potential relevance in cancer patients. These findings paved the way to a series of studies investigating additional deleterious effects of tumor exosomes on effector cells [79–81]. The presence of FasL was also reported to mediate CD3-ζ chain downmodulation and subsequent TCR signaling impairment in patients with ovarian carcinoma [82]. More recently, T-cell apoptosis has been described in Epstein-Barr Virus (EBV)-infected nasopharyngeal carcinoma, whose exosomes eliminate EBV-specific CD4$^+$ lymphocytes through galectin-9 binding to the cognate membrane receptor Tim-3, suggesting a role in the suppression of Th1 responses at both tumor and systemic levels [83]. Another important pathway was revealed by Clayton and coworkers, who demonstrated that tumor exosomes, by the dephosphorylation of exogenous ATP and 5'AMP by functional

CD39 and CD73, mediate a rise in adenosine levels within the tumor microenvironment, thereby negatively regulating local immune responses [84].

B. Inhibition of NK cells

Tumor-derived exosomes can also promote tumor immune evasion by interfering with NK cells. Indeed, NKG2D ligand-containing exosomes derived from human breast cancer and mesothelioma cell lines were reported to directly interact with NK cells, leading to a significant reduction in NKG2D expression and a consequent NK functional defect [22,85,86]. Additionally, it has been reported that treatment of NK cells with exosomes containing MICA*008 molecules mediated the downregulation of NKG2D and a marked reduction in NK cytotoxicity [87], while exosomes produced by human breast cancer and melanoma cell lines were found to inhibit NK-cell proliferation [88]. Studies performed in murine models showed that exosomes produced by TS/A or 4T.1 murine mammary tumor cells can favor the growth of implanted tumor cells in both syngeneic BALB/c and nude mice by blocking IL-2-mediated NK cell activation and perforin/granzyme B-mediated effector functions [88]. These pathways were confirmed using exosome-like microvesicles isolated from sera of acute myeloid leukemia patients [89]. In such setting, *ex vivo* exosomes mediated NKG2D downregulation and NK activity suppression through the expression of TGFβ.

C. Effects on the generation of myeloid-derived suppressor and regulatory T cells

Tumor exosomes can also impact on the functional properties of innate immunity. Indeed, we reported that melanoma-derived and colon carcinoma-derived exosomes skew the CD14$^+$ monocyte differentiation from dendritic cells into immunosuppressive elements highly resembling the well-known population of myeloid-derived suppressor cells (MDSC) [90]. The hallmark of this *in vitro*-induced new MDSC was represented by a CD11b$^+$CD14$^+$HLA-DR$^{-/lo}$ phenotype, associated with TGFβ-mediated suppressive activity on T-cell proliferation and function [91].

Interestingly, cells echoing this phenotype could be detected in the peripheral blood of advanced melanoma patients; in fact, a significant expansion of TGFβ-secreting cells in association with the reduced ability to mount CD8$^+$ T-cell-mediated immune response upon cancer-vaccine administration could be found [92]. These findings led to the hypothesis that melanoma exosomes might be involved in driving MDSC expansion by possibly accumulating in the elective sites of myelopoiesis (e.g., the bone marrow), where they might influence the initiation of immunosuppressive cell subsets [93]. CD14$^+$HLA-DR$^{-/lo}$ MDSC have also been found in peripheral blood of patients affected by other types of cancer, including hepatocellular carcinoma [94], bladder cancer [95] and multiple myeloma [96]. In these latter studies a direct link between tumor exosomes and the generation of monocyte-derived MDSC has not been investigated. However, it is likely that exosomes secreted by tumor cells might contribute to this phenomenon.

T-regulatory cells (Treg) expansion and activity can also be boosted by tumor exosomes. In a recent study, Szajnik et al. reported that microvesicles, isolated from ascites and blood of cancer patients, induce the transition of CD4$^+$CD25$^-$ T cells into CD4$^+$CD25$^+$Foxp3$^+$ Treg via phosphorylation of Smad2/3 and Stat3, thereby upregulating their suppressor functions and resistance to apoptosis through a TGFβ- and IL-10-dependent mechanism [97]. Similarly, exosomes expressing TGFβ derived from human malignant effusions were reported to promote increased Treg number and function in *in vitro* studies [98]. Similarly, Clayton et al. showed that exosomes isolated from different tumor cell lines favor IL-2-mediated Treg expansion thanks to their surface expression of TGFβ [41]. It is worth mentioning that TGFβ^+ exosomes are also involved in physiological immune homeostasis, as depicted by a recent study indicating that TGFβ expressed in thymic exosomes is required for the generation of

523

Foxp3$^+$ Treg in peripheral tissues, such as lung and liver, and participate in the maintenance of immune tolerance [99].

The role of tumor exosomes in promoting the expansion of immunoregulatory cell components are beginning to be investigated in *in vivo* murine models as well, to prove the actual involvement of this pathway in immunosuppression and tumor progression. One major hurdle of this type of studies has been so far to trace the fate of injected exosomes, an issue still poorly investigated.

Nevertheless, immunosuppressive pathways generated by adoptively transferred tumor exosomes have been observed in the TS/A mammary tumor murine model, where injected nanovesicles were found to interact with CD11b$^+$ myeloid precursors in the bone marrow (BM) and to block BMDC differentiation by inducing IL-6 production and Stat3 phosphorylation [100]. Similarly, in a breast carcinoma model, tumor exosomes were demonstrated to skew BMDC differentiation toward an MDSC phenotype promoting tumor progression, through a prostaglandin E2 and TGFβ-mediated pathway [101]. Recent data also demonstrated that MyD88 is required for the MDSC accumulation and lung metastasis promotion induced by tumor exosome in C57BL/6j (B6) mice [102]. Likewise, Chalmin et al. [103] reported, in both murine and human settings, that Hsp72 expressed on the surface of colon cancer-derived exosomes induces IL-6 release from MDSC in a Toll-like receptor 2/MyD88/Stat3-dependent manner, even if the role of Toll-like receptor 2 in this process remains unclear [104,105].

VI. ROLE OF TUMOR-DERIVED EXOSOMES IN CANCER PROGRESSION

Tumor exosomes can promote disease progression not only by promoting immune escape but also by feeding autocrine loops, stimulating angiogenesis, modulating stromal cells and remodeling the extracellular matrix [106]. Indeed, thanks to the ever-growing number of proteins and genetic material being discovered to comprise their cargo, tumor exosomes have the potential of exerting marvelously variegated functions, all merging to promote tumor growth (Figure 30.3B).

A. Tumor exosomes as protein and genetic messengers

In their study on melanoma-derived exosomes, Hood et al. [107] described pro-angiogenic potential that could rapidly stimulate the formation of endothelial spheroids and sprouts in a dose-dependent manner. The same group reported later that melanoma-derived exosomes share the ability to condition sentinel lymph nodes to become niches conducive to melanoma cell deposition, growth, extracellular matrix synthesis and vascular proliferation [108]. One class of molecules that has been hypothesized to confer pro-angiogenic activity to tumor exosomes are the tetraspanins [109,110], which were shown recently to promote tumor growth by inducing systemic angiogenesis in tumor and tumor-free tissues [43]. In particular, in a rat adenocarcinoma model, the tetraspanin Tspan8 contributed to a selective recruitment of proteins and mRNA into exosomes, including CD106 and CD49d, both of which were implicated in the binding and internalization of exosomes by endothelial cells. Upon internalization of Tspan8-CD49d complex—containing exosomes, Nazarenko and collaborators observed an induction of several angiogenesis-related genes (von Willebrand factor, Tspan8, VEGF, chemokines CXCL5 and MIF, chemokine receptors CCR1, and VEGF receptor 2). Moreover, the uptake of Tspan8-CD49d—containing exosomes by endothelial cells (EC) was accompanied by enhanced EC proliferation, migration, sprouting and maturation of EC progenitors [111]. There is also evidence that tumor exosomes containing the Notch ligand Delta-like 4 (Dll4) can participate in vascular development and angiogenesis. These Dll4-containing exosomes confer a tip cell phenotype to EC, resulting in a high Dll4/Notch-receptor ratio, low Notch signaling and filopodia formation. This reversal in phenotype appears to enhance vessel density *in vitro* and branching *in vivo* [43]. In human glioblastoma, Skog and colleagues [52] demonstrated that exosomes containing angiogenic proteins, including angiogenin, FGFα, IL-6, IL-8, TIMP-1, VEGF and TIMP-2, with related mRNAs and miRNAs, are taken up by brain microvascular endothelial cells, thereby stimulating endothelial tubule formation or proliferation of other glioma cells.

Exosomes can also manipulate the tumor microenvironment to influence the growth of neighboring cells by other pathways. For instance, EBV-infected tumor cells can transfer viral oncoproteins, signal transduction molecules and virus-encoded miRNAs into multiple cell types by means of exosomes, as reported for nasopharyngeal carcinoma (NPC) cells harboring latent EBV [112]. Recent data have evidenced that exosomes produced by other cells in the tumor microenvironment can be exploited to drive tumor progression. Indeed, macrophage-derived exosomes are able to shuttle proteins or miRNAs into adjacent cells within the tumor microenvironment. In particular, the study published by Yang et al. demonstrates that exogenous miRNA (miR-223) transfected into IL-4-activated M2 macrophages is internalized by co-cultivated breast cancer cells, thus promoting the invasiveness of breast cancer cells *in vitro* [113].

B. Modulation of stroma and extracellular matrix

Another relevant feature of exosomes derived from different cancer cell lines, including mesothelioma, bladder, breast and colorectal cancer cells, is the capability to modulate stromal cell differentiation. Particularly intriguing results show that the complex TGFβ-transmembrane proteoglycan betaglycan, expressed at the tumor exosome surface, is able to elicit Smad-dependent signaling and to trigger fibroblast differentiation toward a myofibroblastic phenotype leading to an altered stroma, tumor growth, vascularization and metastasis [114]. Likewise, a role for breast cancer exosomes in conversion of adipose tissue-derived mesenchymal stem cells into myofibroblast-like cells has been reported, again through a TGFβ-mediated process and the activation of Smad-related pathway [115]. Recently, exosomes derived from gynecologic neoplasias were found to contain metalloproteinases that increase extracellular matrix degradation and tumor invasion into the stroma [116]. Notably, in a rat pancreatic adenocarcinoma model, tumor-derived exosomes could contribute to metastatic niches, together with soluble factors. This process is dependent on CD44v6, which is required for assembling a soluble matrix that, in cooperation with exosomes, promotes leukocyte, stroma and endothelial cell activation in the (pre) metastatic organ [117].

C. Autocrine role of tumor exosomes

The secretion of soluble factors, such as growth factors, cytokines and chemokines, by the growing tumor to sustain its own growth is well established [118–121]. The subsequent discovery of exosomes raised questions about their benefit to the secreting tumor cell (Figure 30.3C). It has been noticed that the secretion pathways involved in autocrine growth loops may also transfer molecules bound to exosomes. One key study concerning the potential for exosome signaling illustrated intercellular transfer of the oncogenic receptor EGFRvIII by tumor exosomes to glioma cells lacking this receptor, thereby contributing to morphological transformation and anchorage-independent growth [66]. Another recent report describes a role for amphiphiregulin (AREG), an EGFR ligand, in human colorectal and breast cancer cell invasion. Here the authors showed that full-length AREG carried by tumor exosomes increased invasiveness five-fold over equivalent amounts of recombinant AREG [122].

Like all exosomes, tumor exosomes are enriched in the expression of the so-defined canonical exosome markers, which include members of the tetraspan family of transmembrane proteins (CD9, CD81 and CD63), but also small Rab GTPases which act as master regulators of vesicle traffic. Among the latter proteins, two isoforms of Rab27 have

525

been shown to control exosome secretion in HeLa cervical cancer cells [58]. In breast cancer cells, Rab27B appears as a key factor for invasive tumor growth. Hendrix et al. have proposed that this particular GTPase mediates vesicle exocytosis and subsequent HSP90α release into the microenvironment, thereby facilitating the binding of growth factors to their receptors and ultimately leading to cell cycle transition from the growth-factor-sensitive G1-S-phase [123].

VII. MECHANISMS OF INTERACTION WITH TARGET CELLS

If the functional outcome of exosome interaction with target cells is only beginning to be unraveled, even less may be known about the selectivity and specificity of defined exosomes for their targets. Studies dissecting the regulation of exosomes with different cell types have so far shown that exosomes may interact with target cells by different modes: phagocytosis, receptor-ligand interaction, fusion and attachment to the membrane [124]. The type of interaction appears to depend on the recipient cell type (phagocytes and nonphagocytic cells) as well as on the surface molecules expressed by the exosome and/or the cell.

A role for exosomes as vehicles in intercellular homotypic and heterotypic interactions has at first become evident after finding functional MHC class I and II, co-stimulatory and cell adhesion molecules on the outer membrane of APC-derived exosomes [125]. This evidence unravelled that exosomes could be part of the APC-immunostimulating machinery, being involved in recruiting T helper cells and promoting isotype switching and differentiation in B lymphocytes. The recent finding of functional genetic material in exosomes opened new horizons for cross-talk studies. As previously mentioned, Valadi et al. showed in an elegant study that exosomes secreted by mast cells carry RNA into the extracellular milieu. The targeting of exosomes to the recipient cells appears to play a fundamental role, as mast cell-derived RNA bearing exosomes were "accepted" only by other mast cells but not by T cells[51], suggesting indeed that upon the encounter of a cell with exosome its uptake is not compulsory in all cases. Feng et al. evaluated the interaction of exosomes from K562 human erythroleukemia cell line and MT4 HTLV-transformed T-cell leukemia cell line with a variety of different cell lines derived from human and nonhuman cells, including monocytes, macrophages, T cells and fibroblasts. The results showed that all phagocytic cells were able to internalize exosomes and phagocytosis appeared not to be species-specific. On the other hand, exosomes can also attach to the surface of nonphagocytic cells through receptor-ligand interactions with consequent triggering of intracellular signalling cascades [36,124]. In this context the expression of particular integrins and adhesion molecules (such as LFA1 and ICAM1) by exosomes and/or recipient cells appear to be fundamental [31,111].

A role for lipid components commonly expressed by exosomes, like phosphatidylserine, has been also recently been reported [126]. Live cell microscopy studies indicated that exosomes secreted by PC12 rat pheochromocytoma cells are internalized by endocytosis by the same cells, trapped in vesicles and transported to perinuclear regions. Here the exosomal proteins were targeted to endosomes and lysosomes, whereas the nanovesicular lipids were recycled to the plasma membrane, suggesting that exosomes can function as intercellular transporters [127]. Internalization by fusion was instead reported for melanoma exosomes uptaken by melanoma cells and this process was increased at low pH [23]. Finally, a very elegant study recently performed on normal cells showed that exosomes derived from B, T and DC contain repertoires of microRNAs that are different from those of their parental cells. With the help of CD63-GFP expressed by exosomes these authors discovered that exosomes can function as a highly efficient mechanism for unidirectional transfer of regulatory genetic information, represented by exosomal microRNAs, exclusively in the microenvironment of the immunologic synapse during cognate immune reactions. This genetic communication was antigen driven and linked to the formation of the immunological synapse [128].

VIII. TUMOR-DERIVED EXOSOMES AND CANCER THERAPIES

Tumor exosomes appear to have found their way into different mechanisms exploited by cancer cells to counter therapeutic agents (Figure 30.3D). A pioneer study by Luciani and collaborators [129], subsequently confirmed by other groups [130], suggested several years ago that endosomal vesicles of melanoma, adenocarcinoma and lymphoma cells could be responsible for sequestering cytotoxic drugs such as cisplatin, 5-fluorouracil and vinblastine, thus reducing the antitumor potential of chemotherapy. Similarly, Safei and coworkers showed that cisplatin-resistant ovarian cancer cells were able to expel this chemotherapeutic drug through enhanced release of exosomes, which expressed higher levels of the cisplatin export transporters MRP2, ATP7A and ATP7B. In these tumor cells, resistance to cisplatin was accompanied by higher levels of genes whose products function in membrane fusion and vesicle trafficking, a reduction of the lysosomal compartment, where this drug usually becomes concentrated, and an abnormal export of the drug by exosomes [131]. Resistance to cisplatin, associated to increased expression of annexin A3 in ovarian cancer cells, was also found to be linked to the increased production of annexin A3-expressing exosomes, providing additional evidence for exosome-mediated countering of cisplatin cytotoxicity [130].

Potential effects on tumor exosome production were also evaluated in radiation-treated cancer cells, as in prostate carcinoma, where radiotherapy induces premature cellular senescence accounting for most of the death of tumor cells. In this context, treatment-induced senescent cells enhance exosome secretion, though a p53-dependent process [132,133]. Therefore, exosomes may comprise an important and previously unrecognized feature of premature cellular senescence [134]. Interestingly, Khan et al. showed that tumor cell irradiation leads to changes in exosome composition rather than in the secretion rate, as shown by the enhanced survivin content in exosomes produced by irradiated cells [135].

A participation of tumor exosomes has been also described in countering antibody-mediated cancer therapies, in particular for the HER2 antibody trastuzumab in breast cancer treatment. In this regard, HER2-expressing exosomes isolated from sera of breast cancer patients bound to this antibody and autologous exosomes inhibited trastuzumab activity on SKBR3 proliferation [21]. By binding of tumor-reactive antibodies, breast cancer exosomes were also shown to reduce antibody-dependent cytotoxicity (ADCC) of immune effector cells, one of the fundamental antitumor reactions of the immune system [136]. Similarly, in an *in vitro* model of aggressive B-cell lymphoma, CD20-expressing tumor exosomes were able to consume complement and shield target cells from antibody attack, resulting in protection from complement-dependent cytolysis (CDC) as well as ADCC [137].

Although the vast majority of exosome features suggests a prevalent role of these nanovesicles in promoting tumor progression, some of their characteristics could still be exploited for therapeutic purposes. Indeed, thanks to their high content of antigenic proteins (i.e., Mart-1, gp100, TRP-1, HER2 and CEA) and MHC-peptide complexes, tumor exosomes could represent an effective tool for T-cell cross-priming [64,138,139]. Indeed, it was reported that melanoma-specific T lymphocytes could be efficiently expanded by pulsing DC with ascites-derived exosomes from the same patients [64]. In addition, tumor exosomes presenting Hsp70/Bag-4 have been reported to promote NK-cell activity [140], and to activate macrophages [141]. The efficacy of exosomes from heat-stressed tumor cells in the induction of antitumor immunity was also demonstrated by Dai and colleagues, who isolated exosomes from heat-shocked CEA-positive tumor cells that shared the ability to induce DC maturation and T-cell activation [142]. Interestingly, a recent study shows that immunoprotective immunity, in terms of tumor-specific CTL, could be generated *in vitro* using DC pulsed with leukemia-derived exosomes [143]. While several studies in mice have revealed that tumor-derived exosomes can serve as antigen delivery systems and promote antitumor immune responses [40,45,138], methods for the production and purification of clinical GMP-grade exosomes have recently been developed to be used in human clinical trials [68,28,144]. In this regard, Dai et al. report that advanced colorectal carcinoma (CRC) patients (HLA-A0201+CEA+), enrolled in a Phase I clinical trial of ascites-derived exosomes in combination with the granulocyte-macrophage colony-stimulating factor (GM-CSF), documented an in vivo induction of tumor-specific CTL responses [67]. Other Phase I clinical trials, involving the application of exosomes to elicit an immune response against established tumors, foresee the use of autologous DC-derived exosomes (Dex) harboring functional MHC/peptide and loaded with tumor antigens. These studies provide evidence that Dex may also stimulate non-MHC restricted-antitumor effectors and induce tumor regression *in vivo* [145–147].

IX. TUMOR-DERIVED EXOSOMES AS DIAGNOSTIC AGENTS

The discovery of tumor exosomes by electron microscopy in biological fluids is lately receiving great attention. Blood, saliva, nasal secretions and urine are easily accessible and the collection does not require invasive manipulations. Thus, body fluid-derived exosomes could function as biomarkers for a great variety of pathological conditions, including cancer. Here, the presence of tumor exosomes in the circulation and malignant effusions of cancer patients could be exploited as tumor marker for characterization studies and during follow up of patients undergoing surgery or other therapies [5,148,149]. However, the premise for any study on tumor exosomes in body fluids, such as plasma, is the identification of exosomes of tumor origin among the multitude of exosomes normally present in the circulation of any healthy person [150,151]. The expression of tumor antigens by tumor exosomes appeared suitable for detection as well as quantification purposes, leading to the development of rapid techniques for the detection of tumor exosomes in small volumes [152,153]. The analysis of samples from large numbers of patients showed a correlation between the quantity of detectable tumor exosomes and the disease stage and prognosis [154], greatly raising the interest of body fluid-derived exosomes of different cancer histologies, including prostate cancer [38].

The recent finding of microRNA profiling of circulating tumor exosomes (plasma and/or sera) has greatly enhanced their potential to provide surrogate diagnostic markers for biopsy profiling and possible utility to screen asymptomatic populations [155].

X. CONCLUSION AND FUTURE NEEDS

Tumor exosomes are receiving increasing attention for their role in intercellular communication. Nowadays, technical advances in this field and agreements on standardized isolation protocols reached by the scientific community should allow robust phenotypic and functional studies about the biological and therapeutic implications of these organelles in cancer patients. Many secrets of these fascinating vesicles have been recently revealed, but no doubt many others remain to be told. As outlined in this chapter, observed features and effects mediated by tumor exosomes appear to merge into a common multifaceted theme. In fact, to cite some examples, the elimination of activated T cells by pro-apoptotic molecules together with immunosuppressive effects transmitted by TGFβ-containing exosomes are recurrent findings of different groups working on distinct cancer histologies and experimental settings, underlining the importance of understanding the different facets of exosomes in promoting cancer growth and progression. In conclusion, we would like to highlight the enormous potential of tumor exosomes as mediators of immunosuppression and disease progression in cancer patients. Dissection of the pathways leading to these protumorigenic features will greatly enhance our understanding while offering at the same time the opportunity to identify new targets for cancer therapy.

References

[1] Harding C, Heuser J, Stahl P. Endocytosis and intracellular processing of transferrin and colloidal gold-transferrin in rat reticulocytes: demonstration of a pathway for receptor shedding. Eur J Cell Biol 1984;35(2):256−63.

[2] Pan BT, Teng K, Wu C, Adam M, Johnstone RM. Electron microscopic evidence for externalization of the transferrin receptor in vesicular form in sheep reticulocytes. J Cell Biol 1985;101(3):942−8.

[3] Johnstone RM, Adam M, Hammond JR, Orr L, Turbide C. Vesicle formation during reticulocyte maturation. Association of plasma membrane activities with released vesicles (exosomes). J Biol Chem 1987;262(19):9412−20.

[4] Huotari J, Helenius A. Endosome maturation. EMBO J 2011;30(17):3481−500.

[5] Simpson RJ, Lim JW, Moritz RL, Mathivanan S. Exosomes: proteomic insights and diagnostic potential. Expert Rev Proteomics 2009;6(3):267−83.

[6] Fevrier B, Raposo G. Exosomes: endosomal-derived vesicles shipping extracellular messages. Curr Opin Cell Biol 2004;16(4):415−21.

[7] Bobrie A, Colombo M, Raposo G, Thery C. Exosome secretion: molecular mechanisms and roles in immune responses. Traffic 2011;12(12):1659−68.

[8] Thery C, Amigorena S, Raposo G, Clayton A. Isolation and characterization of exosomes from cell culture supernatants and biological fluids. Curr Protoc Cell Biol 2006. Chapter 3: Unit 3.22.

[9] Caby MP, Lankar D, Vincendeau-Scherrer C, Raposo G, Bonnerot C. Exosomal-like vesicles are present in human blood plasma. Int Immunol 2005;17(7):879−87.

[10] Admyre C, Grunewald J, Thyberg J, Gripenback S, Tornling G, Eklund A, et al. Exosomes with major histocompatibility complex class II and co-stimulatory molecules are present in human BAL fluid. Eur Respir J 2003;22(4):578−83.

[11] Pisitkun T, Shen RF, Knepper MA. Identification and proteomic profiling of exosomes in human urine. Proc Natl Acad Sci U S A 2004;101(36):13368−73.

[12] Poliakov A, Spilman M, Dokland T, Amling CL, Mobley JA. Structural heterogeneity and protein composition of exosome-like vesicles (prostasomes) in human semen. Prostate 2009;69(2):159−67.

[13] Asea A, Jean-Pierre C, Kaur P, Rao P, Linhares IM, Skupski D, et al. Heat shock protein-containing exosomes in mid-trimester amniotic fluids. J Reprod Immunol 2008;79(1):12−7.

[14] Gonzalez-Begne M, Lu B, Han X, Hagen FK, Hand AR, Melvin JE, et al. Proteomic analysis of human parotid gland exosomes by multidimensional protein identification technology (MudPIT). J Proteome Res 2009;8(3):1304−14.

[15] Masyuk AI, Huang BQ, Ward CJ, Gradilone SA, Banales JM, Masyuk TV, et al. Biliary exosomes influence cholangiocyte regulatory mechanisms and proliferation through interaction with primary cilia. Am J Physiol Gastrointest Liver Physiol 2010;299(4):G990−9.

[16] Potolicchio I, Carven GJ, Xu X, Stipp C, Riese RJ, Stern LJ, et al. Proteomic analysis of microglia-derived exosomes: metabolic role of the aminopeptidase CD13 in neuropeptide catabolism. J Immunol 2005;175(4):2237−43.

[17] Zhang HG, Liu C, Su K, Yu S, Zhang L, Zhang S, et al. A membrane form of TNF-alpha presented by exosomes delays T cell activation-induced cell death. J Immunol 2006;176(12):7385−93.

[18] Chavez-Munoz C, Morse J, Kilani R, Ghahary A. Primary human keratinocytes externalize stratifin protein via exosomes. J Cell Biochem 2008;104(6):2165−73.

[19] Kesimer M, Scull M, Brighton B, DeMaria G, Burns K, O'Neal W, et al. Characterization of exosome-like vesicles released from human tracheobronchial ciliated epithelium: a possible role in innate defense. FASEB J 2009;23(6):1858−68.

[20] Lai RC, Arslan F, Lee MM, Sze NS, Choo A, Chen TS, et al. Exosome secreted by MSC reduces myocardial ischemia/reperfusion injury. Stem Cell Res 2010;4(3):214−22.

[21] Ciravolo V, Huber V, Ghedini GC, Venturelli E, Bianchi F, Campiglio M, et al. Potential role of HER2-overexpressing exosomes in countering trastuzumab-based therapy. J Cell Physiol 2012;227(2):658−67.

[22] Hedlund M, Nagaeva O, Kargl D, Baranov V, Mincheva-Nilsson L. Thermal- and oxidative stress causes enhanced release of NKG2D ligand-bearing immunosuppressive exosomes in leukemia/lymphoma T and B cells. PLoS One 2011;6(2):e16899.

[23] Parolini I, Federici C, Raggi C, Lugini L, Palleschi S, De Milito A, et al. Microenvironmental pH is a key factor for exosome traffic in tumor cells. J Biol Chem 2009;284(49):34211−22.

[24] Lv LH, Wan YL, Lin Y, Zhang W, Yang M, Li GL, et al. Anticancer drugs cause release of exosomes with heat shock proteins from human hepatocellular carcinoma cells that elicit effective natural killer cell anti-tumor responses in vitro. J Biol Chem 2012.

[25] Koumangoye RB, Sakwe AM, Goodwin JS, Patel T, Ochieng J. Detachment of breast tumor cells induces rapid secretion of exosomes which subsequently mediate cellular adhesion and spreading. PLoS One 2011;6(9):e24234.

[26] van Niel G, Raposo G, Candalh C, Boussac M, Hershberg R, Cerf-Bensussan N, et al. Intestinal epithelial cells secrete exosome-like vesicles. Gastroenterology 2001;121(2):337–49.

[27] Wubbolts R, Leckie RS, Veenhuizen PT, Schwarzmann G, Mobius W, Hoernschemeyer J, et al. Proteomic and biochemical analyses of human B cell-derived exosomes. Potential implications for their function and multivesicular body formation. J Biol Chem 2003;278(13):10963–72.

[28] Lamparski HG, Metha-Damani A, Yao JY, Patel S, Hsu DH, Ruegg C, et al. Production and characterization of clinical grade exosomes derived from dendritic cells. J Immunol Methods 2002;270(2):211–26.

[29] Thery C, Regnault A, Garin J, Wolfers J, Zitvogel L, Ricciardi-Castagnoli P, et al. Molecular characterization of dendritic cell-derived exosomes. Selective accumulation of the heat shock protein hsc73. J Cell Biol 1999;147(3):599–610.

[30] Van Niel G, Mallegol J, Bevilacqua C, Candalh C, Brugiere S, Tomaskovic-Crook E, et al. Intestinal epithelial exosomes carry MHC class II/peptides able to inform the immune system in mice. Gut 2003;52(12):1690–7.

[31] Clayton A, Turkes A, Dewitt S, Steadman R, Mason MD, Hallett MB. Adhesion and signaling by B cell-derived exosomes: the role of integrins. FASEB J 2004;18(9):977–9.

[32] McLellan AD. Exosome release by primary B cells. Crit Rev Immunol 2009;29(3):203–17.

[33] Ludwig AK, Giebel B. Exosomes: small vesicles participating in intercellular communication. Int J Biochem Cell Biol 2012;44(1):11–5.

[34] Segura E, Nicco C, Lombard B, Veron P, Raposo G, Batteux F, et al. ICAM-1 on exosomes from mature dendritic cells is critical for efficient naive T-cell priming. Blood 2005;106(1):216–23.

[35] Mears R, Craven RA, Hanrahan S, Totty N, Upton C, Young SL, et al. Proteomic analysis of melanoma-derived exosomes by two-dimensional polyacrylamide gel electrophoresis and mass spectrometry. Proteomics 2004;4(12):4019–31.

[36] Andreola G, Rivoltini L, Castelli C, Huber V, Perego P, Deho P, et al. Induction of lymphocyte apoptosis by tumor cell secretion of FasL-bearing microvesicles. J Exp Med 2002;195(10):1303–16.

[37] Huber V, Fais S, Iero M, Lugini L, Canese P, Squarcina P, et al. Human colorectal cancer cells induce T-cell death through release of proapoptotic microvesicles: role in immune escape. Gastroenterology 2005;128(7):1796–804.

[38] Mitchell PJ, Welton J, Staffurth J, Court J, Mason MD, Tabi Z, et al. Can urinary exosomes act as treatment response markers in prostate cancer? J Transl Med 2009;7:4.

[39] Bergmann C, Strauss L, Wieckowski E, Czystowska M, Albers A, Wang Y, et al. Tumor-derived microvesicles in sera of patients with head and neck cancer and their role in tumor progression. Head Neck 2009;31(3):371–80.

[40] Graner MW, Alzate O, Dechkovskaia AM, Keene JD, Sampson JH, Mitchell DA, et al. Proteomic and immunologic analyses of brain tumor exosomes. FASEB J 2009;23(5):1541–57.

[41] Clayton A, Mitchell JP, Court J, Mason MD, Tabi Z. Human tumor-derived exosomes selectively impair lymphocyte responses to interleukin-2. Cancer Res 2007;67(15):7458–66.

[42] Chairoungdua A, Smith DL, Pochard P, Hull M, Caplan MJ. Exosome release of beta-catenin: a novel mechanism that antagonizes Wnt signaling. J Cell Biol 2010;190(6):1079–91.

[43] Sheldon H, Heikamp E, Turley H, Dragovic R, Thomas P, Oon CE, et al. New mechanism for Notch signaling to endothelium at a distance by Delta-like 4 incorporation into exosomes. Blood 2010;116(13):2385–94.

[44] Geminard C, De Gassart A, Blanc L, Vidal M. Degradation of AP2 during reticulocyte maturation enhances binding of hsc70 and Alix to a common site on TFR for sorting into exosomes. Traffic 2004;5(3):181–93.

[45] Chaput N, Thery C. Exosomes: immune properties and potential clinical implementations. Semin Immunopathol 2011;33(5):419–40.

[46] Choi DS, Yang JS, Choi EJ, Jang SC, Park S, Kim OY, et al. The protein interaction network of extracellular vesicles derived from human colorectal cancer cells. J Proteome Res 2012;11(2):1144–51.

[47] De Gassart A, Trentin B, Martin M, Hocquellet A, Bette-Bobillo P, Mamoun R, et al. Exosomal sorting of the cytoplasmic domain of bovine leukemia virus TM Env protein. Cell Biol Int 2009;33(1):36–48.

[48] de Gassart A, Geminard C, Fevrier B, Raposo G, Vidal M. Lipid raft-associated protein sorting in exosomes. Blood 2003;102(13):4336–44.

[49] Staubach S, Razawi H, Hanisch FG. Proteomics of MUC1-containing lipid rafts from plasma membranes and exosomes of human breast carcinoma cells MCF-7. Proteomics 2009;9(10):2820–35.

[50] Laulagnier K, Motta C, Hamdi S, Roy S, Fauvelle F, Pageaux JF, et al. Mast cell- and dendritic cell-derived exosomes display a specific lipid composition and an unusual membrane organization. Biochem J 2004;380(Pt 1):161–71.

[51] Valadi H, Ekstrom K, Bossios A, Sjostrand M, Lee JJ, Lotvall JO. Exosome-mediated transfer of mRNAs and microRNAs is a novel mechanism of genetic exchange between cells. Nat Cell Biol 2007;9(6):654—9.

[52] Skog J, Wurdinger T, van Rijn S, Meijer DH, Gainche L, Sena-Esteves M, et al. Glioblastoma microvesicles transport RNA and proteins that promote tumour growth and provide diagnostic biomarkers. Nat Cell Biol 2008;10(12):1470—6.

[53] Pegtel DM, Cosmopoulos K, Thorley-Lawson DA, van Eijndhoven MA, Hopmans ES, Lindenberg JL, et al. Functional delivery of viral miRNAs via exosomes. Proc Natl Acad Sci U S A 2010;107(14):6328—33.

[54] Mathivanan S, Fahner CJ, Reid GE, Simpson RJ. ExoCarta 2012: database of exosomal proteins, RNA and lipids. Nucleic Acids Res 2012;40(Database issue):D1241—4.

[55] Dragovic RA, Gardiner C, Brooks AS, Tannetta DS, Ferguson DJ, Hole P, et al. Sizing and phenotyping of cellular vesicles using Nanoparticle Tracking Analysis. Nanomedicine 2011;7(6):780—8.

[56] Kim JW, Wieckowski E, Taylor DD, Reichert TE, Watkins S, Whiteside TL. Fas ligand-positive membranous vesicles isolated from sera of patients with oral cancer induce apoptosis of activated T lymphocytes. Clin Cancer Res 2005;11(3):1010—20.

[57] Taylor DD, Gercel-Taylor C, Lyons KS, Stanson J, Whiteside TL. T-cell apoptosis and suppression of T-cell receptor/CD3-zeta by Fas ligand-containing membrane vesicles shed from ovarian tumors. Clin Cancer Res 2003;9(14):5113—9.

[58] Ostrowski M, Carmo NB, Krumeich S, Fanget I, Raposo G, Savina A, et al. Rab27a and Rab27b control different steps of the exosome secretion pathway. Nat Cell Biol 2010;12(1):1—13. 19, 30sup.

[59] Logozzi M, De Milito A, Lugini L, Borghi M, Calabro L, Spada M, et al. High levels of exosomes expressing CD63 and caveolin-1 in plasma of melanoma patients. PLoS One 2009;4(4):e5219.

[60] Gajewski TF, Meng Y, Blank C, Brown I, Kacha A, Kline J, et al. Immune resistance orchestrated by the tumor microenvironment. Immunol Rev 2006;213:131—45.

[61] van Niel G, Porto-Carreiro I, Simoes S, Raposo G. Exosomes: a common pathway for a specialized function. J Biochem 2006;140(1):13—21.

[62] Iero M, Valenti R, Huber V, Filipazzi P, Parmiani G, Fais S, et al. Tumour-released exosomes and their implications in cancer immunity. Cell Death Differ 2008;15(1):80—8.

[63] Rupp AK, Rupp C, Keller S, Brase JC, Ehehalt R, Fogel M, et al. Loss of EpCAM expression in breast cancer derived serum exosomes: role of proteolytic cleavage. Gynecol Oncol 2011;122(2):437—46.

[64] Andre F, Schartz NE, Movassagh M, Flament C, Pautier P, Morice P, et al. Malignant effusions and immunogenic tumour-derived exosomes. Lancet 2002;360(9329):295—305.

[65] Taylor DD, Gercel-Taylor C. MicroRNA signatures of tumor-derived exosomes as diagnostic biomarkers of ovarian cancer. Gynecol Oncol 2008;110(1):13—21.

[66] Al-Nedawi K, Meehan B, Micallef J, Lhotak V, May L, Guha A, et al. Intercellular transfer of the oncogenic receptor EGFRvIII by microvesicles derived from tumour cells. Nat Cell Biol 2008;10(5):619—24.

[67] Dai S, Wei D, Wu Z, Zhou X, Wei X, Huang H, et al. Phase I clinical trial of autologous ascites-derived exosomes combined with GM-CSF for colorectal cancer. Mol Ther 2008;16(4):782—90.

[68] Navabi H, Croston D, Hobot J, Clayton A, Zitvogel L, Jasani B, et al. Preparation of human ovarian cancer ascites-derived exosomes for a clinical trial. Blood Cells Mol Dis 2005;35(2):149—52.

[69] André F, Schartz NE, Chaput N, Flament C, Raposo G, Amigorena S, et al. Tumor-derived exosomes: a new source of tumor rejection antigens. Vaccine 2002;20(Suppl 4):A28—31.

[70] Zhang Y, Luo CL, He BC, Zhang JM, Cheng G, Wu XH. Exosomes derived from IL-12-anchored renal cancer cells increase induction of specific antitumor response in vitro: a novel vaccine for renal cell carcinoma. Int J Oncol 2010;36(1):133—40.

[71] Van Parijs L, Abbas AK. Role of Fas-mediated cell death in the regulation of immune responses. Curr Opin Immunol 1996;8(3):355—61.

[72] Osborne BA. Apoptosis and the maintenance of homoeostasis in the immune system. Curr Opin Immunol 1996;8(2):245—54.

[73] Alderson MR, Tough TW, Davis-Smith T, Braddy S, Falk B, Schooley KA, et al. Fas ligand mediates activation-induced cell death in human T lymphocytes. J Exp Med 1995;181(1):71—7.

[74] Suda T, Okazaki T, Naito Y, Yokota T, Arai N, Ozaki S, et al. Expression of the Fas ligand in cells of T cell lineage. J Immunol 1995;154(8):3806—13.

[75] O'Connell J, O'Sullivan GC, Collins JK, Shanahan F. The Fas counterattack: Fas-mediated T cell killing by colon cancer cells expressing Fas ligand. J Exp Med 1996;184(3):1075—82.

[76] Hahne M, Rimoldi D, Schroter M, Romero P, Schreier M, French LE, et al. Melanoma cell expression of Fas(Apo-1/CD95) ligand: implications for tumor immune escape. Science 1996;274(5291):1363—6.

[77] Abusamra AJ, Zhong Z, Zheng X, Li M, Ichim TE, Chin JL, et al. Tumor exosomes expressing Fas ligand mediate CD8+ T-cell apoptosis. Blood Cells Mol Dis 2005;35(2):169—73.

531

[78] Martinez-Lorenzo MJ, Anel A, Alava MA, Pineiro A, Naval J, Lasierra P, et al. The human melanoma cell line MelJuSo secretes bioactive FasL and APO2L/TRAIL on the surface of microvesicles. Possible contribution to tumor counterattack. Exp Cell Res 2004;295(2):315−29.

[79] Qu JL, Qu XJ, Qu JL, Qu XJ, Zhao MF, Teng YE, et al. The role of cbl family of ubiquitin ligases in gastric cancer exosome-induced apoptosis of Jurkat T cells. Acta Oncol 2009;48(8):1173−80.

[80] Wieckowski EU, Visus C, Szajnik M, Szczepanski MJ, Storkus WJ, Whiteside TL. Tumor-derived microvesicles promote regulatory T cell expansion and induce apoptosis in tumor-reactive activated CD8+ T lymphocytes. J Immunol 2009;183(6):3720−30.

[81] Peng P, Yan Y, Keng S. Exosomes in the ascites of ovarian cancer patients: origin and effects on anti-tumor immunity. Oncol Rep 2011;25(3):749−62.

[82] Taylor DD, Gercel-Taylor C. Tumour-derived exosomes and their role in cancer-associated T-cell signalling defects. Br J Cancer 2005;92(2):305−11.

[83] Klibi J, Niki T, Riedel A, Pioche-Durieu C, Souquere S, Rubinstein E, et al. Blood diffusion and Th1--suppressive effects of galectin-9-containing exosomes released by Epstein-Barr virus-infected nasopharyngeal carcinoma cells. Blood 2009;113(9):1957−66.

[84] Clayton A, Al-Taei S, Webber J, Mason MD, Tabi Z. Cancer exosomes express CD39 and CD73, which suppress T cells through adenosine production. J Immunol 2011;187(2):676−83.

[85] Clayton A, Mitchell JP, Court J, Linnane S, Mason MD, Tabi Z. Human tumor-derived exosomes down-modulate NKG2D expression. J Immunol 2008;180(11):7249−58.

[86] Clayton A, Tabi Z. Exosomes and the MICA-NKG2D system in cancer. Blood Cells Mol Dis 2005;34(3):206−13.

[87] Ashiru O, Boutet P, Fernandez-Messina L, Aguera-Gonzalez S, Skepper JN, Vales-Gomez M, et al. Natural killer cell cytotoxicity is suppressed by exposure to the human NKG2D ligand MICA*008 that is shed by tumor cells in exosomes. Cancer Res 2010;70(2):481−9.

[88] Liu C, Yu S, Zinn K, Wang J, Zhang L, Jia Y, et al. Murine mammary carcinoma exosomes promote tumor growth by suppression of NK cell function. J Immunol 2006;176(3):1375−85.

[89] Szczepanski MJ, Szajnik M, Welsh A, Whiteside TL, Boyiadzis M. Blast-derived microvesicles in sera from patients with acute myeloid leukemia suppress natural killer cell function via membrane-associated transforming growth factor-beta1. Haematologica 2011;96(9):1302−9.

[90] Gabrilovich DI, Nagaraj S. Myeloid-derived suppressor cells as regulators of the immune system. Nat Rev Immunol 2009;9(3):162−74.

[91] Valenti R, Huber V, Filipazzi P, Pilla L, Sovena G, Villa A, et al. Human tumor-released microvesicles promote the differentiation of myeloid cells with transforming growth factor-beta-mediated suppressive activity on T lymphocytes. Cancer Res 2006;66(18):9290−8.

[92] Filipazzi P, Valenti R, Huber V, Pilla L, Canese P, Iero M, et al. Identification of a new subset of myeloid suppressor cells in peripheral blood of melanoma patients with modulation by a granulocyte-macrophage colony-stimulation factor-based antitumor vaccine. J Clin Oncol 2007;25(18):2546−53.

[93] Filipazzi P, Huber V, Rivoltini L. Phenotype, function and clinical implications of myeloid-derived suppressor cells in cancer patients. Cancer Immunol Immunother 2012;61(2):255−63.

[94] Hoechst B, Ormandy LA, Ballmaier M, Lehner F, Kruger C, Manns MP, et al. A new population of myeloid-derived suppressor cells in hepatocellular carcinoma patients induces CD4(+)CD25(+)Foxp3(+) T cells. Gastroenterology 2008;135(1):234−43.

[95] Yuan XK, Zhao XK, Xia YC, Zhu X, Xiao P. Increased circulating immunosuppressive CD14(+)HLA-DR(-/low) cells correlate with clinical cancer stage and pathological grade in patients with bladder carcinoma. J Int Med Res 2011;39(4):1381−91.

[96] Brimnes MK, Vangsted AJ, Knudsen LM, Gimsing P, Gang AO, Johnsen HE, et al. Increased level of both CD4+FOXP3+ regulatory T cells and CD14+HLA-DR/low myeloid-derived suppressor cells and decreased level of dendritic cells in patients with multiple myeloma. Scand J Immunol 2010;72(6):540−7.

[97] Szajnik M, Czystowska M, Szczepanski MJ, Mandapathil M, Whiteside TL. Tumor-derived microvesicles induce, expand and up-regulate biological activities of human regulatory T cells (Treg). PLoS One 2010;5(7):e11469.

[98] Wada J, Onishi H, Suzuki H, Yamasaki A, Nagai S, Morisaki T, et al. Surface-bound TGF-beta1 on effusion-derived exosomes participates in maintenance of number and suppressive function of regulatory T-cells in malignant effusions. Anticancer Res 2010;30(9):3747−57.

[99] Wang GJ, Liu Y, Qin A, Shah SV, Deng ZB, Xiang X, et al. Thymus exosomes-like particles induce regulatory T cells. J Immunol 2008;181(8):5242−8.

[100] Yu S, Liu C, Su K, Wang J, Liu Y, Zhang L, et al. Tumor exosomes inhibit differentiation of bone marrow dendritic cells. J Immunol 2007;178(11):6867−75.

532

[101] Xiang X, Liu Y, Zhuang X, Zhang S, Michalek S, Taylor DD, et al. TLR2-mediated expansion of MDSCs is dependent on the source of tumor exosomes. Am J Pathol 2010;177(4):1606—10.

[102] Liu Y, Xiang X, Zhuang X, Zhang S, Liu C, Cheng Z, et al. Contribution of MyD88 to the tumor exosome-mediated induction of myeloid derived suppressor cells. Am J Pathol 2010;176(5):2490—9.

[103] Chalmin F, Ladoire S, Mignot G, Vincent J, Bruchard M, Remy-Martin JP, et al. Membrane-associated Hsp72 from tumor-derived exosomes mediates STAT3-dependent immunosuppressive function of mouse and human myeloid-derived suppressor cells. J Clin Invest 2010;120(2):457—71.

[104] Xiang X, Liu Y, Zhuang X, Zhang S, Michalek S, Taylor DD, et al. TLR2-mediated expansion of MDSCs is dependent on the source of tumor exosomes. Am J Pathol 2010;177(4):1606—10.

[105] Mignot G, Chalmin F, Ladoire S, Rebe C, Ghiringhelli F. Tumor exosome-mediated MDSC activation. Am J Pathol 2011;178(3):1404—5. 1403,4; author reply.

[106] Muralidharan-Chari V, Clancy JW, Sedgwick A, D'Souza-Schorey C. Microvesicles: mediators of extracellular communication during cancer progression. J Cell Sci 2010;123(Pt 10):1603—11.

[107] Hood JL, Pan H, Lanza GM, Wickline SA. Consortium for Translational Research in Advanced Imaging and Nanomedicine (C-TRAIN). Paracrine induction of endothelium by tumor exosomes. Lab Invest 2009;89(11):1317—28.

[108] Hood JL, San RS, Wickline SA. Exosomes released by melanoma cells prepare sentinel lymph nodes for tumor metastasis. Cancer Res 2011;71(11):3792—801.

[109] Richardson MM, Jennings LK, Zhang XA. Tetraspanins and tumor progression. Clin Exp Metastasis 2011;28(3):261—70.

[110] Gesierich S, Berezovskiy I, Ryschich E, Zoller M. Systemic induction of the angiogenesis switch by the tetraspanin D6.1A/CO-029. Cancer Res 2006;66(14):7083—94.

[111] Nazarenko I, Rana S, Baumann A, McAlear J, Hellwig A, Trendelenburg M, et al. Cell surface tetraspanin Tspan8 contributes to molecular pathways of exosome-induced endothelial cell activation. Cancer Res 2010;70(4):1668—78.

[112] Meckes Jr DG, Shair KH, Marquitz AR, Kung CP, Edwards RH, Raab-Traub N. Human tumor virus utilizes exosomes for intercellular communication. Proc Natl Acad Sci U S A 2010;107(47):20370—5.

[113] Yang M, Chen J, Su F, Yu B, Su F, Lin L, et al. Microvesicles secreted by macrophages shuttle invasion-potentiating microRNAs into breast cancer cells. Mol Cancer 2011;10:117.

[114] Webber J, Steadman R, Mason MD, Tabi Z, Clayton A. Cancer exosomes trigger fibroblast to myofibroblast differentiation. Cancer Res 2010;70(23):9621—30.

[115] Cho JA, Park H, Lim EH, Lee KW. Exosomes from breast cancer cells can convert adipose tissue-derived mesenchymal stem cells into myofibroblast-like cells. Int J Oncol 2012;40(1):130—8.

[116] Nieuwland R, van der Post JA, Lok CA, Kenter G, Sturk A. Microparticles and exosomes in gynecologic neoplasias. Semin Thromb Hemost 2010;36(8):925—9.

[117] Jung T, Castellana D, Klingbeil P, Cuesta Hernandez I, Vitacolonna M, Orlicky DJ, et al. CD44v6 dependence of premetastatic niche preparation by exosomes. Neoplasia 2009;11(10):1093—105.

[118] Raman D, Baugher PJ, Thu YM, Richmond A. Role of chemokines in tumor growth. Cancer Lett 2007;256(2):137—65.

[119] Lu T, Sathe SS, Swiatkowski SM, Hampole CV, Stark GR. Secretion of cytokines and growth factors as a general cause of constitutive NFkappaB activation in cancer. Oncogene 2004;23(12):2138—45.

[120] Daughaday WH, Deuel TF. Tumor secretion of growth factors. Endocrinol Metab Clin North Am 1991;20(3):539—63.

[121] Goustin AS, Leof EB, Shipley GD, Moses HL. Growth factors and cancer. Cancer Res 1986;46(3):1015—29.

[122] Higginbotham JN, Demory Beckler M, Gephart JD, Franklin JL, Bogatcheva G, Kremers GJ, et al. Amphiregulin exosomes increase cancer cell invasion. Curr Biol 2011;21(9):779—86.

[123] Hendrix A, Westbroek W, Bracke M, De Wever O. An ex(o)citing machinery for invasive tumor growth. Cancer Res 2010;70(23):9533—7.

[124] Feng D, Zhao WL, Ye YY, Bai XC, Liu RQ, Chang LF, et al. Cellular internalization of exosomes occurs through phagocytosis. Traffic 2010;11(5):675—87.

[125] Raposo G, Nijman HW, Stoorvogel W, Liejendekker R, Harding CV, Melief CJ, et al. B lymphocytes secrete antigen-presenting vesicles. J Exp Med 1996;183(3):1161—72.

[126] Miyanishi M, Tada K, Koike M, Uchiyama Y, Kitamura T, Nagata S. Identification of Tim4 as a phosphatidylserine receptor. Nature 2007;450(7168):435—9.

[127] Tian T, Wang Y, Wang H, Zhu Z, Xiao Z. Visualizing of the cellular uptake and intracellular trafficking of exosomes by live-cell microscopy. J Cell Biochem 2010;111(2):488—96.

533

[128] Mittelbrunn M, Gutierrez-Vazquez C, Villarroya-Beltri C, Gonzalez S, Sanchez-Cabo F, Gonzalez MA, et al. Unidirectional transfer of microRNA-loaded exosomes from T cells to antigen-presenting cells. Nat Commun 2011;2:282.

[129] Luciani F, Spada M, De Milito A, Molinari A, Rivoltini L, Montinaro A, et al. Effect of proton pump inhibitor pretreatment on resistance of solid tumors to cytotoxic drugs. J Natl Cancer Inst 2004;96(22):1702–13.

[130] Yin J, Yan X, Yao X, Zhang Y, Shan Y, Mao N, et al. Secretion of annexin A3 from ovarian cancer cells and its association with platinum resistance in ovarian cancer patients. J Cell Mol Med 2012;16:337–48.

[131] Safaei R, Larson BJ, Cheng TC, Gibson MA, Otani S, Naerdemann W, et al. Abnormal lysosomal trafficking and enhanced exosomal export of cisplatin in drug-resistant human ovarian carcinoma cells. Mol Cancer Ther 2005;4(10):1595–604.

[132] Lehmann BD, McCubrey JA, Jefferson HS, Paine MS, Chappell WH, Terrian DM. A dominant role for p53-dependent cellular senescence in radiosensitization of human prostate cancer cells. Cell Cycle 2007;6(5):595–605.

[133] Yu X, Harris SL, Levine AJ. The regulation of exosome secretion: a novel function of the p53 protein. Cancer Res 2006;66(9):4795–801.

[134] Lehmann BD, Paine MS, Brooks AM, McCubrey JA, Renegar RH, Wang R, et al. Senescence-associated exosome release from human prostate cancer cells. Cancer Res 2008;68(19):7864–71.

[135] Khan S, Jutzy JM, Aspe JR, McGregor DW, Neidigh JW, Wall NR. Survivin is released from cancer cells via exosomes. Apoptosis 2011;16(1):1–12.

[136] Battke C, Ruiss R, Welsch U, Wimberger P, Lang S, Jochum S, et al. Tumour exosomes inhibit binding of tumour-reactive antibodies to tumour cells and reduce ADCC. Cancer Immunol Immunother 2011;60(5):639–48.

[137] Aung T, Chapuy B, Vogel D, Wenzel D, Oppermann M, Lahmann M, et al. Exosomal evasion of humoral immunotherapy in aggressive B-cell lymphoma modulated by ATP-binding cassette transporter A3. Proc Natl Acad Sci U S A 2011;108(37):15336–41.

[138] Wolfers J, Lozier A, Raposo G, Regnault A, Thery C, Masurier C, et al. Tumor-derived exosomes are a source of shared tumor rejection antigens for CTL cross-priming. Nat Med 2001;7(3):297–303.

[139] Napoletano C, Rughetti A, Landi R, Pinto D, Bellati F, Rahimi H, et al. Immunogenicity of allo-vesicle carrying ERBB2 tumor antigen for dendritic cell-based anti-tumor immunotherapy. Int J Immunopathol Pharmacol 2009;22(3):647–58.

[140] Gastpar R, Gehrmann M, Bausero MA, Asea A, Gross C, Schroeder JA, et al. Heat shock protein 70 surface-positive tumor exosomes stimulate migratory and cytolytic activity of natural killer cells. Cancer Res 2005;65(12):5238–47.

[141] Vega VL, Rodriguez-Silva M, Frey T, Gehrmann M, Diaz JC, Steinem C, et al. Hsp70 translocates into the plasma membrane after stress and is released into the extracellular environment in a membrane-associated form that activates macrophages. J Immunol 2008;180(6):4299–307.

[142] Dai S, Wan T, Wang B, Zhou X, Xiu F, Chen T, et al. More efficient induction of HLA-A*0201-restricted and carcinoembryonic antigen (CEA)-specific CTL response by immunization with exosomes prepared from heat-stressed CEA-positive tumor cells. Clin Cancer Res 2005;11(20):7554–63.

[143] Shen C, Hao SG, Zhao CX, Zhu J, Wang C. Antileukaemia immunity: effect of exosomes against NB4 acute promyelocytic leukaemia cells. J Int Med Res 2011;39(3):740–7.

[144] Viaud S, Ploix S, Lapierre V, Théry C, Commere PH, Tramalloni D, et al. Updated technology to produce highly immunogenic dendritic cell-derived exosomes of clinical grade: a critical role of interferon-γ. J Immunother 2011;34(1):65–75.

[145] Escudier B, Dorval T, Chaput N, Andre F, Caby MP, Novault S, et al. Vaccination of metastatic melanoma patients with autologous dendritic cell (DC) derived-exosomes: results of the first phase I clinical trial. J Transl Med 2005;3(1):10.

[146] Viaud S, Terme M, Flament C, Taieb J, Andre F, Novault S, et al. Dendritic cell-derived exosomes promote natural killer cell activation and proliferation: a role for NKG2D ligands and IL-15Ralpha. PLoS One 2009;4(3):e4942.

[147] Morse MA, Garst J, Osada T, Khan S, Hobeika A, Clay TM, et al. A phase I study of dexosome immunotherapy in patients with advanced non-small cell lung cancer. J Transl Med 2005;3(1):9.

[148] Bard MP, Hegmans JP, Hemmes A, Luider TM, Willemsen R, Severijnen LA, et al. Proteomic analysis of exosomes isolated from human malignant pleural effusions. Am J Respir Cell Mol Biol 2004;31(1):114–21.

[149] Runz S, Keller S, Rupp C, Stoeck A, Issa Y, Koensgen D, et al. Malignant ascites-derived exosomes of ovarian carcinoma patients contain CD24 and EpCAM. Gynecol Oncol 2007;107(3):563–71.

[150] Hunter MP, Ismail N, Zhang X, Aguda BD, Lee EJ, Yu L, et al. Detection of microRNA expression in human peripheral blood microvesicles. PLoS One 2008;3(11):e3694.

[151] Keller S, Ridinger J, Rupp AK, Janssen JW, Altevogt P. Body fluid derived exosomes as a novel template for clinical diagnostics. J Transl Med 2011;9:86.

[152] Hoen EN, van der Vlist EJ, Aalberts M, Mertens HC, Bosch BJ, Bartelink W, et al. Quantitative and qualitative flow cytometric analysis of nanosized cell-derived membrane vesicles. Nanomedicine 2011.

[153] Grant R, Ansa-Addo E, Stratton D, Antwi-Baffour S, Jorfi S, Kholia S, et al. A filtration-based protocol to isolate human plasma membrane-derived vesicles and exosomes from blood plasma. J Immunol Methods 2011;371(1−2):143−51.

[154] Silva J, Garcia V, Rodriguez M, Compte M, Cisneros E, Veguillas P, et al. Analysis of exosome release and its prognostic value in human colorectal cancer. Genes Chromosomes Cancer 2012;51(4):409−18.

[155] Kosaka N, Iguchi H, Ochiya T. Circulating microRNA in body fluid: a new potential biomarker for cancer diagnosis and prognosis. Cancer Sci 2010;101(10):2087−92.

CHAPTER 31

Galectins: Key Players in the Tumor Microenvironment

Victoria Sundblad[1], Veronique Mathieu[2], Robert Kiss[2],*, Gabriel A. Rabinovich[1,3],*
[1]Laboratorio de Inmunopatología, Instituto de Biología y Medicina Experimental (IBYME), Consejo Nacional de Investigaciones Científicas y Técnicas (CONICET), Buenos Aires, Argentina
[2]Laboratory of Toxicology, Faculty of Pharmacy, Université Libre de Bruxelles, Brussels, Belgium
[3]Laboratorio de Glicómica Estructural y Funcional, IQUIBICEN-CONICET, Departamento de Química Biológica, Facultad de Ciencias Exactas y Naturales, Universidad de Buenos Aires, Ciudad de Buenos Aires, Argentina
*R.K. and G.A.R. contributed equally to this chapter

I. GALECTINS: DEFINITION, STRUCTURE AND FUNCTION

Galectins are a family of evolutionarily conserved carbohydrate-binding proteins with affinity for β-galactosides [1–2]. These lectins are defined by a common consensus sequence of approximately 130 amino acids in the carbohydrate recognition domain (CRD), which is responsible for their ability to recognize the disaccharide N-acetyllactosamine [Galβ(1–4)-GlcNAc; LacNAc] in N- and O-glycans [3]. To date, 15 mammalian galectins have been identified which can be subdivided into the following three groups: a) "prototype" galectins (galectin-1, 2, 5, 7, 10, 11, 13, 14 and 15) which have one CRD and can dimerize; b) "tandem-repeat" galectins (galectin-4, 6, 8, 9 and 12) which contain two homologous CRDs in tandem in a single polypeptide chain; and c) chimera type galectins, with the unique member galectin-3 that contains a CRD connected to a nonlectin N-terminal region responsible for oligomerization. A schematic representation of different subfamilies of galectins is illustrated in Figure 31.1.

For decades, galectins were considered proteins that functioned only in the extracellular milieu by interacting through their CRD with glycoproteins and glycolipids on the cell surface and extracellular matrix. However, several intracellular functions of galectins have emerged recently, including modulation of signaling and splicing machineries, survival and proliferation. Notably, most intracellular activities of this lectin family involve protein–protein interactions and not protein–glycan interactions [4]. The intracellular signaling pathways controlled by galectins in the tumor microenvironment have recently been reviewed [5].

Given their dual extracellular and intracellular functions, galectins are regarded as major players in normal physiology as well as in oncogenic processes. However, their elevated or attenuated expression in tumor microenvironments allows the identification of different members of this protein family as attractive targets for cancer therapy. In fact, an increasing

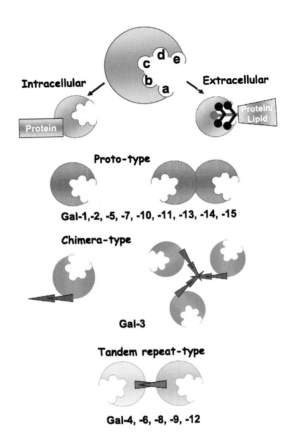

FIGURE 31.1

Galectin structure. Galectins are subdivided into *proto-type* galectins, which contain one carbohydrate recognition domain (CRD) and can form homodimers; *tandem-repeat* galectins that contain two distinct CRDs in tandem connected by a linker of up to 70 amino acids; and the unique *chimera-type* galectin-3, which consists of unusual tandem repeats of proline and glycine-rich short stretches fused onto the CRD.

number of studies have addressed the expression of galectins in several types of cancer [6], unveiling multiple roles of these glycan-binding proteins in tumorigenic and metastatic processes [1,7]. In addition, as galectins are expressed by different immune and inflammatory cells and regulate the functions of these cells [8], it is conceivable they may influence the inflammatory and immune responses in tumor microenvironments. In this chapter, we aim to review and discuss available data on the role of galectins in modulating immune cell networks in the tumor microenvironment. In addition, we will discuss additional nonimmunological functions of galectins, which may contribute to tumor development, growth and metastasis. Understanding the balance of immune-related and nonimmune functions of galectins may contribute to predicting the overall function of these endogenous lectins in tumor biology.

II. GALECTIN–GLYCAN INTERACTIONS AS KEY MODULATORS OF TUMOR IMMUNITY

Several observations in the past decade led to the realization that the greatest obstacles for harnessing the immune system against tumors may be the complex mechanisms that tumors exploit to establish T-cell tolerance against self-tumor antigens. Experimental evidence demonstrated that antigen-specific CD4$^+$ T cells are rendered tolerant during tumor growth *in vivo*. Whereas tumor antigen recognition by antigen-specific T cells indeed occurs *in vivo*, anergy rather than T-cell priming is the default outcome of such an encounter in tumor-bearing hosts [9]. Even though it was initially thought that the entire tumor-specific T-cell population was rendered anergic, a more detailed study demonstrated that *in vivo* interaction with tumor cells led to a heterogeneous T-cell population composed by antigen-experienced T cells (among them anergic T cells), naïve T cells, and tumor-specific regulatory T (T_{reg}) cells displaying immunosuppressive activity [10]. Since then, great efforts have been invested in an attempt to elucidate how different effector and regulatory cell populations are induced and what are the molecular and cellular mechanisms that influence the final composition of these combinations of tumor-specific T cells. In this context, dendritic cells (DCs) have been shown to play a critical role in the decision leading to T-cell tolerance versus T-cell priming *in vivo*. Such a decision is greatly influenced by the environmental context in which DCs encounter the antigen. While antigen encounter by DCs in an inflammatory context triggers their maturation toward a phenotype capable of generating robust immune responses, antigen capture by DCs in a noninflammatory environment would fail to elicit productive T-cell responses, leading instead to the development of T-cell tolerance [11]. Interestingly, as a tumor progresses, its microenvironment not only fails to provide suitable inflammatory signals needed for efficient DC activation, but also provides immunosuppressive mechanisms such as IL-10 [12] and vascular endothelial growth factor (VEGF) [13] which dampen activation and immunogenicity of these cells.

Despite major advances in understanding the mechanisms leading to tumor immunity, a number of obstacles hinder the successful translation of mechanistic insights into effective tumor immunotherapy. Such obstacles include the ability of tumors to display multiple immunosuppressive mechanisms aimed either at avoiding immune recognition or disabling effector T cells [14—16]. These include alterations of components of the antigen presentation machinery, defects in proximal TCR signaling, secretion of immunosuppressive or pro-apoptotic factors, expression of inhibitory molecules (PD-L1, CTLA-4, IDO) and specific recruitment of regulatory cell populations [14,17—18]. These multiple immunosuppressive mechanisms displayed by tumors to evade immune response are discussed in detail elsewhere [19]. Herein, we will integrate recent and pioneer findings on the critical role of galectin—glycan interactions in shaping antitumor immune responses. These observations are summarized in Figure 31.2. Whether these bewildering molecules became allied actors merely exploited by tumors or are induced by tumors as an additional strategy to thwart immune responses still remains to be ascertained.

A. Galectin—glycan interactions in the physiology of dendritic cells

DCs are critically important for orchestrating antitumor immune responses [20]. Tumor cells express a large number of antigens that can be recognized by the host immune system. DCs can take up, process, and present tumor antigens to activate a tumor-specific T-cell response. However, instead of being eradicated, tumors progress, metastasize, and ultimately kill the host. Notably, through secretion of a number of tumor-derived factors, including interleukin (IL)-6, IL-10, granulocyte macrophage-colony stimulating factor (GM-CSF), transforming growth factor (TGF)-β, macrophage colony-stimulating factor (M-CSF) or vascular endothelial growth factor (VEGF), tumors alter DC differentiation, increase expansion and promote accumulation of immature and regulatory DCs [19]. In addition, as discussed above, the environmental context in which DC encounter the antigen strongly influences the decision leading to T-cell tolerance versus T-cell priming. Indeed, a delicate balance between activating and inhibitory pathways influencing these cells certainly plays a key role in such divergent T-cell outcomes [19].

In this context, lectin—glycan interactions play fundamental roles in determining the nature and magnitude of inflammatory or tolerogenic APC programs [8]. Interestingly, examination of the "glycosylation signature" of DCs during maturation revealed profound changes in glycan expression profiles, including upregulation of LacNAc and sialylated structures and

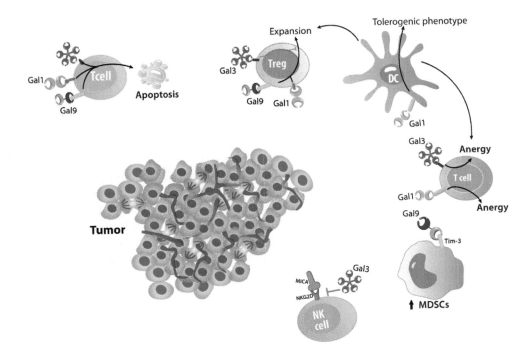

FIGURE 31.2

Role of galectins in tumor immunity. Malignant transformation and metastasis is often associated with altered glycosylation of tumor and tumor-associated inflammatory cells. Galectins, including galectin (Gal)1, Gal3 and Gal9, secreted by tumor or stromal cells, modulate tumor-immune escape by targeting the survival of effector cytotoxic T lymphocytes (CTLs), Th1 and Th17 cells, skewing the balance toward a Th2 cytokine profile and/or inducing the differentiation and/or expansion of T regulatory (T$_{Reg}$) cells. Alternatively, Gal3 induces T-cell dysfunction by distancing the T-cell receptor (TCR) from its coreceptor CD8 in anergic infiltrating CTLs, thus contributing to T-cell tolerance in the tumor microenvironment. On the other hand, Gal9-Tim-3 interactions drive the differentiation of myeloid-derived suppressor cells (MDSCs). Also, Gal3 impairs natural killer (NK) cell function by reducing the magnitude of interactions between the heavily O-glycosylated tumor-derived MICA and the activating receptor NKG2D.

downregulation of core-2 O-glycans [21]. In addition, DCs treated with recombinant galectin-1 showed enhanced migratory capacity through extracellular matrix along with increased phenotypic maturation [22]. This effect appears to be mediated by co-clustering of CD43 and CD45, and engagement of Syk and protein kinase C (PKC) signaling pathways [23]. Moreover, *in vivo* administration of recombinant galectin-1 favored the recruitment of a population of DCs with a regulatory cell surface phenotype to the uterine mucosal tissue [24]. In addition, DCs engineered to overexpress galectin-1 induced apoptosis of activated T cells [25]. Through binding to poly-LacNAc-containing glycans expressed on CD43+ DCs, we found that galectin-1 initiates a tolerogenic circuit involving the differentiation of IL-27-producing DCs, which in turn promote the expansion of IL-10-producing regulatory type 1 (Tr1) cells [26]. When transferred *in vivo*, these DCs promoted IL-10-mediated T-cell tolerance, blunted T helper (Th)1 and Th17 responses and suppressed autoimmune inflammation. Moreover, these DCs differentiated in a galectin-1-enriched microenvironment were unable to elicit an effective T-cell response against tumor challenge, instead skewing the cytokine balance to foster a tolerant milieu that allowed tumor growth [26]. Consistently, DCs lacking galectin-1 or galectin-3 are more immunogenic than wild-type DCs and favor polarization toward Th1 and Th17 profiles [26–27]. Recently, Soldati and colleagues found that galectin-1 released by neuroblastoma cells, promotes the development of immature dendritic cells [28]. Furthermore, galectin-1 produced by lung adenocarcinoma induces release of IL-10 and shedding of mature heparin-binding EGF-like growth factor (HB-EGF) from tumor-associated DCs as a result of the action of the disintegrins ADAM9 and ADAM17 [29]. In addition, purified CD11c+ DCs from galectin-3-deficient (*Lgals3*-/-) mice produced higher amounts of IL-12 than WT DCs, possibly explaining the higher Th1 response verified in response to antigen stimulation by those DCs [30]. Interestingly, while

IFN-γ-producing Th1 cells are generally believed to be important for eradicating tumors, it is still not clear whether IL-17-producing Th17 cells play positive or negative roles in tumor immunity.

On the other hand, galectin-9 has been demonstrated to promote the maturation of DCs at similar levels as lipopolysaccharides [31]. Galectin-9-matured DCs secreted IL-12 but not IL-10 and selectively elicited the production of Th1 cytokines (IL-2 and IFN-γ) by allogeneic CD4$^+$ T cells. This effect did not appear to be dependent on the lectin properties of this protein as it was only slightly inhibited by lactose, and a lectin mutant lacking β-galactoside-binding activity retained its immunostimulatory properties [31]. This "tandem-repeat" galectin has been identified as a major binding partner of the T-cell immunoglobulin- and mucin-domain-containing molecule-3 (TIM-3) [32]. Ligation of Tim-3 by galectin-9 induces divergent functions on APCs and T cells, leading to initiation or termination of Th1-dependent immunity [32]. These contrasting effects have been recently scrutinized at the molecular level, showing that the galectin-9 C-terminal domain is much more potent in inducing T-cell death, while the N-terminal domain is more effective in activating DCs [33]. Thus, different members of the galectin family differentially modulate differentiation, maturation, migration and/or immunogenic potential of DCs.

B. Galectin—glycan interactions in the physiology of monocytes and macrophages

Tumor-associated macrophages (TAMs) are significant for fostering tumor progression. The protumoral properties of TAMs derive from production of soluble mediators that support survival and invasion of malignant cells, direct and indirect suppression of cytotoxic T-cell activity and modulation of angiogenic programs. These varied activities are dependent on the polarization state of TAMs. Targeting molecular pathways that regulate TAM polarization offers great promise for anticancer therapy [34]. Although not studied in the context of tumor biology, galectin-1 has been shown to influence monocyte and macrophage physiology through many different mechanisms [35—37]. In general, galectin-1 has been proposed as a regulatory signal which deactivates inflammatory macrophages [36]. In keeping with its anti-inflammatory functions, this lectin inhibited interferon (IFN)-γ-induced Fcγ receptor type 1-dependent phagocytosis and major histocompatibility complex (MHC) II-dependent T-cell stimulation [36]. In addition, galectin-1 inhibits arachidonic acid release [38], blocks nitric oxide synthesis and increases arginase activity [35], thereby modulating alternative activation of cells of the monocyte/macrophage lineage. Nevertheless, interactions between galectin-1 and monocytes do not always lead to anti-inflammatory effects. In fact, a recent report demonstrated that galectin-1 stimulates monocyte migration in a dose- and saccharide-dependent manner through mechanisms involving mitogen-activated protein kinase (MAPK) pathways [37].

Interestingly, galectin-3 facilitates adhesive interactions between T cells and dendritic cells (DCs) or macrophages [39] and induces CD13-mediated homotypic aggregation of monocytes [40]. Alternatively, galectin-3 can also promote migration of human monocytes/macrophages [41], and induces IL-1 production by human monocytes [42]. When compared to macrophages from wild type mice, macrophages lacking galectin-3 were defective in phagocytosis of opsonized erythrocytes and apoptotic thymocytes [43], and also more prone to apoptosis when treated with apoptotic stimuli [44]. On the other hand, galectin-9 has been shown to induce apoptosis both in monocytic (THP-1) and in myelocytic (HL-60) cell lines through carbohydrate-dependent mechanisms [45]. By functioning intracellularly in human monocytes, galectin-9 induced transcription of the pro-inflammatory cytokines IL-1α, IL-1β, and IFN-γ, whereas exogenously added galectin-9 did not promote the synthesis of these cytokines [46]. Interestingly, while galectin-1, galectin-3 and galectin-9 all favor the differentiation of "alternatively activated" macrophages [36,47—48], poly-LacNAc-deficient macrophages were highly sensitive to agonist-induced activation [49]. Altogether, these observations support the essential role of lectin—glycan lattices in tuning APC functions that tailor adaptive immunity. Whether these interactions modulate the frequency and function of TAMs and the balance between inflammatory or regulatory macrophages in tumor microenvironments remains to be elucidated.

C. Galectin—glycan interactions in the physiology of myeloid-derived suppressor cells

Among the rather elaborate strategies employed by tumors to subvert APC functions, tumor-derived factors stimulate the generation of myeloid-derived suppressor cells (MDSCs) that induce antigen-specific T-cell tolerance via the production of reactive oxygen species (ROS) and direct cell—cell contact [19,50]. MDSCs are a heterogeneous population of myeloid cells composed of immature macrophages, granulocytes, DCs, and other myeloid cells at early stages of differentiation, although, in healthy mice, MDSCs are present in the bone marrow and spleens and differentiate into mature myeloid cells (granulocytes, macrophages, and DCs). In tumor-bearing mice they accumulate in the spleen and, to some extent, in the lymph nodes [51]. Through presentation of antigenic epitopes on their surface, MDSCs induce antigen-specific T-cell anergy [50]. In addition, they inhibit IFN-γ production by CD8+ T cells [52], and can suppress T-cell proliferation *in vitro* as well as inducing the development of Foxp3+ T$_{reg}$ cells *in vivo* [53].

Interestingly, interactions between galectin-9 and Tim-3 have been reported to modulate the frequency of granulocytic MDSC [54]. Overexpression of galectin-9 resulted in an increase in MDSC number and inhibition of tumor-specific immune responses, whereas loss of Tim-3 restored normal levels of MDSC and normal immune response. Thus, promotion of MDSCs via the Tim-3/galectin-9 pathway represents a novel mechanism to regulate antitumor immune responses.

D. The role of galectins in shaping the B-cell compartment

Although compelling evidence supports the function of galectin—saccharide interactions in the control of T-cell fate and of DC physiology, limited information is available on how these proteins could shape B-cell compartment. Galectin-1 has been shown to regulate B-cell function by influencing B-cell development, differentiation, and survival. Within the bone marrow, galectin-1 is highly expressed in stromal cells surrounding pre-B cells, where it binds to the pre-B-cell receptor (pre-BCR) and contributes to synapse formation between pre-B cells and stromal cells [55] to influence pre-BCR signaling and activation [56]. Indeed, galectin-1-deficient (*Lgals1*$^{-/-}$) mice showed an arrest in B-cell development in the pre-BII cell stage [57]. Once in the periphery, galectin-1 is upregulated by activation signals [58] and contributes to differentiation of activated B cells into antibody-secreting plasma cells [59]. Nevertheless, galectin-1 was also shown to negatively regulate B-cell proliferation and BCR-mediated signal transduction [60]. In addition, recent work demonstrated that overexpression of galectin-1 can facilitate death of memory B cells [61], thus confirming the role of this protein in favoring the plasma cell phenotype.

In addition, endogenous galectin-3 favors B-cell survival and mediates IL-4-induced differentiation towards a memory B-cell phenotype [62]. Moreover, recent work has shown that *Lgals1* and *Lgals3* genes are over-represented in anergic compared with conventional B cells [63], which suggests a role of these lectins in the regulation of B-cell tolerance. Given the novel role of B cells in modulating tumor progression and the emergence of regulatory B cells [64], further studies are required to elucidate the role of these proteins in regulating B-cell dependent inflammation and tolerance during tumorigenesis.

542

E. Galectin—glycan interactions as modulators of T-cell effector function

As discussed above, anergy rather than T-cell priming is the default outcome of *in vivo* tumor antigen recognition by antigen-specific T cells [9]. Indeed, a mixture of heterogeneous tumor-specific T cells, composed by antigen-experienced T cells (among them, anergic T cells), naïve cells, and tumor-specific T_{reg} cells, is the final result of such interaction [10]. Galectin—glycan interactions may be one of several molecular and/or cellular mechanisms that influence the final composition of these mixtures of tumor-specific T cells. In addition to their effects on DC differentiation and functionality, which indirectly compromise T-cell responses, galectins directly influence T-cell physiology. Accumulating evidence indicates that galectins contribute to immunoregulation by acting as silencers or turners of T-cell responses. In fact, these endogenous lectins can modulate T-cell effector functions by regulating T-cell survival, extravasation to sites of tumor growth and the balance between pro-inflammatory and anti-inflammatory cytokines. In addition, galectins can profoundly affect TCR signaling thresholds by interacting with specific glycosylated receptors [65].

1. CONTROLLING T-CELL SURVIVAL

Galectins are unique in their capacity to act both extracellularly and intracellularly to control cell death. Extracellularly, galectins cross-link a preferred set of glycosylated receptors to transduce signals that directly lead to T-cell apoptosis. Intracellularly, galectins can interfere with signaling pathways that control cell viability. Thus, the susceptibility of T cells to the pro-apoptotic effects of extracellular galectins is regulated by a selected repertoire of glycoprotein receptors (e.g., CD45 and CD43) and the spatio-temporal expression of selected glycosyl-transferases [8,65].

Galectin-1 has been shown to induce apoptosis of activated but not resting T cells through cross-linking specific glyco-receptors, promoting their segregation into membrane micro-domains and selectively triggering pro-apoptotic signaling pathways [66]. Undoubtedly, one of the most consistent observations in the literature is the ability of galectin-1 to blunt Th1- and Th17-mediated responses and skew the balance toward a Th2-polarized cytokine profile. *In vitro* exposure of activated T cells to recombinant galectin-1 resulted in selective suppression of Th1-type cytokines, including IFN-γ, TNF, and IL-2, and enhanced secretion of Th2 cytokines, including IL-4, IL-5, IL-10, and IL-13 [67—71]. In search for potential mechanisms that could explain these Th1/Th17-specific immunoregulatory effects, we have provided a link among differential glycosylation of T helper cells, susceptibility to galectin-1-induced cell death, and termination of the inflammatory response [72]. While Th1- and Th17-differentiated cells express the repertoire of cell surface glycans that are critical for galectin-1 binding and cell death, Th2 cells are protected from galectin-1 through masking galactosyl moieties through differential α2—6 sialylation of cell surface glycoproteins. The physiologic relevance of galectin-1-mediated effects was demonstrated in galectin-1-deficient ($Lgals1^{-/-}$) mice which display augmented T-cell responses *in vivo* [72—73]. In addition, it has been demonstrated that galectin-1 directly kills activated T cells through binding and clustering of CD45, CD43 and CD7 [74], although it can also sensitize T cells to the canonical Fas/caspase-8-mediated pathway [75]. The ability of galectin-1 to negatively regulate T-cell survival has been extensively studied in the context of the tumor microenvironment demonstrating its pivotal role in tumor cell evasion of T-cell responses [8].

In addition, other members of the galectin family affect T-cell survival and activation. Galectin-2 promotes T-cell apoptosis through mechanisms involving binding to cell surface β-integrins, caspases-3 and -9 activation, cytochrome *c* release, disruption of the mitochondrial membrane potential, and increase of the Bax/Bcl-2 ratio [76]. The "chimera-type" galectin-3, on the other hand, acts in a dual manner either protecting T cells from apoptosis or stimulating T-cell death, depending on whether it functions intracellularly or is added exogenously to T-cell cultures [74,77—78]. T-cell transfectants overexpressing galectin-3 are protected from apoptosis induced by a variety of agents, including Fas ligand and staurosporine [77]. In contrast, through binding to CD45, CD71[74] or CD29[78], extracellular galectin-3 has been shown to induce T-cell apoptosis [74], through mechanisms involving caspase-3, but not caspase-8 activation [78]. As mice lacking galectin-3 frequently show attenuated T-cell responses [79–80], it seems that dominant anti-apoptotic and pro-inflammatory activities of endogenous galectin-3 prevail. Interestingly, intracellular expression of galectin-3 inhibited galectin-1-induced cell death [81]. The pathophysiologic role of galectin-3 in tumor microenvironments has been studied in tumor settings. Using a mouse tumor model, Peng and coworkers [82] showed that delivery of high doses of galectin-3 inhibited tumor-reactive T cells and promoted tumor growth in mice receiving tumor-reactive CD8+ T cells, suggesting that this lectin may function as an immune regulator to inhibit T-cell immune responses and promote tumor growth. In addition, Demotte and colleagues [83] found that a galectin-3 ligand corrects the impaired function of human CD4$^+$ and CD8$^+$ tumor-infiltrating lymphocytes and favors tumor rejection in mice. More recently, a galectin-3-dependent pathway has been identified that upregulates IL-6 production in the neuroblastoma microenvironment [84].

Galectin-9 promotes death of peripheral fully activated CD4$^+$ and CD8$^+$ T cells via mechanisms involving activation of caspase-1, but not caspase-8, 9, and 10 [45]. In an elegant study, Zhu et al. demonstrated that galectin-9 act as a binding partner for Tim-3 and induce selective apoptosis of Th1 cells [85]. The association of this effect with attenuation of autoimmune inflammation [85] as well as with prolongation of allograft survival [86] confirmed the pathophysiologic relevance of these findings. Interestingly, a comparative study revealed that "tandem-repeat" galectins, such as galectin-9, are much more potent than "prototype" galectins, such as galectin-1, in triggering T-cell death. This effect does not relate to different saccharide-binding specificities, but reflects the ability of the linker domain of "tandem-repeat" galectins to permit intermolecular CRD interactions that lead to the formation of higher-order multimers [87]. Interestingly, Nagahara and colleagues [88] found that galectin-9 prolongs the survival of tumor-bearing mice in a dose- and time-dependent manner. Although galectin-9 did not prolong the survival of tumor-bearing nude mice, transfer of naive spleen cells restored prolonged galectin-9-induced survival in nude mice, indicating possible involvement of T-cell-mediated immune responses in galectin-9-mediated antitumor activity. Galectin-9 administration increased the number of IFN-γ-producing Tim-3$^+$ CD8$^+$ T cells with enhanced granzyme B and perforin expression, although it induced CD4$^+$ T-cell apoptosis.

Although their physiologic relevance awaits further examination, other family members including galectin-4 and galectin-8 also display pro-apoptotic activity in *in vitro* settings [89–91], suggesting that galectins may have evolved as cytokines that act in an autocrine or paracrine fashion to regulate thresholds of immune cell survival. In addition, some members of the galectin family (galectin-1, 3, 4 and 8) do not trigger full apoptotic programs, but instead promote reversible phosphatidylserine exposure, thereafter preparing living leukocytes for phagocytic removal [92].

2. MODULATION OF T-CELL SIGNALING, ACTIVATION AND ANERGY

T-cell activation requires stable contacts with APCs to assemble the immunological synapse. Several molecular contacts, including those elicited by lectins and glycans, contribute to defining the nature and magnitude of APC–T-cell interactions as well as the balance between immune cell responsiveness and tolerance [93]. In this regard, multivalent interactions between endogenous lectins and glycosylated receptors profoundly affect signaling thresholds by reducing the rate of receptor trafficking, bridging association with other glycoproteins, limiting receptor clustering and/or preventing receptor endocitosis [8]. Indeed, the T-cell receptor (TCR) is "decorated" by β1,6 N-glycan branch structures that are generated by the glycosyltransferase N–acetylglucosaminyltransferase-5 (GnT5). Elegant studies demonstrated that galectin-3 can modulate T-cell activation and signaling. By forming multivalent complexes with N-glycans on the TCR, galectin-3 potentially restricts the lateral mobility of TCR complexes, raising the threshold for ligand-dependent receptor clustering and signal transduction, thus preventing uncontrolled activation of T cells [94]. Accordingly, deficiency in GnT5 lowers the threshold for T-cell activation by enabling TCR clustering and signaling, which results in augmented Th1-cell responses and enhanced susceptibility to autoimmune disease [94–95].

A further mechanistic analysis revealed that N-glycan branching coordinates homeostatic setpoints in T-cell activation and signaling to modulate TCR clustering [96]. Additional studies aimed at dissecting the mechanistic basis of this effect revealed that galectin–glycan lattices and actin microfilaments act on opposing sides of the plasma membrane to regulate receptor distribution and signaling [97]. In the absence of TCR engagement, galectin binding to N-glycans prevents filamentous actin-dependent targeting of the TCR, CD4 and the protein tyrosine kinase Lck to GM1-enriched membrane microdomains [97]. Moreover, galectin–glycan lattices contribute to the inactivation of Lck by specifically retaining the CD45 phosphatase at these membrane areas, thereby preventing spontaneous TCR activation in the absence of specific ligands [97]. In addition, galectin-1 regulates T-cell fate by modulating T-cell receptor (TCR)/co-stimulator-dependent clustering and signaling [98]. By limiting required protein segregation and lipid raft reorganization at the TCR contact site, galectin-1 prevents processive and sustained TCR signal transduction and allows the establishment of appropriate T-cell activation thresholds for signaling distinct functional responses. Thus, cell surface glycoprotein receptors can bind galectins in proportion to the degree of GlcNAc branching, forming a functional lattice that controls the T-cell signaling threshold. Reinforcing this likelihood, cell surface galectin–glycoprotein lattices can also play an integral role in the control of the effector activity of antitumor cytotoxic T lymphocytes (CTLs). After several days of antigenic stimulation, CTLs become anergic and lose colocalization of the TCR with the glycoprotein CD8. Demotte and colleagues found that during this anergic state, extracellular galectin-3 plays a key role through binding to TCR N-glycans and sequestering the TCR from CD8 molecules in both mouse models and human tumor-infiltrating lymphocytes [99].

Interestingly, recent evidence further demonstrated that, in addition to forming extracellular lattices, galectin-3 also acts intracellularly by promoting TCR downmodulation at sites of immunological synapse via interaction with regulatory/endocytic proteins [100]. Likewise, galectin-1 produced by antigen-experienced CD8$^+$ T cells can function as an autocrine regulator that negatively controls TCR signaling [101]. These results support the essential role of galectin-glycan interactions in discriminating TCR signaling thresholds and tuning T-cell fate, thus modulating the activation or anergic state of tumor-specific T cells.

F. Galectin–glycan interactions in the control of regulatory T cells

Considerable attention has been placed on the premise that tumors may subvert tumor immunity by promoting the expansion, recruitment and activation of T_{reg} cells [102,103]. Undeniably, T_{reg} cells play a key role in restraining antitumor immunity [103]. Indeed, many CD4$^+$CD25$^+$+Foxp3$^+$ cells are found either in the circulation or in the tumor itself in lung, pancreatic, breast, ovary, and skin cancer patients [104]. Curiel and colleagues [104] have provided proof-of-principle of the critical role of CD4$^+$CD25$^+$Foxp3$^+$ cells in promoting tumor-immune privilege. Not only naturally occurring CD4$^+$CD25$^+$Foxp3$^+$ Tregs, but also other regulatory cell populations may contribute to impaired tumor surveillance. In this regard, IL-10-producing Tr1 cells have attracted considerable attention [105–106]. Exposure of DCs to myeloma cell lysates results in increased IL-10 production, which favors the expansion of Tr1 cells [107]. Endowed with the capacity to suppress T-cell responses, different regulatory cell populations are recruited and activated at sites of tumor growth to disarm T-cell effector mechanisms and thwart successful antitumor immunity.

Importantly, at least part of the immunosuppressive function of T regulatory (T_{reg}) cells is mediated by galectin-1. This lectin is overexpressed in T_{reg} cells as compared to effector T cells [108]. Strikingly, the inhibitory activity of human and mouse $CD4^+CD25^+FoxP3^+$ T_{reg} cells is significantly diminished upon galectin-1 blockade [108]. In addition, *in vitro* exposure of T cells to galectin-1 expands a population of $CD4^+CD25^{high}$ T_{reg} cells that highly express FoxP3, the transcription factor that is a hallmark of these cells [109]. Notably, in a model of stress-induced pregnancy failure, treatment with galectin-1 restored tolerance and mitigated inflammation by promoting the differentiation of uterine regulatory DCs and IL-10-producing T_{reg} cells. These tolerogenic effects were hierarchically regulated by progesterone and abrogated in mice depleted of T_{reg} cells or deficient in IL-10, suggesting a hormone-lectin synergism in the induction of immune tolerance [24].

Interestingly, while galectin-1 [110] and galectin-9 [111] contribute to T_{reg} cell expansion *in vivo*, galectin-3 appears to counteract this effect [112]. In an experimental model of autoimmune arthritis, galectin-9 inhibited the development of Th17 cells and increased the frequency of T_{reg} cells [111]. Mice lacking galectin-9 showed decreased number of FoxP3+ T_{reg} cells with an exacerbation of autoimmune pathology [111], whereas galectin-3-deficient mice exhibited higher number of T_{reg} cells and attenuated disease [112].

An essential role for intracellular galectin-10 in controlling T_{reg}-cell function was revealed by Kubach and coworkers [113]. While expression of this lectin was almost absent in resting and activated $CD4^+$ T cells, galectin-10 was found constitutively expressed in human $CD4^+CD25^+Foxp3^+$ T_{reg} cells, with a restricted intracellular expression. Notably, siRNA-mediated silencing of endogenous galectin-10 in T_{reg} cells dramatically restored their proliferative capacity and abrogated their immunosuppressive activity. Hence, T_{reg} cells may confer immune privilege to tumors by synthesizing high amounts of galectin-1 and galectin-10, which counteract effector T-cell responses in tumor microenvironments.

G. Natural killer cells: novel targets of the inhibitory activity of galectins

As previously discussed, different innate and adaptive immune cell populations serve as targets of the immunosuppressive activity of galectins. Recently, a novel glycosylation-dependent strategy has been described that contributes to tumor cell evasion of natural killer (NK) cell immunity. This mechanism occurs in tumors expressing core 2 O-glycans by overexpression of the enzyme core 2 β-6-N-acetylglucosaminyltransferase (C2GnT1) [114]. In bladder cancer cells, interactions between galectin-3 and poly-LacNAc-branched core-2 O-glycans decorating tumor-associated major histocompatibility complex class I-related chain A (MICA) reduces the affinity of MICA for the activating NK-cell receptor NKG2D, thereby impairing NK-cell activation and antitumor activity [114]. Thus, lectin—glycan interactions may also contribute to tumor-immune escape by inhibiting NK-cell effector functions.

H. Integrating the immunoregulatory functions of galectins

As discussed in previous sections, different members of the galectin family can positively or negatively regulate the fate and function of innate and adaptive immune cells. As a result of specific interactions with glycosylated or nonglycosylated binding partners, galectins contribute to create a complex tumor microenvironment that influences tumor growth and metastasis. This microenvironment composed by soluble components (cytokines, chemokines) and cellular networks fails to provide inflammatory signals needed for efficient DC activation, instead supplying immunosuppressive mediators that negatively impact DC maturation and function [12,13]. Galectin-1 has been incorporated into the growing list of immunosuppressive tumor-derived factors that contribute to this tolerogenic microenvironment. Thus, DCs differentiated in a galectin-1-enriched microenvironment acquire a regulatory phenotype and initiate a tolerogenic circuit which in turn promotes the expansion of Tr1 cells [26,28,29]. Notably, tumor-secreted galectin-1 modulates T-cell effective responses not only through its indirect effect on DC differentiation and function, but also through its direct effects on T-cell fate. Through interaction with a particular repertoire of *N*- and *O*-glycans on the surface of effector T cells, galectin-1 differentially regulates the viability of different T-cell populations, thereby blunting Th1- and Th17-mediated responses and skewing the balance toward a Th2-polarized cytokine profile [72]. As a result of these direct and indirect inhibitory mechanisms, galectin-1 contributes to tumor-immune escape. In fact, we found that blockade of galectin-1 counteracted the immunosuppressive activity of melanoma cells and potentiated effective antitumor responses [115]. These findings were further substantiated in head and neck squamous carcinoma [116], Hodgkin's lymphoma [109,117], pancreatic adenocarcinoma [118], neuroblastoma [28], and lung adenocarcinoma [29,119]. Thus, galectin-1 represents an important gear of the complex machinery responsible for tumor-induced immunosuppression.

As mentioned above, galectin-3 contributes to tumor-immune escape by modulating T-cell apoptosis [82], favoring T-cell anergy [99], interrupting TCR signaling at sites of immunological synapse [94, 100] and impairing NK-cell effector functions [114]. On the other hand, galectin-9 contributes to tumor immunosuppression by promoting the differentiation of MDSCs [54] and expanding M2-type anti-inflammatory macrophages [48]. Thus, galectin–glycan interactions play key roles in cancer immunoediting by modulating different immune cell compartments.

III. GALECTINS IN THE TUMOR MICROENVIRONMENT: NON-IMMUNE RELATED FUNCTIONS

In addition to their role in tumor-immune escape, galectins contribute to other biological processes in tumor microenvironments, including homotypic and heterotypic cell adhesion, migration and invasiveness, angiogenesis and tumor chemoresistance [1,120]. Taking these nonimmunological functions into account when assessing the overall effects of these glycan-binding proteins may contribute to predicting the final outcome of modulating galectins gene expression in tumor microenvironments, while providing new clues for the rational design of galectin-related therapeutics. Although most galectins are ubiquitously expressed in various human normal tissues, these glycan-binding proteins are either silenced or upregulated in neoplastic tissues. There is an extensive number of published studies reporting the role for galectins in cancer; most of them demonstrate an altered expression of these lectins in transformed tissues and cancer-associated stroma. This abnormal expression reflects the established roles of galectins in key stages of tumor progression and growth, including tumor transformation, apoptosis and cell-cycle progression, as well as the involvement of these lectins in several steps of tumor metastasis, including tumor cell adhesion, migration and angiogenesis [1,121]. In the following sections we will summarize some of the most important information on the relevance of galectins in these processes. As this chapter is mainly focused on immunological functions of galectins, we will only provide some examples of non-immune-related activities of individual members of this family, with the final goal of validating in full the effect of silencing or stimulating the expression and activity of these proteins in tumor microenvironments.

A. Galectin-3

Undoubtedly, the best studied member of the galectin family is the "chimera-type" galectin-3, a ubiquitously distributed protein responsible for multiple biological functions [122]. Almost 60% of available literature in the galectins field refers to this family member. Indeed, accumulating evidence indicates that galectin-3 is involved in each step of tumor cell development, including cell transformation, proliferation, adhesion, migration, invasion and angiogenesis.

There is direct evidence indicating that galectin-3 expression is necessary for the initiation of the transformed phenotype in tumors. Upon inhibition of galectin-3 expression, breast carcinoma cells and thyroid papillary carcinoma cells lose their characteristic transformed phenotypes in cell culture [123,124]; conversely, in a normal thyroid follicular cell line ectopic expression of galectin-3 induces a transformed phenotype [125]. It was demonstrated that galectin-3 is able to bind oncogenic Ras proteins, preferentially K-RAS, and might thereafter have an important role in RAS-mediated cell transformation [126]. In addition, it was clearly demonstrated that galectin-3 displays an anti-apoptotic activity within a range of tumor cell types exposed to diverse apoptotic stimuli [4]. Following exposure to apoptotic stimuli, galectin-3 has been shown to translocate either from the cytosol or from the nucleus to the mitochondria [127], where it interacts with other apoptosis regulators, thereby preventing apoptosis [128]. Indeed, it is possible that galectin-3 exerts its anti-apoptotic effects through binding to BCL2 or by mediating the transport of BCL2 to the mitochondria [129]. Current evidence indicates that the mechanisms through which galectin-3 inhibits apoptosis are complex and are dependent on galectin-3 subcellular compartmentalization. Specifically, galectin-3 localized in the cytosolic compartment protects the cell from apoptosis, while galectin-3 localized in the nucleus has the opposite effect [130].

The role of galectin-3 in the regulation of tumor growth has been studied by several groups [131]. Most results agree to conclude that galectin-3 is a positive growth regulator. However, some controversial findings have been reported. The prostate cancer cell line LNCaP transfected with galectin-3 was found to grow slower than controls both *in vitro* and *in vivo* [132]. The effect of endogenous galectin-3 on tumor growth may also depend on the subcellular localization of the protein [130]. Finally, galectin-3 might regulate tumorigenesis by controlling cell-cycle progression. In breast cancer cells galectin-3 affects known cell-cycle regulators, including the downregulation of cyclin E and cyclin A, both involved in cycle progression, the upregulation of the cell-cycle inhibitors p21 (WAF1) and p27 (KIP1), and the induction of cyclin D1 (a cyclin expressed in early G1 phase) [133].

As discussed above, several galectins have been shown to contribute to metastasis-related processes. Galectin-3 is involved in homotypic tumor cell adhesion, as originally concluded from staining of cancer cell aggregates which showed clusters of this lectin at sites of cell–cell contact [134]. In addition, highly metastatic human breast carcinoma cells express higher levels of galectin-3 and have significantly increased adhesion to monolayers of endothelial cells *in vitro* compared with their nonmetastatic counterparts [135]. Interestingly, the effects of galectin-3 on cell adhesion described above could be mediated through its binding to integrin $\alpha_1\beta_1$ [136]. In addition, galectin-3 can upregulate integrin expression on tumor cells to influence their adhesive properties [137]. Moreover, galectin-3 affect the invasiveness and migration of tumor cells [138,139,140]. Interestingly, galectin-3 was the first galectin shown to have pro-angiogenic activity *in vitro* [141]. When transplanted into immunocompromised mice, human breast tumor cells that overexpress galectin-3 show an increase in the density of capillaries that surround the tumor compared with control transfectants [141]. Similar results have been documented in LNCaP cells that express transgenic galectin-3 [130]. Notably, there is evidence that galectin-3 is cleaved by matrix metalloproteases, and its biological activity appears to be controlled by these enzymes in the various steps of the metastatic process [142].

In accordance with the role of galectin-3 in different steps of tumor metastasis, an extensive number of published studies report the existence of an altered expression of this lectin in transformed tissues and cancer-associated stroma [143,144]. In fact, expression of galectin-3 has emerged as a potential diagnostic/prognostic marker of disease progression in many cancer types [145]. In addition, galectin-3 expression has been documented to be a useful marker for lymph node metastasis in certain types of cancer [146]. Remarkably, thyroid cancer represents the most studied cancer type regarding the differential expression of galectin-3 and its potential diagnostic and prognostic value. In spite of considerable discrepancies, in a recent review, Chiu and colleagues [147] proposed the expression of this endogenous lectin as a promising marker of diagnostic and prognostic value in thyroid cancer. Interestingly, not only the intensity of galectin-3 expression, but also its subcellular distribution was found to be altered in a variety of tumor types. Strikingly, in elegant studies nuclear localization of galectin-3 has been found to be associated with its antitumor effects, whereas its cytoplasmic localization correlated with neoplastic progression [130,148–152]. Thus, the outcome of galectin-3 blockade might be dependent on the subcellular localization of this protein.

In addition to the expression of galectin-3 in tumor microenvironments, serum levels of galectin-3 were studied in certain types of cancers, suggesting their diagnostic potential and prognostic value to monitor tumor progression and response to therapy in different types of human cancer [153–157]. Thus, in addition to its immunoregulatory functions (induction of CTL anergy, tuning of TCR signaling, regulation of cytokine production and promotion of T-cell apoptosis), galectin-3 also plays key roles in tumor transformation, angiogenesis, cell adhesion and migration in tumor microenvironments.

B. Galectin-1

Gene and protein expression profiles have recurrently led to the identification of galectin-1, the prototypical member of the galectin family, as a protein predominantly upregulated in primary tumors and metastatic lesions [2]. Given its major role in tumor-immune escape, this glycan-binding protein has been proposed as an emerging and multifunctional cancer target [158]. In fact, current evidence indicates a major role of this lectin in several crucial steps of cancer progression. Galectin-1 is present in a broad range of tumors of diverse histopathological types [159], including melanoma and glioma, where it modulates cancer cell aggressiveness and prognosis [5, 160].

Similarly to galectin-3, galectin-1 is essential for the initiation of the transformed phenotype of tumors. Blockade of galectin-1 expression suppresses the transformed phenotype of human glioma cells, as determined by cell morphology [161]. Even though the mechanisms by which galectins are involved in cell transformation are not yet fully understood, it was demonstrated that galectin-1 interacts with oncogenic Ras [162 126]. Overexpression of galectin-1 in tumor cells results in an increase of both membrane association of oncogenic Ras and cell transformation [162].

549

Galectin-1 also functions as an autocrine cell growth suppressor [163]. When added exogenously it inhibits the growth of neuroblastoma cells [164]. Targeting galectin-1 expression in human glioma cells suppresses anchorage-independent growth of these cells [161], in the absence of detectable apoptosis, suggesting that this galectin acts as a tumor cell growth suppressor.

Changes in tumor cell adhesion, migration, motility and invasiveness, as well as promotion of angiogenesis are key factors involved in tumor metastasis. Through its ability to form bridges between cells or between cells and the extracellular matrix, galectin-1 facilitates cell adhesion. This endogenous lectin promotes the adhesion of ovarian and prostate cancer cell lines to the extracellular matrix [152]. Moreover, recent studies indicated a role for galectin-1 in modulating hepatocellular carcinoma cell adhesion, polarization, and *in vivo* tumor growth [165]. In addition, Thijssen and coworkers [166] demonstrated that galectin-1 is also essential for tumor angiogenesis, a key process essential for tumor growth, invasiveness and metastasis. Of note, tumor-secreted galectin-1 enhances endothelial cell activity [167]. In addition, tumor hypoxia induces galectin-1 expression [116] and initiates multiple signaling pathways, including galectin-1-mediated maturation of vascular endothelial growth factor (VEGF) by the oxygen-regulated protein ORP150 [168] and the brain-expressed X-linked gene, BEX2 [169]. Thus, in addition to its role in promoting tumor-immune escape through modulation of T cell and DC physiology, galectin-1 also controls tumor cell transformation, cell adhesion, migration and angiogenesis, suggesting multiple functional targets for this endogenous lectin in the tumor microenvironment.

C. Galectin-9

First cloned as a T-cell-derived eosinophil chemoattractant protein [170], galectin-9 is also expressed in tumor microenvironments, although its role in tumor progression is less clear than galectin-1 or galectin-3. This endogenous lectin can regulate cell adhesion and proliferation. Nobumoto and coworkers [171] reported that galectin-9 inhibits the binding of tumor cells to extracellular matrix components, resulting in the suppression of tumor cell migration. This lectin suppressed the binding of hyaluronic acid to CD44 on both B16-F10 melanoma and Colon-26 cells, and also inhibited the binding of vascular cell adhesion molecule-1 (VCAM-1) to very late antigen-4 (VLA-4) on B16-F10 cells [171]. In contrast, Kasamatsu and coworkers [172] reported that cellular adherence on fibronectin and collagen I is increased in Ca9-22 oral squamous cell carcinoma cells overexpressing galectin-9. In addition, this lectin can inhibit cancer cell proliferation by reducing the expression levels of several cyclins, cyclin-associated proteins and c-Myc [173].

From a clinical standpoint, galectin-9 has been proposed to be an independent prognostic factor with antimetastatic potential in breast cancer [174,175]. Decreased galectin-9 expression is inversely associated with the malignant potential of cervical squamous cell carcinoma [176], and increased galectin-9 expression in primary melanoma lesions is associated with better prognosis [177]. These observations contrast with the positive correlation observed between tumor aggressiveness and galectin-1 or galectin-3 expression. Hence, in addition to its role as a ligand of the immune inhibitory molecule Tim-3 and its ability to regulate Th1- and Th17-dependent immunity, galectin-9 mediates other processes in tumor microenvironments including tumor cell adhesion and proliferation.

D. Galectin-4

Although expressed preferentially in the gastrointestinal tract during development and in adult normal tissues, strong expression of galectin-4 can be induced in some tumor tissues including breast and liver [178]. In fact, expression of this lectin was detected in a wide range of cancers including mucinous epithelial ovarian cancers [179], carcinoid tumors [180], gastro-enteropancreatic neuroendocrine tumors [181] and sinonasal adenocarcinomas [182]. However, decreased galectin-4 mRNA expression was found to be an early event in colon carcinogenesis, suggesting that this lectin may play a major role in colon cancer biology [183]. In line with these findings, significant prognostic values were associated with galectin-1, -3 and -4 in Dukes A and B colon tumors, leading to the hypothesis that these three galectins might be involved in early stages of human colon carcinogenesis [184]. Recently, It was demonstrated that galectin-4 could function as a tumor suppressor of human colorectal cancer through the downregulation of Wnt signaling target genes [185]. In addition, plasma levels of galectin-4 have been postulated as tumor markers to follow-up colorectal cancer patients, in addition to markers already used (CEA/CA19-9) [186]. Indeed, while circulating levels of galectin-4 significantly decreased after surgery, falling below the cut-off value in most patients, its levels significantly increased as tumor growth progressed [186]. Although the role of galectin-4 in tumor immunity has not yet been examined, it is apparent that this lectin may play a role in different events of tumor biology.

E. Galectin-7

Galectin-7, another "prototype" galectin, contributes to different events that are associated with the differentiation and development of pluristratified epithelia, including epithelial cell migration. In addition, through JNK activation and mitochondrial cytochrome *c* release, galectin-7 regulates apoptosis [187–188]. Although the role of galectin-7 in tumor immunity has not yet been studied, this lectin has been found to regulate apoptosis of tumor cells, probably by functioning inside the cells. Tumor cells that overexpress galectin-7 are more likely than control cells to undergo apoptosis induced by a number of apoptotic stimuli [189–190].

Galectin-7 can also regulate cell growth, through a mechanism that is independent of its pro-apoptotic activity; when added exogenously, it inhibits the growth of neuroblastoma cells [164,191]. In addition, a colon carcinoma cell line that expresses transgenic galectin-7 grows slower than controls, in the absence of detectable apoptosis [192]. Moreover, in SCID mice, tumors derived from galectin-7-expressing cells exhibited a dramatically reduced growth rate compared with control cells [192]. This result is probably a consequence of the combination of the pro-apoptotic and growth-suppressing effects of galectin-7.

Similarly to other galectins, galectin-7 can act as either a positive or negative regulatory factor in tumor development, depending on the histological type of the tumor [187]. Even though expression of galectin-7 in human colon carcinoma xenografts accounts for a greater suppressive effect of galectin-7 on tumor growth *in vivo* [192], in two preclinical mouse models, high levels of galectin-7 expression in breast cancer cells drastically increased their ability to metastasize to the lungs and bones [193]. In human breast tissues, high expression levels of galectin-7 were restricted to high-grade breast carcinomas, and in HER2$^+$ cases, galectin-7 expression was associated with lymph node axillary metastasis [193]. In squamous cell carcinomas, high levels of galectin-7 expression were associated with bad prognoses [194–196].

Galectin-7 appears to be a relevant actor in lymphoma biology. Upregulation of this lectin in murine lymphoma cells is associated with progression toward an aggressive phenotype [197]. In mice, blockade of galectin-7 expression significantly inhibited the dissemination and invasion of lymphoma cells to peripheral organs [198]. Interestingly, abnormal expression of galectin-7 in lymphoma cells was not dependent on p53 but was instead associated with DNA hypomethylation [199]. Notably, galectin-7 can also modulate the aggressive behavior of lymphoma cells by controlling the expression of metastatic genes, such as MMP-9 [200].

F. Galectin-8

Several articles have been published to date describing the association between galectin-8 and tumor development [201]. This galectin is expressed by various types of tumors, including laryngeal squamous cell carcinomas [202], thyroid tumors [203], and colon cancers [184,204] and modulates their behavior. While galectin-1, -3 and -4 may be involved in the early stages of colon cancers, galectin-8 appears to be involved in later stages of tumor progression [184]. In colon cancers [204] and urothelial carcinomas of the bladder [205] galectin-8 expression decreases as the disease progresses, suggesting that this protein may act as a tumor suppressor gene.

Notably, Delgado and coworkers [206] provided the first evidence demonstrating an essential role for galectin-8 in the regulation of angiogenesis. Functional assays revealed a critical play for this lectin in the regulation of capillary-tube formation and EC migration, and clearly showed that galectin-8 is endowed with pro-angiogeneic properties. Interestingly, galectin-8 recognizes, in a carbohydrate-dependent manner, β_1 integrins and triggers integrin-mediated signaling cascades, resulting in cytoskeletal changes and cell spreading [207,208], thus regulating cell adhesion and survival [209]. Galectin-8 is also a modulator of cellular growth through upregulation of p21, a process that involves both the activation of Jun kinase (JNK), which enhances the synthesis of p21, and the activation of protein kinase (PK) B, which inhibits p21 degradation [210]. Thus, in addition to its roles in T-cell apoptosis, in tumor settings galectin-8 modulates cell-cycle progression, cellular adhesion, migration, signaling and angiogenesis.

G. Galectin-2

Even though galectin-2 shares 43% amino acid identity with galectin-1, it exhibits a distinct intracellular localization pattern and shares only some functional properties [211]. In fact, emerging information suggests that these two galectin family members do have different roles in tumor cell biology. While tumor grading in urothelial transitional cancer cells correlates with immunoreactivity for galectin-1, -2 and -8, disease-dependent mortality correlates with the expression of galectin-2 and -8 [212]. Although galectin-1 plays a major role in glioma cell biology, transcripts of human galectin-2 are less frequently found in this type of tumor [213] this is also the case in tumor-associated endothelial cells [214]. In contrast, galectin-2 participates in the aggressiveness of gastric cancer [215]. Serum galectin-2 (as well as galectin-4 and -8) levels are greatly increased in colon and breast cancer patients and promote cancer cell adhesion to the vascular endothelium [216]. Although not studied in the context of the tumor immunity, given the pro-inflammatory role of galectin-2 during myocardial infarction [217], we might speculate that this endogenous lectin could contribute to inflammation-induced tumor growth.

IV. EMERGING ROLES OF GALECTINS IN TUMOR CHEMORESISTANCE

In addition to the above-mentioned properties, galectins have recently emerged as novel regulators of tumor chemoresistance. In papillary thyroid cancer cells, galectin-3 exhibits anti-apoptotic effects and confers chemoresistance, which can be partially reversed through inhibition of the PI3K-Akt pathway [218]. Notably, anaplastic thyroid carcinomas (ATCs), which express galectin-3, are highly resistant to apoptosis. Upon cisplatin treatment of ATC cells, galectin-3 expression levels are increased, and interference with galectin-3 expression in the ATC cells in turn stimulates their chemosensitivity [219]. The cellular levels of galectin-3 may contribute to the anti-apoptotic activity and chemoresistance of cholangiocarcinoma cells [220]. In an attempt to identify the mechanisms underlying drug resistance induced by galectin-3 in various types of cancers, Fukumori and collaborators [221] demonstrated that the NWGR anti-death motif of the Bcl-2 family present in galectin-3 may be responsible for its ability to resist chemotherapeutic agents, such as cisplatin and etoposide. In addition, nuclear export of phosphorylated galectin-3 in response to chemotherapeutic drugs may also regulate its anti-apoptotic activity [221]. Thus, targeting galectin-3 could improve the efficacy of anticancer drug chemotherapies in several types of cancers.

Galectin-1 is also implicated in cancer chemoresistance, at least in melanoma and glioma models. Knocking down galectin-1 increased *in vivo* sensitivity to the pro-autophagic alkylating agent, temozolomide, in a mouse metastatic melanoma model; the decrease in galectin-1 expression induces heat shock protein 70-mediated lysosomal membrane permeabilization, a process that was associated with cathepsin B release into the cytosol. This process was hypothesized to sensitize melanoma cells to the pro-autophagic effects of temozolomide [222]. Decreasing galectin-1 expression *in vitro* and *in vivo* also augmented the therapeutic benefits of temozolomide in experimental gliomas [223]. The decrease in galectin-1 expression in glioma cells did not induce apoptotic or autophagic features, but instead decreased the expression levels of several genes that are implicated in cancer drug resistance, such as ORP150, HERP, GRP78/Bip, TRA1, BNIPL3, GADD45B and CYR61 [223].

Recent reports indicated the role of other galectins in cancer drug resistance. For example, in chronic myelogenous leukemia targeting of the activating transcription factor 3 (ATF3) by galectin-9 induced apoptosis and overcame various types of treatment resistance [224]. On the other hand, galectin-7 has been reported as a candidate predictive marker of chemosensitivity against *cis*-diamminedichloroplatinum (CDDP) in urothelial cancers, and the targeted expression of galectin-7 has been proposed to overcome chemoresistance of urothelial cancer [225].

V. GALECTIN INHIBITORS AS POTENTIAL ANTICANCER AGENTS

Galectins have emerged as promising molecular targets for cancer therapy, and galectin inhibitors have the potential to be used as antitumor and antimetastatic agents [1,145,226].

Since the pioneering studies of Raz and Lotan [227] which showed the presence of galactoside-specific binding lectins (galectins) on tumor cells, a growing body of experimental evidence has suggested different inhibitory agents to block expression of these lectins and antagonize their function. In fact, the galectin-3 C-terminal domain fragment significantly suppressed tumor growth and inhibited metastasis in a mouse model of human breast cancer [228]. In addition, peptides specific to the galectin-3 CRD significantly inhibited the adhesion of a human breast carcinoma cell line to endothelial cells *in vitro* [1,228] and administration of an anti-galectin-3 antibody specifically suppressed liver metastasis by adenocarcinoma cell lines [229]. Challenges for the future will be to employ more potent and selective small inhibitors of galectins, and, in fact, molecules with such properties have already been developed. Pioneer studies reported the effects of two synthetic low molecular weight glycoamine analogs (Fru-D-Leu and Lac-L-Leu) on the metastasis of human breast carcinoma xenografts growing in the mammary fat pads of nude mice [230]. The treated animals had no apparent toxicity from chronic daily injection of synthetic glycoamines up to 17 weeks of treatment. However, the molecular mechanisms involved in this antimetastatic effect have not been clearly identified. Moreover, other studies [231] examined the effects of modified citrus pectin, a water-soluble polysaccharide fiber derived from citrus fruit that specifically inhibits galectin-3, in tumor growth and metastasis. Interestingly, the authors found that citrus pectin, given orally, inhibits carbohydrate-mediated tumor growth, angiogenesis, and metastasis by disrupting the interactions between galectin-3 and its specific carbohydrate ligands [231]. Interestingly, GCS-100 is a modified citrus pectin carbohydrate that has recently reached clinical trials for patients with solid tumors [232].

In addition, previous findings described the synthesis of Wedgelike glycodendrimers with two, four, and eight lactose moieties using 3,5 di-(2-aminoethoxy) benzoic acid as the branching unit [233]. These compounds were tested in solid-phase competition assays with lactose maxiclusters and various N-glycans branching profiles (miniclusters) and successfully inhibited the binding of galectin-1 to this glycosylated matrix with a relative inhibitory potency of 150 regarding free lactose [233]. Furthermore, during the past few years, Nilsson and colleagues designed a variety of efficient, stable, and high affinity galectin inhibitors, including low micromolar inhibitors of galectin-3 based on 3'-derivatization of N-acetyllactosamine with an inhibitory potency of about 50 times better than N-acetyllactosaminide [234], O-galactosyl aldoximes [235] and a collection of thio-digalactoside derivatives [236, 237]. In this regard, generation of synthetic lactulosamines (SLA) successfully inhibited galectin-1- and galectin-3-mediated homotypic cell aggregation, tumor-cell apoptosis, and endothelial cell morphogenesis, three critical events linked to tumor metastasis. In this regard, Oberg and colleagues [238] recently reviewed different strategies used to develop efficient and selective small-molecule galectin inhibitors through derivatization of monosaccharides, mainly galactosides.

A successful example of a galectin inhibitor is farnesylthiosalicylic acid (FTS). This molecule was discovered by the Kloog group, who demonstrated that FTS disrupts H-Ras/galectin-1 interactions and thereby Ras membrane binding and oncogenic activity, supporting the concept that Ras anchorage to the membrane relies upon galectin-1 [162]. FTS (salirasib) has been translated to clinical trials for patients with pancreatic cancer [239] and is also currently being tested in a Phase II clinical trial for patients with K-RAS containing lung adenocarcinomas [240]. In this regard, a galectin-1-specific neutralizing monoclonal antibody selectively inhibited galectin-1-mediated apoptosis of tumor-specific CD8$^+$ T cells in posttransplant lymphoproliferative disorders [241], suggesting its potential therapeutic benefit in counteracting the immune inhibitory activities of this lectin. Thus, targeting galectin—glycan interactions may represent a novel immunotherapeutic approach, either alone or in combination with other chemotherapeutic or immunotherapeutic regimens, for treating galectin-expressing tumors. However, for those galectins that are downregulated in certain tumors or correlate with tumor regression, strategies are required to upregulate their expression and stimulate their function.

VI. CONCLUSIONS

During the past decade, a better understanding of the cellular and molecular mechanisms underlying tolerance induction to tumor antigens provided the appropriate framework for the development of therapeutic strategies for cancer immunotherapy. Under this complex scenario, galectins have emerged as promising molecular targets of cancer therapy, and galectin inhibitors have the potential to be used as antitumor and antimetastatic agents in those cases in which galectins are upregulated in tumor microenvironments. In the first section of this chapter, we provided an overview of the role of galectins in different processes implicated in tumor immunity. In the second section we integrated these immunoregulatory properties with nonimmunological functions played by these glycan-binding proteins in an attempt to appreciate in full their multifunctional activities in tumor microenvironments. The emerging data promise a future scenario in which the selective blockade of individual members of the galectin family, either alone or in combination with other therapeutic regimens, will contribute to halt tumor progression by inhibiting tumor cell adhesion, migration, invasiveness, proliferation, angiogenesis and tumor-immune escape.

CONFLICT OF INTEREST

The authors disclose no potential conflicts of interest

ACKNOWLEDGMENTS

The authors wish to express special thanks to Diego Croci for help in figure design. Work in G.A.R's laboratory is supported by grants from Agencia Nacional de Promoción Científica y Tecnológica Argentina (ANPCyT; 2010-870), Mizutani Foundation for Glycoscience (Japan), National Multiple Sclerosis Society (USA), Prostate Action (UK), Fundación Sales (Argentina), University of Buenos Aires (Argentina), and Consejo Nacional de Investigaciones Científicas y Técnicas (CONICET). Work in R.K's laboratory is supported by grants from the Fonds National de la Recherche Scientifique (FRS-FNRS; Belgium).

References

[1] Liu FT, Rabinovich GA. Galectins as modulators of tumour progression. Nat Rev Cancer 2005;5:29—41.

[2] Camby I, Le Mercier M, Lefranc F, Kiss R. Galectin-1: A small protein with major functions. Glycobiology 2006:16.

[3] Barondes SH, Castronovo V, Cooper DN, Cummings RD, Drickamer K, Feizi T, et al. Galectins: a family of animal beta-galactoside-binding lectins. Cell 1994;76:597—8.

[4] Liu FT, Patterson RJ, Wang JL. Intracellular functions of galectins. Biochim Biophys Acta 2002;1572:263—73.

[5] Lefranc F, Mathieu V, Kiss R. Galectin-1-mediated biochemical controls of melanoma and glioma aggressive behavior. World J Biol Chem 2011;2:193—201.

[6] Hassan SS, Ashraf GM, Banu N. Galectins - potencial targets for cancer therapy. Cancer Lett 2007;253:25—33.

[7] Salatino M, Rabinovich GA. Fine-tuning antitumor responses through the control of galectin-glycan interactions: an overview. Methods Mol Biol 2011;677:355—74.

[8] Rabinovich GA, Croci DO. Regulatory circuits mediated by lectin-glycan interactions in autoimmunity and cancer. Immunity 2012;36:322—35.

[9] Staveley-O'Carroll K, Sotomayor E, Montgomery J, Borrello I, Hwang L, Fein S, et al. Induction of antigen-specific T cell anergy: An early event in the course of tumor progression. Proc Natl Acad Sci U S A 1998;95:1178—83.

[10] Zhou G, Drake CG, Levitsky HI. Amplification of tumor-specific regulatory T cells following therapeutic cancer vaccines. Blood 2006;107:628—36.

[11] Steinman RM, Hawiger D, Nussenzweig MC. Tolerogenic dendritic cells. Annu Rev Immunol 2003;21:685—711.

[12] Gerlini G, Tun-Kyi A, Dudli C, Burg G, Pimpinelli N, Nestle FO. Metastatic melanoma secreted IL-10 down-regulates CD1 molecules on dendritic cells in metastatic tumor lesions. Am J Pathol 2004;165:1853—63.

[13] Gabrilovich DI, Chen HL, Girgis KR, Cunningham HT, Meny GM, Nadaf S, et al. Production of vascular endothelial growth factor by human tumors inhibits the functional maturation of dendritic cells. Nat Med 1996;2:1096−103.

[14] Drake CG, Jaffee E, Pardoll DM. Mechanisms of immune evasion by tumors. Adv Immunol 2006;90:51−81.

[15] Igney FH, Krammer PH. Immune escape of tumors: apoptosis resistance and tumor counterattack. J Leukoc Biol 2002;71:907−20.

[16] Whiteside TL. Immune suppression in cancer: effects on immune cells, mechanisms and future therapeutic intervention. Sem Cancer Biol 2006;16:3−15.

[17] Khong HT, Restifo NP. Natural selection of tumor variants in the generation of "tumor escape" phenotypes. Nat Immunol 2002;3:999−1005.

[18] Blank C, Gajewski TF, Mackensen A. Interaction of PD-L1 on tumor cells with PD-1 on tumor-specific T cells as a mechanism of immune evasion: implications for tumor immunotherapy. Cancer Immunol Immunother 2005;54:307−14.

[19] Rabinovich GA, Gabrilovich D, Sotomayor EM. Immunosuppressive Strategies that are Mediated by Tumor Cells. Annu Rev Immunol 2007;25:267−96.

[20] Guermonprez P, Valladeau J, Zitvogel L, Thery C, Amigorena S. Antigen presentation and T cell stimulation by dendritic cells. Annu Rev Immunol 2002;20:621−67.

[21] Bax M, Garcia-Vallejo JJ, Jang-Lee J, North SJ, Gilmartin TJ, Hernandez G, et al. Dendritic cell maturation results in pronounced changes in glycan expression affecting recognition by siglecs and galectins. J Immunol 2007;179:8216−24.

[22] Fulcher JA, Hashimi ST, Levroney EL, Pang M, Gurney KB, Baum LG, et al. Galectin-1-matured human monocyte-derived dendritic cells have enhanced migration through extracellular matrix. J Immunol 2006;177:216−26.

[23] Fulcher JA, Chang MH, Wang S, Almazan T, Hashimi ST, Eriksson AU, et al. Galectin-1 co-clusters CD43/CD45 on dendritic cells and induces cell activation and migration through Syk and protein kinase C signaling. J Biol Chem 2009;284:26860−70.

[24] Blois SM, Ilarregui JM, Tometten M, Garcia M, Orsal AS, Cordo-Russo I, et al. A pivotal role for galectin-1 in fetomaternal tolerance. Nat Med 2007;13:1450−7.

[25] Perone MJ, Bertera S, Tawadrous ZS, Shufesky WJ, Piganelli JD, Baum LG, et al. Dendritic cells expressing transgenic galectin-1 delay onset of autoimmune diabetes in mice. J Immunol 2006;177:5278−89.

[26] Ilarregui JM, Croci DO, Bianco GA, Toscano MA, Salatino M, Vermeulen ME, et al. Tolerogenic signals delivered by dendritic cells to T cells through a galectin-1-driven immunoregulatory circuit involving interleukin 27 and interleukin 10. Nat Immunol 2009;10:981−91.

[27] Mobergslien A, Sioud M. Galectin-1 and -3 gene silencing in immature and mature dendritic cells enhances T cell activation and interferon-gamma production. J Leukoc Biol 2012;91:461−7.

[28] Soldati R, Berger E, Zenclussen AC, Jorch G, Lode HN, Salatino M, et al. Neuroblastoma triggers an immunoevasive program involving galectin-1-dependent modulation of T cell and dendritic cell compartments. Int J Cancer 2011.

[29] Kuo PL, Huang MS, Cheng DE, Hung JY, Yang CJ, Chou SH. Lung cancer-derived galectin-1 enhances tumorigenic potentiation of tumor-associated dendritic cells by expressing heparin-binding EGF-like growth factor. J Biol Chem 2012;287:9753−64.

[30] Bernardes ES, Silva NM, Ruas LP, Mineo JR, Loyola AM, Hsu DK, et al. Toxoplasma gondii infection reveals a novel regulatory role for galectin-3 in the interface of innate and adaptive immunity. Am J Pathol 2006;168:1910−20.

[31] Dai SY, Nakagawa R, Itoh A, Murakami H, Kashio Y, Abe H, et al. Galectin-9 induces maturation of human monocyte-derived dendritic cells. J Immunol 2005;175:2974−81.

[32] Anderson AC, Anderson DE, Bregoli L, Hastings WD, Kassam N, Lei C, et al. Promotion of tissue inflammation by the immune receptor Tim-3 expressed on innate immune cells. Science 2007;318:1141−3.

[33] Li Y, Feng J, Geng S, Wei H, Chen G, Li X, et al. The N- and C-terminal carbohydrate recognition domains of galectin-9 contribute differently to its multiple functions in innate immunity and adaptive immunity. Mol Immunol 2011;48:670−7.

[34] Ruffell B, Affara NI, Coussens LM. Differential macrophage programming in the tumor microenvironment. Trends Immunol 2012;33:119−26.

[35] Correa SG, Sotomayor CE, Aoki MP, Maldonado CA, Rabinovich GA. Opposite effects of galectin-1 on alternative metabolic pathways of L-arginine in resident, inflammatory, and activated macrophages. Glycobiology 2003;13:119−28.

[36] Barrionuevo P, Beigier-Bompadre M, Ilarregui JM, Toscano M, Bianco GA, Isturiz MA, et al. A novel function for galectin-1 a the crossroad of innate and a adaptive immunity: galectin-1 regulates monocyte/macrophage physiology through a nonapoptotic ERK-dependent pathway. J Immunol 2007;178:436−45.

555

[37] Malik RK, Ghurye RR, Lawrence-Watt DJ, Stewart HJ. Galectin-1 stimulates monocyte chemotaxis via the p44/42 MAP kinase pathway and a pertussis toxin-sensitive pathway. Glycobiology 2009;19:1402–7.

[38] Rabinovich GA, Sotomayor CE, Riera CM, Bianco I, Correa SG. Evidence of a role for galectin-1 in acute inflammation. Eur J Immunol 2000;30:1331–9.

[39] Swarte VV, Mebius RE, Joziasse DH, Van den Eijnden DH, Kraal G. Lymphocyte triggering via L-selectin leads to enhanced galectin-3-mediated binding to dendritic cells. Eur J Immunol 1998;28:2864–71.

[40] Mina-Osorio P, Soto-Cruz I, Ortega E. A role for galectin-3 in CD13-mediated homotypic aggregation of monocytes. Biochem Biophys Res Commun 2007;353:605–10.

[41] Sano H, Hsu DK, Yu L, Apgar JR, Kuwabara I, Yamanaka T, et al. Human galectin-3 is a novel chemoattractant for monocytes and macrophages. J Immunol 2000;165:2156–64.

[42] Liu FT, Hsu DK, Zuberi RI, Kuwabara I, Chi EY, Henderson Jr WR. Expression and function of galectin-3, a beta-galactoside-binding lectin, in human monocytes and macrophages. Am J Pathol 1995;147:1016–28.

[43] Sano H, Hsu DK, Apgar JR, Yu L, Sharma BB, Kuwabara I, et al. Critical role of galectin-3 in phagocytosis by macrophages. J Clin Invest 2003;112:389–97.

[44] Hsu DK, Yang RY, Pan Z, Yu L, Salomon DR, Fung-Leung WP, et al. Targeted disruption of the galectin-3 gene results in attenuated peritoneal inflammatory responses. Am J Pathol 2000;156:1073–83.

[45] Kashio Y, Nakamura K, Abedin MJ, Seki M, Nishi N, Yoshida N, et al. Galectin-9 induces apoptosis through the calcium-calpain-caspase-1 pathway. J Immunol 2003;170:3631–6.

[46] Matsuura A, Tsukada J, Mizobe T, Higashi T, Mouri F, Tanikawa R, et al. Intracellular galectin-9 activates inflammatory cytokines in monocytes. Genes Cells 2009;14:511–21.

[47] MacKinnon AC, Farnworth SL, Hodkinson PS, Henderson NC, Atkinson KM, Leffler H, et al. Regulation of alternative macrophage activation by galectin-3. J Immunol 2008;180:2650–8.

[48] Arikawa T, Saita N, Oomizu S, Ueno M, Matsukawa A, Katoh S, et al. Galectin-9 expands immunosuppressive macrophages to ameliorate T-cell-mediated lung inflammation. Eur J Immunol 2010;40:548–58.

[49] Togayachi A, Kozono Y, Ishida H, Abe S, Suzuki N, Tsunoda Y, et al. Polylactosamine on glycoproteins influences basal levels of lymphocyte and macrophage activation. Proc Natl Acad Sci U S A 2007;104:15829–34.

[50] Kusmartsev S, Nefedova Y, Yoder D, Gabrilovich DI. Antigen-specific inhibition of CD8+ T cell response by immature myeloid cells in cancer is mediated by reactive oxygen species. J Immunol 2004;172:989–99.

[51] Youn JI, Gabrilovich DI. The biology of myeloid-derived suppressor cells: the blessing and the curse of morphological and functional heterogeneity. Eur J Immunol 2010;40:2969–75.

[52] Gabrilovich DI, Velders M, Sotomayor E, Kast WM. Mechanism of immune dysfunction in cancer mediated by immature Gr-1+ myeloid cells. J Immunol 2001;166:5398–406.

[53] Huang B, Pan PY, Li Q, Sato AI, Levy DE, Bromberg J, et al. Gr-1+CD115+ immature myeloid suppressor cells mediate the development of tumor-induced T regulatory cells and T-cell anergy in tumor-bearing host. Cancer Res 2006;66:1123–31.

[54] Dardalhon V, Anderson AC, Karman J, Apetoh L, Chandwaskar R, Lee DH, et al. Tim-3/galectin-9 pathway: regulation of Th1 immunity through promotion of CD11b+Ly-6G+ myeloid cells. J Immunol 2010;185:1383–92.

[55] Gauthier L, Rossi B, Roux F, Termine E, Schiff C. Galectin-1 is a stromal cell ligand of the pre-B cell receptor (BCR) implicated in synapse formation between pre-B and stromal cells and in pre-BCR triggering. Proc Natl Acad Sci U S A 2002;99:13014–9.

[56] Rossi B, Espeli M, Schiff C, Gauthier L. Clustering of pre-B cell integrins induces galectin-1-dependent pre-B cell receptor relocalization and activation. J Immunol 2006;177:796–803.

[57] Espeli M, Mancini SJ, Breton C, Poirier F, Schiff C. Impaired B-cell development at the pre-BII-cell stage in galectin-1-deficient mice due to inefficient pre-BII/stromal cell interactions. Blood 2009;113:5878–86.

[58] Zuniga E, Rabinovich GA, Iglesias MM, Gruppi A. Regulated expression of galectin-1 during B-cell activation and implications for T-cell apoptosis. J Leukoc Biol 2001;70:73–9.

[59] Tsai CM, Chiu YK, Hsu TL, Lin IY, Hsieh SL, Lin KI. Galectin-1 promotes immunoglobulin production during plasma cell differentiation. J Immunol 2008;181:4570–9.

[60] Yu X, Siegel R, Roeder RG. Interaction of the B cell-specific transcriptional coactivator OCA-B and galectin-1 and a possible role in regulating BCR-mediated B cell proliferation. J Biol Chem 2006;281:15505–16.

[61] Tabrizi SJ, Niiro H, Masui M, Yoshimoto G, Iino T, Kikushige Y, et al. T cell leukemia/lymphoma 1 and galectin-1 regulate survival/cell death pathways in human naive and IgM+ memory B cells through altering balances in Bcl-2 family proteins. J Immunol 2009;182:1490–9.

[62] Acosta-Rodriguez EV, Montes CL, Motran CC, Zuniga EI, Liu FT, Rabinovich GA, et al. Galectin-3 mediates IL-4-induced survival and differentiation of B cells: functional cross-talk and implications during Trypanosoma cruzi infection. J Immunol 2004;172:493–502.

[63] Clark AG, Chen S, Zhang H, Brady GF, Ungewitter EK, Bradley JK, et al. Multifunctional regulators of cell growth are differentially expressed in anergic murine B cells. Mol Immunol 2007;44:1274—85.

[64] DiLillo DJ, Matsushita T, Tedder TF. B10 cells and regulatory B cells balance immune responses during inflammation, autoimmunity, and cancer. Ann N Y Acad Sci 2010;1183:38—57.

[65] Rabinovich GA, Toscano M. Turning "sweet" on immunity: Galectin-glycan interactions in immune tolerance and inflammation. Nat Rev Immunol 2009;9:338—52.

[66] Hernandez JD, Baum LG. Ah, sweet mystery of death! Galectins and control of cell fate. Glycobiology 2002;12:127R—36R.

[67] Rabinovich GA, Ramhorst RE, Rubinstein N, Corigliano A, Daroqui MC, Kier-Joffe EB, et al. Induction of allogenic T-cell hyporesponsiveness by galectin-1-mediated apoptotic and non-apoptotic mechanisms. Cell Death Differ 2002;9:661—70.

[68] Stowell SR, Qian Y, Karmakar S, Koyama NS, Dias-Baruffi M, Leffler H, et al. Differential roles of galectin-1 and galectin-3 in regulating leukocyte viability and cytokine secretion. J Immunol 2008;180:3091—102.

[69] Rabinovich GA, Ariel A, Hershkoviz R, Hirabayashi J, Kasai KI, Lider O. Specific inhibition of T-cell adhesion to extracellular matrix and proinflammatory cytokine secretion by human recombinant galectin-1. Immunology 1999;97:100—6.

[70] van der Leij J, van den Berg A, Harms G, Eschbach H, Vos H, Zwiers P, et al. Strongly enhanced IL-10 production using stable galectin-1 homodimers. Mol Immunol 2007;44:506—13.

[71] Motran CC, Molinder KM, Liu SD, Poirier F, Miceli MC. Galectin-1 functions as a Th2 cytokine that selectively induces Th1 apoptosis and promotes Th2 function. Eur J Immunol 2008;38:3015—27.

[72] Toscano M, Bianco GA, Ilarregui JM, Croci DO, Correale J, Hernandez JD, et al. Differential glycosylation of TH1, TH2 and TH-17 effector cells selectively regulates susceptibility to cell death. Nat Immunol 2007;8:825—34.

[73] Norling LV, Sampaio AL, Cooper D, Perretti M. Inhibitory control of endothelial galectin-1 on in vitro and in vivo lymphocyte trafficking. FASEB J 2008;22:682—90.

[74] Stillman BN, Hsu DK, Pang M, Brewer CF, Johnson P, Liu FT, et al. Galectin-3 and galectin-1 bind distinct cell surface glycoprotein receptors to induce T cell death. J Immunol 2006;176:778—89.

[75] Matarrese P, Tinari A, Mormone E, Bianco GA, Toscano MA, Ascione B, et al. Galectin-1 sensitizes resting human T lymphocytes to Fas (CD95)-mediated cell death via mitochondrial hyperpolarization, budding, and fission. J Biol Chem 2005;280:6969—85.

[76] Sturm A, Lensch M, Andre S, Kaltner H, Wiedenmann B, Rosewicz S, et al. Human galectin-2: novel inducer of T cell apoptosis with distinct profile of caspase activation. J Immunol 2004;173:3825—37.

[77] Yang RY, Hsu DK, Liu FT. Expression of galectin-3 modulates T-cell growth and apoptosis. Proc Natl Acad Sci U S A 1996;93:6737—42.

[78] Fukumori T, Takenaka Y, Yoshii T, Kim HR, Hogan V, Inohara H, et al. CD29 and CD7 mediate galectin-3-induced type II T-cell apoptosis. Cancer Res 2003;63:8302—11.

[79] Hsu DK, Chernyavsky AI, Chen HY, Yu L, Grando SA, Liu FT. Endogenous galectin-3 is localized in membrane lipid rafts and regulates migration of dendritic cells. J Invest Dermatol 2009;129:573—83.

[80] Hsu DK, Chen HY, Liu FT. Galectin-3 regulates T-cell functions. Immunol Rev 2009;230:114—27.

[81] Hahn HP, Pang M, He J, Hernandez JD, Yang RY, Li LY, et al. Galectin-1 induces nuclear translocation of endonuclease G in caspase- and cytochrome c-independent T cell death. Cell Death Differ 2004;11:1277—86.

[82] Peng W, Wang HY, Miyahara Y, Peng G, Wang RF. Tumor-associated galectin-3 modulates the function of tumor-reactive T cells. Cancer Res 2008;68:7228—36.

[83] Demotte N, Wieers G, Van Der Smissen P, Moser M, Schmidt C, Thielemans K, et al. A galectin-3 ligand corrects the impaired function of human CD4 and CD8 tumor-infiltrating lymphocytes and favors tumor rejection in mice. Cancer Res 2010;70:7476—88.

[84] Silverman AM, Nakata R, Shimada H, Sposto R, Declerck YA. A galectin-3-dependent pathway upregulates interleukin-6 in the microenvironment of human neuroblastoma. Cancer Res 2012;72:2228—38.

[85] Zhu C, Anderson AC, Schubart A, Xiong H, Imitola J, Khoury SJ, et al. The Tim-3 ligand galectin-9 negatively regulates T helper type 1 immunity. Nat Immunol 2005;6:1245—52.

[86] Wang F, He W, Yuan J, Wu K, Zhou H, Zhang W, et al. Activation of Tim-3-Galectin-9 pathway improves survival of fully allogeneic skin grafts. Transpl Immunol 2008;19:12—9.

[87] Earl LA, Bi S, Baum LG. Galectin multimerization and lattice formation are regulated by linker region structure. Glycobiology 2011;21:6—12.

[88] Nagahara K, Arikawa T, Oomizu S, Kontani K, Nobumoto A, Tateno H, et al. Galectin-9 increases Tim-3+ dendritic cells and CD8+ T cells and enhances antitumor immunity via galectin-9-Tim-3 interactions. J Immunol 2008;181:7660—9.

[89] Paclik D, Danese S, Berndt U, Wiedenmann B, Dignass A, Sturm A. Galectin-4 controls intestinal inflammation by selective regulation of peripheral and mucosal T cell apoptosis and cell cycle. PLoS One 2008;3:e2629.

[90] Tribulatti MV, Mucci J, Cattaneo V, Aguero F, Gilmartin T, Head SR, et al. Galectin-8 induces apoptosis in the CD4(high)CD8(high) thymocyte subpopulation. Glycobiology 2007;17:1404—12.

[91] Norambuena A, Metz C, Vicuna L, Silva A, Pardo E, Oyanadel C, et al. Galectin-8 induces apoptosis in Jurkat T cells by phosphatidic acid-mediated ERK1/2 activation supported by protein kinase A down-regulation. J Biol Chem 2009;284:12670—9.

[92] Stowell SR, Karmakar S, Arthur CM, Ju T, Rodrigues LC, Riul TB, et al. Galectin-1 induces reversible phosphatidylserine exposure at the plasma membrane. Mol Biol Cell 2009;20:1408—18.

[93] Dustin ML. T-cell activation through immunological synapses and kinapses. Immunol Rev 2008;221:77—89.

[94] Demetriou M, Granovsky M, Quaggin S, Dennis JW. Negative regulation of T-cell activation and autoimmunity by Mgat5 N-glycosylation. Nature 2001;409:733—9.

[95] Morgan R, Gao G, Pawling J, Dennis JW, Demetriou M, Li B, et al. (Mgat5)-mediated N-glycosylation negatively regulates Th1 cytokine production by T cells. J Immunol 2004;173:7200—8.

[96] Grigorian A, Lee SU, Tian W, Chen IJ, Gao G, Mendelsohn R, et al. Control of T Cell-mediated autoimmunity by metabolite flux to N-glycan biosynthesis. J Biol Chem 2007;282:20027—35.

[97] Chen IJ, Chen HL, Demetriou M. Lateral compartmentalization of T cell receptor versus CD45 by galectin-N-glycan binding and microfilaments coordinate basal and activation signaling. J Biol Chem 2007;282:35361—72.

[98] Chung CD, Patel VP, Moran M, Lewis LA, Miceli MC. Galectin-1 induces partial TCR zeta-chain phosphorylation and antagonizes processive TCR signal transduction. J Immunol 2000;165:3722—9.

[99] Demotte N, Stroobant V, Courtoy PJ, Van Der Smissen P, Colau D, Luescher IF, et al. Restoring the association of the T cell receptor with CD8 reverses anergy in human tumor-infiltrating lymphocytes. Immunity 2008;28:414—24.

[100] Chen HY, Fermin A, Vardhana S, Weng IC, Lo KF, Chang EY, et al. Galectin-3 negatively regulates TCR-mediated CD4+ T-cell activation at the immunological synapse. Proc Natl Acad Sci U S A 2009;106:14496—501.

[101] Liu SD, Tomassian T, Bruhn KW, Miller JF, Poirier F, Miceli MC. Galectin-1 tunes TCR binding and signal transduction to regulate CD8 burst size. J Immunol 2009;182:5283—95.

[102] Sakaguchi S. Naturally arising CD4+ regulatory t cells for immunologic self-tolerance and negative control of immune responses. Annu Rev Immunol 2004;22:531—62.

[103] Zou W. Immunosuppressive networks in the tumour environment and their therapeutic relevance. Nat Rev Cancer 2005;5:263—74.

[104] Curiel TJ, Coukos G, Zou L, Alvarez X, Cheng P, Mottram P, et al. Specific recruitment of regulatory T cells in ovarian carcinoma fosters immune privilege and predicts reduced survival. Nature Med 2004;10:942—9.

[105] O'Garra A, Vieira PL, Vieira P, Goldfeld AE. IL-10-producing and naturally occurring CD4+ Tregs: limiting collateral damage. J Clin Invest 2004;114:1372—8.

[106] Taams LS, Palmer DB, Akbar AN, Robinson DS, Brown Z, Hawrylowicz CM. Regulatory T cells in human disease and their potential for therapeutic manipulation. Immunology 2006;118:1—9.

[107] Fiore F, Nuschak B, Peola S, Mariani S, Muraro M, Foglietta M, et al. Exposure to myeloma cell lysates affects the immune competence of dendritic cells and favors the induction of Tr1-like regulatory T cells. Eur J Immunol 2005;35:1155—63.

[108] Garin MI, Chu CC, Golshayan D, Cernuda-Morollon E, Wait R, Lechler RI. Galectin-1: a key effector of regulation mediated by CD4+CD25+ T cells. Blood 2007;109:2058—65.

[109] Juszczynski P, Ouyang J, Monti S, Rodig SJ, Takeyama K, Abramson J, et al. The AP1-dependent secretion of galectin-1 by reed Sternberg cells fosters immune privilege in classical Hodgkin lymphoma. Proc Natl Acad Sci USA 2007;104:13134—9.

[110] Toscano M, Commodaro AG, Ilarregui JM, Bianco GA, Liberman A, Serra HM, et al. Galectin-1 suppresses autoimmune retinal disease by promoting concomitant Th2- and T regulatory-mediated anti-inflammatory responses. J Immunol 2006;176:6323—32.

[111] Seki M, Oomizu S, Sakata KM, Sakata A, Arikawa T, Watanabe K, et al. Galectin-9 suppresses the generation of Th17, promotes the induction of regulatory T cells, and regulates experimental autoimmune arthritis. Clin Immunol 2008;127:78—88.

[112] Jiang HR, Al Rasebi Z, Mensah-Brown E, Shahin A, Xu D, Goodyear CS, et al. Galectin-3 deficiency reduces the severity of experimental autoimmune encephalomyelitis. J Immunol 2009;182:1167—73.

[113] Kubach J, Lutter P, Bopp T, Stoll S, Becker C, Huter E, et al. Human CD4+CD25+ regulatory T cells: proteome analysis identifies galectin-10 as a novel marker essential for their anergy and suppressive function. Blood 2007;110:1550—8.

[114] Tsuboi S, Sutoh M, Hatakeyama S, Hiraoka N, Habuchi T, Horikawa Y, et al. A novel strategy for evasion of NK cell immunity by tumours expressing core2 O-glycans. EMBO J 2011;30:3173−85.

[115] Rubinstein N, Alvarez M, Zwirner NW, Toscano MA, Ilarregui JM, Bravo A, et al. Targeted inhibition of galectin-1 gene expression in tumor cells results in heightened T cell-mediated rejection; A potential mechanism of tumor-immune privilege. Cancer Cell 2004;5:241−51.

[116] Le QT, Shi G, Cao H, Nelson DW, Wang Y, Chen EY, et al. Galectin-1: a link between tumor hypoxia and tumor immune privilege. J Clin Oncol 2005;23:8932−41.

[117] Gandhi MK, Moll G, Smith C, Dua U, Lambley E, Ramuz O, et al. Galectin-1 mediated suppression of Epstein-Barr virus specific T-cell immunity in classic Hodgkin lymphoma. Blood 2007;110:1326−9.

[118] Tang D, Yuan Z, Xue X, Lu Z, Zhang Y, Wang H, et al. High expression of Galectin-1 in pancreatic stellate cells plays a role in the development and maintenance of an immunosuppressive microenvironment in pancreatic cancer. Int J Cancer 2012;130:2337−48.

[119] Banh A, Zhang J, Cao H, Bouley DM, Kwok S, Kong C, et al. Tumor galectin-1 mediates tumor growth and metastasis through regulation of T-cell apoptosis. Cancer Res 2011;71:4423−31.

[120] Ingrassia L, Camby I, Lefranc F, Mathieu V, Nshimyumukiza P, Darro F, et al. Anti-galectin compounds as potential anti-cancer drugs. Curr Med Chem 2006;13:3513−27.

[121] van den Brule F, Califice S, Castronovo V. Expression of galectins in cancer: a critical review. Glycoconj J 2004;19:537−42.

[122] Sundblad V, Croci DO, Rabinovich GA. Regulated expression of galectin-3, a multifunctional glycan-binding protein, in haematopoietic and non-haematopoietic tissues. Histol Histopathol 2011;26:247−65.

[123] Honjo Y, Nangia-Makker P, Inohara H, Raz A. Down-regulation of galectin-3 suppresses tumorigenicity of human breast carcinoma cells. Clin Cancer Res 2001;7:661−8.

[124] Yoshii T, Inohara H, Takenaka Y, Honjo Y, Akahani S, Nomura T, et al. Galectin-3 maintains the transformed phenotype of thyroid papillary carcinoma cells. Int J Oncol 2001;18:787−92.

[125] Takenaka Y, Inohara H, Yoshii T, Oshima K, Nakahara S, Akahani S, et al. Malignant transformation of thyroid follicular cells by galectin-3. Cancer Lett 2003;195:111−9.

[126] Elad-Sfadia G, Haklai R, Balan E, Kloog Y. Galectin-3 augments K-Ras activation and triggers a Ras signal that attenuates ERK but not phosphoinositide 3-kinase activity. J Biol Chem 2004;279:34922−30.

[127] Yu F, Finley Jr RL, Raz A, Kim HR. Galectin-3 translocates to the perinuclear membranes and inhibits cytochrome c release from the mitochondria. A role for synexin in galectin-3 translocation. J Biol Chem 2002;277:15819−27.

[128] Matarrese P, Tinari N, Semeraro ML, Natoli C, Iacobelli S, Malorni W. Galectin-3 overexpression protects from cell damage and death by influencing mitochondrial homeostasis. FEBS Lett 2000;473:311−5.

[129] Akahani S, Nangia-Makker P, Inohara H, Kim HR, Raz A. Galectin-3: a novel antiapoptotic molecule with a functional BH1 (NWGR) domain of Bcl-2 family. Cancer Res 1997;57:5272−6.

[130] Califice S, Castronovo V, Bracke M, van den Brule F. Dual activities of galectin-3 in human prostate cancer: tumor suppression of nuclear galectin-3 vs tumor promotion of cytoplasmic galectin-3. Oncogene 2004;23:7527−36.

[131] Yang RY, Liu FT. Galectins in cell growth and apoptosis. Cell Mol Life Sci 2003;60:267−76.

[132] Ellerhorst JA, Stephens LC, Nguyen T, Xu XC. Effects of galectin-3 expression on growth and tumorigenicity of the prostate cancer cell line LNCaP. Prostate 2002;50:64−70.

[133] Kim HR, Lin HM, Biliran H, Raz A. Cell cycle arrest and inhibition of anoikis by galectin-3 in human breast epithelial cells. Cancer Res 1999;59:4148−54.

[134] Glinsky VV, Glinsky GV, Glinskii OV, Huxley VH, Turk JR, Mossine VV, et al. Intravascular metastatic cancer cell homotypic aggregation at the sites of primary attachment to the endothelium. Cancer Res 2003;63:3805−11.

[135] Khaldoyanidi SK, Glinsky VV, Sikora L, Glinskii AB, Mossine VV, Quinn TP, et al. MDA-MB-435 human breast carcinoma cell homo- and heterotypic adhesion under flow conditions is mediated in part by Thomsen-Friedenreich antigen-galectin-3 interactions. J Biol Chem 2003;278:4127−34.

[136] Ochieng J, Leite-Browning ML, Warfield P. Regulation of cellular adhesion to extracellular matrix proteins by galectin-3. Biochem Biophys Res Commun 1998;246:788−91.

[137] Matarrese P, Fusco O, Tinari N, Natoli C, Liu FT, Semeraro ML, et al. Galectin-3 overexpression protects from apoptosis by improving cell adhesion properties. Int J Cancer 2000;85:545−54.

[138] Le Marer N, Hughes RC. Effects of the carbohydrate-binding protein galectin-3 on the invasiveness of human breast carcinoma cells. J Cell Physiol 1996;168:51−8.

[139] Hittelet A, Legendre H, Nagy N, Bronckart Y, Pector JC, Salmon I, et al. Upregulation of galectins-1 and -3 in human colon cancer and their role in regulating cell migration. Int J Cancer 2003;103:370−9.

[140] O'Driscoll L, Linehan R, Liang YH, Joyce H, Oglesby I, Clynes M. Galectin-3 expression alters adhesion, motility and invasion in a lung cell line (DLKP), in vitro. Anticancer Res 2002;22:3117−25.

[141] Nangia-Makker P, Honjo Y, Sarvis R, Akahani S, Hogan V, Pienta KJ, et al. Galectin-3 induces endothelial cell morphogenesis and angiogenesis. Am J Pathol 2000;156:899—909.

[142] Ochieng J, Green B, Evans S, James O, Warfield P. Modulation of the biological functions of galectin-3 by matrix metalloproteinases. Biochim Biophys Acta 1998;1379:97—106.

[143] Califice S, Castronovo V. Van Den Brule F. Galectin-3 and cancer (Review). Int J Oncol 2004;25:983—92.

[144] Newlaczyl AU, Yu LG. Galectin-3—a jack-of-all-trades in cancer. Cancer Lett 2011;313:123—8.

[145] Danguy A, Camby I, Kiss R. Galectins and cancer. Biochim Biophys Acta 2002;1572:285—93.

[146] Takenaka Y, Fukumori T, Raz A. Galectin-3 and metastasis. Glycoconj J 2004;19:543—9.

[147] Chiu CG, Strugnell SS, Griffith OL, Jones SJ, Gown AM, Walker B, et al. Diagnostic utility of galectin-3 in thyroid cancer. Am J Pathol 2010;176:2067—81.

[148] Honjo Y, Inohara H, Akahani S, Yoshii T, Takenaka Y, Yoshida J, et al. Expression of cytoplasmic galectin-3 as a prognostic marker in tongue carcinoma. Clin Cancer Res 2000;6:4635—40.

[149] Lotz MM, Andrews Jr CW, Korzelius CA, Lee EC, Steele Jr GD, Clarke A, et al. Decreased expression of Mac-2 (carbohydrate binding protein 35) and loss of its nuclear localization are associated with the neoplastic progression of colon carcinoma. Proc Natl Acad Sci U S A 1993;90:3466—70.

[150] Puglisi F, Minisini AM, Barbone F, Intersimone D, Aprile G, Puppin C, et al. Galectin-3 expression in non-small cell lung carcinoma. Cancer Lett 2004;212:233—9.

[151] Sanjuan X, Fernandez PL, Castells A, Castronovo V, van den Brule F, Liu FT, et al. Differential expression of galectin 3 and galectin 1 in colorectal cancer progression. Gastroenterology 1997;113:1906—15.

[152] van den Brule F, Califice S, Garnier F, Fernandez PL, Berchuck A, Castronovo V. Galectin-1 accumulation in the ovary carcinoma peritumoral stroma is induced by ovary carcinoma cells and affects both cancer cell proliferation and adhesion to laminin-1 and fibronectin. Lab Invest 2003;83:377—86.

[153] Kim SJ, Lee SJ, Sung HJ, Choi IK, Choi CW, Kim BS, et al. Increased serum 90K and Galectin-3 expression are associated with advanced stage and a worse prognosis in diffuse large B-cell lymphomas. Acta Haematol 2008;120:211—6.

[154] Sakaki M, Oka N, Nakanishi R, Yamaguchi K, Fukumori T, Kanayama HO. Serum level of galectin-3 in human bladder cancer. J Med Invest 2008;55:127—32.

[155] Iacovazzi PA, Notarnicola M, Caruso MG, Guerra V, Frisullo S, Altomare DF. Serum levels of galectin-3 and its ligand 90k/mac-2bp in colorectal cancer patients. Immunopharmacol Immunotoxicol 2010;32:160—4.

[156] Saussez S, Lorfevre F, Lequeux T, Laurent G, Chantrain G, Vertongen F, et al. The determination of the levels of circulating galectin-1 and -3 in HNSCC patients could be used to monitor tumor progression and/or responses to therapy. Oral Oncol 2008;44:86—93.

[157] Vereecken P, Awada A, Suciu S, Castro G, Morandini R, Litynska A, et al. Evaluation of the prognostic significance of serum galectin-3 in American Joint Committee on Cancer stage III and stage IV melanoma patients. Melanoma Res 2009;19:316—20.

[158] Rabinovich GA. Galectin-1 as a potential cancer target. Br J Cancer 2005;92:1188—92.

[159] Demydenko D, Berest I. Expression of galectin-1 in malignant tumors. Exp Oncol 2009;31:74—9.

[160] Verschuere T, De Vleeschouwer S, Lefranc F, Kiss R, Van Gool SW. Galectin-1 and immunotherapy for brain cancer. Expert Rev Neurother 2011;11:533—43.

[161] Yamaoka K, Mishima K, Nagashima Y, Asai A, Sanai Y, Kirino T. Expression of galectin-1 mRNA correlates with the malignant potential of human gliomas and expression of antisense galectin-1 inhibits the growth of 9 glioma cells. J Neurosci Res 2000;59:722—30.

[162] Paz A, Haklai R, Elad-Sfadia G, Ballan E, Kloog Y. Galectin-1 binds oncogenic H-Ras to mediate Ras membrane anchorage and cell transformation. Oncogene 2001;20:7486—93.

[163] Wells V, Davies D, Mallucci L. Cell cycle arrest and induction of apoptosis by beta galactoside binding protein (beta GBP) in human mammary cancer cells. A potential new approach to cancer control. Eur J Cancer 1999;35:978—83.

[164] Kopitz J, von Reitzenstein C, Andre S, Kaltner H, Uhl J, Ehemann V, et al. Negative regulation of neuroblastoma cell growth by carbohydrate-dependent surface binding of galectin-1 and functional divergence from galectin-3. J Biol Chem 276:35917—23, 32001.

[165] Espelt MV, Croci DO, Bacigalupo ML, Carabias P, Manzi M, Elola MT, et al. Novel roles of galectin-1 in hepatocellular carcinoma cell adhesion, polarization, and in vivo tumor growth. Hepatology 2011;53:2097—106.

[166] Thijssen VL, Postel R, Brandwijk RJ, Dings RP, Nesmelova I, Satijn S, et al. Galectin-1 is essential in tumor angiogenesis and is a target for antiangiogenesis therapy. Proc Natl Acad Sci U S A 103:15975—15980, 12006.

[167] Thijssen VL, Barkan B, Shoji H, Aries IM, Mathieu V, Deltour L, et al. Tumor cells secrete galectin-1 to enhance endothelial cell activity. Cancer Res 2010;70:6216—24.

[168] Le Mercier M, Mathieu V, Haibe-Kains B, Bontempi G, Mijatovic T, Decaestecker C, et al. Knocking down galectin 1 in human hs683 glioblastoma cells impairs both angiogenesis and endoplasmic reticulum stress responses. J Neuropathol Exp Neurol 2008;67:456—69.

[169] Le Mercier M, Fortin S, Mathieu V, Roland I, Spiegl-Kreinecker S, Haibe-Kains B, et al. Galectin 1 proangiogenic and promigratory effects in the Hs683 oligodendroglioma model are partly mediated through the control of BEX2 expression. Neoplasia 2009;11:485—96.

[170] Hirashima M, Kashio Y, Nishi N, Yamauchi A, Imaizumi TA, Kageshita T, et al. Galectin-9 in physiological and pathological conditions. Glycoconj J 2004;19:593—600.

[171] Nobumoto A, Nagahara K, Oomizu S, Katoh S, Nishi N, Takeshita K, et al. Galectin-9 suppresses tumor metastasis by blocking adhesion to endothelium and extracellular matrices. Glycobiology 2008;18:735—44.

[172] Kasamatsu A, Uzawa K, Nakashima D, Koike H, Shiiba M, Bukawa H, et al. Galectin-9 as a regulator of cellular adhesion in human oral squamous cell carcinoma cell lines. Int J Mol Med 2005;16:269—73.

[173] Makishi S, Okudaira T, Ishikawa C, Sawada S, Watanabe T, Hirashima M, et al. A modified version of galectin-9 induces cell cycle arrest and apoptosis of Burkitt and Hodgkin lymphoma cells. Br J Haematol 2008;142:583—94.

[174] Irie A, Yamauchi A, Kontani K, Kihara M, Liu D, Shirato Y, et al. Galectin-9 as a prognostic factor with antimetastatic potential in breast cancer. Clin Cancer Res 2005;11:2962—8.

[175] Yamauchi A, Kontani K, Kihara M, Nishi N, Yokomise H, Hirashima M. Galectin-9, a novel prognostic factor with antimetastatic potential in breast cancer. Breast J 2006;12:S196—200.

[176] Liang M, Ueno M, Oomizu S, Arikawa T, Shinonaga R, Zhang S, et al. Galectin-9 expression links to malignant potential of cervical squamous cell carcinoma. J Cancer Res Clin Oncol 2008;134:899—907.

[177] Kageshita T, Kashio Y, Yamauchi A, Seki M, Abedin MJ, Nishi N, et al. Possible role of galectin-9 in cell aggregation and apoptosis of human melanoma cell lines and its clinical significance. Int J Cancer 2002;99:809—16.

[178] Huflejt ME, Leffler H. Galectin-4 in normal tissues and cancer. Glycoconj J 2004;20:247—55.

[179] Heinzelmann-Schwarz VA, Gardiner-Garden M, Henshall SM, Scurry JP, Scolyer RA, Smith AN, et al. A distinct molecular profile associated with mucinous epithelial ovarian cancer. Br J Cancer 2006;94:904—13.

[180] Rumilla KM, Erickson LA, Erickson AK, Lloyd RV. Galectin-4 expression in carcinoid tumors. Endocr Pathol 2006;17:243—9.

[181] Duerr EM, Mizukami Y, Ng A, Xavier RJ, Kikuchi H, Deshpande V, et al. Defining molecular classifications and targets in gastroenteropancreatic neuroendocrine tumors through DNA microarray analysis. Endocr Relat Cancer 2008;15:243—56.

[182] Tripodi D, Quemener S, Renaudin K, Ferron C, Malard O, Guisle-Marsollier I, et al. Gene expression profiling in sinonasal adenocarcinoma. BMC Med Genomics 2009;2:65.

[183] Rechreche H, Mallo GV, Montalto G, Dagorn JC, Iovanna JL. Cloning and expression of the mRNA of human galectin-4, an S-type lectin down-regulated in colorectal cancer. Eur J Biochem 1997;248:225—30.

[184] Nagy N, Legendre H, Engels O, Andre S, Kaltner H, Wasano K, et al. Refined prognostic evaluation in colon carcinoma using immunohistochemical galectin fingerprinting. Cancer 2003;97:1849—58.

[185] Satelli A, Rao PS, Thirumala S, Rao US. Galectin-4 functions as a tumor suppressor of human colorectal cancer. Int J Cancer 2011;129:799—809.

[186] Watanabe M, Takemasa I, Kaneko N, Yokoyama Y, Matsuo E, Iwasa S, et al. Clinical significance of circulating galectins as colorectal cancer markers. Oncol Rep 2011;25:1217—26.

[187] Saussez S, Kiss R. Galectin-7. Cell Mol Life Sci 2006;63:686—97.

[188] St-Pierre Y, Campion CG, Grosset AA. A distinctive role for galectin-7 in cancer? Front Biosci 2012;17:438—50.

[189] Bernerd F, Sarasin A, Magnaldo T. Galectin-7 overexpression is associated with the apoptotic process in UVB-induced sunburn keratinocytes. Proc Natl Acad Sci U S A 1999;96:11329—34.

[190] Kuwabara I, Kuwabara Y, Yang RY, Schuler M, Green DR, Zuraw BL, et al. Galectin-7 (PIG1) exhibits proapoptotic function through JNK activation and mitochondrial cytochrome c release. J Biol Chem 2002;277:3487—97.

[191] Kopitz J, Andre S, von Reitzenstein C, Versluis K, Kaltner H, Pieters RJ, et al. Homodimeric galectin-7 (p53-induced gene 1) is a negative growth regulator for human neuroblastoma cells. Oncogene 2003;22:6277—88.

[192] Ueda S, Kuwabara I, Liu FT. Suppression of tumor growth by galectin-7 gene transfer. Cancer Res 2004;64:5672—6.

[193] Demers M, Rose AA, Grosset AA, Biron-Pain K, Gaboury L, Siegel PM, et al. Overexpression of galectin-7, a myoepithelial cell marker, enhances spontaneous metastasis of breast cancer cells. Am J Pathol 2010;176:3023—31.

561

[194] Saussez S, Cucu DR, Decaestecker C, Chevalier D, Kaltner H, Andre S, et al. Galectin 7 (p53-induced gene 1): a new prognostic predictor of recurrence and survival in stage IV hypopharyngeal cancer. Ann Surg Oncol 2006;13:999—1009.

[195] Zhu X, Ding M, Yu ML, Feng MX, Tan LJ, Zhao FK. Identification of galectin-7 as a potential biomarker for esophageal squamous cell carcinoma by proteomic analysis. BMC Cancer 2010;10:290.

[196] Alves PM, Godoy GP, Gomes DQ, Medeiros AM, de Souza LB, da Silveira EJ, et al. Significance of galectins-1, -3, -4 and -7 in the progression of squamous cell carcinoma of the tongue. Pathol Res Pract 2011;207:236—40.

[197] Moisan S, Demers M, Mercier J, Magnaldo T, Potworowski EF, St-Pierre Y. Upregulation of galectin-7 in murine lymphoma cells is associated with progression toward an aggressive phenotype. Leukemia 2003;17:751—9.

[198] Demers M, Biron-Pain K, Hebert J, Lamarre A, Magnaldo T, St-Pierre Y. Galectin-7 in lymphoma: elevated expression in human lymphoid malignancies and decreased lymphoma dissemination by antisense strategies in experimental model. Cancer Res 2007;67:2824—9.

[199] Demers M, Couillard J, Giglia-Mari G, Magnaldo T, St-Pierre Y. Increased galectin-7 gene expression in lymphoma cells is under the control of DNA methylation. Biochem Biophys Res Commun 2009;387:425—9.

[200] Demers M, Magnaldo T, St-Pierre Y. A novel function for galectin-7: promoting tumorigenesis by up-regulating MMP-9 gene expression. Cancer Res 2005;65:5205—10.

[201] Bidon-Wagner N, Le Pennec JP. Human galectin-8 isoforms and cancer. Glycoconj J 2004;19:557—63.

[202] Dong GW, Kim J, Park JH, Choi JY, Cho SI, Lim SC. Galectin-8 expression in laryngeal squamous cell carcinoma. Clin Exp Otorhinolaryngol 2009;2:13—9.

[203] Savin S, Cvejic D, Jankovic M, Isic T, Paunovic I, Tatic S. Evaluation of galectin-8 expression in thyroid tumors. Med Oncol 2009;26:314—8.

[204] Nagy N, Bronckart Y, Camby I, Legendre H, Lahm H, Kaltner H, et al. Galectin-8 expression decreases in cancer compared with normal and dysplastic human colon tissue and acts significantly on human colon cancer cell migration as a suppressor. Gut 2002;50:392—401.

[205] Kramer MW, Waalkes S, Serth J, Hennenlotter J, Tezval H, Stenzl A, et al. Decreased galectin-8 is a strong marker for recurrence in urothelial carcinoma of the bladder. Urol Int 2011;87:143—50.

[206] Delgado VM, Nugnes LG, Colombo LL, Troncoso MF, Fernandez MM, Malchiodi EL, et al. Modulation of endothelial cell migration and angiogenesis: a novel function for the "tandem-repeat" lectin galectin-8. FASEB J 2011;25:242—54.

[207] Levy Y, Arbel-Goren R, Hadari YR, Eshhar S, Ronen D, Elhanany E, et al. Galectin-8 functions as a matri-cellular modulator of cell adhesion. J Biol Chem 2001;276:31285—95.

[208] Carcamo C, Pardo E, Oyanadel C, Bravo-Zehnder M, Bull P, Caceres M, et al. Galectin-8 binds specific beta1 integrins and induces polarized spreading highlighted by asymmetric lamellipodia in Jurkat T cells. Exp Cell Res 2006;312:374—86.

[209] Hadari YR, Arbel-Goren R, Levy Y, Amsterdam A, Alon R, Zakut R, et al. Galectin-8 binding to integrins inhibits cell adhesion and induces apoptosis. J Cell Sci 2000;113(Pt 13):2385—97.

[210] Arbel-Goren R, Levy Y, Ronen D, Zick Y. Cyclin-dependent kinase inhibitors and JNK act as molecular switches, regulating the choice between growth arrest and apoptosis induced by galectin-8. J Biol Chem 2005;280:19105—14.

[211] Dvorankova B, Lacina L, Smetana Jr K, Lensch M, Manning JC, Andre S, et al. Human galectin-2: nuclear presence in vitro and its modulation by quiescence/stress factors. Histol Histopathol 2008;23:167—78.

[212] Langbein S, Brade J, Badawi JK, Hatzinger M, Kaltner H, Lensch M, et al. Gene-expression signature of adhesion/growth-regulatory tissue lectins (galectins) in transitional cell cancer and its prognostic relevance. Histopathology 2007;51:681—90.

[213] Camby I, Belot N, Rorive S, Lefranc F, Maurage CA, Lahm H, et al. Galectins are differentially expressed in supratentorial pilocytic astrocytomas, astrocytomas, anaplastic astrocytomas and glioblastomas, and significantly modulate tumor astrocyte migration. Brain Pathol 2001;11:12—26.

[214] Thijssen VL, Hulsmans S, Griffioen AW. The galectin profile of the endothelium: altered expression and localization in activated and tumor endothelial cells. Am J Pathol 2008;172:545—53.

[215] Jung JH, Kim HJ, Yeom J, Yoo C, Shin J, Yoo J, et al. Lowered expression of galectin-2 is associated with lymph node metastasis in gastric cancer. J Gastroenterol 2012;47:37—48.

[216] Barrow H, Guo X, Wandall HH, Pedersen JW, Fu B, Zhao Q, et al. Serum galectin-2, -4, and -8 are greatly increased in colon and breast cancer patients and promote cancer cell adhesion to blood vascular endothelium. Clin Cancer Res 2011;17:7035—46.

[217] Ozaki K, Inoue K, Sato H, Iida A, Ohnishi Y, Sekine A, et al. Functional variation in LGALS2 confers risk of myocardial infarction and regulates lymphotoxin-alpha secretion in vitro. Nature 2004;429:72—5.

[218] Lin CI, Whang EE, Donner DB, Jiang X, Price BD, Carothers AM, et al. Galectin-3 targeted therapy with a small molecule inhibitor activates apoptosis and enhances both chemosensitivity and radiosensitivity in papillary thyroid cancer. Mol Cancer Res 2009;7:1655–62.

[219] Lavra L, Ulivieri A, Rinaldo C, Dominici R, Volante M, Luciani E, et al. Gal-3 is stimulated by gain-of-function p53 mutations and modulates chemoresistance in anaplastic thyroid carcinomas. J Pathol 2009;218:66–75.

[220] Wongkham S, Junking M, Wongkham C, Sripa B, Chur- S, Araki N. Suppression of galectin-3 expression enhances apoptosis and chemosensitivity in liver fluke-associated cholangiocarcinoma. Cancer Sci 2009;100:2077–84.

[221] Fukumori T, Kanayama HO, Raz A. The role of galectin-3 in cancer drug resistance. Drug Resist Update 2007;10:101–8.

[222] Mathieu V, Le Mercier M, De Neve N, Sauvage S, Gras T, Roland I, et al. Galectin-1 knockdown increases sensitivity to temozolomide in a B16F10 mouse metastatic melanoma model. J Invest Dermatol 2007;127:2399–410.

[223] Le Mercier M, Lefranc F, Mijatovic T, Debeir O, Haibe-Kains B, Bontempi G, et al. Evidence of galectin-1 involvement in glioma chemoresistance. Toxicol Appl Pharmacol 2008;229:172–83.

[224] Kuroda J, Yamamoto M, Nagoshi H, Kobayashi T, Sasaki N, Shimura Y, et al. Targeting activating transcription factor 3 by Galectin-9 induces apoptosis and overcomes various types of treatment resistance in chronic myelogenous leukemia. Mol Cancer Res 2010;8:994–1001.

[225] Matsui Y, Ueda S, Watanabe J, Kuwabara I, Ogawa O, Nishiyama H. Sensitizing effect of galectin-7 in urothelial cancer to cisplatin through the accumulation of intracellular reactive oxygen species. Cancer Res 2007;67:1212–20.

[226] Lahm H, Andre S, Hoeflich A, Kaltner H, Siebert HC, Sordat B, et al. Tumor galectinology: insights into the complex network of a family of endogenous lectins. Glycoconj J 2004;20:227–38.

[227] Raz A, Lotan R. Lectin-like activities associated with human and murine neoplastic cells. Cancer Res 1981;41:3642–7.

[228] John CM, Leffler H, Kahl-Knutsson B, Svensson I, Jarvis GA. Truncated galectin-3 inhibits tumor growth and metastasis in orthotopic nude mouse model of human breast cancer. Clin Cancer Res 2003;9:2374–83.

[229] Inufusa H, Nakamura M, Adachi T, Aga M, Kurimoto M, Nakatani Y, et al. Role of galectin-3 in adenocarcinoma liver metastasis. Int J Oncol 2001;19:913–9.

[230] Glinsky GV, Price JE, Glinsky VV, Mossine VV, Kiriakova G, Metcalf JB. Inhibition of human breast cancer metastasis in nude mice by synthetic glycoamines. Cancer Res 1996;56:5319–24.

[231] Nangia-Makker P, Hogan V, Honjo Y, Baccarini S, Tait L, Bresalier R, et al. Inhibition of human cancer cell growth and metastasis in nude mice by oral intake of modified citrus pectin. J Natl Cancer Inst 2002;94:1854–62.

[232] Streetly MJ, Maharaj L, Joel S, Schey SA, Gribben JG, Cotter FE. GCS-100, a novel galectin-3 antagonist, modulates MCL-1, NOXA, and cell cycle to induce myeloma cell death. Blood 2010;115:3939–48.

[233] Andre S, Pieters RJ, Vrasidas I, Kaltner H, Kuwabara I, Liu FT, et al. Wedgelike glycodendrimers as inhibitors of binding of mammalian galectins to glycoproteins, lactose maxiclusters, and cell surface glycoconjugates. Chembiochem 2001;2:822–30.

[234] Sorme P, Qian Y, Nyholm PG, Leffler H, Nilsson UJ. Low micromolar inhibitors of galectin-3 based on 3′-derivatization of N-acetyllactosamine. Chembiochem 2002;3:183–9.

[235] Tejler J, Leffler H, Nilsson UJ. Synthesis of O-galactosyl aldoximes as potent LacNAc-mimetic galectin-3 inhibitors. Bioorg Med Chem Lett 2005;15:2343–5.

[236] Cumpstey I, Sundin A, Leffler H, Nilsson UJ. C2-symmetrical thiodigalactoside bis-benzamido derivatives as high-affinity inhibitors of galectin-3: efficient lectin inhibition through double arginine-arene interactions. Angew Chem Int Ed Engl 2005;44:5110–2.

[237] Salameh BA, Leffler H, Nilsson UJ. 3-(1,2,3-Triazol-1-yl)-1-thio-galactosides as small, efficient, and hydrolytically stable inhibitors of galectin-3. Bioorg Med Chem Lett 2005;15:3344–6.

[238] Oberg CT, Leffler H, Nilsson UJ. Inhibition of galectins with small molecules. Chimia (Aarau) 2011;65:18–23.

[239] Bustinza-Linares E, Kurzrock R, Tsimberidou AM. Salirasib in the treatment of pancreatic cancer. Future Oncol 2010;6:885–91.

[240] Riely GJ, Johnson ML, Medina C, Rizvi NA, Miller VA, Kris MG, et al. A phase II trial of Salirasib in patients with lung adenocarcinomas with KRAS mutations. J Thorac Oncol 2011;6:1435–7.

[241] Ouyang J, Juszczynski P, Rodig SJ, Green MR, O'Donnell E, Currie T, et al. Viral induction and targeted inhibition of galectin-1 in EBV+ posttransplant lymphoproliferative disorders. Blood 2011;117:4315–22.

CHAPTER 32

IDO in Immune Escape: Regulation and Therapeutic Inhibition

Alexander J. Muller[1], Courtney Smith[1], Richard Metz[2], George C. Prendergast[1,3]

[1]Lankenau Institute for Medical Research, Wynnewood, PA USA
[2]NewLink Genetics Corporation, Wynnewood, PA USA
[3]Department of Pathology, Anatomy & Cell Biology, Jefferson Medical School, Thomas Jefferson University, Philadelphia, PA USA

I. INTRODUCTION

The treatment of advanced, metastatic cancers remains a major clinical challenge. Current regimens of chemotherapy and other systemic modalities are still not able to provide more than a limited benefit to many of the ~50% of cancer patients in developed countries who present with advanced disease at diagnosis. Similarly, these regimens ultimately fail patients that relapse with disseminated disease following the initial treatment of primary tumors. It has long been recognized that tumors display immunogenic tumor antigens yet escape immune rejection, somehow evading, subverting, or perhaps even reprogramming the immune system for their own benefit. This phenomenon of immune escape is central to tumor cell survival, but its basis has remained poorly understood, in part because its role as a critical trait of cancer was not fully appreciated by cancer geneticists until recently [1].

While an appropriately activated immune system can eradicate cancer, even when it is aggressive and disseminated, spontaneous occurrences of such events are rare. This has prompted development of numerous peptide- and cell-based immunotherapy strategies aimed at stimulating an antitumor immune response, for example, through administration of cytokines, tumor-associated antigen peptide vaccines, dendritic cell (DC) vaccines, and adoptive transfer of tumor antigen-specific effector T cells expanded *ex vivo* from cancer patients [2—8]. In contrast to passive immunotherapies involving the administration of defined antibodies, these active immunotherapies are conceptually based on stimulating components of the host immune system to elicit an effective response. This type of approach may not, however, be sufficient to overcome tumoral immune escape if pathological immune tolerance is dominant in cancer patients as has been proposed [9]. In cases where escape hinges on active principles of immune tolerance, relieving these suppression mechanisms may first be required to achieve therapeutic efficacy. In short, to "get on the gas" of immune activation against tumors it may be necessary to "get off the brakes" of tumor-associated immune suppression.

In recent years, there have been significant advances in understanding how tumors escape the immune system [10,11]. Intriguingly, many immune escape mechanisms are configured as active immune suppression by the tumor or by stromal cells under the influence of the tumor, implying that continuous activity is required. This is provocative, because it implies that

Cancer Immunotherapy. http://dx.doi.org/10.1016/B978-0-12-394296-8.00032-4

disrupting these mechanisms of immune suppression could de-repress (activate) the immune system, enabling it to attack the tumor. Such mechanisms may offer particularly attractive targets for therapeutic intervention with small molecule drugs [12], which have distinct advantages over biological agents that are currently the norm for immunotherapeutic strategies. Of the mechanisms which have been described to date, one with considerable practical appeal involves the tryptophan catabolizing enzyme IDO [13].

II. TRYPTOPHAN CATABOLISM BY IDO: A HISTORICAL CONUNDRUM

While most early studies of IDO were not related to cancer, the discovery of this enzyme is actually rooted in initial observations made in cancer patients. Elevated tryptophan catabolism was first reported in patients with bladder cancer in the 1950s [14]. By the 1960s, elevated levels of tryptophan catabolites had been documented in the urine of patients with a variety of malignancies including leukemia, Hodgkin's disease, prostate cancer, and breast cancer [15—20]. The hepatic enzyme tryptophan dioxygenase (TDO2; EC 1.13.11.11), which was the first inducible mammalian enzyme ever to be isolated, had been known since the 1930s to initiate the metabolism of dietary tryptophan [21,22]. However, no increase in TDO2 activity was detected in cancer patients who presented with elevated tryptophan catabolites [23], implying the existence of a second enzyme.

The isolation of the extra-hepatic tryptophan catabolizing enzyme termed indoleamine 2,3-dioxygenase (IDO; EC 1.13.11.42; originally D-tryptophan pyrrolase) was first reported in 1963 [24,25]. Notably, while IDO catalyzes the same reaction as its hepatic relative TDO2—the conversion of tryptophan to N-formyl-kynurenine—these two enzymes are otherwise remarkably dissimilar [26]. Whereas active TDO2 is a homotetramer of 320 kD, IDO is a monomeric enzyme of 41 kD that is antigenically distinct from TDO2 [27] and lacking in amino acid sequence similarity. Additionally, IDO has less stringent substrate specificity, cleaving a number of indole-containing compounds not recognized by the hepatic enzyme. Lastly, while both enzymes contain heme, IDO utilizes superoxide anion for activity whereas TDO2 does not use superoxide to donate oxygen in the tryptophan catabolic reaction.

Structural and enzymological studies have revealed several interesting features about IDO. Enzymological studies indicate that an electron donor such as methylene blue is critical to achieve full activity *in vitro*, a role that *in vivo* is thought to be assumed by tetrahydrobiopterin or flavin cofactors. The binding site on the enzyme for the putative cofactor is distinct from the substrate binding site [28], implying the potential for allosteric regulation and possibly opportunities for developing noncompetitive enzymatic inhibitors (in addition to the more classical substrate-competitive inhibitors). Crystallographic studies of human IDO reveal a two-domain structure of alpha-helical domains with the heme group located in between [29]. Notably, these findings suggest that strict shape requirements in the catalytic site are required, not for substrate binding but instead for abstraction of a proton from the substrate by iron-bound dioxygen in the first step of the reaction [29]. This detail of the reaction mechanism is important because it is distinct from that used by other monooxygenases (e.g., cytochrome P450), filling a gap in understanding of heme chemistry. In terms of small molecule inhibitor development, the biochemical differences that distinguish IDO from TDO2 and other monooxygenases are useful because they increase the likelihood of identifying IDO-specific inhibitors.

Mammalian genomes include not only the IDO-encoding gene *IDO1* (formerly designated *INDO*) but also a newly identified relative termed *IDO2* (formerly *INDOL1*) [30,31]. Human *IDO1*, located at 8p12-11, comprises 10 exons spanning ~15 kb that encode a 403 amino acid polypeptide of ~41 kD [32,33]. Mouse *Ido1* is syntenic and similar in its genomic organization; however, the gene diverges somewhat at the primary sequence level from human *IDO1*, sharing only 63% identity. The likely existence of a related *IDO2* gene became apparent to us while inspecting sequences immediately downstream of *IDO1* in the human genome [31]. At the time, the genome database in that region was erroneously annotated, referring to a set of partial *IDO1*-related sequences by the anonymous nomenclature *LOC169355*. Correction of the erroneous annotation by trial-and-error exon searches revealed the presence of a 420 amino acid open-reading frame that is 44% identical to IDO at the primary sequence level. The protein encoded by the *IDO2* ORF conserves all the residues in IDO that have been defined as critical for tryptophan binding and catabolism [29]. The IDO2 proteins in mouse and human are more closely conserved than the mouse and human IDO proteins, displaying 73% identity at the primary sequence level. The presence of the two IDO-related proteins in such close proximity is likely the result of a gene duplication event and phylogenetic analysis has been interpreted to indicate that *IDO2* may actually be the ancestral gene [34]. As in the human genome, the mouse *Ido2* gene is located immediately downstream of *Ido1*. Expression of *IDO2* message was detected in a more limited range of tissues than *IDO1* [31]. At the cellular level, evaluation of the NCBI SAGEmap database identified the top hits for *IDO2* expression to be bone marrow derived DCs [31], which is intriguing given the evidence that IDO-based activity profoundly influences the immunogenic nature of DCs.

In contrast to the biochemical and genetic knowledge about IDO that accumulated relatively quickly in the years since its discovery, a precise understanding of its physiological function remained obscure due to the fact that mammals mostly salvage rather than synthesize NAD to meet their metabolic needs. Why then was IDO evolutionarily conserved in mammals? Initial clues as to its function were suggested in the late 1970s by findings from Hayaishi and his colleagues that IDO expression was strongly stimulated in the lungs of mice by viral infection, or exposure to bacterial lipopolysaccharide (LPS) or interferon-γ (IFN-γ) [35]. These findings prompted the interpretation that elevated tryptophan catabolism by IDO at sites of inflammation might provide an antimicrobial benefit. Given the antitumor properties of IFN-γ, this concept was extended to encompass the notion that IDO acted functionally in the manner of a tumor suppressor, contributing to the antitumor effects of IFN-γ activity by starving growing tumor cells of tryptophan [36].

It was not until the late 1990s that a conceptual breakthrough emerged from work by Munn, Mellor and their colleagues, establishing the possibility that IDO might mediate an immunosuppressive function based on the preferential sensitivity of T cells to tryptophan deprivation. In this radical reconceptualization of the biological role of IDO-based metabolic activity, impaired antigen-dependent T-cell activation occurs in microenvironments where IDO activation results in reduced tryptophan levels [37,38]. The ability of IDO to promote immune tolerance to "foreign" antigens was supported by evidence that the specific bioactive IDO inhibitor 1-methyl-tryptophan (1MT) [39] could elicit MHC-restricted T-cell-mediated rejection of allogeneic mouse concepti [40,41]. In cancer, these findings implied that IDO could be pro-oncogenic by limiting the eradication of tumor cells that occurs through immune-based recognition of "foreign" tumor antigens.

In the last few years, the concept that tryptophan catabolism regulates T-cell immunity has now been corroborated in many laboratories, with regulatory functions identified for both tryptophan depletion and the production of downstream catabolites. In particular, there has been a keen focus on the immune regulatory role of IDO expressed in dendritic cells (DCs), an important class of "professional" antigen-presenting cell. IDO expression in a small minority population of DCs enables them to dominantly suppress the activation of T cells that occurs through antigen presentation [42,43]. Tryptophan depletion has been shown to promote T-cell anergy by signaling through the integrated stress response kinase GCN2, which is also required for IDO-induced differentiation of CD4$^+$ T cells into Tregs [44]. Likewise, tryptophan catabolites can block T-cell activation and trigger T-cell apoptosis while also promoting the emergence of Tregs through a TGF-β dependent mechanism, and evidence of synergistic consequences of both depleting tryptophan and elevating tryptophan catabolites has been described [45].

Most of the signaling and mechanistic data surrounding the IDO proteins have come from studies of IDO and not the more recently identified IDO2. Due to the more restricted localization of IDO2 compared to IDO, it is conjectured that these two molecules do not serve a redundant function. This view is supported by a divergence in signaling between these two molecules through the integrated stress response pathway. Local tryptophan depletion due to IDO activity engages this pathway resulting in the elevated expression of LIP [31], a truncated isoform of the transcription factor NF-IL6/CEBPß which alters expression of key immune modulatory factors including IL-6, TGF-ß, and IL-10. Supplementing with additional tryptophan after depletion quickly abolished the LIP response induced by IDO but not by IDO2[31]. Thus, after IDO2 induction, LIP expression is maintained in a tryptophan-independent manner, indicating a stable effect of tryptophan catabolic signaling unique to IDO2. While the significance of this distinction has yet to be evaluated *in vivo*, one implication is that IDO2 might differ from IDO in its ability to transmit a stable immune regulatory signal. LIP-mediated signaling initiated by IDO2 could alter distal immunity, since the signal could persist in microenvironments where tryptophan levels are normal. Alternately, IDO2 might produce a stable differentiation signal.

Another unique aspect of IDO2 is the considerable genetic variability that exists among different individuals for expressing the active enzyme. This variability is due the presence of two commonly occurring, nonsynonymous single nucleotide polymorphisms in the *IDO2* gene that ablate its enzymatic activity [31]. Indeed, as many as 50% of individuals of European or Asian descent and 25% of individuals of African descent appear to lack functional *IDO2* alleles [31]. The frequent occurrence of inactive genetic variants in human populations suggests that there may be some evolutionary benefit to attenuating IDO2 activity, perhaps reflecting competing selective pressures to establish an optimal degree of immunological responsiveness under differing conditions of infection, autoimmunity and malignancy. In this vein, one clinical study provides evidence that active IDO2 alleles may be disproportionately represented among younger individuals with aggressive pancreatic cancer [46].

A. Complex control of IDO by immune regulatory factors

Initial clues regarding the involvement of IDO in inflammation originated with the finding that its expression and activity are strongly stimulated by the cytokine IFN-γ [47]. IFN-γ is now recognized as a major inducer of IDO, especially in antigen presenting cells including macrophages and DCs [48–51]. Transcriptional induction of the *IDO1* gene through IFN-γ is mediated through the JAK/STAT pathway, in particular JAK1 and STAT1α [52]. STAT1α appears to act to induce *IDO1* gene expression both directly through binding of GAS sites within the *IDO1* promoter as well as indirectly through induction of IRF-1 which binds the *IDO1* promoter at two ISRE sites [52–56]. The upregulation of IDO in antigen-presenting cells that occurs in response to IFN-γ, which is produced by activated T cells, suggests that IDO participates in a negative feedback loop that regulates T-cell activation.

The transcription factor NF-κB, which has a central role in directing inflammatory processes, has also been identified as a key factor controlling the induction of IDO. The precise mechanisms for NF-κB mediated control of *IDO1* expression have yet to be fully elucidated and may be contextually based as both canonical and noncanonical pathways have been found to be important under different experimental conditions [57–59]. IRF-1 may be a common element through which both STAT1α and NF-κB contribute to the induction of *IDO1*, as both IFN-γ and TNF-α (which signals through NF-κB) can synergistically induce expression of IRF-1 through a novel composite binding element for both STAT1α and NF-κB in the IRF-1 promoter (termed a GAS/κB element) that combines a GAS element overlapped by a nonconsensus site for NF-κB [60].

In DCs, interferons (both type 1 and type 2) have been found to act at a central interface between IDO and other components of inflammation and immunity. TLR9 ligands such as CpG were found to induce IDO expression in a subset of DCs through a type 1 interferon-dependent signaling pathway [61]. Interactions with immune cells are also implicated in IDO regulation. The first of these interactions to be characterized was an intriguing reverse signaling mechanism described for the inhibitory T-cell coreceptor CTLA-4, which is constitutively expressed on T regulatory (Treg) cells. By binding to B7 ligands (CD80 and CD86) on DCs, CTLA-4 was shown to elicit the IFN-γ-dependent induction of IDO [62]. The stimulatory T-cell coreceptor CD28 also binds the same B7 ligands but fails to similarly induce IDO because of the concomitant induction of IL-6 which interferes with IFN-γ elicited STAT signaling through upregulation of SOCS3 [63]. Other cell surface proteins including CD40, CD200 and GITR have since been shown to induce IDO through similar reverse signaling mechanisms all of which appear to share the noncanonical NF-κB pathway as a common point of convergence [64].

The pro-inflammatory prostaglandin PGE-2, which is frequently elevated during cancer progression as a result of activation of cyclooxygenase-2 (COX-2), has also been implicated as an important inducer of IDO activity. In support of the concept that IDO acts downstream of COX-2, induction of IDO activity can be blocked *in vitro* by COX-2 inhibitors such as aspirin, indomethacin, and phenylbutazone but not by anti-inflammatory agents that do not affect prostaglandin production [65]. This signaling mechanism may be relevant to the biological activity of upstream regulators of *COX2* expression as well. For instance, HGF, which is known to be able to elevate COX2 activity, has been found to also elevate IDO in monocyte-derived DCs [66]. The relationship between PGE-2 and IDO is clearly complex insofar as IDO activity can affect the ratio of prostaglandin synthesis [67]. Interestingly, while PGE-2 is employed widely as an *in vitro* maturation factor for dendritic cells, treatment of these cells with PGE-2 has been reported to elevate IDO expression ~100-fold [68]. Although the induction of IDO enzymatic activity does appear to require an additional signal(s), (i.e., exposure to TNF or agonists of TLRs), these findings raise the concern that such preparations may inadvertently compromise the desired immune stimulatory activity of the DCs used in the setting of cancer vaccines.

More recently, interconnections identified between IDO and the xenobiotic aryl hydrocarbon receptor (AhR) have been generating particular interest due to a developing appreciation for the importance of AhR in modulating immune function especially at the level of mucosal immunity [69] where IDO may also be particularly relevant. AhR activation by 2,3,7,8-tetrachlorodibenzo-p-dioxin (TCCD) resulted in the induction of both IDO1 and IDO2 *in vitro* [70]. Furthermore, it was shown that TCDD treatment of mouse splenic T cells resulted in increased levels of Foxp3, an effect that was abrogated in *Ahr*-null mice suggesting that AhR is important for the development of Tregs possibly through the induction of IDO [70]. Conversely, several tryptophan catabolites have been implicated as physiological ligands for AhR including kynurenine [71,72], produced by the ubiquitous arylformamidase enzyme following IDO or TDO initiated catabolism of tryptophan. Further biological ramifications can be inferred from studies by DiNatale et al. showing that kynurenic acid, another downstream tryptophan catabolite, induces AhR-mediated induction of IL-6 [73], an important inflammatory cytokine for promoting tumor progression. Interestingly, *Ido1*-nullizygous mice exhibited a marked reduction in IL-6 levels in primary lung tumors and pulmonary metastases which was functionally linked to increased tumor resistance [74]. As noted earlier in this section, IL-6 has been demonstrated to antagonize IDO expression, suggesting its involvement in an important negative regulatory feedback loop that may go awry during the development of cancer.

In addition to IL-6, other important negative regulators of IDO have been identified. Inducible nitric oxide synthase (iNOS) and IDO appear to be mutually antagonistic in DC-based studies [75–77]. The production of NO by iNOS prevents the IFN-γ-induced expression of IDO [78], interferes directly with its enzymatic activity [78–80] and promotes its proteolytic degradation [81]. NO can directly inactivate IDO by binding to the heme iron, which under lowered pH conditions induces iron-His bond rupture and the formation of a 5C NO-bound derivative that is associated with protein conformational changes that may be sufficient to target the protein for ubiquitination and proteosomal degradation [82]. In the NOD mouse model of diabetes, *in vivo* evidence suggests that IFN-γ signaling is impaired as the result of nitration of the downstream STAT1 transcription factor by peroxynitrate, which is derived from NO and superoxide. This impairment can be overcome by CTLA-4-Ig treatment, which, by promoting PTEN activity, relieves the negative regulation that phosphorylated Akt imposes on FOXO3a-mediated transcription of superoxide dismutase (SOD2) which degrades peroxynitrate [83]. Through this complex route, the blockade to activation of IDO gene expression, to which iNOS contributes through peroxynitrate-mediated nitration of STAT1, is relieved. Two implications of the configuration of this mechanism are the following. First, NO agonists will tend to reverse immunosuppression at the level of DCs in cancer, which should benefit treatment. Second, small molecule inhibitors of Akt that are being developed as anticancer therapeutics will tend to heighten immunosuppression by phenocopying this effect of CTLA-4-Ig on IDO expression. Other findings suggest that Akt inhibition may also heighten the invasive capability of cancer cells [84]. Thus, for cancer treatment, the desirable pro-apoptotic quality of Akt inhibitors may be balanced by their undesirable pro-invasive and immuno-suppressive properties.

TGF-β was initially reported to antagonize IFN-γ-mediated induction of IDO expression [85]. These experiments, carried out in fibroblasts, appear to run counter to immunosuppressive activity ascribed to TGF-β but are consistent with its ability to antagonize positively regulated targets of IFN-γ. More recently, the opposite relationship between IDO and TGF-β has been reported in experiments carried out in DCs suggesting that the regulatory impact of TGF-β on IDO expression may be complex and contextual. In these experiments, autocrine TGF-β sustained the activation of IDO in a tolerogenic subpopulation of CD8$^+$ DCs while exogenous TGF-β could convert immunogenic CD8$^-$ DCs into tolerogenic cells in conjunction with induction of IDO [86]. In this milieu, it was found that even DCs that lack expression of IDO could be rendered tolerogenic by exposure to tryptophan catobolites produced by IDO-expressing cells [87] as part of a feedforward expansion of IDO-elicited immune suppression described as "infectious tolerance" [88].

III. IDO DYSREGULATION IN THE PATHOGENESIS OF CANCER

Several epidemiological studies suggest that IDO overexpression is generally associated with poor prognosis in many different cancers [89]. Tumor transplant studies in mice have likewise linked IDO expression with enhanced tumor outgrowth in the context of an active immune system [58,90,91]. Loss of the *Bin1* tumor suppressor gene has been identified as a possible mechanism whereby tumor cells can intrinsically activate IDO activity through dysregulation of *Ido1* expression [58]. This mechanism is summarized in Figure 32.1. Targeted deletion of *Bin1* in mouse cells resulted in superinduction of IDO gene expression by IFN-γ. Transformation of *Bin1*-null and *Bin1*-expressing mouse embryo keratinocytes with *c-Myc+Ras* oncogenes produced cell lines with similar *in vitro* growth properties. However, when these cells were introduced into syngeneic animals, the *Bin1*-null cells formed large tumors whereas the *Bin1*-expressing cells formed only indolent nodules. This dichotomy reflected a difference in immune response to the cells, as *Bin1*-expressing cells produced rapidly growing tumors when introduced into T-cell-deficient mice. Treatment with the IDO inhibitor 1MT suppressed the outgrowth of *Bin1*-null tumors in syngeneic mice but this effect was absent in T-cell-deficient animals. Taken together, these findings showed how the dysregulation of IDO by *Bin1* loss promoted tumorigenicity by enabling IDO-based immune escape. Given the

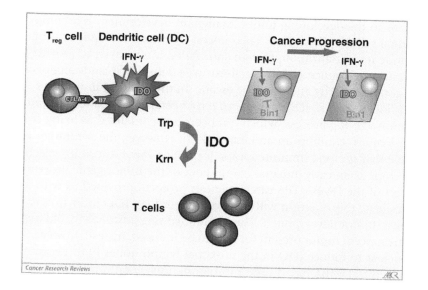

FIGURE 32.1

Mechanisms of IDO-induced tumoral immune escape. IDO expression in local immune stroma or tumor cells themselves has been implicated in promoting immune tolerance. IDO is upregulated in antigen-presenting dendritic cells (*DC*) by autocrine IFN-γ released as a result of Treg cell–induced CTLA–4/B7-dependent cell–cell signaling. Local tryptophan catabolism limits the proliferation and survival of T cells that would otherwise be activated by tumor antigens on the DC. This mechanism may operate in tumor-draining lymph nodes. In tumor cells, attenuation of the suppressor gene Bin1 leads to superactivation of IDO expression by IFN-γ, directly suppressing activation of T cells in the local tumor environment. Blocking IDO activity systemically with small molecule inhibitors (e.g., 1-methyl-tryptophan) reverses T-cell suppression that occurs as a result of tryptophan catabolism in both settings. *Taken from Muller and Prendergast (2005)*, Cancer Res. 65: 8065-8068.

frequent attenuation of *Bin1* expression and the frequent overexpression of IDO in human cancers, it will be important to further evaluate the relationship between these two events.

Unlike a conventional proto-oncogene, the role of IDO in cancer is predominantly to create a more hospitable environment for the tumor rather than enhancing malignant properties intrinsic to the tumor cells. Therefore, it is not surprising that normal cells outside the tumor have also been found to be a relevant source of IDO expression. In particular, a subset of DCs, with characteristics indicative of the B-cell lineage [92], express high levels of IDO in the proximal lymph nodes of mice with subcutaneous melanoma tumor grafts that exhibited no expression of IDO in the tumor cells themselves [93]. Elevated levels of IDO can often be found in tumor draining lymph nodes of human cancer patients as well [93]. Studies based on the classical 2-stage DMBA/TPA skin carcinogenesis protocol demonstrated that mice in which both alleles of the *Ido1* gene were genetically disrupted (*Ido1*-nullizygous) are quite resistant to the development of tumors [94]. In this model, tumors are initiated with a single application of the carcinogen 7, 12-dimethylbenz[*a*]anthracene (DMBA) followed by multiple rounds of exposure to the pro-inflammatory phorbol ester 12-O-tetradecanoyl phorbol-13-acetate (TPA; a.k.a. phorbol 12-myristate 13-acetate or PMA) which elicits a state of chronic inflammation in the skin that promotes tumor outgrowth. These studies have provided the first direct genetic validation that IDO has an important effector role in the process of *de novo* tumorigenesis, but, at least under these circumstances, apparently not as a consequence of IDO expressed intrinsically within the developing tumor cells. Instead, elevated IDO was found in a T-cell suppressive population of DCs localized within the tumor draining lymph nodes that had the same characteristics as those previously observed in the melanoma tumor graft model [93,94]. These findings highlight the complexity of interpreting IDO in biological systems, as its expression can be either intrinsic or extrinsic to the tumor and its immunoregulatory impact is most likely directed externally in a non-cell-autonomous manner.

With regard to the immunoregulatory role of IDO in cancer, recent findings have produced an even more complex and nuanced interpretation of what elevated tryptophan catabolism means to the developing tumor. Malignant development is accompanied by a breakdown of normal cellular physiology. This process involves the acquisition of cell-intrinsic traits that include immortalization, growth sufficiency, insensitivity to growth inhibitory signals and apoptosis resistance as well as cell-extrinsic traits that include angiogenesis, invasive capability, metastatic capacity and immune escape. In this context, immune escape mechanisms utilized by tumors, such as IDO induction, have been postulated to be a terminal feature of the immunoediting process, which has been conceptualized as being comprised of three phases: elimination, equilibrium and escape [95]. However, the contrarian argument has also been made that tumoral immune escape is not late-event driven by selective pressure but instead develops as an early, integral component of the tumorigenic process [96]. The multistage aspect of the DMBA/TPA carcinogenesis protocol provided us with a unique opportunity to investigate this question with regard to the role of IDO induction in the contextual setting of *de novo* tumor development. The immunoediting postulate would require that there be at least some nascent tumor present for IDO to be induced. Instead, however, TPA treatment alone was sufficient to induce IDO in the proximal lymph nodes [94]. Because these mice were never exposed to DMBA-based tumor initiation, this elevation of IDO occurred in the absence of cancer, as TPA alone is not able to drive the development of neoplasia in the absence of an initiating agent. This outcome, therefore, is more in line with the elevation of IDO being an early event driven by TPA-elicited inflammation rather than a late event driven by immune selection.

Based on the generally accepted characterization of IDO as an immunosuppressive enzyme, inflammation might be expected to run rampant in an *Ido1*-nullizygous mouse in which this immunosuppressive check is no longer in place. However, when the severity of the inflammation that develops in *Ido1*-nullizygous mice treated with TPA was evaluated, it was not discernibly different than in wild type control animals receiving the same treatment [97]. So, rather than IDO simply being an immunosuppressive counterbalance in inflammatory reactions, these data instead suggest a more nuanced interpretation whereby IDO, acting as an integral component of inflammation, shapes its pathogenic capacity to promote tumor development. Our most recent findings further elucidate how IDO contributes to cancer development by altering the inflammatory milieu. The loss of *Ido1* was shown to significantly reduce lung tumor burden in mouse models of pulmonary adenocarcinoma and breast cancer metastasis development which correlated with improved survival of the $Ido1^{-/-}$ mice in both models [74]. In both these cancer models, IL-6 levels were attenuated in the $Ido1^{-/-}$ mice leading to an impairment of myeloid-derived suppressor cell (MDSC)-mediated suppression of T cells. The importance of these findings to pulmonary tumor development was demonstrated in the metastatic model where restoration of IL-6 overcame the MDSC impairment and allowed metastatic disease to progress at the rate observed in *Ido1*-competent mice [74]. The implication that IL-6 serves as a key regulator of tumor growth downstream of IDO has therapeutic value as increased IL-6 levels are associated with recurring tumors in patients [98].

The conceptual realization that IDO may act as an integral component within the inflammatory milieu to shape its pathogenic capacity to support tumor development led us to consider the broader question of whether IDO might likewise contribute to the development of other pathologies associated with chronic inflammation. Indeed, evidence that elevated tryptophan degradation correlates with disease activity in both rheumatoid arthritis and systemic lupus erythematosus patients suggested that increased IDO activity might play an activating role in the autoimmune response in humans [99,100]. Direct corroborative evidence for this idea came from studies we performed in the KxB/N spontaneous mouse model of arthritis [101]. IDO activity was elevated at the onset of disease and treatment of these animals with the small molecule inhibitor of IDO, 1MT, resulted in significant alleviation of the joint inflammation that develops in this model, with 1MT-treated animals exhibiting minimal synovial expansion and fewer infiltrating inflammatory cells [102]. 1MT treatment had no apparent effect on the percentage of Tregs or the levels of Th1/Th2/Th17 cytokines but did greatly diminish the autoreactive B-cell response, indicative of a novel role for IDO in contributing to the development of autoimmune disease by supporting the activation of autoreactive B cells. In conjunction with the cancer models, these data argue strongly that the role of IDO in chronic inflammation is more complex than simply to act as an immuno-suppressive brake. Rather, IDO appears to alter inflammatory pathogenesis in these models, exacerbating the development of tumors in the cancer models and contributing to the severity of autoimmune arthritis in the K/BxN model.

IV. 1MT AS A THERAPEUTIC PROTOTYPE

Several studies have now provided evidence that IDO inhibition with 1MT or other small molecule inhibitors of the IDO pathway can exert antitumor effects. Initial evidence was offered in 2002 that the IDO inhibitor 1MT could partly retard the growth of mouse lung carcinoma cells engrafted onto a syngeneic host [90]. Similar results were obtained as part of an investigation to assess the ramifications of IDO overexpression, which was detected in a wide range of human tumors [91]. In this study, ectopic overexpression of IDO in an established tumor cell line was shown to be sufficient to enable tumor formation in animals pre-immunized against a specific tumor antigen and 1MT partially suppressed tumor outgrowth in this context as well. Against established, autochthonous (spontaneously arising) mammary tumors in the MMTV-neu/HER2 transgenic mouse model of breast cancer, we found that 1MT could likewise retard tumor outgrowth [58]. By itself, however, 1MT was unable to elicit tumor regression in this model, as shown previously in the tumor cell graft models, suggesting that IDO inhibition may produce limited antitumor efficacy when applied as a monotherapy.

In contrast, the delivery of 1MT in combination with a variety of classical cytotoxic chemo-therapeutic agents elicited regression of established MMTV-neu/HER2 tumors which responded poorly to any single-agent therapy [58]. In each case, the observed regressions were unlikely to result from a drug–drug interaction—that is, by 1MT acting to raise the effective dose of the cytotoxic agent—because efficacy was increased in the absence of increased side effects (e.g., neuropathy produced by paclitaxel, which is displayed by hind leg dragging in affected mice). Immunodepletion of CD4$^+$ or CD8$^+$ T cells from the mice before treatment abolished the combinatorial antitumor effect, confirming the expectation that 1MT acted indirectly through activation of T-cell-mediated antitumor immunity. We have observed that combinatorial effi-cacy in achieving tumor regressions can be replicated by oral dosing of 1MT at 400 mg/kg on a b.i.d. schedule, again in the absence of any detectable side effects [103]. These striking findings, while seemingly counterintuitive at the time, were a harbinger of the now popular concept of combining conventional chemotherapy with treatment modalities that interfere with mecha-nisms of tumoral immune escape as a novel approach for improving therapeutic outcomes [104,105] and helped propel 1MT onto a select list of 12 immunotherapeutic agents identified by an NCI workshop panel as having high potential for use in cancer therapy [106]. Early stage clinical trials with 1MT were initiated in 2008 and are currently ongoing.

A. Discovery and development of alternative inhibitors

IDO has a number of appealing features as a target for drug development. First, IDO is a single-chain catalytic enzyme with a well-defined biochemistry. Unlike many proposed therapeutic targets in cancer, this means that IDO is very tractable for discovery and development of small molecule inhibitors. Second, the other known tryptophan catabolizing enzyme on the kynur-enine pathway, TDO2, is structurally distinct from IDO and has a much more restricted pattern of expression and substrate specificity, which mitigates "off-target" issues usually posed by novel agents. Third, bioactive and orally bioavailable "lead" inhibitors exist which can serve as useful tools for preclinical validation studies. Fourth, the *Ido1* gene "knockout" mouse that has been constructed is viable and healthy [107], and further analysis encourages the notion that IDO

573

inhibitors will not produce unmanageable, mechanism-based toxicities [108]. Fifth, pharmacodynamic evaluation of IDO inhibitors can be performed by examining blood serum levels of tryptophan and kynurenine, the chief substrate and downstream product of the IDO reaction, respectively. Lastly, small molecule inhibitors of IDO offer logistical and cost advantages compared to biological or cell-based therapeutic alternatives to modulating T-cell immunity.

While early phase clinical trials with 1MT are currently ongoing, legitimate concerns regarding its inhibitory potency against the IDO enzyme leave open the possibility for the development of pharmacologically superior IDO inhibitory compounds. The rational design and development of new inhibitory compounds require understanding the IDO active site and catalytic mechanism. Proposed models for the processes at work in the active site have been developed based on mechanistic studies [109]. The publication of an X-ray crystal structure for IDO complexed with a simple inhibitor [29] has greatly facilitated this work. Alternately, screening for novel inhibitors is likely to identify novel structural series to evaluate. Through this route, our group initially identified the natural product brassinin as an IDO inhibitor and evaluated brassinin derivatives for *in vitro* potency and cell-based activity [110]. Brassinin is a phytoalexin-type compound found in cruciferous vegetables that has potent chemopreventative activity against breast and colon cancer in rodent models [111,112]. In order to probe the relationship between inhibitors and the active site, that is, to perform a structure-activity relationship (SAR) analysis, we synthesized a series of derivatives from the core brassinin structure [110]. Among the conclusions drawn, we determined that the indole core is not essential for enzyme inhibitory activity, consistent with the known promiscuity of the active site in IDO [39], thus broadening the spectrum of potential inhibitory compounds. In addition, we found that the dithiocarbamate segment of brassinin is an optimized moiety for inhibition, probably on the basis of chelation of the heme iron at the active site. Of the large number of derivatives evaluated, the most potent were only ~1 μM, suggesting that it may be difficult to achieve significant improvements in potency within this simple structural class.

High-throughput screening of comprehensive compound libraries remains the most effective way to identify new structural series. A unique yeast screen has been used to identify IDO inhibitory compounds representing diverse structural classes [113] including several complex natural products with potent IDO inhibitory activity [114,115]. The insight that a naphthoquininone pharmacophore might be at the core of several of the most potent IDO inhibitory compounds led us to conduct an SAR-driven study that yielded a promising series of pyranonapthoquinone-based IDO inhibitory compounds, some with inhibition constants of less than 100 nM, [116]. Similar studies based on the phenylamidazole pharmacophore have likewise yielded a series of IDO inhibitory compounds, though not achieving the degree of inhibitory potency seen with pyranonapthoquinones [117].

In 2010, a new IDO inhibitor, INCB024360, entered Phase I trials for advanced malignancies. INCB024360 is a hydrozyamidine that competitively blocks the degradation of tryptophan to kynurenine by IDO with an IC_{50} of approximately 72 nM [118]. Oral administration of this compound in mice and dogs reduced kynurenine levels in the plasma as well as in tumors and tumor draining lymph nodes [119]. Using several mouse models, INCB024360 delayed tumor growth in wildtype mice but not in nude mice or $Ido1^{-/-}$ mice, indicating not only that this drug targets IDO1 but also that it mediates its antitumor effects through the immune system [118,119]. The *in vivo* data complement *in vitro* experiments showing that INCB024360 does not inhibit IDO2 or TDO2 activity [118]. An important mechanistic observation is the ability of INCB024360 to increase the survival and decrease the apoptosis of DCs, suggesting that this drug may improve the number of functional DCs thereby allowing T cells to be more effectively primed against tumor cell antigens [118].

Possible alternative targeting strategies include inhibiting IDO expression (upstream) or inhibiting the signaling pathway through which IDO acts (downstream). As mentioned earlier, some NSAIDs have been shown to indirectly block IDO activity by inhibiting

COX2[65], and the anti-inflammatory compound, ethyl pyruvate, previously found to inhibit NF-κB activity, has been shown in mouse models to be an effective inhibitor of IDO expression and to produce robust antitumor responses that were both T-cell and IDO dependent [59]. Inadvertent targeting of IDO expression may already be providing a clinical benefit, as recent investigations into the therapeutic role of Gleevec in treating GIST found that the inhibition of oncogenic Kit signaling could potentiate antitumor T-cell responses by interfering with the induction of IDO [120]. Downstream of IDO, the integrated stress response kinase GCN2 has been identified as responding to tryptophan depletion to limit T-cell responses [121] and thus might represent an alternative target. Recent attention has also focused on the aryl hydrocarbon receptor (AhR) in mediating the downstream response to tryptophan catabolites, including kynurenine and kynurenic acid [71,73]. The liver enzyme TDO2 catalyzes the same reaction as IDO, and recent reports indicate that TDO2 elevation in some cancers may serve as an alternate mechanism for eliciting the same immune escape mechanism [72,122]. Thus, while targeting the IDO pathway has clearly been established as an attractive approach for leveraging cancer treatment, it remains to be determined how this will be translated to provide the greatest benefit to patients.

V. CONCLUSIONS

In a relatively short period, IDO has become recognized as a major regulator of the immune system. Pathophysiologically, IDO has been strongly implicated in tumoral immune tolerance and immune escape and appears to be widely overexpressed in cancer at the level of tumor cells and/or tumor-associated immune regulatory cells. IDO has a variety of characteristics that make it an appealing target for cancer drug development. To date, preclinical validation of IDO inhibitors suggests they may offer the greatest promise in combination with classical cytotoxic drugs, but their potential to heighten the response to active immunotherapeutic agents such as TLR ligands or tumor vaccines is also important to consider. Given the provocative preclinical findings that have emerged from studies of agents targeting IDO and the IDO pathway, one would expect therapeutic interest in this pathway to continue to grow.

ACKNOWLEDGMENTS

Work in the authors' laboratories is supported by the Susan G. Komen for the Cure and the W. W. Smith Foundation (A.J.M.), NIH grants R01 CA109542, R21 CA159337 and R03 CA159315 (G.C.P.), with additional support from NewLink Genetics Corporation, the Sharpe-Strumia Foundation, the Lankenau Medical Center Foundation and the Main Line Health System. C.S. is the recipient of a Postdoctoral Fellowship through the Department of Defense Breast Cancer Research Program. The authors declare competing financial interests. G.C.P. and A.J.M. are significant stockholders and G.C.P. is a member of the scientific advisory board at New Link Genetics Corporation, a biotechnology company that has licensed IDO intellectual property created by the authors, described in patents US 7,705,022, US 7,714,139 and US 8,008,281.

RECOMMENDED RESOURCES

Websites

Science Signal Transduction Virtual Journal (STKE). D.H. Munn, M.D. Sharma, J.R. Lee, K.G. Jhaver, T.S. Johnson, et al,.Potential regulatory function of human dendritic cell expressing indoleamine 2,3-dioxygenase. http://stke.sciencemag.org/cgi/content/abstract/sci;297/5588/1867.

Human Protein Reference Database. Indoleamine 2,3-dioxygenase. http://www.hprd.org/protein/00935.

SwissProt: *In silico* analysis of proteins. Indoleamine 2,3-dioxygenase. http://ca.expasy.org/uniprot/P14902.

Further Reading

Fallarino F, Puccetti P. Toll-like receptor 9-mediated induction of the immunosuppressive pathway of tryptophan catabolism. Eur. J. Immunol 2006;36:8–11. * Discusses how activation of Toll-like receptor 9 (TLR9) signaling by CpG oligonucleotides can lead to IDO activation and immunosuppression. This review highlights how IDO induction by CpG oligonucleotides may limit their potential as adjuvants for cancer therapeutics and vaccines.

Gajewski TF. Identifying and overcoming immune resistance mechanisms in the melanoma tumor microenvironment. Clin Cancer Res 2006;12:2326s–30s. *Highlights melanoma as an illustration of how immunosuppression can thwart the activity of tumor antigen-specific T cells, through the influence of T-cell anergy, CD25+ regulatory T cells, and overexpression of immune suppressive genes such as PD-L1 and IDO.

Kim, R., Emi, M., Tanabe, K., and Arihiro, K. Tumor-driven evolution of immunosuppression networks during malignant progression. Cancer Res. 66, 5527–5536 *Along with the additional information provided by Zou (2005), this review provides an excellent general overview of immune suppressive mechanisms in cancer.

Liu X, Newton RC, Friedman SM, Scherle PA. Indoleamine 2,3-dioxygenase, an emerging target for anti-cancer therapy. Curr Cancer Drug Targets 2009;9:938–52. *Along with Malachowski et al. (2005), this review focuses on the current state of medicinal chemistry development of IDO inhibitory compounds as potential pharmaceutical agents.

Malachowski WB, Metz R, Prendergast GC, Muller AJ. A new cancer immunosuppression target: indoleamine 2,3-dioxygenase (IDO). A review of the IDO mechanism, inhibition, and therapeutic applications. Drugs Fut 2005;30:897–905. * Along with Liu et al. (2009), this review focuses on the development of IDO inhibitory compounds as potential pharmaceutical agents in the context of proposed catalytic mechanisms.

Muller AJ, Scherle PA. Targeting the mechanisms of tumoral immune tolerance with small-molecule inhibitors. Nature Rev Cancer 2006;6:613–25. *General overview of the use of small molecule inhibitors of IDO and other immune suppressive targets to overcome tumoral immune tolerance for therapeutic benefit.

Munn DH. Indoleamine 2,3-dioxygenase, tumor-induced tolerance and counter-regulation. Curr Opin Immunol 2006;18:220–5. *Discusses possible consequence of IDO expression within the tumor itself versus within host stromal cells, as well as how IDO may counter pro-inflammatory signals such as those provided by IFN-γ, IFN-α, CpG oligonucleotides, and 4–1BB ligation.

Prendergast GC, Metz R, Muller AJ. Towards a genetic definition of cancer-associated inflammation: role of the IDO pathway. Am J Pathol 2010;176:2082–7. *Based on genetic evidence for the role of IDO in contributing to cancer development, discusses how genetic pathways of immune escape may be the defining properties of tumor-promoting inflammation.

Schrocksnadel K, Wirleitner B, Winkler C, Fuchs D. Monitoring tryptophan metabolism in chronic immune activation. Clin Chim Acta 2006;364:82–90. *Discusses how IDO activation in cancer and other chronic immune suppressed states may, by decreasing serum tryptophan, also affect serotonin biosynthesis, thereby contributing to impaired quality of life and depressed moods.

Zou W. Immunosuppressive networks in the tumour environment and their therapeutic relevance. Nature Rev Cancer 2005;5:263–74. *Along with the additional information provided by Kim et al. (2006), this review provides an excellent general overview of immune suppressive mechanisms in cancer.

References

[1] Prendergast GC, Jaffee EM. Cancer immunologists and cancer biologists: why we didn't talk then but need to now. Cancer Res 2007;67(8):3500–4.

[2] Melief CJ, Toes RE, Medema JP, van der Burg SH, Ossendorp F, Offringa R. Strategies for immunotherapy of cancer. Adv Immunol 2000;75:235–82.

[3] Finn OJ. Cancer vaccines: between the idea and the reality. Nat Rev Immunol 2003;3(8):630–41.

[4] Gilboa E. The promise of cancer vaccines. Nat Rev Cancer 2004;4(5):401–11.

[5] O'Neill DW, Adams S, Bhardwaj N. Manipulating dendritic cell biology for the active immunotherapy of cancer. Blood 2004;104(8):2235–46.

[6] Figdor CG, de Vries IJ, Lesterhuis WJ, Melief CJ. Dendritic cell immunotherapy: mapping the way. Nat Med 2004;10(5):475–80.

[7] Rosenberg SA, Packard BS, Aebersold PM, Solomon D, Topalian SL, Toy ST, et al. Use of tumor-infiltrating lymphocytes and interleukin-2 in the immunotherapy of patients with metastatic melanoma. A preliminary report. N Engl J Med 1988;319(25):1676–80.

[8] Dudley ME, Wunderlich JR, Robbins PF, Yang JC, Hwu P, Schwartzentruber DJ, et al. Cancer regression and autoimmunity in patients after clonal repopulation with antitumor lymphocytes. Science 2002;298(5594):850–4.

[9] Zou X, Rudchenko S, Wong K, Calame K. Induction of c-myc transcription by the v-Abl tyrosine kinase requires Ras, Raf1, and cyclin-dependent kinases. Genes and Development 1997;11:654–62.

[10] Zou W. Immunosuppressive networks in the tumour environment and their therapeutic relevance. Nat Rev Cancer 2005;5(4):263−74.

[11] Kim R, Emi M, Tanabe K, Arihiro K. Tumor-driven evolution of immunosuppressive networks during malignant progression. Cancer Res 2006;66(11):5527−36.

[12] Muller AJ, Scherle PA. Targeting the mechanisms of tumoral immune tolerance with small-molecule inhibitors. Nat Rev Cancer 2006;6(8):613−25.

[13] Muller AJ, Prendergast GC. Marrying immunotherapy with chemotherapy: why say IDO? Cancer Res 2005;65(18):8065−8.

[14] Boyland E, Williams DC. The metabolism of tryptophan. 2. The metabolism of tryptophan in patients suffering from cancer of the bladder. Biochem J 1956;64(3):578−82.

[15] Ivanova VD. [Studies on tryptophan metabolites in the blood and urine of patients with leukemia.]. Probl Gematol Pereliv Krovi 1959;4:18−21.

[16] Ivanova VD. Disorders of Tryptophan Metabolism in Leukaemia. Acta Unio Int Contra Cancrum 1964;20:1085−6.

[17] Ambanelli U, Rubino A. Some aspects of tryptophan−nicotinic acid chain in Hodgkin's disease. Relative roles of tryptophan loading and vitamin supplementation on urinary excretion of metabolites. Haematol Lat 1962;5:49−73.

[18] Chabner BA, DeVita VT, Livingston DM, Oliverio VT. Abnormalities of tryptophan metabolism and plasma pyridoxal phosphate in Hodgkin's disease. N Engl J Med 1970;282(15):838−43.

[19] Wolf H, Madsen PO, Price JM. Studies on the metabolism of tryptophan in patients with benign prostatic hypertrophy or cancer of the prostate. J Urol 1968;100(4):537−43.

[20] Rose DP. Tryptophan metabolism in carcinoma of the breast. Lancet 1967;1(7484):239−41.

[21] Kotake Y, Masayama T. Uber den mechanismus der kynurenine-bildung aus tryptophan. Hoppe-Seyler's Z Physiol Chem 1937;243:237−44.

[22] Taylor MW, Feng GS. Relationship between interferon-gamma, indoleamine 2,3-dioxygenase, and tryptophan catabolism. FASEB J 1991;5(11):2516−22.

[23] Gailani S, Murphy G, Kenny G, Nussbaum A, Silvernail P. Studies on tryptophen metabolism in patients with bladder cancer. Cancer Res 1973;33(5):1071−7.

[24] Higuchi K, Kuno S, Hayaishi O. Enzymatic formation of D-kynurenine. Federation Proc 1963;22:243 (abstr.).

[25] Higuchi K, Hayaishi O. Enzymic formation of D-kynurenine from D-tryptophan. Arch Biochem Biophys 1967;120(2):397−403.

[26] Shimizu T, Nomiyama S, Hirata F, Hayaishi O. Indoleamine 2,3-dioxygenase. Purification and some properties. J Biol Chem 1978;253(13):4700−6.

[27] Watanabe Y, Yoshida R, Sono M, Hayaishi O. Immunohistochemical localization of indoleamine 2,3-dioxygenase in the argyrophilic cells of rabbit duodenum and thyroid gland. J Histochem Cytochem 1981;29(5):623−32.

[28] Sono M. Enzyme kinetic and spectroscopic studies of inhibitor and effector interactions with indoleamine 2,3-dioxygenase. 2. Evidence for the existence of another binding site in the enzyme for indole derivative effectors. Biochemistry 1989;28(13):5400−7.

[29] Sugimoto H, Oda SI, Otsuki T, Hino T, Yoshida T, Shiro Y. Crystal structure of human indoleamine 2,3-dioxygenase: Catalytic mechanism of O2 incorporation by a heme-containing dioxygenase. Proc Natl Acad Sci USA 2006;103:2311−6.

[30] Ball HJ, Sanchez-Perez A, Weiser S, Austin CJ, Astelbauer F, Miu J, et al. Characterization of an indoleamine 2,3-dioxygenase-like protein found in humans and mice. Gene 2007;396(1):203−13.

[31] Metz R, Duhadaway JB, Kamasani U, Laury-Kleintop L, Muller AJ, Prendergast GC. Novel tryptophan catabolic enzyme IDO2 is the preferred biochemical target of the antitumor indoleamine 2,3-dioxygenase inhibitory compound D-1-methyl-tryptophan. Cancer Res 2007;67(15):7082−7.

[32] Kadoya A, Tone S, Maeda H, Minatogawa Y, Kido R. Gene structure of human indoleamine 2,3-dioxygenase. Biochem Biophys Res Commun 1992;189(1):530−6.

[33] Najfeld V, Menninger J, Muhleman D, Comings DE, Gupta SL. Localization of indoleamine 2,3-dioxygenase gene (INDO) to chromosome 8p12(-)->p11 by fluorescent in situ hybridization. Cytogenet Cell Genet 1993;64(3-4):231−2.

[34] Yuasa HJ, Ball HJ, Ho YF, Austin CJ, Whittington CM, Belov K, et al. Characterization and evolution of vertebrate indoleamine 2, 3-dioxygenases IDOs from monotremes and marsupials. Comp Biochem Physiol B Biochem Mol Biol 2009;153(2):137−44.

[35] Hayaishi O, Ryotaro Y, Takikawa O, Yasui H. Indoleamine-dioxygenase − a possible biological function. Progress in Tryptophan and Serotonin Research. Berlin: Walter De Gruyter and Co.; 1984. p. 33−42.

[36] Ozaki Y, Edelstein MP, Duch DS. Induction of indoleamine 2,3-dioxygenase: a mechanism of the antitumor activity of interferon gamma. Proc Natl Acad Sci USA 1988;85(4):1242−6.

[37] Mellor AL, Munn DH. Tryptophan catabolism and T-cell tolerance: immunosuppression by starvation? Immunol Today 1999;20:469–73.

[38] Munn DH, Shafizadeh E, Attwood JT, Bondarev I, Pashine A, Mellor AL. Inhibition of T cell proliferation by macrophage tryptophan catabolism. J Exp Med 1999;189:1363–72.

[39] Cady SG, Sono M. 1-methyl-DL-tryptophan, beta-(3-benzofuranyl)-DL-alanine (the oxygen analog of tryptophan), and beta-[3-benzo(b)thienyl]-DL-alanine (the sulfur analog of tryptophan) are competitive inhibitors for indoleamine 2,3-dioxygenase. Arch Biochem Biophys 1991;291:326–33.

[40] Munn DH, Zhou M, Attwood JT, Bondarev I, Conway SJ, Marshall B, et al. Prevention of allogeneic fetal rejection by tryptophan catabolism. Science 1998;281:1191–3.

[41] Mellor AL, Sivakumar J, Chandler P, K.S., Molina H, Mao D, et al. Prevention of T cell-driven complement activation and inflammation by tryptophan catabolism during pregnancy. Nat Immunol 2001;2:64–8.

[42] Grohmann U, Fallarino F, Puccetti P. Tolerance, DCs and tryptophan: much ado about IDO. Trends Immunol 2003;24(5):242–8.

[43] Mellor AL, Munn DH. IDO expression by dendritic cells: tolerance and tryptophan catabolism. Nat Rev Immunol 2004;4(10):762–74.

[44] Munn DH, Mellor AL. Indoleamine 2,3-dioxygenase and tumor-induced tolerance. J Clin Invest 2007;117(5):1147–54.

[45] Fallarino F, Grohmann U, You S, McGrath BC, Cavener DR, Vacca C, et al. The combined effects of tryptophan starvation and tryptophan catabolites down-regulate T cell receptor zeta-chain and induce a regulatory phenotype in naive T cells. J Immunol 2006;176(11):6752–61.

[46] Witkiewicz AK, Costantino CL, Metz R, Muller AJ, Prendergast GC, Yeo CJ, et al. Genotyping and expression analysis of IDO2 in human pancreatic cancer: a novel, active target. J Am Coll Surg 2009;208(5):781–7. discussion 7–9.

[47] Yoshida R, Imanishi J, Oku T, Kishida T, Hayaishi O. Induction of pulmonary indoleamine 2,3-dioxygenase by interferon. Proc Natl Acad Sci USA 1981;78(1):129–32.

[48] Carlin JM, Borden EC, Sondel PM, Byrne GI. Biologic-response-modifier-induced indoleamine 2,3-dioxygenase activity in human peripheral blood mononuclear cell cultures. J Immunol 1987;139(7):2414–8.

[49] Carlin JM, Borden EC, Sondel PM, Byrne GI. Interferon-induced indoleamine 2,3-dioxygenase activity in human mononuclear phagocytes. J Leukoc Biol 1989;45(1):29–34.

[50] Takikawa O, Tagawa Y, Iwakura Y, Yoshida R, Truscott RJ. Interferon-gamma-dependent/independent expression of indoleamine 2,3-dioxygenase. Studies with interferon-gamma-knockout mice. Adv Exp Med Biol 1999;467:553–7.

[51] Hwu P, Du MX, Lapointe R, Do M, Taylor MW, Young HA. Indoleamine 2,3-dioxygenase production by human dendritic cells results in the inhibition of T cell proliferation. J Immunol 2000;164(7):3596–9.

[52] Du MX, Sotero-Esteva WD, Taylor MW. Analysis of transcription factors regulating induction of indoleamine 2,3-dioxygenase by IFN-gamma. J Interferon Cytokine Res 2000;20(2):133–42.

[53] Chon SY, Hassanain HH, Pine R, Gupta SL. Involvement of two regulatory elements in interferon-gamma-regulated expression of human indoleamine 2,3-dioxygenase gene. J Interferon Cytokine Res 1995;15(6):517–26.

[54] Chon SY, Hassanain HH, Gupta SL. Cooperative role of interferon regulatory factor 1 and p91 (STAT1) response elements in interferon-gamma-inducible expression of human indoleamine 2,3-dioxygenase gene. J Biol Chem 1996;271(29):17247–52.

[55] Konan KV, Taylor MW. Importance of the two interferon-stimulated response element (ISRE) sequences in the regulation of the human indoleamine 2,3-dioxygenase gene. J Biol Chem 1996;271(32):19140–5.

[56] Robinson CM, Hale PT, Carlin JM. The role of IFN-gamma and TNF-alpha-responsive regulatory elements in the synergistic induction of indoleamine dioxygenase. J Interferon Cytokine Res 2005;25(1):20–30.

[57] Grohmann U, Volpi C, Fallarino F, Bozza S, Bianchi R, Vacca C, et al. Reverse signaling through GITR ligand enables dexamethasone to activate IDO in allergy. Nat Med 2007;13(5):579–86.

[58] Muller AJ, DuHadaway JB, Donover PS, Sutanto-Ward E, Prendergast GC. Inhibition of indoleamine 2,3-dioxygenase, an immunoregulatory target of the cancer suppression gene Bin1, potentiates cancer chemotherapy. Nat Med 2005;11(3):312–9.

[59] Muller AJ, DuHadaway JB, Jaller D, Curtis P, Metz R, Prendergast GC. Immunotherapeutic suppression of indoleamine 2,3-dioxygenase and tumor growth with ethyl pyruvate. Cancer Res 2010;70(5):1845–53.

[60] Pine R. Convergence of TNFalpha and IFNgamma signalling pathways through synergistic induction of IRF-1/ISGF-2 is mediated by a composite GAS/kappaB promoter element. Nucleic Acids Res 1997;25(21):4346–54.

[61] Mellor AL, Baban B, Chandler PR, Manlapat A, Kahler DJ, Munn DH. Cutting edge: CpG oligonucleotides induce splenic CD19+ dendritic cells to acquire potent indoleamine 2,3-dioxygenase-dependent T cell regulatory functions via IFN Type 1 signaling. J Immunol 2005;175(9):5601–5.

[62] Grohmann U, Orabona C, Fallarino F, Vacca C, Calcinaro F, Falorni A, et al. CTLA-4-Ig regulates tryptophan catabolism in vivo. Nat Immunol 2002;3(11):1097—101.

[63] Orabona C, Belladonna ML, Vacca C, Bianchi R, Fallarino F, Volpi C, et al. Cutting edge: silencing suppressor of cytokine signaling 3 expression in dendritic cells turns CD28-Ig from immune adjuvant to suppressant. J Immunol 2005;174(11):6582—6.

[64] Puccetti P, Grohmann U. IDO and regulatory T cells: a role for reverse signalling and non-canonical NF-kappaB activation. Nat Rev Immunol 2007;7(10):817—23.

[65] Sayama S, Yoshida R, Oku T, Imanishi J, Kishida T, Hayaishi O. Inhibition of interferon-mediated induction of indoleamine 2,3-dioxygenase in mouse lung by inhibitors of prostaglandin biosynthesis. Proc Natl Acad Sci USA 1981;78(12):7327—30.

[66] Rutella S, Bonanno G, Procoli A, Mariotti A, de Ritis DG, Curti A, et al. Hepatocyte growth factor favors monocyte differentiation into regulatory interleukin (IL)-10++IL-12low/neg accessory cells with dendritic-cell features. Blood 2006;108(1):218—27.

[67] Marshall B, Keskin DB, Mellor AL. Regulation of prostaglandin synthesis and cell adhesion by a tryptophan catabolizing enzyme. BMC Biochem 2001;2:5.

[68] Braun D, Longman RS, Albert ML. A two-step induction of indoleamine 2,3 dioxygenase (IDO) activity during dendritic-cell maturation. Blood 2005;106(7):2375—81.

[69] Lawrence BP, Sherr DH. You AhR what you eat? Nat Immunol 2012;13(2):117—9.

[70] Vogel CF, Goth SR, Dong B, Pessah IN, Matsumura F. Aryl hydrocarbon receptor signaling mediates expression of indoleamine 2,3-dioxygenase. Biochem Biophys Res Commun 2008;375(3):331—5.

[71] Mezrich JD, Fechner JH, Zhang X, Johnson BP, Burlingham WJ, Bradfield CA. An interaction between kynurenine and the aryl hydrocarbon receptor can generate regulatory T cells. J Immunol 2010;185(6):3190—8.

[72] Opitz CA, Litzenburger UM, Sahm F, Ott M, Tritschler I, Trump S, et al. An endogenous tumour-promoting ligand of the human aryl hydrocarbon receptor. Nature 2011;478(7368):197—203.

[73] DiNatale BC, Murray IA, Schroeder JC, Flaveny CA, Lahoti TS, Laurenzana EM, et al. Kynurenic acid is a potent endogenous aryl hydrocarbon receptor ligand that synergistically induces interleukin-6 in the presence of inflammatory signaling. Toxicol Sci 2010;115(1):89—97.

[74] Smith C, Chang MY, Parker KH, Beury DW, DuHadaway JB, Flick HE, et al. IDO is a nodal pathogenic driver of lung cancer and metastasis development July 19, 2012:2159—8290. Cancer Discovery, 10.1158/2159—8290.CD-12-0014.

[75] Fujigaki S, Saito K, Takemura M, Maekawa N, Yamada Y, Wada H, et al. L-tryptophan-L-kynurenine pathway metabolism accelerated by Toxoplasma gondii infection is abolished in gamma interferon-gene-deficient mice: cross-regulation between inducible nitric oxide synthase and indoleamine-2,3-dioxygenase. Infect Immun 2002;70(2):779—86.

[76] Fujigaki H, Saito K, Lin F, Fujigaki S, Takahashi K, Martin BM, et al. Nitration and inactivation of IDO by peroxynitrite. J Immunol 2006;176(1):372—9.

[77] Chiarugi A, Rovida E, Dello Sbarba P, Moroni F. Tryptophan availability selectively limits NO-synthase induction in macrophages. J Leukoc Biol 2003;73(1):172—7.

[78] Alberati-Giani D, Malherbe P, Ricciardi-Castagnoli P, Kohler C, Denis-Donini S, Cesura AM. Differential regulation of indoleamine 2,3-dioxygenase expression by nitric oxide and inflammatory mediators in IFN-gamma-activated murine macrophages and microglial cells. J Immunol 1997;159(1):419—26.

[79] Daubener W, Posdziech V, Hadding U, MacKenzie CR. Inducible anti-parasitic effector mechanisms in human uroepithelial cells: tryptophan degradation vs. NO production. Med Microbiol Immunol (Berl) 1999;187(3):143—7.

[80] Thomas SR, Mohr D, Stocker R. Nitric oxide inhibits indoleamine 2,3-dioxygenase activity in interferon-gamma primed mononuclear phagocytes. J Biol Chem 1994;269(20):14457—64.

[81] Hucke C, MacKenzie CR, Adjogble KD, Takikawa O, Daubener W. Nitric oxide-mediated regulation of gamma interferon-induced bacteriostasis: inhibition and degradation of human indoleamine 2,3-dioxygenase. Infect Immun 2004;72(5):2723—30.

[82] Samelson-Jones BJ, Yeh SR. Interactions between nitric oxide and indoleamine 2,3-dioxygenase. Biochemistry 2006;45(28):8527—38.

[83] Fallarino F, Bianchi R, Orabona C, Vacca C, Belladonna ML, Fioretti MC, et al. CTLA-4-Ig activates forkhead transcription factors and protects dendritic cells from oxidative stress in nonobese diabetic mice. J Exp Med 2004;200(8):1051—62.

[84] Yoeli-Lerner M, Toker A. Akt/PKB signaling in cancer: a function in cell motility and invasion. Cell Cycle 2006;5(6):603—5.

[85] Yuan W, Collado-Hidalgo A, Yufit T, Taylor M, Varga J. Modulation of cellular tryptophan metabolism in human fibroblasts by transforming growth factor-beta: selective inhibition of indoleamine 2,3-dioxygenase and tryptophanyl-tRNA synthetase gene expression. J Cell Physiol 1998;177(1):174—86.

[86] Belladonna ML, Volpi C, Bianchi R, Vacca C, Orabona C, Pallotta MT, et al. Cutting edge: Autocrine TGF-beta sustains default tolerogenesis by IDO-competent dendritic cells. J Immunol 2008;181(8):5194–8.

[87] Belladonna ML, Grohmann U, Guidetti P, Volpi C, Bianchi R, Fioretti MC, et al. Kynurenine pathway enzymes in dendritic cells initiate tolerogenesis in the absence of functional IDO. J Immunol 2006;177(1):130–7.

[88] Belladonna ML, Orabona C, Grohmann U, Puccetti P. TGF-beta and kynurenines as the key to infectious tolerance. Trends Mol Med 2009;15(2):41–9.

[89] Liu X, Newton RC, Friedman SM, Scherle PA. Indoleamine 2,3-dioxygenase, an emerging target for anti-cancer therapy. Curr Cancer Drug Targets 2009;9(8):938–52.

[90] Friberg M, Jennings R, Alsarraj M, Dessureault S, Cantor A, Extermann M, et al. Indoleamine 2,3-dioxygenase contributes to tumor cell evasion of T cell-mediated rejection. Int J Cancer 2002;101(2):151–5.

[91] Uyttenhove C, Pilotte L, Theate I, Stroobant V, Colau D, Parmentier N, et al. Evidence for a tumoral immune resistance mechanism based on tryptophan degradation by indoleamine 2,3-dioxygenase. Nat Med 2003;9(10):1269–74.

[92] Johnson 3rd BA, Kahler DJ, Baban B, Chandler PR, Kang B, Shimoda M, et al. B-lymphoid cells with attributes of dendritic cells regulate T cells via indoleamine 2,3-dioxygenase. Proc Natl Acad Sci USA 2010;107(23):10644–8.

[93] Munn DH, Sharma MD, Hou D, Baban B, Lee JR, Antonia SJ, et al. Expression of indoleamine 2,3-dioxygenase by plasmacytoid dendritic cells in tumor-draining lymph nodes. J Clin Invest 2004;114(2):280–90.

[94] Muller AJ, Sharma MD, Chandler PR, Duhadaway JB, Everhart ME, Johnson 3rd BA, et al. Chronic inflammation that facilitates tumor progression creates local immune suppression by inducing indoleamine 2,3 dioxygenase. Proc Natl Acad Sci USA 2008;105(44):17073–8.

[95] Dunn GP, Old LJ, Schreiber RD. The immunobiology of cancer immunosurveillance and immunoediting. Immunity 2004;21(2):137–48.

[96] Willimsky G, Czeh M, Loddenkemper C, Gellermann J, Schmidt K, Wust P, et al. Immunogenicity of premalignant lesions is the primary cause of general cytotoxic T lymphocyte unresponsiveness. J Exp Med 2008;205(7):1687–700.

[97] Muller AJ, Duhadaway JB, Chang MY, Ramalingam A, Sutanto-Ward E, Boulden J, et al. Non-hematopoietic expression of IDO is integrally required for inflammatory tumor promotion. Cancer Immunol Immunother 2010;59(11):1655–63.

[98] Kita H, Shiraishi Y, Watanabe K, Suda K, Ohtsuka K, Koshiishi Y, et al. Does postoperative serum interleukin-6 influence early recurrence after curative pulmonary resection of lung cancer? Ann Thorac Cardiovasc Surg 2011;17(5):454–60.

[99] Pertovaara M, Hasan T, Raitala A, Oja SS, Yli-Kerttula U, Korpela M, et al. Indoleamine 2,3-dioxygenase activity is increased in patients with systemic lupus erythematosus and predicts disease activation in the sunny season. Clin Exp Immunol 2007;150(2):274–8.

[100] Schroecksnadel K, Winkler C, Duftner C, Wirleitner B, Schirmer M, Fuchs D. Tryptophan degradation increases with stage in patients with rheumatoid arthritis. Clin Rheumatol 2006;25(3):334–7.

[101] Mandik-Nayak L, Allen PM. Initiation of an autoimmune response: insights from a transgenic model of rheumatoid arthritis. Immunol Res 2005;32(1-3):5–13.

[102] Scott GN, DuHadaway J, Pigott E, Ridge N, Prendergast GC, Muller AJ, et al. The immunoregulatory enzyme IDO paradoxically drives B cell-mediated autoimmunity. J Immunol 2009;182(12):7509–17.

[103] Hou DY, Muller AJ, Sharma MD, DuHadaway J, Banerjee T, Johnson M, et al. Inhibition of indoleamine 2,3-dioxygenase in dendritic cells by stereoisomers of 1-methyl-tryptophan correlates with antitumor responses. Cancer Res 2007;67(2):792–801.

[104] Peggs KS, Segal NH, Allison JP. Targeting immunosupportive cancer therapies: accentuate the positive, eliminate the negative. Cancer Cell 2007;12(3):192–9.

[105] Ramakrishnan R, Antonia S, Gabrilovich DI. Combined modality immunotherapy and chemotherapy: a new perspective. Cancer Immunol Immunother 2008;57(10):1523–9.

[106] Cheever MA. Twelve immunotherapy drugs that could cure cancers. Immunol Rev 2008;222:357–68.

[107] Baban B, Chandler P, McCool D, Marshall B, Munn DH, Mellor AL. Indoleamine 2,3-dioxygenase expression is restricted to fetal trophoblast giant cells during murine gestation and is maternal genome specific. J Reprod Immunol 2004;61(2):67–77.

[108] Chang MY, Smith C, Duhadaway JB, Pyle JR, Boulden J, Peralta Soler A, et al. Cardiac and gastrointestinal liabilities caused by deficiency in the immune modulatory enzyme indoleamine 2,3-dioxygenase. Cancer Biol Ther 2011;12(12).

[109] Malachowski WP, Metz R, Prendergast GC, Muller AJ. A new cancer immunosuppression target: indoleamine 2,3-dioxygenase (IDO). A review of the IDO mechanism, inhibition, and therapeutic applications. Drugs Fut 2005;30:897–813.

[110] Gaspari P, Banerjee T, Malachowski WP, Muller AJ, Prendergast GC, Duhadaway J, et al. Structure-activity study of brassinin derivatives as indoleamine 2,3-dioxygenase inhibitors. J Med Chem 2006;49(2):684—92.

[111] Mehta RG, Liu J, Constantinou A, Thomas CF, Hawthorne M, You M, et al. Cancer chemopreventive activity of brassinin, a phytoalexin from cabbage. Carcinogenesis 1995;16(2):399—404.

[112] Park EJ, Pezzuto JM. Botanicals in cancer chemoprevention. Cancer Metastasis Rev 2002;21(3-4):231—55.

[113] Vottero E, Balgi A, Woods K, Tugendreich S, Melese T, Andersen RJ, et al. Inhibitors of human indoleamine 2,3-dioxygenase identified with a target-based screen in yeast. Biotech J 2006;1:282—8.

[114] Brastianos HC, Vottero E, Patrick BO, Van Soest R, Matainaho T, Mauk AG, et al. Exiguamine A, an indole-amine-2,3-dioxygenase (IDO) inhibitor isolated from the marine sponge Neopetrosia exigua. J Am Chem Soc 2006;128(50):16046—7.

[115] Pereira A, Vottero E, Roberge M, Mauk AG, Andersen RJ. Indoleamine 2,3-dioxygenase inhibitors from the Northeastern Pacific Marine Hydroid Garveia annulata. J Nat Prod 2006;69(10):1496—9.

[116] Kumar S, Malachowski WP, Duhadaway JB, Lalonde JM, Carroll PJ, Jaller D, et al. Indoleamine 2,3-Dioxygenase Is the Anticancer Target for a Novel Series of Potent Naphthoquinone-Based Inhibitors. J Med Chem 2008;51(6):1706—18.

[117] Kumar S, Jaller D, Patel B, LaLonde JM, DuHadaway JB, Malachowski WP, et al. Structure based development of phenylimidazole-derived inhibitors of indoleamine 2,3-dioxygenase. J Med Chem 2008;51(16):4968—77.

[118] Liu X, Shin N, Koblish HK, Yang G, Wang Q, Wang K, et al. Selective inhibition of IDO1 effectively regulates mediators of antitumor immunity. Blood 2010;115(17):3520—30.

[119] Koblish HK, Hansbury MJ, Bowman KJ, Yang G, Neilan CL, Haley PJ, et al. Hydroxyamidine inhibitors of indoleamine-2,3-dioxygenase potently suppress systemic tryptophan catabolism and the growth of IDO-expressing tumors. Mol Cancer Ther 2010;9(2):489—98.

[120] Balachandran VP, Cavnar MJ, Zeng S, Bamboat ZM, Ocuin LM, Obaid H, et al. Imatinib potentiates anti-tumor T cell responses in gastrointestinal stromal tumor through the inhibition of Ido. Nat Med 2011;17(9):1094—100.

[121] Munn DH, Sharma MD, Baban B, Harding HP, Zhang Y, Ron D, et al. GCN2 kinase in T cells mediates proliferative arrest and anergy induction in response to indoleamine 2,3-dioxygenase. Immunity 2005;22(5):633—42.

[122] Pilotte L, Larrieu P, Stroobant V, Colau D, Dolusic E, Frederick R, et al. Reversal of tumoral immune resistance by inhibition of tryptophan 2,3-dioxygenase. Proc Natl Acad Sci USA 2012;109(7):2497—502.

CHAPTER 33

IDO Pathway: Effect on Foxp3+ Tregs and Cancer

David H. Munn[1], Andrew L. Mellor[2]
[1]Cancer Immunotherapy Program and Department of Pediatrics, Medical College of Georgia, Georgia Health Sciences University, Augusta, GA USA
[2]Immunotherapy Center and Department of Medicine, Medical College of Georgia, Georgia Health Sciences University, Augusta, GA USA

I. INTRODUCTION

Tumors acquire numerous potentially antigenic mutations as they develop [1]. The immune system plays an important surveillance role in detecting and eliminating these malignant cells as they arise. This means that in order to grow, tumors must evade the host immune response [2]. In essence, the host immune system must be rendered functionally tolerant to tumor-associated antigens. A phenomenon as complex as systemic tolerance cannot be orchestrated simply by a few random genetic mutations in the tumor cells; rather, the tumor must enlist the natural array of host regulatory pathways that already exist in the immune system, and co-opt them to create tolerance to itself.

Of these natural tolerogenic mechanisms, one of the most potent and far-reaching is the Foxp3+ regulatory T-cell (Treg) system [3]. Tregs are an essential component of self-tolerance, as witness the rapid onset of autoimmune disorders when Tregs are artificially ablated. Therefore, it is not surprising that tumors recruit Tregs to the site of the developing tumor [4], activate these Tregs for suppressive function [5], and use Tregs to shield the tumor from immune attack [6]. However, Tregs do not function in isolation: they depend on additional control signals from the immune system to instruct resting Tregs when to become suppressive, how suppressive to be, and even (in the case of inducible Tregs) whether naïve CD4 T cells should differentiate into new Tregs. Thus, in order to understand how tumors exploit the Treg system, it is necessary to understand how tumors enlist and manipulate these upstream pathways that control Treg function. This chapter considers the role of the indoleamine 2,3-dioxygenase (IDO) pathway as a regulator of Treg function, and how IDO interacts with other regulatory pathways in the tumor microenvironment.

II. IDO IS A NATURAL MECHANISM OF PERIPHERAL TOLERANCE

IDO is a molecular mechanism in the innate immune system that contributes to immune regulation in several important settings [7]. The IDO pathway includes two closely-related genes, IDO1 and IDO2 [8,9], both of which catalyze the degradation of tryptophan along the kynurenine pathway. (In this chapter, we will use the term "IDO" to include both genes, unless otherwise specified.) The tryptophan depletion produced by IDO activates the GCN2 kinase pathway [10], a stress-response pathway sensitive to depletion of amino acids. GCN2 activation inhibits effector cell proliferation and differentiation, and biases naive CD4+ T cells toward Treg differentiation [10,11]. The kynurenine metabolites produced by IDO bind to the

583

Cancer Immunotherapy. http://dx.doi.org/10.1016/B978-0-12-394296-8.00033-6

aryl hydrocarbon receptor (AhR) [12], which can promote both Treg differentiation [12] and generation of immunosuppressive DCs [13].

The IDO pathway is not primarily a regulator of constitutive self-tolerance; rather, it is a selective pathway that contributes to local control of inflammation, and participates in creation of acquired peripheral tolerance. Thus, for example, IDO is expressed in the placenta during gestation, and mice treated with an IDO-inhibitor drug spontaneously reject genetically disparate fetuses (i.e., they fail to become tolerant to fetal alloantigens) [14–16]. In experimental models of acquired peripheral tolerance, pharmacologic or genetic ablation of IDO prevents induction of mucosal tolerance [17,18], tolerance created by CTLA–4-Ig or CD40 blockade [19–22], and other forms of induced peripheral tolerance [23,24]. Tissue allografts engineered to overexpress the IDO gene are accepted across full haplo-mismatched MHC barriers without additional immunosuppression [22,25,26]. Thus, the IDO pathway is able to create tolerance *de novo* in certain settings, and participates as a downstream suppressive mechanism in tolerance created by several other mechanisms.

Conversely, blocking or ablating endogenous IDO makes autoimmunity and inflammation markedly worse. Ablating IDO in mouse models of graft-versus-host disease increases lethality [27,28]. Similarly, ablating or blocking IDO in models of autoimmunity [29–32] or chronic infection [33,34] markedly increases inflammation and exacerbates disease severity. Finally, blocking IDO in splenic marginal-zone macrophages prevents the immune system from creating tolerance to self antigens taken up with apoptotic cells, leading to development of a lethal lupus-like autoimmunity [35]. Thus, taken together, these studies implicate IDO as an important natural mechanism of acquired peripheral tolerance. It is therefore perhaps not surprising that the IDO pathway is induced in host cells by many types of tumors.

III. IDO EXPRESSION IN HUMAN TUMORS AND TUMOR-DRAINING LNS

In tumor-bearing hosts, IDO can either be expressed directly by the tumor cells themselves, or induced indirectly in host cells by the presence of tumor. In the former setting, IDO expression by tumor cells has been demonstrated in malignant melanoma [36,37], pancreatic cancer [38,39], ovarian cancer [40,41], acute myelogenous leukemia [42–44], colorectal cancer [45,46], prostate cancer [47] and others [48–51]. In a number of these reports, expression of IDO by the tumor has been associated with significantly worse clinical outcomes. The mechanism of this association is not yet known, but it is tempting to speculate that at least part of the effect is immunologic. (As one caveat, however, it is also possible that there might be an autocrine tumor-promoting effect of IDO, e.g., via endogenous kynurenine production [52].)

IDO can also be expressed by cells of the host immune system that are associated with tumors. In sentinel LNs draining human malignant melanoma, IDO-expressing cells with a plasmacytoid morphology are frequently seen [53,54], and many of these IDO[+] cells have been shown to express BDCA2, a marker of human plasmacytoid dendritic cells [55]. In other studies, IDO has been found in human tumor-associated macrophages [56] and tumor-associated DCs [41,57]. In the absence of tumors, IDO would not normally be expressed by the DCs or macrophages in these locations, so the presence of tumor appears to actively induce or recruit IDO-expressing antigen-presenting cells. The mechanism of this induction/recruitment is not known, but may be related to similar recruitment in mouse tumor models [4].

If tumors induce expression of IDO in host APCs, this raises the question of whether these cells participate functionally in creating tolerance to the tumor. Host APCs (dendritic cells) are key regulators of the immune response to tumors, because the initial encounter of resting T cells with tumor antigen occurs primarily through cross presentation on host DCs [58,59]. Thus, it becomes critical whether this cross presentation is immunizing or tolerizing. In other contexts, DCs that express IDO have been shown to be tolerogenic [17], and the IDO+ DCs isolated from mouse tumor-draining LNs suppress T-cell proliferation *in vitro*, and create antigen-specific anergy *in vivo* [10,54]. Thus, it is not unreasonable to speculate that IDO may contribute to the tolerogenic activity of DCs in tumor-bearing hosts. It is fairly easy to envision how IDO might create local immune suppression, but an unresolved key question is whether IDO promotes systemic tolerance.

IV. IDO AND TREGS

A. Tregs and cancer

One mechanism by which IDO may contribute to systemic tolerance is via activation of the Tregs system [17,60]. In cancer, Tregs are a potent component of tumor-induced immune suppression (and thus a major impediment to successful immunotherapy). Tumors have been found to activate local Tregs for immune suppression within a few days of tumor emergence [5]. By the time a growing tumor has been in place for 4–5 days it becomes highly resistant to immunotherapy, due in large part to Treg-mediated immunosuppression [6]. In hosts with established tumors, antitumor CD8+ T-cell responses may be weak or nonexistent unless Tregs are first depleted [61]. These observations are based on mouse models, but analogous findings appear to occur in humans as well [62]. Thus, if IDO-expressing APCs were to expand or activate tumor-associated Tregs then this might be a potent suppressive pathway in malignancy.

B. IDO drives inducible Tregs

IDO can influence naive CD4+ T cells to differentiate into new ("inducible") Foxp3+ Tregs. This was first demonstrated by Fallarino and colleagues, using mouse CD4+ T cells activated in the presence of IDO-expressing DCs [11]. The role of IDO+ DCs could be replaced by culture conditions of low tryptophan and high downstream kynurenine metabolites (to simulate the biochemical effects of IDO). Similar effects were seen when mouse CD4+ T cells were activated in the presence of IDO+ DCs from tumor-draining LNs [63]. *In vivo*, IDO expression by CD103+ DCs in the gut was required for *de novo* generation of Tregs from naive CD4+ T cells in the gut [17]. In the human system, plasmacytoid DCs (sorted from peripheral blood) upregulate IDO *in vitro* when they are activated with CpG oligonucleotides [64] or infected with HIV [65]. In both of these models, the IDO+ pDCs induce differentiation of CD4+ cells into Foxp3+ Treg-like cells. Similar findings have been reported using human monocyte-derived DCs [66,67]. Thus, IDO is able to drive differentiation of inducible Tregs from naive CD4+ T cells.

However, in tumors the role of inducible Tregs is still somewhat controversial. In mice, tumors may drive the conversion of naive CD4+ cells into Tregs [68–71], and presumably this is the mechanism by which Tregs arise against unique, tumor-specific neo-antigens [72]. However, it is not yet clear to what extent such *de novo* generation of Tregs represents a major route by which tumors enlist Tregs, or whether most tumor-associated Tregs are simply the natural pool of Tregs recruited, activated (and perhaps expanded) by the tumor. More research is needed to define the antigen specificity and origins of tumor-associated Tregs [73,74]. However, one recent finding that may be important in this regard is that even thymically-derived (natural) Tregs will still undergo extensive activation and expansion in the periphery, in response to encounter with cognate antigen [75,76].

This latter observation raises an important point. While the original commitment to the Treg lineage may have occurred in the thymus, the actual functional properties of Tregs may be controlled by local conditions in peripheral tissues—such as those created by the tumor.

C. IDO activates pre-existing mature Tregs

One key point at which Tregs could be regulated by tumors might be the step of functional activation. This terminal activation step has been less well studied than the initial Treg differentiation process [77], but it is clear that some such activation step must be necessary because resting (unactivated) Tregs are not spontaneously suppressive. Quiescent Tregs isolated from noninflamed tissues typically require some form of activation signal before they become suppressive *in vitro*; this signal may be TCR cross-linking, artificial mitogen or cognate antigen [78]. *In vivo*, the physiologic signals that activate Tregs are less clear, but for self-reactive Tregs may be provided by cognate antigen in tissues [75,76,79,80]. Additional activation signals may be delivered to Tregs by innate inflammation, since in one model Tregs required migration into inflamed tissues in order to acquire full effector function [81]. At the molecular level, maturation of suppressive function may involve transcription factors such as Blimp−1 and IRF4 [82], although this is still a subject of active investigation.

How tumors activate the suppressive function of resting Tregs is currently incompletely understood. However, it is clear that highly activated Tregs rapidly appear in growing tumors [5]. The Tregs isolated from mouse tumor-draining LNs are constitutively pre-activated for *in vitro* suppression, without requiring any additional signals [63]. Similar Treg activation appears to occur in human tumors as well [83]. Thus, by some mechanism, tumors activate Treg function.

We have previously shown that plasmacytoid DCs isolated from tumor-draining LNs are able to potently activate the suppressor function of resting Tregs *in vitro*, in an IDO-dependent fashion [63]. This was a direct activation, occurring within hours and affecting mature pre-existing Tregs (not a long-term process involving cell division and differentiation of new Tregs). The resulting IDO-activated Tregs were potent, showing suppression of effector cells at very low Treg: Teff ratios (<1:100). Mechanistically, the form of suppression elicited by IDO was characterized by a strict dependence on PD1/PD-ligand binding and lack of dependence on IL-10 and TGFβ during the effector phase [63], which distinguishes IDO-induced Treg activation from other forms of Treg-mediated suppression.

In vivo, the Tregs isolated from mouse tumor-draining LNs displayed a similar potent, constitutive suppressor activity. Consistent with the high levels of IDO present in these draining LNs, most of the suppressor activity in tumor-activated Tregs occurred via the characteristic PD−1-dependent effector mechanism (i.e., the same characteristic mechanism elicited by IDO *in vitro*) [63]. This IDO-induced/PD-1-dependent component of Treg activation was selectively lost in IDO1−KO mice, or in mice treated with the IDO-pathway inhibitor drug D-1MT. (Other forms of Treg-mediated suppression requiring IL−10 and TGFβ were still present, but the IDO-induced component of Treg activity was lost.) This characteristic IDO--induced Treg activation was not confined only to the tumor system, because IDO-activated Tregs with identical characteristics could be elicited in mice treated *in vivo* with IDO-inducing ligands [60]. Just as with tumors, the IDO-induced component of Treg activation was selectively lost in IDO1-KO mice, or when mice were treated with the D-1MT. Thus, IDO can directly activate the suppressor function of mature, pre-existing Tregs. While IDO is only one of several pathways by which Tregs may become activated, the particular IDO-induced form of Treg activation is very potent, and, in the models studied, appears to be a major component of the Treg activation elicited tumors.

D. IDO stabilizes the suppressive Treg phenotype and inhibits reprogramming

In addition to enhancing functional suppression, IDO can also stabilize the phenotype of Tregs and prevent their loss of suppressor activity under inflammatory conditions (a phenomenon sometimes termed plasticity or "reprogramming"). There is some controversy in the literature regarding the degree to which Tregs are able to alter their phenotype and change into pro-inflammatory effector cells. Two seemingly contradictory sets of observations have been described. One set of studies suggests that Tregs may be more plastic than previously thought [84]: e.g., when Tregs are transferred into lymphopenic hosts a substantial fraction may lose their suppressor phenotype and acquire a pro-inflammatory "helper-like" phenotype or become pathogenic effector cells [85,86]; and several different pro-inflammatory stimuli have been shown to drive Treg reprogramming *in vivo* [87–89]. However, these models examined abnormal or pathogenic states (lymphopenia, sepsis, autoimmunity), and the reprogrammed Tregs had lost their expression of Foxp3. In contrast to these studies, several genetic tracking studies have suggested that true, lineage-committed Tregs almost never lose expression of Foxp3 [90,91], and the authors of these studies concluded that the apparent loss of Foxp3 may represent uncommitted (non-Treg) cells with transient ectopic expression of Foxp3, rather than reprogramming of committed Tregs [91]. It is somewhat unclear to what degree these differences may relate to the experimental conditions under which the Tregs are studied [92].

To help resolve some of these apparent contradictions, we asked whether Tregs might undergo a change in functional attributes (loss of suppression and gain of pro-inflammatory function) but without any loss of Foxp3 expression. Using an *in vitro* model, we found that many Tregs exposed to the pro-inflammatory combination of antigen-activated effector T cells plus TLR-activated DCs underwent extensive upregulation of inflammatory (T-helper) molecules (CD40L, IL–2, IL17 and TNFα) [93]. A contribution from both the activated effector cells and the activated DCs was required for conversion of Tregs, which was dependent on IL–6 production by the DCs. Importantly, the Treg expression of Foxp3 remained unchanged despite the marked alteration in Treg phenotype and function. Similar inflammation-induced conversion of Tregs was observed *in vivo* in response to vaccination [94], and this likewise occurred without loss of Foxp3. Functionally, these converted ("reprogrammed") Tregs not only lost regulatory attributes but also supplied helper activity essential for the initial priming of naive hosts to a new cross-presented antigen [94]. Thus, alteration in Treg phenotype, with biologically important consequences, can occur under pro-inflammatory settings such as in vaccine-draining LNs.

When this Treg reprogramming pathway was studied in mice with tumors, the Tregs in tumor-draining LNs proved highly resistant to conversion following vaccination, and remained in their suppressive phenotype [94]. This lack of Treg reprogramming resulted in sustained suppression and a deficiency in CD40L-mediated helper activity, and consequent poor responses to vaccination and endogenous tumor antigens. Treg reprogramming could be restored if vaccinated hosts were treated with IDO-inhibitor drugs *in vivo* [94]. The ability of IDO to suppress Treg reprogramming during activation was confirmed using *in vitro* culture systems. In other experimental systems (using IDO induction *in vivo* via mechanisms other than tumors), a similar effect of IDO on Treg reprogramming was seen: i.e., rapid acquisition of a T-helper phenotype by Tregs in response to TLR9 ligands was blocked when IDO was active [60]. Mechanistically, IDO appeared to exert its effects on Treg reprogramming at least in part by antagonizing the production of IL–6 by DCs [60,93]. IL–6 is known to drive the differentiation of pro-inflammatory TH17 cells, and it can also drive reprogramming of Foxp3⁺ Tregs into IL–17-expressing cells *in vitro* [95,96] and perhaps *in vivo* [97,98]. IDO has been shown to suppress IL–6 production both *in vitro* and *in vivo* [33,60,93]. The mechanism by which IDO suppresses IL–6 is not fully elucidated, but may include its effect on the transcription factor NF–IL6 (CEBPβ) [8,93].

V. DOWNSTREAM MECHANISMS OF IDO

A. Effects of IDO mediated via GCN2 kinase

IDO degrades the amino acid tryptophan, thus depriving the IDO-expressing cells (and any neighboring cells in close contact) of an essential nutrient. Cells have sensing mechanisms to detect deficiency in any amino acid, thus allowing them to transiently suspend noncritical protein synthesis and coordinate a recovery response. One such amino-acid sensing mechanism is the kinase known as GCN2 [99]. GCN2 contains a regulatory domain that binds transfer-RNA (tRNA) when not charged with an amino acid (as would occur when the level of cognate amino acid became insufficient for charging). When GCN2 binds uncharged tRNA this activates the GCN2 kinase domain, which phosphorylates the ribosomal initiation factor eIF2α [100]. In its phosphorylated configuration, p-eIF2α prevents the translation of most mRNA species; however, it selectively increases translation of small number of mRNAs that contain a specific IRES sequence [101]. These targeted mRNAs include transcription factors such as ATF4 and other genes involved in compensation responses to the inciting stress [100]. Selective translation of these transcripts orchestrate a cellular response to protect and recover from the nutrient deficiency or other stress [102]. Tryptophan deprivation created by IDO activates this GCN2-mediated stress-response pathway in affected cells.

In T cells, GCN2 serves as one of the signaling pathways mediating response to IDO. CD8$^+$ T cells appear highly sensitive to IDO-induced activation of GCN2 [103], which in these cells causes cell cycle arrest and induction of anergy [10,104,105]. CD8$^+$ T cells that lack GCN2 are resistant to many (although not all) effects of IDO. The ability to suppress T-cell activation via GCN2 is not unique to the IDO/tryptophan pathway: similar GCN2-mediated effects occur when T cells are deprived of arginine by cells expressing the enzyme arginase (such as tumor-associated macrophages and myeloid-derived suppressor cells) [106]. Within the immune system, the effects of GCN2 are cell-type specific. While GCN2 causes cell-cycle arrest and anergy in CD8$^+$ T cells, in CD4$^+$ cells it appears to primarily affect differentiation [107]. Thus, pharmacologic activation of GCN2 using the drug halofuginone blocks the differentiation of naive T cells into TH17 cells [108], while activation of GCN2 during CD4 differentiation upregulates Foxp3 and helps bias the cells to become Tregs [11]. In mature Tregs, the ability of IDO to trigger enhanced suppressor activity is lost in GCN2-deficient Tregs, suggesting that GCN2-mediated signals are important for IDO-induced Treg functional activation as well [63].

Hence, the IDO pathway functions as a selective signaling mechanism, rather than a general response to nutrient "starvation." It remains to be elucidated whether the GCN2 pathway is more responsive (or responds differently) to certain specific amino acids such as tryptophan and arginine. For example, T cells activated in medium lacking isoleucine/leucine entered S-phase before eventual metabolic arrest, whereas T cells activated in tryptophan-free medium failed to enter S-phase at all [104], suggesting that access to particular amino acids may be an essential checkpoint for S-phase entry by T cells.

To date, most studies of amino-acid withdrawal created by IDO have focused on the GCN2 pathway. However, amino-acid deficiency might also affect signaling via the mTOR pathway. mTOR is an important regulator of immune responses, including responses by Tregs [109–111]. At present little is known about the effects (if any) that IDO may have on the mTOR pathway. However, this area is worth investigating, because IDO, arginase, and other enzymes that degrade amino acids might affect mTOR as well as GCN2 [112].

B. Effects of IDO mediated via kynurenine

In addition to depleting tryptophan, IDO generates a series of bioactive downstream metabolites along the kynurenine pathway. Kynurenine metabolites have suppressive effects on inflammation and immune responses in a variety of experimental models [33,113,114]. The cellular receptor for these compounds has previously been elusive, but recent evidence now implicates the aryl hydrocarbon receptor (AhR). AhR is a ligand-activated transcription factor that responds to toxic xenobiotics such as dioxin, but also responds to a suite of natural endogenous and exogenous ligands with potent biologic effects on immunologic function [115–117]. AhR-mediated signaling is important for normal immune development and function [118,119]. Depending on the ligands and conditions, AhR signaling can promote either Treg differentiation [120] or TH17 development [121]. Kynurenine is a natural ligand for the AhR, and in T cells, binding of kynurenine to the AhR drives upregulation of Foxp3 and differentiation of inducible Tregs [12]. This is consistent with the known role of kynurenine-pathway metabolites in helping drive Treg differentiation *in vitro* and *in vivo* [11,31]. The AhR is also expressed in DCs [13], and kynurenine metabolites can drive an immunosuppressive/tolerogenic DCs phenotype [122]. Biologically, tryptophan/kynurenine metabolites appear to act as an important immunomodulatory pathway in settings as diverse as HIV [114], tuberculosis [113] and autoimmunity [31]. This pathway has now been implicated in the immunobiology of tumors as well [52]. Additional research will be needed to elucidate the specific role of the kynurenine/AhR pathway in differentiation and activation of Tregs in tumor-bearing hosts.

C. Cell-intrinsic effects of IDO in the APCs

Finally, an important but neglected pathway is the cell-intrinsic (autocrine) effect of IDO on the IDO-expressing APCs themselves. Logically, the cell that is most exposed to low tryptophan and high kynurenine is the cell that expresses the IDO, so autocrine effects would be expected. The existence of such effects was originally implied by the observation that brief (overnight) treatment of mouse DCs *in vitro* with an IDO inhibitor drug could cause long-lasting change in their subsequent immunogenicity *in vivo* (e.g., converting them from tolerogenic to immunogenic after adoptive transfer) [123]. An effect of IDO on the phenotype of human DCs has also been reported [124]. Such autocrine/paracrine effects might be mediated via GCN2 or kynurenine metabolites (or both), since DCs are affected by both pathways [13,125]. In addition, a recent study suggests that the IDO molecule in DCs can itself bind directly to intracellular regulatory molecules such as SHP1 and SOCS3, thus participating as part of a signaling complex to maintain a TGFβ-induced tolerogenic DC phenotype [126]. At present it is unknown how these various autocrine effects of IDO may alter the properties of an IDO⁺ APC when it interacts with Tregs, but it seems likely that there is an impact.

VI. INDUCTION OF IDO BY TREGS

The previous sections of this chapter have focused on the ways in which IDO can activate Tregs. But the converse pathway may also play an important immunoregulatory role: Tregs can activate IDO. This response was originally described by Fallarino and colleagues, who showed that when the CTLA−4 molecule expressed on Tregs binds to B7 molecules (CD80/CD86) on DCs, this transduces a signal in the DCs ("reverse-signaling") that upregulates expression of IDO [127]. A similar intracellular signal can be generated by artificially cross-linking B7 molecules on the DC using recombinant CTLA−4-Ig [20,128,129]; in some models this IDO induction via reverse-signaling is an important mechanism of the tolerogenic properties of CTLA−4-Ig in transplantation [19]. At the molecular level, this CTLA−4 → B7 reverse-signaling may be mediated via activation and translocation of the Foxo3 transcription factor in the DCs [130,131]. The ability of Tregs (via cell-surface CTLA−4 expression) to upregulate IDO in APCs has been suggested as one downstream molecular mechanism by which Tregs create immune suppression [132]. Indeed, IDO expression may be one part of a more general "tolerogenic DC phenotype" that is induced when Foxo3 is activated in DCs [133]. Consistent with this, one recent study suggests that Foxo3 activation (and the Foxo3-induced IDO activation) are important contributors to the immunosuppressive DC phenotype found in human and mouse tumors [57]. Exactly how Foxo3 and IDO are induced in these tumors is still unknown, but it is tempting to speculate that one possible mechanism might be via CTLA−4 expressed on tumor-infiltrating Tregs. Indeed, mAb-mediated blockade of either CTLA−4 or PD−1/PD−L pathways prevented IDO induction in DCs following treatment with TLR9 ligands [134], suggesting that signals from CTLA−4 or PD−1 expressed by Tregs may be essential to maintain the competence of DCs to express IDO.

VII. IDO-PATHWAY INHIBITOR DRUGS AS A POTENTIAL STRATEGY TO REDUCE TREG-MEDIATED SUPPRESSION

Drugs to inhibit the IDO pathway are currently in clinical trials or in preclinical development as immune adjuvants for cancer immunotherapy. Such drugs include

1-methyl-D-tryptophan [135,136], INCB024360 [137], and other compounds still in the development pipeline. Conceptually, these inhibitors are usually thought of as targeting the tumor milieu—i.e., removing the local immune suppression created by IDO within the tumor [48]. However, in addition to this local mechanism, IDO-pathway inhibitors may also help to reduce systemic immune suppression by reducing the tumor-induced activation of Tregs, in tumor-draining lymph nodes and systemically.

At present the clinical relevance of this IDO/Treg link in humans is still unknown. However, the need to reduce Treg-mediated suppression in cancer is clearly an important goal for successful immunotherapy [138]. Tumors doubtless have many ways to activate Tregs, so it would be naive to think that blocking IDO by itself would remove all Treg-mediated suppression. However, there may be specific times when tumors become more dependent on IDO. For example. when tumors are treated with chemotherapy, their hold on global immune suppression may become transiently more tenuous [139,140]. In this post-chemotherapy window, there is a race between desirable immune activation and re-establishment of immunosuppression and tolerance by the tumor. Speculatively, this might be a time when tumors become dependent on IDO to help them activate Tregs and re-create suppression. It is known that IDO-inhibitor drugs are frequently synergistic with chemotherapy, and that this is an immune-mediated process [15,135]. Additional preclinical studies will be needed to ask whether a component of this effect may be reduced Treg activation when IDO is blocked. Future studies may also wish to address whether antitumor vaccines or other forms of active immunotherapy might benefit by blocking IDO—perhaps thereby reducing Treg activation (and perhaps even allowing inflammation-induced conversion of Tregs into a nonsuppressive state). Given the potent effects of the IDO pathway on certain forms of acquired tolerance, and the relatively nontoxic nature of IDO-pathway inhibitor drugs in early clinical trials, these speculations may be worthwhile to explore.

CONFLICT OF INTEREST

The authors hold intellectual property interest in the therapeutic use of IDO and IDO inhibitors, and receive consulting income and research support from NewLink Genetics, Inc., which holds a license to develop the technology for clinical trials.

References

[1] Schreiber H, Rowley DA. Cancer. Quo vadis, specificity? Science 2008 Jan 11;319:164—5.

[2] Schreiber RD, Old LJ, Smyth MJ. Cancer immunoediting: integrating immunity's roles in cancer suppression and promotion. Science 2011;331:1565—70.

[3] Wing K, Sakaguchi S. Regulatory T cells exert checks and balances on self tolerance and autoimmunity. Nat Immunol 2010 Jan;11:7—13.

[4] Shields JD, Kourtis IC, Tomei AA, Roberts JM, Swartz MA. Induction of Lymphoidlike Stroma and Immune Escape by Tumors That Express the Chemokine CCL21. Science 2010 Mar 25;328:749—52.

[5] Darrasse-Jeze G, Bergot AS, Durgeau A, Billiard F, Salomon BL, Cohen JL, et al. Tumor emergence is sensed by self-specific CD44hi memory Tregs that create a dominant tolerogenic environment for tumors in mice. J Clin Invest 2009 Aug 3.

[6] Quezada SA, Peggs KS, Simpson TR, Shen Y, Littman DR, Allison JP. Limited tumor infiltration by activated T effector cells restricts the therapeutic activity of regulatory T cell depletion against established melanoma. J Exp Med 2008;205:2125—38.

[7] Mellor AL, Munn DH. Creating immune privilege: active local suppression that benefits friends, but protects foes. Nat Rev Immunol 2008;8:74—80.

[8] Metz R, Duhadaway JB, Kamasani U, Laury-Kleintop L, Muller AJ, Prendergast GC. Novel tryptophan catabolic enzyme IDO2 is the preferred biochemical target of the antitumor indoleamine 2,3-dioxygenase inhibitory compound D-1-methyl-tryptophan. Cancer Res 2007;67:7082—7.

[9] Ball HJ, Yuasa HJ, Austin CJ, Weiser S, Hunt NH. Indoleamine 2,3-dioxygenase-2; a new enzyme in the kynurenine pathway. Int J Biochem Cell Biol 2009 Mar;41:467—71.

[10] Munn DH, Sharma MD, Baban B, Harding HP, Zhang Y, Ron D, et al. GCN2 kinase in T cells mediates proliferative arrest and anergy induction in response to indoleamine 2,3-dioxygenase. Immunity 2005;22:633—42.

[11] Fallarino F, Grohmann U, You S, McGrath BC, Cavener DR, Vacca C, et al. The combined effects of tryptophan starvation and tryptophan catabolites down-regulate T cell receptor zeta-chain and induce a regulatory phenotype in naive T cells. J Immunol 2006;176(11):6752—61.

[12] Mezrich JD, Fechner JH, Zhang X, Johnson BP, Burlingham WJ, Bradfield CA. An interaction between kynurenine and the aryl hydrocarbon receptor can generate regulatory T cells. J Immunol 2010;185:3190—8.

[13] Quintana FJ, Murugaiyan G, Farez MF, Mitsdoerffer M, Tukpah AM, Burns EJ, et al. An endogenous aryl hydrocarbon receptor ligand acts on dendritic cells and T cells to suppress experimental autoimmune encephalomyelitis. Proc Natl Acad Sci USA 2010;107:20768—73.

[14] Munn DH, Zhou M, Attwood JT, Bondarev I, Conway SJ, Marshall B, et al. Prevention of allogeneic fetal rejection by tryptophan catabolism. Science 1998;281:1191—3.

[15] Muller AJ, Duhadaway JB, Donover PS, Sutanto-Ward E, Prendergast GC. Inhibition of indoleamine 2,3-dioxygenase, an immunoregulatory target of the cancer suppression gene Bin1, potentiates cancer chemotherapy. Nat Med 2005;11:312—9.

[16] Mellor AL, Sivakumar J, Chandler P, Smith K, Molina H, Mao D, et al. Prevention of T cell-driven complement activation and inflammation by tryptophan catabolism during pregnancy. Nat Immunol 2001;2:64—8.

[17] Matteoli G, Mazzini E, Iliev ID, Mileti E, Fallarino F, Puccetti P, et al. Gut CD103+ dendritic cells express indoleamine 2,3-dioxygenase which influences T regulatory/T effector cell balance and oral tolerance induction. Gut 2010;59:595—604.

[18] van der Marel AP, Samsom JN, Greuter M, van Berkel LA, O'Toole T, Kraal G, et al. Blockade of IDO inhibits nasal tolerance induction. J Immunol 2007;179:894—900.

[19] Sucher R, Fischler K, Oberhuber R, Kronberger I, Margreiter C, Ollinger R, et al. IDO and regulatory T cell support are critical for cytotoxic T lymphocyte-associated Ag-4 Ig-mediated long-term solid organ allograft survival. J Immunol 2012;188:37—46.

[20] Grohmann U, Orabona C, Fallarino F, Vacca C, Calcinaro F, Falorni A, et al. CTLA-4-Ig regulates tryptophan catabolism in vivo. Nat Immunol 2002;3:1097—101.

[21] Mellor AL, Baban B, Chandler P, Marshall B, Jhaver K, Hansen A, et al. Cutting Edge: Induced indoleamine 2,3 dioxygenase expression in dendritic cell subsets suppresses T cell clonal expansion. J Immunol 2003;171:1652—5.

[22] Guillonneau C, Hill M, Hubert FX, Chiffoleau E, Herve C, Li XL, et al. CD40Ig treatment results in allograft acceptance mediated by CD8CD45RC T cells, IFN-gamma, and indoleamine 2,3-dioxygenase. J Clin Invest 2007;117:1096—106.

[23] Tsai S, Shameli A, Yamanouchi J, Clemente-Casares X, Wang J, Serra P, et al. Reversal of autoimmunity by boosting memory-like autoregulatory T cells. Immunity 2010;32:568—80.

[24] Lan Z, Ge W, Arp J, Jiang J, Liu W, Gordon D, et al. Induction of kidney allograft tolerance by soluble CD83 associated with prevalence of tolerogenic dendritic cells and indoleamine 2,3-dioxygenase. Transplant 2010;90:1286—93.

[25] Swanson KA, Zheng Y, Heidler KM, Mizobuchi T, Wilkes DS. CDllc+ cells modulate pulmonary immune responses by production of indoleamine 2,3-dioxygenase. Am J Respir Cell Mol Biol 2004;30:311—8.

[26] Liu H, Liu L, Fletcher BS, Visner GA. Novel action of indoleamine 2,3-dioxygenase attenuating acute lung allograft injury. Am J Respir Crit Care Med 2006;173:566—72.

[27] Jasperson LK, Bucher C, Panoskaltsis-Mortari A, Taylor PA, Mellor AL, Munn DH, et al. Indoleamine 2,3-dioxygenase is a critical regulator of acute GVHD lethality. Blood 2008;111:3257—65.

[28] Lu Y, Giver CR, Sharma A, Li JM, Darlak KA, Owens LM, et al. IFN-gamma and indoleamine 2,3-dioxygenase signaling between donor dendritic cells and T cells regulates graft versus host and graft versus leukemia activity. Blood 2012;119:1075—85.

[29] Gurtner GJ, Newberry RD, Schloemann SR, McDonald KG, Stenson WF. Inhibition of indoleamine 2,3-dioxygenase augments trinitrobenzene sulfonic acid colitis in mice. Gastroenterology 2003;125:1762—73.

[30] Szanto S, Koreny T, Mikecz K, Glant TT, Szekanecz Z, Varga J. Inhibition of indoleamine 2,3-dioxygenase-mediated tryptophan catabolism accelerates collagen-induced arthritis in mice. Arthritis Res Ther 2007;9:R50.

[31] Yan Y, Zhang GX, Gran B, Fallarino F, Yu S, Li H, et al. IDO upregulates regulatory T cells via tryptophan catabolite and suppresses encephalitogenic T cell responses in experimental autoimmune encephalomyelitis. J Immunol 2010;185:5953—61.

[32] Fallarino F, Volpi C, Zelante T, Vacca C, Calvitti M, Fioretti MC, et al. IDO mediates TLR9-driven protection from experimental autoimmune diabetes. J Immunol 2009;183:6303—12.

[33] Romani L, Fallarino F, De Luca A, Montagnoli C, D'Angelo C, Zelante T, et al. Defective tryptophan catabolism underlies inflammation in mouse chronic granulomatous disease. Nature 2008;451:211—5.

591

[34] Grohmann U, Volpi C, Fallarino F, Bozza S, Bianchi R, Vacca C, et al. Reverse signaling through GITR ligand enables dexamethasone to activate IDO in allergy. Nat Med 2007;13:579—86.

[35] Ravishankar B, Liu H, Shinde R, Chandler P, Baban B, Tanaka M, et al. Tolerance to apoptotic cells is regulated by indoleamine 2,3-dioxygenase. Proc Natl Acad Sci USA 2012;109:3909—14.

[36] Brody JR, Costantino CL, Berger AC, Sato T, Lisanti MP, Yeo CJ, et al. Expression of indoleamine 2,3-dioxygenase in metastatic malignant melanoma recruits regulatory T cells to avoid immune detection and affects survival. Cell Cycle 2009 Jun 15;8:1930—4.

[37] Polak ME, Borthwick NJ, Gabriel FG, Johnson P, Higgins B, Hurren J, et al. Mechanisms of local immuno-suppression in cutaneous melanoma. Br J Cancer 2007;96:1879—87.

[38] Witkiewicz A, Williams TK, Cozzitorto J, Durkan B, Showalter SL, Yeo CJ, et al. Expression of indoleamine 2,3-dioxygenase in metastatic pancreatic ductal adenocarcinoma recruits regulatory T cells to avoid immune detection. J Am Coll Surg 2008 May;206:849—54. discussion 54—6.

[39] Witkiewicz AK, Costantino CL, Metz R, Muller AJ, Prendergast GC, Yeo CJ, et al. Genotyping and expression analysis of IDO2 in human pancreatic cancer: a novel, active target. J Am Coll Surg 2009 May;208:781—7. discussion 7—9.

[40] Okamoto A, Nikaido T, Ochiai K, Takakura S, Saito M, Aoki Y, et al. Indoleamine 2,3-dioxygenase serves as a marker of poor prognosis in gene expression profiles of serous ovarian cancer cells. Clin Cancer Res 2005;11(16):6030—9.

[41] Qian F, Villella J, Wallace PK, Mhawech-Fauceglia P, Tario Jr JD, Andrews C, et al. Efficacy of Levo-1-Methyl Tryptophan and Dextro-1-Methyl Tryptophan in Reversing Indoleamine-2,3-Dioxygenase-Mediated Arrest of T-Cell Proliferation in Human Epithelial Ovarian Cancer. Cancer Res 2009 Jun 2;69:5498—504.

[42] Curti A, Pandolfi S, Valzasina B, Aluigi M, Isidori A, Ferri E, et al. Modulation of tryptophan catabolism by human leukemic cells results in the conversion of CD25- into CD25+ T regulatory cells. Blood 2007;109:2871—7.

[43] Chamuleau ME, van de Loosdrecht AA, Hess CJ, Janssen JJ, Zevenbergen A, Delwel R, et al. High INDO (indoleamine 2,3-dioxygenase) mRNA level in blasts of acute myeloid leukemic patients predicts poor clinical outcome. Haematologica 2008 Dec;93:1894—8.

[44] Corm S, Berthon C, Imbenotte M, Biggio V, Lhermitte M, Dupont C, et al. Indoleamine 2,3-dioxygenase activity of acute myeloid leukemia cells can be measured from patients' sera by HPLC and is inducible by IFN-gamma. Leuk Res 2009 Mar;33:490—4.

[45] Brandacher G, Perathoner A, Ladurner R, Schneeberger S, Obrist P, Winkler C, et al. Prognostic value of indoleamine 2,3-dioxygenase expression in colorectal cancer: effect on tumor-infiltrating T cells. Clin Cancer Res 2006;12(4):1144—51.

[46] Huang A, Fuchs D, Widner B, Glover C, Henderson DC, Allen-Mersh TG. Serum tryptophan decrease correlates with immune activation and impaired quality of life in colorectal cancer. Br J Cancer 2002;86(11):1691—6.

[47] Feder-Mengus C, Wyler S, Hudolin T, Ruszat R, Bubendorf L, Chiarugi A, et al. High expression of indole-amine 2,3-dioxygenase gene in prostate cancer. Eur J Cancer 2008 Oct;44:2266—75.

[48] Uyttenhove C, Pilotte L, Theate I, Stroobant V, Colau D, Parmentier N, et al. Evidence for a tumoral immune resistance mechanism based on tryptophan degradation by indoleamine 2,3-dioxygenase. Nat Med 2003;9:1269—74.

[49] Ino K, Yoshida N, Kajiyama H, Shibata K, Yamamoto E, Kidokoro K, et al. Indoleamine 2,3-dioxygenase is a novel prognostic indicator for endometrial cancer. Br J Cancer 2006;95:1555—61.

[50] Ino K, Yamamoto E, Shibata K, Kajiyama H, Yoshida N, Terauchi M, et al. Inverse correlation between tumoral indoleamine 2,3-dioxygenase expression and tumor-infiltrating lymphocytes in endometrial cancer: its association with disease progression and survival. Clin Cancer Res 2008 Apr 15;14:2310—7.

[51] Balachandran VP, Cavnar MJ, Zeng S, Bamboat ZM, Ocuin LM, Obaid H, et al. Imatinib potentiates antitumor T cell responses in gastrointestinal stromal tumor through the inhibition of Ido. Nat Med 2011;17:1094—100.

[52] Opitz CA, Litzenburger UM, Sahm F, Ott M, Tritschler I, Trump S, et al. An endogenous tumour-promoting ligand of the human aryl hydrocarbon receptor. Nature 2011;478:197—203.

[53] Lee JR, Dalton RR, Messina JL, Sharma MD, Smith DM, Burgess RE, et al. Pattern of recruitment of immu-noregulatory antigen presenting cells in malignant melanoma. Lab Invest 2003;83:1457—66.

[54] Munn DH, Sharma MD, Hou D, Baban B, Lee JR, Antonia SJ, et al. Expression of indoleamine 2,3-dioxygenase by plasmacytoid dendritic cells in tumor-draining lymph nodes. J Clin Invest 2004;114:280—90.

[55] Gerlini G, Di Gennaro P, Mariotti G, Urso C, Chiarugi A, Pimpinelli N, et al. Indoleamine 2,3-dioxygenase+ cells correspond to the BDCA2+ plasmacytoid dendritic cells in human melanoma sentinel nodes. J Invest Dermatol 2010 Mar;130:898—901.

[56] Duluc D, Delneste Y, Tan F, Moles MP, Grimaud L, Lenoir J, et al. Tumor-associated leukemia inhibitory factor and IL-6 skew monocyte differentiation into tumor-associated-macrophage-like cells. Blood 2007;110:4319—30.

592

[57] Watkins SK, Zhu Z, Riboldi E, Shafer-Weaver KA, Stagliano KE, Sklavos MM, et al. FOXO3 programs tumor-associated DCs to become tolerogenic in human and murine prostate cancer. J Clin Invest 2011;121:1361–72.

[58] Sotomayor EM, Borrello I, Rattis FM, Cuenca AG, Abrams J, Staveley-O'Carroll K, et al. Cross-presentation of tumor antigens by bone marrow-derived antigen-presenting cells is the dominant mechanism in the induction of T-cell tolerance during B-cell lymphoma progression. Blood 2001;98(4):1070–7.

[59] Hildner K, Edelson BT, Purtha WE, Diamond M, Matsushita H, Kohyama M, et al. Batf3 deficiency reveals a critical role for CD8alpha+ dendritic cells in cytotoxic T cell immunity. Science 2008 Nov 14;322:1097–100.

[60] Baban B, Chandler PR, Sharma MD, Pihkala J, Koni PA, Munn DH, et al. IDO activates regulatory T cells and blocks their conversion into Th17-like T cells. J Immunol 2009 Aug 15;183:2475–83.

[61] Ercolini AM, Ladle BH, Manning EA, Pfannenstiel LW, Armstrong TD, Machiels JP, et al. Recruitment of latent pools of high-avidity CD8(+) T cells to the antitumor immune response. J Exp Med 2005;201(10):1591–602.

[62] Curiel TJ. Regulatory T cells and treatment of cancer. Curr Opin Immunol 2008 Apr;20:241–6.

[63] Sharma MD, Baban B, Chandler P, Hou DY, Singh N, Yagita H, et al. Plasmacytoid dendritic cells from mouse tumor-draining lymph nodes directly activate mature Tregs via indoleamine 2,3-dioxygenase. J Clin Invest 2007;117:2570–82.

[64] Chen W, Liang X, Peterson AJ, Munn DH, Blazar BR. The indoleamine 2,3-dioxygenase pathway is essential for human plasmacytoid dendritic cell-induced adaptive T regulatory cell generation. J Immunol 2008;181:5396–404.

[65] Manches O, Munn D, Fallahi A, Lifson J, Chaperot L, Plumas J, et al. HIV-activated human plasmacytoid DCs induce Tregs through an indoleamine 2,3-dioxygenase-dependent mechanism. J Clin Invest 2008;118:3431–9.

[66] Chung DJ, Rossi M, Romano E, Ghith J, Yuan J, Munn DH, et al. Indoleamine 2,3-dioxygenase-expressing mature human monocyte-derived dendritic cells expand potent autologous regulatory T cells. Blood 2009 Jul 16;114:555–63.

[67] Jurgens B, Hainz U, Fuchs D, Felzmann T, Heitger A. Interferon-gamma-triggered indoleamine 2,3-dioxygenase competence in human monocyte-derived dendritic cells induces regulatory activity in allogeneic T cells. Blood 2009 Oct 8;114:3235–43.

[68] Valzasina B, Piconese S, Guiducci C, Colombo MP. Tumor-induced expansion of regulatory T cells by conversion of CD4+CD25- lymphocytes is thymus and proliferation independent. Cancer Res 2006;66(8):4488–95.

[69] Wang L, Pino-Lagos K, de Vries VC, Guleria I, Sayegh MH, Noelle RJ. Programmed death 1 ligand signaling regulates the generation of adaptive Foxp3+CD4+ regulatory T cells. Proc Natl Acad Sci U S A 2008;105:9331–6.

[70] Zhou G, Levitsky HI. Natural regulatory T cells and de novo-induced regulatory T cells contribute independently to tumor-specific tolerance. J Immunol 2007;178:2155–62.

[71] Olkhanud PB, Damdinsuren B, Bodogai M, Gress RE, Sen R, Wejksza K, et al. Tumor-evoked regulatory B cells promote breast cancer metastasis by converting resting CD4 T cells to T-regulatory cells. Cancer Res 2011;71:3505–15.

[72] Wang HY, Peng G, Guo Z, Shevach EM, Wang RF. Recognition of a new ARTC1 peptide ligand uniquely expressed in tumor cells by antigen-specific CD4+ regulatory T cells. J Immunol 2005;174(5):2661–70.

[73] Hindley JP, Ferreira C, Jones E, Lauder SN, Ladell K, Wynn KK, et al. Analysis of the T-cell receptor repertoires of tumor-infiltrating conventional and regulatory T cells reveals no evidence for conversion in carcinogen-induced tumors. Cancer Res 2011;71:736–46.

[74] Kuczma M, Kopij M, Pawlikowska I, Wang CY, Rempala GA, Kraj P. Intratumoral convergence of the TCR repertoires of effector and Foxp3+ CD4+ T cells. PLoS ONE 2010;5:e13623.

[75] Rosenblum MD, Gratz IK, Paw JS, Lee K, Marshak-Rothstein A, Abbas AK. Response to self antigen imprints regulatory memory in tissues. Nature 2011;480:538–42.

[76] Thompson LJ, Valladao AC, Ziegler SF. Cutting edge: De novo induction of functional Foxp3+ regulatory CD4 T cells in response to tissue-restricted self antigen. J Immunol 2011;186:4551–5.

[77] Campbell DJ, Koch MA. Phenotypical and functional specialization of FOXP3+ regulatory T cells. Nat Rev Immunol 2011;11:119–30.

[78] Thornton AM, Piccirillo CA, Shevach EM. Activation requirements for the induction of CD4+CD25+ T cell suppressor function. Eur J Immunol 2004;34:366–76.

[79] Samy ET, Parker LA, Sharp CP, Tung KS. Continuous control of autoimmune disease by antigen-dependent polyclonal CD4+CD25+ regulatory T cells in the regional lymph node. J Exp Med 2005;202(6):771–81.

[80] Setiady YY, Ohno K, Samy ET, Bagavant H, Qiao H, Sharp C, et al. Physiologic self antigens rapidly capacitate autoimmune disease-specific polyclonal CD4+ CD25+ regulatory T cells. Blood 2006;107(3):1056–62.

[81] Zhang N, Schroppel B, Lal G, Jakubzick C, Mao X, Chen D, et al. Regulatory T cells sequentially migrate from inflamed tissues to draining lymph nodes to suppress the alloimmune response. Immunity 2009;30:458–69.

[82] Cretney E, Xin A, Shi W, Minnich M, Masson F, Miasari M, et al. The transcription factors Blimp-1 and IRF4 jointly control the differentiation and function of effector regulatory T cells. Nat Immunol 2011;12:304—11.

[83] Menetrier-Caux C, Gobert M, Caux C. Differences in tumor regulatory T-cell localization and activation status impact patient outcome. Cancer Res 2009;69:7895—8.

[84] O'Shea JJ, Paul WE. Mechanisms Underlying Lineage Commitment and Plasticity of Helper CD4+ T Cells. Science 2010 Feb 26;327:1098—102.

[85] Duarte JH, Zelenay S, Bergman ML, Martins AC, Demengeot J. Natural Treg cells spontaneously differentiate into pathogenic helper cells in lymphopenic conditions. Eur J Immunol 2009 Apr;39:948—55.

[86] Komatsu N, Mariotti-Ferrandiz ME, Wang Y, Malissen B, Waldmann H, Hori S. Heterogeneity of natural Foxp3+ T cells: a committed regulatory T-cell lineage and an uncommitted minor population retaining plasticity. Proc Natl Acad Sci USA 2009 Feb 10;106:1903—8.

[87] Osorio F, LeibundGut-Landmann S, Lochner M, Lahl K, Sparwasser T, Eberl G, et al. DC activated via dectin-1 convert Treg into IL-17 producers. Eur J Immunol 2008 Dec;38:3274—81.

[88] Oldenhove G, Bouladoux N, Wohlfert EA, Hall JA, Chou D, Dos Santos L, et al. Decrease of Foxp3+ Treg cell number and acquisition of effector cell phenotype during lethal infection. Immunity 2009 Nov 20;31:772—86.

[89] Zhou X, Bailey-Bucktrout SL, Jeker LT, Penaranda C, Martinez-Llordella M, Ashby M, et al. Instability of the transcription factor Foxp3 leads to the generation of pathogenic memory T cells in vivo. Nat Immunol 2009 Jul 26;10:1000—7.

[90] Rubtsov YP, Niec RE, Josefowicz S, Li L, Darce J, Mathis D, et al. Stability of the regulatory T cell lineage in vivo. Science 2010;329:1667—71.

[91] Miyao T, Floess S, Setoguchi R, Luche H, Fehling HJ, Waldmann H, et al. Plasticity of Foxp3(+) T Cells Reflects Promiscuous Foxp3 Expression in Conventional T Cells but Not Reprogramming of Regulatory T Cells. Immunity 2012.

[92] Sakaguchi S. Immunology: Conditional stability of T cells. Nature 2010;468:41—2.

[93] Sharma MD, Hou DY, Liu Y, Koni PA, Metz R, Chandler P, et al. Indoleamine 2,3-dioxygenase controls conversion of Foxp3+ Tregs to TH17-like cells in tumor-draining lymph nodes. Blood 2009;113:6102—11.

[94] Sharma MD, Hou DY, Baban B, Koni PA, He Y, Chandler PR, et al. Reprogrammed Foxp3(+) Regulatory T Cells Provide Essential Help to Support Cross-presentation and CD8(+) T Cell Priming in Naive Mice. Immunity 2010;33:942—54.

[95] Zhou X, Kong N, Wang J, Fan H, Zou H, Horwitz D, et al. Cutting edge: all-trans retinoic acid sustains the stability and function of natural regulatory T cells in an inflammatory milieu. J Immunol 2010;185:2675—9.

[96] Yang XO, Nurieva R, Martinez GJ, Kang HS, Chung Y, Pappu BP, et al. Molecular antagonism and plasticity of regulatory and inflammatory T cell programs. Immunity 2008 Jul;29:44—56.

[97] Vokaer B, Van Rompaey N, Lemaitre PH, Lhomme F, Kubjak C, Benghiat FS, et al. Critical role of regulatory T cells in Th17-mediated minor antigen-disparate rejection. J Immunol 2010;185:3417—25.

[98] Addey C, White M, Dou L, Coe D, Dyson J, Chai JG. Functional plasticity of antigen-specific regulatory T cells in context of tumor. J Immunol 2011;186:4557—64.

[99] Kilberg MS, Shan J, Su N. ATF4-dependent transcription mediates signaling of amino acid limitation. Trends in endocrinology and metabolism: TEM 2009;20:436—43.

[100] Wek RC, Jiang HY, Anthony TG. Coping with stress: eIF2 kinases and translational control. Biochem Soc Trans 2006;34:7—11.

[101] Harding HP, Novoa I, Zhang Y, Zeng H, Wek R, Schapira M, et al. Regulated translation initiation controls stress-induced gene expression in mammalian cells. Mol Cell 2000;6(5):1099—108.

[102] Peng W, Robertson L, Gallinetti J, Mejia P, Vose S, Charlip A, et al. Surgical stress resistance induced by single amino acid deprivation requires Gcn2 in mice. Sci Transl Med 2012;4:118ra11.

[103] Jalili RB, Forouzandeh F, Moeenrezakhanlou A, Rayat GR, Rajotte RV, Uludag H, et al. Mouse pancreatic islets are resistant to indoleamine 2,3 dioxygenase-induced general control nonderepressible-2 kinase stress pathway and maintain normal viability and function. Am J Pathol 2009 Jan;174:196—205.

[104] Lee GK, Park HJ, Macleod M, Chandler P, Munn DH, Mellor AL. Tryptophan deprivation sensitizes activated T cells to apoptosis prior to cell division. Immunol 2002;107:1—9.

[105] Forouzandeh F, Jalili RB, Germain M, Duronio V, Ghahary A. Differential immunosuppressive effect of indoleamine 2,3-dioxygenase (IDO) on primary human CD4+ and CD8+ T cells. Mol Cell Biochem 2008 Feb;309:1—7.

[106] Rodriguez PC, Quiceno DG, Ochoa AC. L-arginine availability regulates T-lymphocyte cell-cycle progression. Blood 2007;109:1568—73.

[107] Blander JM, Amsen Immunology D. Amino acid addiction. Science 2009 Jun 5;324:1282—3.

[108] Sundrud MS, Koralov SB, Feuerer M, Calado DP, Kozhaya AE, Rhule-Smith A, et al. Halofuginone inhibits TH17 cell differentiation by activating the amino acid starvation response. Science 2009 Jun 5;324:1334–8.

[109] Powell JD, Pollizzi KN, Heikamp EB, Horton MR. Regulation of Immune Responses by mTOR. Ann Rev Immunol 2012;30:39–68.

[110] Delgoffe GM, Kole TP, Zheng Y, Zarek PE, Matthews KL, Xiao B, et al. The mTOR kinase differentially regulates effector and regulatory T cell lineage commitment. Immunity 2009;30:832–44.

[111] Procaccini C, Galgani M, De Rosa V, Matarese G. Intracellular metabolic pathways control immune tolerance. Trends Immunol 2012;33:1–7.

[112] Cobbold SP, Adams E, Farquhar CA, Nolan KF, Howie D, Lui KO, et al. Infectious tolerance via the consumption of essential amino acids and mTOR signaling. Proc Natl Acad Sci USA 2009 Jul 21;106:12055–60.

[113] Desvignes L, Ernst JD. Interferon-gamma-responsive nonhematopoietic cells regulate the immune response to Mycobacterium tuberculosis. Immunity 2009 Dec 18;31:974–85.

[114] Favre D, Mold J, Hunt PW, Kanwar B, Loke P, Seu L, et al. Tryptophan catabolism by indoleamine 2,3-dioxygenase 1 alters the balance of TH17 to regulatory T cells in HIV disease. Sci Transl Med 2010;2:32ra6.

[115] Barouki R, Coumoul X, Fernandez-Salguero PM. The aryl hydrocarbon receptor, more than a xenobiotic-interacting protein. FEBS Let 2007;581:3608–15.

[116] Kiss EA, Vonarbourg C, Kopfmann S, Hobeika E, Finke D, Esser C, et al. Natural aryl hydrocarbon receptor ligands control organogenesis of intestinal lymphoid follicles. Science 2011;334:1561–5.

[117] Li Y, Innocentin S, Withers DR, Roberts NA, Gallagher AR, Grigorieva EF, et al. Exogenous stimuli maintain intraepithelial lymphocytes via aryl hydrocarbon receptor activation. Cell 2011;147:629–40.

[118] Stockinger B, Hirota K, Duarte J, Veldhoen M. External influences on the immune system via activation of the aryl hydrocarbon receptor. Sem Immunol 2011;23:99–105.

[119] Korn T. How T cells take developmental decisions by using the aryl hydrocarbon receptor to sense the environment. Proc Natl Acad Sci USA 2010;107:20597–8.

[120] Singh NP, Singh UP, Singh B, Price RL, Nagarkatti M, Nagarkatti PS. Activation of aryl hydrocarbon receptor (AhR) leads to reciprocal epigenetic regulation of FoxP3 and IL-17 expression and amelioration of experimental colitis. PLoS ONE 2011;6:e23522.

[121] Quintana FJ, Basso AS, Iglesias AH, Korn T, Farez MF, Bettelli E, et al. Control of T(reg) and T(H)17 cell differentiation by the aryl hydrocarbon receptor. Nature 2008;453:65–71.

[122] Nguyen NT, Kimura A, Nakahama T, Chinen I, Masuda K, Nohara K, et al. Aryl hydrocarbon receptor negatively regulates dendritic cell immunogenicity via a kynurenine-dependent mechanism. Proc Natl Acad Sci USA 2010;107:19961–6.

[123] Grohmann U, Fallarino F, Bianchi R, Belladonna ML, Vacca C, Orabona C, et al. IL-6 inhibits the tolerogenic function of CD8alpha(+) dendritic cells expressing indoleamine 2,3-dioxygenase. J Immunol 2001;167(2):708–14.

[124] Brenk M, Scheler M, Koch S, Neumann J, Takikawa O, Hacker G, et al. Tryptophan deprivation induces inhibitory receptors ILT3 and ILT4 on dendritic cells favoring the induction of human CD4+CD25+ Foxp3+ T regulatory cells. J Immunol 2009 Jul 1;183:145–54.

[125] Manlapat AK, Kahler DJ, Chandler PR, Munn DH, Mellor AL. Cell-autonomous control of interferon type I expression by indoleamine 2,3-dioxygenase in regulatory CD19(+) dendritic cells. Eur J Immunol 2007;37:1064–71.

[126] Pallotta MT, Orabona C, Volpi C, Vacca C, Belladonna ML, Bianchi R, et al. Indoleamine 2,3-dioxygenase is a signaling protein in long-term tolerance by dendritic cells. Nat Immunol 2011;12:870–8.

[127] Fallarino F, Grohmann U, Hwang KW, Orabona C, Vacca C, Bianchi R, et al. Modulation of tryptophan catabolism by regulatory T cells. Nat Immunol 2003;4:1206–12.

[128] Mellor AL, Chandler P, Baban B, Hansen AM, Marshall B, Pihkala J, et al. Specific subsets of murine dendritic cells acquire potent T cell regulatory functions following CTLA4-mediated induction of indoleamine 2,3 dioxygenase. Int Immunol 2004;16:1391–401.

[129] Munn DH, Sharma MD, Mellor AL. Ligation of B7-1/B7-2 by human CD4+ T cells triggers indoleamine 2,3-dioxygenase activity in dendritic cells. J Immunol 2004;172:4100–10.

[130] Fallarino F, Bianchi R, Orabona C, Vacca C, Belladonna ML, Fioretti MC, et al. CTLA-4-Ig Activates forkhead transcription factors and protects dendritic cells from oxidative stress in nonobese diabetic mice. J Exp Med 2004;200:1051–62.

[131] Dejean AS, Beisner DR, Ch'en IL, Kerdiles YM, Babour A, Arden KC, et al. Transcription factor Foxo3 controls the magnitude of T cell immune responses by modulating the function of dendritic cells. Nat Immunol 2009;10:504–13.

[132] Wing K, Yamaguchi T, Sakaguchi S. Cell-autonomous and -non-autonomous roles of CTLA-4 in immune regulation. Trends Immunol 2011;32:428–33.

[133] Kerdiles YM, Stone EL, Beisner DL, McGargill MA, Ch'en IL, Stockmann C, et al. Foxo transcription factors control regulatory T cell development and function. Immunity 2010;33:890–904.

[134] Baban B, Chandler PR, Johnson 3rd BA, Huang L, Li M, Sharpe ML, et al. Physiologic control of IDO competence in splenic dendritic cells. J Immunol 2011;187:2329–35.

[135] Hou DY, Muller AJ, Sharma MD, Duhadaway JB, Banerjee T, Johnson M, et al. Inhibition of IDO in dendritic cells by stereoisomers of 1-methyl-tryptophan correlates with anti-tumor responses. Cancer Res 2007;67:792–801.

[136] Soliman HH, Antonia SJ, Sullivan D, Vanahanian N, Link C. Overcoming tumor antigen anergy in human malignancies using the novel indeolamine 2,3-dioxygenase (IDO) enzyme inhibitor, 1-methyl-D-tryptophan (1MT). J Clin Oncol 2009;27:3004 (meeting abstract).

[137] Liu X, Shin N, Koblish HK, Yang G, Wang Q, Wang K, et al. Selective inhibition of indoleamine 2,3-dioxygenase (IDO1) effectively regulates mediators of anti-tumor immunity. Blood 2010 Mar 2.

[138] Jacobs JF, Nierkens S, Figdor CG, de Vries IJ, Adema GJ. Regulatory T cells in melanoma: the final hurdle towards effective immunotherapy? The lancet oncology 2012;13:e32–42.

[139] McDonnell AM, Nowak AK, Lake RA. Contribution of the immune system to the chemotherapeutic response. Seminars in immunopathology 2011;33:353–67.

[140] Sistigu A, Viaud S, Chaput N, Bracci L, Proietti E, Zitvogel L. Immunomodulatory effects of cyclophosphamide and implementations for vaccine design. Seminars in immunopathology 2011;33:369–83.

CHAPTER 34

Arginase, Nitric Oxide Synthase, and Novel Inhibitors of L-arginine Metabolism in Immune Modulation

Mariacristina Chioda[1], Ilaria Marigo[2], Susanna Mandruzzato[3], Simone Mocellin[4], Vincenzo Bronte[5]

[1]Istituto Oncologico Veneto, Padova, Italy
[2]Stem Cell Biology, Department of Medicine, Division of Experimental Medicine, Hammersmith Hospital, London, UK
[3]Department of Surgery, Oncology and Gastroenterology, Oncology and Immunology Section, University of Padova, Italy
[4]Department of Surgery, Oncology and Gastroenterology, Surgery Section, University of Padova, Italy
[5]University Hospital and Department of Pathology, Immunology Section, Verona, Italy

I. INTRODUCTION

A successful immune response against offending insults to the body relies on the orderly interaction between cells of the innate and adaptive immune system. Although T lymphocytes bearing a clonotypic receptor for the antigen are needed for the complete elimination of the offending insult, other cells assist them in antigen clearance, destruction of intracellular pathogens, triggering of vascular and inflammatory responses, production of collagen, and tissue remodeling. These "accessory cells" are also important in guiding lymphocyte activation, and in this regard one can schematically picture two main classes of accessory cells: those deciding whether an immune response needs to be generated and naïve T lymphocytes need to be activated by the antigen (gatekeepers), and those assuring that activated T lymphocytes are correctly turned off at the end of their job to avoid damage and accumulation of useless cells (caretakers). Dendritic cells (DCs) are the perfect gatekeepers since they are strategically placed at the ports of antigen entry and express an array of molecules that can aid the priming of naïve T lymphocytes. On the other hand, they can employ L-tryptophan (L-Trp) metabolism via indoleamine 2,3-deoxygenase (IDO) to limit T-lymphocyte reactivity if necessary, to tolerize rather than activate. The myelomonocytic system, on the other hand, possesses the qualities to accomplish the caretaker role. Cells belonging to this differentiation lineage are released from pools circulating in the blood and from hematopoietic organs in a number proportional to the offending insult and are equipped with a number of tools that are extremely efficient in killing invading pathogens but are also useful to silence activated T lymphocytes. A pathological

Cancer Immunotherapy. http://dx.doi.org/10.1016/B978-0-12-394296-8.00034-8

expansion of myelomonocytic cells in the bone marrow, secondary lymphoid organs, and blood can be seen under different pathological conditions: during acute and chronic immune responses to pathogens, immune stress leading to extensive T-lymphocyte activation such as exposure to superantigens or certain parasite products; altered hematopoiesis by radiation, graft-vs-host reaction, or chemotherapy; autoimmune diseases; and, during tumor growth/ development. These cells have been termed myeloid-derived suppressor cells (MDSCs) and they have an uncanny ability to impair T-lymphocyte functions or to limit their access to inflammatory sites [85,224,271,272].

Amino-acid degradation is crucial for restoring nitrogen levels and the availability of essential amino acids. The pathways of amino-acid catabolism are evolutionary conserved between higher organisms and pathogens; this makes them an ideal ground for competition between microbes and hosts. Disease outbreak or successful immune responses might thus rely on winning the competition for essential compounds. Tumors exploit the very same strategy by educating myelomonocytic cells to use the metabolism of L-Arginine (L-Arg) to restrain lymphocyte activation [131]. There are two classes of enzymes metabolizing L-Arg critical for this function, the nitric oxide synthase (NOS) and arginase (ARG). These activities can be induced by Th1- and Th2-type cytokines that control cellular and humoral adaptive immune responses, respectively. The other two enzymes catabolizing L-Arg, arginine: glycine amidi-notransferase and arginine decarboxylase, have not been shown to possess immunoregulatory properties to date. L-Arg is not an essential amino acid for adult mammals but its demand can exceed the endogenous biosynthesis in situations such as intense stress, in cancer patients, following liver transplantation, or in severe trauma [16,99]. Recent findings suggest that L-Arg metabolism in myeloid cells can result in the impairment of lymphocyte responses to antigen [87]. Moreover, tumor cells themselves can alter L-Arg metabolism within the microenvironment to their own advantage [317].

598

II. NITRIC OXIDE SYNTHASE (NOS): GENES, REGULATION, AND ACTIVITY

Nitric oxide production by NOS has been extensively reviewed [4,26,34,230, 265,329] so we will discuss in this section only basic aspects that are relevant to understanding the NOS immunoregulatory activity in cancer. There are four isoforms of the heme-containing enzymes catalyzing the synthesis of NO from L-Arg, namely, the neuronal (nNOS/NOS1), inducible (iNOS/NOS2), endothelial (eNOS/NOS3) NO synthases [4,189] and a mitochondrial-specific isoform (mtNOS), which has an important role in bioenergetics of mitochondria [74]. Two main domains can be identified in all NOS isoforms: an N-terminal oxygenase domain and a C-terminal reductase domain. Electrons donated by conversion of NADPH to NADP are transferred to the oxygenase domain through the redox chain involving the electron carriers FAD and FMN. The oxygenase domain uses the iron heme and BH_4 to catalyze the reaction between O_2 and L-Arg to generate citrulline and NO. These isoforms share about 50% sequence similarity and are differentially regulated, making the catalytic activity specific for each of them. The expression of NOS1 and NOS3 is constitutive in a restricted number of cell types, mainly neurons and endothelial cells, respectively. Their enzymatic activity is dependent on calcium/calmodulin and yields NO in a picomolar-nanomolar range for a limited time window of seconds/minutes [141]. They may also be activated and/or inhibited by phosphorylation through various protein kinases. For example, the catalytic activity of NOS3 is augmented by phosphorylation of a C-terminal serine residue through the Akt pathway [65,66] which is often activated in malignant cells.

On the other hand, NOS2 can be potentially induced in all cell types and its expression is not dependent on calcium levels. Indeed NOS2 displays a high affinity for calmodulin, which, at physiological calcium concentrations, is normally tightly bound to it and therefore insensitive to calcium signals [189]. The presence of bound calmodulin is necessary to assure electron flow [4]. NOS2 is mainly induced by pro-inflammatory cytokines (e.g., interferons (IFN), interleukin (IL)—1, IL-2, tumor necrosis factor (TNF)) [139]. Once expressed, NOS2 can locally produce large amounts of NO in the micromolar range; its activity persists until enzyme degradation (hours/days) [139,165].

Regulation of NOS2 expression occurs preferentially at the transcriptional level rather than through the modulation of its enzymatic activity as is the case for NOS1 and NOS3. The promoter sequence of NOS2 contains a number of binding sites for transcription factors basically regulating all the aspects of cellular processes ranging from cell proliferation, apoptosis and cell differentiation; amongst these are AP-1, C/EBP, CREB, HIF, IRF-1, NF-kB, Oct-1, PARP-1, p53, STAT-1α [230]. However, NF-kB seems to represent the central target for both activators and inhibitors of NOS2: for example, NF-kB activation mediated by LPS, IL-1β TNF-α, INF-γ, pathogen-associated molecular pattern (PAMP) or oxidative stress, has been shown to determine NOS2 expression in different cell types [26,45,130]. All the mammalian NOS2 promoters contain also interferon regulatory factor-1 (IRF-1) and signal transducer and activator of transcription-1 (STAT-1) binding sites [230]. INF-α, β and γ by activating IRF-1, mediate NOS2 induction. A physical interaction between NF-κB and IRF-1 can probably stimulate the maximal induction of NOS2 gene expression. LPS can induce NOS2 expression through stimulation of the mitogen-activated protein kinase (MAPK) pathway [332]. Hypoxia is another relevant factor in induction of NOS2 transcription due to the presence of hypoxia-responsive enhancer (HRE) on NOS2 promoter [185]. Further, scaffolding proteins such as HMG-Y(I) and transcriptional activators as CBP have been shown to increase NOS2 transcription [233]. NOS2 is instead downregulated by steroids [278], anti-inflammatory cytokines (e.g., transforming growth factor-beta—TGF-β—and IL-10) [46,326], p53 [7], and NO itself [114].

Besides transcriptional regulation NOS2 can be modulated by controlling its mRNA or protein stability. For example, the absence of the mRNA stabilizing protein HuR causes the decrease of NOS2 expression [250] and src-mediated tyrosine phosphorylation has been shown to increase NOS2 half-life [107].

Others strategies controlling NOS2 enzymatic activity target its dimerization or the bioavailability of its substrate, L-Arg. The interaction of NOS2 with NOS-associated protein 110 kDa (NAP110) prevents the homodimerization of the enzyme and therefore inhibits its function [247]. A particularly important factor regulating NOS2 expression is the availability of L-Arg, that affects both NOS2 catalitic activity and the translation of NOS2 mRNA. To a lesser degree, NOS1 and NOS3 can also be regulated at the transcriptional level, but the main mechanisms controlling their enzymatic activities depend on Ca^{2+} binding and the calcium/calmodulin axis [83,192]. Recently, some evidence emerged linking NOS2 regulation to noncoding RNA (ncRNA) such as anti-sense RNA (asRNA) [180] and micro-RNAs (miR) [314]. The biovalability of L-Arg is also greatly influenced by the activity of another class of enzymes metabolizing it: arginases (ARG). Given the immune-regulatory effect of this interaction, this issue will be discussed later in this section.

Although several cell types (e.g., neutrophils, hepatocytes, cardiac myocytes) can express NOS2, mouse macrophages represent the typical source of this enzyme [26]. NOS2 activation is considered a hallmark of classically activated macrophages, i.e., macrophages that are mediators of the delayed type hypersensitivity response and are endowed with antitumor properties, as opposed to alternatively activated macrophages [92,240]. Differences have been described between human and mouse cells with respect to NOS2 activity. The promoter of human NOS2 is quite different from the mouse Nos2, despite many transcription factors binding sites being conserved between the two species; the human promoter contains regulatory sequences enhancing LPS/cytokine stimulation even at 16Kb upstream of the transcriptional start site (TSS). This is in sharp contrast with Nos2 promoter in mice, where basically all regulatory elements are within 1Kb of the 5'UTR and are sufficient for strong induction of cytokine mediated transcriptional activity [230]. Apparently, human macrophages respond to stimuli other than LPS + IFN-γ (very active on rodent macrophages) since they are rather susceptible to IFN-α, chemokines, or the combination of CD23 + IL-4 [274,309,311]; however, in light of the very different promoter organization it might be a matter of different sensitivity to various stimuli [230]. Further, expression of NOS2 mRNA and/or protein has been also detected in human blood mononuclear cells and neutrophils under different conditions [26].

NOS2 knockout (NOS2$^{-/-}$) mice are viable, fertile, and without evident histopathological abnormalities but are susceptible to infection with the parasite *Leishmania major*. However, they are capable of developing a stronger Th1 type immune response than wild-type mice. Moreover, NOS2$^{-/-}$ mice were resistant to lipopolysaccharide-induced mortality [315].

Importantly, polymorphisms of the promoter regions of both NOS2 and NOS3 have been linked to higher risk of cancer development, greater tumor aggressiveness, and poorer survival in humans, although to date a strict correlation between gene polymorphism and cancer progression has not been clearly identified [184,230,293].

III. ARGINASE (ARG): GENES, REGULATION, AND ACTIVITY

ARG is a manganese metalloenzyme that catalyzes the hydrolysis of L-Arg to form L-ornithine and urea. L-ornithine is further processed to give rise to L-proline via ornithine aminotransferase (OAT) and polyamines via the ornithine decarboxylase (ODC) pathway [26,329]. In mammals, two genetically distinct isoenzymes have been identified that differ in tissue distribution and subcellular location. Arginase I (ARG1, also known as liver-type) is found predominantly in hepatocytes, where it catalyzes the final cytosolic step of the urea cycle, whereas arginase II (ARG2, also known as kidney-type) is more widely distributed in numerous tissue (e.g., kidneys, small intestine, brain, skeletal muscle, liver), is localized to the mitochondrial matrix within the cell, and does not appear to function in the urea cycle [9]. The human type I and type II arginases are related by 58% sequence identity. The human *ARG1* gene gives rise, by alternative splicing, to 12 different transcripts, putatively encoding 11 different protein isoforms, while the *ARG2* gene encodes 4 different transcripts by alternative splicing, putatively encoding 4 different protein isoforms. The function and relevance of these variants have not been investigated in detail.

The family of arginases is highly conserved across species and arginase activity from pathogens can interfere with host L-Arg metabolism and vice versa. For example, the *Helycobacter pylori* gene *rocF* encodes a constitutively active ARG that consumes L-Arg from the medium and completely prevents NO production by NOS2 in macrophages, conferring an advantage for bacterial growth [90]. In fact, whereas wild type *H. pylori* is resistant to macrophage-derived NO, the *rocF*-deficient strain is efficiently killed and eliminated by activated macrophages. On the other hand, *Leishmania major*-infected BALB/c macrophages exposed to Th2-type cytokines express ARG (likely ARG1) and support the intracellular growth of the parasites, a permissive status that was reversed by the addition of the physiologic ARG inhibitor NOHA [122].

ARG1 is expressed in mammalian cells of the innate immune system where it might have assumed important biological functions during evolution. Whereas ARG1 expression in mouse hepatocytes is constitutive, in resting rodent macrophages *Arg1* mRNA, protein- and enzymatic activity are undetectable but could be upregulated several orders of magnitude by cytokines such as IL-4 and IL-13 activating a signaling pathway involving the transcription factors STAT6 and CEBP/β [191,208,209]. The 5′ flanking region of the mouse *Arg1* gene is responsible for the transcriptional response to IL-4, cAMP, TGF-β, dexamethasone, and LPS [202]. On the enhancer element, about 3 kb from the basal *Arg1* promoter, a multimeric complex assembles comprising STAT6, PU.1, CEBP-β transcription factors and as yet unidentified proteins synthesized *ex novo* following STAT6 activation [229]. In particular, STAT6 binding to the promoter requires an adjacent CEBP-β to confer responsiveness to IL-4 in mouse macrophages [96]. CEBP-β is also the transcription factor regulating ARG1 induction by glucocorticoids and glucan in rat hepatocytes [93] and it is also essential for mediating the activity of cAMP, LPS, and hypoxia on ARG1 expression [2].

Although the STAT6 pathway is considered the main one controlling ARG1 expression, recent data showed ARG1 induction in a STAT6 independent manner through the TLR and MyD88 (myeloid differentiation factor 88) in macrophages of mice infected with endoparasites such as *Toxoplasma gondii* and *Mycobacterium tubercolosis*. Albeit STAT6 independent, ARG1 expression resulted CEBP/β dependent [73]. The requirement for CEBP/β in these two pathways might be consistent with the observation that CEBP/β is required for LPS-driven ARG1 expression in macrophages [286].

An important role for macrophage-ARG1 in inflammation has been supported by evidence such as the upregulation in response to LPS, or lipoproteins [86,202], a variety of inflammatory stimuli [116] and in rat alveolar macrophages by hydrogen peroxide (H_2O_2) [181].

A third circuit resulting in STAT6-independent ARG1 induction involves the macrophage stimulating protein (MSP) and the RON kinase, through the binding of an AP-1 binding site located at -433bp from the TSS [275]. Given the specific expression of *Ron* in tissue-resident macrophages, the activation of ARG1 through this signaling could be a way to restrict its action to a particular cellular subset. The *Arg1* promoter contains other functional AP-1 sites necessary for transcriptional regulation driven by different stimuli, such as thrombin, for its expression in endothelial cells [336]. This emphasizes how the combination of different factors might eventually result in *Arg1* regulation. ARG1 activation is now considered as one of the specific markers of alternatively activated mouse macrophages, which are important mediators of allergic responses, control of parasitic infections, wound repair and fibrosis, and have been found in tumor infiltrates of various human tumors where they have been suspected to promote tumorigenesis [92,172,240]. The mechanism restraining ARG1 expression in macrophages depends on the Src-homology 2 (SH2)-containing inositol-5'-phosphatase 1 (SHIP1) whose STAT6-dependent degradation is necessary for IL-4 mediated ARG1 induction [321]. The properties of tumor-infiltrating macrophages are discussed in detail in Chapter 27.

Other cytokines including TGF-β [29], the macrophage stimulating protein (MSP) acting on the receptor RON [203], and GM-CSF [128] can induce the enzyme activity in different cell types of the innate immune system. ARG1 is also regulated by phosphodiesterase (PDE) inhibitors with rather divergent effects. Inhibitors of PDE4, the predominant PDE in macrophages, elevate cAMP levels and results in ARG1 (and to a lesser extent ARG2) induction in RAW 264.7 cells and human alveolar macrophages stimulated with IL-4 or TGF-β [76]. Conversely, PDE5 inhibitors such as sildenafil, vardenafil, and tadalafil increase intracellular concentrations of cGMP and downregulate ARG1 activity and expression in tumor-infiltrating CD11b$^+$ MDSCs [87]. LPS, dexamethasone and hypoxia induce ARG expression with a certain variability in terms of induced isoforms (i.e., ARG1 vs. ARG2) in various cell types [202]. The cAMP-mediated ARG1 expression in murine cells is mediated by protein kinase A type I (PKAI) by mechanisms involving chromatin decondensation at the promoter sequence requiring histone deacetylation [104].

ARG1 regulation by IL-4 and IL-13 in human macrophages has been disputed on the account that IL-4/IL-13 do not induce an increase of *ARG1* transcripts in monocytes isolated from the buffy coat of healthy volunteers [243]. However, human alveolar macrophages can respond to IL-4 in the presence of increased cAMP levels [76] suggesting that rather than a general difference between mice and humans, a difference in anatomic localization and/or stimuli responsiveness account for the diversity between the species, analogous to the observations for NO production (see above). In patients with different types of cancers the activity of ARG1 was found to be restricted to cellular subsets characterized by a distinct combination of surface markers [251,334]. In freshly isolated bone marrow cells, ARG1 expression was also described in a peculiar promyelocytic-like population of CD11b$^{low/neg}$CD16^{neg} cells displaying the strongest suppressor effect on effector T-cell functions [285].

A divergence in ARG localization during evolution might indeed exist, since ARG1 has been shown to be constitutively present in human granulocytes [210] whereas mouse granulocyte-like MDSCs express only low levels of *Arg1* mRNA, and a higher amount of *Arg2* mRNA. Moreover, this population exerts suppressive function towards T cells only at very high suppressor to lymphocyte ratio *in vitro*; lastly, also the *in vivo* suppressive activity of this subset is inferior to monocyte-like MDSCs [67]. Although the stimuli and the cell populations expressing ARG1 might be different between humans and mice, it appears that the immu-noregulatory mechanisms associated with ARG1 activity might be conserved.

ARG2, indicated originally as kidney-type, has been considered for a long time to be a mitochondrial enzyme constitutively expressed in different cell types and dedicated to L-proline synthesis because of its close proximity to OAT, also located in the mitochondria. Recent investigations have challenged this division and it is now clear that both ARG1 and 2 regulate polyamine synthesis and can be both constitutive and inducible in cells of the innate immune system. ARG2 is activated in macrophages by infection with *Helicobacter pylori* where it suppresses host immune system by reducing NOS2 activity that is crucial for pathogen clearance. This is achieved by imparing *Nos2* mRNA translation which derives from intracellular L-Arg depletion and leads to a reduction in NO levels [157]. ARG2 is also induced in Jurkat cells and macrophages infected with Sendai virus through a mechanism independent of type I IFN production but requiring control by the interferon regulatory factor 3 (IRF3) [94]. It was advanced that increased spermine production after ARG2 activation inhibited viral replication and induced apoptosis of infected cells, but this mechanism was in apparent contrast to the known ability of polyamines to promote rather than inhibit cell proliferation. However, a very recent work on infections by *H. pylori* showed how this pathogen can inactivate NOS2-mediated NO synthesis by upregulating its own arginase and, at the same time, inducing host macrophage ARG2 and ODC. Generation of spermine by ODC inhibits NOS2 translation and NO-mediated *H. pylori* killing. Macrophage apoptosis is mediated by the oxidation of spermine by spermine oxidase (SMO), which generates oxidative stress by H$_2$O$_2$ production. In gastric epithelial cells, the oxidative stress by *H. pylori* is dependent on SMO expression and results in DNA damage and apoptosis [44].

ARG1 might be part of a functional unit including membrane transporters of L-Arg. In various responses both proteins are, in fact, coregulated by the same signals and stimuli. Mouse cationic amino acid transporters (mCATs) are integral membrane proteins with the function of transporting L-Arg, L-lysine, and L-ornithine from the extracellular to intracellular environment. This transport is pH-independent, sensitive to stimulation, and saturable at circulating plasma concentrations of cationic amino acids. Among the four related proteins, CAT-2A, CAT-2B, CAT-3, and CAT4, identified in different mammalian species, CAT-2A is predominantly expressed in liver, whereas CAT-2B is usually induced under inflammatory conditions in a variety of cells and tissues including T cells, macrophages, lung, and testis [170].

ARG1 knockout mice carrying a nonfunctional *Arg1* gene lacked liver arginase activity and died between postnatal days 10 and 14 with severe symptoms of hyperammonemia [124]. For this reason, conditional knockout mice have been generated with a system allowing specific depletion of the *Arg1* gene in a cell type specific manner. Targeted ARG1 depletion in mice macrophages confirmed that the main role of this enzyme, at least in these cells, is to control NOS2 activity, thus NO levels [73]. On the other hand, targeted disruption of the *Arg2* gene showed that homozygous *Arg2*-deficient mice were viable and apparently normal, but had elevated plasma L-Arg levels, which suggests that this enzyme also plays a role in L-Arg homeostasis [276].

IV. IMMUNOREGULATORY ACTIVITIES OF ARG AND NOS

Depending on the local tissue involved in an immune response, the genetic background of the mouse, skewing of Th1/Th2 balance, and the disease state, the products of L-Arg metabolism not only exert either protective or damaging effects on tissues but also regulate activities of innate and specific immune compartments. It is clear that this regulatory role can strongly influence the outcome of infectious and inflammatory pathologies, autoimmune disorders, and cancer. In this sense, NOS and ARG can enter immunoregulatory circuits independently but they can also collaborate, especially under circumstances related to cancer growth. The prevalence of one enzyme pathway over the other appears to be related to the type of tumor and the genetic background of the mice, which dictates the Th1 vs. Th2 orientation of the immune response. As a rule of thumb, when one of the two enzymes is active, the net effect on T lymphocytes can be attributed to cell cycle arrest whereas the concomitant activation of both enzymes within the same environment can lead to T-cell death by apoptosis. Moreover, immune regulation by L-Arg metabolism is not antigen specific but requires that T cells are activated through their clonotypic T-cell receptor (TCR) in order to be susceptible to the inhibitory activity of ARG- and NOS-dependent pathways. Exceptions to these simple rules do exist and will be discussed below.

An intriguing aspect of L-Arg metabolism is the number of molecules and products that can be released extracellularly: NO, N^G-hydroxy-L-arginine (NOHA), L-ornithine, polyamines, L-NMMA, and even the ARG enzyme itself can be found in the extracellular space, where they act as messengers or biological response modifiers that modulate the functions of nearby cells [329]. NOHA can be released by macrophages during intense NOS2 activity [109], inhibiting ARG and stimulating further release of NO by either NOS [37], or hemeproteins such as peroxidases and cytochrome p450 [329] in neighboring cells during inflammatory reactions. NO causes S-nitrosylation of the cysteine present in the ODC active site [19] resulting in its enzymatic inhibition, arrest of polyamine production, and polyamine-driven cell proliferation [37]. Conversely, polyamines produced by ODC are known NOS inhibitors [24]. L-ornithine and eosinophil-derived cationic proteins can impede CAT2B-dependent transport of L-Arg, leading to decreased NO production in asthma [188].

V. MECHANISMS OF NOS-DEPENDENT IMMUNOREGULATION

NO is an uncharged molecule containing an unpaired electron which determines its ability to interact with a number of organic and inorganic molecules including oxygen, superoxide, DNA and proteins; thus it is straightforward why the modulation of its levels might influence virtually all cellular processes [156]. NO at high concentrations reacts with other oxidants generating reactive nitrogen species (RNS), which can directly cause apoptosis or mutagenesis by damaging DNA and proteins. Interaction of NO with oxygen or superoxide forms intermediates that will produce S-nitrosylation of cysteine residues or nitration of aromatic amino acid (such as tyrosine or tryptophan residues), respectively [282]. Posttranslational modification of various target molecules represents one of the mechanisms by which NOS2 might modulate their activity. For example, NOS2 can directly modify ARG1 by S-nitrosylation which results in the enhancement of ARG1 enzymatic activity, thus to depletion of L-Arg which in turn causes NOS2 inhibition [70]. Although so far this phenomenon has been shown only in rat endothelial cells, it might represent a regulatory feedback loop to control excessive NO levels and therefore their damage on cellular structures [70]. S-nytrosilated proteins can be rapidly reduced by the GSH/GSSG redox system, which ensures that cellular proteins keep a reduced state. In this process GSH can be S-nitrosilated turning into nitrosoglutathione (GSNO) which represents a potent transfer agent of NO to other thiols by trans-nitrosylation [323].

NO, produced at high levels in the immune system by NOS2, has protective effects during infection but also damaging properties during autoimmune responses. To date, there is no doubt that NO is a critical player in different immunological responses other than pathogens and tissue assault since it regulates cytokine production, leukocyte chemotactic responses, cell survival, and thymic education [26,28,165]. This multifunctional molecule is also involved in the pathogenesis of infectious diseases, the degenerative effects of chronic inflammatory diseases and the growth of tumors [85,198,282].

NOS2-derived NO (the term NO is used here collectively for all its reactive intermediates) plays a dual role in an immune response, by exerting protective and toxic effects in parallel. The first immunoregulatory activity assigned to NO was the ability to impair the proliferation of T lymphocytes. For many years, in fact, NO production was considered the key mechanism by which macrophages inhibited T-lymphocyte proliferative responses to antigens and mitogens [165,318]. This inhibition might account, at least partially, for the immunosuppressed state seen in certain infectious diseases, malignancies, and graft-vs-host reactions, but it is also important for the control of inflammatory processes or to delete autoreactive T lymphocytes [25,142,144].

A direct pro-apoptotic effect of NO on T lymphocytes has been observed at high NO concentrations and it has been considered important for the regulation of T-cell maturation in the thymus as well as T-cell growth in the periphery [144]. NO-induced T-cell death has been associated with different mechanisms such as p53 accumulation, Fas- or TNF-receptor activated signaling, as well as caspase-independent pathways [113,166,171].

The immunoregulatory role of NO has been further unveiled by the use of NOS inhibitors such as N^G-monomethyl-L-arginine monoacetate (L-NMMA) or by experiments making use of transgenic mice in which *Nos2* was deleted. These sets of experiments revealed that NOS2 could also be expressed by T lymphocytes where it played a major role in trophic signal withdrawal death (TSWD) following T-cell activation. As a consequence, after antigen challenge, $Nos2^{-/-}$ mice displayed higher frequency of memory T cells, since activated effector cells failing to undergo apoptosis become memory T cells. This process is independent from the NOS2 activity of antigen-presenting cells since back addition of these cells from wild-type animals did not restore the normal levels of postactivation apoptotic events following IL-2 withdrawal in $Nos2^{-/-}$ T cells. The mechanism underlying this phenomenon involves the anti-apoptotic protein Bcl-2, whose levels fail to decrease upon IL-2 deprivation in $Nos2^{-/-}$ T cells, therefore activated T cells were protected from TSWD [308]. The Bcl-2 pathway, involving mitochondrial death route, is distinct from the one triggered by NO produced by macrophages and myeloid cells, which instead requires TNF, p53 and CD95.

The expression of NOS2 has been described in mouse T lymphoblasts, Jurkat cells, and human T lymphocytes infiltrating grafts in immunodeficient mice [143,171,308]. In many human studies, the cells analyzed were of neoplastic derivation, raising the question whether NO production could depend on the acquisition of a malignant phenotype, a rather frequent possibility as discussed in the next paragraphs. Indeed, human T cells and peripheral lymphocytes were shown to express *NOS2* mRNA only upon infection with human T-cell leukemia virus [200]. However, this controversial debate is still open since it has been shown that human T cells produce NO via NOS3 following TCR-mediated Ca^{2+} release and phosphoinositide 3-kinase activation [120]. Interestingly, NOS3 overexpression increased ERK phosphorylation, altered CD3 distribution within the immunological synapse and stimulated IFN-γ release while repressing IL-2 production [120]. Given the data obtained from $Nos2^{-/-}$ mice, it is possible that in human the effect of NO on T cells could be ascribed to the differential expression of NOS enzymes in immune cells, though the net result of NO on T-cell biology is still conserved between the two species.

Further, NO interferes not only with the survival of T lymphocytes but also it impairs their activation by altering the signaling cascade downstream of IL-2 binding to the IL-2 receptor (IL-2R). This activity might depend on both S-nitrosylation of critical cysteine residues or activation of soluble guanylate cyclase (sGC) and cGMP-dependent protein kinase (cGK)

[23,69,81]. The final results of this process are that the phosphorylation and activation of signaling intermediates in the IL-2R pathway (JAK1, JAK3, STAT5, Erk, and Akt) are inhibited in T lymphocytes by NO [23,182]. NO can also affect the stability of IL-2 mRNA and its release by activated human T lymphocytes [81,166], again suggesting that NO action on T lymphocytes translates into a reversible proliferative arrest.

NO secretion by MDSCs is also required for the recruitment of immunoregulatory T cells (NO-Treg) characterized by specific surface markers (CD25$^+$CD27$^+$FoxP3$^-$GITR$^+$ T-bet^{low} GATA3^{high}) and functionally similar to natural Treg lymphocytes [78]. Recently, it was shown that also subsets of antigen-induced regulatory T cells may be a source of NO necessary for their inhibitory effect on activated T lymphocytes [45]. Therefore, with respect to Treg functions NO might be required for both induction and suppressive function in some cell subsets.

Although macrophages are the main source of NOS2/NO the facility of NO, to diffuse through cell membranes explains its effects also on different immune cell types such as B lymphocytes, where it impairs immunoglobulin expression [26,127], and NK cells, where it is required for IFN-γ mediated cytotoxic activity [64].

The ability to influence the production of pro-inflammatory cytokines (including IFN-γ) by various cell types represents a third immunoregulatory property of NO [27]. For several cytokines, however, conflicting results have been reported and the pathway subjected to NO regulation remains to be defined. Controversy also exists with respect to the net effect of NO on Th1/Th2 balance, even though different studies have indicated a possible selective activity of exogenous NO on the cytokine released by established Th1 lines. By interfering prevalently with the IL-2-dependent signaling pathways, low levels of NO mainly control Th1-lymphocyte proliferation/function [18,218]. In particular INF-γ mediated NO production can inhibit the adhesion of Th1 lymphocytes to endothelial cells during inflammation, a process that can be considered as a feedback mechanism to limit excessive accumulation of Th1 cells at sites of inflammation [219]. Under these conditions, NO could also favor Th2-cell functions by upregulating IL-4 production. The controversy in establishing a sharp effect of NO on the Th1/Th2 balance is also further complicated by the reciprocal regulation between NOS2 and ARG1 activities, thus making the scenario a sort of yin-yang system [70].

In acute bacterial or parasitic infections, NO is described as a resistance factor elaborated by the host to fight pathogens whereas persistent infection with parasites, such as *Tripanosoma*, *Chlamidya*, *Schistosoma*, or *Leishmania*, are commonly characterized by an increase in ARG expression concomitantly with the prevalent production of IL-4, IL-10, and TGF-β [310]. On the other hand, results obtained in models of *Candida albicans* and *Tripanosoma cruzi* infections demonstrated the existence of an immunosuppressive mechanism depending on IFN-γ-induced secretion of NO by myeloid cells that colonize the spleen during the acute phase of infection [91,186,295].

Despite apparently divergent data, high levels of NO can affect both Th1 and Th2 lymphocytes and induce their apoptosis, possibly in conjunction with other NO- and O$_2$-derived metabolites, as discussed in the next sections.

VI. MECHANISMS OF ARG-DEPENDENT IMMUNOREGULATION

An unexpected role of ARG has also been demonstrated in the suppression of the immune response. Although in recent years this field of research produced a large amount of experimental evidence, the first observation that arginase can suppress an immune response under certain conditions dates back to 1977 [147]. Since then, the mechanisms exhibited by ARG to induce suppression of T lymphocytes have been extensively reviewed [31,99].

The bulk of evidence accumulated so far indicates that the effect of ARG on the immune system depends mostly on the depletion of L-Arg from the intracellular and extracellular environment rather than on production of metabolites through the downstream metabolic pathways involving ODC and OAT. Mouse macrophages stimulated *in vitro* with IL-4/IL-13 upregulate ARG1 and CAT2B transporter leading to enhanced consumption of extracellular L-Arg levels [254,256]. Decreased levels of L-Arg have been detected in wounds, in liver transplanted individuals, after surgery, in patients with acute bacterial peritonitis, and in tumors [255]. ARG1 activation in tumor-infiltrating CD11b$^+$, Gr-1$^-$, CD16/32$^+$, and F4/80$^-$ myeloid cells, also expressing high levels of CAT2B transporter, consumed L-Arg and inhibited the re-expression of CD3 ζ chain in T cells stimulated by antigen, thus impairing their proliferation [254,256]. The CD3 ζ chain is the main signal transduction element of the TCR and is required for the correct assembly of the receptor complex [15]. Loss of CD3 ζ chain in circulating peripheral blood lymphocytes, in fact, is a hallmark of patients that experience a reduction in blood L-Arg, possibly through ARG activation, in pathologies as varied as cancer, chronic infections, liver transplantation, and trauma [15,255]. Alteration of CD3 ζ chain levels in T cells could thus represent an important mechanism for tumor escape *in vivo*.

ARG1 is expressed in immunosuppressive granulocytes expanded in patients with renal cell carcinomas [335], and in a mouse lung carcinoma model, the ARG inhibitor N-hydroxy-nor-L-Arg (Nor-NOHA) was shown to slow the growth of an experimental lung carcinoma in a dose-dependent fashion [254]. Genetic and pharmacological inhibition of cyclooxygenase 2 (COX-2), but not COX-1, also blocked ARG1 activity in tumor-infiltrating cells. COX-2 was expressed in lung cancer cells and generated PGE2, which ultimately induced ARG1 in myeloid cells through the PGE2 receptor E-prostanoid 4. Analogously to Nor-NOHA, COX-2 inhibitors enhanced a lymphocyte-mediated antitumor response [252].

ARG1 in human granulocytes [210] can be released in the cellular milieu inducing a profound suppression of T-cell proliferation and cytokine synthesis [211]. Interestingly, ARG1, released from gelatinase granules by human granulocytes is inactive at physiological pH unless activated by factor(s) stored in azurophil granules. Whereas ARG1 exocytosis was induced by either TNF-α or ionomycin, only the latter mediated the release of both granules, resulting in extracellular ARG enzyme activation at physiological pH and inhibition of T-cell activation [261]. It thus appears that, despite the different prevalent localization in mouse and human cells of the innate immune system, the immunoregulatory properties of ARG1 were conserved during evolution.

Analogously to tumors, parasites might also have developed strategies to overcome T-lymphocyte recognition by altering L-Arg metabolism. Patients infected with *H. pylori* can develop a chronic gastritis in the absence of protective immunity. Human T lymphocytes stimulated in the presence of a crude extract of *H. pylori* had a reduced proliferation that correlated with a decreased CD3 ζ chain expression [333]. Interestingly, when the extract was derived from the mutant strain of *H. pylori* rocF(−), lacking the arginase gene, alterations of T lymphocytes were absent, indicating a close relationship between *H. pylori*-induced lymphocyte dysfunction and *H. pylori* arginase [333].

The biochemical bases for linking T-lymphocyte proliferative arrest, loss of CD3 ζ chain, and L-Arg starvation are only partially known. The signaling elements GCN2 kinase and mTOR function as amino acid sensors in mammalian cells and it was suggested that they might play a role in regulating mRNA stability of crucial molecules in T cells, including the CD3 ζ chain [31]. GCN2 kinase phosphorylation via L-Arg deprivation was shown to occur in astrocytes, similar to how activation of GCN2 kinase mediates proliferative arrest and T-cell anergy induction in response to L-tryptophan deprivation by IDO [155,212]. T cells stimulated and cultured in the absence of L-Arg undergo a proliferative arrest at the G_0-G_1 phase of the cell cycle. L-Arg consumption by ARG1 in tumor-conditioned macrophages mediated GCN2 kinase-dependent cell cycle arrest in the G_0-G_1 phase and downregulation of the ζ chain of the TCR/CD3 complex in antigen-activated T cells [253,254]. The anergic status of T cells is associated with the impairment of cyclin D3 and cyclin-dependent kinase 4 upregulation, decreased phosphorylation of retinoblastoma protein and a low expression and binding of E2F1. These findings might explain how GCN2 can control T lymphocyte proliferation; to date, however, no direct link between L-Arg deprivation and CD3 ζ chain dowregulation by the GCN2 and/or mTOR pathways has been established.

B lymphocytes are also severely affected by chronic L-Arg deficiency. Transgenic mice that overexpress ARG1 in their enterocytes suffer from a 30—35% reduction in serum L-Arg levels, retardation of hair and muscle growth, and irregular development of the lymphoid tissues. Whereas T-cell number is not affected, B cells undergo a maturation block at the transition from the pro- to pre-B-cell stage in the bone marrow [59]. As a result, the number of B lymphocytes is reduced in peripheral lymphoid organs and small intestine, serum IgM levels are decreased and the architecture of lymphoid organs, especially Peyer's patches, is profoundly compromised. The reason for this selective effect on B-lymphocyte maturation is not known and models in which ARG1 expression is targeted to other immunological sites are required to understand the effects of more localized L-Arg consumption.

VII. ARG AND NOS COOPERATION IN IMMUNOREGULATION: AN EMERGING CONCEPT

ARG and NOS can cooperate to restrain T-lymphocyte functions in tumor-bearing hosts by altering the production of reactive nitrogen and oxygen species (RNS and ROS, respectively). The dual co-expression of ARG and NOS might be a singular property of MDSCs, or at least a part of this heterogeneous population of myeloid suppressors induced by tumors [31]. The molecular bases for the synergism between these enzymes are still not yet entirely known. Even though it is still under debate whether ARG and NOS could be active in the same cell, in the tumor microenvironment the co-existence of classically activated (NOS2$^+$) and alternatively activated (ARG1$^+$) macrophages in tumor environment has been accepted [240]. Further, the hypoxic microenvironment in growing tumor lesions has been shown to induce both enzymes through the stabilization of HIF1α [36,56], thus representing the ideal biological system where MDSCs might exploit NOS2/ARG1 co-activation in order to achieve a powerful control of T-cell effector functions thus promoting cancer outgrowth.

On the other hand, a number of cross-regulatory circuits might limit the activity of one enzyme when the other is functional (reviewed in [31]). For example, NOHA, an intermediate during the biosynthesis of NO by NOS, is a physiologic inhibitor of ARG. Despite the plethora of regulatory pathways, there is no definitive conclusion on whether induction of ARG activity limits the availability of L-Arg as a substrate for NOS to the point of impairing NO production. IL-13 pretreatment of mouse peritoneal macrophages stimulated by IFN-γ and LPS caused downregulation of NOS2 protein (but not mRNA), a process dependent on L-Arg depletion by IL-13-induced ARG1 [72]. Low extracellular L-Arg concentration, overexpression of ARG1, or reduction of L-Arg uptake can decrease intracellular L-Arg concentration and halt translation of *Nos2* mRNA, a phenomenon known as the *arginine paradox* [155]. However, in other studies carried out in macrophages, ARG1 induction and depletion of the cytosolic L-Arg content did not affect the NO generation [82].

At first sight, this evidence may seem contradictory, although this dichotomy could be simply due to the combination of stimuli present in a given cellular microenvironment, which can overcome the apparent incompatibility of the ARG1/NOS2 metabolic pathways [108].

VIII. PEROXYNITRITE GENERATION

ARG and NOS2 co-expression could actually have important supplementary effects: i.e., the possible production of superoxide (O_2^-) from the NOS2 reductase domain. At low local L-Arg concentration, NOS2 activity shifts from a prevalent NO production to O_2^- production [33,330,331]. ARG1 might thus function as controller of NOS2 activity by modulating L-Arg

607

content in the microenvironment where T cells are activated, a hypothesis substantiated by a number of findings in mouse and human tumors [31,32,60,254,256,335]. Once generated, O_2^- reacts immediately with the residual NO leading to the formation of peroxynitrite ($ONOO^-$), a highly reactive oxidizing agent with the potential of damaging different biological targets [242,267]. Peroxynitrite is no longer considered simply a toxic byproduct but is currently viewed as an intra- and intercellular messenger since it can diffuse through cell membranes and induce posttranslational protein modifications by nitrating protein-associated tyrosines [242,267]. Peroxynitrite can either stimulate or inhibit tyrosine phosphorylation depending on its concentration: inhibition of phosphatases mainly occurs at low and acute doses, while prolonged high-dose treatments cause massive modification of proteins, receptors and protein tyrosin kinase (PTK) inhibition [145].

In vitro treatment of human T cells with peroxynitrite induced impairment of T-cell functions. Peroxynitrite was found to induce a TCR-independent tyrosine phosphorylation of several proteins, including the CD3 ζ chain of the TCR complex, and release of Ca^{2+} from intracellular stores. However, prolonged exposure to this RNS caused a state of T-cell refractoriness to stimulation, characterized by downregulation of membrane proteins including CD4, CD8, and chemokine receptors [131]. Strikingly, at least *in vitro*, this RNS-mediated T-cell anergy was irreversible. Thus, oxidative stress mediated by RNS directly might cause downregulation of co-receptors by triggering abortive signals. Nitrotyrosines are also detected in apoptotic thymocytes suggesting that peroxynitrite can be involved in thymic-dependent T-cell education *in vivo* [206]. Nitrotyrosines are also found in tissue sections of hyperplastic human lymph nodes obtained from surgical resections of patients with lung and colon cancer [30] and in human prostate adenocarcinomas [31]. Recently, it was shown that production of RNS by both cancer cells and tumor-infiltrating MDSCs is responsible for limiting $CD8^+$ T-cell infiltration within the tumor mass. This is due to the local nitration/nytrosylation of CCL2, an inflammatory chemokine fostering both CTL and myeloid cell recruitment to tumors. The presence of nitrated/nitrosylated-CCL2 (N-CCL2) within human prostate and colon cancer correlated with the accumulation of T lymphocytes at the periphery of tumors. On the other hand, myeloid cells were still recruited to the inner part of tumor lesions even in presence of N-CCL2. This is explained by the fact that RNS-induced posttranslational modification of the chemokine changes its affinity for the corresponding receptor, CCR2, differentially expressed on T cells with respect to MDSCs. Thus N-CCL2 still attracts MDSCs expressing higher levels of CCR2 than T cells [197].

Activated T lymphocytes are more prone to $ONOO^-$-induced death than resting T cells. Peroxynitrite-induced apoptosis of T cells activated by PHA or anti-CD3 (but not by phorbol esters) likely requires inhibition of protein tyrosine phosphorylation via nitration of tyrosine residues [30]. At high doses, peroxynitrite can directly control cell death by nitration of the protein voltage-dependent anion channel, a component of the mitochondrial permeability transition pore [10,35]. However, peroxynitrite-induced inhibition of T lymphocytes is not invariably associated with cell apoptosis. In human prostate cancer, the neoplastic but not the normal prostate epithelium overexpressed ARG2 and NOS1 and addition of a combination of enzyme-specific inhibitors to prostate cultures was sufficient to decrease the nitrotyrosine content in tumor-infiltrating lymphocytes (TILs) and restore their local responsiveness to various stimuli [33]. This is an important finding for the development of therapeutic interventions aimed at restoring lymphocyte responsiveness in tumor-bearing hosts.

IX. PEROXYNITRITE AND AUTOIMMUNITY

Paradoxically, findings in non-obese diabetic (NOD) mice also suggest that excessive nitrotyrosine formation might be linked to autoimmune disease. NOD mice develop progressive autoimmune diabetes that shares some similarity with the human disease. From 4 weeks of age, mononuclear cells start to infiltrate the islet of the pancreas (insulitis) causing a progressive destruction of insulin-secreting β cells, which ultimately leads to clinical signs of diabetes at 12 weeks of age. Macrophages are among the first cells to seed the pancreata and together with autoreactive T lymphocytes are considered the first offensive line for tissue destruction. Among various disorders described in NOD mice, some appear to be related to L-Arg and L-Trp metabolism including the propensity of NOD mouse bone marrow to produce CD11b$^+$/Gr-1$^+$ (putative MDSCs) rather than DCs in response to GM-CSF [201], the overexpression of ARG during insulitis [259], and the increased production of peroxynitrite by myeloid cells, including the cells infiltrating the pancreas [100,289]. These abnormalities have a direct link with the pathology. Administration of the peroxynitrite scavenger guanidinoe-thyldisuplphide (GED) at 5 weeks of age decreased the incidence of diabetes from 80% to 17% [288]. Peroxynitrite is also produced in response to IFN-γ by CD8$^+$ DCs isolated from NOD mice at 4 but not at 8 weeks of age [101]. CD8$^+$ DCs constitute a peculiar regulatory popu-lation exploiting L-Trp metabolism to induce T-cell tolerance. In normal mice, INF-γ activates the enzyme IDO in CD8$^+$ DCs through a STAT1-dependent pathway [98,102]. In NOD mice, STAT1 is nitrated by peroxynitrite and is not able to properly drive IDO expression in response to IFN-γ. The peroxynitrite inhibitor GED but not the NOS2 inhibitor L-NMMA restored the normal pathway, raising the question about the route of peroxynitrite production in these cells. Since L-NMMA does not reduce O$_2^-$ generation by the NOS2 reductase domain, an effect that can be obtained only by increasing L-Arg concentrations [330,331], it would be interesting to examine the role of ARG-driven depletion of L-Arg in this model. However, it is clear that at an age (4 weeks) critical for shaping the repertoire of autoreactive T cells, DCs are impaired in their ability to activate IDO-dependent tolerogenic pathways.

These findings suggest that L-Arg and L-Trp metabolism cannot operate in the same cell due to the existence of cross-inhibitory circuits. IDO is inhibited by NO and peroxynitrite, terminal effector molecules generated by L-Arg metabolism, whereas L-Trp cytosolic depletion by IDO blocks IFN-γ-dependent NOS2 expression in macrophages [47,100,117]. These findings might help to explain the association between cancer and autoimmune paraneoplastic syndromes where an extensive production of peroxynitrite by myeloid cells (or tumor them-selves) might inhibit the tolerogenic pathways and unleash autoreactive lymphocytes.

X. HYDROGEN PEROXIDE GENERATION

ARG activation was associated with hydrogen peroxide (H$_2$O$_2$) production by MDSCs isolated from the spleen of mice bearing a transplantable fibrosarcoma. In this model, MDSCs presented class I-restricted epitopes directly to CD8$^+$ T lymphocytes and caused the inhibition of their IFN-γ release through contact-dependent production of H$_2$O$_2$ [151]. Although the molecular mechanisms are still under investigation, the link between ARG1 and H$_2$O$_2$ has been confirmed in other tumor models [150,283]. A possible explanation would link ARG1 activity to the simultaneous expression of various NOS isoforms: under L-Arg starvation NOS2 but also NOS1 and NOS3 generate O$_2^-$ although with differences in the kinetics of this NADPH-dependent oxidation. At low L-Arg concentrations NOS2 can produce NO and O$_2^-$ while NOS1 produces O$_2^-$ and H$_2$O$_2$. Differential enzymatic activity and expression profiles in MDSC subsets [67] of NOS2 (monocytes-like) with respect to NOS1 and NOS3 (granulocytes-like), might therefore influence the outcome of the suppressive mechanisms operated by these cells under conditions of L-Arg deprivation generated by ARG1 of either TAMs or cancer cells. ROS released from CD11b$^+$/Gr-1$^+$ cells were shown to alter CD3 ζ chain expression and function in mice [225] and in patients with advanced-stage cancer, where H$_2$O$_2$ was found to be produced by an expanded pool of circulating, low-density granulocytes [266]. These granulocytes are also positive for ARG1 [168,169]. H$_2$O$_2$ originates from the conversion of superoxide in contact with protons in water according to the simple formula: $2\,O_2^- + 2H^+ \leftrightarrow H_2O_2 + O_2$ [248]. This spontaneous reaction occurs any time superoxide is produced by both oxygen dependent and independent pathways. H$_2$O$_2$ is electrically neutral, relatively stable, and diffuses across membranes, thus representing another potential intra- and intercellular messenger [248]. Analogously to peroxynitrite, H_2O_2 can induce apoptosis of antigen-activated T lymphocytes although through different mechanisms, for example by down-regulating intracellular Bcl-2 and increasing plasma membrane levels of Fas-L via NF-κB [111]. Human central memory and effector memory T cells ($CD45RA^-CCR7^+$ and $CD45RA^-CCR7^-$, respectively) are more sensitive to H_2O_2 than naïve T cells and respond to lower concentrations of this oxidative molecule by undergoing mitochondrial and caspase-dependent apoptosis in the absence of stimulation [229]. Cancer cells and cell population infiltrating the tumor such as TAMs, activated granulocytes and MDSCs produce a large amount of ROS and NO which, as previously mentioned, can drive apoptosis of T and NK cells [158,167,266]. Paradoxically, the number of regulatory T (Treg) lymphocytes and NK ($CD56^{bright}$) cells is higher within the tumor lesions. Tumor can induce Tregs through factors secreted in the microenvironment such as NO, $COX-2/PGE_2$ or IL-10 [21,217]. Treg and NK $CD56^{bright}$ are less sensitive to H_2O_2 induced oxidative stress than their effector counterparts mainly because they are naturally protected by ROS through a higher thiols density of the plasma membranes and a higher intracellular anti-oxidative potential [106,205,302]. In particular Tregs express and secrete high levels of thyoredoxin, which helps neutralize the effect of H_2O_2 [204].

A similar strategy is also used physiologically by DCs to protect T-cell survival from premature inactivation and apoptosis driven by oxidative stress conditions such as microbial infections. Myeloid DCs have been shown to neutralize H_2O_2 by maintaining high levels of membrane associated thiols and by upregulating the expression/secretion of thioredoxin upon interaction with antigen-specific T lymphocytes [8]. Further, *in vitro* co-culture of myeloid DCs and T cells produced an increase of thiol density also on the cellular membrane of the lymphocytes [301]. Although the mechanisms underlying this phenomenon are not fully understood yet, it is clear that controlling the ability of surviving in a hostile redox environment can push the balance towards either immune response or tolerance.

In this scenario it is clear that ARG1 and H_2O_2 create a positive loop aimed at selectively eliminating effector cells from the tumor microenvironment while progressively favoring the accumulation of regulatory elements. ROS produced by MDSCs inhibit both T- and NK-reactivity by causing downregulation of the CD3 ζ chain [80,179] and the CD16 ζ [106], respectively, and by forcing them to undergo apoptosis [238]. The association between H_2O_2 and ARG1 requires further studies since ARG1 was shown to be upregulated after treating porcine coronary arterioles with H_2O_2 through a process requiring the formation of hydroxyl radicals from H_2O_2 [297]. This finding suggests that ARG1 activation might also follow and not precede H_2O_2 generation.

XI. IS THERE A PHYSIOLOGICAL ROLE FOR L-ARG METABOLISM IN THE CONTROL OF IMMUNITY?

Much of the data discussed in previous paragraphs were obtained in pathological settings. However, the impact of ROS and RNS on T-lymphocyte functions can be important in controlling normal responses to antigen. Indeed, some evidence points to a specific role in modulating the contraction of $CD8^+$ T cells during normal immune responses. The contraction phase follows the massive clonal expansion of naïve $CD8^+$ T cells that encountered pathogen that was captured, processed, and presented by antigen-presenting cells. During antigen-driven activation, quiescent cells are turned into effector T cells that secrete cytokines and eliminate infected host cells within a few weeks. In the contraction phase, the majority of antigen-specific effector cells die by apoptosis over the next 2—3 weeks and only a minority of cells ($\sim$5—10%) survives as the long-lived memory cell population.

Memory T cells have an increased ability to survive *in vivo* compared with naïve T cells that arises from the ability to bind and respond to the homeostatic cytokine IL-7 [264]. Selective expression of IL-7Rα on effector $CD8^+$ T cells identifies memory cell precursors. Whereas the molecular bases for the long-term survival of memory cells have been partially unveiled, the factor(s) regulating contraction of CD8$^+$ effectors still remains obscure. The contraction phase is not dependent on antigen clearance, as one can intuitively guess, but it appears to be an event programmed during the initial phases of infection [11,12]. The contraction phase is impaired in mice lacking either IFN-γ or its receptor and requires the acquisition of suppressive functions by a population of CD11b$^+$ cells that counter-regulate CD8$^+$ T cells [11,12,273]. How CD11b$^+$ cells conditioned by IFN-γ contribute to the contraction phase is still not completely clear but several lines of evidence point to RNS and ROS released by these cells as final mediators. T-cell death during the contraction phase is also inhibited in mice lacking NOS2, resulting in a higher frequency of memory T cells following immunization [49,85,308]. Further, CD11b$^+$/Gr-1$^+$ MDSCs activated by IFN-γ produce reactive species which then affect T cells during apoptosis induced by superantigens [39]. In agreement with a role for ROS/RNS in controlling the execution of the program leading to immunological memory, the peroxynitrite scavenger Mn(III)tetrakis(4-benzoic acid)porphyrin chloride (MnTBAP) enhanced memory responses by blocking postactivation death and contraction of CD8$^+$ T cells in mice immunized either with the antigen ovalbumin or infected with lymphocytic choriomeningitis virus [153,308]. ARG mediated T-cell impairment is also involved in the suppression of the maternal immune response against the fetus. Arginase activity is strongly upregulated in the placenta and increased in the peripheral blood of pregnant women [146]. While the placental ARG might be an important source of polyamines, ARG of the polymorphonuclear leukocytes depletes locally L-Arg and thus promotes T-cell anergy [146].

It must be pointed out, however, that activation also increases the amount of reactive species (H$_2$O$_2$, NO and O$_2^-$) within the very same T lymphocytes [63,113] and that ROS produced by T lymphocytes can regulate their apoptosis during the contraction phase, possibly via modulation of Bcl-2 and Fas-L [112]. Interestingly enough, in one of these studies, MnTABP protected T lymphocytes from apoptotic death [113]. Production of ROS/RNS might thus be the major rheostat regulating adaptive immune responses. It is not entirely clear which population is the most important contributor to ROS/RNS production: T lymphocytes (inner rheostat) or myeloid cells (external rheostat). For this reason, the use of inhibitors that can act both on T cells and myeloid cells, such as MnTABP, certainly cannot help to address this issue.

XII. NOS IN CANCER

Several investigators have reported the expression of NOS2 by malignant cells or within the tumor microenvironment, both at the mRNA and protein level. In breast carcinoma, an initial study suggested that NOS2 activity was higher in less differentiated tumors [300] and was detected predominantly in tumor-infiltrating macrophages. Subsequently, other studies have demonstrated that NOS2 is expressed also by breast carcinoma cells and it correlates with tumor stage and microvessel density [159,160,249,305].

In addition to breast cancer, NOS2 is markedly expressed in approximately 60% of human colon adenomas and in 20—25% of colon carcinomas, while expression is either low or absent in the surrounding normal tissues [7,220]. Similarly, in human ovarian cancer and melanoma, NOS2 activity was localized to tumor cells but not to normal ovarian tissue and melanocytes, respectively [177,298]. Other cancers that express NOS2 are head and neck [227], esophagus [325], lung [6], bladder [291] and pancreatic carcinomas [105], brain tumors [53], Kaposi's sarcoma [322], mesothelioma [176], prostate carcinoma [31,140] and hematological malignancies [187,257]. Regarding the other two NOS isoenzymes, in a series of 54 cases of breast carcinoma, NOS3 was expressed in 33 samples (61%), and its degree of expression strongly correlated with that of NOS2 [160]. In another series (n = 80), both NOS2 and NOS3 were found not only in the surrounding stroma, but also within carcinoma cells [305]. Finally, NOS1 has been detected in some oligodendroglioma and neuroblastoma cell lines [53].

612

These findings, together with the observation that NOS (particularly NOS2) expression levels correlate with poor clinical outcome of patients affected with different types of cancer, such as melanoma [71], breast [159], ovarian [246], head and neck [88], and colorectal [221] carcinoma, have led several investigators to consider NO as a potential mediator of tumor development/progression. Indeed, various RNS can damage DNA through a variety of different mechanisms [77,175,326]. N_2O_3 is a strong nitrosylating agent mediating the addition of NO^+ to nucleophiles and able to deaminate DNA bases (e.g., cytosine to uracil, guanine to xanthine), eventually causing a variety of point mutations. N_2O_3 can also react with secondary amines to form carcinogenic N–nitrosamines, which can damage DNA by alkylation. Peroxynitrite, as previously discussed, represent highly reactive nitrating species, that can directly induce DNA mutations and single-strand breaks [175,262]. RNS-mediated DNA damage can be measured as conversion of guanine into 8-nitroguanine and 8-oxoguanine involved in inflammation-related carcinogenesis. In humans, *H. Pylori* infection—which is recognized as an etiologic factor for human gastric lymphoma and carcinoma—has been associated with high levels of 8–oxoguanine in urine [327] and gastric mucosa [163]. Moreover, 8-oxoguanine levels are higher in gastric cancer rather than normal surrounding tissues [43]. An increased level of 8-nitroguanine by immunohistochemical analysis was frequently found at tumor sites in patients with various inflammatory disease and in asbestos-exposed mice [115]. Nitrotyrosine is the footprint of peroxynitrite-mediated nitration and the presence of nitrotyrosine has been identified by immunohistochemistry in *H. Pylori* gastritis [129] and several human cancers including cholangiocarcinoma [126], pancreatic cancer [307], prostate carcinoma [31], esophageal carcinoma [133], breast carcinomas [215], head and neck cancer [20], mesothelioma [137], and melanoma [97]. Similarly, patients with lung cancer not only exhale more NO but also have higher plasma levels of nitrated proteins compared to controls [138,234].

The production of NO within the tumor microenvironment is believed to promote tumor growth by stimulating angiogenesis [22,199], a multistep process regulated by the release of angiogenic factors (e.g., vascular endothelial growth factor (VEGF), integrins, basic-fibroblast growth factor (b-FGF), and hypoxia-inducible factor-1 (HIF-1)) produced by malignant cells, stromal fibroblasts, and TAMs. A functional NO/cGMP pathway is required for VEGF to promote angiogenesis [88,337]. Accordingly, *in vitro* NOS inhibition decreases endothelial cell proliferation [194] while L-Arg depletion inhibits endothelial cell tubularization and capillary formation [228]. NO-dependent upregulation of VEGF, likely by mRNA stabilization [48], yields increased vascularization in xenograft tumors [6]. Additionally, in human colon and gastric carcinoma specimens *NOS2* expression correlate with both VEGF mRNA levels and microvessel density [51,121]. Moreover, human carcinoma cells transfected with a murine *Nos2* cDNA show an increased tumor growth and neo-vascularization in a nude mouse xenograft model [299].

Another mechanism by which angiogenesis could be influenced by NO is through the modulation of prostaglandins production. NO can activate COX-2 [50,176,196,228] that, by generating prostaglandins, promotes angiogenesis and inhibits apoptosis [303]. HIF-1, an O_2 regulated transcriptional activator plays a central role in tumor angiogenesis and it is known to regulate the expression of several angiogenesis-related genes, including *NOS2* [270]. In a positive feedback circuit, NO can activate HIF-1, thus potentiating *NOS2* transcription [136]. Since NO induces HIF-1 expression under nonhypoxic conditions [132], it has been postulated that high levels of NO within the tumor microenvironment might have the same effect as hypoxia in inducing angiogenesis [269]. Furthermore, in macrophages, the hypoxia-driven activation of HIF-1α directly upregulates *NOS2* and *ARG* transcription [3,279] and in the tumor microenvironment promotes differentiation of MDSC into TAMs. These TAMs, characterized by high levels of ARG1 and NO but not of ROS, were stronger inhibitors of antigen-specific T-cell functions than splenic MDSCs but were also able to suppress T cells in an antigen-independent manner [56,279].

TABLE 34.1 Nitric oxide and cancer: knockout models*

Gene	Experimental model	Findings	Comments/interpretation	Reference
NOS2	Animal: mice C57BL Tumor: B16 melanoma, M5076 ovarian sarcoma (syngeneic)	NOS2$^{-/-}$: tumor regression (melanoma) or progression (sarcoma), ↓ VEGF, ↓ angiogenesis (melanoma) NOS2$^{+/+}$: macrophages kill sarcoma but not melanoma cells Sarcoma (but not melanoma) cells produce NO	NOS2 is crucial in macrophage-mediated killing of sensitive tumors (sarcoma) and in cancer progression of resistant tumors (melanoma)	[277] [313]
NOS2	Animal: mice B6/129P Tumor: urethane-induced lung cancer	NOS2$^{-/-}$: ↓ tumor development, ↓ VEGF, ↓ angiogenesis; COX expression: unaffected by NOS2	NOS2 is important in lung cancerogenesis and favors tumor angiogenesis through VEGF (but not COX) overexpression	[138]
NOS2	Animal: APC$^{MIN/+}$ (polyposis-prone) mice Tumor: colon adenomas (colon carcinoma precursors)	NOS2$^{-/-}$: ↓ tumor development NOS2$^{+/+}$ treated with NOS2-inhibitor (aminoguanidine): ↓ tumor development	NOS2 favors colon tumorigenesis	[1]
NOS2	Animal: APC$^{MIN/+}$ (polyposis-prone) mice Tumor: colon adenomas (colon carcinoma precursors)	NOS2$^{-/-}$: ↑ tumor development COX expression: unaffected by NOS2	NOS2 plays a protective role with respect to colon tumorigenesis	[268]
NOS2	Animal: mice (C57BL) Tumor: NOS2$^{-/-}$ MDA-induced fibrosarcoma cell lines injected s.c. and i.v.	NOS2$^{-/-}$: ↑ tumor progression NOS2$^{+/+}$: NOS2 is expressed within tumor nodules by stromal cells	Physiological expression of NOS2 in host cells (mainly macrophages) inhibits tumor growth and metastasis	[315]
NOS2	Animal: mice (C57BL) Tumor: polyomavirus middle T antigen-mediated breast cancerogenesis	NOS2$^{-/-}$: ↓ tumor development, no effect on tumor progression (angiogenesis, metastatization rate)	NOS2 plays an important role only in the early events of breast tumorigenesis	[75]
NOS2	Animal: mice C57BL Tumor: H7 pancreatic carcinoma (syngeneic) transfected with IFN-β	NOS2−/−: ↑ tumor progression	Antitumor effects of IFN-β are NO-dependent	[313]
NOS2, p53	Animal: mice (C57BL) Tumor: spontaneously developing lymphoma (p53−/−) & sarcoma (p53+/−)	NOS2$^{-/-}$: ↑ tumor development, ↑ p21/waf1 (↓ proliferation), ↑ TRAIL & FAS-L (↑ apoptosis) p53$^{+/+}$: ↓ NOS2 (NOS2 is transcriptionally repressed by p53)	Functional NOS2 protects from tumorigenesis p53-knockout mice are an animal model of the cancer-prone human Li–Fraumeni syndrome	[119]
NOS2, p53	Animal: mice (C57BL) Tumor: spontaneously developing thymic and non-thymic lymphomas	NOS2$^{-/-}$: ↓ thymic lymphoma development, ↑ non-thymic lymphoma development	Microenvironment profoundly affects the relationship between NO and lymphomagenesis	[294]
eNOS	Animal: mice C57BL Tumor: B16F1 melanoma (syngeneic)	eNOS$^{-/-}$ (and L-NAME treatment): ↓ lung metastases	Endothelial cells have a role in controlling tumor metastasis	[241]

613

Continued

TABLE 34.1	Nitric oxide and cancer: knockout models*—continued			
Gene	Experimental model	Findings	Comments/ interpretation	Reference
eNOS	Animal: C57BL Tumor: Lewis lung carcinoma	eNOS$^{-/-}$: ↓ antitumor activity of cavtratin (antiangiogenic agent)	Cavtratin antitumor effects depend upon eNOS inhibition	[95]
p53	Animal: athymic mice Tumor: p53-/- human colon carcinoma transfected with NOS2	p53$^{-/-}$: ↓ antitumor activity of radiotherapy	NO and ionizing radiation act synergistically to induce p53-dependent apoptosis	[55]
IFN-γ	Animal: mice C57BL Tumor: H7 pancreatic carcinoma (syngeneic)	IFN-γ$^{-/-}$: ↑ tumor progression, ↓ NOS2 expression	IFN-γ secretion by host cells mediates tumor killing via NOS2 expression	[313]

*Adapted from "Nitric oxide, a double edged sword in cancer biology: searching for therapeutic opportunities," by [192].

A third mechanism by which NO may favor tumor progression is represented by the ability to enhance tissue invasion [152]. Studies examining the signaling mechanisms underlying this phenomenon show that both tumor and endothelial cell migration is reduced by NOS2 inhibition/knockdown [125,161,280]. RNS appear to be involved in NO-mediated induction of matrix metalloproteinase activation/overexpression [123,223], a key signature of cancer invasiveness. Although some knockout models support these findings, others demonstrate that macrophage-derived NO can contribute to control of tumor growth and that NO might be fundamental in tumor development but not in tumor progression (Table 34.1). These sometimes conflicting results indicate that the role of NOS2 during tumor development is highly complex and still not completely understood. Both promoting and deterring actions can be observed, presumably depending upon the local concentration of NO within the tumor microenvironment. NO at low concentrations could have a premalignant effect, and at very high concentrations could instead act as a potent anticancer agent [282].

XIII. ARG IN CANCER

Although ARG analysis in mouse and human cancers was initiated more recently in comparison to NOS, it appears that ARG1 and ARG2 are both found within the tumor microenvironment but are distributed in different compartments. From an overall scrutiny of the available literature, the emerging picture is that generally ARG1 is mainly expressed in tumor-infiltrating myeloid cells [251,260] whereas ARG2 is detected primarily in cancerous cells [287]. However, this distinction cannot be taken as absolute since now ARG1 is also used as a marker for some tumors such as hepatocarcinoma [183] and prostate cancer [89], while ARG2 has also been found expressed in murine macrophages [17,44]. The frequent finding of ARG in cancer underlies its important role in tumor biology and development. ARG-dependent tumor-promoting actions can range from pro-angiogenetic activity, lymphocyte suppression, assistance in tumor cell proliferation, and stroma remodeling, all properties that have been assigned to tumor-associated macrophages with an alternative activation profile [13,172]. Several examples, both in preclinical tumor models and in clinical studies, emphasize this multifaceted ARG activity [178].

Intratumoral ARG induction can help tumor growth basically in two ways: by suppressing TIL response and by providing cancerous cells with polyamines. L-ornithine produced by arginase is used by ODC to form polyamines, essential nutrients for mammalian cell proliferation and differentiation. In a mouse model, macrophages transfected with the rat *Arg1* gene enhanced *in vitro* and *in vivo* proliferation of co-cultured tumor cells [42] and ARG-driven polyamine synthesis in macrophages was shown to enhance tumor vascularization [58]. The *Arg1* gene was found, by a genome-wide approach, to be overexpressed in two murine cell lines that are highly metastatic, and consistently elevated in pulmonary metastases compared to the primary tumor in two different mouse metastatic models, suggesting that ARG1 may also be important for tumor colonization of the lungs [173]. Additional evidence supporting involvement of ARG1 in mechanisms of immune system suppression in cancer patients came from the work of Zea and collaborators, showing that peripheral blood mononuclear cells from renal cell carcinoma patients have a significant increase in ARG activity. Moreover, they showed that this increase in activity was restricted to a specific subset of cells with polymorphonuclear granulocyte morphology and surface phenotype [335].

In recent years, a significant association between arginase and cancer has been documented in human tumors. Since polyamines are needed by rapidly dividing cells and tissues, the reaction catalyzed by ARG might meet the requirement for increased metabolism; in fact, increased ARG2 activity has been found in human cell lines [37,281], as well as in human breast [236] and gastric cancers [328]. High ARG activity has been described also in patients with various malignancies including gastric, colon, breast, prostate, and lung cancers either in the serum or in the tumor tissue. In these studies ARG activity has been determined by enzymatic assays that do not discriminate between the different isoforms of the enzyme, and therefore it is not known whether ARG activity can be ascribed to ARG1 or ARG2. The increase in serum ARG activity has been associated with disease progression in colorectal and breast cancer, and, moreover, ARG activity has been proposed as a diagnostic tool to monitor patients with colorectal carcinoma [40,62,134,190,235,236,237,290].

As already anticipated, the role of ARG2 is even more obscure. Using a genomic approach, ARG2 was found to be differentially expressed between follicular thyroid carcinoma (FTC) and benign follicular thyroid adenoma (FTA), with an average increase in expression of at least five-fold in nearly all the FTCs tested [41]. Moreover, in this study, ARG2 was one of the four genes found to be statistically the most consistent marker for FTC. Interestingly, ARG2 knockdown in a follicular thyroid carcinoma cell line by using a siRNA-based approach changed the tumor properties enhancing nitic oxide and ROS production and promoting apoptosis [287].

Deregulated ARG expression and activity have been associated with a number of pathological conditions other than cancer. One of the most interesting developments concerning L-Arg homeostasis is the recent discovery of an increase in the expression and activity of ARG in many tissues and cell types in response to a variety of cytokines, in particular Th2-derived. Increased ARG activity has been recently associated with several inflammatory conditions, such as infections, asthma, arthritis, hyperoxic lung injury, psoriasis, and autoimmune disease [188,207,231]. *In vivo* administration of a pegylated form of human ARG1 and *in vitro* derived MDSCs in a mouse model of GVHD resulted in L-Arg depletion and reduction of disease severity [110].

XIV. ARG AND NOS INHIBITORS: A NOVEL CLASS OF IMMUNE ADJUVANTS?

Although many cancers arise *de novo* without an identifiable predisposing disease, chronic inflammation strongly favors tumor development [5,14,52,57,118,148]. Several *in vitro* models have shown mutagenic and carcinogenic effects of ROS and RNS produced by activated immune cells (e.g., macrophages, neutrophils, eosinophils) expressing enzymes such as myeloperoxidase, eosinophil peroxidase, and NOS2 [222]. The epidemiological association between inflammatory diseases (e.g., chronic gastritis, bowel inflammatory disease, interstitial lung disease) and gastrointestinal or lung cancers further supports this pathogenetic hypothesis [149,164]. These findings—together with the promising results obtained with nonsteroidal anti-inflammatory drugs (NSAID) in colon cancer chemo-prevention [263]—strengthen the notion that inflammation and cancerogenesis share some

615

metabolic pathways, such as those generating high levels of ROS and RNS [118]. As NOS2 overexpression and NO production are cardinal features of inflamed tissues [54,103,154,162], these observations suggest that NO may play a fundamental role in the initiation of cancer arising within a background of chronic inflammation, thereby supporting the rationale for the use of anti-NO agents as antineoplastic drugs [244]. A similar role for ARG is currently suspected but not yet proven due to the absence of complete $Arg1^{-/-}$ mice. However, the possibility of selective depletion *in vivo* of *Arg1* in cells of the myeloid compartment will help in solving this issue [78].

Selective NOS and ARG inhibitors or molecules interfering with the generation of RNS/ROS from the combined activities of NOS/ARG have been proven beneficial in controlling myeloid-dependent suppression *in vitro* [32,60,149,254,283]. However, several considerations motivated increasing interest in combining two or multiple inhibitors. Many of the inhibitors are not selective, plagued by important side effects when administered *in vivo*, and difficult to bring to the clinic. Moreover, we cannot exclude that inhibiting only one arm of L-Arg metabolic pathways might not be sufficient to exert a therapeutic effect in all the different tumors. Additionally, the contemporaneous biosynthesis of NO and prostaglandins (PGs) in various tissues and cells has received much attention in the last few years, because of the possible involvement of the metabolites of these pathways in pathophysiological mechanisms of various chronic inflammatory disorders including cancer. In fact, increasing evidence suggests that there is a substantial cross-talk between NO and PG biosynthetic circuits involving both negative and positive feedback loops mediated by reaction end-products, including the very same NO, PGs, and other cyclic nucleotides. This strict link was further confirmed by the demonstration that NOS2 binds specifically to COX2 and activates it by S-nitrosylation of critical cysteine residues [135]. Together, these results suggest that drugs blocking NOS2-COX2 activities and/or their interaction domain might have a therapeutic benefit greater than the single inhibitors.

The idea of coupling aspirin and a NO-donating moiety in the same structure was originally inspired by the need for reducing the side effects of the former [312]. NO-donating aspirin was shown to possess both antiproliferative and cytocidal effects on colon cancer cell lines depending on the concentration tested [296]. *In vivo*, NO-donating aspirin was also able to reduce gastrointestinal tumorigenesis in transgenic Min mice, chemically induced colon carcinogenesis in rats, and pancreatic cancer development in hamsters [226,245,324]. Interestingly, NO-donating aspirin was shown to inhibit both NOS and ARG activity, *in vitro* and *in vivo*, suppress generation of RNS/ROS at the tumor site and abrogate myeloid cell-dependent suppression *in vivo*. In some mouse tumor models, NO-aspirin did not show any direct antitumor activity but synergized with a recombinant cancer vaccine in inducing prevention and even treatment of established tumors [61]. NO-releasing drugs might thus represent a potent and completely novel immune adjuvant, acting by relieving the suppressive mechanisms negatively affecting T lymphocytes in tumor-bearing hosts.

Prostate cancer represents an interesting target for NO-donating drug therapy for several reasons. Prostate inflammation and prostate cancer development have been related to each other [216]. Moreover, identified prostate-specific antigens could represent suitable targets for immunotherapy but, unfortunately, T lymphocytes infiltrating human prostate cancers are rendered unresponsive within the tumor site, by the combined expression of ARG1 and NOS2 [34]. In fact, prostate cancer is one of the many tumors overexpressing both ARG1 and NOS2 within the cancerous cells. This inhibitory mechanism can be corrected *in vitro* by drugs inhibiting ARG1 and NOS2, thus allowing full rescue of T-cell cytotoxic activity against prostate cancer cells [31]. Preliminary studies indicated that NO-donating aspirin and derivatives could exert the same effect in human prostate cancer cultures (V.B., unpublished).

The mechanism of NO-donating aspirin acting as a modulator of ARG1 and NOS2 activity has not been completely clarified yet. Negative feedback inhibition of both NOS2 enzymatic activity and expression by NO-aspirin [174] likely depends on the NO donation, since this negative feedback was lost upon treatment with a denitrated derivative unable to deliver NO because the nitroester group on the linker had been removed. ARG1 inhibition, on the other hand, could be attributed to the aspirin and aromatic spacer portion of the compound. NO-donating aspirin inhibited ARG1 enzymatic activity *in vitro* but the IC_{50} was greater than ten-fold the dose administered to tumor-bearing mice, a dose too high to hypothesize was produced on direct *in vivo* activity of the salicylic portion of the NO-donating aspirin on ARG enzyme. Perhaps more likely, salicylates operate indirectly by inhibiting the intracellular STAT6-mediated signals triggered by some ARG inducers such as IL-4 and IL-13 [232]. We also demonstrated that expression of IL-4Rα and the binding of IL-13 are critically required for ARG induction and suppressive activity of splenic and tumor-infiltrating MDSCs [87].

As discussed above, regulation of ARG at the tumor site is likely to be more composite since other factors, such as hypoxia and cycloxygenase activity, can sustain the enzyme activity. ARG expression and function in tumor-infiltrating myeloid cells is also controlled by COX-2, an enzyme overexpressed in different human and mouse tumors. In a mouse model of lung cancer, signaling through the PGE_2 receptor in tumor-infiltrating myeloid cells was necessary for ARG induction and pharmacological interference by COX-2 inhibitors resulted in ARG downregulation and stimulation of an otherwise silent lymphocyte-mediated antitumor response [252]. Treatment of breast-cancer 4T1-tumor bearing mice with the COX-2 inhibitors reduces MDSC accumulation and delays tumor growth factor by restraining MDSC accumulation [284].

Selective inhibitors of COX-2 enzyme activity have shown chemopreventive activity in carcinogen-induced and transgenic tumor models and clinically for colon cancer by reducing the expansion of MDSC [292]. In a mouse model of mesothelioma the treatment with the COX-2 inhibitor celecoxib not only prevented the MDSC expansion but also their function as shown by the reduced levels of ROS and NO and the improved survival when the inhibitor was used in combination with a dendritic cell-based immunotherapy [306].

CSF-1 signaling through its receptor CSF1R (CD115, c-fms) is a critical regulator of the survival, differentiation, and proliferation of monocytes and macrophages. Recently, CSF1R expression was observed on MDSCs. The use of GW2580, a selective kinase inhibitor of CSF1R, showed that the recruitment of TAMs and monocytic-MDSCs to lung, melanoma, and prostate tumors is also regulated by CSF1R signaling. The block of this pathway not only caused a reduction in the accumulation of these populations but also modulated the expression of VEGF-A, MMP-9, and ARG1, thus reducing the pro-angiogenic and immunosuppressive environment within the tumor [239].

Given the ability of PDE5 inhibitors (sildenafil, tadalafil, and vardenafil) to inhibit ARG1 and NOS2 activity in MDSCs, these compounds were tested as potential adjuvants for immunotherapy. PDE5 inhibition reverted tumor-induced immunosuppressive mechanisms, restored immune surveillance in mice and allowed the spontaneous generation of a measurable antitumor immune response that significantly delayed tumor progression in the absence of any immunotherapeutic approach. Moreover, by removing MDSC-dependent suppression, PDE5 inhibitors enhanced intratumoral T-cell infiltration and activation and improved the antitumor efficacy of adoptive T-cell therapy. When tested *in vitro*, sildenafil restored T-cell proliferation of PBMCs from multiple myeloma and head and neck cancer patients [271]. These results have a potential clinical translation since PDE5 inhibitors are safe and effective agents already in the clinic.

RNS/ROS inhibitors also represent effective strategies for decreasing MDSC-mediated immune suppression in tumor-bearing mice. Nitroaspirin effect has been associated with an inhibition of the activity of ARG1 and NOS2 in splenic MDSC. In combination with a protocol of vaccination using an endogenous tumor antigen, nitroaspirin inhibited MDSC function and increased the number and function of specific antitumor T cells [60]. Despite these positive results, nitroaspirin was not effective as an adjuvant for adoptive cell transfer therapies (ACT) (V. Bronte, unpublished data). However, a novel NO-donor based on furoxan molecule was identified—AT38—that regulated the generation of RNS at the tumor microenvironment following *in vivo* administration. By removing the chemical barriers raised by the tumor, AT38 facilitated the infiltration of low-affinity, tumor-antigen specific CTLs used in the ACT protocols [197].

An alternative option for enhancing the effect of cancer immunotherapies based on impairing the immunosuppressive function of MDSC is represented by the anti-inflammatory triterpenoids. These compounds are potent activators of the nuclear factor (erythroid-derived 2)-like 2 (NRF2) trascription factor, which controls the upregulation of antioxidant genes including NAD(P)H:quinone oxidoreductase 1, catalase, superoxide dismutase and heme oxygenase, resulting in reduction of intracellular ROS produced by MDSCs. The treatment of tumor-bearing mice with the synthetic triterpenoid C-28 methyl ester of 2-cyano-3,12-dioxooleana-1,9-dien-28-oic acid did not affect the subset composition of the MDSC population but completely abrogated their suppressive activity with consequent reduction of tumor growth [214]. Moreover, synthetic triterpenoids are well tolerated *in vivo*, as demonstrated by the treatment of pancreatic cancer patients in a phase I clinical trial in combination with gencitabine: after two weeks of treatment, a significant improvement of the immune response against tumors was observed without affecting the number of MDSCs in the peripheral blood [214].

It must be pointed out that the use of some adjuvants in immunotherapy may, by itself, lead to the accumulation of myeloid cells with immunosuppressive effect in tumor-bearing mice and cancer patients. The immune modulatory mechanisms of these substances should be always very well defined, considering not only the immediate effects on tumor growth but also their actions on the various components of the immune system (i.e., effector or regulatory populations). Very small size proteoliposomes (VSSP) constitute an adjuvant based on the combination of outer membrane vesicles (OMPs) from Neisseria meningitidis with GM3 ganglioside. This product is currently under investigation as part of the formulation of cancer vaccine candidates [38,84,304]. VSSP-based adjuvant was able to recruit MDSCs in the spleens of tumor-free mice but these cells had a lower capacity to suppress antigen-specific CTL response than tumor-induced MDSCs. The residual suppressive capacity of VSSP-MDSCs seemed to be more dependent on NOS rather than ARG activity. Moreover, whereas NOS3 was induced more than NOS1 or NOS2 in VSSP-recruited MDSCs, tumor-induced MDSCs showed a prevalent NOS2 expression, indicating potentially different mechanisms of actions between the two types of MDSCs. Since NOS2 is more efficient than NOS3 in generating NO, this might explain why VSSP-MDSCs displayed a lower suppressive activity towards T-cell functions. Further, VSSP treatment of tumor-bearing mice also generated splenic MDSC populations with reduced suppressive ability. Another useful feature of VSSP as adjuvant could be associated with its ability to promote differentiation of tumor-induced MDSCs into mature APCs [79]. Indeed VSSP could be a double-edged sword for reducing MDSC-mediated T-cell suppression by acting both at the level of ARG/NOS metabolism as well as by inducing full differentiation of the immature DCs present in the pool of MDSCs.

Many strategies for cancer treatment use combinations of immunotherapeutic agents for enhanced antitumor responses, resulting in altered balance between intratumoral ARG and NOS. In an orthotopic mouse model of renal cell carcinoma the treatment with the combination of IL-2 and anti-CD40 antibody induced a tumor regression and reduced the number of lung metastases through a process involving IFN-γ and IL-12. The antitumor responses were associated with a shift towards M1-like phenotype in macrophages infiltrating the tumor microenvironment, parallel reduction in suppressive Tregs and MDSCs and a significant reduction in ARG1 expression in TAMs [213,319]. On the contrary, the IL-2/anti-CD40 treatment induced significant increase in NOS2 expression in TAMs. CD8$^+$ effector T cells, activated by the treatment, contributed to the IFN-γ–dependent upregulation of NOS2 expression in macrophages within the tumor microenvironment. Interestingly, the effect of the co-treatment to control primary tumor was independent from NO, whereas the reduction in lung metastases and control of metastatic spread completely relied on NO production [320].

XV. CONCLUSIONS AND PERSPECTIVES

As discussed in different sections above, even though many aspects of the biology of the L-Arg metabolizing enzymes and their role in immune regulation have been discovered, many others need to be further investigated to clarify further the role of the L-Arg metabolizing enzyme in the immune dysfunctions found in tumor-bearing hosts. In fact, a mouse model which targets ARG1 depletion in various cell populations and tissues has been only recently described [73]. This tool would be fundamental to conclusively confirm the data obtained with small inhibitors, which of course might have effects on other intracellular pathways. However, the initial observations discussed in this chapter contributed to defining the potential benefit of modulating L-Arg metabolism in cancer patients. The use of novel adjuvants is perceived as a major improvement in the field of cancer immunotherapy. Active and passive immunotherapy have been exploited in the past years as a rational approach based on the exquisite selectivity of the immune system against tumor-associated antigens. An unprecedented number of clinical trials have definitely shown that T and B lymphocytes recognizing tumors can be activated, both *in vitro* and *in vivo*, in patients bearing solid and hematological tumors. Unfortunately, the number of objective clinical responses remains unsatisfactory [193,195,258]

Immunotherapy adjuvants can be defined not only as those molecules affecting the priming of the immune response (i.e., the classic meaning of the word "adjuvant") but, in a broader sense, all the substances and treatments that enhance the efficacy of immunotherapy. Many of these adjuvants are being developed presently to relieve the restraints on the antitumor immune response. Molecules affecting the metabolism of either L-Arg or L-Trp amino acid certainly belong to this category and they could soon be tested in clinical trials. The impact of these combined approaches—i.e., the combination of novel adjuvants with immunotherapy—will be quite significant as anticipated in mouse models by the combined use of ACT and AT38 [197]. Another example is offered by the demonstration that lymphodepletion followed by adoptive cell transfer of tumor-specific T lymphocytes can induce about 50% clinical response in melanoma patients, likely dependent on the elimination of Treg lymphocytes and/or interference with negative regulatory signals to T cells [68]. These findings offer a harbinger of the impact that reversing immunosuppression in cancer may ultimately exert.

Glossary

Reactive oxygen species (ROS) Reduction of oxygen is necessary to generate energy for the cells in aerobic conditions but this process (especially reduction through the mitochondrial electron transfer chain) also generates some byproducts such as superoxide (O_2^-), hydrogen peroxide (H_2O_2), and hydroxyl radical (OH$\cdot$). These moieties and the unstable intermediates formed by their interaction with lipids (lipid peroxidation) are usually termed Reactive Oxygen Species (ROS). ROS can basically interact chemically and damage all the key intracellular molecules including DNA, carbohydrates, and proteins.

Reactive nitrogen species (RNS or RNOS) NO is a gas with a complex reactivity, which can give rise to different reactive nitrogen species (RNS) including nitric oxide radical (NO), peroxynitrite (ONOO$^-$), nitrogen dioxide radical (NO$_2$), other oxides of nitrogen, and products arising when NO reacts with O_2^-, RO, and RO$_2$. The critical factor governing the molecular species is the amount of NO produced by cells. At low concentrations, NO reacts directly with metals and radicals whereas at higher concentrations, indirect effects are prominent. Among these, particularly relevant are the oxidative or nitrosative reactions with O_2 that can generate highly reactive species, sometimes defined as reactive nitrogen oxide species (RNOS). NO and related RNS/RNOS are effective antimicrobial agents and signal-transducing molecules.

SELECTED INTERNET URLS

ARG in the web:

http://www.hprd.org/protein/01947

http://www.godatabase.org/cgi-bin/amigo/go.cgi?action=query&view=query&query=arginase&search_constraint=gp

http://www.brenda.uni-koeln.de/php/result_flat.php4?ecno=3.5.3.1

http://www.ncbi.nlm.nih.gov/IEB/Research/Acembly/av.cgi?db=35g&c=Gene&l=ARG1

http://www.ncbi.nlm.nih.gov/IEB/Research/Acembly/av.cgi?exdb=AceView&db=35g&term=ARG2&submit=Go

ARG inhibitors:

http://cgmp.blauplanet.com/tool/arginase.html

Arginine metabolism:

KEGG pathway: http://www.ergo-light.com/ERGO/CGI/show_kegg_map.cgi?request=PAINT_MAP_WITH_ECS&user=&map=map00330&ecgroup=2.6.1.21

KEGG pathway website:

http://www.genome.ad.jp/kegg/metabolism.html

NOS on the web:

http://metallo.scripps.edu/PROMISE/NOS.html

http://www.wxumac.demon.co.uk/

http://www.ihop-net.org/UniPub/iHOP/

http://www.godatabase.org/cgi-bin/amigo/go.cgi?action=query&view=query&query=nitric+oxide+synthase&search_constraint=gp

http://www.ncbi.nlm.nih.gov/Structure/mmdb/mmdbsrv.cgi?form=6&db=t&Dopt=s&uid=12498

NOS knockout mice:

http://www.bioscience.org/knockout/inos.htm

http://www.jax.org/

http://sageke.sciencemag.org/resources/experimental/transgenic/

Genes and gene expression profiles:

http://www.nslij-genetics.org/search_omim.html

http://www.ncbi.nlm.nih.gov/entrez/query.fcgi?db=geo

http://www.ihop-net.org/UniPub/iHOP/

Nitroaspirin:

http://ctd.mdibl.org/voc.go;jsessionid=7DC23382D6A5FF4CA8C0A802E55D897E?voc=chem&acc=C102148

DISCLAIMER

The opinions expressed by the authors in this article do not necessarily reflect the opinions of the companies with which the authors have collaborated in the past. The use of trade names is for identification only and does not constitute endorsement by the authors or their institutions. The authors declare no conflicting interests.

ACKNOWLEDGMENTS

This work has been supported by grants from the Italian Ministry of Health, Italian Ministry of Education, University, and Research, Italian Association for Cancer Research (AIRC), Fondazione Cassa di Risparmio di Verona, Vicenza, Belluno e Ancona and Associazione Italiana Ricerca sul Cancro (AIRC; grant 6599).

References

[1] Ahn B, Ohshima H. Suppression of Intestinal Polyposis in Apc(Min/+) Mice by Inhibiting Nitric Oxide Production. Cancer Res 2001;61:8357–60.

[2] Albina JE, Mahoney EJ, Daley JM, Wesche DE, Morris Jr SM, Reichner JS. Macrophage Arginase Regulation by CCAAT/Enhancer-Binding Protein Beta. Shock 2005;23:168–72.

[3] Albina JE, Reichner JS. Oxygen and the Regulation of Gene Expression in Wounds. Wound Repair Regen 2003;11:445–51.

[4] Alderton WK, Cooper CE, Knowles RG. Nitric Oxide Synthases: Structure, Function and Inhibition. Biochem J 2001;357:593–615.

[5] Allavena P, Mantovani A. Immunology in the Clinic Review Series; Focus on Cancer: Tumour-Associated Macrophages: Undisputed Stars of the Inflammatory Tumour Microenvironment. Clin Exp Immunol 2012;167:195–205.

[6] Ambs S, Bennett WP, Merriam WG, Ogunfusika MO, Oser SM, Khan MA, et al. Vascular Endothelial Growth Factor and Nitric Oxide Synthase Expression in Human Lung Cancer and the Relation to p53. Br J Cancer 1998;78:233–9.

[7] Ambs S, Merriam WG, Bennett WP, Felley-Bosco E, Ogunfusika MO, Oser SM, et al. Frequent Nitric Oxide Synthase-2 Expression in Human Colon Adenomas: Implication for Tumor Angiogenesis and Colon Cancer Progression. Cancer Res 1998;58:334–41.

[8] Angelini G, Gardella S, Ardy M, Ciriolo MR, Filomeni G, Di Trapani G, et al. Antigen-Presenting Dendritic Cells Provide the Reducing Extracellular Microenvironment Required for T Lymphocyte Activation. Proc Natl Acad Sci U S A 2002;99:1491–6.

[9] Ash DE. Structure and Function of Arginases. J Nutr 2004;134:2760S–4S. Discussion 5S-7S.

[10] Aulak KS, Miyagi M, Yan L, West KA, Massillon D, Crabb JW, et al. Proteomic Method Identifies Proteins Nitrated in Vivo During Inflammatory Challenge. Proc Natl Acad Sci U S A 2001;98:12056–61.

[11] Badovinac VP, Porter BB, Harty JT. Programmed Contraction of CD8(+) T Cells after Infection. Nat Immunol 2002;3:619–26.

[12] Badovinac VP, Porter BB, Harty JT. CD8+ T Cell Contraction Is Controlled by Early Inflammation. Nat Immunol 2004;5:809–17.

[13] Balkwill F, Charles KA, Mantovani A. Smoldering and Polarized Inflammation in the Initiation and Promotion of Malignant Disease. Cancer Cell 2005;7:211–7.

[14] Balkwill F, Mantovani A. Inflammation and Cancer: Back to Virchow? Lancet 2001;357:539–45.

[15] Baniyash M. Tcr Zeta-Chain Downregulation: Curtailing an Excessive Inflammatory Immune Response. Nat Rev Immunol 2004;4:675–87.

[16] Barbul A, Lazarou SA, Efron DT, Wasserkrug HL, Efron G. Arginine Enhances Wound Healing and Lymphocyte Immune Responses in Humans. Surgery 1990;108:331–6. Discussion 6–7.

[17] Barra V, Kuhn AM, von Knethen A, Weigert A, Brune B. Apoptotic Cell-Derived Factors Induce Arginase II Expression in Murine Macrophages by Activating Erk5/Creb. Cell Mol Life Sci 2011;68:1815–27.

[18] Bauer H, Jung T, Tsikas D, Stichtenoth DO, Frolich JC, Neumann C. Nitric Oxide Inhibits the Secretion of T-Helper 1- and T-Helper 2-Associated Cytokines in Activated Human T Cells. Immunology 1997;90:205–11.

[19] Bauer PM, Fukuto JM, Buga GM, Pegg AE, Ignarro LJ. Nitric Oxide Inhibits Ornithine Decarboxylase by S-Nitrosylation. Biochem Biophys Res Commun 1999;262:355–8.

[20] Bentz BG, Haines 3rd GK, Radosevich JA. Increased Protein Nitrosylation in Head and Neck Squamous Cell Carcinogenesis. Head Neck 2000;22:64–70.

[21] Bergmann C, Strauss L, Zeidler R, Lang S, Whiteside TL. Expansion of Human T Regulatory Type 1 Cells in the Microenvironment of Cyclooxygenase 2 Overexpressing Head and Neck Squamous Cell Carcinoma. Cancer Res 2007;67:8865–73.

[22] Bing RJ, Miyataka M, Rich KA, Hanson N, Wang X, Slosser HD, et al. Nitric Oxide, Prostanoids, Cyclooxygenase, and Angiogenesis in Colon and Breast Cancer. Clin Cancer Res 2001;7:3385–92.

[23] Bingisser R, Tilbrook P, Holt P, Kees U. Macrophage-Derived Nitric Oxide Regulates T-Cell Activation Via Reversible Disruption of the Jak3/Stat5 Signaling Pathway. J Immunol 1998;160:5729–34.

[24] Blachier F, Mignon A, Soubrane O. Polyamines Inhibit Lipopolysaccharide-Induced Nitric Oxide Synthase Activity in Rat Liver Cytosol. Nitric Oxide 1997;1:268–72.

[25] Bobe P, Benihoud K, Grandjon D, Opolon P, Pritchard LL, Huchet R. Nitric Oxide Mediation of Active Immunosuppression Associated with Graft-Versus-Host Reaction. Blood 1999;94:1028–37.

[26] Bogdan C. Nitric Oxide and the Immune Response. Nat Immunol 2001;2:907–16.

[27] Bogdan C, Rollinghoff M, Diefenbach A. Reactive Oxygen and Reactive Nitrogen Intermediates in Innate and Specific Immunity. Curr Opin Immunol 2000;12:64–76.

[28] Bogdan C, Rollinghoff M, Diefenbach A. The Role of Nitric Oxide in Innate Immunity. Immunol Rev 2000;173:17–26.

[29] Boutard V, Havouis R, Fouqueray B, Philippe C, Moulinoux JP, Baud L. Transforming Growth Factor-Beta Stimulates Arginase Activity in Macrophages. Implications for the Regulation of Macrophage Cytotoxicity. J Immunol 1995;155:2077–84.

[30] Brito C, Naviliat M, Tiscornia AC, Vuillier F, Gualco G, Dighiero G, et al. Peroxynitrite Inhibits T Lymphocyte Activation and Proliferation by Promoting Impairment of Tyrosine Phosphorylation and Peroxynitrite-Driven Apoptotic Death. J Immunol 1999;162:3356–66.

[31] Bronte V, Kasic T, Gri G, Gallana K, Borsellino G, Marigo I, et al. Boosting Antitumor Responses of T Lymphocytes Infiltrating Human Prostate Cancers. J Exp Med 2005;201:1257–68.

[32] Bronte V, Serafini P, De Santo C, Marigo I, Tosello V, Mazzoni A, et al. IL-4-Induced Arginase 1 Suppresses Alloreactive T Cells in Tumor-Bearing Mice. J Immunol 2003;170:270–8.

[33] Bronte V, Serafini P, Mazzoni A, Segal DM, Zanovello P. L-Arginine Metabolism in Myeloid Cells Controls T-Lymphocyte Functions. Trends Immunol 2003;24:302–6.

[34] Bronte V, Zanovello P. Regulation of Immune Responses by L-Arginine Metabolism. Nat Rev Immunol 2005;5:641–54.

[35] Brookes PS, Salinas EP, Darley-Usmar K, Eiserich JP, Freeman BA, Darley-Usmar VM, et al. Concentration-Dependent Effects of Nitric Oxide on Mitochondrial Permeability Transition and Cytochrome C. Release. J Biol Chem 2000;275:20474–9.

[36] Brune B, Zhou J. The Role of Nitric Oxide (NO) in Stability Regulation of Hypoxia Inducible Factor-1alpha (HIF-1alpha). Curr Med Chem 2003;10:845–55.

[37] Buga GM, Wei LH, Bauer PM, Fukuto JM, Ignarro LJ. Ng-Hydroxy-L-Arginine and Nitric Oxide Inhibit Caco-2 Tumor Cell Proliferation by Distinct Mechanisms. Am J Physiol 1998;275:R1256–64.

[38] Carr A, Rodriguez E, Arango Mdel C, Camacho R, Osorio M, Gabri M, et al. Immunotherapy of Advanced Breast Cancer with a Heterophilic Ganglioside (Neugcgm3) Cancer Vaccine. J Clin Oncol 2003;21:1015–21.

[39] Cauley L, Miller E, Yen M, Swain S. Superantigen-Induced CD4 T Cell Tolerance Mediated by Myeloid Cells and Ifn-Gamma. J Immunol 2000;165:6056.

[40] Cederbaum SD, Yu H, Grody WW, Kern RM, Yoo P, Iyer RK. Arginases I and II: Do Their Functions Overlap? Mol Genet Metab 2004;81(Suppl. 1):S38–44.

[41] Cerutti JM, Latini FR, Nakabashi C, Delcelo R, Andrade VP, Amadei MJ, et al. Diagnosis of Suspicious Thyroid Nodules Using Four Protein Biomarkers. Clin Cancer Res 2006;12:3311–8.

[42] Chang CI, Liao JC, Kuo L. Macrophage Arginase Promotes Tumor Cell Growth and Suppresses Nitric Oxide-Mediated Tumor Cytotoxicity. Cancer Res 2001;61:1100–6.

[43] Chang CS, Chen WN, Lin HH, Wu CC, Wang CJ. Increased Oxidative DNA Damage, Inducible Nitric Oxide Synthase, Nuclear Factor KappaB Expression and Enhanced Antiapoptosis-Related Proteins in Helicobacter Pylori-Infected Non-Cardiac Gastric Adenocarcinoma. World J Gastroenterol 2004;10:2232–40.

[44] Chaturvedi R, de Sablet T, Coburn LA, Gobert AP, Wilson KT. Arginine and Polyamines in Helicobacter Pylori-Induced Immune Dysregulation and Gastric Carcinogenesis. Amino Acids 2012;42:627–40.

[45] Chen C, Liu CP. Regulatory Function of a Novel Population of Mouse Autoantigen-Specific Foxp3 Regulatory T Cells Depends on IFN-Gamma, NO, and Contact with Target Cells. PLoS One 2009;4:e7863.

[46] Chen YH, Layne MD, Chung SW, Ejima K, Baron RM, Yet SF, et al. Elk-3 Is a Transcriptional Repressor of Nitric-Oxide Synthase 2. J Biol Chem 2003;278:39572–7.

[47] Chiarugi A, Rovida E, Dello Sbarba P, Moroni F. Tryptophan Availability Selectively Limits No-Synthase Induction in Macrophages. J Leukoc Biol 2003;73:172–7.

[48] Chin K, Kurashima Y, Ogura T, Tajiri H, Yoshida S, Esumi H. Induction of Vascular Endothelial Growth Factor by Nitric Oxide in Human Glioblastoma and Hepatocellular Carcinoma Cells. Oncogene 1997;15:437–42.

[49] Choy JC, Wang Y, Tellides G, Pober JS. Induction of Inducible No Synthase in Bystander Human T Cells Increases Allogeneic Responses in the Vasculature. Proc Natl Acad Sci U S A 2007;104:1313–8.

[50] Cianchi F, Cortesini C, Fantappie O, Messerini L, Sardi I, Lasagna N, et al. Cyclooxygenase-2 Activation Mediates the Proangiogenic Effect of Nitric Oxide in Colorectal Cancer. Clin Cancer Res 2004;10:2694–704.

[51] Cianchi F, Cortesini C, Fantappie O, Messerini L, Schiavone N, Vannacci A, et al. Inducible Nitric Oxide Synthase Expression in Human Colorectal Cancer: Correlation with Tumor Angiogenesis. Am J Pathol 2003;162:793–801.

[52] Clevers H. At the Crossroads of Inflammation and Cancer. Cell 2004;118:671–4.

[53] Cobbs CS, Brenman JE, Aldape KD, Bredt DS, Israel MA. Expression of Nitric Oxide Synthase in Human Central Nervous System Tumors. Cancer Res 1995;55:727–30.

[54] Coleman JW. Nitric Oxide in Immunity and Inflammation. Int Immunopharmacol 2001;1:1397–406.

[55] Cook T, Wang Z, Alber S, Liu K, Watkins SC, Vodovotz Y, et al. Nitric Oxide and Ionizing Radiation Synergistically Promote Apoptosis and Growth Inhibition of Cancer by Activating P53. Cancer Res 2004;64:8015–21.

[56] Corzo CA, Condamine T, Lu L, Cotter MJ, Youn JI, Cheng P, et al. Hif-1alpha Regulates Function and Differentiation of Myeloid-Derived Suppressor Cells in the Tumor Microenvironment. J Exp Med 2010;207:2439–53.

[57] Coussens LM, Werb Z. Inflammation and Cancer. Nature 2002;420:860–7.

[58] Davel LE, Jasnis MA, de la Torre E, Gotoh T, Diament M, Magenta G. Sacerdote de Lustig E and Sales ME. Arginine Metabolic Pathways Involved in the Modulation of Tumor-Induced Angiogenesis by Macrophages. FEBS Lett 2002;532:216–20.

[59] de Jonge WJ, Kwikkers KL, te Velde AA, van Deventer SJ, Nolte MA, Mebius RE, et al. Arginine Deficiency Affects Early B Cell Maturation and Lymphoid Organ Development in Transgenic Mice. J Clin Invest 2002;110:1539–48.

[60] De Santo C, Serafini P, Marigo I, Dolcetti L, Bolla M, P DS Melani C, et al. Nitroaspirin Corrects Immune Dysfunction in Tumor-Bearing Hosts and Promotes Tumor Eradication by Cancer Vaccination. Proc Natl Acad Sci U S A 2005;102:4185–90.

[61] De Santo C, Serafini P, Marigo I, Dolcetti L, Bolla M, Del Soldato P, et al. Nitroaspirin Corrects Immune Dysfunction in Tumor-Bearing Hosts and Promotes Tumor Eradication by Cancer Vaccination. Proc Natl Acad Sci U S A 2005;102:4185–90.

[62] del Ara RM, Gonzalez-Polo RA, Caro A, del Amo E, Palomo L, Hernandez E, et al. Diagnostic Performance of Arginase Activity in Colorectal Cancer. Clin Exp Med 2002;2:53–7.

[63] Devadas S, Zaritskaya L, Rhee SG, Oberley L, Williams MS. Discrete Generation of Superoxide and Hydrogen Peroxide by T Cell Receptor Stimulation: Selective Regulation of Mitogen-Activated Protein Kinase Activation and Fas Ligand Expression. J Exp Med 2002;195:59–70.

[64] Diefenbach A, Schindler H, Rollinghoff M, Yokoyama WM, Bogdan C. Requirement for Type 2 NO Synthase for IL-12 Signaling in Innate Immunity. Science 1999;284:951–5.

[65] Dimmeler S, Fleming I, Fisslthaler B, Hermann C, Busse R, Zeiher AM. Activation of Nitric Oxide Synthase in Endothelial Cells by Akt-Dependent Phosphorylation. Nature 1999;399:601–5.

[66] Dimmeler S, Zeiher AM. Nitric Oxide-an Endothelial Cell Survival Factor. Cell Death Differ 1999;6:964–8.

[67] Dolcetti L, Peranzoni E, Ugel S, Marigo I, Fernandez Gomez A, Mesa C, et al. Hierarchy of Immunosuppressive Strength among Myeloid-Derived Suppressor Cell Subsets Is Determined by GM-CSF Eur J Immunol 2010;40:22–35.

[68] Dudley ME, Wunderlich JR, Yang JC, Sherry RM, Topalian SL, Restifo NP, et al. Adoptive Cell Transfer Therapy Following Non-Myeloablative but Lymphodepleting Chemotherapy for the Treatment of Patients with Refractory Metastatic Melanoma. J Clin Oncol 2005;23:2346–57.

[69] Duhe RJ, Evans GA, Erwin RA, Kirken RA, Cox GW, Farrar WL. Nitric Oxide and Thiol Redox Regulation of Janus Kinase Activity. Proc Natl Acad Sci U S A 1998;95:126–31.

[70] Dunn J, Gutbrod S, Webb A, Pak A, Jandu SK, Bhunia A, et al. S-Nitrosation of Arginase 1 Requires Direct Interaction with Inducible Nitric Oxide Synthase. Mol Cell Biochem 2011;355:83–9.

[71] Ekmekcioglu S, Ellerhorst J, Smid CM, Prieto VG, Munsell M, Buzaid AC, et al. Inducible Nitric Oxide Synthase and Nitrotyrosine in Human Metastatic Melanoma Tumors Correlate with Poor Survival. Clin Cancer Res 2000;6:4768–75.

[72] El-Gayar S, Thuring-Nahler H, Pfeilschifter J, Rollinghoff M, Bogdan C. Translational Control of Inducible Nitric Oxide Synthase by IL-13 and Arginine Availability in Inflammatory Macrophages. J Immunol 2003;171:4561–8.

[73] El Kasmi KC, Qualls JE, Pesce JT, Smith AM, Thompson RW, Henao-Tamayo M, et al. Toll-Like Receptor-Induced Arginase 1 in Macrophages Thwarts Effective Immunity against Intracellular Pathogens. Nat Immunol 2008;9:1399–406.

[74] Elfering SL, Sarkela TM, Giulivi C. Biochemistry of Mitochondrial Nitric-Oxide Synthase. J Biol Chem 2002;277:38079–86.

[75] Ellies LG, Fishman M, Hardison J, Kleeman J, Maglione JE, Manner CK, et al. Mammary Tumor Latency Is Increased in Mice Lacking the Inducible Nitric Oxide Synthase. Int J Cancer 2003;106:1–7.

[76] Erdely A, Kepka-Lenhart D, Clark M, Zeidler-Erdely P, Poljakovic M, Calhoun WJ, et al. Inhibition of Phosphodiesterase 4 Amplifies Cytokine-Dependent Induction of Arginase in Macrophages. Am J Physiol Lung Cell Mol Physiol 2006;290:L534–9.

[77] Felley-Bosco E. Role of Nitric Oxide in Genotoxicity: Implication for Carcinogenesis. Cancer Metastasis Rev 1998;17:25–37.

[78] Feng G, Gao W, Strom TB, Oukka M, Francis RS, Wood KJ, et al. Exogenous Ifn-Gamma Ex Vivo Shapes the Alloreactive T-Cell Repertoire by Inhibition of Th17 Responses and Generation of Functional FoxP3[+] Regulatory T Cells. Eur J Immunol 2008;38:2512–27.

[79] Fernandez A, Mesa C, Marigo I, Dolcetti L, Clavell M, Oliver L, et al. Inhibition of Tumor-Induced Myeloid-Derived Suppressor Cell Function by a Nanoparticulated Adjuvant. J Immunol 2011;186:264–74.

[80] Finke JH, Zea AH, Stanley J, Longo DL, Mizoguchi H, Tubbs RR, et al. Loss of T-Cell Receptor Zeta Chain and P56lck in T-Cells Infiltrating Human Renal Cell Carcinoma. Cancer Res. 1993;53:5613–6.

[81] Fischer TA, Palmetshofer A, Gambaryan S, Butt E, Jassoy C, Walter U, et al. Activation of Cgmp-Dependent Protein Kinase Ibeta Inhibits Interleukin 2 Release and Proliferation of T Cell Receptor-Stimulated Human Peripheral T Cells. J Biol Chem 2001;276:5967–74.

[82] Fligger J, Blum J, Jungi TW. Induction of Intracellular Arginase Activity Does Not Diminish the Capacity of Macrophages to Produce Nitric Oxide in Vitro. Immunobiology 1999;200:169–86.

[83] Forstermann U, Boissel JP, Kleinert H. Expressional Control of the Constitutive Isoforms of Nitric Oxide Synthase (Nos I and Nos III). FASEB J 1998;12:773–90.

[84] Gabri MR, Mazorra Z, Ripoll GV, Mesa C, Fernandez LE, Gomez DE, et al. Complete Antitumor Protection by Perioperative Immunization with GM3/VSSP Vaccine in a Preclinical Mouse Melanoma Model. Clin Cancer Res 2006;12:7092–8.

[85] Gabrilovich DI, Ostrand-Rosenberg S, Bronte V. Coordinated Regulation of Myeloid Cells by Tumours. Nat Rev Immunol 2012;12:253–68.

[86] Gallardo-Soler A, Gomez-Nieto C, Campo ML, Marathe C, Tontonoz P, Castrillo A, et al. Arginase I Induction by Modified Lipoproteins in Macrophages: A Peroxisome Proliferator-Activated Receptor-Gamma/Delta-Mediated Effect That Links Lipid Metabolism and Immunity. Mol Endocrinol 2008;22:1394–402.

[87] Gallina G, Dolcetti L, Serafini P, De Santo C, Marigo I, Colombo MP, et al. Tumors Induce a Subset of Inflammatory Monocytes with Immunosuppressive Activity on CD8[+] T Cells. J Clin Invest 2006;116:2777–90.

[88] Gallo O, Masini E, Morbidelli L, Franchi A, Fini-Storchi I, Vergari WA, et al. Role of Nitric Oxide in Angiogenesis and Tumor Progression in Head and Neck Cancer. J Natl Cancer Inst 1998;90:587–96.

[89] Gannon PO, Godin-Ethier J, Hassler M, Delvoye N, Aversa M, Poisson AO, et al. Androgen-Regulated Expression of Arginase 1, Arginase 2 and Interleukin-8 in Human Prostate Cancer. PLoS One 2010;5:e12107.

[90] Gobert AP, McGee DJ, Akhtar M, Mendz GL, Newton JC, Cheng Y, et al. Helicobacter Pylori Arginase Inhibits Nitric Oxide Production by Eukaryotic Cells: A Strategy for Bacterial Survival. Proc Natl Acad Sci U S A 2001;98:13844–9.

[91] Goni O, Alcaide P, Fresno M. Immunosuppression During Acute Trypanosoma Cruzi Infection: Involvement of Ly6G (Gr1(+))Cd11b(+) Immature Myeloid Suppressor Cells. Int Immunol 2002;14:1125–34.

[92] Gordon S. Alternative Activation of Macrophages. Nat Rev Immunol 2003;3:23–35.

[93] Gotoh T, Chowdhury S, Takiguchi M, Mori M. The Glucocorticoid-Responsive Gene Cascade. Activation of the Rat Arginase Gene through Induction of C/EBPbeta. J Biol Chem 1997;272:3694–8.

[94] Grandvaux N, Gaboriau F, Harris J, tenOever BR, Lin R, Hiscott J. Regulation of Arginase Ii by Interferon Regulatory Factor 3 and the Involvement of Polyamines in the Antiviral Response. FEBS J 2005;272:3120–31.

[95] Gratton JP, Lin MI, Yu J, Weiss ED, Jiang ZL, Fairchild TA, et al. Selective Inhibition of Tumor Microvascular Permeability by Cavtratin Blocks Tumor Progression in Mice. Cancer Cell 2003;4:31–9.

[96] Gray MJ, Poljakovic M, Kepka-Lenhart D, Morris Jr SM. Induction of Arginase I Transcription by IL-4 Requires a Composite DNA Response Element for STAT6 and C/Ebpbeta. Gene 2005;353:98–106.

[97] Grimm EA, Ellerhorst J, Tang C-H, Ekmekcioglu S. Constitutive Intracellular Production of Inos and No in Human Melanoma: Possible Role in Regulation of Growth and Resistance to Apoptosis. Nitric Oxide 2008;19:133–7.

[98] Grohmann U, Bianchi R, Belladonna ML, Silla S, Fallarino F, Fioretti MC, et al. Ifn-Gamma Inhibits Presentation of a Tumor/Self Peptide by CD8 Alpha- Dendritic Cells Via Potentiation of the CD8 Alpha+ Subset. J Immunol 2000;165:1357–63.

[99] Grohmann U, Bronte V. Control of Immune Response by Amino Acid Metabolism. Immunol Rev 2010;236:243–64.

[100] Grohmann U, Fallarino F, Bianchi R, Orabona C, Vacca C, Fioretti MC, et al. Defect in Tryptophan Catabolism Impairs Tolerance in Nonobese Diabetic Mice. J Exp Med 2003;198:153–60.

[101] Grohmann U, Fallarino F, Bianchi R, Vacca C, Orabona C, Belladonna ML, et al. Tryptophan Catabolism in Nonobese Diabetic Mice. Adv Exp Med Biol 2003;527:47–54.

[102] Grohmann U, Orabona C, Fallarino F, Vacca C, Calcinaro F, Falorni A, et al. CTLA-4-Ig Regulates Tryptophan Catabolism in Vivo. Nat Immunol 2002;3:1097–101.

[103] Guzik TJ, Korbut R, Adamek-Guzik T. Nitric Oxide and Superoxide in Inflammation and Immune Regulation. J Physiol Pharmacol 2003;54:469–87.

[104] Haffner I, Teupser D, Holdt LM, Ernst J, Burkhardt R, Thiery J. Regulation of Arginase-1 Expression in Macrophages by a Protein Kinase a Type I and Histone Deacetylase Dependent Pathway. J Cell Biochem 2008;103:520–7.

[105] Hajri A, Metzger E, Vallat F, Coffy S, Flatter E, Evrard S, et al. Role of Nitric Oxide in Pancreatic Tumour Growth: In Vivo and in Vitro Studies. Br J Cancer 1998;78:841–9.

[106] Harlin H, Hanson M, Johansson CC, Sakurai D, Poschke I, Norell H, et al. The CD16⁻ CD56(Bright) NK Cell Subset Is Resistant to Reactive Oxygen Species Produced by Activated Granulocytes and Has Higher Anti-oxidative Capacity Than the CD16⁺ CD56(Dim) Subset. J Immunol 2007;179:4513–9.

[107] Hausel P, Latado H, Courjault-Gautier F, Felley-Bosco E. Src-Mediated Phosphorylation Regulates Subcellular Distribution and Activity of Human Inducible Nitric Oxide Synthase. Oncogene 2006;25:198–206.

[108] Haverkamp JM, Crist SA, Elzey BD, Cimen C, Ratliff TL. Vivo Suppressive Function of Myeloid-Derived Suppressor Cells Is Limited to the Inflammatory Site. Eur J Immunol 2011;41:749–59.

[109] Hecker M, Nematollahi H, Hey C, Busse R, Racke K. Inhibition of Arginase by Ng-Hydroxy-L-Arginine in Alveolar Macrophages: Implications for the Utilization of L-Arginine for Nitric Oxide Synthesis. FEBS Lett 1995;359:251–4.

[110] Highfill SL, Rodriguez PC, Zhou Q, Goetz CA, Koehn BH, Veenstra R, et al. Bone Marrow Myeloid-Derived Suppressor Cells (MDSCs) Inhibit Graft-Versus-Host Disease (GVHD) Via an Arginase-1-Dependent Mechanism That Is up-Regulated by Interleukin-13. Blood 2010;116:5738–47.

[111] Hildeman DA, Mitchell T, Aronow B, Wojciechowski S, Kappler J, Marrack P. Control of Bcl-2 Expression by Reactive Oxygen Species. Proc Natl Acad Sci U S A 2003;100:15035–40.

[112] Hildeman DA, Mitchell T, Kappler J, Marrack PT. Cell Apoptosis and Reactive Oxygen Species. J Clin Invest 2003;111:575–81.

[113] Hildeman DA, Mitchell T, Teague TK, Henson P, Day BJ, Kappler J, et al. Reactive Oxygen Species Regulate Activation-Induced T Cell Apoptosis. Immunity 1999;10:735–44.

[114] Hinz B, Brune K, Pahl A. Nitric Oxide Inhibits Inducible Nitric Oxide Synthase mRNA Expression in RAW 264.7 Macrophages. Biochem Biophys Res Commun 2000;271:353–7.

[115] Hiraku Y, Kawanishi S, Ichinose T, Murata M. The Role of iNOS-Mediated DNA Damage in Infection- and Asbestos-Induced Carcinogenesis. Ann N Y Acad Sci 2010;1203:15–22.

[116] Hrabak A, Bajor T, Csuka I. The Effect of Various Inflammatory Agents on the Alternative Metabolic Pathways of Arginine in Mouse and Rat Macrophages. Inflamm Res 2006;55:23–31.

[117] Hucke C, MacKenzie CR, Adjogble KD, Takikawa O, Daubener W. Nitric Oxide-Mediated Regulation of Gamma Interferon-Induced Bacteriostasis: Inhibition and Degradation of Human Indoleamine 2,3-Dioxygenase. Infect Immun 2004;72:2723–30.

[118] Hussain SP, Hofseth LJ, Harris CC. Radical Causes of Cancer. Nat Rev Cancer 2003;3:276–85.

[119] Hussain SP, Trivers GE, Hofseth LJ, He P, Shaikh I, Mechanic LE, et al. Nitric Oxide, a Mediator of Inflammation, Suppresses Tumorigenesis. Cancer Res 2004;64:6849–53.

[120] Ibiza S, Victor VM, Bosca I, Ortega A, Urzainqui A, O'Connor JE, et al. Endothelial Nitric Oxide Synthase Regulates T Cell Receptor Signaling at the Immunological Synapse. Immunity 2006;24:753–65.

625

[121] Ichinoe M, Mikami T, Shiraishi H, Okayasu I. High Microvascular Density Is Correlated with High VEGF, iNOS and COX-2 Expression in Penetrating Growth-Type Early Gastric Carcinomas. Histopathology 2004;45:612—8.

[122] Iniesta V, Gomez-Nieto LC, Corraliza I. The Inhibition of Arginase by N(Omega)-Hydroxy-L-Arginine Controls the Growth of Leishmania inside Macrophages. J Exp Med 2001;193:777—84.

[123] Ishii Y, Ogura T, Tatemichi M, Fujisawa H, Otsuka F, Esumi H. Induction of Matrix Metalloproteinase Gene Transcription by Nitric Oxide and Mechanisms of MMP-1 Gene Induction in Human Melanoma Cell Lines. Int J Cancer 2003;103:161—8.

[124] Iyer RK, Yoo PK, Kern RM, Rozengurt N, Tsoa R, O'Brien WE, et al. Mouse Model for Human Arginase Deficiency. Mol Cell Biol 2002;22:4491—8.

[125] Jadeski LC, Chakraborty C, Lala PK. Nitric Oxide-Mediated Promotion of Mammary Tumour Cell Migration Requires Sequential Activation of Nitric Oxide Synthase, Guanylate Cyclase and Mitogen-Activated Protein Kinase. Int J Cancer 2003;106:496—504.

[126] Jaiswal M, LaRusso NF, Burgart LJ, Gores GJ. Inflammatory Cytokines Induce DNA Damage and Inhibit DNA Repair in Cholangiocarcinoma Cells by a Nitric Oxide-Dependent Mechanism. Cancer Res 2000;60: 184—90.

[127] Jayasekera JP, Vinuesa CG, Karupiah G, King NJ. Enhanced Antiviral Antibody Secretion and Attenuated Immunopathology During Influenza Virus Infection in Nitric Oxide Synthase-2-Deficient Mice. J Gen Virol 2006;87:3361—71.

[128] Jost MM, Ninci E, Meder B, Kempf C, Van Royen N, Hua J, et al. Divergent Effects of GM-CSF and TGFbeta1 on Bone Marrow-Derived Macrophage Arginase-1 Activity, MCP-1 Expression, and Matrix Metalloproteinase-12: A Potential Role During Arteriogenesis. FASEB J 2003;17:2281—3.

[129] Kai H, Ito M, Kitadai Y, Tanaka S, Haruma K, Chayama K. Chronic Gastritis with Expression of Inducible Nitric Oxide Synthase Is Associated with High Expression of Interleukin-6 and Hypergastrinaemia. Aliment Pharmacol Ther 2004;19:1309—14.

[130] Karin M, Greten FR. NF-KappaB: Linking Inflammation and Immunity to Cancer Development and Progression. Nat Rev Immunol 2005;5:749—59.

[131] Kasic T, Colombo P, Soldani C, Wang CM, Miranda E, Roncalli M, et al. Modulation of Human T-Cell Functions by Reactive Nitrogen Species. Eur J Immunol 2011;41:1843—9.

[132] Kasuno K, Takabuchi S, Fukuda K, Kizaka-Kondoh S, Yodoi J, Adachi T, et al. Nitric Oxide Induces Hypoxia-Inducible Factor 1 Activation That Is Dependent on MAPK and Phosphatidylinositol 3-Kinase Signaling. J Biol Chem 2004;279:2550—8.

[133] Kato H, Miyazaki T, Yoshikawa M, Nakajima M, Fukai Y, Tajima K, et al. Nitrotyrosine in Esophageal Squamous Cell Carcinoma and Relevance to p53 Expression. Cancer Lett 2000;153:121—7.

[134] Keskinege A, Elgun S, Yilmaz E. Possible Implications of Arginase and Diamine Oxidase in Prostatic Carcinoma. Cancer Detect Prev 2001;25:76—9.

[135] Kim SF, Huri DA, Snyder SH. Inducible Nitric Oxide Synthase Binds, S-Nitrosylates, and Activates Cyclo-oxygenase-2. Science 2005;310:1966—70.

[136] Kimura H, Weisz A, Kurashima Y, Hashimoto K, Ogura T, D'Acquisto F, et al. Hypoxia Response Element of the Human Vascular Endothelial Growth Factor Gene Mediates Transcriptional Regulation by Nitric Oxide: Control of Hypoxia-Inducible Factor-1 Activity by Nitric Oxide. Blood 2000;95:189—97.

[137] Kinnula VL, Torkkeli T, Kristo P, Sormunen R, Soini Y, Paakko P, et al. Ultrastructural and Chromosomal Studies on Manganese Superoxide Dismutase in Malignant Mesothelioma. Am J Respir Cell Mol Biol 2004;31:147—53.

[138] Kisley LR, Barrett BS, Bauer AK, Dwyer-Nield LD, Barthel B, Meyer AM, et al. Genetic Ablation of Inducible Nitric Oxide Synthase Decreases Mouse Lung Tumorigenesis. Cancer Res 2002;62:6850—6.

[139] Kleinert H, Schwarz PM, Forstermann U. Regulation of the Expression of Inducible Nitric Oxide Synthase. Biol Chem 2003;384:1343—64.

[140] Klotz T, Bloch W, Volberg C, Engelmann U, Addicks K. Selective Expression of Inducible Nitric Oxide Synthase in Human Prostate Carcinoma. Cancer 1998;82:1897—903.

[141] Knowles RG, Moncada S. Nitric Oxide Synthases in Mammals. Biochem J 1994;298(Pt 2):249—58.

[142] Koblish HK, Hunter CA, Wysocka M, Trinchieri G, Lee WM. Immune Suppression by Recombinant Interleukin (rIL)-12 Involves Interferon Gamma Induction of Nitric Oxide Synthase 2 (iNOS) Activity: Inhibitors of NO Generation Reveal the Extent of rIL-12 Vaccine Adjuvant Effect. J Exp Med 1998;188: 1603—10.

[143] Koh KP, Wang Y, Yi T, Shiao SL, Lorber MI, Sessa WC, et al. T Cell-Mediated Vascular Dysfunction of Human Allografts Results from Ifn-Gamma Dysregulation of NO Synthase. J Clin Invest 2004;114:846—56.

[144] Kolb H, Kolb-Bachofen V. Nitric Oxide in Autoimmune Disease: Cytotoxic or Regulatory Mediator? Immunol Today 1998;19:556—61.

626

[145] Kong SK, Yim MB, Stadtman ER, Chock PB. Peroxynitrite Disables the Tyrosine Phosphorylation Regulatory Mechanism: Lymphocyte-Specific Tyrosine Kinase Fails to Phosphorylate Nitrated Cdc2(6-20)Nh2 Peptide. Proc Natl Acad Sci U S A 1996;93:3377–82.

[146] Kropf P, Baud D, Marshall SE, Munder M, Mosley A, Fuentes JM, et al. Arginase Activity Mediates Reversible T Cell Hyporesponsiveness in Human Pregnancy. Eur J Immunol 2007;37:935–45.

[147] Kung JT, Brooks SB, Jakway JP, Leonard LL, Talmage DW. Suppression of in Vitro Cytotoxic Response by Macrophages Due to Induced Arginase. J Exp Med 1977;146:665–72.

[148] Kuraishy A, Karin M, Grivennikov SI. Tumor Promotion Via Injury- and Death-Induced Inflammation. Immunity 2011;35:467–77.

[149] Kusmartsev S, Gabrilovich DI. STAT1 Signaling Regulates Tumor-Associated Macrophage-Mediated T Cell Deletion. J Immunol 2005;174:4880–91.

[150] Kusmartsev S, Li Y, Chen S- H. Gr-1$^+$ Myeloid Cells Derived from Tumor-Bearing Mice Inhibit Primary T Cell Activation Induced through CD3/CD28 Costimulation. J Immunol 2000;165:779–85.

[151] Kusmartsev S, Nefedova Y, Yoder D, Gabrilovich DI. Antigen-Specific Inhibition of CD8$^+$ T Cell Response by Immature Myeloid Cells in Cancer Is Mediated by Reactive Oxygen Species. J Immunol 2004;172:989–99.

[152] Lala PK, Chakraborty C. Role of Nitric Oxide in Carcinogenesis and Tumour Progression. Lancet Oncol 2001;2:149–56.

[153] Laniewski NG, Grayson JM. Antioxidant Treatment Reduces Expansion and Contraction of Antigen-Specific CD8$^+$ T Cells During Primary but Not Secondary Viral Infection. J Virol 2004;78:11246–57.

[154] Laroux FS, Pavlick KP, Hines IN, Kawachi S, Harada H, Bharwani S, et al. Role of Nitric Oxide in Inflammation. Acta Physiol Scand 2001;173:113–8.

[155] Lee J, Ryu H, Ferrante RJ, Morris Jr SM, Ratan RR. Translational Control of Inducible Nitric Oxide Synthase Expression by Arginine Can Explain the Arginine Paradox. Proc Natl Acad Sci U S A 2003;100:4843–8.

[156] Leon L, Jeannin JF, Bettaieb A. Post-Translational Modifications Induced by Nitric Oxide (NO): Implication in Cancer Cells Apoptosis. Nitric Oxide 2008;19:77–83.

[157] Lewis ND, Asim M, Barry DP, Singh K, de Sablet T, Boucher JL, et al. Arginase II Restricts Host Defense to Helicobacter Pylori by Attenuating Inducible Nitric Oxide Synthase Translation in Macrophages. J Immunol 2010;184:2572–82.

[158] Li W, Lidebjer C, Yuan XM, Szymanowski A, Backteman K, Ernerudh J, et al. Cell Apoptosis in Coronary Artery Disease: Relation to Oxidative Stress. Atherosclerosis 2008;199:65–72.

[159] Loibl S, Buck A, Strank C, von Minckwitz G, Roller M, Sinn HP, et al. The Role of Early Expression of Inducible Nitric Oxide Synthase in Human Breast Cancer. Eur J Cancer 2005;41:265–71.

[160] Loibl S, von Minckwitz G, Weber S, Sinn HP, Schini-Kerth VB, Lobysheva I, et al. Expression of Endothelial and Inducible Nitric Oxide Synthase in Benign and Malignant Lesions of the Breast and Measurement of Nitric Oxide Using Electron Paramagnetic Resonance Spectroscopy. Cancer 2002;95:1191–8.

[161] Lopez-Rivera E, Lizarbe TR, Martinez-Moreno M, Lopez-Novoa JM, Rodriguez-Barbero A, Rodrigo J, et al. Matrix Metalloproteinase 13 Mediates Nitric Oxide Activation of Endothelial Cell Migration. Proc Natl Acad Sci U S A 2005;102:3685–90.

[162] Lundberg JO, Lundberg JM, Alving K, Weitzberg E. Nitric Oxide and Inflammation: The Answer Is Blowing in the Wind. Nat Med 1997;3:30–1.

[163] Ma N, Adachi Y, Hiraku Y, Horiki N, Horiike S, Imoto I, et al. Accumulation of 8-Nitroguanine in Human Gastric Epithelium Induced by Helicobacter Pylori Infection. Biochem Biophys Res Commun 2004;319:506–10.

[164] Macarthur M, Hold GL, El-Omar EM. Inflammation and Cancer Ii. Role of Chronic Inflammation and Cytokine Gene Polymorphisms in the Pathogenesis of Gastrointestinal Malignancy. Am J Physiol Gastrointest Liver Physiol 2004;286:G515–20.

[165] MacMicking J, Xie QW, Nathan C. Nitric Oxide and Macrophage Function. Annu Rev Immunol 1997;15:323–50.

[166] Macphail SE, Gibney CA, Brooks BM, Booth CG, Flanagan BF, Coleman JW. Nitric Oxide Regulation of Human Peripheral Blood Mononuclear Cells: Critical Time Dependence and Selectivity for Cytokine Versus Chemokine Expression. J Immunol 2003;171:4809–15.

[167] Malmberg K, Arulampalam V, Ichihara F, Petersson M, Seki K, Andersson T, et al. Inhibition of Activated/Memory (CD45RO(+)) T Cells by Oxidative Stress Associated with Block of NF-KB Activation. J Immunol 2001;167:2595–601.

[168] Mandruzzato S, Callegaro A, Turcatel G, Francescato S, Montesco MC, Chiarion-Sileni V, et al. Gene Expression Signature Associated with Survival in Metastatic Melanoma. J Transl Med 2006;4:50.

[169] Mandruzzato S, Solito S, Falisi E, Francescato S, Chiarion-Sileni V, Mocellin S, et al. IL4Ralpha$^+$ Myeloid-Derived Suppressor Cell Expansion in Cancer Patients. J Immunol 2009;182:6562–8.

627

[170] Mann GE, Yudilevich DL, Sobrevia L. Regulation of Amino Acid and Glucose Transporters in Endothelial and Smooth Muscle Cells. Physiol Rev 2003;83:183−252.

[171] Mannick JB, Hausladen A, Liu L, Hess DT, Zeng M, Miao QX, et al. Fas-Induced Caspase Denitrosylation. Science 1999;284:651−4.

[172] Mantovani A, Sozzani S, Locati M, Allavena P, Sica A. Macrophage Polarization: Tumor-Associated Macrophages as a Paradigm for Polarized M2 Mononuclear Phagocytes. Trends Immunol 2002;23:549−55.

[173] Margalit O, Eisenbach L, Amariglio N, Kaminski N, Harmelin A, Pfeffer R, et al. Overexpression of a Set of Genes, Including WISP-1, Common to Pulmonary Metastases of Both Mouse D122 Lewis Lung Carcinoma and B16-F10.9 Melanoma Cell Lines. Br J Cancer 2003;89:314−9.

[174] Mariotto S, Cuzzolin L, Adami A, Del Soldato P, Suzuki H, Benoni G. Effect of a New Non-Steroidal Anti-Inflammatory Drug, Nitroflurbiprofen, on the Expression of Inducible Nitric Oxide Synthase in Rat Neutrophils. Br J Pharmacol 1995;115:225−6.

[175] Marnett LJ, Riggins JN, West JD. Endogenous Generation of Reactive Oxidants and Electrophiles and Their Reactions with DNA and Protein. J Clin Invest 2003;111:583−93.

[176] Marrogi A, Pass HI, Khan M, Metheny-Barlow LJ, Harris CC, Gerwin BI. Human Mesothelioma Samples Overexpress Both Cyclooxygenase-2 (COX-2) and Inducible Nitric Oxide Synthase (NOS2): In Vitro Antiproliferative Effects of a COX-2 Inhibitor. Cancer Res 2000;60:3696−700.

[177] Massi D, Franchi A, Sardi I, Magnelli L, Paglierani M, Borgognoni L, et al. Inducible Nitric Oxide Synthase Expression in Benign and Malignant Cutaneous Melanocytic Lesions. J Pathol 2001;194:194−200.

[178] Massi D, Marconi C, Franchi A, Bianchini F, Paglierani M, Ketabchi S, et al. Arginine Metabolism in Tumor-Associated Macrophages in Cutaneous Malignant Melanoma: Evidence from Human and Experimental Tumors. Hum Pathol 2007;38:1516−25.

[179] Matsuda M, Petersson M, Lenkei R, Taupin JL, Magnusson I, Mellstedt H, et al. Alterations in the Signal-Transducing Molecules of T Cells and NK Cells in Colorectal Tumor-Infiltrating, Gut Mucosal and Peripheral Lymphocytes: Correlation with the Stage of the Disease. Int J Cancer 1995;61:765−72.

[180] Matsui K, Nishizawa M, Ozaki T, Kimura T, Hashimoto I, Yamada M, et al. Natural Antisense Transcript Stabilizes Inducible Nitric Oxide Synthase Messenger Rna in Rat Hepatocytes. Hepatology 2008;47:686−97.

[181] Matthiesen S, Lindemann D, Warnken M, Juergens UR, Racke K. Inhibition of NADPH Oxidase by Apocynin Inhibits Lipopolysaccharide (LPS) Induced up-Regulation of Arginase in Rat Alveolar Macrophages. Eur J Pharmacol 2008;579:403−10.

[182] Mazzoni A, Bronte V, Visintin A, Spitzer JH, Apolloni E, Serafini P, et al. Myeloid Suppressor Lines Inhibit T Cell Responses by an NO-Dependent Mechanism. J Immunol 2002;168:689−95.

[183] McKnight R, Nassar A, Cohen C, Siddiqui MT. Arginase-1: A Novel Immunohistochemical Marker of Hepatocellular Differentiation in Fine Needle Aspiration Cytology. Cancer Cytopathol 2012.

[184] Medeiros R, Morais A, Vasconcelos A, Costa S, Pinto D, Oliveira J, et al. Endothelial Nitric Oxide Synthase Gene Polymorphisms and Genetic Susceptibility to Prostate Cancer. Eur J Cancer Prev 2002;11:343−50.

[185] Melillo G, Musso T, Sica A, Taylor LS, Cox GW, Varesio LA. Hypoxia-Responsive Element Mediates a Novel Pathway of Activation of the Inducible Nitric Oxide Synthase Promoter. J Exp Med 1995;182:1683−93.

[186] Mencacci A, Montagnoli C, Bacci A, Cenci E, Pitzurra L, Spreca A, et al. CD80$^+$Gr-1$^+$ Myeloid Cells Inhibit Development of Antifungal Th1 Immunity in Mice with Candidiasis. J Immunol 2002;169:3180−90.

[187] Mendes RV, Martins AR, de Nucci G, Murad F, Soares FA. Expression of Nitric Oxide Synthase Isoforms and Nitrotyrosine Immunoreactivity by B-Cell Non-Hodgkin's Lymphomas and Multiple Myeloma. Histopathology 2001;39:172−8.

[188] Meurs H, Maarsingh H, Zaagsma J. Arginase and Asthma: Novel Insights into Nitric Oxide Homeostasis and Airway Hyperresponsiveness. Trends Pharmacol Sci 2003;24:450−5.

[189] Michel T, Feron O. Nitric Oxide Synthases: Which, Where, How, and Why? J Clin Invest 1997;100:2146−52.

[190] Mielczarek M, Chrzanowska A, Scibior D, Skwarek A, Ashamiss F, Lewandowska K, et al. Arginase as a Useful Factor for the Diagnosis of Colorectal Cancer Liver Metastases. Int J Biol Markers 2006;21:40−4.

[191] Mills CD, Kincaid K, Alt JM, Heilman MJ, Hill AM. M-1/M-2 Macrophages and the Th1/Th2 Paradigm. J Immunol 2000;164:6166−73.

[192] Mocellin S, Bronte V, Nitti D. Nitric Oxide, a Double Edged Sword in Cancer Biology: Searching for Therapeutic Opportunities. Med Res Rev 2007;27:317−52.

[193] Mocellin S, Mandruzzato S, Bronte V, Lise M, Nitti D. Vaccines for Solid Tumours. Part I: Lancet Oncol 2004;5:681−9.

[194] Mocellin S, Provenzano M, Rossi CR, Pilati P, Scalerta R, Lise M, et al. Induction of Endothelial Nitric Oxide Synthase Expression by Melanoma Sensitizes Endothelial Cells to Tumor Necrosis Factor-Driven Cytotoxicity. Clin Cancer Res 2004;10:6879−86.

[195] Mocellin S, Semenzato G, Mandruzzato S, Riccardo Rossi C. Vaccines for Haematological Malignant Disorders. Part II: Lancet Oncol 2004;5:727—37.

[196] Mollace V, Muscoli C, Masini E, Cuzzocrea S, Salvemini D. Modulation of Prostaglandin Biosynthesis by Nitric Oxide and Nitric Oxide Donors. Pharmacol Rev 2005;57:217—52.

[197] Molon B, Ugel S, Del Pozzo F, Soldani C, Zilio S, Avella D, et al. Chemokine Nitration Prevents Intratumoral Infiltration of Antigen-Specific T Cells. J Exp Med 2011;208:1949—62.

[198] Moncada S, Palmer RM, Higgs EA. Nitric Oxide: Physiology, Pathophysiology, and Pharmacology. Pharmacol Rev 1991;43:109—42.

[199] Morbidelli L, Donnini S, Ziche M. Role of Nitric Oxide in Tumor Angiogenesis. Cancer Treat Res 2004;117:155—67.

[200] Mori N, Nunokawa Y, Yamada Y, Ikeda S, Tomonaga M, Yamamoto N. Expression of Human Inducible Nitric Oxide Synthase Gene in T-Cell Lines Infected with Human T-Cell Leukemia Virus Type-I and Primary Adult T-Cell Leukemia Cells. Blood 1999;94:2862—70.

[201] Morin J, Chimenes A, Boitard C, Berthier R, Boudaly S. Granulocyte-Dendritic Cell Unbalance in the Non-Obese Diabetic Mice. Cell Immunol 2003;223:13—25.

[202] Morris Jr SM. Regulation of Enzymes of the Urea Cycle and Arginine Metabolism. Annu Rev Nutr 2002;22:87—105.

[203] Morrison AC, Correll PH. Activation of the Stem Cell-Derived Tyrosine Kinase/Ron Receptor Tyrosine Kinase by Macrophage-Stimulating Protein Results in the Induction of Arginase Activity in Murine Peritoneal Macrophages. J Immunol 2002;168:853—60.

[204] Mougiakakos D, Johansson CC, Jitschin R, Bottcher M, Kiessling R. Increased Thioredoxin-1 Production in Human Naturally Occurring Regulatory T Cells Confers Enhanced Tolerance to Oxidative Stress. Blood 2011;117:857—61.

[205] Mougiakakos D, Johansson CC, Kiessling R. Naturally Occurring Regulatory T Cells Show Reduced Sensitivity Towards Oxidative Stress Induced Cell Death. Blood 2008.

[206] Moulian N, Truffault F, Gaudry-Talarmain YM, Serraf A, Berrih-Aknin S. Vivo and in Vitro Apoptosis of Human Thymocytes Are Associated with Nitrotyrosine Formation. Blood 2001;97:3521—30.

[207] Munder M. Arginase: An Emerging Key Player in the Mammalian Immune System. Br J Pharmacol 2009;158:638—51.

[208] Munder M, Eichmann K, Modolell M. Alternative Metabolic States in Murine Macrophages Reflected by the Nitric Oxide Synthase/Arginase Balance: Competitive Regulation by CD4$^+$ T Cells Correlates with Th1/Th2 Phenotype. J Immunol 1998;160:5347—54.

[209] Munder M, Eichmann K, Moran JM, Centeno F, Soler G, Modolell M. Th1/Th2-Regulated Expression of Arginase Isoforms in Murine Macrophages and Dendritic Cells. J Immunol 1999;163:3771—7.

[210] Munder M, Mollinedo F, Calafat J, Canchado J, Gil-Lamaignere C, Fuentes JM, et al. Arginase I Is Constitutively Expressed in Human Granulocytes and Participates in Fungicidal Activity. Blood 2005;105:2549—56.

[211] Munder M, Schneider H, Luckner C, Giese T, Langhans CD, Fuentes J, et al. Suppression of T Cell Functions by Human Granulocyte Arginase. Blood 2006.

[212] Munn DH, Sharma MD, Baban B, Harding HP, Zhang Y, Ron D, et al. GCN2 Kinase in T Cells Mediates Proliferative Arrest and Anergy Induction in Response to Indoleamine 2,3-Dioxygenase. Immunity 2005;22:633—42.

[213] Murphy WJ, Welniak L, Back T, Hixon J, Subleski J, Seki N, et al. Synergistic Anti-Tumor Responses after Administration of Agonistic Antibodies to CD40 and IL-2: Coordination of Dendritic and CD8$^+$ Cell Responses. J Immunol 2003;170:2727—33.

[214] Nagaraj S, Youn JI, Weber H, Iclozan C, Lu L, Cotter MJ, et al. Anti-Inflammatory Triterpenoid Blocks Immune Suppressive Function of MDSCs and Improves Immune Response in Cancer. Clin Cancer Res 2010;16:1812—23.

[215] Nakamura Y, Yasuoka H, Tsujimoto M, Yoshidome K, Nakahara M, Nakao K, et al. Nitric Oxide in Breast Cancer: Induction of Vascular Endothelial Growth Factor-C and Correlation with Metastasis and Poor Prognosis. Clin Cancer Res 2006;12:1201—7.

[216] Nelson WG, De Marzo AM, DeWeese TL, Isaacs WB. The Role of Inflammation in the Pathogenesis of Prostate Cancer. J Urol 2004;172:S6—11. Discussion S-2.

[217] Niedbala W, Cai B, Liu H, Pitman N, Chang L, Liew FY. Nitric Oxide Induces CD4$^+$CD25$^+$ FoxP3 Regulatory T Cells from CD4$^+$CD25 T Cells Via p53, IL-2, and OX40. Proc Natl Acad Sci U S A 2007;104:15478—83.

[218] Niedbala W, Wei XQ, Piedrafita D, Xu D, Liew FY. Effects of Nitric Oxide on the Induction and Differentiation of Th1 Cells. Eur J Immunol 1999;29:2498—505.

[219] Norman MU, Zbytnuik L, Kubes P. Interferon-Gamma Limits Th1 Lymphocyte Adhesion to Inflamed Endothelium: A Nitric Oxide Regulatory Feedback Mechanism. Eur J Immunol 2008;38:1368—80.

629

[220] Nosho K, Yamamoto H, Adachi Y, Endo T, Hinoda Y, Imai K. Gene Expression Profiling of Colorectal Adenomas and Early Invasive Carcinomas by cDNA Array Analysis. Br J Cancer 2005;92:1193—200.

[221] Nozoe T, Yasuda M, Honda M, Inutsuka S, Korenaga D. Immunohistochemical Expression of Cytokine Induced Nitric Oxide Synthase in Colorectal Carcinoma. Oncol Rep 2002;9:521—4.

[222] Ohshima H, Tatemichi M, Sawa T. Chemical Basis of Inflammation-Induced Carcinogenesis. Arch Biochem Biophys 2003;417:3—11.

[223] Okamoto T, Akaike T, Sawa T, Miyamoto Y, van der Vliet A, Maeda H. Activation of Matrix Metalloproteinases by Peroxynitrite-Induced Protein S-Glutathiolation Via Disulfide S-Oxide Formation. J Biol Chem 2001;276:29596—602.

[224] Ostrand-Rosenberg S, Sinha P, Beury DW, Clements VK. Cross-Talk between Myeloid-Derived Suppressor Cells (MDSC), Macrophages, and Dendritic Cells Enhances Tumor-Induced Immune Suppression. Semin Cancer Biol 2012.

[225] Otsuji M, Kimura Y, Aoe T, Okamoto Y, Saito T. Oxidative Stress by Tumor-Derived Macrophages Suppresses the Expression of CD3 Zeta Chain of T-Cell Receptor Complex and Antigen-Specific T- Cell Responses. Proc Natl Acad Sci U S A 1996;93:13119—24.

[226] Ouyang N, Williams JL, Tsioulias GJ, Gao J, Iatropoulos MJ, Kopelovich L, et al. Nitric Oxide-Donating Aspirin Prevents Pancreatic Cancer in a Hamster Tumor Model. Cancer Res 2006;66:4503—11.

[227] Park IS, Kang SW, Shin YJ, Chae KY, Park MO, Kim MY, et al. Arginine Deiminase: A Potential Inhibitor of Angiogenesis and Tumour Growth. Br J Cancer 2003;89:907—14.

[228] Park SW, Lee SG, Song SH, Heo DS, Park BJ, Lee DW, et al. The Effect of Nitric Oxide on Cyclooxygenase-2 (COX-2) Overexpression in Head and Neck Cancer Cell Lines. Int J Cancer 2003;107:729—38.

[229] Pauleau AL, Rutschman R, Lang R, Pernis A, Watowich SS, Murray PJ. Enhancer-Mediated Control of Macrophage-Specific Arginase I Expression. J Immunol 2004;172:7565—73.

[230] Pautz A, Art J, Hahn S, Nowag S, Voss C, Kleinert H. Regulation of the Expression of Inducible Nitric Oxide Synthase. Nitric Oxide 2010;23:75—93.

[231] Peranzoni E, Marigo I, Dolcetti L, Ugel S, Sonda N, Taschin E, et al. Role of Arginine Metabolism in Immunity and Immunopathology. Immunobiology 2007;212:795—812.

[232] Perez GM, Melo M, Keegan AD, Zamorano J. Aspirin and Salicylates Inhibit the IL-4- and IL-13-Induced Activation of STAT6. J Immunol 2002;168:1428—34.

[233] Perrella MA, Pellacani A, Wiesel P, Chin MT, Foster LC, Ibanez M, et al. High Mobility Group-I(Y) Protein Facilitates Nuclear Factor-Kappab Binding and Transactivation of the Inducible Nitric-Oxide Synthase Promoter/Enhancer. J Biol Chem 1999;274:9045—52.

[234] Pignatelli B, Li CQ, Boffetta P, Chen Q, Ahrens W, Nyberg F, et al. Nitrated and Oxidized Plasma Proteins in Smokers and Lung Cancer Patients. Cancer Res 2001;61:778—84.

[235] Polat MF, Taysi S, Polat S, Boyuk A, Bakan E. Elevated Serum Arginase Activity Levels in Patients with Breast Cancer. Surg Today 2003;33:655—61.

[236] Porembska Z, Luboinski G, Chrzanowska A, Mielczarek M, Magnuska J, Baranczyk-Kuzma A. Arginase in Patients with Breast Cancer. Clin Chim Acta 2003;328:105—11.

[237] Porembska Z, Skwarek A, Mielczarek M, Baranczyk-Kuzma A. Serum Arginase Activity in Postsurgical Monitoring of Patients with Colorectal Carcinoma. Cancer 2002;94:2930—4.

[238] Poschke I, Mougiakakos D, Kiessling R. Camouflage and Sabotage: Tumor Escape from the Immune System. Cancer Immunol Immunother 2011;60:1161—71.

[239] Priceman SJ, Sung JL, Shaposhnik Z, Burton JB, Torres-Collado AX, Moughon DL, et al. Targeting Distinct Tumor-Infiltrating Myeloid Cells by Inhibiting CSF-1 Receptor: Combating Tumor Evasion of Antiangiogenic Therapy. Blood 2010;115:1461—71.

[240] Qian BZ, Pollard JW. Macrophage Diversity Enhances Tumor Progression and Metastasis. Cell 2010;141:39—51.

[241] Qiu H, Orr FW, Jensen D, Wang HH, McIntosh AR, Hasinoff BB, et al. Arrest of B16 Melanoma Cells in the Mouse Pulmonary Microcirculation Induces Endothelial Nitric Oxide Synthase-Dependent Nitric Oxide Release That Is Cytotoxic to the Tumor Cells. Am J Pathol 2003;162:403—12.

[242] Radi R. Nitric Oxide, Oxidants, and Protein Tyrosine Nitration. Proc Natl Acad Sci U S A 2004;101:4003—8.

[243] Raes G, Van den Bergh R, De Baetselier P, Ghassabeh GH, Scotton C, Locati M, et al. Arginase-1 and YM1 Are Markers for Murine, but Not Human, Alternatively Activated Myeloid Cells. J Immunol 2005;174:6561.

[244] Rao CV. Nitric Oxide Signaling in Colon Cancer Chemoprevention. Mutat Res 2004;555:107—19.

[245] Rao CV, Reddy BS, Steele VE, Wang CX, Liu X, Ouyang N, et al. Nitric Oxide-Releasing Aspirin and Indomethacin Are Potent Inhibitors against Colon Cancer in Azoxymethane-Treated Rats: Effects on Molecular Targets. Mol Cancer Ther 2006;5:1530—8.

[246] Raspollini MR, Amunni G, Villanucci A, Boddi V, Baroni G, Taddei A, et al. Expression of Inducible Nitric Oxide Synthase and Cyclooxygenase-2 in Ovarian Cancer: Correlation with Clinical Outcome. Gynecol Oncol 2004;92:806—12.

[247] Ratovitski EA, Bao C, Quick RA, McMillan A, Kozlovsky C, Lowenstein CJ. An Inducible Nitric-Oxide Synthase (NOS)-Associated Protein Inhibits Nos Dimerization and Activity. J Biol Chem 1999;274:30250—7.

[248] Reth M. Hydrogen Peroxide as Second Messenger in Lymphocyte Activation. Nat Immunol 2002;3:1129—34.

[249] Reveneau S, Arnould L, Jolimoy G, Hilpert S, Lejeune P, Saint-Giorgio V, et al. Nitric Oxide Synthase in Human Breast Cancer Is Associated with Tumor Grade, Proliferation Rate, and Expression of Progesterone Receptors. Lab Invest 1999;79:1215—25.

[250] Rodriguez-Pascual F, Hausding M, Ihrig-Biedert I, Furneaux H, Levy AP, Forstermann U, et al. Complex Contribution of the 3′-Untranslated Region to the Expressional Regulation of the Human Inducible Nitric-Oxide Synthase Gene. Involvement of the RNA-Binding Protein HuR. J Biol Chem 2000;275: 26040—9.

[251] Rodriguez PC, Ernstoff MS, Hernandez C, Atkins M, Zabaleta J, Sierra R, et al. Arginase I-Producing Myeloid-Derived Suppressor Cells in Renal Cell Carcinoma Are a Subpopulation of Activated Granulocytes. Cancer Res 2009;69:1553—60.

[252] Rodriguez PC, Hernandez CP, Quiceno D, Dubinett SM, Zabaleta J, Ochoa JB, et al. Arginase I in Myeloid Suppressor Cells Is Induced by COX-2 in Lung Carcinoma. J Exp Med 2005;202:931—9.

[253] Rodriguez PC, Ochoa AC. T Cell Dysfunction in Cancer: Role of Myeloid Cells and Tumor Cells Regulating Amino Acid Availability and Oxidative Stress. Semin Cancer Biol 2006;16:66—72.

[254] Rodriguez PC, Quiceno DG, Zabaleta J, Ortiz B, Zea AH, Piazuelo MB, et al. Arginase I Production in the Tumor Microenvironment by Mature Myeloid Cells Inhibits T-Cell Receptor Expression and Antigen-Specific T-Cell Responses. Cancer Res 2004;64:5839—49.

[255] Rodriguez PC, Zea AH, Culotta KS, Zabaleta J, Ochoa JB, Ochoa AC. Regulation of T Cell Receptor Cd3zeta Chain Expression by L-Arginine. J Biol Chem 2002;277:21123—9.

[256] Rodriguez PC, Zea AH, DeSalvo J, Culotta KS, Zabaleta J, Quiceno DG, et al. L-Arginine Consumption by Macrophages Modulates the Expression of CD3 Zeta Chain in T Lymphocytes. J Immunol 2003;171:1232—9.

[257] Roman V, Zhao H, Fourneau JM, Marconi A, Dugas N, Dugas B, et al. Expression of a Functional Inducible Nitric Oxide Synthase in Hairy Cell Leukaemia and ESKOL Cell Line. Leukemia 2000;14:696—705.

[258] Rosenberg SA, Yang JC, Restifo NP. Cancer Immunotherapy: Moving Beyond Current Vaccines. Nat Med 2004;10:909—15.

[259] Rothe H, Hausmann A, Kolb H. Immunoregulation During Disease Progression in Prediabetic Nod Mice: Inverse Expression of Arginase and Prostaglandin H Synthase 2 Vs. Interleukin-15. Horm Metab Res 2002;34:7—12.

[260] Rotondo R, Barisione G, Mastracci L, Grossi F, Orengo AM, Costa R, et al. IL-8 Induces Exocytosis of Arginase 1 by Neutrophil Polymorphonuclears in Nonsmall Cell Lung Cancer. Int J Cancer 2009;125:887—93.

[261] Rotondo R, Bertolotto M, Barisione G, Astigiano S, Mandruzzato S, Ottonello L, et al. Exocytosis of Azurophil and Arginase 1-Containing Granules by Activated Polymorphonuclear Neutrophils Is Required to Inhibit T Lymphocyte Proliferation. J Leukoc Biol 2011;89:721—7.

[262] Routledge MN. Mutations Induced by Reactive Nitrogen Oxide Species in the Supf Forward Mutation Assay. Mutat Res 2000;450:95—105.

[263] Sandler RS, Halabi S, Baron JA, Budinger S, Paskett E, Keresztes R, et al. Randomized Trial of Aspirin to Prevent Colorectal Adenomas in Patients with Previous Colorectal Cancer. N Engl J Med 2003;348:883—90.

[264] Schluns KS, Lefrancois L. Cytokine Control of Memory T-Cell Development and Survival. Nat Rev Immunol 2003;3:269—79.

[265] Schmidt N, Pautz A, Art J, Rauschkolb P, Jung M, Erkel G, et al. Transcriptional and Post-Transcriptional Regulation of iNOS Expression in Human Chondrocytes. Biochem Pharmacol 2010;79:722—32.

[266] Schmielau J, Finn OJ. Activated Granulocytes and Granulocyte-Derived Hydrogen Peroxide Are the Underlying Mechanism of Suppression of T-Cell Function in Advanced Cancer Patients. Cancer Res 2001;61:4756—60.

[267] Schopfer FJ, Baker PR, Freeman BA. NO-Dependent Protein Nitration: A Cell Signaling Event or an Oxidative Inflammatory Response? Trends Biochem Sci 2003;28:646—54.

[268] Scott DJ, Hull MA, Cartwright EJ, Lam WK, Tisbury A, Poulsom R, et al. Lack of Inducible Nitric Oxide Synthase Promotes Intestinal Tumorigenesis in the Apc(Min/+) Mouse. Gastroenterology 2001;121:889—99.

[269] Semenza GL. HIF-1 and Mechanisms of Hypoxia Sensing. Curr Opin Cell Biol 2001;13:167—71.

[270] Semenza GL. Targeting HIF-1 for Cancer Therapy. Nat Rev Cancer 2003;3:721—32.

[271] Serafini P, Borrello I, Bronte V. Myeloid Suppressor Cells in Cancer: Recruitment, Phenotype, Properties, and Mechanisms of Immune Suppression. Semin Cancer Biol 2006;16:53—65.

[272] Serafini P, De Santo C, Marigo I, Cingarlini S, Dolcetti L, Gallina G, et al. Derangement of Immune Responses by Myeloid Suppressor Cells. Cancer Immunol Immunother 2004;53:64−72.

[273] Sercan O, Hammerling GJ, Arnold B, Schuler T. Innate Immune Cells Contribute to the IFN-Gamma-Dependent Regulation of Antigen-Specific CD8$^+$ T Cell Homeostasis. J Immunol 2006;176:735−9.

[274] Sharara AI, Perkins DJ, Misukonis MA, Chan SU, Dominitz JA, Weinberg JB. Interferon (IFN)-Alpha Activation of Human Blood Mononuclear Cells in Vitro and in Vivo for Nitric Oxide Synthase (NOS) Type 2 mRNA and Protein Expression: Possible Relationship of Induced NOS2 to the Anti-Hepatitis C Effects of IFN-Alpha in Vivo. J Exp Med 1997;186:1495−502.

[275] Sharda DR, Yu S, Ray M, Squadrito ML, De Palma M, Wynn TA, et al. Regulation of Macrophage Arginase Expression and Tumor Growth by the Ron Receptor Tyrosine Kinase. J Immunol 2011;187:2181−92.

[276] Shi O, Morris Jr SM, Zoghbi H, Porter CW, O'Brien WE. Generation of a Mouse Model for Arginase II Deficiency by Targeted Disruption of the Arginase II Gene. Mol Cell Biol 2001;21:811−3.

[277] Shi Q, Xiong Q, Wang B, Le X, Khan NA, Xie K. Influence of Nitric Oxide Synthase II Gene Disruption on Tumor Growth and Metastasis. Cancer Res 2000;60:2579−83.

[278] Shinoda J, McLaughlin KE, Bell HS, Swaroop GR, Yamaguchi S, Holmes MC, et al. Molecular Mechanisms Underlying Dexamethasone Inhibition of iNOS Expression and Activity in C6 Glioma Cells. Glia 2003;42:68−76.

[279] Sica A, Bronte V. Altered Macrophage Differentiation and Immune Dysfunction in Tumor Development. J Clin Invest 2007;117:1155−66.

[280] Siegert A, Rosenberg C, Schmitt WD, Denkert C, Hauptmann S. Nitric Oxide of Human Colorectal Adenocarcinoma Cell Lines Promotes Tumour Cell Invasion. Br J Cancer 2002;86:1310−5.

[281] Singh R, Pervin S, Karimi A, Cederbaum S, Chaudhuri G. Arginase Activity in Human Breast Cancer Cell Lines: N(Omega)-Hydroxy-L-Arginine Selectively Inhibits Cell Proliferation and Induces Apoptosis in MDA-MB-468 Cells. Cancer Res 2000;60:3305−12.

[282] Singh S, Gupta AK. Nitric Oxide: Role in Tumour Biology and iNOS/NO-Based Anticancer Therapies. Cancer Chemother Pharmacol 2011;67:1211−24.

[283] Sinha P, Clements V, Ostrand-Rosenberg S. Reduction of Myeloid-Derived Suppressor Cells and Induction of M1 Macrophages Facilitate the Rejection of Established Metastatic Disease. J Immunol 2005;174:636−45.

[284] Sinha P, Clements VK, Fulton AM, Ostrand-Rosenberg S. Prostaglandin E2 Promotes Tumor Progression by Inducing Myeloid-Derived Suppressor Cells. Cancer Res 2007;67:4507−13.

[285] Solito S, Falisi E, Diaz-Montero CM, Doni A, Pinton L, Rosato A, et al. Human Promyelocytic-Like Population Is Responsible for the Immune Suppression Mediated by Myeloid-Derived Suppressor Cells. Blood 2011;118:2254−65.

[286] Sonoki T, Nagasaki A, Gotoh T, Takiguchi M, Takeya M, Matsuzaki H, et al. Coinduction of Nitric-Oxide Synthase and Arginase I in Cultured Rat Peritoneal Macrophages and Rat Tissues in Vivo by Lipopolysaccharide. J Biol Chem 1997;272:3689−93.

[287] Sousa MS, Latini FR, Monteiro HP, Cerutti JM. Arginase 2 and Nitric Oxide Synthase: Pathways Associated with the Pathogenesis of Thyroid Tumors. Free Radic Biol Med 2010;49:997−1007.

[288] Suarez-Pinzon WL, Mabley JG, Strynadka K, Power RF, Szabo C, Rabinovitch A. An Inhibitor of Inducible Nitric Oxide Synthase and Scavenger of Peroxynitrite Prevents Diabetes Development in NOD Mice. J Autoimmun 2001;16:449−55.

[289] Suarez-Pinzon WL, Szabo C, Rabinovitch A. Development of Autoimmune Diabetes in Nod Mice Is Associated with the Formation of Peroxynitrite in Pancreatic Islet Beta-Cells. Diabetes 1997;46:907−11.

[290] Suer Gokmen S, Yoruk Y, Cakir E, Yorulmaz F, Gulen S. Arginase and Ornithine, as Markers in Human Non-Small Cell Lung Carcinoma. Cancer Biochem Biophys 1999;17:125−31.

[291] Swana HS, Smith SD, Perrotta PL, Saito N, Wheeler MA, Weiss RM. Inducible Nitric Oxide Synthase with Transitional Cell Carcinoma of the Bladder. J Urol 1999;161:630−4.

[292] Talmadge JE, Hood KC, Zobel LC, Shafer LR, Coles M, Toth B. Chemoprevention by Cyclooxygenase-2 Inhibition Reduces Immature Myeloid Suppressor Cell Expansion. Int Immunopharmacol 2007;7:140−51.

[293] Tatemichi M, Sawa T, Gilibert I, Tazawa H, Katoh T, Ohshima H. Increased Risk of Intestinal Type of Gastric Adenocarcinoma in Japanese Women Associated with Long Forms of CCTTT Pentanucleotide Repeat in the Inducible Nitric Oxide Synthase Promoter. Cancer Lett 2005;217:197−202.

[294] Tatemichi M, Tazawa H, Masuda M, Saleem M, Wada S, Donehower LA, et al. Suppression of Thymic Lymphomas and Increased Nonthymic Lymphomagenesis in Trp53-Deficient Mice Lacking Inducible Nitric Oxide Synthase Gene. Int J Cancer 2004;111:819−28.

[295] Terrazas LI, Walsh KL, Piskorska D, McGuire E, Harn Jr DA. The Schistosome Oligosaccharide Lacto-N-Neotetraose Expands Gr1(+) Cells That Secrete Anti-Inflammatory Cytokines and Inhibit Proliferation of Naive CD4(+) Cells: A Potential Mechanism for Immune Polarization in Helminth Infections. J Immunol 2001;167:5294−303.

[296] Tesei A, Ricotti L, Ulivi P, Medri L, Amadori D, Zoli W. Ncx 4016, a Nitric Oxide-Releasing Aspirin Derivative, Exhibits a Significant Antiproliferative Effect and Alters Cell Cycle Progression in Human Colon Adenocarcinoma Cell Lines. Int J Oncol 2003;22:1297—302.

[297] Thengchaisri N, Hein TW, Wang W, Xu X, Li Z, Fossum TW, et al. Upregulation of Arginase by H2o2 Impairs Endothelium-Dependent Nitric Oxide-Mediated Dilation of Coronary Arterioles. Arterioscler Thromb Vasc Biol 2006.

[298] Thomsen LL, Lawton FG, Knowles RG, Beesley JE, Riveros-Moreno V, Moncada S. Nitric Oxide Synthase Activity in Human Gynecological Cancer. Cancer Res 1994;54:1352—4.

[299] Thomsen LL, Miles DW. Role of Nitric Oxide in Tumour Progression: Lessons from Human Tumours. Cancer Metastasis Rev 1998;17:107—18.

[300] Thomsen LL, Miles DW, Happerfield L, Bobrow LG, Knowles RG, Moncada S. Nitric Oxide Synthase Activity in Human Breast Cancer. Br J Cancer 1995;72:41—4.

[301] Thoren FB, Betten A, Romero AI, Hellstrand K. Cutting Edge: Antioxidative Properties of Myeloid Dendritic Cells: Protection of T Cells and NK Cells from Oxygen Radical-Induced Inactivation and Apoptosis. J Immunol 2007;179:21—5.

[302] Thoren FB, Romero AI, Hermodsson S, Hellstrand K. The CD16⁻/CD56^{bright} Subset of Nk Cells Is Resistant to Oxidant-Induced Cell Death. J Immunol 2007;179:781—5.

[303] Thun MJ, Henley SJ, Patrono C. Nonsteroidal Anti-Inflammatory Drugs as Anticancer Agents: Mechanistic, Pharmacologic, and Clinical Issues. J Natl Cancer Inst 2002;94:252—66.

[304] Torrens I, Mendoza O, Batte A, Reyes O, Fernandez LE, Mesa C, et al. Immunotherapy with Ctl Peptide and Vssp Eradicated Established Human Papillomavirus (HPV) Type 16 E7-Expressing Tumors. Vaccine 2005;23:5768—74.

[305] Vakkala M, Kahlos K, Lakari E, Paakko P, Kinnula V, Soini Y. Inducible Nitric Oxide Synthase Expression, Apoptosis, and Angiogenesis in in Situ and Invasive Breast Carcinomas. Clin Cancer Res 2000;6:2408—16.

[306] Veltman JD, Lambers ME, van Nimwegen M, Hendriks RW, Hoogsteden HC, Aerts JG, et al. COX-2 Inhibition Improves Immunotherapy and Is Associated with Decreased Numbers of Myeloid-Derived Suppressor Cells in Mesothelioma. Celecoxib Influences Mdsc Function. BMC Cancer 2010;10:464.

[307] Vickers SM, MacMillan-Crow LA, Green M, Ellis C, Thompson JA. Association of Increased Immunostaining for Inducible Nitric Oxide Synthase and Nitrotyrosine with Fibroblast Growth Factor Transformation in Pancreatic Cancer. Arch Surg 1999;134:245—51.

[308] Vig M, Srivastava S, Kandpal U, Sade H, Lewis V, Sarin A, et al. Inducible Nitric Oxide Synthase in T Cells Regulates T Cell Death and Immune Memory. J Clin Invest 2004;113:1734—42.

[309] Villalta F, Zhang Y, Bibb KE, Kappes JC, Lima MF. The Cysteine-Cysteine Family of Chemokines Rantes, MIP-1alpha, and MIP-1beta Induce Trypanocidal Activity in Human Macrophages Via Nitric Oxide. Infect Immun 1998;66:4690—5.

[310] Vincendeau P, Gobert AP, Daulouede S, Moynet D, Djavad Mossalayi M. Arginases in Parasitic Diseases. Trends Parasitol 2003;19:9—12.

[311] Vouldoukis I, Riveros-Moreno V, Dugas B, Ouaaz F, Becherel P, Debre P, et al. The Killing of Leishmania Major by Human Macrophages Is Mediated by Nitric Oxide Induced after Ligation of the Fc Epsilon RII/CD23 Surface Antigen. Proc Natl Acad Sci U S A 1995;92:7804—8.

[312] Wallace JL, Ignarro LJ, Fiorucci S. Potential Cardioprotective Actions of No-Releasing Aspirin. Nat Rev Drug Discov 2002;1:375—82.

[313] Wang B, Xiong Q, Shi Q, Le X, Abbruzzese JL, Xie K. Intact Nitric Oxide Synthase Ii Gene Is Required for Interferon-Beta-Mediated Suppression of Growth and Metastasis of Pancreatic Adenocarcinoma. Cancer Res 2001;61:71—5.

[314] Wang X, Zhao Q, Matta R, Meng X, Liu X, Liu CG, et al. Inducible Nitric-Oxide Synthase Expression Is Regulated by Mitogen-Activated Protein Kinase Phosphatase-1. J Biol Chem 2009;284:27123—34.

[315] Wei D, Richardson EL, Zhu K, Wang L, Le X, He Y, et al. Direct Demonstration of Negative Regulation of Tumor Growth and Metastasis by Host-Inducible Nitric Oxide Synthase. Cancer Res 2003;63:3855—9.

[316] Wei XQ, Charles IG, Smith A, Ure J, Feng GJ, Huang FP, et al. Altered Immune Responses in Mice Lacking Inducible Nitric Oxide Synthase. Nature 1995;375:408—11.

[317] Weigert A, Brune B. Nitric Oxide, Apoptosis and Macrophage Polarization During Tumor Progression. Nitric Oxide 2008;19:95—102.

[318] Weinberg JB. Nitric Oxide Production and Nitric Oxide Synthase Type 2 Expression by Human Mononuclear Phagocytes: A Review. Mol Med 1998;4:557—91.

[319] Weiss JM, Back TC, Scarzello AJ, Subleski JJ, Hall VL, Stauffer JK, et al. Successful Immunotherapy with IL-2/Anti-CD40 Induces the Chemokine-Mediated Mitigation of an Immunosuppressive Tumor Microenvironment. Proc Natl Acad Sci U S A 2009;106:19455—60.

633

[320] Weiss JM, Ridnour LA, Back T, Hussain SP, He P, Maciag AE, et al. Macrophage-Dependent Nitric Oxide Expression Regulates Tumor Cell Detachment and Metastasis after IL-2/Anti-CD40 Immunotherapy. J Exp Med 2010;207:2455–67.

[321] Weisser SB, McLarren KW, Voglmaier N, van Netten-Thomas CJ, Antov A, Flavell RA, et al. Alternative Activation of Macrophages by IL-4 Requires SHIP Degradation. Eur J Immunol 2011;41:1742–53.

[322] Weninger W, Rendl M, Pammer J, Mildner M, Tschugguel W, Schneeberger C, et al. Nitric Oxide Synthases in Kaposi's Sarcoma Are Expressed Predominantly by Vessels and Tissue Macrophages. Lab Invest 1998;78:949–55.

[323] West MB, Hill BG, Xuan YT, Bhatnagar A. Protein Glutathiolation by Nitric Oxide: An Intracellular Mechanism Regulating Redox Protein Modification. FASEB J 2006;20:1715–7.

[324] Williams JL, Kashfi K, Ouyang N, del Soldato P, Kopelovich L, Rigas B. No-Donating Aspirin Inhibits Intestinal Carcinogenesis in Min (Apc(Min/+)) Mice. Biochem Biophys Res Commun 2004;313:784–8.

[325] Wilson KT, Fu S, Ramanujam KS, Meltzer SJ. Increased Expression of Inducible Nitric Oxide Synthase and Cyclooxygenase-2 in Barrett's Esophagus and Associated Adenocarcinomas. Cancer Res 1998;58:2929–34.

[326] Wink DA, Vodovotz Y, Laval J, Laval F, Dewhirst MW, Mitchell JB. The Multifaceted Roles of Nitric Oxide in Cancer. Carcinogenesis 1998;19:711–21.

[327] Witherell HL, Hiatt RA, Replogle M, Parsonnet J. Helicobacter Pylori Infection and Urinary Excretion of 8-Hydroxy-2-Deoxyguanosine, an Oxidative DNA Adduct. Cancer Epidemiol Biomarkers Prev 1998;7:91–6.

[328] Wu CW, Chung WW, Chi CW, Kao HL, Lui WY, P'Eng FK, et al. Immunohistochemical Study of Arginase in Cancer of the Stomach. Virchows Arch 1996;428:325–31.

[329] Wu G, Morris Jr SM. Arginine Metabolism: Nitric Oxide and Beyond. Biochem J 1998;336(Pt 1):1–17.

[330] Xia Y, Roman LJ, Masters BS, Zweier JL. Inducible Nitric-Oxide Synthase Generates Superoxide from the Reductase Domain. J Biol Chem 1998;273:22635–9.

[331] Xia Y, Zweier JL. Superoxide and Peroxynitrite Generation from Inducible Nitric Oxide Synthase in Macrophages. Proc Natl Acad Sci U S A 1997;94:6954–8.

[332] Xie QW, Kashiwabara Y, Nathan C. Role of Transcription Factor NF-Kappa B/Rel in Induction of Nitric Oxide Synthase. J Biol Chem 1994;269:4705–8.

[333] Zabaleta J, McGee DJ, Zea AH, Hernandez CP, Rodriguez PC, Sierra RA, et al. Helicobacter Pylori Arginase Inhibits T Cell Proliferation and Reduces the Expression of the Tcr Zeta-Chain (CD3zeta). J Immunol 2004;173:586–93.

[334] Zea AH, Culotta KS, Ali J, Mason C, Park HJ, Zabaleta J, et al. Decreased Expression of CD3zeta and Nuclear Transcription Factor Kappa B in Patients with Pulmonary Tuberculosis: Potential Mechanisms and Reversibility with Treatment. J Infect Dis 2006;194:1385–93.

[335] Zea AH, Rodriguez PC, Atkins MB, Hernandez C, Signoretti S, Zabaleta J, et al. Arginase-Producing Myeloid Suppressor Cells in Renal Cell Carcinoma Patients: A Mechanism of Tumor Evasion. Cancer Res 2005;65:3044–8.

[336] Zhu W, Chandrasekharan UM, Bandyopadhyay S, Morris Jr SM, DiCorleto PE, Kashyap VS. Thrombin Induces Endothelial Arginase through AP-1 Activation. Am J Physiol Cell Physiol 2010;298:C952–60.

[337] Ziche M, Morbidelli L, Choudhuri R, Zhang HT, Donnini S, Granger HJ, et al. Nitric Oxide Synthase Lies Downstream from Vascular Endothelial Growth Factor-Induced but Not Basic Fibroblast Growth Factor-Induced Angiogenesis. J Clin Invest 1997;99:2625–34.

Note: Page numbers followed by "f" or "t" indicate figure or table respectively

641

650